Brenner and Stevens'
PHARMACOLOGY

Brenner and Stevens'
PHARMACOLOGY

SIXTH EDITION

Craig W. Stevens, PhD

Professor of Pharmacology
Oklahoma State University
Center for Health Sciences
Tulsa, Oklahoma

ELSEVIER

Elsevier
1600 John F. Kennedy Blvd.
Ste 1800
Philadelphia, PA 19103-2899

BRENNER AND STEVENS' PHARMACOLOGY, SIXTH EDITION

ISBN: 978-0-323-75898-7

Notice

Previous editions copyrighted 2018, 2013, 2010, 2006, and 2000

Content Strategist: Alexandra Mortimer
Content Development Specialist: Akanksha Marwah
Publishing Services Manager: Deepthi Unni
Project Manager: Aparna Venkatachalam
Design Direction: Margaret Reid

Printed in India

Last digit is the print number: 9 8 7 6 5 4 3 2

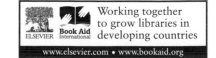

Working together
to grow libraries in
developing countries

www.elsevier.com • www.bookaid.org

Preface

Medical pharmacology is primarily concerned with the mechanisms by which drugs treat disease processes, relieve symptoms, and counteract the molecular manifestations of pathological states. Pharmacology is also concerned with the factors that determine the time course of drug action, including drug absorption, distribution, metabolism, and excretion. Students are often overwhelmed by the vast amount of pharmacological information available today. This textbook provides the essential concepts and drug information that students need to be successful in their courses without an overwhelming amount of detail.

This text is primarily intended for students who are taking their first course in pharmacology, but it will also be useful for those who are preparing to take medical boards or licensing examinations. Because of the large number of drugs available today, this text emphasizes the general properties of drug categories and prototypical drugs. The chapters begin with a drug classification box to familiarize students with drug categories, subcategories, and specific drugs to be presented in the chapter. Additionally, all FDA-approved drugs are listed along with the emphasized drugs to enhance the value of this textbook as a reference volume.

In the four years since the publication of the previous edition of *Brenner and Stevens' Pharmacology*, major trends in the development and marketing of new medications and new formulations were apparent. First, there was an explosion of combination drugs released onto the market in recent years. This is a good thing, as there is often pharmacological synergy between combined agents, but also because patient compliance is greatly improved. It is easier to take one pill than two, or three, or four. The usual product combines two successful and effective single agents for the treatment of a disorder. These newly approved combination drugs are included in this 6th edition of *Brenner & Stevens' Pharmacology*.

Second, the market is flush with immunopharmacology drug products. Immunopharmacology products are rampant and apparent to both the physician and consumer by the numerous monoclonal antibody drugs touted in TV commercials. Pharmaceutical manufacturing of monoclonal antibody drugs that target enzymes, receptors, or other proteins is a rapidly growing sector of biologicals. Many therapeutic classes of pharmacological agents now have one or two drugs that work via antibodies or that target immune system factors. Because of the exponential growth of immunopharmacology drugs, a new Chapter 46 was added to close the book.

Third, the development and marketing of small molecule inhibitors skyrocketed in the last five years. Small molecule inhibitors were developed to go inside of cells and inhibit particular kinases or other enzymes and proteins. By contrast, more traditional drugs target receptor or enzymes on the cell membrane, like morphine acting on opioid receptors. Small molecule inhibitors are effective in many neoplastic (cancer) diseases and other pathological states with a well-defined molecular pathway. This new class of drugs with intracellular targets was added to Chapter 45.

The book has been meticulously organized to include extensive cross-referencing of many drugs that have more than one therapeutic use or multiple classifications. This will aid the reader in following a particular drug that is included in different chapters. Additionally, to aid the reader in drug recognition, drug names are followed by trade (brand) names in SMALL CAPS FONT. This helps because the trade name of many drugs are heavily advertised and the reader may already have some knowledge of their drug uses. As all medications are indexed under both their generic and brand names, this book is also a valuable reference for a quick review of drugs encountered in the reader's personal or professional life. However the student reader will bear in mind that for purposes of examination and boards, the unbranded generic drug name is exclusively used.

The book now in your hands was extensively revised for the 6th edition to include all new drugs on the market since the last edition (more than 200), and to exclude older drugs that were withdrawn from the market. Much ancillary drug information, such as chemical structures and unremarkable pharmacokinetics, was shortened or deleted. The figures that were retained were updated and new figures added, with an emphasis on illustrating drug mechanisms of action. A modern graphic style was developed for the figures to improve understanding and to entice the eye.

This new edition is sadly noted by the recent passing of Dr. George M. Brenner, my mentor, my friend, and co-author on previous editions of this textbook. George hired me 30 years ago as a young Assistant Professor of Pharmacology, collaborated on research projects, and encouraged my career as an academic scientist. Dr. Brenner had an encyclopedic knowledge of medications and his expertise is greatly missed. On another sad note, this book was written during the COVID-19 pandemic which took hundreds of thousands of lives due to infection with the SARS-CoV-2 virus. Although at the time of this writing there are no fully-approved FDA treatments for the pandemic virus, special sections on the emergency use drugs and developing vaccines are included in *Chapter 43* and *Chapter 46*.

I thank my numerous offspring and their mates for their constant love and attention which inspires me to undertake such massive projects like this textbook. I especially want to thank my OB/GYN wife, Dr. Timmeni L. Stevens, D.O., (*'the real doctor'*) for her help on *Chapter 34, Drugs Affecting Fertility and Reproduction*. I also appreciate the fine people at Elsevier, who bring it all together to produce the nicely designed textbook now in your hands. The interactions with

Alexandra Mortimer, Meghan Andress, and Kevin Travers were especially professional and pleasant. They seem to really enjoy their career and know what they are doing.

Finally, I am a pharmacologist who spent most of my career as a preclinical researcher using animals and cell cultures as models for understanding the human condition. I am not a physician or medical consultant. Therefore none of the following text should be taken as medical advice.

Craig W. Stevens, PhD
Professor of Pharmacology
OSU-Center for Health Sciences
Tulsa, Oklahoma

Contents

Section

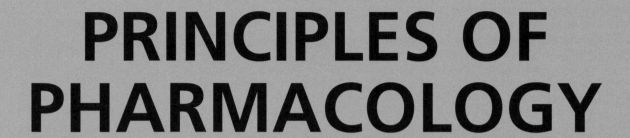

PRINCIPLES OF PHARMACOLOGY

Introduction to Pharmacology and Drug Names

PHARMACOLOGY AND RELATED SCIENCES

Pharmacology is the **study of drugs and their effects** on living organisms, whether it be whole organisms, tissues, or cells. Pharmacology is a fundamental biomedical science that sprang to the forefront of modern medicine with a demonstrated success in using drugs to treat disease and save human lives. Pharmacology is also the scientific discipline that drives the international **pharmaceutical industry** to multibillion-dollar sales. This chapter reviews the history of pharmacology, identifies its major subdivisions, and introduces the types of drugs, formulations, and routes of administration.

History and Definition of Pharmacology

Since the beginning of our species, people have treated pain and disease with substances derived from plants, animals, and minerals. However, the **science of pharmacology** is less than 150 years old, ushered in by the ability to isolate pure compounds from plants and the establishment of the scientific method.

Initially, drug use for aiding the sick consisted of crude plant and animal preparations given in a ritualistic manner to rid the body of the evil spirits believed to cause illness. Their effectiveness was probably due as much to beliefs or a placebo effect as it was to any medicinal property of the substances administered. Many cultures relied on a magic-man or *shaman* to perform the healing rituals. Indeed, the Greek word *pharmakon*, from which the term *pharmacology* is derived, originally meant a magic charm for treating disease. Later, *pharmakon* came to mean a remedy or drug.

In the next phase of pharmacology, accrued knowledge from generations of medicinal rituals enabled people to correlate natural substances with treatment of particular diseases or symptoms. The **first effective drugs** were probably simple external preparations, such as cool mud for sunburn or a soothing mixture of plant leaves for an insect bite. The earliest known prescriptions, dating from 2100 BCE, included salves containing the spice thyme. In the ensuing centuries, people learned the **therapeutic value of natural products** through trial and error. By 1500 BCE, Egyptian prescriptions called for **castor oil, opium,** and other drugs still used today. In China, ancient scrolls from that time listed prescriptions for **herbal medicines** for more than 50 diseases. *Dioscorides,* a Greek army surgeon who lived in the 1st century, described more than 600 medicinal plants that he collected and studied as he traveled with the Roman army. *Susruta,* a Hindu healer, described the principles of Ayurvedic medicine in the 5th century. During the Middle Ages, Islamic physicians (most famously *Avicenna*) and Christian monks cultivated and studied the use of herbal medicines.

The current phase of pharmacology gradually evolved with important advances in **chemistry and physiology** that gave rise to modern pharmacology. At the same time, a more rational understanding of disease mechanisms provided a scientific basis for using drugs whose physiologic actions and effects were understood. The advent of pharmacology was particularly dependent on the isolation of pure drug compounds from natural sources and on the development of experimental physiology methods to study these compounds. The **isolation of morphine** from opium in 1804 was rapidly followed by the extraction of many other drugs from plant sources, providing a diverse array of pure drugs for **pharmacologic experimentation.** Advances in physiology allowed pioneers, such as François Magendie and Claude Bernard, to conduct some of the earliest pharmacologic investigations, including studies that localized the site of action of curare to the neuromuscular junction. The first medical school pharmacology laboratory was started by Rudolf Buchheim in Estonia. Buchheim and one of his students, Oswald Schmiedeberg, trained many other pharmacologists, including John Jacob Abel, who established the first pharmacology department at the University of Michigan in 1891 and is considered the father of American pharmacology.

The goal of pharmacology is to **understand the mechanisms by which drugs interact** with biologic systems to enable the rational use of effective agents in the diagnosis and treatment of disease. The success of pharmacology in this task has led to an explosion of new drug development, particularly in the past 50 years. Significant drug development includes the isolation and use of insulin for diabetes, the discovery of antimicrobial and antineoplastic drugs, and the advent of modern psychopharmacology. Recent advances in molecular biology, genetics, and computer-aided drug design suggest that new drug development and pharmacologic innovations will provide even greater advances in the treatment of medical disorders in the coming years.

The history of many significant events in pharmacology, as highlighted by selected Nobel Prize recipients, is presented in Table 1.1.

Pharmacology and Its Subdivisions

Pharmacology is the biomedical science concerned with the interaction of chemical substances with living cells, tissues, and organisms. It is particularly concerned with the mechanisms by which drugs counteract the manifestations of disease and affect fertility. Pharmacology is not primarily focused on the methods of synthesis, isolation of drugs, or with the preparation of pharmaceutical products. The disciplines that deal with these subjects are described later.

Pharmacology is divided into two main subdivisions, **pharmacokinetics** and **pharmacodynamics.** The relationship between these subdivisions is shown in Fig. 1.1. Pharmacokinetics is concerned with the processes that determine the concentration of drugs in body fluids and tissues over time, including drug **absorption, distribution, metabolism,**

TABLE 1.1 The Nobel Prize and the History of Pharmacology*

PERSON(S) AND YEAR AWARDED	SIGNIFICANT DISCOVERY IN PHARMACOLOGY
Ilya Metchnikoff and Paul Ehrlich (1908)	First antimicrobial drugs *(magic bullet)*
Frederick Banting and John Macleod (1923)	Isolation and discovery of insulin and its application in the treatment of diabetes
Sir Henry Dale and Otto Loewi (1936)	Chemical transmission of nerve impulses
Sir Alexander Fleming, Ernst Chain, and Sir Howard Florey (1945)	Discovery of penicillin and its curative effect in various infectious diseases
Daniel Bovet (1957)	Antagonists that block biologically active amines, including the first antihistamine
Sir Bernard Katz, Ulf von Euler, and Julius Axelrod (1970)	Transmitters in the nerve terminals and the mechanism for storage, release, and inactivation
Sune Bergström, Bengt Samuelsson, and John Vane (1982)	Discovery of prostaglandins and the mechanism of action of aspirin that inhibits prostaglandin synthesis
Sir James Black, Gertrude Elion, and George Hitchings (1988)	Development of the first β-blocker, propranolol, and anticancer agents that block nucleic acid synthesis
Alfred Gilman and Martin Rodbell (1994)	Discovery of G proteins and the role of these proteins in signal transduction in cells
Robert Furchgott, Louis Ignarro, and Ferid Murad (1998)	Recognition of nitric oxide as a signaling molecule in the cardiovascular system
Arvid Carlsson, Paul Greengard, and Eric Kandel (2000)	Role of dopamine in schizophrenia and signal transduction in the nervous system leading to long-term potentiation
Robert J. Lefkowitz and Brian K. Kobilka (2012)	The structural basis of G protein–coupled receptor signaling

*Selected from the list of recipients of the Nobel Prize for Physiology or Medicine, or the Nobel Prize for Chemistry; note that many other discoveries pertinent to pharmacology have been made by other Nobel Prize winners and that the original discovery was often made many years before the Nobel Prize was awarded.

and **excretion (ADME).** Pharmacodynamics is the study of the actions of drugs on target receptors and tissues. A shorthand way of thinking about it is that pharmacodynamics is what the drug does to the body, and pharmacokinetics is what the body does to the drug. Modern pharmacology is focused on the biochemical and molecular mechanisms by which drugs produce their physiologic effects and with the **dose-response relationship,** defined as the relationship between the concentration of a drug in a tissue and the magnitude of the tissue's response to that drug. Most drugs produce their effects by binding to protein **receptors** in target tissues, a process that activates a cascade of events known as **signal transduction.** Pharmacokinetics and pharmacodynamics are discussed in greater detail in Chapters 2 and 3, respectively.

Toxicology
Toxicology is the study of **poisons** and **organ toxicity.** It focuses on the **harmful effects of drugs** and other chemicals and on the mechanisms by which these agents produce pathologic changes, disease, and death. As with pharmacology, toxicology is concerned with the relationship between the dose of an agent and the resulting tissue concentration and biologic effects that the agent produces. Most drugs have **toxic effects** at high enough doses and may have **adverse effects** related to toxicity at therapeutic doses.

Pharmacotherapeutics
Pharmacotherapeutics is the medical science concerned with the **use of drugs in the treatment of disease.** Pharmacology provides a rational basis for pharmacotherapeutics by explaining the mechanisms and effects of drugs on the body and the relationship between dose and drug response. A cadre of research pharmacologists around the world does much preclinical research before drug candidates emerge. Human studies known as **clinical trials** are then used to determine the efficacy and safety of drug therapy in human subjects. The purpose, design, and evaluation of human drug studies are discussed in Chapter 4.

Pharmacy and Related Sciences
Pharmacy is the science and profession concerned with the **preparation, storage, dispensing,** and **proper use** of drug products. Related sciences include pharmacognosy, medicinal chemistry, and pharmaceutical chemistry. **Pharmacognosy** is the study of drugs isolated from natural

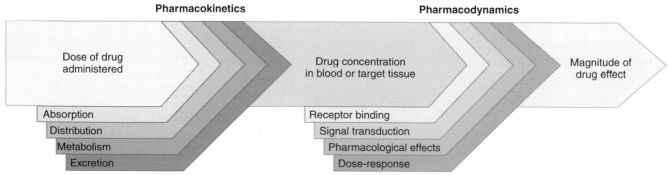

FIG. 1.1 Relationship between pharmacokinetics and pharmacodynamics.

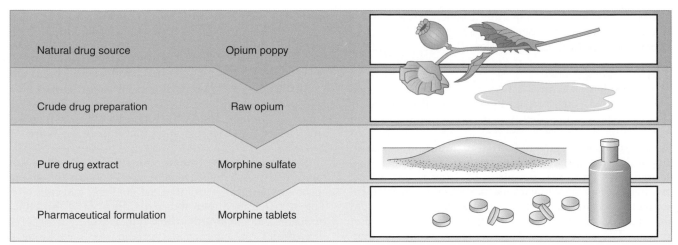

Natural drug source	Opium poppy
Crude drug preparation	Raw opium
Pure drug extract	Morphine sulfate
Pharmaceutical formulation	Morphine tablets

FIG. 1.2 Types of drug preparations. A crude drug preparation retains most or all of the active and inactive compounds contained in the natural source from which it was derived. After a pure drug compound (e.g., morphine) is extracted from a crude drug preparation (in this case, opium), it is possible to manufacture pharmaceutical preparations that are suitable for administration of a particular dose to the patient.

sources, including plants, microbes, animal tissues, and minerals. **Medicinal chemistry** is a branch of organic chemistry that specializes in the design and chemical synthesis of drugs used in medicine. **Pharmaceutical chemistry,** or **pharmaceutics,** is concerned with the formulation and chemical properties of pharmaceutical products, such as tablets, liquid solutions and suspensions, and aerosols.

DRUG SOURCES AND PREPARATIONS

A **drug** can be defined as a natural product, chemical substance, or pharmaceutical preparation intended for administration to a human or animal to diagnose or treat a disease. A drug can also be a *biologic* (e.g., a preparation of monoclonal antibodies). The word *drug* is derived from the French *drogue*, which originally meant dried herbs and was applied to herbs in the marketplace used for cooking rather than for any medicinal reason. Ironically, the medical use of the drug **marijuana,** a dried herb, is hotly debated in many societies nowadays. Drugs may be **hormones, neurotransmitters,** or **peptides** produced by the body; conversely, a **xenobiotic** is a drug produced outside the body, either synthetic or natural. A **poison** is a drug that can kill, whereas a **toxin** is a drug that can kill and is produced by a living organism. The terms **medication** and, used less frequently, **medicament** are synonymous with the word *drug*.

Natural Sources of Drugs

Drugs have been obtained from plants, microbes, animal tissues, and minerals. Among the various types of drugs derived from plants are **alkaloids,** which are substances that contain nitrogen groups and produce an alkaline reaction in aqueous solution. Examples of alkaloids include morphine, cocaine, atropine, and quinine. **Antibiotics** have been isolated from numerous microorganisms, including *Penicillium* and *Streptomyces* species. **Hormones** are the most common type of drug obtained from animals, whereas **minerals** have yielded a few useful therapeutic agents, including the lithium compounds used to treat bipolar mental illness.

Synthetic Drugs

Modern chemistry in the 19th century enabled scientists to synthesize new compounds and to modify naturally occurring drugs. Aspirin, barbiturates, and local anesthetics (e.g., **procaine**) were among the first drugs to be synthesized in the laboratory. Semisynthetic derivatives of naturally occurring compounds have led to new drugs with different properties, such as the morphine derivative **oxycodone.**

In some cases, new drug uses were discovered by accident when drugs were used for another purpose, or by actively screening a huge number of related molecules for a specific pharmacologic activity. Medicinal chemists now use molecular modeling software to discern the **structure-activity relationship,** which is the relationship among the drug molecule, its target receptor, and the resulting pharmacologic activity. In this way a virtual model for the receptor of a particular drug is created, and drug molecules that best fit the three-dimensional conformation of the receptor are synthesized. This approach has been used, for example, to design agents that inhibit angiotensin synthesis, treat hypertension, and inhibit the maturation of the human immunodeficiency virus (HIV).

Drug Preparations

Drug preparations include **crude drug** preparations obtained from natural sources, **pure drug** compounds isolated from natural sources or synthesized in the laboratory, and **pharmaceutical preparations** of drugs intended for administration to patients. The relationship among these types of drug preparations is illustrated in Fig. 1.2.

Natural Sources of Drugs

The natural source of drugs is often a plant well known for its medicinal use and taken as is. Nicotine and marijuana plants are usually administered as drugs in their raw form as dried leaves. Other natural sources of drugs include *Amanita* mushrooms, which yield the plant alkaloid muscarine, and peyote cacti with the active ingredient of mescaline.

Crude Drug Preparations

Some **crude drug preparations** are made by drying or pulverizing a plant or animal tissue. Others are made by extracting substances from a natural product with the aid of hot water or a solvent such as alcohol. Familiar examples of crude drug preparations are **coffee** and **tea,** made from distillates of the beans and leaves of *Coffea arabica* and *Camellia sinensis* plants, respectively, and **opium,** which is the dried juice of the unripe poppy capsule of the plant *Papaver somniferum.*

Pure Drug Compounds

It is difficult to identify and quantify the pharmacologic effects of crude drug preparations because these products contain multiple ingredients with varying amounts from batch to batch. Therefore the development of methods to isolate **pure drug compounds from natural sources** was an important step in the growth of pharmacology and rational therapeutics. Frederick Sertürner, a German pharmacist, isolated the first pure drug from a natural source in 1804. He extracted and tested a potent **analgesic** agent from opium and named it **morphine,** from Morpheus, the Greek god of dreams. The subsequent isolation of many other drugs from natural sources provided pharmacologists with a number of pure compounds for study and characterization. One of the greatest medical achievements of the early 20th century was the isolation of insulin from the pancreas. This achievement led to the development of **insulin** preparations for treating **diabetes mellitus.**

Pharmaceutical Preparations

Pharmaceutical preparations or dosage forms are drug products suitable for administration of a specific dose of a drug to a patient by a **particular route of administration.** Most of these preparations are made from pure drug compounds, but a few are made from crude drug preparations and sold as herbal remedies. By far, the most common formulation of drugs is for the **oral route** of administration, followed by formulations used for **injections.**

Tablets and Capsules. Tablets and capsules are the most common preparations for oral administration because they are suitable for mass production, are stable and convenient to use, and can be formulated to release the drug immediately after ingestion or to release it over a period of hours.

In the manufacture of tablets, a machine with a punch and die mechanism compresses a mixture of powdered drug and inert ingredients into a hard pill. The **inert ingredients** include specific components that provide bulk, prevent sticking to the punch and die during manufacture, maintain tablet stability in the bottle, and facilitate solubilization of the tablet when it reaches gastrointestinal fluids. These ingredients are called **fillers, lubricants, adhesives,** and **disintegrants,** respectively.

A tablet must disintegrate after it has been ingested, and then the drug must **dissolve in gastrointestinal fluids** before it can be absorbed into the circulation. Variations in the rate and extent of tablet disintegration and drug dissolution can give rise to differences in *bioavailability* of drugs from different tablet formulations (see Chapter 2).

Tablets may have various types of coatings. **Enteric coatings** consist of polymers that will not disintegrate in gastric acid but will break down in the more basic pH of the intestines. Enteric coatings are used to protect drugs that would otherwise be destroyed by gastric acid and to slow the release and absorption of a drug when a large dose is given at one time, for example, in the formulation of the antidepressant **fluoxetine,** called PROZAC WEEKLY.

Sustained-release products, or **extended-release products,** release the drug from the preparation over many hours. The two methods used to extend the release of a drug are **controlled diffusion** and **controlled dissolution.** With controlled diffusion, a rate-controlling membrane regulates release of the drug from the pharmaceutical product. Inert polymers gradually break down in body fluids creating a controlled dissolution. These polymers may be part of the tablet matrix, or they may be used as coatings over small pellets of drug enclosed in a capsule. In either case, the drug is gradually released into the gastrointestinal tract as the polymers dissolve.

Some products use **osmotic pressure** to provide a sustained release of a drug. These products contain an osmotic agent that attracts gastrointestinal fluid at a constant rate. The attracted fluid then forces the drug out of the tablet through a small laser-drilled hole (Fig. 1.3A).

Capsules are hard or soft gelatin shells enclosing a powdered or liquid medication. **Hard capsules** are used to enclose powdered drugs, whereas **soft capsules** enclose a drug in solution. The gelatin shell quickly dissolves in gastrointestinal fluids to release the drug for absorption into the circulation.

Solutions and Suspensions. Drug solutions and particle suspensions, the most common liquid pharmaceutical preparations, can be formulated for oral, parenteral, or other routes of administration. Solutions and suspensions provide a convenient method for administering drugs to pediatric and other patients who cannot easily swallow pills or tablets. However, they are less convenient than solid dosage forms because the liquid must be measured each time a dose is given.

Solutions and suspensions for oral administration are often sweetened and flavored to increase palatability. Sweetened aqueous solutions are called **syrups,** whereas sweetened aqueous-alcoholic solutions are known as **elixirs.** Alcohol is included in elixirs as a solvent for drugs that are not sufficiently soluble in water alone.

Sterile solutions and suspensions are available for **parenteral** administration with a needle and syringe or with an intravenous infusion pump. Many drugs are formulated as sterile powders for reconstitution with sterile liquids at the time the drug is to be injected, because the drug is not stable for long periods of time in solution. Sterile ophthalmic solutions and suspensions are suitable for administration with an eyedropper into the conjunctival sac.

Skin Patches. Transdermal skin patches are drug preparations in which the drug is slowly released from the patch for absorption through the skin into the circulation. Most skin patches use a **rate-controlling membrane** to regulate the diffusion of the drug from the patch (see Fig. 1.3B). Such devices are most suitable for potent drugs, which are therefore effective at relatively low doses and that have **sufficient lipid solubility** to enable skin penetration.

Aerosols. Aerosols are a type of drug preparation administered by inhalation through the **nose or mouth.** They are particularly useful for treating respiratory disorders because they deliver the drug directly to the site of action and may thereby minimize the risk of systemic side effects. Some aerosol devices contain the drug dispersed in a pressurized gas and are designed to deliver a precise dose each time they are activated by the patient. **Nasal sprays,** another type of aerosol preparation, can be used either to deliver drugs that have a localized effect on the nasal mucosa or to deliver

A

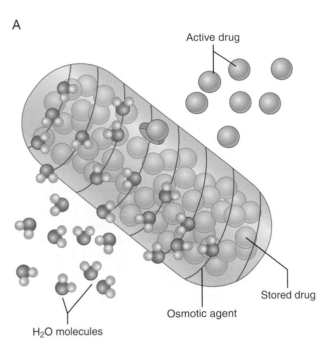

Active drug

Osmotic agent

Stored drug

H₂O molecules

B

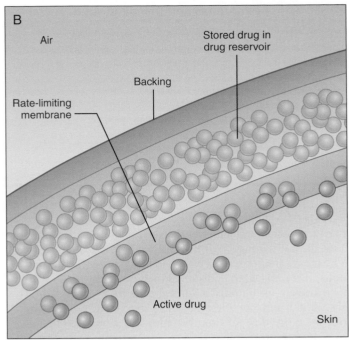

Air

Stored drug in drug reservoir

Backing

Rate-limiting membrane

Active drug

Skin

FIG. 1.3 Mechanisms of sustained-release drug products. In the sustained-release tablet (A). Water is attracted by an osmotic agent in the tablet, and this forces the drug out through a small orifice. In the transdermal skin patch (B). The drug diffuses through a rate-controlling membrane and is absorbed through the skin into the circulation.

drugs that are absorbed through the mucosa and exert an effect on another organ. For example, **butorphanol,** an opioid analgesic, is available as a nasal spray (STADOL NS) for the treatment of pain.

Ointments, Creams, Lotions, and Suppositories. Ointments and creams are semisolid preparations intended for **topical application** of a drug to the skin or mucous membranes. These products contain an active drug incorporated into a vehicle (e.g., polyethylene glycol or petrolatum), which enables the drug to adhere to the tissue for a sufficient length of time to exert its effect. Lotions are liquid preparations often formulated as oil-in-water emulsions and are used to treat dermatologic conditions. Suppositories are products in which the drug is incorporated into a solid base that melts or dissolves at body temperature. Suppositories are used for **rectal, vaginal,** or **urethral administration** and may provide either localized or systemic drug therapy.

ROUTES OF DRUG ADMINISTRATION

Some routes of drug administration, such as the **enteral** and common **parenteral** routes compared in Table 1.2, are intended to elicit systemic effects and are therefore called **systemic routes.** Other routes of administration, such as the inhalational route, can elicit either localized effects or systemic effects, depending on the drug being administered.

Enteral Administration

The enteral routes of administration are those in which the drug is absorbed from the gastrointestinal tract. These include the **sublingual, buccal, oral,** and **rectal** routes.

In **sublingual administration,** a drug product is placed under the tongue. In **buccal administration,** the drug is placed between the cheek and the gum. Both the sublingual and the buccal routes of administration enable the rapid absorption of certain drugs and are not affected by first-pass

drug metabolism in the liver. Drugs for sublingual and buccal administration are given in a relatively low dose and must have good solubility in water and lipid membranes. Larger doses might be irritating to the tissue and would likely be washed away by saliva before the drug could be absorbed. Two examples of drugs available for sublingual administration are **nitroglycerin** for treating ischemic heart disease and **hyoscyamine** for treating bowel cramps. **Fentanyl,** a potent opioid analgesic, is available in an oral transmucosal formulation (ACTIQ) with a lozenge on a stick ("lollypop") for rapid absorption from the buccal mucosa in the treatment of breakthrough cancer pain.

In medical orders and prescriptions, **oral administration** is designated as *per os* (PO), which means to administer "by mouth." The medication is swallowed, and the drug is absorbed from the stomach and small intestine. The oral route of administration is convenient, relatively safe, and the most economical. However, it does have some disadvantages. Absorption of orally administered drugs can vary widely because of the interaction of drugs with food and gastric acid and the varying rates of gastric emptying, intestinal transit, and tablet disintegration and dissolution. Moreover, some drugs are inactivated by the liver after their absorption from the gut, called **first-pass metabolism** (see Chapter 2), and oral administration is not suitable for use by patients who are sedated, comatose, or experiencing nausea and vomiting.

Rectal administration of drugs in suppository form can result in either a localized effect or a systemic effect. Suppositories are useful when patients cannot take medications by mouth, as in the treatment of nausea and vomiting. They can also be administered for localized conditions such as hemorrhoids. Drugs absorbed from the lower rectum undergo relatively little first-pass metabolism in the liver.

TABLE 1.2 **Advantages and Disadvantages of Four Common Routes of Drug Administration**

ROUTE	ADVANTAGES	DISADVANTAGES
Oral	Convenient, relatively safe, and economical.	Cannot be used for drugs inactivated by gastric acid, for drugs with a large first-pass effect, or for drugs that irritate the gut.
Intramuscular	Suitable for suspensions and oily vehicles. Absorption is rapid from solutions and is slow and sustained from suspensions.	May be painful. Can cause bleeding if the patient is receiving an anticoagulant.
Subcutaneous	Suitable for suspensions and pellets. Absorption is similar to that in the intramuscular route but is usually somewhat slower.	Cannot be used for drugs that irritate cutaneous tissues or for drugs that must be given in large volumes.
Intravenous	Bypasses absorption to give an immediate effect. Allows for rapid titration of drug. Achieves 100% bioavailability.	Poses more risks for toxicity and tends to be more expensive than other routes.

Parenteral Administration

Parenteral administration refers to drug administration with a needle and syringe or with an intravenous infusion pump. The most commonly used parenteral routes are the **intravenous, intramuscular,** and **subcutaneous** routes.

Intravenous administration bypasses the process of drug absorption and provides the greatest reliability and control over the dose of drug reaching the systemic circulation. Because the drug is delivered directly into the blood, it has 100% **bioavailability** (see Chapter 2). The route is often preferred for administration of drugs with short half-lives and drugs whose dose must be carefully titrated to the physiologic response, such as agents used to treat hypotension, shock, and acute heart failure. The intravenous route is widely used to administer antibiotics and antineoplastic drugs to critically ill patients, as well as to treat various types of medical emergencies. The intravenous route is potentially the **most dangerous** because rapid administration of drugs by this route can cause serious toxicity.

Intramuscular administration and **subcutaneous administration** are suitable for treatment with drug solutions and particle suspensions. Solutions are absorbed more rapidly than particle suspensions, so suspensions are often used to extend the duration of action of a drug over many hours or days. Most drugs are absorbed more rapidly after intramuscular than after subcutaneous administration because of the greater circulation of blood to the muscle.

Intrathecal administration refers to injection of a drug through the thecal covering of the spinal cord and into the subarachnoid space. In cases of meningitis, the intrathecal route is useful in administering antibiotics that do not cross the blood-brain barrier. **Epidural administration,** common in labor and delivery, targets analgesics into the space above the dural membranes of the spinal cord.

Other, less common parenteral routes include **intra-articular administration** of drugs used to treat arthritis, **intradermal administration** for allergy tests, and **insufflation (intranasal administration)** for sinus medications.

Transdermal Administration

Transdermal administration is the application of drugs to the skin for absorption into the circulation. Application can be via a **skin patch** or, less commonly, via an ointment. Transdermal administration, which bypasses first-pass metabolism, is a reliable route of administration for drugs that are effective when given at a relatively low dosage and that are highly soluble in lipid membranes. Transdermal skin patches slowly release medication for periods of time that typically range from 1 to

7 days. Two examples of transdermal preparations are the skin patches called **fentanyl transdermal** (DURAGESIC), used to treat severe chronic pain, and **nitroglycerin** ointment, used to treat heart failure and angina pectoris.

Inhalational Administration

Inhalational administration can be used to produce either a localized or a systemic drug effect. A localized effect on the respiratory tract is achieved with drugs used to treat **asthma** or **rhinitis,** whereas a systemic effect is observed when a general anesthetic such as **sevoflurane** is inhaled.

Topical Administration

Topical administration refers to the application of drugs to the **surface** of the body to produce a localized effect. It is often used to treat disease and trauma of the skin, eyes, nose, mouth, throat, rectum, and vagina.

DRUG NAMES

A drug often has several names, including a **chemical** name, a **nonproprietary (generic)** name, and a **proprietary** name (or **trade** or **brand** name).

The **chemical name,** which specifies the chemical structure of the drug, uses standard chemical nomenclature. Some chemical names are short and easily pronounceable (e.g., the chemical name of aspirin is acetylsalicylic acid). Others are long and hard to pronounce owing to the size and complexity of the drug molecule. For most drugs, medicinal chemists primarily use the chemical name.

The **generic name** (nonproprietary name) is the type of drug name **most suitable for use by health care professionals.** In the United States, the generic names of drugs are the **United States Adopted Name** (USAN) designations. These designations, which are often derived from the chemical names of drugs, provide some indication of the class to which a particular drug belongs. For example, oxacillin can be easily recognized as a type of penicillin. The designations are selected by the USAN Council, which is a nomenclature committee representing the medical and pharmacy professions and the *United States Pharmacopeial Convention* (see Chapter 4). Students taking various board examinations including pharmacology (e.g., nursing boards, medical boards) will also be **most attentive to the generic** names of drugs.

The **brand name** (proprietary name, trade name) for a drug is the registered trademark belonging to a particular drug manufacturer and is used to designate a drug product marketed by that manufacturer. Heavily marketed brand names become common knowledge to patients, such as PROZAC and

VIAGRA. Many drugs are marketed under two or more brand names, especially after the manufacturer loses patent exclusivity. For example, ibuprofen (generic name) is marketed in the United States with the brand names of ADVIL, MOTRIN, and MIDOL. Drugs can also be marketed under their USAN designation. For these reasons, it is often less confusing and more precise to use the USAN rather than a brand name for a drug. However, the brand name may provide a better indication of the drug's pharmacologic or therapeutic effect. For example, DIURIL is a brand name for **chlorothiazide,** a diuretic; FLOMAX for **tamsulosin,** a drug used to increase urine flow; and MAXAIR for **pirbuterol,** a drug used to treat asthma.

Generic Drug Substitution for Branded Drugs

When a new drug is developed and brought to market by a pharmaceutical manufacturer, the US Food and Drug Administration (FDA) approval comes with an exclusivity patent for the next 17 to 20 years. During this time, no other company can manufacture or sell the same drug. When the original drug loses exclusivity, generic drug manufacturers can file for a brief form of drug approval, limited to showing that the generic formulation exhibits the same **absorption** and **bioavailability** as the original, branded drug. Generic drugs are much cheaper because the second manufacturer does not have to recoup the costs of drug discovery, development, clinical trials, and the FDA new drug application.

Although the FDA does not regulate when to use generic drugs, most states have passed laws on **generic substitution.** Because use of generic medications instead of branded drugs can save millions of dollars in health care costs, some states mandate generic substitution without patient or physician approval, although physicians can override generic substitutions in some cases. Other states need the approval of the patient or physician to switch from a branded drug prescription to a generic substitute.

Both patient and physician misconceptions affect the underutilization of generic drugs. Scientific studies show that the overwhelming majority of generic medicines are **bioequivalent** to the branded, originator drug. The FDA has identified certain drugs that may be more dangerous to switch, called **narrow therapeutic index** (NTI) drugs, which may warrant further drug blood monitoring after a generic to branded drug substitution.

In this textbook, the generic name of a drug is given in the normal-sized font and its brand name in SMALL CAPS font. Note that not all generic drugs have a brand name counterpart.

SUMMARY OF IMPORTANT POINTS

- The development of pharmacology was made possible by important advances in chemistry and physiology that enabled scientists to isolate and synthesize pure chemical compounds (drugs) and to design methods for identifying and quantifying the physiologic actions of the compounds.
- Pharmacology has two main subdivisions. Pharmacodynamics is concerned with the mechanisms of drug action and the dose-response relationship, whereas pharmacokinetics is concerned with the relationship between the drug dose and the plasma drug concentration over time.

- The sources of drugs are natural products (including plants, microbes, animal tissues, and minerals) and chemical synthesis. Drugs can exist as crude drug preparations, pure drug compounds, or pharmaceutical preparations used to administer a specific dose to a patient.
- The primary routes of administration are enteral (e.g., oral ingestion), parenteral (e.g., intravenous, intramuscular, and subcutaneous injection), transdermal, inhalational, and topical. Most routes produce systemic effects. Topical administration produces a localized effect at the site of administration.
- All drugs (pure compounds) have a nonproprietary name (or generic name, such as a USAN designation) and a chemical name. Some drugs also have one or more proprietary names (trade names or brand names) under which they are marketed by their manufacturer.

Review Questions

1. Which route of drug administration is used with potent and lipophilic drugs in a patch formulation and avoids first-pass metabolism?
   - (A) topical
   - (B) sublingual
   - (C) rectal
   - (D) oral
   - (E) transdermal
2. Which one of the following routes of administration does not have an absorption phase?
   - (A) subcutaneous
   - (B) intramuscular
   - (C) intravenous
   - (D) sublingual
   - (E) inhalation
3. Which of the following correctly describes the intramuscular route of parenteral drug administration?
   - (A) drug absorption is erratic and unpredictable
   - (B) used to administer drug suspensions that are slowly absorbed
   - (C) bypasses the process of drug absorption to achieve an immediate effect
   - (D) cannot be used for drugs that undergo a high degree of first-pass metabolism
   - (E) poses more risks than intravenous administration
4. An elderly patient has problems remembering to take her medication 3 times a day. Which one of the drug formulations might be particularly useful in this case?
   - (A) extended release
   - (B) suspension
   - (C) suppository
   - (D) skin patch
   - (E) enteric coated
5. Which form of a drug name is most likely known by patients from exposure to drug advertisements?
   - (A) nonproprietary name
   - (B) British Approved Name
   - (C) chemical name
   - (D) generic name
   - (E) trade name

Pharmacokinetics or What the Body Does to the Drug

OVERVIEW

Pharmacokinetics is the study of drug disposition in the body and focuses on the changes in **drug plasma concentration.** For any given drug and dose, the plasma concentration of the drug will rise and fall according to the rates of four processes: **absorption, distribution, metabolism,** and **excretion** (ADME). *Absorption* is the movement of drug from the site of administration to the bloodstream. The rate and extent of absorption are dependent on the physical characteristics of the drug and its formulation. *Distribution* is the process of a drug leaving the bloodstream and being distributed throughout the body, into the organs and tissues. **Metabolism,** also called **biotransformation,** is the process of converting a drug to one or more metabolites, primarily in the liver. **Excretion** is the removal of a drug or its metabolites from the body, primarily by the kidneys and urination. Sometimes the term **elimination** of a drug is used; this refers to the processes of metabolism and excretion combined. The relationship between these pharmacokinetic processes is explained more fully later and is shown in Fig. 2.1.

DRUG ABSORPTION

Drug absorption refers to the **passage of drug molecules** from the site of administration into the circulation. The process of drug absorption applies to all routes of administration, except for the topical route, in which drugs are applied directly on the target tissue, and intravenous administration, in which the drug is given directly in the bloodstream. Drug absorption requires that drugs cross one or more layers of cells and cell membranes. Drugs injected into the subcutaneous tissue and muscle bypass the epithelial barrier and are more easily absorbed through spaces between capillary endothelial cells. In the gut, lungs, and skin, drugs must first be absorbed through a layer of epithelial cells that have tight junctions. For this reason, drugs face a greater **barrier** to absorption after oral administration than after parenteral administration.

Processes of Absorption

Most drugs are absorbed by **passive diffusion** across a biologic barrier and into the circulation. The rate of absorption is proportional to the drug concentration gradient across the barrier and the surface area available for absorption at that site, known as **Fick's law.** Drugs can be absorbed passively through cells either by lipid diffusion or by aqueous diffusion. **Lipid diffusion** is a process by which the drug dissolves in the lipid components of the cell membranes. This process is facilitated by a high degree of lipid solubility of the drug. **Aqueous diffusion** occurs by passage through aqueous pores in cell membranes. Because aqueous diffusion is restricted to drugs with low molecular weights, many drugs are too large to be absorbed by this process.

A few drugs are absorbed by **active transport** or by **facilitated diffusion.** Active transport requires a **carrier molecule** and a form of **energy,** provided by hydrolysis of the terminal high-energy phosphate bond of adenosine triphosphate (ATP). Active transport can transfer drugs against a concentration gradient. For example, the antineoplastic drug **5-fluorouracil** undergoes active transport. Facilitated diffusion also requires a carrier molecule, but no energy is needed. Thus drugs or substances cannot be transferred against a concentration gradient but diffuse faster than without a carrier molecule present. Some cephalosporin antibiotics, such as **cephalexin,** undergo facilitated diffusion by an oligopeptide transporter protein located in intestinal epithelial cells.

Effect of pH on Absorption of Weak Acids and Bases

Many drugs are weak acids or bases that exist in both ionized and nonionized forms in the body. Only the **nonionized form** of these drugs is sufficiently soluble in membrane lipids to cross cell membranes (Box 2.1). The ratio of the two forms at a particular site influences the **rate of absorption** and is also a factor in distribution and elimination.

The protonated form of a weak acid is nonionized, whereas the protonated form of a weak base is ionized. The ratio of the protonated form to the nonprotonated form of these drugs can be calculated using the **Henderson-Hasselbalch equation** (see Box 2.1). The pK_a is the negative log of the ionization constant, particular for each acidic or basic drug. At a pH equal to the pK_a, **equal** amounts of the protonated and nonprotonated forms are present. If the pH is less than the pK_a, the protonated form predominates. If the pH is greater than the pK_a, the nonprotonated form predominates.

In the stomach, with a pH of 1, weak acids and bases are highly protonated. At this site, the nonionized form of weak acids (pK_a = 3–5) and the ionized form of weak bases (pK_a = 8–10) will predominate. Hence weak acids are more readily absorbed from the stomach than are weak bases. In the intestines, with a pH of 7, weak bases are also mostly ionized but much less so than in the stomach, and weak bases are absorbed more readily from the intestines than from the stomach.

However, weak acids can also be absorbed more readily from the intestines than from the stomach, despite their greater ionization in the intestines, because the intestines have a greater surface area than the stomach for absorption of the nonionized form of a drug, and this outweighs the influence of greater ionization in the intestines.

DRUG DISTRIBUTION

Drugs are distributed to organs and tissues via the circulation, diffusing into interstitial fluid and into cells from the bloodstream. Most drugs are not uniformly distributed throughout total body water, and some drugs are restricted to the extracellular fluid or the plasma compartment. Drugs

Pill taken   Drug concentration in blood   Removed in urine

Plasma protein binding

Absorption
Distribution

Excretion
Metabolism

Tissues
and organs   Liver

Fig. 2.1   The absorption, distribution, biotransformation (metabolism), and excretion of a typical drug after its oral administration.

BOX 2.1 EFFECT OF PH ON THE ABSORPTION OF A WEAK ACID AND A WEAK BASE

Weak **acids** (HA) donate a proton (H^+) to form anions (A^-), whereas **weak bases** (B) accept a proton to form cations (HB^+).

$$HA \rightleftharpoons H^+ + A^-$$

For weak acids, the protonated form is nonionized.

$$B + H^+ \rightleftharpoons HB^+$$

For weak bases, the protonated form is ionized.

Only the **nonionized form** of a drug can readily penetrate cell membranes.

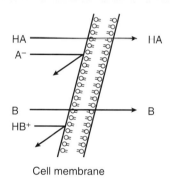

Cell membrane

The **pK_a** of a weak acid or weak base is the **pH** at which there are equal amounts of the protonated form and the nonprotonated form. The **Henderson-Hasselbalch equation** can be used to determine the ratio of the two forms:

$$\log \frac{[\text{protonate form}]}{[\text{non protonate form}]} = pK_a - pH$$

For **salicylic acid,** which is a weak acid with a pK_a of 3, log $[HA]/[A^-]$ is 3 minus the pH. At a pH of 2, then, log $[HA]/[A^-] = 3 - 2 = 1$. Therefore $[HA]/[A^-] = 10/1$.

COOH
OH
Protonated

$\rightleftharpoons$

COO⁻
OH   + H⁺
Nonprotonated

For **amphetamine,** which is a weak base with a pK_a of 10, log $[HB^+]/[B]$ is 10 minus the pH. At a pH of 8, then, log $[HB^+]/[B] = 10 - 8 = 2$. Therefore $[HB^+]/[B] = 100/1$.

CH₂ — CH — NH₂
     |
     CH₃   + H⁺

Nonprotonated

$\rightleftharpoons$

CH₂ — CH — NH₃⁺
     |
     CH₃

Protonated

The following are the ratios of the protonated form to the nonprotonated form at different pH levels:

	Salicylic acid					Amphetamine			
Protonated	10	1	1	1	1	1000	100	10	1
pH	2	3	4	5	6	7	8	9	10
Nonprotonated	1	1	10	100	1000	1	1	1	1

with sufficient lipid solubility can simply diffuse through membranes into cells. Other drugs are concentrated in cells by the phenomenon of **ion trapping,** which is described later. Drugs can also be actively transported into cells. For example, some drugs are actively transported into hepatic cells, where they undergo metabolism.

Opposing the distribution of drugs to tissues are a number of ATP-driven drug efflux pumps, known as **ABC transporters** (ABC is an acronym for "ATP-binding cassette"). The most studied of these proteins, called *permeability glycoprotein* or simply **P-glycoprotein (Pgp),** is expressed on the luminal side of endothelial cells lining the intestines, brain capillaries, and a number of other tissues. Drug transport in the blood-to-lumen direction leads to a secretion of various drugs into the intestinal tract, thereby serving as a detoxifying mechanism. Pgp also serves to exclude drugs from the brain. The Pgp proteins may exclude drugs from tissues throughout the body, including anticancer agents from tumors, leading to **chemotherapeutic drug resistance.** Inhibition of Pgp by amiodarone, erythromycin, propranolol, and other agents can increase tissue levels of these drugs and augment their pharmacologic effects (see Fig. 45.2).

Factors Affecting Distribution
Organ Blood Flow
The rate at which a drug is distributed to various organs after a drug dose is administered depends largely on the proportion of **cardiac output** received by the organs. Drugs are rapidly distributed to highly perfused tissues, namely the brain, heart, liver, and kidney. This enables a rapid onset of action of drugs affecting these tissues. Drugs are distributed more slowly to less perfused tissues such as skeletal muscle and even more slowly to those with the lowest blood flow, such as skin, bone, and adipose (fat) tissue.

Plasma Protein Binding
Almost all drugs are reversibly bound to plasma proteins, primarily **albumin,** but also lipoproteins, glycoproteins, and β-globulins. The extent of binding depends on the affinity of a particular drug for protein-binding sites and ranges from less than 10% to as high as 99% of the plasma concentration. As the free (unbound) drug diffuses into interstitial fluid and cells, drug molecules dissociate from plasma proteins to maintain the equilibrium between free drug and bound drug. In general, **acidic drugs bind to albumin** and **basic drugs to glycoproteins and β-globulins.**

Plasma protein binding is **saturable,** and a drug can be displaced from binding sites by other drugs that have a high affinity for such sites. However, most drugs are not used at high enough plasma concentrations to occupy the vast number of plasma protein binding sites. There are a few agents that may cause drug interactions by competing for plasma protein binding sites, as highlighted in Chapter 4.

Molecular Size
Molecular size is a factor affecting the distribution of extremely large molecules, such as those of the anticoagulant **heparin.** Heparin is largely confined to the plasma compartment, although it does undergo some biotransformation in the liver.

Lipid Solubility. Lipid solubility is a major factor affecting the extent of drug distribution, particularly to the brain, where the **blood-brain barrier** restricts the penetration of polar and ionized molecules. The barrier is formed by tight junctions between the capillary endothelial cells and also by the glial cells that surround the capillaries, which inhibit the penetration of polar molecules into brain neurons.

DRUG METABOLISM
Drug metabolism (biotransformation) and **excretion** are the two processes responsible for the decline of the plasma drug concentration over time. Both of these processes contribute to the **elimination** of active drug from the body. As discussed later in the chapter, **clearance** is a measure of the rate of elimination. Drug metabolism is the enzyme-catalyzed conversion of drugs to their metabolites. Most drug biotransformation takes place in the liver, but drug-metabolizing enzymes are found in many other tissues, including the gut, kidneys, brain, lungs, and skin.

Role of Drug Biotransformation
The fundamental role of drug-metabolizing enzymes is to **inactivate** and **detoxify** drugs and other foreign substances (xenobiotics) that can enter the body. Drug metabolites are usually more water soluble than is the parent molecule, and therefore they are more readily excreted by the kidneys. No particular relationship exists between metabolism and pharmacologic activity. Some drug metabolites are active, whereas others are inactive. Many drug molecules undergo attachment of polar groups, a process called **conjugation,** for more rapid excretion. As a general rule, most conjugated drug metabolites are inactive, but a few exceptions exist.

Formation of Active Metabolites
Many pharmacologically active drugs, such as the sedative-hypnotic agent **diazepam** (VALIUM), are biotransformed to active metabolites. Some agents, known as **prodrugs,** are administered as inactive compounds and then biotransformed to active metabolites. This type of agent is usually developed because the prodrug is better absorbed than its active metabolite. For example, the antiglaucoma agent **dipivefrin** (PROPINE) is a prodrug converted to its active metabolite, epinephrine, by corneal enzymes after topical ocular administration. Orally administered prodrugs, such as the antihypertensive agent **enalapril** (VASOTEC), are converted to their active metabolite by hepatic enzymes during their first pass through the liver.

First-Pass Biotransformation
Drugs that are absorbed from the gut reach the liver via the hepatic portal vein before entering the systemic circulation (Fig. 2.2). Many drugs, such as the antihypertensive agent **felodipine** (PLENDIL), are extensively converted to inactive metabolites during their first pass through the gut wall and liver and have low **bioavailability** (see later) after oral administration. This phenomenon is called the **first-pass effect.** Drugs administered by the sublingual or rectal route undergo less first-pass metabolism and have a higher degree of bioavailability than do drugs administered by the oral route.

Phases of Drug Biotransformation
Drug biotransformation can be divided into two phases, each carried out by a unique set of metabolic enzymes. In many cases, phase I enzymatic reactions create or unmask a

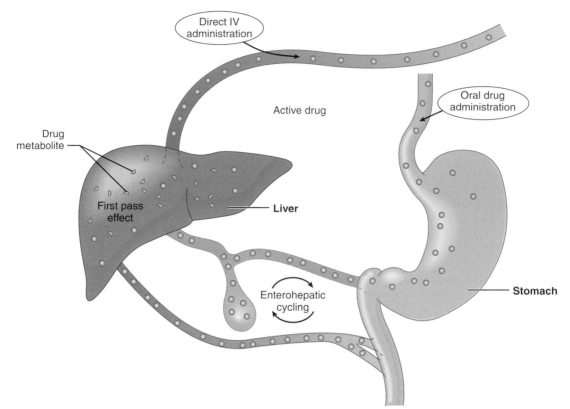

Fɪɢ. 2.2 First-pass drug biotransformation. Drugs that are absorbed from the gut can be biotransformed by enzymes in the gut wall and liver before reaching the systemic circulation. This process lowers their degree of bioavailability. Enterohepatic cycling can occur when drugs and drug metabolites with molecular weights greater than 300 are excreted via the bile, stored in the gallbladder, delivered to the intestines by the bile duct, and then reabsorbed into the hepatic portal system. This process reduces the elimination of a drug and prolongs its half-life and duration of action in the body.

chemical group required for a phase II reaction. However, in some cases, drugs bypass phase I biotransformation and go directly to phase II. Although some phase I drug metabolites are pharmacologically active, most phase II drug metabolites are inactive.

Phase I Biotransformation

Phase I biotransformation includes oxidative, hydrolytic, and reductive reactions (Fig. 2.3).

Oxidative Reactions. Oxidative reactions are the most common type of phase I biotransformation. They are catalyzed by enzymes isolated in the microsomal fraction of liver homogenates (the fraction derived from the endoplasmic reticulum) and by cytoplasmic enzymes.

The **microsomal cytochrome P450 (CYP) monooxygenase system** is a family of enzymes that catalyze the biotransformation of drugs with a wide range of chemical structures. The microsomal **monooxygenase reaction** requires the following: CYP (a hemoprotein); a flavoprotein reduced by nicotinamide adenine dinucleotide phosphate (NADPH), called *NADPH CYP reductase*; and membrane lipids in which the system is embedded. In the drug-oxidizing reaction, one atom of oxygen is used to form a hydroxylated metabolite of a drug, whereas the other atom of oxygen forms water when combined with electrons contributed by NADPH. The hydroxylated metabolite may be the end product of the reaction or serve as an intermediate that leads to the formation of another metabolite.

The most common chemical reactions catalyzed by CYP enzymes are aliphatic hydroxylation, aromatic hydroxylation, *N*-dealkylation, and *O*-dealkylation.

Many **CYP isozymes** have been identified and cloned, and their role in metabolizing specific drugs elucidated. Each isozyme catalyzes a different but overlapping spectrum of oxidative reactions. Most drug metabolism is catalyzed by three CYP families named *CYP1, CYP2,* and *CYP3.* The different CYP families are likely related by gene duplication, and each family is divided into subfamilies, also clearly related by homologous protein sequences. The **CYP3A** subfamily catalyzes more than half of all microsomal drug oxidation reactions.

Many drugs alter drug metabolism by inhibiting or inducing CYP enzymes, and **drug interactions** can occur when these drugs are administered concurrently with other drugs that are metabolized by CYP (see Chapter 4). Two examples of **inducers of CYP** are the barbiturate **phenobarbital** and the antitubercular drug **rifampin.** The inducers stimulate the transcription of genes encoding CYP enzymes, resulting in increased messenger RNA (mRNA) and protein synthesis. Drugs that induce CYP enzymes activate the binding of **transcription factors** to the promoter domains of CYP genes, increasing their rate of gene transcription.

A few drugs are oxidized by **cytoplasmic enzymes.** For example, **ethanol** is oxidized to aldehyde by alcohol dehydrogenase, and **caffeine** and the bronchodilator **theophylline** are metabolized by xanthine oxidase. Other cytoplasmic oxidases include **monoamine oxidase,** a site of action for some psychotropic medications.

Hydrolytic Reactions. Esters and amides are hydrolyzed by a variety of enzymes. These include cholinesterase and other plasma esterases that inactivate choline esters, local anesthetics, and drugs such as **esmolol** (Bʀᴇᴠɪʙʟᴏᴄ), an

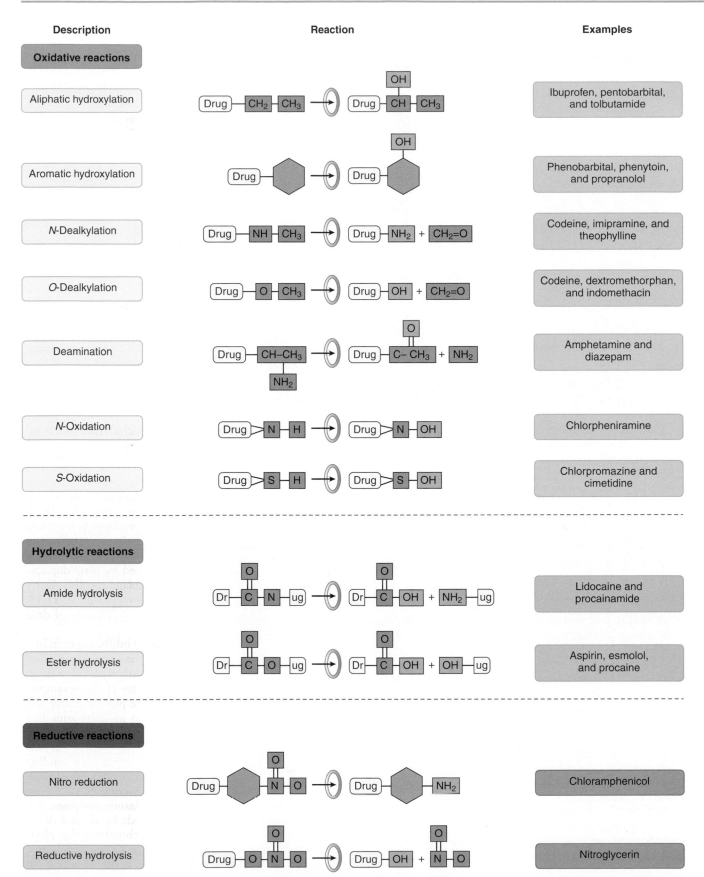

Fig. 2.3 Phase I drug biotransformation. Many drugs are biotransformed by oxidative, hydrolytic, or reductive reactions and then undergo conjugation with endogenous substances. A few drugs bypass phase I reactions and directly enter phase II biotransformation.

Description | Reaction | Examples

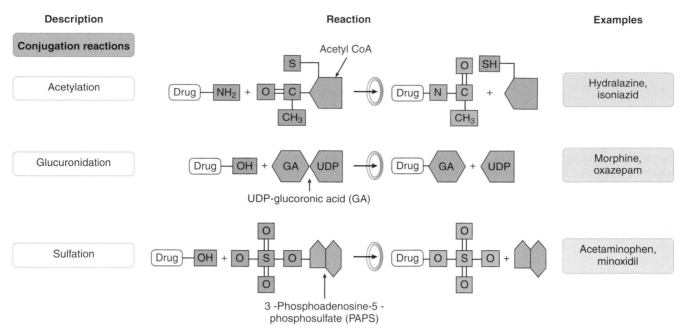

FIG. 2.4 Phase II drug biotransformation. Many drugs undergo conjugation with endogenous substances as shown in the figure. *UDP,* Uridine diphosphate.

agent for the treatment of tachycardia that blocks cardiac β_1-adrenoceptors. There are few CYP enzymes that carry out hydrolytic reactions.

Reductive Reactions. Reductive reactions are less common than are oxidative and hydrolytic reactions. **Chloramphenicol,** an antimicrobial agent, and a few other drugs are partly metabolized by a hepatic nitroreductase, and this process involves CYP enzymes. **Nitroglycerin,** a vasodilator, undergoes reductive hydrolysis catalyzed by glutathione-organic nitrate reductase.

Phase II Biotransformation

In phase II biotransformation, drug molecules undergo **conjugation reactions** with an endogenous substance such as **acetate, glucuronate, sulfate,** or **glycine** (Fig. 2.4). Conjugation enzymes, which are present in the liver and other tissues, join various drug molecules with one of these endogenous substances to form water-soluble metabolites that are more easily excreted. Except for microsomal **glucuronosyltransferases,** these enzymes are located in the cytoplasm. Most conjugated drug metabolites are pharmacologically inactive.

Glucuronide Formation. Glucuronide formation, the most common conjugation reaction, uses **glucuronosyltransferases** to conjugate a glucuronate molecule with the parent drug molecule.

Acetylation. Acetylation is accomplished by **N-acetyltransferase** enzymes that use acetyl coenzyme A (acetyl CoA) as a source of the acetate group.

Sulfation. **Sulfotransferases** catalyze the conjugation of several drugs, including the vasodilator **minoxidil** and the potassium-sparing diuretic **triamterene,** whose sulfate metabolites are pharmacologically active.

Pharmacogenomics

Since the completion of the Human Genome Project, it is now fully realized that there is a great degree of individual variation, called **polymorphism,** in the genes coding for

drug-metabolizing enzymes. Modern genetic studies were triggered by rare fatalities in children being treating for leukemia using the thiopurine agent 6-mercaptopurine (6-MP). It was discovered that the children died as a result of drug toxicity because they expressed a faulty variant of thiopurine methyltransferase, the enzyme that metabolizes 6-MP.

Variations in Acetyltransferase Activity

Individuals exhibit slow or fast acetylation of some drugs because of genetically determined differences in *N*-acetyltransferase. Slow acetylators (SAs) were first identified by neuropathic effects of **isoniazid,** a drug to treat tuberculosis (see Chapter 41). These patients had higher plasma levels of isoniazid compared with other patients classified as rapid acetylators (RAs). The SA phenotype is autosomal recessive, although more than 20 allelic variants of the gene for *N*-acetyltransferase have been identified. In individuals with one wild-type enzyme and one faulty variant, an intermediate phenotype is observed. The **distribution** of these phenotypes varies from population to population. Approximately 15% of Asians, 50% of Whites and Africans, and more than 80% of Mideast populations have the SA phenotype. Other drugs that may cause toxicity in the SA patient are **sulfonamide antibiotics,** the antidysrhythmic agent **procainamide,** and the antihypertensive agent **hydralazine.**

Variations in CYP2D6 and CYP2C19 Activity

Variations in oxidation of some drugs have been attributed to genetic differences in certain CYP enzymes. Genetic polymorphisms of CYP2D6 and CYP2C19 enzymes are well characterized, and human populations of "extensive metabolizers" and "poor metabolizers" have been identified. These differences are caused by more than 70 identified variants in the *CYP2D6* gene and more than 25 variants of the *CYP2C19* genes, resulting from point mutations, deletions, or additions; gene rearrangements; or deletion or duplication of the entire gene. This gives rise to an increase, reduction, or complete loss of enzyme activity and to different levels of enzyme expression that result in **altered rates** of enzymatic reactions.

Most individuals are extensive metabolizers of CYP2D6 substrates, but 10% of Whites and a smaller fraction of Asians and Africans are poor metabolizers of substrates for CYP2D6. Psychiatric patients who are poor metabolizers of CYP2D6 drugs have been found to have a higher rate of adverse drug reactions than do those who are extensive metabolizers, because of higher psychotropic drug plasma levels. In addition, poor metabolizers of CYP2D6 drugs have a reduced ability to metabolize **codeine** to **morphine** sufficiently to obtain adequate pain relief when codeine is administered for analgesia.

Poor metabolizers of CYP2C19 substrates have higher plasma levels of proton pump inhibitors, such as **omeprazole** (PRILOSEC), whereas some extensive metabolizers of CYP2C19 drugs require larger doses of omeprazole to treat peptic ulcer.

Other Variations in Drug Metabolism Enzymes

Approximately 1 in 3000 individuals exhibits a familial **atypical cholinesterase** that will not metabolize **succinylcholine,** a neuromuscular blocking agent, at a normal rate. Affected individuals are subject to prolonged apnea after receiving the usual dose of the drug. For this reason, patients should be screened for atypical cholinesterase before receiving succinylcholine.

There are many more **polymorphisms** in both phase I and phase II metabolic enzymes. With more than 30 families of drug-metabolizing enzymes, all with genetic variants, a major development in pharmacotherapy will be the individual tailoring of drug and dose to each patient's genomic identity.

DRUG EXCRETION

Excretion is the removal of drug from body fluids and occurs primarily in the **urine.** Other routes of excretion from the body include in bile, sweat, saliva, tears, feces, breast milk, and exhaled air.

Renal Drug Excretion

Most drugs are excreted in the urine, either as the parent compound or as a drug metabolite. Drugs are handled by the kidneys in the same manner as are endogenous substances, undergoing processes of glomerular filtration, active tubular secretion, and passive tubular reabsorption. The amount of drug excreted is the sum of the amounts filtered and secreted minus the amount reabsorbed. The relationship among these processes, the rate of drug excretion, and renal clearance is shown in Box 2.2.

Glomerular Filtration

Glomerular filtration is the first step in renal drug excretion. In this process, the free drug enters the renal tubule as a dissolved solute in the plasma filtrate (see Box 2.2). If a drug has a large fraction bound to plasma proteins, as is the case with the anticoagulant **warfarin,** it will have a low rate of glomerular filtration.

Active Tubular Secretion

Some drugs, particularly weak acids and bases, undergo active tubular secretion by transport systems located primarily in proximal tubular cells. This process is competitively inhibited by other drugs of the same chemical class. For example, the secretion of penicillins and other weak acids is inhibited by **probenecid,** an agent used to treat gout.

Active tubular secretion is not affected by plasma protein binding. This is a result of the equilibrium of free drug and bound drug, such that when free drug is actively transported across the renal tubule, this fraction of free drug is replaced by a fraction that dissociates from plasma proteins.

Passive Tubular Reabsorption

The extent to which a drug undergoes passive reabsorption across renal tubular cells and into the circulation depends on the **lipid solubility** of the drug. Drug biotransformation facilitates drug elimination by forming polar drug metabolites that are not as readily reabsorbed as the less-polar parent molecules.

Most nonelectrolytes, including **ethanol,** are passively reabsorbed across tubular cells. Ionized weak acids and bases are not reabsorbed across renal tubular cells, and they are more rapidly excreted in the urine than are nonionized drugs that undergo passive reabsorption. The proportion of ionized and nonionized drugs is affected by **renal tubular pH,** which can be manipulated to increase the excretion of a drug after a drug overdose (Box 2.3).

Biliary Excretion and Enterohepatic Cycling

Many drugs are excreted in the bile as the parent compound or a drug metabolite. Biliary excretion favors compounds with molecular weights greater than 300 and with both polar and lipophilic groups; smaller molecules are excreted only in negligible amounts. Conjugation, particularly with **glucuronate,** increases biliary excretion.

Numerous conjugated drug metabolites, including both the glucuronate and sulfate metabolites of steroids, are excreted in the bile. After the bile empties into the intestines, a fraction of the drug may be reabsorbed into the circulation and eventually return to the liver. This phenomenon is called **enterohepatic cycling** (see previous Fig. 2.2). Excreted conjugated drugs can be hydrolyzed back to the parent drug by intestinal bacteria, and this facilitates the drug's reabsorption. Thus biliary excretion eliminates substances from the body only to the extent that enterohepatic cycling is incomplete (i.e., when some of the excreted drug is not reabsorbed from the intestine).

Other Routes of Excretion

Sweat and saliva are minor routes of excretion for some drugs. In pharmacokinetic studies, saliva measurements are sometimes used because the saliva concentration of a drug often reflects the intracellular concentration of the drug in target tissues.

QUANTITATIVE PHARMACOKINETICS

To derive and use expressions for pharmacokinetic parameters, the first step is to establish a mathematical model that accurately relates the plasma drug concentration to the rates of drug absorption, distribution, and elimination. The **one-compartment model** is the simplest model of drug disposition, but the **two-compartment model** provides a more accurate representation of the pharmacokinetic behavior of many drugs (Fig. 2.5). With the one-compartment model, a

BOX 2.2 THE RENAL EXCRETION AND CLEARANCE OF A WEAK ACID, PENICILLIN G

DESCRIPTION AND CHEMICAL STRUCTURE

Penicillin G (benzylpenicillin) is an example of a weak acid. It has a **pK$_a$** of 2.8 and is primarily excreted via renal tubular secretion. Approximately 60% of penicillin G is bound to plasma proteins. The pharmacokinetic calculations that follow are based on a urine **pH** of 5.8, a **plasma drug concentration** of 3 mg/mL, a **glomerular filtration rate** of 100 mL/min, and a **measured drug excretion rate** of 1200 mg/min. Because 40% of penicillin G is free (unbound), the **free drug plasma concentration** is 0.4 × 3 mg/mL = 1.2 mg/mL.

RENAL EXCRETION

The discussion and accompanying figure illustrate the relationship among the rates of glomerular filtration, active tubular secretion, passive tubular reabsorption, and excretion.

1. **Filtration.** The **drug filtration rate** is calculated by multiplying the glomerular filtration rate by the free drug plasma concentration: 100 mL/min × 1.2 mg/mL = 120 mg/min.
2. **Secretion.** The **drug secretion rate** is calculated by subtracting the drug filtration rate from the drug excretion rate: 1200 mg/min – 120 mg/min = 1080 mg/min. This amount indicates that 90% of the drug's excretion occurs by the process of tubular secretion.
3. **Reabsorption.** The ratio of the nonionized form to the ionized form of the drug in the urine is equal to the antilog of the pK$_a$ minus the pH: antilog of 2.8 – 5.8 = antilog of –3 = 1:1000. Because most of the drug is ionized in the urine, the **drug reabsorption rate** is probably less than 1 mg/min.
4. **Excretion.** The drug excretion rate was initially given as 1200 mg/min. It was determined by measuring the drug concentration in urine and multiplying it by the urine flow rate. Note that the drug excretion rate is equal to the drug filtration rate (120 mg/min) plus the drug secretion

rate (1080 mg/min) minus the drug reabsorption rate (<1 mg/min).

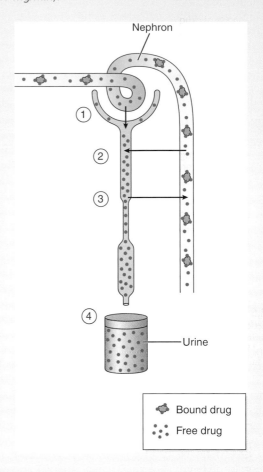

RENAL CLEARANCE

Renal clearance is calculated by dividing the excretion rate (1200 mg/min) by the plasma drug concentration (3 mg/mL). The result is 400 mL/min, which is equal to 24 L/h.

BOX 2.3 URINE ACIDIFICATION AND ALKALINIZATION IN THE TREATMENT OF DRUG OVERDOSE

If a drug or other compound is a weak acid or base, its degree of ionization and rate of renal excretion will depend on its pK$_a$ and on the pH of the renal tubular fluid. The rate of excretion of a **weak acid** can be accelerated by **alkalinizing the urine,** whereas the rate of excretion of a **weak base** can be accelerated by **acidifying the urine.** These procedures have been used to enhance the excretion of drugs and poisons, but they are not without risk to the patient, and their benefits have been established for only a few drugs.

To make manipulation of the urine pH worthwhile, a drug must be excreted to a large degree by the kidneys. The short-acting barbiturates (e.g., secobarbital) are eliminated almost entirely via biotransformation to inactive metabolites, so modification of the urine pH has little effect on their excretion. In contrast, phenobarbital is excreted to a large degree by the

kidneys, so urine alkalinization is useful in treating an overdose of this drug. Urine acidification to enhance the elimination of weak bases (e.g., amphetamine) has been largely abandoned because it does not significantly increase the elimination of these drugs and poses a serious risk of metabolic acidosis.

In cases involving an overdose of aspirin or other salicylate, alkalinization of the urine produces the dual benefits of increasing drug excretion and counteracting the metabolic acidosis that occurs with serious aspirin toxicity. For patients with phenobarbital overdose or herbicide 2,4-dichlorophenoxyacetic acid poisoning, alkalinization of the urine is also helpful; this is accomplished by administering sodium bicarbonate intravenously every 3 to 4 hours to increase the urinary pH to 7 to 8.

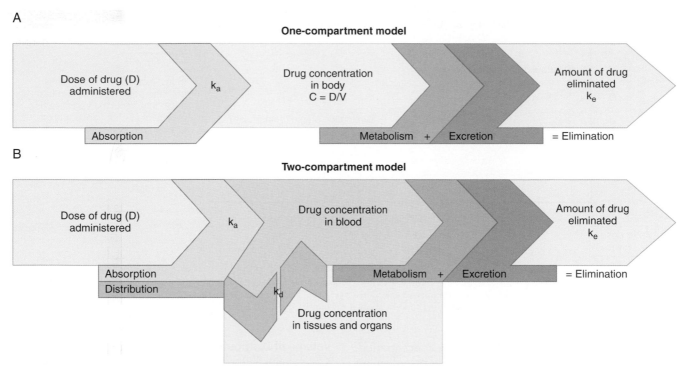

FIG. 2.5 Two models of the processes of drug absorption, distribution, and elimination: k_a, k_d, and k_e are the rate constants, representing the fractional completion of each process per unit of time. (A) In the one-compartment model, the drug concentration at any time, C, is the amount of drug in the body at that time, D, divided by the volume of the compartment, V. Thus D is a function of the dose administered and the rates of absorption and elimination represented by k_a and k_e, respectively. (B) In the two-compartment model, the drug concentration in the central compartment (the blood) is a function of the dose administered and the rates of drug absorption, distribution to the peripheral compartment (the tissues), and elimination from the central compartment.

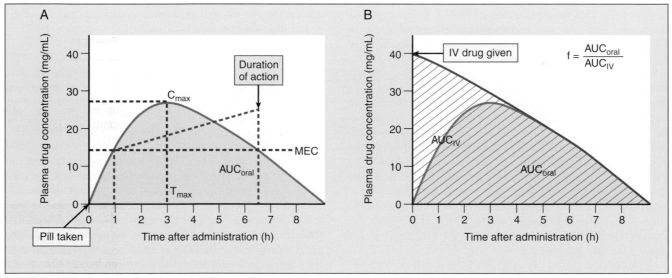

FIG. 2.6 Plasma drug concentration and drug bioavailability. The plasma drug concentration curve for a single dose of a drug given orally (A) shows maximum concentration (C_{max}), the time needed to reach the maximum (T_{max}), the minimum effective concentration (MEC), the duration of action, and the area under the curve (AUC). (B) To determine bioavailability, F, the AUC of the AUC_{oral} is divided by the AUC of the intravenously administered drug, AUC_{IV}.

drug undergoes absorption into the blood according to the rate constant k_a and elimination from the blood with the rate constant k_e. In the two-compartment model, drugs are absorbed into the central compartment (blood), distributed from the central compartment to the peripheral compartment (the tissues), and eliminated from the central compartment. Regardless of the model used, rate constants can be determined for each process and used to derive expressions

for other pharmacokinetic parameters, such as the **elimination half-life (t½)** of a drug. In this section, the most important parameters of pharmacokinetics are explained in greater detail.

Drug Plasma Concentration Curves
Fig. 2.6A shows a standardized **drug plasma concentration curve** over time after oral administration of a typical drug.

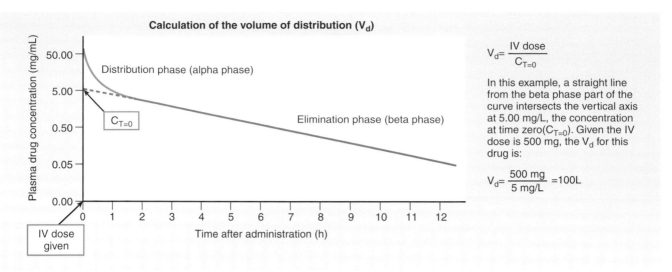

FIG. 2.7   Calculating the volume of distribution (V_d) of a drug. The graph provides an example of how the V_d is calculated. A dose of 500 mg was injected intravenously at time zero, and plasma drug concentrations were measured over time. The terminal elimination curve (β elimination phase) was extrapolated back to time zero to determine that the plasma drug concentration at time zero, $C_{T=0}$, was 5 mg/L. Then the V_d was calculated by dividing the dose by the $C_{T=0}$. In this case the result was 100 L.

The y-axis is a linear scale of drug plasma concentration, often expressed in micrograms per milliliter or milligrams per liter, and the x-axis is a scale of time, usually expressed in hours. Parameters of the plasma drug concentration curve are the **maximum concentration (Cmax)**, the time needed to reach the maximum **(Tmax)**, the **minimum effective concentration (MEC)**, and the **duration of action.** A measure of the total amount of drug during the time course is given by the **area under the curve (AUC).** These measures are useful for comparing the **bioavailability** of different pharmaceutical formulations or of drugs given by different routes of administration.

Bioavailability

Bioavailability is defined as the **fraction (F)** of the administered dose of a drug that reaches the systemic circulation in an active form. As shown in Fig. 2.6B, the oral bioavailability of a particular drug is determined by dividing the AUC of an orally administered dose of the drug (AUC_{oral}) by the AUC of an intravenously administered dose of the same drug (AUC_{IV}). By definition, an intravenously administered drug has 100% bioavailability. The bioavailability of drugs administered intramuscularly or via other routes can be determined in the same manner as the bioavailability of drugs administered orally.

The bioavailability of orally administered drugs is of particular concern because it can be reduced by many pharmaceutical and biologic factors. Pharmaceutical factors include the **rate and extent of tablet disintegration** and drug dissolution. Biologic factors include the effects of food, which can sequester or inactivate a drug; the effects of gastric acid, which can inactivate a drug; and the effects of gut and liver enzymes, which can metabolize a drug during its absorption and first pass through the liver. The CYP3A4 isozyme found in intestinal enterocytes and hepatic cells is a particularly important catalyst of first-pass drug metabolism. CYP3A4 works in conjunction with Pgp (described in the section discussing drug distribution), as the 3A4 isozyme located in enterocytes inactivates drugs transported into the intestinal lumen by Pgp.

Volume of Distribution

The volume of distribution (V_d) is defined as the volume of fluid in which a dose of a drug would need to be dissolved to have the **same concentration** as it does in plasma. The V_d does not necessarily represent the volume in a particular body fluid compartment. Instead, the V_d is an apparent volume that represents the relationship between the dose of a drug and the resulting plasma concentration of the drug, to account for the immediate distribution of the drug out of the blood after absorption.

Calculation of the Volume of Distribution

After intravenous drug administration, the plasma drug concentration falls rapidly at first as the drug is distributed from the central compartment to the peripheral compartment. The V_d is calculated by dividing the dose of a drug given intravenously by the plasma drug concentration immediately after the initial or *alpha* (α) distribution phase. As shown in Fig. 2.7, this drug concentration can be determined by extrapolating the plasma drug concentration back to time zero from the linear part of the latter or *beta* (β) elimination phase. Note that the y-axis in this case is plotted on a **log scale** so that the exponential decay curve of the elimination phase is converted to a straight line. The plasma **drug concentration at time zero ($C_{T=0}$)** represents the plasma concentration of a drug that would be obtained if it were instantaneously dissolved in its V_d. The equation for calculating V_d is rearranged to determine the dose of a drug required to establish a specified plasma drug concentration and to calculate a loading dose (Box 2.4).

Interpretation of the Volume of Distribution

Although the V_d does not correspond to an actual body fluid compartment, it does provide a measure of the extent of distribution of a drug. A low V_d that approximates plasma volume or extracellular fluid volume usually indicates that the drug's distribution is restricted to a particular compartment (the plasma or extracellular fluid). The anticoagulant **warfarin** has a V_d of approximately 8 L, which reflects a high degree of plasma protein binding. When the V_d of a drug

BOX 2.4 DRUG DOSAGE CALCULATIONS

LOADING DOSE

The loading dose, or priming dose, of a drug is determined by multiplying the **volume of distribution** (V_d) of the drug by the **desired plasma drug concentration** (desired C). (This information can be found in the medical literature.) For example, for theophylline, the estimated V_d for an adult weighing 70 kg is 35 L, and the desired C is 15 mg/L. The calculation is as follows:

$$\text{Loading dose} = V_d \times C$$
$$= 35 \text{ L} \times 15 \text{ mg/L}$$
$$= 525 \text{ mg}$$

As is discussed in Chapter 4 (see Table 4.5), the patient's age can affect the V_d and therefore should be considered in determining the appropriate loading dose for a particular patient.

MAINTENANCE DOSE

Calculations of the maintenance dose must take into consideration the **intended frequency of drug administration.** With intermittent administration, the fluctuations in C increase as the dosage interval increases. A twofold fluctuation in C will occur when the dosage interval is equal to the drug's half-life. This is because the C will fall 50% between doses. For many drugs, the half-life is a convenient and acceptable dosage interval.

The maintenance dose is designed to establish or maintain a **desired steady state C.** The amount of drug to be given is based on the principle that at the steady state, the rate of drug administration equals the rate of drug elimination. The rate of elimination is equal to the clearance multiplied by the steady-state drug concentration. For example, if the steady-state gentamicin concentration is 2 mg/L and the clearance rate for gentamicin is 100 mL/min (0.1 L/min), then the elimination rate is 0.1 L/min × 2 mg/L = 0.2 mg/min. If the drug is to be administered every 8 hours, then the dosage would be calculated as follows:

$$\text{Maintenance dose} = \text{Hourly rate} \times \text{dosage interval in hours}$$
$$= 0.2 \text{ mg/min} \times 60 \text{ minutes in an hour}$$
$$\times 8 \text{ hours}$$
$$= 96 \text{ mg every 8 hours}$$

If a drug is to be administered orally, the calculated dose must be divided by the fractional bioavailability to determine the administered dose.

DOSAGE ADJUSTMENT USING PHARMACOKINETIC VALUES

First, choose the target C and administer the initial dose on the basis of the standard published values (general population values) for clearance or V_d. Second, measure the patient's plasma drug levels and calculate the patient's V_d and clearance. Third, revise the dosage based on the patient's V_d and clearance.

---

is equivalent to total body water (approximately 40 L, as occurs with ethanol), this usually indicates that the drug has reached the intracellular fluid as well.

Some drugs have a V_d that is much larger than total body water. A large V_d may indicate that the drug is concentrated intracellularly, with a resulting low concentration in the plasma. Many weak bases, such as the antidepressant **fluoxetine** (PROZAC), have a large V_d (40–55 L) because of the phenomenon of intracellular **ion trapping.** Weak bases are less ionized within plasma than they are within cells because intracellular fluid usually has a lower pH than extracellular fluid. After a weak base diffuses into a cell, a larger fraction is ionized in the more acidic intracellular fluid. This restricts its diffusion out of a cell and results in a large V_d.

A large V_d may also result from sequestration into fat tissue, such as occurs with the antimalarial agent **chloroquine.**

Drug Clearance

Clearance (Cl) is the most fundamental expression of drug elimination. It is defined as the volume of body fluid (blood) from which a drug is removed per unit of time. Although the clearance of a particular drug is **constant,** it is important to note that the amount of drug contained in the clearance volume will **vary** with the plasma drug concentration.

Renal Clearance

Renal clearance can be calculated as the renal excretion rate divided by the plasma drug concentration (see Box 2.2). Drugs that are eliminated primarily by glomerular filtration, with little tubular secretion or reabsorption, will have a renal clearance approximately **equal to the creatinine clearance,** which is normally approximately 100 mL/min

in an adult. A renal drug clearance higher than the creatinine clearance indicates that the drug is a substance that undergoes tubular secretion. A renal drug clearance lower than the creatinine clearance suggests that the drug is highly bound to plasma proteins or that it undergoes passive reabsorption from the renal tubules.

Hepatic Clearance

Hepatic clearance is more difficult to determine than renal clearance. This is because hepatic drug elimination includes the biotransformation and biliary excretion of parent compounds. For this reason, hepatic clearance is usually determined by multiplying hepatic blood flow by the arteriovenous drug concentration difference.

SINGLE-DOSE PHARMACOKINETICS
First-Order Kinetics

Most drugs exhibit **first-order kinetics,** in which the rate of drug elimination (amount of drug eliminated per unit time) is proportional to the plasma drug concentration and follows an exponential decay function. Note that the rate of drug elimination is not the same as the elimination rate constant, k_e (fraction of drug eliminated per unit time). A few drugs (e.g., ethanol) exhibit **zero-order kinetics,** in which the rate of drug elimination is constant and independent of plasma drug concentration (Fig. 2.8).

For drugs that exhibit first-order kinetics, the plasma drug concentration can be determined from the dose of a drug and its clearance. Because the plasma drug concentration is often correlated with the magnitude of a drug's effect, it is possible to use pharmacokinetic expressions to determine and adjust drug dosages to achieve a desired therapeutic effect (see Box 2.4).

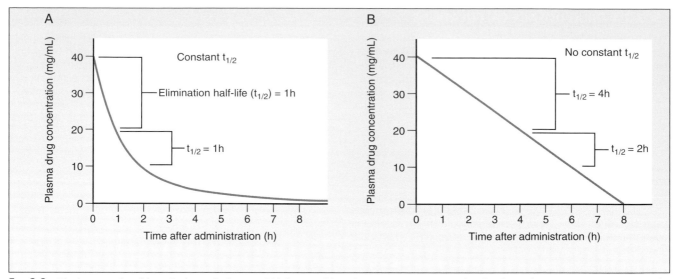

FIG. 2.8 The kinetic order of drugs. In first-order kinetics (A) the rate of drug elimination is proportional to the plasma drug concentration. In zero-order kinetics (B) the rate of drug elimination is constant. The kinetic order of a drug is derived from the exponent n in the following expression:

$$\Delta[\text{Drug}]/\Delta t = -k_e\,[\text{Drug}]^n$$

where Δ represents change, [Drug] represents the plasma drug concentration, and t is time. If n is 1, then $\Delta[\text{Drug}]/\Delta t$ is proportional to [Drug]. If n is 0, then $\Delta[\text{Drug}]/\Delta t$ is constant (k_e), because $[\text{Drug}]^0$ equals 1.

The following principles pertain to first-order kinetics: A drug's **rate of elimination is equal to the plasma drug concentration multiplied by the drug clearance;** the elimination rate declines as the plasma concentration declines; and the half-life and clearance of the drug remain constant as long as renal and hepatic function do not change.

Elimination Half-Life

Elimination half-life ($t_{1/2}$) is the time required to **reduce the plasma drug concentration by 50%.** It can be calculated from the elimination rate constant, but it is usually determined from the plasma drug concentration curve (Fig. 2.9). The half-life can also be expressed in terms of the drug's clearance and V_d, indicating that the drug's half-life will change when either of these factors is altered. The formula for relating half-life to clearance and V_d is given in the legend of Fig. 2.9. Disease, age, and other physiologic variables can alter drug clearance or V_d and thereby change the elimination half-life (see Chapter 4).

Zero-Order Kinetics

The following principles pertain to zero-order kinetics: The rate of drug elimination is constant (see Fig. 2.8B); the drug's elimination half-life is **proportional** to the plasma drug concentration; the clearance is **inversely proportional** to the drug concentration; and a small increase in dosage can produce a disproportionate increase in the plasma drug concentration.

In many cases, the reason that the rate of drug elimination is constant is that the elimination process becomes **saturated.** This occurs, for example, at most plasma concentrations of **ethanol.** In some cases, drugs exhibit zero-order elimination when high doses are administered, which occurs, for example, with **aspirin** and the anticonvulsant **phenytoin** (DILANTIN) or when a hepatic or renal disease has impaired the drug elimination processes.

CONTINUOUS-DOSE AND MULTIPLE-DOSE KINETICS

Drug Accumulation and the Steady-State Principle

When a drug that exhibits first-order pharmacokinetics is administered to a patient continuously or intermittently, the drug will accumulate until it reaches a plateau or steady-state plasma drug concentration.

The basis for this accumulation to a steady state is shown in Fig. 2.10. When the drug is first administered, the rate of administration is much greater than the rate of elimination because the plasma concentration is so low. As the drug continues to be administered, the rate of drug elimination gradually increases, whereas the rate of administration remains constant. Eventually, as the plasma concentration rises sufficiently, the rate of drug elimination equals the rate of drug administration. At this point, the **steady-state equilibrium** is achieved.

Time Required to Reach the Steady-State Condition

Drug accumulation to a steady state is a **first-order process** and therefore obeys the rule that half of the process is completed in a defined time. Because the time to reach the steady state is dependent on the time it takes for the rate of drug elimination to equal to the rate of drug administration, the time to reach the steady state is a function of the elimination half-life of the drug. Any first-order process requires approximately **five half-lives** to be completed; thus the time to reach the steady-state drug concentration is approximately five drug half-lives. If the half-life of a drug changes, then the time required to reach the steady state also changes. Note that the time required to reach the steady state is independent both of the drug dose and the rate or frequency of drug administration.

Steady-State Drug Concentration

The steady-state drug concentration depends on the drug dose administered per unit of time and on the half-life of the

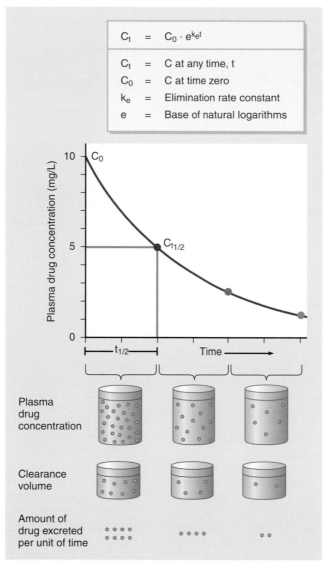

$$C_t = C_0 \cdot e^{k_e t}$$

C_t	=	C at any time, t
C_0	=	C at time zero
k_e	=	Elimination rate constant
e	=	Base of natural logarithms

FIG. 2.9 Drug half-life and clearance. The elimination half-life ($t_{1/2}$) is the time required to reduce the plasma drug concentration (C) by 50%. The formula is as follows:

$$t_{1/2} = 0.693 / k_e$$

where 0.693 is the natural logarithm of 2, and k_e is the elimination rate constant. The half-life is often determined from the plasma drug concentration curve shown here. The clearance (Cl) is the volume of fluid from which a drug is eliminated per unit of time. It can be calculated as the product of the volume of distribution, V_d, and k_e. If $0.693/t_{1/2}$ is substituted for k_e, the equation is as follows:

$$Cl = 0.693 V_d / t_{1/2}$$

Thus a drug's clearance is directly proportional to its volume of distribution and is inversely proportional to its half-life.

drug. Fig. 2.11 illustrates typical plasma concentration curves after drugs are **administered continuously** or **intermittently.** If the dose is doubled, the steady-state concentration is also doubled (Fig. 2.11A). Likewise, if the half-life is doubled, the steady-state concentration is doubled (Fig. 2.11B).

A drug administered intermittently will **accumulate to a steady state at the same rate** as a drug given by continuous infusion, but the plasma drug concentration will fluctuate as each dose is absorbed and eliminated. The average steady-state plasma drug concentration with intermittent intravenous administration will be the same as if the equivalent dose were administered by continuous infusion (Fig. 2.11C). A comparison of the steady-state drug levels following continuous intravenous infusion, multiple oral doses, and a single oral dose is shown in Fig. 2.11D. With intermittent oral administration, the bioavailability of the drug will also influence the steady-state plasma concentration.

Dosage Calculations
The methods for calculating both the loading dose and the maintenance dose are given in Box 2.4.

Loading Dose
A loading dose, or **priming dose,** is given to rapidly establish a therapeutic plasma drug concentration. The loading dose can be calculated by multiplying the V_d by the desired plasma drug concentration. The loading dose, which is larger than the maintenance dose, is generally administered

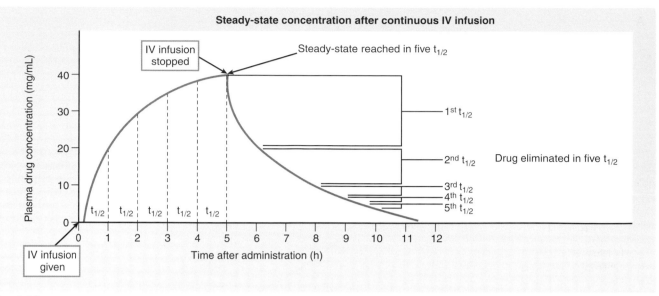

FIG. 2.10 Drug accumulation to the steady state. The time required to reach the steady state depends on the half-life ($t_{1/2}$); it does not depend on the dose or dosage interval. The steady-state drug concentration depends on the drug dose administered per unit of time and on the drug's clearance or $t_{1/2}$.

as a single dose, but it can be divided into fractions that are given over several hours. A **divided loading dose** is sometimes used for drugs that are more toxic (e.g., **digitalis glycosides** used to treat congestive heart failure).

Maintenance Dose

A **maintenance dose** is given to establish or maintain the **desired steady-state** plasma drug concentration. For drugs given intermittently, the maintenance dose is one of a series of doses administered at regular intervals. The amount of drug to be given is based on the principle that, at the steady state, the rate of drug administration equals the rate of drug elimination. To determine the rate of drug elimination, the drug clearance is multiplied by the average steady-state plasma drug concentration. The maintenance dose is then calculated as the rate of drug elimination multiplied by the dosage intervals. If the drug is administered orally, its bioavailability must also be included in the equation.

SUMMARY OF IMPORTANT POINTS

- Most drugs are absorbed by passive diffusion across cell membranes or between cells. The rate of passive diffusion of a drug across cell membranes is proportional to the drug's lipid solubility and the surface area available for absorption. Only the nonionized form of weak acids and bases is lipid soluble.
- The ratio of the ionized form to the nonionized form of a weak acid or base can be determined from the pK_a of the drug and the pH of the body fluid in which the drug is dissolved.
- The distribution of a drug is influenced by organ blood flow and by the plasma protein binding, molecular size, and lipid solubility of the drug. Only drugs with high lipid solubility can penetrate the blood-brain barrier.
- The volume of distribution is the volume of fluid in which a drug would need to be dissolved to have the same concentration in that volume as it does in

plasma. It is calculated by dividing the drug dose by the plasma drug concentration at time zero.
- Many drugs are metabolized (biotransformed) before excretion. Drug metabolites can be pharmacologically active or inactive. Phase I reactions include oxidative, reductive, and hydrolytic reactions, whereas phase II reactions conjugate a drug with an endogenous substance. The CYP enzymes located in the endoplasmic reticulum of liver cells are the most important oxidative metabolic enzymes.
- Most drugs are excreted in the urine, either as the parent compound and/or as drug metabolites, and undergo the processes of glomerular filtration, active tubular secretion, and passive tubular reabsorption. The renal clearance of a drug can be calculated by dividing the renal excretion rate by the plasma drug concentration.
- Most drugs exhibit first-order kinetics, in which the rate of drug elimination is proportional to the plasma drug concentration at any given time. If drug elimination mechanisms (biotransformation and excretion) become saturated, a drug can exhibit zero-order kinetics, in which the rate of drug elimination is constant.
- In first-order kinetics, a drug's half-life and clearance are constant as long as elimination processes are constant. The half-life is the time required for the plasma drug concentration to decrease by 50%. The clearance is the volume of plasma from which a drug is eliminated per unit of time.
- The oral bioavailability of a drug is the fraction of the administered dose that reaches the bloodstream in an active form. It is determined by dividing the AUC after oral administration by the AUC after intravenous administration. Factors that reduce bioavailability include incomplete tablet disintegration and first-pass and gastric inactivation of a drug.
- With continuous or intermittent drug administration, the plasma drug concentration increases until it reaches a steady-state condition, in which the rate of

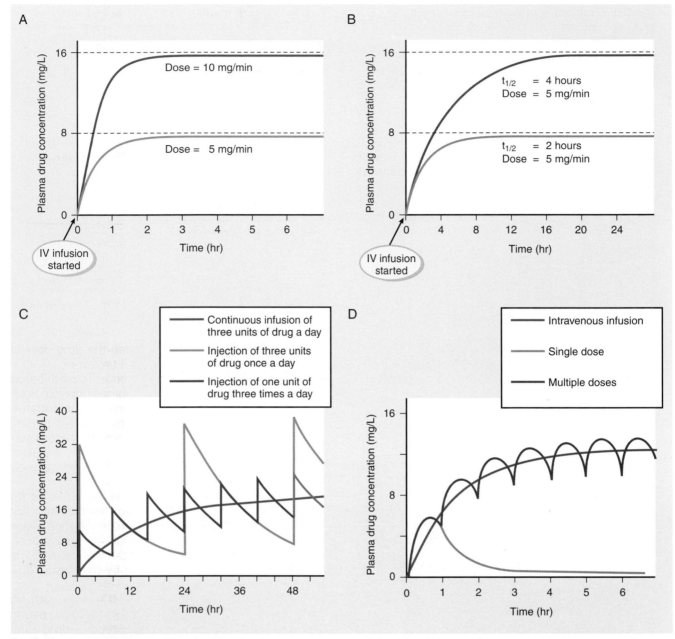

FIG. 2.11 Plasma drug concentrations after continuous or intermittent drug administration. (A) The steady-state plasma drug concentration is proportional to the dose administered per unit of time. (B) The steady-state plasma drug concentration is directly proportional to the half-life (and is inversely related to clearance). (C) The average steady-state concentration is the same for intermittent infusion as it is for continuous infusion. However, with intermittent drug administration, the plasma concentrations fluctuate between doses, and the size of fluctuations increases as the dosage interval increases. (D) Plasma drug concentrations after intermittent oral administration are affected by the rates of drug absorption, distribution, and elimination. If only one dose is given, the peak in plasma drug concentration is followed by a continuous decline in the curve.

drug elimination is equal to the rate of drug administration. It takes approximately four to five drug half-lives to achieve the steady-state condition.

- The steady-state drug concentration can be calculated as the dose per unit of time divided by the clearance, and this equation can be rearranged to determine the dose per unit of time required to establish a specified steady-state drug concentration.
- A loading dose is a single or divided dose given to rapidly establish a therapeutic plasma drug concentration. The dose can be calculated by multiplying the volume of distribution by the desired plasma drug concentration.

Review Questions

1. If food decreases the rate but not the extent of the absorption of a particular drug from the gastrointestinal tract, then taking the drug with food will result in a smaller
   (A) area under the plasma drug concentration time curve.
   (B) maximal plasma drug concentration.
   (C) time at which the maximal plasma drug concentration occurs.
   (D) fractional bioavailability.
   (E) total clearance.

2. If a drug exhibits first-order elimination, then
   (A) the elimination half-life is proportional to the plasma drug concentration.
   (B) the drug is eliminated at a constant rate.
   (C) hepatic drug metabolizing enzymes are saturated.
   (D) drug clearance will increase if the plasma drug concentration increases.
   (E) the rate of drug elimination (mg/min) is proportional to the plasma drug concentration.

3. After a person ingests an overdose of an opioid analgesic, the plasma drug concentration is found to be 32 mg/L. How long will it take to reach a safe plasma concentration of 2 mg/L if the drug's half-life is 6 hours?
   (A) 12 hours
   (B) 24 hours
   (C) 48 hours
   (D) 72 hours
   (E) 1 week

4. What dose of a drug should be injected intravenously every 8 hours to obtain an average steady-state plasma drug concentration of 5 mg/L if the drug's volume of distribution is 30 L and its clearance is 8 L/h?
   (A) 40 mg
   (B) 80 mg
   (C) 160 mg
   (D) 320 mg
   (E) 400 mg

5. The volume of distribution of a drug will be greater if the drug
   (A) is more ionized inside cells than in plasma.
   (B) is administered very rapidly.
   (C) is highly ionized in plasma.
   (D) has poor lipid solubility.
   (E) has a high molecular weight.

CHAPTER 3

Pharmacodynamics or What the Drug Does to the Body

OVERVIEW

Pharmacodynamics is the study of the detailed **mechanism of action** by which drugs produce their pharmacologic effects. This study of a drug's mechanism of action begins with the binding of a drug to its target receptor, enzyme, or other protein. With some drugs, such as a receptor antagonist, this simple action may be the complete description of the drug's mechanism of action. For other drugs, binding to a receptor or other target initiates a molecular chain of events, called the **signal transduction pathway.** The signal transduction pathway may activate **second messenger** molecules, which then activate or inhibit other molecules. In this case, the mechanism of action is complex and complete only when an ultimate description of all intracellular processes altered by a drug are known. Pharmacodynamics provides a **scientific basis for the selection and use of drugs** to counteract specific pathologic changes caused by disease, trauma, or genetic anomalies.

There is also a quantitative aspect to pharmacodynamics in characterizing the **dose-response curve,** which is the relationship between the drug dose and the magnitude of the pharmacologic effect. This dose-response curve translates a drug's mechanism of action into an observable effect that can be measured in tissues and the whole patient.

NATURE OF DRUG RECEPTORS

Drugs produce their effects by interacting with specific cell molecules called *receptors*. By far, most **ligands** (drugs or neurotransmitters) **bind to protein molecules,** although some agents act directly on DNA or membrane lipids (Table 3.1).

Types of Drug Receptors

The largest family of receptors for pharmaceutical agents is **G protein–coupled receptors (GPCRs).** These membrane-spanning proteins consist of four extracellular, seven transmembrane, and four intracellular domains (Fig. 3.1). Extracellular domains and, to some extent, transmembrane regions determine ligand binding and selectivity. Intracellular loops, especially the third one, mediate the receptor interaction with its effector molecule, a guanine nucleotide binding protein (G protein).

A number of ligands inhibit the function of specific enzymes by **competitive** or **noncompetitive inhibition.** A ligand that binds to the same active, catalytic site as the endogenous substrate is called a *competitive inhibitor.* Ligands that bind at a different site on the enzyme and alter the shape of the molecule, thereby reducing its catalytic activity, are called *noncompetitive inhibitors.*

Drugs also target **membrane transport proteins,** including ligand- and voltage-gated ion channels and neurotransmitter transporters. At **ligand-gated ion channels,** drugs can bind at the same site as the endogenous ligand (called an **orthosteric site**) and directly compete for the receptor.

Drugs can also bind at a different site, called an **allosteric site,** which alters the response of the endogenous ligand at the ligand-gated ion channel and increases or decreases the flow of ions. Some drugs directly bind and inactivate **voltage-gated ion channels;** these are ion-channel proteins that do not have an endogenous ligand (as ligand-gated ion channels do) but open or close as a function of the membrane voltage potential. **Neurotransmitter transporter proteins** are large, 12-transmembrane domain proteins that transfer neurotransmitter molecules out of the synapse and back into the neuron. A large group of agents, known generally as **reuptake inhibitors,** target these transport proteins.

Steroid hormone receptors are **intracellular proteins** that **translocate to the nucleus** on ligand (steroid) binding. In the nucleus, the steroid-receptor complex alters the transcription rate of specific genes (Fig. 3.2). **DNA** is also a receptor site for ligands that bind directly to nucleic acids, most notably the antineoplastic agents. Other macromolecules that serve as receptors include the various lipids and phospholipids that make up the membrane. Some of the effects of general anesthetics and alcohol are caused by interaction with membrane lipids.

Receptor Classification

Drug receptors are classified according to **drug specificity, tissue location,** and, more recently, their **primary amino acid sequence.** For example, **adrenoceptors** were initially divided into two types (α and β) based on their affinity for norepinephrine, epinephrine, and other agents in different tissues. Subsequently, the distinction between the types was confirmed by the development of selective antagonists that blocked either α-adrenoceptors or β-adrenoceptors. Later, the two types of receptors were divided into **subtypes** (α_1, α_2, β_1, β_2, etc.) based on more subtle differences in agonist potency, tissue distribution, and varying effects.

At present, most receptors for drug targets and endogenous ligands are cloned and their amino acid sequences determined. There are also numerous other receptor-like proteins predicted from the human genome for which an endogenous ligand is not identified, called **orphan receptors.** The orphan receptors are of great interest to pharmaceutical companies as they represent **targets for the development of new drugs.** Families of receptor types are grouped by their sequence similarity using bioinformatics, and this classification supports results from earlier *in vivo* and *in vitro* functional studies. In many cases, each type of receptor corresponds to a single, unique gene with subtypes of receptors arising from different transcripts of the same gene by the process of **alternative splicing.**

DRUG-RECEPTOR INTERACTIONS
Receptor Binding and Affinity

To initiate a cellular response, a drug must first bind to a receptor. In most cases, drugs bind to their receptor by

TABLE 3.1   Drug Receptors

TYPES OF DRUG RECEPTORS	EXAMPLES OF DRUGS THAT BIND RECEPTORS
Hormone and Neurotransmitter Receptors	
Adrenoceptors	Epinephrine and propranolol
Histamine receptors	Cimetidine and diphenhydramine
5-Hydroxytryptamine (serotonin) receptors	Lysergic acid diethylamide (LSD) and sumatriptan
Insulin receptors	Insulin
Muscarinic receptors	Atropine and bethanechol
Opioid receptors	Morphine and naltrexone
Steroid receptors	Cortisol and tamoxifen
Enzymes	
Carbonic anhydrase	Acetazolamide
Cholinesterase	Donepezil and physostigmine
Cyclooxygenase	Aspirin and celecoxib
DNA polymerase	Acyclovir and zidovudine
DNA topoisomerase	Ciprofloxacin
Human immunodeficiency virus (HIV) protease	Indinavir
Monoamine oxidase	Phenelzine
Na^+K^+-adenosine triphosphatase	Digoxin
Xanthine oxidase	Allopurinol
Membrane Transport Proteins	
Ligand-gated ion channels	Diazepam and ondansetron
Voltage-gated ion channels	Lidocaine and verapamil
Ion transporters	Furosemide and hydrochlorothiazide
Neurotransmitter transporters	Fluoxetine and cocaine
Other Macromolecules	
Membrane lipids	Alcohol and amphotericin B
Nucleic acids	Cyclophosphamide and doxorubicin

forming **hydrogen, ionic,** or **hydrophobic** (van der Waals) bonds with a receptor site. These weak bonds are reversible and enable the drug to dissociate from the receptor as the tissue concentration of the drug declines. The binding of drugs to receptors often exhibits **stereospecificity,** so that only one of the **stereoisomers (R- or L-enantiomers)** of a drug with a chiral center will bind to the receptor and activate its signaling. In a few cases, drugs form relatively permanent covalent bonds with a specific receptor. This occurs, for example, with antineoplastic drugs that bind to DNA and with drugs that irreversibly inhibit the enzyme cholinesterase.

The ability of a drug to bind with its receptor or target is called **affinity,** which is a measure of the strength of the drug-receptor complex. According to the law of mass action, the number of receptors (R) occupied by a drug depends on the drug concentration (D) and the drug-receptor **association and dissociation rate constants** (k_1 and k_2):

$$[D]+[R] \underset{k_2}{\overset{k_1}{\rightleftharpoons}} [D\text{-}R] \rightarrow Effect$$

The **ratio of k_2 to k_1** is known as the drug's **dissociation constant (K_D)** and represents the drug concentration required to occupy 50% of its receptors in a controlled *in vitro* tissue or cell preparation. The lower the K_D, the greater the drug's affinity for the receptor, as it takes less drug to occupy 50% of its receptors. Most drugs have a K_D in the micromolar to nanomolar (10^{-6} to 10^{-9} M) range of drug concentrations. As discussed later, receptor affinity is the **primary determinant of drug** potency.

Signal Transduction

Signal transduction describes the pathway from ligand binding to conformational changes in the receptor, receptor interaction with an effector molecule (if present), and other downstream molecules called second messengers. This cascade of receptor-mediated biochemical events ultimately leads to one or more pharmacologic effects (Table 3.2).

G Protein–Coupled Receptors

The signal transduction pathway for GPCRs is well understood. These receptors constitute a superfamily of receptors

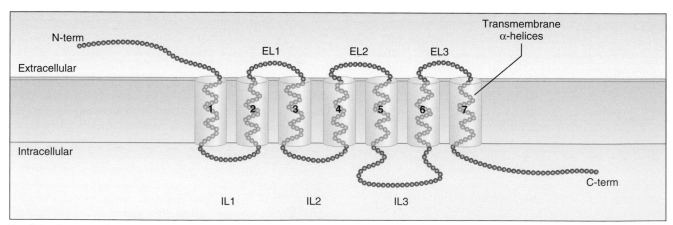

Fig. 3.1   Structure of a typical G protein–coupled receptor (GPCR). All GPCRs consist of a long polypeptide chain of amino acids threaded through the cell membrane with seven transmembrane (TM) domains. These TM domains are arranged in α-helices composed of hydrophobic residues. The N-terminal of the receptor protein is outside the cell and the C-terminal is on the inside. Three extracellular loops (EL) and three intracellular loops (IL) are formed by this configuration. The protein in the cell membrane forms a circle with TM1 and TM7 in close proximity but is shown here in a two-dimensional view for clarity.

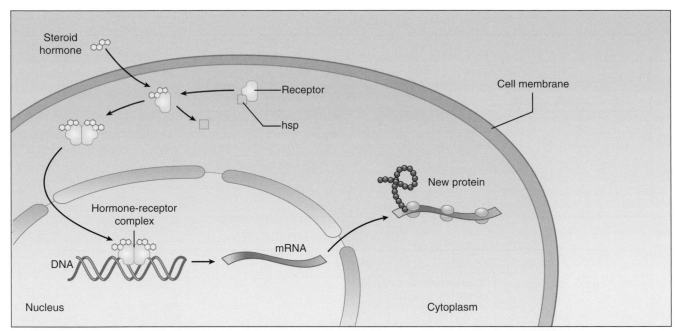

Fig. 3.2 Signal transduction with a steroid hormone receptor. Steroid hormones diffuse through the cell membrane and bind to steroid receptors in the cytoplasm. Binding of the steroid ligand displaces accessory heat-shock proteins (hsp) and allows steroid receptor dimerization. The dimerized steroid hormone–receptor complex is translocated to the nucleus and binds to specific sequences on the DNA upstream of a gene, leading to increased transcription of a gene, messenger RNA (mRNA), and translation of proteins.

TABLE 3.2   Examples of Receptors and Signal Transduction Pathways

FAMILY AND TYPE OF RECEPTOR	MECHANISM OF SIGNAL TRANSDUCTION	EXAMPLE OF EFFECT IN TISSUE OR CELL
G Protein–Coupled Receptors		
α_1-Adrenoceptor	Activation of phospholipase C	Vasoconstriction
α_2-Adrenoceptor	Inhibition of adenylyl cyclase	Release of norepinephrine decreased
β-Adrenoceptor	Stimulation of adenylyl cyclase	Heart rate increased
Muscarinic receptor	Activation of phospholipase C	Glandular secretion increased
Ligand-Gated Ion Channels		
$GABA_A$ receptors	Chloride ion flux	Hyperpolarization of neuron
Nicotinic receptors	Sodium ion flux	Skeletal muscle contraction
Membrane-Bound Enzymes		
Atrial natriuretic factor receptors	Stimulation of guanylyl cyclase	Sodium excretion increased
Insulin receptors	Activation of tyrosine kinase	Glucose uptake stimulated
Nuclear Receptors		
Steroid receptors	Activation of gene transcription	Reduced cytokine production
Thyroid hormone receptors	Activation of gene transcription	Oxygen consumption increased

GABA, Gamma-aminobutyric acid.

for many endogenous ligands and drugs, including receptors for acetylcholine, epinephrine, histamine, opioids, and serotonin. Fig. 3.3 illustrates the inactive state and the active state with signal transduction for a typical GPCR, the *mu* **opioid receptor.**

The **heterotrimeric G proteins** have three subunits, known as G_α, G_β and G_γ. The G_α subunit serves as the site of guanosine triphosphate (GTP) hydrolysis, a process catalyzed by **innate GTPase activity,** which acts to terminate the signal. Several types of G_α subunits exist, each of which determines a specific cellular response. For example, the $G_{\alpha s}$ (stimulating) subunit **increases** adenylyl cyclase activity

and thereby stimulates the production of cyclic adenosine monophosphate (cyclic AMP, or cAMP). The $G_{\alpha i}$ (inhibitory) subunit **decreases** adenylyl cyclase activity and inhibits the production of cAMP. Another G protein ($G_{\alpha q}$) activates phospholipase C and leads to the formation of **inositol triphosphate** (IP_3) and **diacylglycerol** (DAG) from membrane phospholipids. IP_3 and DAG further cause an **elevation of** Ca^{+2} **ions** inside the cell. Several other types of G_α subunits are also present in cells and activated by receptors. The G_β and G_γ subunits are so tightly bound together that they do not dissociate and are therefore written as $G_{\beta\gamma}$. The $G_{\beta\gamma}$ subunit also has signaling function when separated from G_α

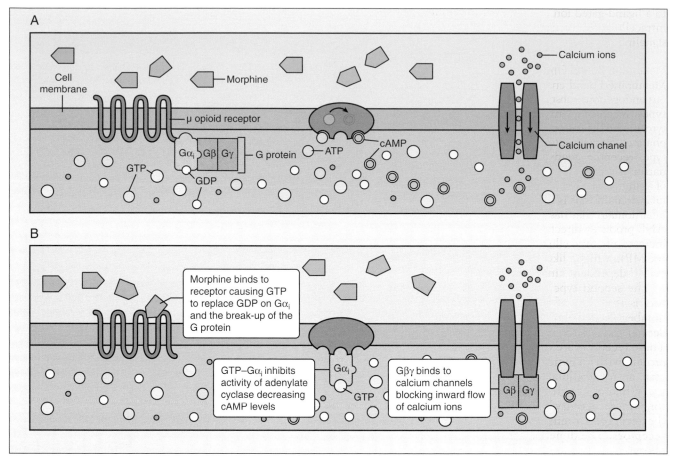

Fig. 3.3 Signal transduction with a G protein–coupled receptor. (A) The inactive state of a GPCR using the example of a *mu* opioid receptor. The receptor is shown in a linear pose; it exists as an enclosed circle in real life. The G protein is next with its heterotrimeric structure, in this case containing an inhibitory $G_{\alpha i}$ subunit, bound to GDP. Other molecules in the signal transduction pathway include adenylate cyclase, which converts ATP to cAMP, and a calcium channel protein. (B) When an agonist ligand (morphine in this example) binds to the receptor, the receptor interacts with the G protein, enabling the dissociation of GDP and facilitation of GTP binding. The extra power of the additional phosphate bond on GTP causes $G_{\alpha i}$ to separate from the G_{β} and G_{γ} subunits. The inhibitory $G_{\alpha i}$ subunit then inhibits adenylate cyclase activity and decreases levels of cAMP. The conjoined G_{β} and G_{γ} subunits inhibit the inward flow of Ca^{2+} at calcium channel proteins. GTP hydrolysis, catalyzed by G_{α} subunit GTPase, leads to reassociation of $G_{\alpha i}$ with G_{β} and G_{γ} subunits and returns the receptor to an inactive state.

on ligand-receptor activation, for example, by altering K^+ or Ca^{+2} channel conductance (see Fig. 3.3B). The receptor sequence of its C-terminal inside the cell determines which type of G-protein will interact with a given GPCR. Additionally, *beta*-arrestins are intracellular protein partners with GPCRs and are activated by agonist binding to produce their own signaling pathways.

Recently, the demonstration that some receptor agonists will shunt the signaling pathway of GPCRs to either the G-protein pathway or *beta*-arrestin signaling pathway led to the concept of **biased agonism**. Drugs that show selective bias towards one signaling pathway or the other may have increased clinical efficacy with reduced adverse effects. For example, it is thought that G-protein biased agonists at the opioid receptor may increase the G_{α} pathway to produce **analgesia with reduced stimulation of the *beta*-arrestin pathways** which is associated with respiratory depression and constipation (see Chapter 23).

The **second messengers** cAMP, IP_3, DAG, and Ca^{+2} activate or inhibit unique cellular enzymes in each target cell. cAMP activates a number of tissue-specific **cAMP-dependent protein kinases.** These kinases phosphorylate other enzymes or proteins that ultimately affect intracellular

processes such as ion channel activity, release of neurotransmitter, regulation of transcription, and numerous other processes. For example, one of the best studied kinases, protein kinase A, is activated by the increase of cAMP produced by epinephrine binding to β_2-adrenoceptors in muscle. Protein kinase A phosphorylates the enzyme glycogen phosphorylase, which then increases the breakdown of glycogen to free glucose, providing the fuel needed by the muscles to respond to the event that initiated the release of epinephrine.

IP_3 and DAG evoke the release of calcium from intracellular storage sites and thereby augment calcium-mediated processes such as muscle contraction, glandular secretion, and neurotransmitter release. The increased intracellular Ca^{+2} ions also **activate calcium-dependent kinases** and a number of other enzyme cascades.

Ligand-Gated Ion Channels

Ligand-gated ion channels are a **large class of membrane proteins** that share similar subunit structure and are assembled in **tetrameric** or **pentameric** structures. Drugs that bind to ligand-gated ion channels alter the conductance (g) of ions through the channel protein. In this case, there are **no second messengers** directly activated by the drug binding to a ligand-gated ion channel, but the resulting changes in intracellular ion concentrations may regulate other enzyme signaling cascades.

Membrane-Bound Enzymes

Membrane-bound enzymes that serve as receptors for various endogenous substances and drugs are classified into **five types:** receptor guanylate cyclase, receptor tyrosine kinase, tyrosine kinase–associated receptor, receptor tyrosine phosphatase, and receptor serine/threonine kinase. The first type, **receptor guanylate cyclase,** is the target for atrial natriuretic factor (ANF) and related peptides and consists of a single transmembrane domain protein with an extracellular domain that is the binding site for ANF and intracellular domain that has guanylate cyclase activity. Binding of ANF produces direct **activation of guanylate cyclase** and increase of intracellular cyclic guanosine monophosphate (cGMP), which, like cAMP signaling, activates specific cGMP-dependent kinases.

The second type of membrane-bound enzyme receptors is the class of **receptor tyrosine kinases.** A large number of ligands activate these receptors, including epidermal growth factor, nerve growth factor, and insulin. These receptors are composed of a single transmembrane protein with an extracellular binding domain and, in this case, an intracellular domain with tyrosine kinase activity. When a growth factor or insulin binds to its receptor, kinase activity phosphorylates tyrosine residues of the receptor protein itself, causing **dimerization of two receptors.** The dimerized receptor then goes on to phosphorylate a number of intracellular enzymes and proteins at tyrosine residues and alters the activity of resulting enzyme cascades.

The other types of membrane-bound enzyme receptors initiate signaling in much the same way but have different ligands and different substrates as their signaling targets.

Nuclear Receptors

The nuclear receptor family consists of **two types** of receptors that have similar protein structure. Parts of the receptor protein, called *domains,* are homologous (contain similar amino acid sequence) among all nuclear receptor family members and include an N-terminal variable domain, a DNA binding domain, a hinge region, and a C-terminal hormone binding domain. **Type I nuclear receptors** include targets for sex hormones (androgen, estrogen, and progesterone receptors), glucocorticoid receptors, and mineralocorticoid receptors. These steroid receptors are located inside the cell, bound to accessory heat-shock proteins, and activated by steroids that diffuse through the cell membrane. On activation, the heat shock protein dissociates and two steroid-receptor proteins dimerize and translocate to the nucleus. **Type II nuclear receptors** include receptors for nonsteroid ligands including thyroid hormone, vitamin A and D receptors, and retinoid receptors. These receptors are already present in the nucleus and are activated by the ligand entering the nucleus through nuclear pores.

Once activated, both types of receptors bind to specific DNA sequences (promoters) upstream of genes and **initiate transcription.** A schematic of steroid hormone signaling is shown in Fig. 3.2.

Drug Efficacy

The ability of a drug to initiate a cellular effect is called **efficacy** (also known as intrinsic activity). Efficacy is not directly related to receptor affinity and differs among various drugs that bind to a receptor and start the signal transduction pathway. Drugs that have **both receptor affinity and efficacy are called agonists,** whereas drugs that have **receptor affinity but lack efficacy are called antagonists.** With a few classes of drugs, such as agonists and antagonists at the β-adrenoceptor, the specific molecular structures responsible for affinity and efficacy are identified. Both agonists and antagonists have common components sufficient for receptor affinity, but only agonists have the structure required for efficacy.

There are **three types of agonists. Full agonists** can produce the **maximal response** obtainable in a tissue and therefore have maximal efficacy. **Partial agonists** can produce only a **submaximal response.** In the presence of a full agonist, a partial agonist will act like an antagonist because it will prevent the full agonist from binding to the receptor and exerting a maximal response. **Inverse agonists,** which are also called *negative antagonists,* are involved in a special type of drug-receptor interaction. The effect of inverse agonists is based on the finding, in some cases, that signal transduction proceeds at a basal rate in the absence of any ligand binding to the receptor. A full agonist increases the rate of signal transduction when it binds to the receptor, whereas an **inverse agonist decreases** the rate of signal transduction. Only a few inverse agonists are identified, and some drugs that bind to the *gamma*-aminobutyric acid (GABA)$_A$ receptor located in the central nervous system are examples (see Chapter 19). **Antagonists** can prevent the action of agonists and inverse agonists by occupying binding sites on the receptor. Although antagonists do not "do" anything but block an agonist from binding and activating its receptor, they can be useful therapeutically in blocking excess endogenous ligand. **Competitive antagonists** bind to the same site as the agonist on the receptor but are reversibly bound. **Noncompetitive antagonists** block the agonist site irreversibly, usually by forming a covalent bond.

Receptor Regulation and Drug Tolerance

Receptors can undergo **dynamic changes** with respect to their density (number per cell) and their affinity for drugs and other ligands. The continuous or repeated exposure to agonists can **desensitize receptors,** usually by phosphorylating serine or threonine residues in the C-terminal domain of GPCRs. Phosphorylation of the receptor reduces the G protein–coupling efficiency and alters the binding affinity. This short-term effect of agonist exposure is called **desensitization** or **tachyphylaxis.** Phosphorylation also signals the cell to internalize the membrane receptor. Through internalization and regulation of the receptor gene, the number of receptors on the cell membrane decreases. This longer-term adaptation is called **down-regulation.** In contrast, continuous or repeated exposure to antagonists initially can increase the response of the receptor, called **supersensitivity.** With chronic exposure to antagonists, the number of receptors on the membrane surface (density) increases via **up-regulation.**

Drug tolerance is seen when the same dose of drug given repeatedly loses its effect or when greater doses are needed

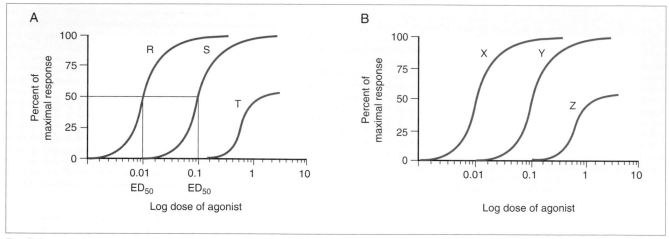

FIG. 3.4 Graded dose-response relationships. (A) The dose-response curves of three agonists (R, S, and T) are compared. Drugs R and S are full agonists. Both have maximal efficacy, but R is more potent than S. Drug T is a partial agonist and therefore is incapable of producing the same magnitude of effect as a full agonist. T is also less potent than R and S. (B) The effects that antagonists have on an agonist's dose-response curve are compared. ED_{50}, Median effective dose; X, Agonist alone; Y, agonist in the presence of a competitive antagonist; Z, agonist in the presence of a noncompetitive antagonist.

to achieve a previously obtained effect. Receptor down-regulation is often responsible for **pharmacodynamic tolerance,** which describes adaptations to chronic drug exposure at the tissue and receptor level. Pharmacodynamic tolerance is distinct from **pharmacokinetic tolerance** in that the latter is caused by accelerated drug elimination, usually resulting from an up-regulation of the enzymes that metabolize the drug.

Disease states can alter the number and function of receptors and thereby affect the response to drugs. For example, **myasthenia gravis** is an autoimmune disorder in which **antibodies destroy the nicotinic receptors** in skeletal muscle, leading to impaired neurotransmission and muscle weakness. This condition is treated by administration of nicotinic receptor agonists (see Chapter 6).

DOSE-RESPONSE RELATIONSHIPS
In pharmacodynamic studies, **different doses of a drug** can be tested in a group of subjects or in isolated organs, tissues, or cells. The relationship between the concentration of a drug at the receptor site and the magnitude of the response is called the **dose-response relationship.** Depending on the purpose of the studies, this relationship can be described in terms of a **graded** (continuous) response or a **quantal** (all-or-none) response.

Graded Dose-Response Relationships
In graded dose-response relationships, the response elicited with each dose of a drug is described in terms of a **percentage of the maximal response** and is plotted against the log dose of the drug (Fig. 3.4). Graded dose-response curves illustrate the relationship among drug dose, receptor occupancy, and the magnitude of the resulting physiologic effect. For a given drug, the maximal response is produced when all of the receptors are occupied, and the half-maximal response is produced when 50% of the receptors are occupied. In some cases, fewer than 50% of total receptors will be occupied but still give the half-maximal response. This is because only a fraction of the total receptors are needed to produce the maximal response. The remaining unbound receptors are considered to be **spare receptors.**

Potency is a characteristic of drug action useful for comparing different pharmacologic agents. It is usually expressed

in terms of the **median effective dose (ED_{50}),** which is the dose that produces 50% of the maximal response. For *in vitro* experiments, this value may also be expressed as EC_{50} (effective concentration for 50% effect). The **potency of a drug varies inversely** with ED_{50} of a drug, so that a drug with an ED_{50} of 4 mg is 10 times more potent than a drug whose ED_{50} is 40 mg. Potency is largely determined by the affinity of a drug for its receptor, because drugs with greater affinity require a lower dose to occupy 50% of the functional receptors (or less if spare receptors are present).

The maximal response produced by a drug is known as its **efficacy.** A full agonist has maximal efficacy, whereas a partial agonist has less than maximal efficacy and is incapable of producing the same magnitude of effect as a full agonist, even at the very highest doses (see Fig. 3.4A). When a partial agonist is administered with an agonist, the **partial agonist may act as an antagonist** by preventing the agonist from binding to the receptor and thereby reducing its effect. An antagonist, by definition, has no efficacy in this sense but can be an effective medication, as in the use of a β-adrenoceptor antagonist (beta-blocker) to treat hypertension.

The effect that an **antagonist** has on the dose-response curve of an agonist depends on whether the antagonist is competitive or noncompetitive (see Fig. 3.4B). A **competitive antagonist** binds reversibly to a receptor, and its effects are surmountable if the dose of the agonist is increased sufficiently. A competitive antagonist shifts the agonist's dose-response curve to the right, but it does not reduce the maximal response. Although a noncompetitive antagonist also shifts the agonist's dose-response curve to the right, it binds to the receptor in a way that reduces the ability of the agonist to elicit a response. The amount of reduction is in proportion to the dose of the antagonist. The effects of a **noncompetitive antagonist cannot be overcome** or surmounted with greater doses of an agonist.

Quantal Dose-Response Relationship
In **quantal dose-response relationships,** the response elicited with each dose of a drug is described in terms of the cumulative percentage of subjects exhibiting a defined

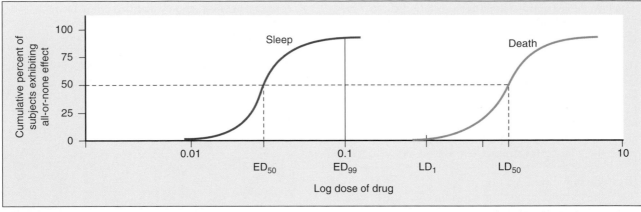

FIG. 3.5   Quantal dose-response relationships. The dose-response curves for a therapeutic effect (sleep) and a toxic effect (death) of a drug are compared. The ratio of the LD_{50} to the ED_{50} is the therapeutic index. The ratio of the LD_1 to the ED_{99} is the certain safety factor. *ED*, Effective dose; *LD*, lethal dose.

all-or-none effect and is plotted against the log dose of the drug (Fig. 3.5). An example of an all-or-none effect is sleep or not-asleep when a sedative-hypnotic agent is given. With quantal dose-response curves, the ED_{50} is the dose that produces the observed effect in 50% of the experimental subjects.

Quantal relationships can be defined for both **toxic and therapeutic** drug effects to allow calculation of the **therapeutic index (TI)** and the **certain safety factor (CSF)** of a drug. The TI and CSF are based on the difference between the toxic dose and the therapeutic dose in a population of subjects. The TI is defined as the **ratio** between the median lethal dose (LD_{50}) and the ED_{50}. It provides a general indication of the margin of safety of a drug, but the CSF is a more realistic estimate of drug safety (see Fig. 3.5). The CSF is defined as the ratio between the dose that is lethal in 1% of subjects (LD_1) and the dose that produces a therapeutic effect in 99% of subjects (ED_{99}). When phenobarbital was tested in animals, for example, it was found to have a TI of 10 and a CSF of 2. Because the dose that will kill 1% of animals is twice the dose that is required to produce the therapeutic effect in 99% of animals, the drug has a good margin of safety.

SUMMARY OF IMPORTANT POINTS

- Most drugs form reversible, stereospecific bonds with macromolecular receptors located in target cells.
- Ligand-gated drug receptors are comprised of multiple receptor subunits and form an inner ion channel which is opened or closed by the actions of drugs.
- GPCRs are a large superclass of membrane receptors targeted by neurotransmitters, hormones, and many types of exogenous drugs. The binding of a drug to a GPCR leads to activation of G-proteins, which are heterotrimeric proteins comprised of G_α, G_β, and G_γ subunits.
- The molecular interactions induced inside the cell by the binding of a drug to its receptor is called the signal transduction pathway. Molecules that carry out the signaling inside the cell are called second messengers.
- The tendency of a drug to bind to a receptor, called *affinity,* is directly related to potency. The affinity of a

drug is often expressed as the K_D, which is the drug concentration required to saturate 50% of the functional receptors.

- The ability of a drug to initiate a response is called *intrinsic activity* or *efficacy.* Agonists have both affinity and efficacy, whereas antagonists only have receptor affinity.
- Graded dose-response curves show the relationship between the dose and the magnitude of the drug effect in a group of subjects or in a particular tissue, organ, or type of cell. The median effective dose (ED_{50}) produces 50% of the maximal response.
- Both a competitive antagonist and a noncompetitive antagonist will cause a rightward shift in the dose-response curve of an agonist, but only a noncompetitive antagonist will reduce the maximal response of the agonist.
- Quantal dose-response curves show the relationship between the dose and the cumulative percentage of subjects exhibiting an all-or-none effect. The ratio of the median lethal dose (toxic dose) to the median effective dose (therapeutic dose) is called the *therapeutic index,* which is an indication of the margin of safety of a drug.

Review Questions

1. The description of molecular events initiated with the ligand binding and ending with a pharmacologic effect is called
   (A) receptor down-regulation.
   (B) signal transduction pathway.
   (C) ligand-receptor binding.
   (D) law of mass action.
   (E) intrinsic activity or efficacy.
2. G protein–coupled receptors that activate an inhibitory G_α subunit alter the activity of adenylate cyclase to
   (A) increase the coupling of receptor to G protein.
   (B) block the ligand from binding.
   (C) initiate the conversion of GTP to GDP.
   (D) generate intracellular inositol triphosphate.
   (E) decrease the production of cAMP.

3. The law of mass action explains the relationship between
   (A) the dose of drug and physiologic response.
   (B) the concentration of drug and the association/dissociation of drug-receptor complex.
   (C) receptors and the rate of signal transduction.
   (D) an enzyme and ligands that inhibit the enzyme.
   (E) graded and quantal dose-response curves.

4. In a log dose-response plot, drug efficacy is determined by the maximal height of the measured response on the effect axis, whereas drug potency is determined by
   (A) the number of animals exhibiting an all-or-none response.
   (B) the signal transduction pathway.
   (C) the formula, including the affinity of the drug and the number of drug receptors.
   (D) the position of the curve along the log-dose axis. ·
   (E) the steepness of the dose-response curve.

5. A partial agonist is best described as an agent that
   (A) has low potency but high efficacy.
   (B) has affinity but lacks efficacy.
   (C) interacts with more than one receptor type.
   (D) cannot produce the full effect, even at high doses.
   (E) blocks the effect of the antagonist.

CHAPTER 4

Drug Development and Drug Safety

OVERVIEW

The market arrival of a new Food and Drug Administration (FDA)-approved drug, launched with a massive advertisement campaign and clever commercials, does little to illuminate the highly regulated process that drugs pass through to make it onto the market. The overwhelming success in modern pharmacotherapy in treating disease states and saving millions of lives attests to the **safety and efficacy of prescribed drugs.** However, drugs can also be poisons, causing unwanted adverse effects, and drugs can kill.

This chapter begins with a description of drug development and the processes for evaluating drug safety and efficacy and then discusses the various types of **adverse effects and interactions** that are caused by drugs. Considerations for specific populations, such as the neonate and the elderly, are highlighted, and the laws relating to drug use and abuse are briefly reviewed.

DRUG DEVELOPMENT

Drug development in most countries has many features in common, beginning with the **discovery** and **characterization** of a new drug and proceeding through the **clinical investigations** that ultimately lead to regulatory approval for marketing the drug. Steps in the process of drug development in the United States are depicted in Fig. 4.1.

Discovery and Characterization

New drug compounds are synthesized *de novo* or are isolated from a **natural product,** or a combination of the two as in semisynthetic compounds. Synthetic drugs may be patterned after other drugs with known pharmacologic activity, or their structure may be designed to bind a particular receptor and based on computer modeling of the drug and receptor. Because the likely activity of some new compounds is relatively uncertain, they must be subjected to a battery of **screening tests** to determine their effects. There are cases in which a particular pharmacologic activity of a drug was discovered accidentally after the drug was administered to patients for other purposes. For example, the antihypertensive effect of **clonidine** was discovered when the drug was tested for treatment of nasal congestion and a profound hypotensive episode ensued. This led to the subsequent development of clonidine for treating hypertension. More recently, the drugs to treat **erectile dysfunction (ED)** (VIAGRA, etc.) started as drug candidates for treating hypertension. The candidate drug was quickly switched to the treatment of ED program after an observant preclinical researcher noted tiny erections on the laboratory mice.

Preclinical Studies

Before a new drug is administered to humans, its pharmacologic effects are thoroughly investigated in studies involving animals, called **preclinical testing.** The studies are designed to (1) ascertain whether the new drug has any harmful or beneficial effects on vital organ function, including cardiovascular, renal, and respiratory function; (2) elucidate the drug's mechanisms and therapeutic effects on target organs; and (3) determine the drug's pharmacokinetic properties, thereby providing some indication of how the drug would be handled by the human body. Although a few people object to using animals, there are even fewer willing to refuse all medical treatment and pharmacotherapy that resulted from animal testing (or to stop wearing leather shoes).

Federal regulations require that extensive toxicity studies in animals be conducted to predict the risks that will be associated with administering the drug to healthy human subjects and patients. The value of the preclinical studies is based on the proven correlation between drug toxicity in animals and humans. As outlined in Table 4.1, the studies involve short-term and long-term administration of the drug and are designed to determine the risk of acute, subacute, and chronic toxicity, as well as the risk of **teratogenesis, mutagenesis,** and **carcinogenesis.** After animals are treated with the new drug, their behavior is assessed and their blood samples are analyzed for indications of tissue damage, metabolic abnormalities, and immunologic effects. Tissues are removed and examined for gross and microscopic pathologic changes. Offspring are also studied for adverse effects.

Studies in animals may not reveal all of the adverse effects that will be found in human subjects, either because of the low incidence of particular effects or because of differences in susceptibility among species. This means that some adverse reactions may not be detected until the drug is administered to patients. However, because studies of chronic toxicity of new drugs in animals may require years for completion, it is usually possible to begin clinical studies while animal studies are being completed if the acute and subacute toxicity studies have not revealed any abnormalities in animals.

THE INVESTIGATIONAL NEW DRUG APPLICATION

The FDA must approve an application for an investigational new drug (IND) before the drug can be distributed for the purpose of conducting studies in human subjects. The IND application includes a complete description of the drug, the results of all preclinical studies completed to date, and a description of the design and methods of the proposed clinical studies and the qualifications of the investigators.

Clinical Trials

Phase I clinical trials seek to determine the pharmacokinetic properties and safety of an IND in healthy human subjects. In the past, most of the subjects were men. Today, women are included in phase I studies to determine whether gender has any influence on the properties of the IND. The

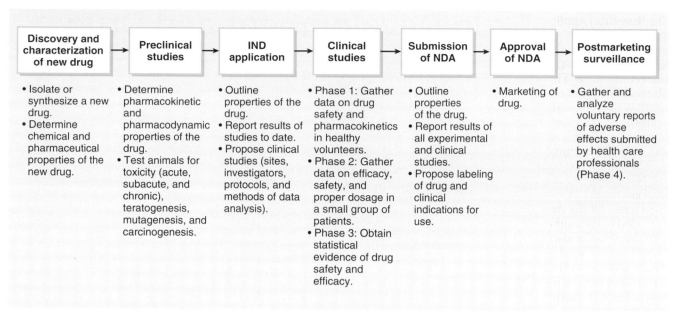

Fig. 4.1   Steps in the process of drug development in the United States. *IND*, Investigational new drug; *NDA*, new drug application.

TABLE 4.1   Drug Toxicity Studies in Animals

TYPE OF STUDY	METHOD	OBSERVATIONS
Acute toxicity	Administer a single dose of the drug in two species via two routes.	Behavioral changes, LD_{50}*, and mortality
Subacute toxicity	Administer the drug for 90 days in two species via a route intended for humans.	Behavioral and physiologic changes, blood chemistry levels, and pathologic findings in tissue samples
Chronic toxicity	Administer the drug for 6–24 months, depending on the type of drug.	Behavioral and physiologic changes, blood chemistry levels, and pathologic findings in tissue samples
Teratogenesis	Administer the drug to pregnant rats and rabbits during organogenesis.	Anatomic defects and behavioral changes in offspring
Mutagenesis	Perform the Ames test in bacteria. Examine cultured mammalian cells for chromosomal defects.	Evidence of chromosome breaks, gene mutations, chromatid exchange, trisomy, or other defects
Carcinogenesis	Administer the drug to rats and mice for their entire lifetime.	Higher than normal rate of malignant neoplasms

*The LD_{50} (the median lethal dose) is the dose that kills half of the animals in a 14-day period after the dose is administered.

subjects typically undergo a complete history and physical examination, diagnostic imaging studies, and chemical and pharmacokinetic analyses of samples of blood and other bodily fluids. The pharmacokinetic analyses provide a basis for estimating doses to be employed in the next phase of trials, and the other examinations seek to determine whether the drug is safe for use in humans.

Phase II clinical trials are the first studies to be performed in human subjects who have the particular disease the IND is targeting. These studies use a small number of patients to obtain a preliminary assessment of the drug's efficacy and safety in diseased individuals and to establish a dosage range for further clinical studies.

Phase III clinical trials are conducted to compare the safety and efficacy of the IND with that of another substance or treatment approach. Phase III studies employ a larger group of subjects, often consisting of hundreds or even thousands of patients and involving multiple clinical sites and investigators. Phase III clinical trials are rigorously designed to prevent investigator bias and include double-blind and placebo-control procedures. In a double-blind study, neither the investigator nor the patient knows if the patient is receiving the new drug or another substance. Placebo-control design includes a group receiving an identical formulation but with no active ingredients. With some diseases, it is unethical to administer a placebo because of the proven benefits of standard drug therapy. In such cases, the new drug is compared with the standard drug for treatment of that disease. Phase III trials often involve crossover studies in which the patients receive one medication or placebo for a period of time and then are switched, after a washout period, to the other medication or placebo.

In many cases, the data are analyzed statistically at various points to determine whether the IND is sufficiently effective or toxic to justify terminating a clinical trial. For example, if a statistically significant greater therapeutic effect can be demonstrated after 6 months in the group of patients who are receiving the new drug, it is unethical to continue giving a placebo or a standard drug to the control group, the members of which could also benefit from receiving the new drug. A clinical trial is also stopped if the new drug causes a significant increase in rate of mortality or serious toxicity.

The New Drug Application and Its Approval

After phase III clinical trials have been completed and analyzed, the drug developer may submit a **new drug application (NDA)** to the FDA to request approval to market the drug. This application includes the results of all preclinical and clinical studies, as well as the proposed labeling and clinical indications for the drug. The NDA typically consists of an enormous amount of printed material, although online submission has now reduced the carbon footprint.

The FDA often requires a number of months to review the NDA before deciding whether to permit the drug to be marketed. Approved drugs are labeled for specific indications based on the data submitted to the FDA. Some drugs are found to have other clinical uses after the drug has been introduced to the market. These non-FDA approved uses are known as unlabeled or "off-label" uses. For example, **gabapentin** (NEURONTIN) was initially approved for treating partial seizures but was used "off-label" for preventing migraine headaches and treating chronic pain. In some cases, manufacturers will seek revised labeling for an approved drug with a new, additional indication and establish a new trade name. This was done for the antidepressant **bupropion,** the exact same drug marketed as WELLBUTRIN for treating depression and ZYBAN for use in smoking cessation.

Postmarketing Surveillance

If a drug is approved for marketing, its safety in the general patient population is monitored by a procedure known as *postmarketing surveillance*, also considered phase IV. The FDA seeks voluntary reporting of adverse drug reactions from health care professionals through its MedWatch program, and standard forms for this purpose are disseminated widely. Post-marketing surveillance is particularly important for detecting drug reactions that are uncommon and are therefore unlikely to be found during clinical trials.

FEDERAL DRUG LAWS AND REGULATIONS

There are two major types of legislation pertaining specifically to drugs. One type concerns **drug safety** and **efficacy** and regulates the processes by which drugs are evaluated, labeled, and marketed. The other type focuses on the **prevention of drug abuse.** In both cases, the laws and regulations reflect the concern of society for minimizing the harm that may result from drug use while permitting the therapeutic use of safe and beneficial agents. Legislation on certifying drug safety and efficacy were slow in coming but are essential to support a lifesaving and thriving pharmaceutical industry. Legislation attempting to curb drug abuse in this country is an abject failure, with a focus on punishment and few treatment opportunities for drug offenders (see Chapter 25).

Drug Safety and Efficacy Laws
Pure Food and Drug Act

The **Pure Food and Drug Act** of 1906 was the **first federal legislation concerning drug product safety and efficacy** in the United States. The Act was passed in response to the increased sales of "patent medicines," often hawked in town squares by "snake-oil salesmen." These totally unregulated concoctions often contained alcohol and/or toxic or other habit-forming drugs. The **Pure Food and Drug Act** required accurate **labeling of the ingredients** in drug products. It also aimed to prevent the adulteration of products through the substitution of inactive or toxic ingredients for the labeled ingredients. Because the Act did not regulate fraudulent advertising, the legislation was only partially successful in eliminating unsafe drug products from the populace.

Food, Drug, and Cosmetic Act

The **Food, Drug, and Cosmetic (FD&C) Act** of 1938 came in response to a tragic incident in which more than 100 people died after ingesting an elixir that contained **sulfanilamide,** used to treat streptococcal infections, in a solution of **ethylene glycol.** The legislation, which is still in force today, made major strides by requiring evidence of drug safety before a drug product could be marketed, by establishing the FDA to enforce this requirement, and by giving legal authority to the **drug product standards** contained in the *United States Pharmacopeia* (**USP**).

First compiled in 1820, the USP has been updated and published at regular intervals by a private organization called the United States Pharmacopeial Convention, which is composed of representatives of medical and pharmacy colleges and societies from each state. The USP contains information on the chemical analysis of drugs and indicates how much variance in drug content is allowable for each drug product. For example, the USP states that aspirin tablets must contain not less than 90% and not more than 110% of the labeled amount of acetylsalicylic acid (aspirin). In addition, the USP outlines standards for tablet disintegration and many other aspects of drug product composition and analysis.

Provisions of the Food, Drug, and Cosmetic Act. The FD&C Act prohibits the distribution of drug products that are **adulterated** or **misbranded** (mislabeled) or that do not have an **approved NDA.** The Act requires that drug product labels contain the name, dosage, and quantity of ingredients, as well as warnings against unsafe use in children or in persons with medical conditions for whom use of the drug might be dangerous. A drug product is said to be adulterated if it does not meet USP standards or if it is not manufactured according to defined "good manufacturing practices."

Amendments to the Food, Drug, and Cosmetic Act. The FD&C Act has been amended many times. The **Durham-Humphrey Amendment** was passed in 1952 and created a legal distinction **between nonprescription and prescription drugs.** Prescription drugs are labeled "Rx Only." Agents that are classified as prescription drugs are those that are determined to be unsafe for use without the supervision of a designated health care professional. After a new drug has been marketed for a period of time, or if it is found to be safe enough to be used without physician supervision, the FDA may reclassify the drug as a nonprescription drug, known as an over-the-counter (OTC) drug. For example, topical cortisone products, antifungal drugs for treating candidiasis, proton pump inhibitors for treating acid reflux such as omeprazole (PRILOSEC), and antihistamines such as loratadine (CLARITIN) were originally classified as prescription drugs but are now available as OTC nonprescription drugs.

The **Kefauver-Harris Amendments** were passed in 1962, largely in response to reports of **severe malformations** in the offspring of women in Europe who took **thalidomide** for sedation during their pregnancy. In fact, thalidomide had not been marketed in the United States because a female scientist at the FDA, Frances Kelsey, held up approval of the drug. Nevertheless, the shocking pictures from Europe of deformed babies spurred Congress to more strongly regulate drug development. Congress passed amendments that required the demonstration of **both safety and efficacy in studies involving animals and humans** before a drug product could be marketed. Although the processes of new drug development and testing have not changed substantially since this amendment was passed, the FDA review of new drugs has been streamlined in recent years.

The **Orphan Drug Act** was passed in 1983 to provide tax benefits and other incentives for drug manufacturers to test and produce drugs that are used in the **treatment of rare diseases** and are therefore unlikely to generate large profits. The Act appears to have been successful as several hundred orphan drugs are now available. Examples are drugs used for the treatment of urea cycle enzyme deficiencies, Gaucher disease, homocystinuria, and other rare metabolic disorders.

Drug Price Competition and Patent Term Restoration Act

The **Drug Price Competition and Patent Term Restoration Act** of 1984 **extended the patent life** of drug products (which at that time was 17 years) by adding the amount of time required for regulatory review of an NDA. It also accelerated the approval of **generic drug products** by allowing investigators to submit an **abbreviated NDA (ANDA)** in which the generic product is shown to be therapeutically equivalent to an approved brand name product. Therapeutic equivalence is demonstrated on the basis of a single-dose oral **bioavailability** study that compares the generic drug with the brand name drug. If the variance is within a specified range (usually ±20%), the generic drug will likely be approved for marketing. The cost of such a study is relatively small compared with the millions of dollars required for the development of a completely new drug.

The HIV-AIDS crisis of the 1980s showed a serious weakness in the federal laws regulating medical use of drugs. Although the pharmaceutical industry responded with vigor in the development of new retroviral medications, the ultimate goal to get them into the growing number of HIV patients was stymied by FDA regulations. Finally, in 1992, legislation for **accelerated drug approval** was passed, authorizing the quicker use of new drugs to **treat life-threatening conditions** such as acquired immunodeficiency syndrome (AIDS) and cancer. Under the new regulations, patients with these conditions can be treated with an investigational drug **before clinical trials have been completed.**

Drug Abuse Prevention Laws
Harrison Narcotics Act
The **Harrison Narcotics Act** of 1914 was the **first major drug abuse legislation** in the United States. It was prompted by the growing problem of heroin abuse, which followed the discovery and commercial success of heroin by the Bayer Company. Heroin is a rapid-acting derivative of morphine, preferred by addicts for its quick action on the brain ("rush"). The Act sought to control narcotics through the use of **tax stamps on legal drug products,** a practice similar to the use of tax stamps on alcoholic beverages today. The Harrison Narcotics Act also had a profound and unfortunate influence on the treatment of substance abuse in that

it **prohibited physicians from administering opioid drugs** to heroin-dependent patients as part of their treatment program.

Comprehensive Drug Abuse Prevention and Control Act
During the 1960s, the prevalence of drug abuse increased, especially among adolescents and young adults. The practitioners of this growing youth movement were using a wide variety of drugs that included prescription stimulants and sedatives ("uppers" and "downers"), lysergic acid diethylamide (LSD, "acid"), marijuana ("grass," "weed"), and other mind-altering substances. Believing that they could solve the "drug abuse problem," the members of Congress passed the Comprehensive Drug Abuse Prevention and Control Act of 1970. This law is often called simply the **Controlled Substances Act (CSA).**

The CSA classified drugs with abuse potential into **five schedules,** based on their degree of potential for abuse and their clinical usage (Fig. 4.2). **Schedule I** drugs are classified as having high abuse potential and no legitimate medical use, and their distribution and possession are prohibited. **Schedule II** drugs have high abuse potential but a legitimate medical use, and their distribution is highly controlled through requirements for inventories and records, and through restrictions on prescriptions. **Schedule III, IV, and V** drugs have lower abuse potential and decreasingly fewer restrictions on distribution. The CSA requires that all manufacturers, distributors, physicians, and medical researchers using controlled drugs register with the **Drug Enforcement Administration (DEA)**, which is responsible for enforcing the Act.

Unfortunately, the Controlled Substances Act also included **mandatory sentencing guidelines for drug offenders,** which swelled the judicial system and led to the incarceration of a great deal of our urban and rural population. Under various additional amendments and legislation, such as the "three strikes law," and the laws passed during the "crack epidemic," sentences for drug offenders continued to evolve from harsh to draconian, leading to more lengthy sentences and the overcrowding of prisons that is the current state today.

ADVERSE EFFECTS OF DRUGS
Adverse effects, or side effects, can be classified with respect to their mechanisms of action and predictability. Those caused by **excessive pharmacologic activity** are the most predictable and are often the easiest to prevent or counteract. Organ toxicity caused by other mechanisms is often unpredictable because its occurrence depends on the drug susceptibility of the individual patient, the drug dosage, and numerous other factors. **Drug hypersensitivity reactions** ("drug allergies") are responsible for a large number of adverse organ system effects. These reactions occur frequently with a few drugs but only rarely with most.

Excessive Pharmacologic Effects
Drugs often produce adverse effects by the same mechanism responsible for their therapeutic effect on the target organ. For example, **atropine** may cause dry mouth and urinary retention by the same mechanism that reduces gastric acid secretion in the treatment of peptic ulcer, namely, by **muscarinic receptor antagonism.** This type of adverse effect

Controlled Substances

Schedule	Symbol	Characteristics	Examples
I (C I)	C_I	High abuse potential. May lead to severe dependence. No accepted medical use.	Heroin Marijuana Peyote
II (C II)	C_{II}	High abuse potential. May lead to severe dependence.	Cocaine Morphine Codeine Methadone Amphetamine
III (C III)	C_{III}	Abuse potential less than Schedules I and II. May lead to moderate dependence.	Drugs that are combinations of opiate and non-narcotic drugs, such as hydrocodone and acetaminophen (VICODIN)
IV (C IV)	C_{IV}	Moderate abuse potential. May lead to limited dependence.	Alprazolam (XANAX) Zolpidem (AMBIEN) Phenobarbital (LUMINAL) Modafinil (PROVIGIL)
V (C V)	C_V	Small abuse potential. May lead to limited dependence.	Cough medications with codeine, certain antidiarrheals.

FIG. 4.2 Schedule of controlled substances and example drugs. Note that many states have legalized the medical use of marijuana, although federally it is still illegal to use marijuana for medicinal purposes.

may be managed by reducing the drug dosage or by substituting a drug that is more selective for the target organ.

Drug Hypersensitivity Reactions

Drug Hypersensitivity Reactions are responsible for a large number of organ toxicities that range in severity from a mild skin rash to major organ system failure. In some cases, a true allergic reaction occurs when the drug, acting as a hapten, combines with an endogenous protein to form an antigen that induces antibody production. The antigen and antibody subsequently interact with body tissues to produce a wide variety of adverse effects.

In the Gell and Coombs classification system, allergic reactions are divided into four general types, each of which can be produced by drugs. **Type I** reactions are **immediate hypersensitivity** reactions that are mediated by immunoglobulin E antibodies. Examples of these reactions are **angioedema** (rapid swelling [edema] of the dermis through submucosal layers of the skin, often most detectable with the swelling of lips and mouth), **urticaria** ("hives"), **dermatitis,** and **anaphylactic shock. Type II** reactions are **cytolytic reactions** that involve immune complement and are mediated by immunoglobulins G and M. Examples are **hemolytic anemia, thrombocytopenia,** and drug-induced **lupus erythematosus. Type III** reactions are mediated by **immune complexes.** The deposition of antigen-antibody complexes in vascular endothelium leads to inflammation, lymphadenopathy, and fever (serum sickness). An example is the severe skin rash seen in patients with a life-threatening form of **drug-induced vasculitis** known as *Stevens-Johnson syndrome*. **Type IV** reactions are **delayed hypersensitivity** reactions that are mediated by **sensitized lymphocytes.** An example is the ampicillin-induced skin rash that occurs in patients with viral mononucleosis.

Adverse Effects on Organs

In some cases, the adverse effects and therapeutic effects of a drug are caused by different mechanisms. For example, in

patients taking aspirin, the adverse reaction such as hyperventilation that leads to respiratory alkalosis is caused by adverse effects that do not appear to be mediated by the drug's primary mechanism of action, which is inhibition of prostaglandin synthesis. A variety of drugs (Table 4.2) produce toxicity of the liver, kidneys, or other vital organs, and this toxicity may not be readily apparent until significant organ damage has occurred. Patients receiving these drugs should be monitored with appropriate laboratory tests. For example, **hepatotoxicity** may be detected by monitoring serum transaminase levels, and hematopoietic toxicity may be detected by periodically performing blood cell counts.

Hematopoietic Toxicity

Bone marrow toxicity, one of the most frequent types of drug-induced toxicity, may manifest as agranulocytosis, anemia, thrombocytopenia, or a combination of these (pancytopenia). The effects are often reversible when the drug is withdrawn, but they may have serious consequences before toxicity can be detected. For example, patients who develop agranulocytosis may succumb to a fatal infection before the problem is recognized.

Many drugs, such as **chloramphenicol,** are believed to cause hematopoietic toxicity by triggering hypersensitivity reactions directed against the stem cells in bone marrow or their derivatives. Chloramphenicol also produces a reversible form of anemia by blocking the action of the enzyme ferrochelatase, thereby preventing the incorporation of iron into heme.

The most serious form of hematopoietic toxicity is **aplastic anemia,** which may be associated with several types of blood cell deficiencies and lead to pancytopenia. Aplastic anemia is probably caused by a hypersensitivity reaction and is often irreversible, although it has recently been treated by administration of hematopoietic growth factors (see Chapter 17).

TABLE 4.2 Drug-Induced Organ Toxicities

ORGAN TOXICITY	EXAMPLES OF ADVERSE EFFECTS	EXAMPLES OF DRUGS
Cardiotoxicity	Cardiomyopathy	Daunorubicin, doxorubicin, and idarubicin
Hematopoietic toxicity	Agranulocytosis*	Captopril, chlorpromazine, chlorpropamide, clozapine, and propylthiouracil
	Aplastic anemia*	Chloramphenicol and phenylbutazone
	Hemolytic anemia*	Captopril, levodopa, and methyldopa
	Thrombocytopenia*	Quinidine, rifampin, and sulfonamides
Hepatotoxicity	Cholestatic jaundice*	Erythromycin estolate and phenothiazines
	Hepatitis*	Amiodarone, captopril, isoniazid, phenytoin, and sulfonamides
Nephrotoxicity	Acute tubular necrosis	Aminoglycoside antibiotics, amphotericin B, and vancomycin
	Interstitial nephritis*	Nonsteroidal anti-inflammatory drugs (NSAIDs) and penicillins (especially methicillin)
Ototoxicity	Vestibular and cochlear disorders	Aminoglycoside antibiotics, furosemide, and vancomycin
Pulmonary toxicity	Inflammatory fibrosis	Methysergide
	Pulmonary fibrosis	Amiodarone, bleomycin, busulfan, and nitrofurantoin
Skin toxicity	All forms of skin rash*	Antibiotics, diuretics, phenytoin, sulfonamides, and sulfonylureas

*Immunologic mechanisms known or suspected.

Hepatotoxicity

A large number of drugs produce liver toxicity, either via an immunologic mechanism or via their direct effect on the hepatocytes. Liver toxicity can be classified as **cholestatic** or **hepatocellular. Cholestatic hepatotoxicity** is often caused by a **hypersensitivity mechanism** producing inflammation and stasis of the biliary system. **Hepatocellular toxicity** is sometimes caused by a **toxic drug metabolite.** For example, **acetaminophen** and **isoniazid** have toxic metabolites that may cause hepatitis. With many hepatotoxic drugs, elevated serum transaminase levels may provide an early indication of liver damage, and levels should be monitored during the first 6 months of therapy and at longer intervals thereafter. Many authorities believe that, if transaminase levels exceed two times the upper normal limit, a physician should consider alternative drug therapy or frequent monitoring of enzyme levels. If transaminase levels exceed three times the upper normal limit, the drug should be discontinued. Unfortunately, some patients have developed acute hepatic failure even when serum transaminase levels have been monitored appropriately. In recent years, several drugs such as **troglitazone,** used to treat diabetes, have been removed from the market as a result of excessive cases of fatal hepatic failure.

Nephrotoxicity

Renal toxicity is caused by various drugs, including several groups of antibiotics. The forms of renal toxicity can be classified according to site and mechanism and include **interstitial nephritis, renal tubular necrosis,** and **crystalluria** (the precipitation of insoluble drug in the renal tubules). **Nephrotoxicity** often reduces drug clearance, thereby elevating plasma drug concentrations and leading to greater toxicity. With some drugs that routinely cause renal toxicity, such as the antineoplastic agent cisplatin, the kidneys can be protected by means of forced diuresis, in which the drug is administered with large quantities of intravenous fluid so as to lower the drug concentration in the renal tubules.

Bladder toxicity is less common than renal toxicity, but it may occur as an adverse effect of a few drugs. One example is **cyclophosphamide,** an antineoplastic drug whose metabolite causes hemorrhagic cystitis. Administering mesna, a sulfhydryl-releasing agent that conjugates the toxic metabolite in the urine, can prevent this disorder.

Other Organ Toxicities

Pulmonary toxicity occurs through a variety of mechanisms. Some drugs, such as opioid analgesics, cause **respiratory depression** via their effects on the brainstem respiratory centers. The drugs bleomycin and amiodarone produce pulmonary fibrosis, so patients who are being treated with these agents should have periodic chest radiographs and blood gas measurements to detect early signs of fibrosis.

Relatively few drugs produce **cardiotoxicity.** Anthracycline anticancer drugs, such as **doxorubicin** (ADRIAMYCIN), produce adverse cardiac effects that resemble congestive heart failure. HMG-CoA reductase inhibitors **(statins)** such as **simvastatin** (ZOCOR) may cause **skeletal muscle damage,** especially at higher doses. This can result in muscle pain and sometimes leads to **rhabdomyolysis** and **renal failure.**

Skin rashes of all varieties, including macular, papular, maculopapular, and urticarial rashes, may be produced by drug hypersensitivity reactions. A mild skin rash may disappear with continued drug administration. Nevertheless, because rashes may lead to more serious skin or organ toxicity, they should be monitored carefully.

Idiosyncratic Reactions

Idiosyncratic reactions are unexpected drug reactions caused by a **genetically determined susceptibility.** For example, patients who have glucose-6-phosphate dehydrogenase deficiency may develop hemolytic anemia when they are exposed to an oxidizing drug, such as primaquine, or to a sulfonamide.

DRUG INTERACTIONS

A **drug interaction** is defined as a change in the pharmacologic effect of a drug that results when it is given **concurrently with another drug or with food.** Drug interactions

TABLE 4.3 Types and Mechanisms of Drug Interactions

TYPE	MECHANISM
Drug interactions with food	Altered drug absorption
Pharmaceutical interactions (drug incompatibilities)	Chemical reaction between drugs before their administration or absorption
Pharmacodynamic interactions	Additive, synergistic, or antagonistic effects on a microbe or tumor cells
	Additive, synergistic, or antagonistic effects on a tissue or organ system
Pharmacokinetic interactions	
Altered drug absorption	Altered gut motility or secretion
	Binding or chelation of drugs
	Competition for active transport
Altered drug distribution	Displacement from plasma protein–binding sites
	Displacement from tissue-binding sites
Altered drug biotransformation	Altered hepatic blood flow
	Enzyme induction
	Enzyme inhibition
Altered drug excretion	Altered biliary excretion or enterohepatic cycling
	Altered urine pH
	Drug-induced renal impairment
	Inhibition of active tubular secretion

may be caused by changes in the pharmaceutical, pharmacodynamic, or pharmacokinetic properties of the affected drug (Table 4.3).

Pharmaceutical Interactions

Pharmaceutical interactions are caused by a chemical reaction between drugs **before their administration or absorption.** Pharmaceutical interactions occur most frequently when drug solutions are combined before they are given intravenously. For example, if a penicillin solution and an aminoglycoside solution are mixed, they will form an insoluble precipitate, because penicillins are negatively charged and aminoglycosides are positively charged. Many other drugs are incompatible and should not be combined before they are administered.

Pharmacodynamic Interactions

Pharmacodynamic interactions occur when two drugs have **additive, synergistic,** or **antagonistic effects** on tissues, organ systems, microbes, or tumor cells. An **additive effect** is equal to the sum of the individual drug effects, whereas a **synergistic effect** is greater than the sum of the individual drug effects. Some pharmacodynamic interactions occur when two drugs act on the same receptor, and others occur when the drugs affect the same physiologic function through actions on different receptors. For example, **epinephrine** and **histamine** affect the same function but have **antagonistic effects.** Epinephrine activates adrenergic receptors to cause bronchial smooth muscle relaxation,

whereas histamine activates histamine receptors to produce bronchial smooth muscle contraction.

Pharmacokinetic Interactions

In **pharmacokinetic interactions,** a drug alters the **absorption, distribution, biotransformation,** or **excretion** of another drug or drugs. Mechanisms and examples of pharmacokinetic interactions are provided in Table 4.4 (see also Table 4.3).

Altered Drug Absorption

There are **several mechanisms** by which a drug may affect the absorption and bioavailability of another drug. One mechanism involves binding to another drug in the gut and preventing its absorption. For example, **cholestyramine,** a bile acid sequestrant, binds to **digoxin** and **prevents its absorption.** Another mechanism involves altering gastric or intestinal motility so as to affect the absorption of another drug. Drugs tend to be absorbed more rapidly from the intestines than from the stomach. Therefore, a drug that slows gastric emptying, such as **atropine,** often **delays the absorption** of another drug. A drug that increases intestinal motility, such as a laxative, may reduce the time available for the absorption of another drug, thereby causing its incomplete absorption.

Altered Drug Distribution

Many drugs **displace other drugs from plasma proteins** and thereby increase the plasma concentration of the free (unbound) drug, but the magnitude and duration of this effect are usually small. As the free drug concentration increases, so does the drug's rate of elimination, and any change in the drug's effect on target tissues is usually short-lived.

The **enterohepatic cycling** of some drugs is dependent on intestinal bacteria that hydrolyze drug conjugates excreted by the bile and thereby enable the more lipid-soluble parent compound to be reabsorbed into the circulation. Antibiotics administered concurrently with these drugs may kill the bacteria and reduce the enterohepatic cycling and plasma drug concentrations. When antibiotics are taken concurrently with **oral contraceptives** containing estrogen, for example, they may reduce the plasma concentration of estrogen and cause contraceptive failure (Fig. 4.3).

Altered Drug Biotransformation

In some cases, **biotransformation** is affected by drugs that alter hepatic blood flow. In many cases, it is affected by drug interactions that either induce or inhibit drug-metabolizing enzymes (see Table 4.4).

Inducers of cytochrome P450 enzymes include **barbiturates, carbamazepine,** and **rifampin,** which bind to regulatory domains of cytochrome P450 (CYP) genes and increase gene transcription. These agents induce the CYP1A2, CYP2C9, CYP2C19, and CYP3A4 isozymes, whereas the CYP2D6 and CYP2E1 isozymes are not readily induced by commonly used drugs. The rate of induction depends on the dose and frequency of administration. Enzyme induction is usually maximal after several days of continuing drug administration. Enzyme induction **increases the clearance** and **reduces the half-life of drugs** biotransformed by the enzyme. When the inducing drug is discontinued, the

TABLE 4.4   Management of Clinically Significant Pharmacokinetic Drug Interactions

EXAMPLES OF INDUCERS OR INHIBITORS	EXAMPLES OF AFFECTED DRUGS	MANAGEMENT
Inducers of Drug Biotransformation		
Barbiturates, carbamazepine, and rifampin	Warfarin	Increase warfarin dosage as indicated by prothrombin time (international normalized ratio).
Carbamazepine	Theophylline	Monitor plasma theophylline concentration and adjust dosage as needed.
Rifampin	Phenytoin	Monitor plasma phenytoin concentration and adjust dosage as needed.
Inhibitors of Drug Absorption		
Aluminum, calcium, and iron	Tetracycline	Give tetracycline 1 h before or 2 h after giving the other agent.
Cholestyramine	Digoxin and warfarin	Give digoxin or warfarin 1 h before or 2 h after giving cholestyramine.
Inhibitors of Drug Biotransformation		
Cimetidine	Benzodiazepines, lidocaine, phenytoin, theophylline, and warfarin	Instead of giving cimetidine, substitute a histamine blocker that does not inhibit drug metabolism.
Disulfiram	Ethanol	Make sure the patient understands that disulfiram is used therapeutically to promote abstinence from alcohol (ethanol).
Erythromycin	Carbamazepine and theophylline	Lower the dose of the affected drug during erythromycin therapy.
Erythromycin, itraconazole, and ketoconazole	Lovastatin and atorvastatin	Avoid concurrent therapy and thereby avoid myopathy.
Monoamine oxidase inhibitors	Levodopa and sympathomimetic drugs	Avoid concurrent therapy, if possible; otherwise, give a subnormal dose of the affected drug.
Inhibitors of Drug Clearance		
Diltiazem, quinidine, and verapamil	Digoxin	Give a subnormal dose of digoxin and monitor the plasma drug concentration.
Probenecid	Cephalosporins and penicillin	Advise the patient that the combination of drugs is intended to increase the plasma concentration of the antibiotic.
Thiazide diuretics	Lithium	Give a subnormal dose of lithium and monitor the plasma drug concentration.

synthesis of P450 enzymes gradually returns to the pretreatment level.

A large number of drugs bind to and **inhibit CYP isozymes.** CYP3A4 is selectively inhibited by **erythromycin, itraconazole,** and **doxycycline,** whereas other drugs such as **cimetidine, ketoconazole,** and **fluoxetine** inhibit several CYP isozymes. Significant interactions occur when these drugs reduce the clearance and increase the plasma concentration of other drugs. For example, **itraconazole** inhibits the biotransformation of **HMG-CoA reductase inhibitors,** such as **lovastatin** and **atorvastatin,** by CYP3A4. This inhibition increases plasma levels severalfold, sometimes leading to severe muscle inflammation and rhabdomyolysis. Grapefruit juice has been found to contain bioflavonoid compounds that inhibit CYP3A4 and thereby elevate concentrations of drugs such as **felodipine** (Plendil) that are metabolized by this enzyme.

Altered Drug Excretion

Drugs can **alter the renal or biliary excretion** of other drugs by several mechanisms. A few drugs, such as **carbonic anhydrase inhibitors,** alter the renal pH. This in turn can change the ratio of another drug's ionized form to its nonionized form and affect its renal excretion. **Probenecid** competes with other organic acids, such as penicillin, for the active transport system in renal tubules. **Quinidine** and **verapamil** decrease the **biliary clearance** of digoxin and thereby **increase serum digoxin levels.** Potentially nephrotoxic drugs, such as the **aminoglycoside antibiotics,** may impair the renal excretion of other drugs via their effect on renal function.

Clinical Significance of Drug Interactions

The clinical significance of drug interactions varies widely. In some cases, **toxicity is severe** and can be prevented only by avoiding the concurrent administration of drugs. In other cases, toxicity can be avoided by proper dosage adjustment and other measures (see Table 4.4). For example, when **quinidine** and **digoxin** are administered concurrently, a subnormal dose of digoxin should be used to prevent adverse effects. Fortunately, many drug interactions are of minor significance, and the interacting drugs can usually be administered concurrently without affecting their efficacy or the patient's safety. Drug interactions are more likely to occur if the affected drug has a low therapeutic index or is being used to treat a critically ill patient. However, **polypharmacy,** which refers to the use of multiple medications by a patient, is linked to many adverse effects and toxicity caused by drug interactions, especially in the elderly.

FACTORS AFFECTING DRUG SAFETY AND EFFICACY

Age, disease, pregnancy, and **lactation** are important biologic variables that can alter the response to drugs in particular patients.

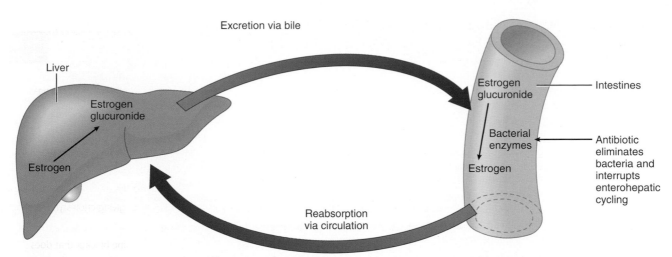

FIG. 4.3 Interaction of antibiotics with estrogens found in oral contraceptives. Estrogen is conjugated with glucuronate and sulfate in the liver, and the conjugates are excreted via the bile into the intestines. Intestinal bacteria hydrolyze the conjugates, and estrogen is reabsorbed into the circulation. The enterohepatic cycling is interrupted if concurrently administered antibiotics destroy the intestinal bacteria. Contraceptive failure may result.

TABLE 4.5 Factors Affecting Drug Disposition in Different Age Populations

PROCESS OF DRUG DISPOSITION	POPULATION		
	NEONATES AND INFANTS	**CHILDREN**	**ELDERLY ADULTS**
Absorption	Altered absorption of some drugs.	No major changes, but first-pass inactivation may be increased.	No major changes.
Distribution	Incomplete blood-brain barrier; higher volumes of distribution for water-soluble drugs.	No major changes.	Higher volumes of distribution for fat-soluble drugs.
Biotransformation	Lower rate of oxidative reactions and glucuronate conjugation.	Biotransformation rate for some drugs higher than in adults.	Reduced oxidative metabolism; relatively unchanged conjugation metabolism.
Excretion	Reduced capacity to excrete drugs.	No major changes.	Reduced capacity to excrete drugs.

Age

Factors affecting drug disposition in different age populations are summarized in Table 4.5.

In **neonates,** and especially in premature infants, the capacity to metabolize and excrete drugs is often greatly reduced because of low levels of drug biotransformation enzymes. Oxidative reactions and glucuronate conjugation occur at a lower rate in neonates than in adults, whereas sulfate conjugation is well developed in neonates. Consequently, some drugs that are metabolized primarily by glucuronate conjugation in adults (drugs such as **acetaminophen**) are metabolized chiefly by sulfate conjugation in neonates. Nevertheless, the overall rate of biotransformation of most drugs is lower in neonates and infants than it is in adults.

In comparison with **children** and **young adults,** elderly adults also tend to have a reduced capacity to metabolize drugs. Biotransformation via oxidative reactions usually declines more than biotransformation via drug conjugation. Therefore, it may be safer to use drugs that are conjugated when the choice is available. For example, benzodiazepines that are metabolized by conjugation, such as **lorazepam** and **temazepam,** are believed to be safer for treatment of the elderly than are benzodiazepines that undergo oxidative biotransformation (e.g., diazepam).

Renal function is lower in neonates and elderly adults than it is in young adults, and this affects the renal excretion of many drugs. For example, the half-lives of aminoglycoside antibiotics are greatly prolonged in neonates. Glomerular filtration declines 35% between the ages of 20 and 90 years with a corresponding reduction in the renal elimination of many drugs.

Because the very young and the very old tend to have **increased sensitivity to drugs,** the dosage per kilogram of body weight should be reduced when most drugs are used in the treatment of these populations.

Disease

Hepatic and renal disease may **reduce the capacity of the liver and kidneys** to biotransform and excrete drugs, thereby reducing drug clearance and necessitating a dosage reduction to avoid toxicity. Heart failure and other conditions that reduce hepatic blood flow may also reduce drug biotransformation. Oxidative drug metabolism is usually impaired in patients with hepatic disease, whereas conjugation processes may be little affected.

Guidelines for dosage adjustment in patients with hepatic or renal disease are available and can be found in clinical references. **Dosage adjustments** are made by reducing the dose, increasing the interval between doses, or both. Adjustments for individual patients are usually based on laboratory measurements of renal or hepatic function and on plasma drug concentration.

TABLE 4.6 Examples of Teratogenic Drugs and Their Effects on the Fetus or Newborn Infant*

DRUG	ADVERSE EFFECTS
Alkylating agents and antimetabolites (anticancer drugs)	Cardiac defects; cleft palate; growth retardation; malformation of ears, eyes, fingers, nose, or skull; and other anomalies.
Carbamazepine	Abnormal facial features; neural tube defects, such as spina bifida; reduced head size; and other anomalies.
Coumarin anticoagulants	Fetal warfarin syndrome (characterized by chondrodysplasia punctata, malformation of ears and eyes, mental retardation, nasal hypoplasia, optic atrophy, skeletal deformities, and other anomalies).
Diethylstilbestrol (DES)	Effects in female offspring: clear cell vaginal or cervical adenocarcinoma; irregular menses; and reproductive abnormalities, including decreased rate of pregnancy and increased rate of preterm deliveries. Effects in male offspring: cryptorchidism, epididymal cysts, and hypogonadism.
Ethanol	Fetal alcohol syndrome (characterized by growth retardation, hyperactivity, mental retardation, microcephaly and facial abnormalities, poor coordination, and other anomalies).
Phenytoin	Fetal hydantoin syndrome (characterized by cardiac defects; malformation of ears, lips, palate, mouth, and nasal bridge; mental retardation; microcephaly; ptosis; strabismus; and other anomalies).
Retinoids (systemic)	Spontaneous abortions. Hydrocephaly; malformation of ears, face, heart, limbs, and liver; microcephaly; and other anomalies.
Tetracycline	Hypoplasia of tooth enamel and staining of teeth.
Thalidomide	Deafness, heart defects, limb abnormalities (amelia or phocomelia), renal abnormalities, and other anomalies.
Valproate	Cardiac defects, central nervous system defects, lumbosacral spina bifida, and microcephaly.

*Other substances known to be teratogenic include lead, lithium, methyl mercury, penicillamine, polychlorinated biphenyls, and trimethadione. Other drugs that should be avoided during the second and third trimester of pregnancy are angiotensin-converting enzyme inhibitors, chloramphenicol, indomethacin, prostaglandins, sulfonamides, and sulfonylureas. Other drugs that should be used with great caution during pregnancy include antithyroid drugs, aspirin, barbiturates, benzodiazepines, corticosteroids, heparin, opioids, and phenothiazines.

Pregnancy and Lactation

Drugs taken by a woman during pregnancy or lactation can cause **adverse effects in the fetus or infant.**

The risk of drug-induced developmental abnormalities known as **teratogenic effects** is the greatest during the period of organogenesis from the 4th to the 10th week of gestation. After the 10th week, the major risk is to the development of the brain and spinal cord. An estimated 1% to 5% of fetal malformations are attributed to drugs. Although only a few drugs have been proven to cause teratogenic effects (Table 4.6), the safety of many other drugs has **not yet been determined.**

The FDA has divided drugs into **five categories** based on their safety in pregnant women. Drugs in Categories A and B are relatively safe. Drugs in **Category A** have been shown in clinical studies to pose no risk to the fetus, whereas those in **Category B** may have shown risk in animal studies but not in human studies. For drugs in **Category C,** adverse effects on the fetus have been demonstrated in animals, but there are insufficient data in pregnant women, so risk to the fetus cannot be ruled out. Drugs in **Category D** show positive evidence of risk to the fetus, and drugs in **Category X** are contraindicated during pregnancy.

Drugs of choice for **pregnant women** are listed in clinical references and are selected on the basis of their safety to the fetus as well as their therapeutic efficacy. For example, **penicillin, cephalosporin,** and **macrolide antibiotics** (all Category B drugs) are preferred for treating many infections in pregnant women, whereas tetracycline antibiotics (Category D) should be avoided. **Acetaminophen** (Category B) is usually the analgesic of choice in pregnancy, but ibuprofen and related drugs are also in Category B and may be used when required. For the treatment of nausea and vomiting of pregnancy, the combination of **pyridoxine** (Category A) and **doxylamine** (Category B) is the only medication specifically labeled for this indication by the FDA. Other drugs considered relatively safe for use in pregnancy include **insulin** and **metformin** (GLUCOPHAGE) for treating diabetes mellitus (both Category B drugs), **famotidine** (PEPCID) and **omeprazole** (PRILOSEC) for reducing gastric acidity (Category B drugs), **diphenhydramine** (BENADRYL) for treating allergic reactions (Category B), and tricyclic antidepressants such as **desipramine** (NORPRAMIN) for treating mood depression (Category B). Most antiepileptic drugs pose some risk to the fetus, and the selection of drugs for treating epilepsy in pregnant women requires careful consideration of the risks and benefits of such medication.

Lactating women can take some drugs without posing a risk to their breast-fed infants. Other drugs place the infant at risk for toxicity. As a general rule, breast-feeding should be avoided if a drug taken by the mother would cause the infant's plasma drug concentration to be greater than 50% of the mother's plasma concentration. Clinical references provide guidelines on the use of specific drugs by lactating women.

Starting in June 2015, the FDA codified new regulations regarding the safety of medication use in pregnancy and lactation. New drug regulations remove the Category A, B, C, D, X system as previously outlined and use mandatory subheadings in the FDA label. These subheadings include Pregnancy, Lactation, and a new section entitled Females and Males of Reproductive Potential. This change was to better assist health care providers in benefit-risk decisions and in giving treatment options to pregnant women and nursing mothers who need to take medications.

SUMMARY OF IMPORTANT POINTS

- The process of drug development includes chemical and pharmacologic characterization, experimental studies to test for toxicity in animals, and clinical studies to determine efficacy and safety in humans.

- The FDA regulates drug development. An IND application must be completed before clinical studies can be started, and an NDA must be submitted and approved before the drug can be marketed.
- Phase I studies provide data about drug safety and pharmacokinetics in healthy subjects; phase II studies provide data about the proper dosage and potential efficacy in a small group of patients; and phase III studies provide statistical evidence of efficacy and safety in a controlled clinical trial.
- The Food, Drug, and Cosmetic Act established the FDA to regulate the development, manufacturing, distribution, and use of drugs. Amendments have established the prescription class of drugs, stricter requirements for human drug testing, incentives for developing orphan drugs for rare diseases, and abbreviated procedures for marketing generic drug products.
- The Comprehensive Drug Abuse Prevention and Control Act, also called the *Controlled Substances Act* (CSA), classifies potentially abused drugs in five categories (Schedules I to V), requires registration of legitimate drug distributors and health care professionals, and limits the prescription and distribution of controlled substances.
- The adverse effects of drugs may be caused by excessive pharmacologic effects, hypersensitivity reactions, or other mechanisms responsible for organ toxicities. The bone marrow, liver, kidney, and skin are frequent sites of drug toxicity.
- Drug interactions occur when one drug alters the pharmacologic properties of another drug. Pharmacokinetic effects, particularly inhibition or induction of drug biotransformation, cause most interactions.
- Age, disease, pregnancy, and lactation are factors that must be considered in drug selection and dosage. The very young and the very old tend to have an increased sensitivity to therapeutic agents, usually because of a reduced capacity to eliminate drugs. Target organs may also be more sensitive to drugs in these populations.

Review Questions

1. An advertisement in a local newspaper seeks to enroll 20 patients with arthritis in a medical study that would be the first time that a new drug would be tested in persons with this disease. The study would therefore be classified as a
   (A) Phase I clinical study.
   (B) Phase II clinical study.
   (C) Phase III clinical study.
   (D) Phase IV clinical study.
   (E) Phase V clinical study.

2. Which one of the following schedules of controlled substances is for drugs with the highest abuse potential that have a legitimate medical use?
   (A) Schedule I
   (B) Schedule II
   (C) Schedule III
   (D) Schedule IV
   (E) Schedule V

3. The 4th to the 10th week of gestation is the period of time when there is the greatest concern about drug-induced
   (A) fetal cardiac arrest.
   (B) fetal hemorrhage.
   (C) fetal malformations.
   (D) labor.
   (E) fetal jaundice.

4. Which of the following drug interaction mechanisms is most likely to lead to sustained elevations of plasma drug concentrations and drug toxicity?
   (A) induction of CYP2C19
   (B) inhibition of CYP3A4
   (C) displacement of a drug from plasma albumin–binding sites
   (D) inhibition of the P-glycoprotein carrier protein
   (E) acceleration of gastric emptying by a "prokinetic" drug

5. Elderly persons may have altered drug disposition because of
   (A) a markedly reduced absorption of many drugs.
   (B) higher volumes of distribution for water-soluble drugs.
   (C) an accelerated renal excretion of ionized drugs.
   (D) an increased permeability of the blood-brain barrier.
   (E) a reduced capacity to oxidize drugs.

Toxicology Principles and the Treatment of Poisoning

Pesticides

Herbicides
- 2,4-Dichlorphenoxyacetic acid (2,4-D)
- Paraquat[a]

Insecticides
Organophosphate insecticides
- Malathion
- Parathion
- Trichlorfon[b]

Carbamate insecticides
- Carbaryl (SEVIN)

Organochlorine insecticides
- Dichloro-diphenyl-trichloroethane (DDT)
- Benzene hexachloride
- Toxaphene

Botanical insecticides
- Pyrethrins
- Allethrin
- Rotenone
- Neonicotinoids

Metals and Chelators

Metals
- Lead
- Mercury
- Arsenic

Chelators
- Calcium disodium EDTA
- Dimercaprol
- Unithiol
- Succimer (CHEMET)[c]

Hydrocarbons
- Benzene
- Toluene

Carbon Monoxide and Air Pollutants
- Carbon monoxide (CO)
- Ozone (O_3)[d]

[a]Also diquat, glyphosate.
[b]Also diazinon, dichlorvos.
[c]Also deferoxamine (Desferal), penicillamine (Cuprimine), and trientine (Syprine).
[d]Also sulfur dioxide (SO_2), nitrogen dioxide (NO_2).

OVERVIEW

Toxicology is the science concerned with the mechanisms of action and physiologic effects of potentially **harmful substances** that are sometimes called **poisons.** These substances include pesticides; industrial, household, and agricultural chemicals; environmental pollutants; substances produced by poisonous plants, animals, and fungi; and any other harmful substance to which animals are exposed in toxic amounts, including pharmaceutical and recreational drugs. As with pharmaceutical drugs, the effects of toxic substances often exhibit a **dose-response relationship** (see Chapter 3), with the magnitude of toxicity increasing proportionally above a threshold dose or concentration to doses that cause maximal toxicity or death.

Toxicology is also concerned with the bodily **disposition and time-course** of harmful substances and with the **treatment and prevention of poisoning.** This chapter will describe the basic principles of the treatment of poisoning and discuss some of the most important and commonly encountered household, occupational, and environmental poisons and pollutants. This chapter will not discuss the adverse reactions to medical or recreational drugs, which are described in other chapters of this book.

TREATMENT OF POISONING

The basic steps in the treatment of poisoning are outlined in Box 5.1 and can be summarized as follows: (1) provide immediate **cardiopulmonary support** as needed; (2) remove the patient from the poison or the poison from the patient; (3) determine the substance causing the poisoning;(4) administer any **antidotes** available to counteract the poison; and (5) continue monitoring and supporting the patient's vital organs as long as required.

The first procedure to employ in a case of poisoning will depend on the nature of the poison and route of exposure, as well as the patient's cardiopulmonary status. For example, a person exposed to carbon monoxide from smoke inhalation during a fire should be evacuated to fresh air and given oxygen immediately. Other cardiopulmonary support can then be provided but may not be required if the patient is conscious and breathing.

Orally ingested poisons can be removed from the gastrointestinal tract by inducing **vomiting** or by giving a **laxative** to evacuate the poison from the intestines. **Activated charcoal** can be given to adsorb certain poisons and prevent their absorption, followed by a laxative to induce elimination from the intestines. The appropriate action for removing orally ingested poisons depends on several factors, including the estimated time of ingestion, the type of poisonous substance ingested, and the patient's neurologic and cardiopulmonary status. For example, **vomiting is contraindicated** in the case of ingested poisons that might be **aspirated into the lungs** during emesis, such as hydrocarbon solvents, and in the case of unconscious patients. **Dilution of the poison** by administering liquids is usually advisable before inducing emesis or giving a laxative. Dilution slows the absorption of the poison and may facilitate vomiting or bowel evacuation.

BOX 5.1 THE TREATMENT OF ACUTE POISONING

The use of these procedures and the order in which they are employed will depend on the condition of the patient, the nature of the poison and route of exposure, and other factors.

I. Provide cardiopulmonary support if needed
    - Assess patient's pulse, respiration, and oxygenation
    - Perform ventricular defibrillation if needed
    - Administer oxygen if needed
    - Provide cardiac life support if needed
II. Remove patient from the poison and poison from the patient
    - Remove patient from the source of an inhaled poison
    - Remove contaminated clothing and vigorously wash the skin after dermal exposure
    - Administer activated charcoal orally when appropriate for an ingested poison
    - Employ gastric lavage, induction of vomiting, or laxative administration when appropriate and safe
III. Determine the cause of poisoning if not already known
    - Obtain physical evidence and history of exposure
    - Obtain blood and urine for analysis
IV. Administer available antidote and provide supportive care
    - Give antidote as soon as possible
    - Continue oxygen and cardiopulmonary support as needed
    - Assess renal function and electrolytes; replace fluids and electrolytes as needed
    - Provide other supportive care as required for as long as needed

Hemodialysis or peritoneal dialysis can be used to remove certain kinds of poisons from the blood.

In the case of **dermal exposure** to a poison, removing contaminated clothing and vigorously washing exposed areas to prevent further absorption of the poison is often the first step and may be the only treatment required in some cases. Other steps will depend on the patient's physiologic status and the nature of the poison. Allergic reactions are often produced by dermal exposure to **poisonous plants** and may require treatments ranging from administration of antihistamines to topical and systemic corticosteroids. **Epinephrine** should be administered as soon as possible if an **anaphylactic reaction** occurs.

Pesticides

Herbicides

The toxicity of herbicides varies considerably with the route and duration of exposure. Acute dermal exposure usually does not cause serious toxicity if the herbicide is rapidly and thoroughly removed from the skin to prevent absorption. In contrast, accidental or intentional ingestion of herbicides can cause serious, irreversible, and life-threatening toxicity. Inhalation of herbicide vapors tends to cause an intermediate degree of toxicity. This section will present the basic toxicology of 2,4-dichlorophenoxyacetic acid (2,4-D), glyphosate, and the bipyridyl herbicides, diquat and paraquat.

2,4-D is the primary chlorophenoxy herbicide used today. It is used to control broad-leafed weeds in lawns and fields without significantly harming grasses. 2,4-D is relatively nontoxic, but sufficient **dermal or inhalational exposure** can cause mild **neurotoxicity and muscle weakness.** Decontamination and supportive care are usually all that is required in these cases. **Oral ingestion** of 2,4-D may cause more **serious toxicity,** including gastrointestinal distress, hypotension, and neurotoxicity manifested as muscle weakness, ataxia, respiratory failure, and coma. About one-third of such exposures reported in the literature have been **fatal.** The agent exerts nonspecific effects that damage cell membranes, uncouple oxidative phosphorylation, and disrupt acetyl-coenzyme-A metabolism. Treatment of oral 2,4-D poisoning is primarily by gastrointestinal decontamination and supportive care. Alkaline diuresis or hemodialysis to enhance herbicide excretion should be considered in seriously poisoned persons. Epidemiologic evidence also indicates that 2,4-D exposure is causally linked with **non-Hodgkin lymphoma,** probably because 2,4-D can be converted to a potent carcinogen called N-nitrosodimethylamine (NDMA).

Paraquat and diquat are closely related contact herbicides with a bipyridyl structure. **Paraquat is more toxic than diquat** and can only be used by **licensed applicators** in the United States and has been banned in the European Union since 2007. In the human body, these agents are converted to **free radicals** that induce lipid peroxidation in cell membranes and can cause widespread organ damage and death. The majority of paraquat fatalities have been suicides following oral ingestion, but accidental exposures have also caused serious toxicity. Ingestion of paraquat initially causes **bloody vomiting and stools,** followed later by respiratory distress and failure due to **pulmonary edema.** Widespread damage to the liver, heart, kidneys, and other organs may also occur. The treatment of paraquat poisoning includes **activated charcoal** administration to prevent its absorption, followed by gut decontamination. Little can be done to ameliorate toxicity once paraquat is absorbed into the body.

Diquat is a moderately toxic contact herbicide that is readily available for home and commercial use. Of the 30 cases of diquat poisoning reported in the literature over several decades, 43% were fatal, and these were invariably associated with oral ingestion of the herbicide. **Severe toxicity** was manifested as gastrointestinal mucosal ulceration, intestinal paralysis, hypovolemic shock, acute renal failure, and coma. The treatment of diquat poisoning includes **gut decontamination** in victims who present within 1 hour of ingestion. Supportive measures include fluid and electrolyte replacement. **Dermal exposure** can cause localized skin reactions, whereas inhalation can lead to nasal irritation, nosebleeds, coughing, and respiratory distress. Diquat also causes **eye injury** if accidental ocular exposure occurs, and chronic exposure may promote cataract formation. A rapid urine test is available to confirm diquat poisoning.

Glyphosate is the most widely used herbicide in the world, produced by the Monsanto Company marketed as ROUNDUP. It is a contact herbicide that kills both grasses and broadleaf plants. Its use in agricultural weed control in conjunction with genetically engineered glyphosate-resistant food crops has been controversial because it has led to significant elimination of milkweeds and other food sources of butterflies and other insects. Because of its wide availability and use, glyphosate poisonings are fairly common, and a number of **fatalities have occurred** following

TABLE 5.1 Toxicology of Pesticides

AGENT	SYMPTOMS OF TOXICITY	TOXIC EFFECTS AND SEQUELA	TREATMENT
Herbicides			
Glyphosate	Skin and eye irritation; mouth throat irritation	Esophageal erosion; aspiration pneumonia; renal failure	Decontamination and supportive care; peritoneal and hemodialysis
Chlorophenoxy herbicides (2,4-D)	Nonspecific	Coma and muscle weakness; liver and kidney damage, non-Hodgkin lymphoma	Decontamination and supportive care
Paraquat	Hematemesis and bloody stools; respiratory distress (delayed)	Hemorrhagic pulmonary edema, hepatic and renal failure; death	Activated charcoal; supportive care; treatment rarely successful
Pesticides			
Organophosphates	Salivation, lacrimation, urination, diarrhea; muscle weakness	Acute and delayed central and peripheral cholinergic toxicity; delayed neuropathy	Atropine and pralidoxime, supportive care
Carbamates	Same as previous entry	Less severe cholinergic toxicity	Atropine and supportive care
Rotenone	Skin and eye irritation, pharyngitis, and gastrointestinal irritation	Localized inflammation	Symptomatic and supportive care
Pyrethrum compounds	Skin and eye irritation; CNS excitation and convulsions; tetanic muscle paralysis	Allergic and irritant effects; neurotoxicity	Symptomatic and supportive care; ivermectin and CNS depressants
DDT and other organochlorine compounds	CNS stimulation; tremor and convulsions	Enhanced carcinogenesis; endocrine disruption	Symptomatic and supportive care

CNS, Central nervous system; *DDT,* dichlorodiphenyltrichloroethane (chlorophenothane); *2,4-D,* 2,4-dichlorophenoxyacetic acid.

intentional oral ingestion. Glyphosate can cause skin and ocular irritation; mouth, throat, and esophageal damage; aspiration pneumonia; and **renal failure.** Treatment focuses on decontamination and supportive care, and hemodialysis can be helpful in cases of renal failure.

Insecticides
Organophosphate and Carbamate Compounds
Organophosphate compounds include the **pesticides** such as **diazinon, dichlorvos, malathion, parathion,** and **trichlorfon,** and the internationally banned **chemical warfare agents** ("weapons of mass destruction") such as **soman** and **sarin.** These agents inhibit **acetylcholinesterase** in both insects and mammals, and their toxicity results from excessive **acetylcholine receptor stimulation** and subsequent **neurotoxicity.** Organophosphates are well absorbed from the skin and by inhalation and ingestion. Treatment includes decontamination and the administration of **atropine** and **pralidoxime.** The toxicology of these agents is summarized in Table 5.1, and the treatment of insecticide poisoning is described fully in Chapter 6. The mechanism of action of organophosphate insecticides and other agents are shown in Fig. 5.1.

The **carbamate** pesticides include **carbaryl** (Sevin) and other insecticides widely used for home and commercial applications. These agents inhibit acetylcholinesterase to a lesser degree and for a shorter period of time than the organophosphates.

Atropine is used in the treatment of carbamate poisoning, but pralidoxime is not employed because of the spontaneous reactivation of acetylcholinesterase after carbamate exposure (see Chapter 6).

Organochlorine Insecticides
Organochlorine compounds include dichloro-diphenyl-trichloroethane **(DDT), benzene hexachloride,** and **toxaphene. Organochlorine insecticides open sodium channels,** causing them to fire continuously, leading to neurotoxicity, spasms, and eventually death in arthropod species (insects). These **neurotoxic insecticides** also cause significant **endocrine disruption** in humans and **increase the risk of certain cancers** (see Table 5.1). DDT and related agents persist in the human body for a lifetime and in the environment for decades, and their use is now prohibited in most countries. DDT remains in use in parts of Africa where it is needed to control mosquito populations in malaria-infested areas. The only treatment for poisoning by this class of pesticides is decontamination and supportive care.

Botanical Pesticides
Pyrethrins are naturally occurring organic compounds produced as a chemical defense by the flowering plant *Chrysanthemum cinerariifolium.* These compounds have neurotoxic effects that are insecticidal. Synthetic pyrethrins known as **pyrethroids** are becoming the **most widely used household insecticides** around the world and have largely replaced organophosphate and organochlorine compounds for this purpose. Pyrethrins are biodegradable and do not persist in the environment. **Pyrethroids** such as **allethrin** (Raid) are generally broken down by sunlight and do not usually affect groundwater quality, though they tend to be more persistent than the natural pyrethrins. Although the human toxicity of pyrethrins and pyrethroids is relatively low, they have the potential to cause serious **central nervous system toxicity** if ingested, including convulsions and tetanic muscle paralysis (see Table 5.1). These effects result from the **inhibition of various ion channels,** including those for sodium, calcium, and chloride. The use of pyrethroids on aircraft has led to respiratory and skin problems. The treatment of pyrethroid exposure is primarily decontamination and supportive care.

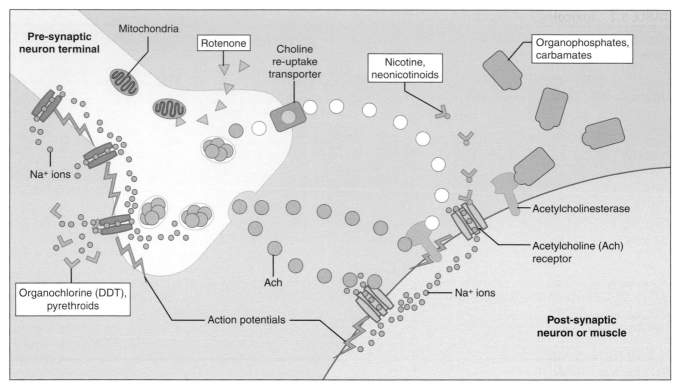

Fig. 5.1 Mechanism of action of different insecticides. Organochlorine (e.g., *DDT*) and pyrethroid insecticides open voltage-gated sodium channels, causing them to fire continuously, leading to neurotoxicity. Organophosphate and carbamate insecticides inhibit acetylcholinesterase, increasing the synaptic concentration of acetylcholine *(Ach)*. The overwhelming amount of Ach produces excessive acetylcholine receptor stimulation and subsequent neurotoxicity. Nicotine and neonicotinoids are Ach receptor agonists that exert a broad-spectrum insecticidal effect due to their excessive acetylcholine receptor stimulation and neurotoxicity. Rotenone's mechanism of action is disruption of the electron transport chain in mitochondria, causing generation of oxygen free radicals and DNA and mitochondrial damage.

Rotenone is another naturally occurring organic pesticide that has **relatively low toxicity** to humans. Its mechanism of action is disruption of the electron transport chain in mitochondria, causing generation of oxygen free radicals and DNA and mitochondrial damage. It has been used to kill insects, lice, and mites and to eliminate alien fish species by wildlife agencies. Skin, eye, and upper respiratory irritation may occur from contact or inhalation, and gastrointestinal irritation results from oral ingestion. Decontamination and symptomatic treatment are usually all that is needed after rotenone exposure.

Nicotine and its synthetic analogs, known as **neonicotinoids,** are **acetylcholine receptor agonists** that exert a broad-spectrum insecticidal effect due to their neurotoxicity. The neonicotinoids generally have lower human toxicity but greater environmental persistence than nicotine. The detrimental effect of neonicotinoids on honeybee populations has been a concern, and these agents are currently under review by the U.S. Environmental Protection Agency. In early 2020, the EPA made interim decisions, for example, to ban their use on crops pollinated by bees. The American Bird Conservancy has called for a ban on the use of neonicotinoids as a seed treatment due to adverse effects on bird populations. The treatment of neonicotinoid exposure in humans consists of decontamination and supportive care.

Metals and Chelators
Lead
Lead has been used since ancient times because of its abundance, easy extraction, and malleability. The Latin word

for lead is *plumbum*, which is the origin of the chemical symbol for lead (*Pb*) and the English word *plumbing* and its derivatives. Lead was used for plumbing in ancient Rome, and some historians believe that the toxic cognitive effects resulting from drinking lead-contaminated water may have contributed to the decline of Rome as a world power. Until recent decades, lead continued to be used as a pigment in paints and as a gasoline additive in the form of tetraethyl lead. The Ethyl Corporation's cover-up of the toxic effects of tetraethyllead in leaded gasoline is a modern tragedy that rivals the tobacco industry's cover-up of the carcinogenic effects of tobacco smoke in cigarettes.

Lead continues to be an **important occupational and environmental toxin** due to its use in the production of storage batteries, ammunition, and a variety of other products. Exposure often results from **drinking water supplied by corroded lead plumbing** and from **leaded paint.** In 2015, the entire city of Flint, Michigan, experienced toxic levels of lead in their drinking water after their water supply was switched and an anticorrosion agent was not added. Some formulations of aviation gasoline still contain lead, and lead is found in various folk remedies and cosmetics available in some countries.

Lead can be absorbed from the respiratory and gastrointestinal tracts. Once absorbed, it is almost entirely **bound to circulating red blood cells,** which slowly distribute lead to soft tissues and bone. Lead is primarily excreted in the **urine** with smaller amounts in other fluids. **Bone** serves as the **storage site** for 90% of the lead in the body, from which it is slowly released over many years.

TABLE 5.2 Toxicology of Metals

AGENT	SYMPTOMS OF TOXICITY	MAJOR TOXIC EFFECTS	PREVENTION AND TREATMENT
Arsenic, acute	Gastrointestinal distress and enteritis	Dehydration, hypotension, shock, death; delirium and coma, respiratory failure; metabolic acidosis	Remove from gut and administer dimercaprol; supportive care
Arsenic, chronic	Fatigue, weight loss	Neuropathy, anemia, skin lesions, cancer	Remove from exposure; supportive care
Beryllium	Skin and lung irritation	Pulmonary fibrosis, cancer, and death; skin irritation and disease	Avoid inhalation of beryllium dust; supportive care
Cadmium	Cough, fever, chills, malaise	Pulmonary fibrosis and cancer, renal failure	Avoid inhalation of cadmium dust and fumes; supportive care
Lead	Irritability, fatigue, anorexia, insomnia, headache, arthralgia, loss of appetite, constipation	Cognitive defects, motor neuropathy, anemia, nephropathy, ataxia, convulsions, coma, death	Terminate exposure; chelation with calcium disodium EDTA, dimercaprol, succimer; supportive care
Mercury, acute	Gastrointestinal distress if ingested; difficult breathing if inhaled	Hemorrhagic gastroenteritis, renal failure if ingested; pneumonitis and edema if inhaled	Avoid inhalation and other exposure; vigorous hydration; succimer or dimercaprol chelation
Mercury, chronic	Memory loss, insomnia, fatigue, anorexia	Tremor, neuropsychiatric changes (anger, depression), gum and mouth inflammation	Chelation with succimer (not dimercaprol); supportive care

EDTA, Ethylenediamine-tetraacetic acid.

Lead has toxic effects on many organs and is particularly toxic to the **developing nervous system,** with low levels causing **cognitive defects** and higher levels leading to various behavioral and cognitive symptoms. Headaches and sleep disturbances, as well as muscle and joint pain, are among the complaints of those exposed to lead. Higher levels of lead may cause stupor, coma, and death, and lead may contribute to dementia. Lead also interferes with heme synthesis, contributing to **hemolysis and anemia.** Various other organs are also affected by lead poisoning, including the kidneys, gastrointestinal, cardiovascular, and reproductive systems.

Lead exposure may be acute or chronic, and the onset and time course of symptoms varies accordingly. **Blood lead levels** can serve to confirm excessive lead exposure but are not a reliable index of cumulative exposure or toxicity. The average blood lead level in developed countries has declined 90% in recent decades, and individuals with levels above the normal range can be easily identified.

The **treatment of symptomatic lead poisoning** is based on **chelation of lead** using **calcium disodium EDTA.** This agent is given intravenously by continuous infusion for up to 5 days and acts to bind lead in the blood and excrete it in the urine. **Dimercaprol** is sometimes used with EDTA for the initial treatment of persons with lead encephalopathy. Parenteral chelation for 5 days is followed by **oral succimer,** which may be continued until blood lead levels return to a safe range, keeping in mind that lead levels may rebound as the lead gradually redistributes from bone. Hence, blood levels should continue to be checked for several months or longer during the treatment of lead poisoning. The US Centers for Disease Control and Prevention recommends chelation for persons with lead levels above 45 mcg/dL (normal is <10 mcg/dL). The benefit of treating asymptomatic persons with blood lead between 25 and 45 mcg/dL is uncertain.

Mercury

Mercury, also known as quicksilver, is the only metallic element that is a liquid at ambient temperatures. It was known to ancient civilizations and was erroneously employed as a folk remedy and in cosmetics. Later, mercury was utilized in the manufacture of thermometers, barometers, sphygmomanometers, and electrical switches. Most of these applications have been phased out, but mercury is still used in **fluorescent light bulbs,** which should be recycled through a hazardous waste disposal center to avoid environmental contamination. Ingestion of either inorganic or organic forms of mercury can result in toxicity, including **methylmercury** in contaminated seafood. **Inhalation** of elemental mercury and mercury compounds can also cause poisoning, which is the primary source of occupational exposure. Some forms of mercury are absorbed through the skin.

Once absorbed into the circulation, mercury is distributed to various organs and tissues, with the highest concentrations found in the **kidneys.** Mercury is slowly excreted over weeks and months, though some remains in the tissues for years. Table 5.2 summarizes the symptoms and effects of mercury poisoning, which includes various gastrointestinal, pulmonary, and neurologic reactions. **Neuropsychiatric changes** are a hallmark of chronic toxicity, as represented by the iconic mad hatter (hat-makers used mercury to make felt for hats) in Lewis Carroll's *Alice's Adventures in Wonderland.* A wide range of other organ system damage can also be observed in many cases of mercury poisoning. The treatment of acute toxicity includes immediate chelation with **unithiol, dimercaprol,** or **succimer,** as well as fluid administration to maintain renal function and other supportive care as needed. For chronic toxicity, the value of chelation is unknown, but **dimercaprol should not be used** because it can redistribute mercury to the central nervous system. Succimer and unithiol might be useful in removing methylmercury from the body.

Arsenic

The 1940s play entitled *Arsenic and Old Lace* exemplifies the popular view of arsenic as an intentional poison, but arsenic toxicity is more likely to result from commercial, industrial, and environmental exposure than the poisoning of suitors by elderly spinsters. Arsenic is used in the manufacture of a wide variety of products, and arsenic-contaminated groundwater is a major source of toxicity in parts of Asia. Organic arsenicals were once employed in the chemotherapy of syphilis (arsphenamine), and melarsoprol is still utilized in the treatment of African trypanosomiasis (see Chapter 44).

Arsenic is well absorbed through the lungs and gastrointestinal tract, and it undergoes methylation in the liver followed by gradual excretion in the urine. Arsenic exerts its toxic effects through a variety of mechanisms, including **enzyme inhibition** and **altered gene expression** that may result from its binding to sulfhydryl groups of amino acids and proteins.

Both acute and chronic toxicity may result from arsenic exposure. Acute toxicity causes **nausea, vomiting, and diarrhea,** contributing to **hypotension, shock, and death.** Life-threatening **pulmonary and cardiac toxicity** are also likely, and **pancytopenia** and basophilic stippling of erythrocytes can be observed within a few days after exposure, as well as **central and peripheral neuropathy,** manifested as delirium and coma. Arsenic is also a known **carcinogen** causing lung, skin, and bladder cancer.

The **treatment of acute arsenic poisoning** includes the elimination of the poison from the gastrointestinal tract and immediate chelation with parenteral **unithiol** or **dimercaprol** to reduce blood levels. Vigorous fluid administration to support renal function is also recommended. Chronic poisoning has no specific treatment except supportive care and possibly administration of **folate** to promote the conversion of arsenic to methylated derivatives that are excreted in the urine.

Other Metals

A large number of other metals are less frequent causes of poisoning, including bismuth, iron, copper, and many others. Occupational exposure to beryllium, cadmium, and manganese can also cause toxicity, and the symptoms, effects, and treatment of beryllium and cadmium exposure are summarized in Table 5.2.

Chelators

In addition to decontamination of the victim and supportive care, the treatment of acute and sometimes chronic exposure to metals may include chelation. Chelators are substances that **bind up metals** in the bloodstream and **increase excretion of the bound metal** in the urine, thereby accelerating the removal of metals from the body. The chelators used today include **disodium calcium EDTA** (ethylenediamine-tetraacetic acid [edetate]) and three sulfhydryl compounds named **dimercaprol, unithiol,** and **succimer.** Unithiol and succimer are derivatives of dimercaprol. Although chelators serve to promote the elimination of metals from the body, they may also redistribute metals to target organs and are therefore contraindicated in treating certain metal intoxications. For example, chelators redistribute cadmium to the kidneys and are not employed in treating cadmium poisoning. Likewise, **dimercaprol redistributes arsenic and mercury to the brain** and **should not be used in treating chronic toxicity.**

Calcium disodium EDTA is a salt of ethylenediamine-tetraacetic acid (EDTA) administered intravenously in the treatment of **lead poisoning** and has potential use for other metal toxicities such as those caused by zinc and manganese

exposure. The calcium disodium salt is employed to avoid serious **depletion of calcium** caused by pure EDTA administration. Adequate urine flow must be maintained during its administration to avoid nephrotoxicity. Several salts of EDTA congeners are available for treating certain radioactive metal intoxications.

Dimercaprol, also known as British antilewisite or BAL, is an oily liquid containing sulfhydryl groups that bind arsenic, lead, and mercury. It reverses arsenic-induced inhibition of sulfhydryl-containing enzymes and has been used alone in treating **acute arsenic and mercury** poisoning. For lead poisoning, dimercaprol is used with edetate calcium disodium. Unfortunately, dimercaprol has a high incidence of **adverse effects,** including nausea, vomiting, fever, tachycardia, and hypertension. For these reasons, water-soluble derivatives of dimercaprol have replaced its use in many situations.

Unithiol is a water-soluble derivative of dimercaprol that can be given orally and intravenously. It increases the excretion of arsenic, mercury, and lead and protects against arsenic and mercury-induced toxicity. It is legally available from compounding pharmacies in the US.

Succimer is a water-soluble derivative of dimercaprol used in treating arsenic and mercury poisoning. It is available for **oral administration** in the United States, but intravenous formulations are employed in some other countries. Succimer appears to **decrease mercury levels in the kidneys,** and it **decreases blood lead levels** while increasing lead excretion.

Penicillamine (CUPRIMINE) is a chelating agent used in the treatment of Wilson's disease, which is characterized by a build-up of copper in the brain. It is also used to treat patients with severe, active rheumatoid arthritis unresponsive to conventional therapy (see Chapter 30). **Trientine** is also a chelating agent used to bind up and remove copper in the body in patients with Wilson's disease, particularly in those who fail on trials of penicillamine.

There is another medically useful metal chelator obtained from soil bacteria called **deferoxamine** (DESFERAL). It is used for the treatment of acute iron toxicity and transfusion-related iron overload. The chemical structures of deferoxamine and other chelators, with their metal-binding sites and targeted ions, are shown in Fig. 5.2.

Environmental and Occupational Poisons
Regulations to Prevent Toxic Workplace Exposure

The toxicology and treatment of selected environmental and occupational poisons are summarized in Table 5.3. These agents are gases or volatile liquids at ambient temperatures, and exposure is usually by inhalation of polluted air. The US **Occupational Safety and Health Administration (OSHA)** has established exposure limits for a number of potentially toxic substances encountered in the workplace. In addition, OSHA requires that information about the **identities and hazards** of chemicals encountered in the workplace is available and disseminated to workers in understandable language and that workers must receive **training in the proper handling** and avoidance of excessive dermal, inhalational, or other exposure to these chemicals.

OSHA has established various types of **Permissible Exposure Limits** for airborne concentrations of various chemicals to protect workers from hazardous exposures. These limits include **ceiling (maximal exposure) limits,**

Chemical structure of metal chelators

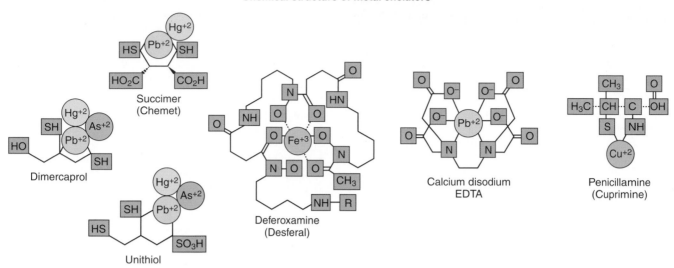

FIG. 5.2   Chemical structure and metal-binding sites of chelators. Calcium disodium EDTA, dimercaprol, unithiol, and succimer bind lead (Pb^{+2}) and are used primarily for the treatment of lead poisoning and lead toxicity. Some of these chelators are used to treat arsenic (As^{+3}) and mercury (Hg^{+2}) toxicity as well. Deferoxamine binds ferric iron (Fe^{+3}) in cases of iron toxicity or iron overload following blood transfusions. Penicillamine and trientine (not shown) bind copper (Cu^{+2}) and are used in the treatment of Wilson's disease.

TABLE 5.3   Toxicology of Occupational and Environmental Poisons

AGENT	SYMPTOM OF TOXICITY	MAJOR TOXIC EFFECTS	PREVENTION AND TREATMENT
Benzene, toluene, xylene	Drowsiness, headache, ataxia, nausea, eye irritation, fainting	Bone marrow depression and cancer (benzene); CNS depression (all)	Prevent occupational exposure; provide supportive care
Carbon monoxide	Headache, confusion, dizziness, vertigo, tachycardia, psychomotor impairment	Loss of consciousness, respiratory failure, cerebral edema, coma, neurologic impairment, death	Immediate removal from source, oxygen, mechanical respiration, hyperbaric oxygen, supportive care
Halogenated hydrocarbons	CNS depression, impaired memory	Liver, kidney, cardiac, and neurotoxicity; cancer	Prevent exposure; supportive care
Nitrogen dioxide	Eye and nose irritation, difficult breathing	Pulmonary edema and fibrosis	Prevent exposure; provide oxygenation, pulmonary ventilation; bronchodilators
Ozone	Respiratory tract irritation, rapid breathing, dyspnea, chest pain	Pulmonary edema, bronchitis, fibrosis, cardiopulmonary disease	Prevent exposure; provide oxygenation; pulmonary ventilation
Sulfur dioxide	Eye, nose, throat, lung irritation	Bronchoconstriction, asthmatic episodes, pulmonary edema	Prevent exposure; provide oxygenation; pulmonary ventilation; bronchodilators

CNS, Central nervous system.

short-term exposure limits (typically for 15–30-minute exposures), and **time-weighted average limits** (usually for 8-hour exposures). These standards are based on recommendations of the **National Institute for Occupational Safety and Health** (NIOSH) as required by law. OSHA has also established requirements for the **use of respirators** to avoid inhalation of toxic chemicals when other air quality measures are not sufficient.

Hydrocarbons

A large number of volatile hydrocarbon compounds are encountered in various industrial and commercial occupations, including **benzene, toluene,** and **halogenated hydrocarbons.** Benzene is also found in premium automobile gasoline and aviation gasoline. Inhalation of sufficient quantities of the vapors of these substances can cause dose-dependent **central nervous system (CNS) depression,** and

benzene is associated with **bone marrow depression** and **cancer.** Controlling occupational and environmental exposure is absolutely essential for preventing long-term toxicity from exposure to these compounds. There is no specific treatment for exposure to these agents other than removal from the source and providing supportive care. A discussion of the many other hydrocarbon compounds found in the workplace is beyond the scope of this text.

Carbon Monoxide and Air Pollutants

Carbon monoxide (CO) is a **colorless, odorless,** and **tasteless gas** produced by the incomplete combustion of carbon compounds found in wood, charcoal, and fossil fuels. Because of the abundance and widespread use of these materials for construction, heating, and powering engines, CO poisoning is a common cause of dysfunction and death, both accidental and intentional.

BOX 5.2 A CASE OF HEADACHE, DIZZINESS, AND TACHYCARDIA

CASE PRESENTATION

A 27-year-old fireman suffered smoke inhalation while rescuing two small children during a house fire. He complained of dizziness, vertigo, and a frontal headache, and another fireman carried him to safety. Paramedics immediately administered oxygen with a nonrebreather mask and then switched to high-flow nasal oxygen. His vital signs included heart rate, 104 beats/minute; blood pressure, 138/84 mm Hg; and respiratory rate, 26 breaths/minute. A finger-tip monitor showed a carboxyhemoglobin concentration of 8%. He responded to rest and oxygen and was transported to the emergency department of a local hospital for further evaluation. His headache slowly resolved, and he was discharged without further treatment. A follow-up evaluation found that he had no neurologic sequela.

CASE DISCUSSION

In addition to causing respiratory irritation and reducing the oxygen concentration of air, fires produce considerable amounts of carbon monoxide (CO) and other toxic gases, particularly when the oxygen supply to the fire is limited by poor ventilation. CO poisoning is the major cause of dysfunction and death due to smoke inhalation during a fire. High-flow oxygen administration is the specific antidote for CO toxicity, serving to increase oxyhemoglobin while causing dissociation of carboxyhemoglobin. Hyperbaric oxygen administration has been used to treat CO poisoning, but its advantage compared with normobaric high-flow oxygen has not been clearly established. In addition to the acute manifestations of toxicity, CO exposure can lead to brain damage and chronic neurologic impairment. Victims should be evaluated and monitored for neurologic sequela, though there is no specific treatment beyond the prompt restoration of tissue oxygenation.

CO is rapidly absorbed from the lungs into the circulation, where it forms carboxyhemoglobin because CO has a **200 times greater affinity for hemoglobin** than oxygen. Carboxyhemoglobin reduces oxygen delivery to the tissues by reducing the concentration of oxyhemoglobin and by shifting the oxygen dissociation curve of oxyhemoglobin to the left, such that less oxygen is delivered to the tissues at any given oxyhemoglobin concentration. These effects rapidly cause tissue hypoxia and symptoms of cerebral dysfunction, including **headache, dizziness, and vertigo.** Higher levels of carboxyhemoglobin lead to loss of consciousness, **coma,** and **death.** Brain damage and **chronic neurologic sequela** can also occur if the victim survives.

The treatment of CO poisoning includes removal from the source of exposure and immediate administration of **high-flow oxygen.** Hyperbaric oxygen administration has been used when it is available, though the advantage of this procedure has not been fully established. Victims should also be assessed and treated for cardiovascular and acid-base abnormalities. Box 5.2 for a case example.

Air pollutants such as **ozone, sulfur dioxide,** and **nitrogen dioxide** are highly irritating to the **eyes** and **respiratory tract,** and sufficient exposure can lead to **irreversible pulmonary damage.** These agents are primarily produced by the burning of fossil fuels in motor vehicles and power plants. Prevention of exposure by controlling air pollution, remaining indoors during environmental alerts, and preventing occupational exposure are of paramount importance in preventing toxicity. There is no specific treatment for exposure to these compounds except to ensure adequate pulmonary ventilation and gas exchange and to treat pulmonary edema if it occurs.

SUMMARY OF IMPORTANT POINTS

- The major steps in the treatment of poisoning include cardiopulmonary support, decontamination, prevention of absorption, administration of any antidote available, and supportive care.
- Pesticides may cause serious and lethal toxicity, especially if ingested, while external exposure can cause skin and eye irritation. Decontamination and supportive care are the primary measures of treatment, though atropine and pralidoxime are useful in treating organophosphate toxicity.
- Toxic metals include arsenic, lead, and mercury. These agents produce a wide range of CNS and organ system toxicity. Chelation with calcium disodium EDTA, dimercaprol, succimer, and unithiol has been useful in reducing the acute toxicity of these agents.
- Environmental and occupational poisons are gases and volatile liquids that can be accidentally or intentionally inhaled. Air pollutants such as sulfur dioxide and nitrogen dioxide typically cause respiratory distress, while aromatic and halogenated hydrocarbons can produce CNS depression, and benzene also increases the risk of cancer.
- Carbon monoxide produced by the incomplete oxidation of wood, fossil fuels, and charcoal forms carboxyhemoglobin that produces tissue hypoxia and various CNS and cardiovascular effects.
- Volatile hydrocarbon compounds such as benzene, toluene, and halogenated hydrocarbons, are common in industrial settings and cause dose-dependent CNS depression, with benzene specifically associated with bone marrow depression and cancer.

Review Questions

1. Calcium disodium EDTA is employed in the treatment of which metal poisoning?
   - (A) lead
   - (B) cadmium
   - (C) mercury
   - (D) arsenic
   - (E) beryllium
2. Which herbicide can cause renal failure after accidental or intentional ingestion?
   - (A) 2,4-dichlorophenoxyacetic acid (2,4-D)
   - (B) glyphosate
   - (C) paraquat
   - (D) diquat
   - (E) diazinon
3. What is the most characteristic feature of chronic mercury poisoning?
   - (A) hypothermia
   - (B) heart failure
   - (C) biliary obstruction and jaundice
   - (D) anger, depression, irrational behavior
   - (E) rhabdomyolysis

4. Which agent is used to reduce the gastrointestinal absorption of ingested poisons?
   (A) succimer
   (B) activated charcoal
   (C) pralidoxime
   (D) dimercaprol
   (E) unithiol

5. An increased risk of which disease has been linked to exposure to 2,4-dichlorophenoxyacetic acid (2,4-D)?
   (A) hypertension
   (B) hyponatremia
   (C) pulmonary fibrosis
   (D) dementia
   (E) non-Hodgkin lymphoma

Section

II

AUTONOMIC AND NEUROMUSCULAR PHARMACOLOGY

CHAPTER 6

Parasympathetic, Neuromuscular Pharmacology, and Cholinergic Agonists

CLASSIFICATION OF ACETYLCHOLINE AGONISTS

Direct-Acting Acetylcholine Receptor Agonists

- Acetylcholine (MIOCHOL-E)
- Bethanechol (URECHOLINE)
- Carbachol (MIOSTAT)
- Cevimeline (EVOXAC)
- Muscarine
- Nicotine
- Pilocarpine (SALAGEN)
- Varenicline (CHANTIX)

Reversible Cholinesterase Inhibitors

- Edrophonium (TENSILON)
- Neostigmine (PROSTIGMIN)
- Physostigmine (ESERINE)
- Pyridostigmine (MESTINON)

Irreversible Cholinesterase Inhibitors

- Echothiophate (PHOSPHOLINE IODIDE)
- Malathion (OVIDE)
- Pralidoxime (PROTOPAM)

Type 5 Phosphodiesterase Inhibitors

- Sildenafil (VIAGRA, REVATIO)
- Tadalafil (CIALIS, ADCIRCA)[a]

Soluble Guanylate Cyclase (SGC) Stimulators

- Riociguat (ADEMPAS)

[a]Also vardenafil (Levitra, Staxyn) and avanafil (Stendra).

OVERVIEW

The nervous system is composed of central and peripheral components. The **central nervous system** (CNS) consists of the brain and spinal cord, and the **peripheral nervous system** comprises the **autonomic** and **somatic** nerves that innervate muscles and tissues throughout the body.

Drugs alter nervous system function primarily by affecting **neurotransmitters** or their **receptors.** In some cases, drugs alter the synthesis, storage, release, inactivation, or neuronal reuptake of neurotransmitters. In other cases, they activate or block neurotransmitter receptors.

ANATOMY AND PHYSIOLOGY OF THE PERIPHERAL NERVOUS SYSTEM

Autonomic Nervous System

The **autonomic nervous system** involuntarily regulates the activity of smooth muscles, exocrine glands, cardiac tissue, and certain endocrine and metabolic activities, whereas the somatic nervous system activates skeletal muscle contraction, enabling voluntary body movements. Both the autonomic and the somatic nervous systems originate in and are controlled by the CNS. The autonomic nervous system is regulated by brainstem centers responsible for cardiovascular, respiratory, and other visceral functions. The somatic nervous system is activated by corticospinal tracts, which originate in the cerebral motor cortex, and by spinal reflexes.

The autonomic nervous system includes the sympathetic, parasympathetic, and enteric nervous systems. In the **sympathetic nervous system,** nerves arise from the thoracic and lumbar spinal cord and have a short preganglionic fiber and a long postganglionic fiber. Most of the ganglia are located in the paravertebral chain adjacent to the spinal cord, but a few prevertebral ganglia (the celiac, splanchnic, and mesenteric ganglia) are located more distally to the spinal cord. The **parasympathetic nervous system** includes portions of cranial nerves III, VII, IX, and X (the oculomotor, facial, glossopharyngeal, and vagus nerves, respectively), as well as some nerves originating from the sacral spinal cord. The parasympathetic nerves have long preganglionic fibers and short postganglionic fibers, with the ganglia often located in the innervated organs.

The origins, neurotransmitters, and receptors of the sympathetic and parasympathetic systems are shown in Fig. 6.1. The sympathetic nervous system tends to discharge as a unit, producing a diffuse activation of target organs. Preganglionic is a sympathetic neuron synapse with a large number of postganglionic neurons, which contributes to the widespread activation of the organs during sympathetic stimulation. In addition, the release of **epinephrine** and **norepinephrine** from the adrenal medulla into the circulation enables the activation of target tissues throughout the body, including some tissues not directly innervated by sympathetic nerves. In contrast, the parasympathetic system can discretely activate specific target tissues. For example, it is possible for parasympathetic nerves to slow the heart rate without simultaneously stimulating gastrointestinal or bladder function. This is partly because of the low ratio of postganglionic fibers to preganglionic fibers in the parasympathetic system.

As shown in Fig. 6.2, the sympathetic and parasympathetic nervous systems often have opposing effects on organ function. Activation of the sympathetic system produces the **"fight or flight"** reaction in response to threatening situations. In this reaction, cardiovascular stimulation provides muscles with oxygen and fuels required to support vigorous physical activity, and activation of glycogenolysis and lipolysis releases the necessary energy substrates. The parasympathetic system is sometimes called the **"rest and digest"** system because it slows the heart rate and promotes vegetative functions, such as digestion, defecation, and

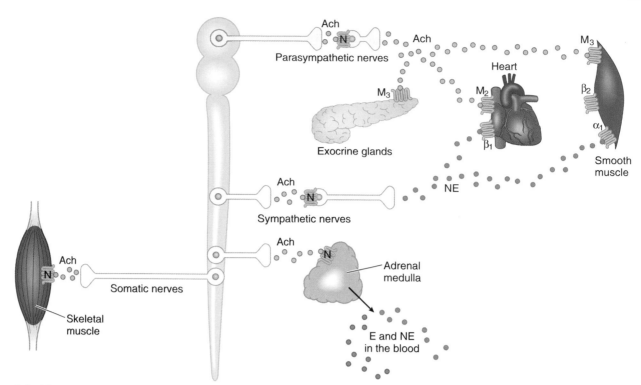

FIG. 6.1   Neurotransmission in the autonomic and somatic nervous systems. The parasympathetic nervous system consists of cranial and sacral nerves with long preganglionic and short postganglionic fibers. The sympathetic nervous system consists of thoracic and lumbar nerves with short preganglionic and long postganglionic fibers. The sympathetic system includes the adrenal medulla, which releases norepinephrine and epinephrine into the blood. The somatic nervous system consists of motor neurons to the skeletal muscle. α, α-Adrenoceptors; *ACh*, acetylcholine; β, β-adrenoceptors; *E*, epinephrine; *M*, muscarinic receptors; *N*, nicotinic receptors; *NE*, norepinephrine.

micturition. Many parasympathetic effects (including pupillary constriction, bronchoconstriction, and stimulation of gut and bladder motility) are caused by smooth muscle contraction. In addition to their effects on innervated tissues, parasympathetic neurons innervate and inhibit neurotransmitter release from sympathetic neurons, and sympathetic neurons innervate and inhibit neurotransmitter release from parasympathetic neurons.

Enteric Nervous System

The enteric nervous system (ENS) is usually considered to be the third division of the autonomic nervous system. The ENS consists of a network of nerves **located in the gut wall** that regulates gastrointestinal motility and secretion. It is innervated by the sympathetic and parasympathetic nervous systems and is composed of the submucosal, myenteric, and subserosal nerve plexuses. Through sensory and motor neurons and interneurons, the ENS integrates autonomic input with localized reflexes so as to synchronize **propulsive contractions of gut muscle (peristalsis)** and regulate glandular secretion. Parasympathetic stimulation typically activates the ENS, whereas sympathetic stimulation inhibits the ENS. Unlike the sympathetic and parasympathetic systems, the ENS can function independently of the CNS after autonomic denervation.

Somatic Nervous System

The somatic nervous system consists of the motor neurons and their efferent nerves that innervate the skeletal muscle. These neurons mediate voluntary movement and release **acetylcholine** at the neuromuscular junction.

NEUROTRANSMISSION AND SITES OF DRUG ACTION

Peripheral neurotransmission involves the synthesis, storage, and release of neurotransmitters in response to nerve stimulation. Most neurotransmitters are synthesized in nerve terminals, stored in membrane-bound vesicles, and released into the synapse in response to nerve stimulation. Peptide neurotransmitters are synthesized in the cell body and then transported to the nerve terminal. After the neurotransmitter is released, it activates postjunctional receptors to initiate a physiologic effect. Neurotransmitter action is terminated either by metabolism or neuronal reuptake. Drugs exert effects on specific steps in neurotransmission.

The sites of action for drugs affecting autonomic neurotransmission are shown in Fig. 6.3, and the mechanisms of action of prototype drugs are listed in Table 6.1.

Neurotransmitters

The primary neurotransmitters found in the sympathetic, parasympathetic, and somatic nervous systems are **acetylcholine** and **norepinephrine** (see Fig. 6.1). The terms *adrenergic* and *cholinergic* refer to neurons that release norepinephrine or acetylcholine, respectively.

Acetylcholine is the transmitter at all autonomic ganglia, at parasympathetic neuroeffector junctions, and at somatic neuromuscular junctions. It is also the transmitter at a few sympathetic neuroeffector junctions, including the junctions of nerves in sweat glands and vasodilator fibers in skeletal muscle. The presence of acetylcholine in several types of autonomic and somatic synapses contributes to the lack of specificity of drugs acting on acetylcholine receptors.

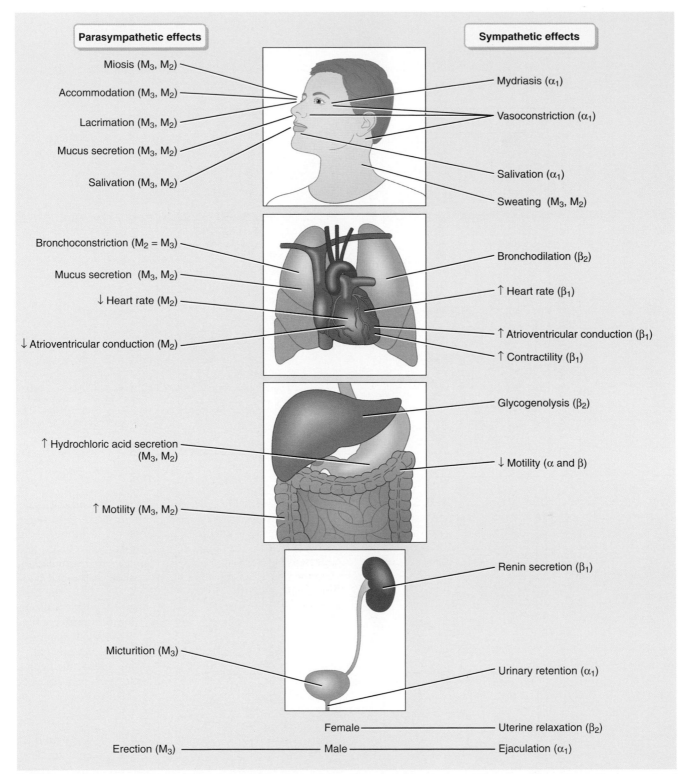

Parasympathetic effects

Miosis (M_3, M_2)

Accommodation (M_3, M_2)

Lacrimation (M_3, M_2)

Mucus secretion (M_3, M_2)

Salivation (M_3, M_2)

Bronchoconstriction ($M_2 = M_3$)

Mucus secretion (M_3, M_2)

↓ Heart rate (M_2)

↓ Atrioventricular conduction (M_2)

↑ Hydrochloric acid secretion (M_3, M_2)

↑ Motility (M_3, M_2)

Micturition (M_3)

Erection (M_3)

Sympathetic effects

Mydriasis (α_1)

Vasoconstriction (α_1)

Salivation (α_1)

Sweating (M_3, M_2)

Bronchodilation (β_2)

↑ Heart rate (β_1)

↑ Atrioventricular conduction (β_1)

↑ Contractility (β_1)

Glycogenolysis (β_2)

↓ Motility (α and β)

Renin secretion (β_1)

Urinary retention (α_1)

Female — Uterine relaxation (β_2)

Male — Ejaculation (α_1)

FIG. 6.2 Autonomic nervous system effects on organs. All parasympathetic effects are mediated by muscarinic receptors. Sympathetic effects are mediated by α-adrenoceptors (α), β-adrenoceptors (β), or muscarinic receptors (M).

Although **norepinephrine** (noradrenaline) is the primary neurotransmitter at most sympathetic postganglionic neuroeffector junctions, **epinephrine** (adrenaline) is the principal catecholamine released from the adrenal medulla in response to activation of the sympathetic nervous system.

Amazingly, the **ENS** utilizes some 30 different neurotransmitters, including acetylcholine, **nitric oxide, serotonin, dopamine,** and several peptides, including **neuropeptide Y, vasoactive intestinal peptide,** and **enkephalin.** In some tissues, adenosine triphosphate (ATP) released by autonomic neurons is converted to **adenosine,** which can

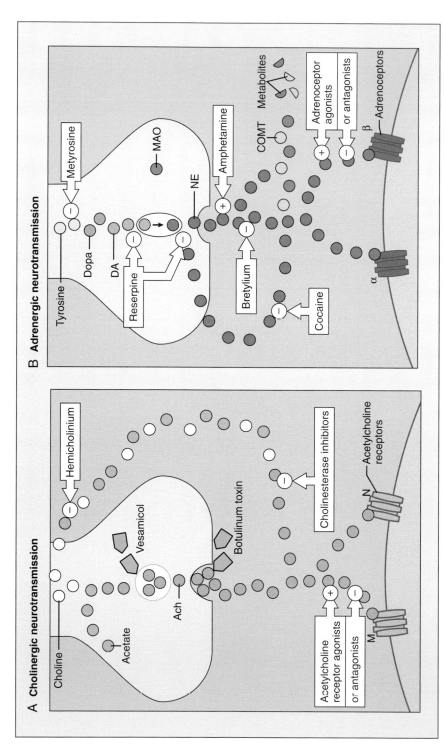

Fig. 6.3 **A.** Cholinergic neurotransmission and sites of drug action. Acetylcholine (ACh) is synthesized from choline and acetate, stored in neuronal vesicles, and released into the synapse by nerve stimulation. Hemicholinium blocks choline uptake by the neuron and inhibits ACh synthesis. Vesamicol blocks ACh storage, and botulinum toxin blocks ACh release. ACh breakdown is inhibited by cholinesterase inhibitors such as physostigmine. Postjunctional acetylcholine receptors are activated or blocked by acetylcholine receptor agonists or antagonists, respectively. M, Muscarinic receptors; N, nicotinic receptors; **B.** Adrenergic neurotransmission and sites of drug action. Norepinephrine, NE, is synthesized from the amino acid tyrosine via formation of Dopa (levodopa) and DA (dopamine) and released into the synapse by nerve stimulation. Metyrosine inhibits the use of tyrosine for NE synthesis, reserpine blocks packaging of NE into vesicles, bretylium inhibits the release of NE, amphetamine increases NE release, and cocaine inhibits the reuptake of NE. Also shown are the adrenergic receptors where adrenergic agonists or antagonists bind; (−), inhibits; (+), stimulates.

TABLE 6.1   Examples of Drugs Affecting Autonomic Neurotransmission

MECHANISM OF ACTION	DRUGS AFFECTING ACETYLCHOLINE NEUROTRANSMISSION	DRUGS AFFECTING SYMPATHETIC NEUROTRANSMISSION
Inhibit synthesis of neurotransmitter	Hemicholinium[a]	Metyrosine (methyl-tyrosine)
Prevent vesicular storage of neurotransmitter	Vesamicol[a]	Reserpine[a]
Inhibit release of neurotransmitter	Botulinum toxin	Bretylium[a]
Increase release of neurotransmitter	Black widow spider venom (α-latrotoxin)[a]	Amphetamine
Inhibit reuptake of neurotransmitter	—	Cocaine
Inhibit metabolism of neurotransmitter	Cholinesterase inhibitors (neostigmine)	Monoamine oxidase inhibitors
Activate postsynaptic receptors	Acetylcholine, pilocarpine	Albuterol, dobutamine, and epinephrine
Block postsynaptic receptors	Atropine and atracurium (block muscarinic and nicotinic receptors, respectively)	Phentolamine and propranolol (block α- and β-adrenoceptors, respectively)

[a]These drugs have no current medical use.

then activate adenosine receptors in a number of tissues (see Chapter 27).

Cholinergic Neurotransmission

Acetylcholine is synthesized from choline and acetate in the neuronal cytoplasm by choline acetyltransferase, and then it is stored in vesicles. When a parasympathetic nerve is stimulated, the action potential induces calcium influx into the neuron, and calcium mediates the release of the neurotransmitter by a process called *exocytosis*. During exocytosis, the vesicle membrane and plasma membrane fuse, and the neurotransmitter is released into the synapse through an opening in the fused membranes. After acetylcholine activates postsynaptic acetylcholine receptors, it is rapidly hydrolyzed by the enzyme **acetylcholinesterase** to form choline and acetate. Choline is recycled through the process of reuptake by the presynaptic neuron. This process is mediated by a membrane protein that transports choline into the neuron. Acetylcholine can also activate presynaptic autoreceptors, which inhibits further release of the neurotransmitter from the neuron.

Drugs Affecting Cholinergic Neurotransmission

Fig. 6.3A shows the sites of various agents that affect cholinergic neurotransmission, including substances affecting acetylcholine synthesis **(hemicholinium)** and storage **(vesamicol)** that are used in pharmacology research but have no clinical use.

Several biologic toxins affect the release of acetylcholine. **Black widow spider venom** containing α-**latrotoxin** stimulates vesicular release of acetylcholine, producing excessive activation of acetylcholine receptors. A black widow spider bite may cause muscle contraction and pain, and abdominal muscles are often affected. Salivation, lacrimation, sweating, and changes in heart rate and blood pressure can occur but are uncommon, and death from a black widow spider bite is rare. Administration of analgesic and anti-inflammatory medication is usually the only treatment required.

Botulinum toxin A, which is produced by *Clostridium botulinum*, blocks the exocytotic release of acetylcholine and inhibits neuromuscular transmission. Botulinum toxin is being used for a number of medical and cosmetic conditions. It is used to treat localized muscle spasms of the eyes, face, hands, and upper limbs, and it is employed

in treating tremor, dystonia, excessive salivation, and other symptoms of Parkinson's disease. In these applications, very small doses of botulinum toxin are injected directly into the affected muscle, causing **muscle relaxation** (see Chapter 24). The specific applications of botulinum toxin include **strabismus** (improper alignment of the eyes), **dysphonia** (vocal cord dysfunction), **bruxism** (grinding of teeth), and **blepharospasm** (spasm of the eyelids). Injection of a preparation of this toxin known as BOTOX is used to reduce facial wrinkles for cosmetic purposes. Botulinum toxin has also been used to treat excessive sweating (hyperhidrosis) of the palms and soles. Irrigation of the urinary bladder with botulinum toxin may provide long-lasting relief of **bladder spasm** and urinary incontinence. The most common side effects of botulinum toxin injections are **dry mouth** and dysphagia (difficult swallowing).

After acetylcholine is released, it can activate postsynaptic muscarinic or nicotinic receptors. Drugs that activate these receptors are called **acetylcholine receptor agonists** and are discussed later in this chapter. Drugs that block acetylcholine receptors (antagonists) are discussed in Chapter 7.

ACETYLCHOLINE RECEPTORS
Muscarinic Receptors

Acetylcholine receptors (cholinergic receptors) are divided into two types, **muscarinic receptors** and **nicotinic receptors,** based on their selective activation by the alkaloids muscarine and nicotine. Muscarinic receptors are found in **smooth muscle, cardiac tissue,** and **glands** at parasympathetic neuroeffector junctions (Table 6.2). They are also found in the CNS, on presynaptic sympathetic and parasympathetic nerves, and at autonomic ganglia. Activation of muscarinic receptors on presynaptic autonomic nerves inhibits further neurotransmitter release. The presence of muscarinic receptors on sympathetic nerve terminals provides for interaction between the parasympathetic and sympathetic nervous systems, wherein the release of acetylcholine from parasympathetic nerves inhibits the release of norepinephrine from sympathetic nerves.

Muscarinic receptors are divided into **five subtypes,** M_1 through M_5, based on their pharmacologic properties and molecular structures. The principal subtypes found in most tissues are M_1, M_2, and M_3 receptors (see Table 6.2).

TABLE 6.2   Properties of Acetylcholine Receptors

TYPE OF RECEPTOR	PRINCIPAL LOCATIONS	MECHANISM OF SIGNAL TRANSDUCTION	EFFECTS
Muscarinic			
M_1 (neural)	Autonomic ganglia, presynaptic nerve terminals, and CNS	Increased IP_3	Modulation of neurotransmission
M_2 (cardiac)	Cardiac tissue (sinoatrial and atrioventricular nodes)	Increased potassium efflux or decreased cAMP	Slowing of heart rate and conduction
M_3 (glandular)	Smooth muscle and glands	Increased IP_3	Contraction of smooth muscles and stimulation of glandular secretions
	Vascular smooth muscle	Increased cGMP as a result of nitric oxide stimulation	Vasodilation
Nicotinic			
Muscle type	Neuromuscular junctions	Increased sodium influx	Muscle contraction
Ganglionic type	Autonomic ganglia	Increased sodium influx	Neuronal excitation
CNS type	CNS	Increased sodium influx	Neuronal excitation

cAMP, Cyclic adenosine monophosphate; *cGMP,* cyclic guanosine monophosphate; *CNS,* central nervous system; *IP₃,* inositol triphosphate.

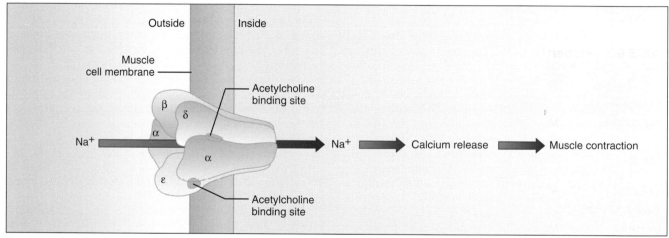

FIG. 6.4   The nicotinic receptor is an acetylcholine-gated sodium channel. The channel is a polypeptide pentamer composed of varying combinations of α, β, δ, and ε subunits. In the muscle type of nicotinic receptor shown here, acetylcholine-binding sites are formed by pockets at the interface of the α and δ subunits and the α and ε subunits. Acetylcholine binding to the receptor causes sodium influx, membrane depolarization, the release of calcium from the sarcoplasmic reticulum, and muscle contraction. Nicotinic receptors at autonomic ganglia and in the brain have a different subunit composition.

Muscarinic receptor stimulation leads to the activation of guanine nucleotide-binding proteins (G proteins), which increases or decreases the formation of other second messengers (see Chapter 3). The M_1, M_3, and M_5 receptors are coupled with G_q **proteins,** and their activation stimulates phospholipase C, leading to the formation of **inositol triphosphate** (IP_3) and **diacylglycerol** (DAG) from membrane phospholipids. In smooth muscles, **IP_3 increases calcium release** from the sarcoplasmic reticulum and promotes **muscle contraction.** In exocrine glands, IP_3 causes calcium release and **glandular secretion.** In vascular endothelial cells, IP_3-activated calcium release stimulates nitric oxide synthesis, leading to **vascular smooth muscle relaxation.**

The M_2 and M_4 receptors are coupled with $G_{\alpha i}$ **proteins;** their activation **decreases cyclic adenosine monophosphate (cAMP) levels** by inhibiting adenylate cyclase and also increases potassium efflux. The effects produced by the activation of muscarinic receptors are summarized in Table 6.1.

Most muscarinic acetylcholine receptor agonists do not selectively activate subtypes of muscarinic receptors, but **cevimeline** shows some selectivity for M_3 receptors.

Nicotinic Receptors

Nicotinic receptors are found at all **autonomic ganglia,** at somatic **neuromuscular junctions,** and in the CNS. These receptors are **ligand-gated sodium channels** whose activation leads to sodium influx and membrane depolarization. At autonomic ganglia, activation of nicotinic receptors produces excitation of postganglionic neurons leading to the release of neurotransmitters at postganglionic neuroeffector junctions. At junctions of somatic nerves and skeletal muscle, activation of nicotinic receptors depolarizes the motor endplate and leads both to the release of calcium from the sarcoplasmic reticulum and to the **contraction of muscles.** In the brain, activation of nicotinic receptors causes **excitation** of presynaptic and postsynaptic neurons.

Nicotinic receptors are pentamers formed by the assembly of five transmembrane polypeptide subunits (Fig. 6.4). These subunits are divided into classes (*alpha* [α] through *epsilon* [ε]) according to their molecular structure. Each type of nicotinic receptor (muscle, ganglionic, brain) is composed of a unique combination of these subunits. All subunits appear to participate in the formation of acetylcholine-binding sites and influence the functional properties of the receptors, but a clear understanding of the unique roles of the different classes of subunits has not yet been obtained.

ACETYLCHOLINE AGONISTS

The acetylcholine agonists can be classified as direct-acting or indirect-acting. The **direct-acting agonists** bind and activate acetylcholine receptors. Most **indirect-acting agonists** increase the synaptic concentration of acetylcholine by inhibiting cholinesterase, whereas others augment acetylcholine signal transduction.

Direct-Acting Acetylcholine Receptor Agonists

The direct-acting agonists include **choline esters, plant alkaloids,** and synthetic drugs called **cevimeline** and **varenicline.** Their properties and uses are listed in Table 6.3. These drugs all bind and activate acetylcholine receptors, but they differ with respect to their affinity for muscarinic and nicotinic receptors and their susceptibility to hydrolysis by cholinesterase.

Choline Esters

The choline esters include **acetylcholine** and synthetic acetylcholine analogs, such as **bethanechol** and **carbachol.** The choline esters are positively charged quaternary ammonium compounds that are poorly absorbed from the gastrointestinal tract and are **not distributed to the CNS. Acetylcholine** and **carbachol** activate both muscarinic and nicotinic receptors, whereas **bethanechol activates only muscarinic receptors.** Because of their lack of specificity for muscarinic receptor subtypes, the muscarinic receptor agonists cause a wide range of effects on many organ systems.

Ocular Effects. Muscarinic receptor agonists increase lacrimal gland secretion and **stimulate contraction of the iris** sphincter muscle and the ciliary muscles. Contraction of the iris sphincter muscle produces pupillary constriction **(miosis),** whereas contraction of the ciliary muscles enables accommodation of the lens to focus on close objects (Fig. 6.5).

Respiratory Tract Effects. Stimulation of muscarinic receptors increases **bronchial muscle contraction** and causes an increase in the secretion of mucus throughout the

TABLE 6.3 Properties and Clinical Uses of Direct-Acting Acetylcholine Receptor Agonists

DRUG	RECEPTOR SPECIFICITY	HYDROLYZED BY CHOLINESTERASE	ROUTE OF ADMINISTRATION	CLINICAL USE
Choline Esters				
Acetylcholine	Muscarinic and nicotinic	Yes	Intraocular	Miosis during ophthalmic surgery
			Intracoronary	Coronary angiography
Bethanechol	Muscarinic	No	Oral or subcutaneous	Gastrointestinal and urinary stimulation
Carbachol	Muscarinic and nicotinic	No	Intraocular	Miosis during ophthalmic surgery
Plant Alkaloids				
Muscarine	Muscarinic	No	None	None
Nicotine	Nicotinic	No	Oral or transdermal	Smoking cessation programs
Pilocarpine	Muscarinic	No	Topical ocular	Glaucoma
			Oral	Xerostomia
Other Drugs				
Cevimeline	Muscarinic	No	Oral	Xerostomia
Varenicline	Nicotinic	No	Oral	Smoking cessation

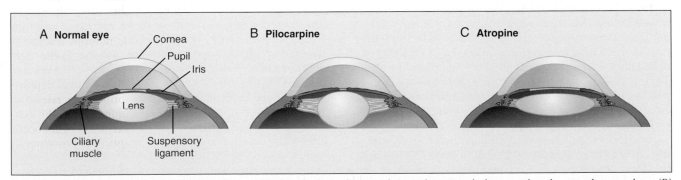

Fig. 6.5 Effects of pilocarpine and atropine on the eye. (A) The relationship between the iris sphincter and ciliary muscle is shown in the normal eye. (B) When pilocarpine, a muscarinic receptor agonist, is administered, contraction of the iris sphincter produces pupillary constriction (miosis). Contraction of the ciliary muscle causes the muscle to be displaced centrally. This relaxes the suspensory ligaments connected to the lens, and the internal elasticity of the lens allows it to increase in thickness. As the lens thickens, its refractive power increases so that it focuses on close objects. (C) When atropine, a muscarinic receptor antagonist, is administered, the iris sphincter and ciliary muscles relax. This produces pupillary dilatation (mydriasis) and increases the tension on the suspensory ligaments so that the lens becomes thinner and focuses on distant objects.

respiratory tract. Because muscarinic receptor agonists can cause **bronchoconstriction,** they should be avoided or used with extreme caution in patients with asthma and other forms of obstructive lung disease.

Cardiac Effects. Muscarinic receptor agonists decrease impulse formation in the sinoatrial node by **reducing the rate of diastolic depolarization.** As a result, they slow the heart rate. In addition, they slow conduction of the cardiac action potential through the atrioventricular node, and this leads to an **increased PR interval** (time between the beginning of the P wave to the beginning of the QRS complex) on the electrocardiogram.

Vascular Effects. Acetylcholine typically causes **vasodilation,** though vasoconstriction may occur under some conditions. The **vasodilative effect** of acetylcholine is mediated by muscarinic M_3 receptors located in vascular endothelial cells, where muscarinic stimulation causes **activation of nitric oxide synthetase** and the formation of nitric oxide. Nitric oxide is a gas that diffuses into vascular smooth muscle cells and activates guanylyl cyclase to increase the formation of **cyclic guanosine monophosphate (cGMP),** leading to vascular smooth muscle relaxation and **vasodilation.** This effect is potentiated by type 5 phosphodiesterase inhibitors used in treating erectile dysfunction.

Gastrointestinal and Urinary Tract Effects. When muscarinic receptor agonists are taken, they stimulate salivary, gastric, and other secretions in the gastrointestinal tract. They also increase the contraction of gastrointestinal smooth muscle (except sphincters) by stimulating the ENS located in the gut wall. This, in turn, **increases gastrointestinal motility.** Whereas muscarinic receptor agonists stimulate the bladder detrusor muscle, they relax the internal sphincter of the bladder, and these effects promote emptying of the bladder **(micturition).** Higher doses of these agonists, therefore, can produce **excessive salivation** and **cause diarrhea,** intestinal **cramps,** and urinary **incontinence** (the "all faucets turned on" syndrome).

Acetylcholine

Acetylcholine is the choline ester of acetic acid. It is rapidly hydrolyzed by cholinesterase and has an extremely short duration of action (see Fig. 6.3). Because of its limited absorption, short duration of action, and lack of specificity for muscarinic or nicotinic receptors, acetylcholine has limited clinical applications. An ophthalmic solution of acetylcholine (MIOCHOL-E) is available for intraocular use during **cataract surgery** and produces miosis after extraction of the lens. The solution is also used in other types of **ophthalmic surgery** that require rapid and complete miosis. Topical ocular administration of acetylcholine is not effective because acetylcholine is hydrolyzed by corneal cholinesterase before it can penetrate to the iris and ciliary muscle.

In patients having **diagnostic coronary angiography,** acetylcholine can be administered by direct intracoronary injection to provoke coronary artery spasm. The **vasospastic effect** of acetylcholine is caused by stimulation of muscarinic M_3 receptors located on vascular smooth muscle that mediate smooth muscle contraction. In most situations, the vasodilation produced by acetylcholine is more pronounced than the vasoconstrictive effect. In patients with vasospastic angina pectoris, however, intracoronary injection of acetylcholine can provoke a localized vasoconstrictive response, and this helps establish the diagnosis of vasospastic angina.

Bethanechol and Carbachol

Bethanechol and **carbachol** are choline esters of carbamic acid. They are resistant to hydrolysis by cholinesterase; their duration of action is relatively short, lasting for several hours after topical ocular or systemic administration. **Bethanechol** selectively activates muscarinic receptors and has been used to **stimulate bladder** or **gastrointestinal muscle** without significantly affecting heart rate or blood pressure. Although it generally has been replaced by more effective treatments, bethanechol can be given postoperatively or postpartum to increase bladder muscle tone in patients with nonobstructive **neurogenic urinary retention** after receiving anesthetics or other drugs administered during childbirth or surgery. Therapeutic doses of bethanechol given orally or subcutaneously have little effect on blood pressure, but the drug should never be administered intravenously because this can cause hypotension and bradycardia.

Carbachol is available as a solution instilled intraocularly to produce **miosis** during **ophthalmic surgery,** such as cataract surgery and iridectomy. It is no longer used in treating open-angle glaucoma, having been replaced by agents with fewer side effects.

Plant Alkaloids

The cholinergic plant alkaloids include **muscarine, nicotine,** and **pilocarpine.** Muscarine is found in **mushrooms** of the genera *Inocybe* and *Clitocybe,* and the consumption of these poisonous mushrooms can cause diarrhea, sweating, salivation, and lacrimation. Muscarine is also found in trace amounts in *Amanita muscaria,* the original source of muscarine, but the toxicity of this mushroom is largely a result of the ibotenic acid it contains. Nicotine is derived from *Nicotiana* plants and is contained in cigarettes and other tobacco products such as vape pens. Nicotine is highly addictive, and the treatment of nicotine dependence is discussed in Chapter 25. Muscarine has no current medical use. **Nicotine** is available in chewing gum, transdermal patches, and other products designed for use in **smoking cessation** programs.

Pilocarpine is a tertiary amine alkaloid that is obtained from *Pilocarpus,* a small shrub. The drug is well absorbed after topical ocular and oral administration. Pilocarpine, which has a greater affinity for muscarinic receptors than for nicotinic receptors, can produce all the effects of muscarinic receptor stimulation. Pilocarpine is a second-line drug for the treatment of **chronic open-angle glaucoma,** in which it lowers intraocular pressure by increasing the outflow of aqueous humor (Box 6.1). It is also used in the treatment of **acute angle-closure glaucoma,** a medical emergency in which blindness can result if the intraocular pressure is not lowered immediately. The main side effects of ocular pilocarpine administration are decreased night vision, which is caused by **miosis,** and difficulty in focusing on distant objects, which occurs because the lens is accommodated for close vision.

In patients with **xerostomia** (dry mouth), pilocarpine is administered orally to stimulate salivary gland secretion. Low doses can be used to produce this effect with minimal side effects in many patients because of the high sensitivity of the salivary glands to muscarinic stimulation.

BOX 6.1 TREATMENT OF CHRONIC OPEN-ANGLE GLAUCOMA

In the normal eye, aqueous humor is secreted by the ciliary processes and flows through the pupillary aperture of the iris and into the anterior chamber. It then drains through the trabecular meshwork in the Schlemm canal. In patients with open-angle glaucoma, persistently elevated intraocular pressure is associated with narrowing of the anterior chamber angle, a decrease in the rate of aqueous outflow, and the gradual loss of peripheral vision. Various types of drugs can be used to reduce intraocular pressure before irreversible optic nerve damage occurs. The sites of action of these drugs are shown later in this box.

Some types of drugs act by enhancing the drainage of aqueous humor. Muscarinic receptor agonists (e.g., pilocarpine) stimulate the contraction of meridional ciliary muscle fibers that insert near the trabecular meshwork. Contraction of these

fibers opens the trabecular spaces so that aqueous humor drains more easily. Prostaglandins (e.g., latanoprost) increase aqueous drainage through an alternative pathway known as the *uveoscleral route*. In this pathway, aqueous humor flows through the ciliary muscles into the suprachoroidal space.

Other types of drugs act by reducing the amount of aqueous humor produced by the ciliary processes. The β-adrenoceptor blockers (e.g., timolol) and the α_2-adrenoceptor agonists (e.g., apraclonidine) reduce the formation of cyclic adenosine monophosphate (cAMP), a substance that stimulates aqueous humor production. Carbonic anhydrase inhibitors (e.g., dorzolamide) block the formation of bicarbonate by carbonic anhydrase, an enzyme that is required for aqueous humor secretion. Epinephrine probably acts by reducing blood flow in the ciliary processes.

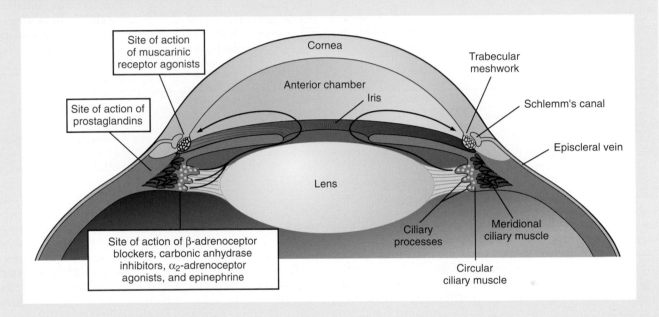

Other Drugs

Cevimeline is a synthetic direct-acting muscarinic receptor agonist that selectively activates M_3 receptors. It is administered orally to treat **dry mouth** in patients who have had radiation therapy for head and neck cancer and to patients with **Sjögren syndrome** (dry eyes, dry mouth, and arthritis) to increase salivary and lacrimal secretion. Adverse effects include increased sweating, nausea, and visual disturbances caused by drug-induced miosis. As with other acetylcholine receptor agonists, **cevimeline** should be used cautiously in persons with asthma or cardiac arrhythmias.

Varenicline is a partial agonist at the nicotinic receptor subtype found in the brain that mediates the reinforcing effects of nicotine in smokers. The drug is used as an aid to **smoking cessation** and has been found to reduce both the craving and withdrawal effects caused by the absence of nicotine (see Chapter 25). Studies show it increases the chances of successful long-term smoking cessation.

Indirect-Acting Acetylcholine Agonists

The indirect-acting acetylcholine receptor agonists include the cholinesterase inhibitors, the type 5 phosphodiesterase inhibitors, and a direct stimulant of guanylate cyclase.

Cholinesterase Inhibitors

The cholinesterase inhibitors prevent the breakdown of acetylcholine at all cholinergic synapses. The shorter-acting drugs are referred to as **reversible cholinesterase inhibitors,** whereas longer-acting compounds are called **quasi reversible cholinesterase inhibitors.** The properties and clinical uses of inhibitors from each group are outlined in Table 6.4.

Reversible Cholinesterase Inhibitors

Edrophonium. Edrophonium is a positively charged alcohol that reversibly binds to a negatively charged (anionic) site on cholinesterase, but it is not a substrate for the enzyme. The reversible binding and rapid renal excretion of the drug are responsible for its short duration of action (about 10 minutes).

Edrophonium prevents the hydrolysis of acetylcholine by cholinesterase, and it **rapidly increases acetylcholine concentrations** at cholinergic synapses such as the somatic neuromuscular junction. **Edrophonium** is used for two purposes. During anesthesia, it is used to reverse the effects of neuromuscular blockade caused by the administration of neuromuscular blocking drugs (see Chapter 7). In this setting, edrophonium increases the synaptic concentration of acetylcholine at the neuromuscular junction, which competitively displaces the blocking agent from the nicotinic receptor.

TABLE 6.4 **Properties and Clinical Uses of Cholinesterase Inhibitors, Phosphodiesterase Inhibitors, and Riociguat**

DRUG	ROUTE OF ADMINISTRATION	DURATION OF ACTION	CLINICAL USE
Donepezil	Oral	24 h	Alzheimer disease
Edrophonium	Intravenous	10 min	Myasthenia gravis (diagnosis)
Neostigmine	Oral, subcutaneous, or intramuscular	2–4 h	Myasthenia gravis; postoperative urinary retention
	Intravenous	2–5 min	Reversal of curariform drug effects
Physostigmine	Intramuscular or intravenous	1–5 h	Reversal of central nervous system effects of antimuscarinic drugs
Pyridostigmine	Oral	3–6 h	Myasthenia gravis
	Intramuscular or intravenous	2–5 min (IV); 15 min (IM)	Reversal of curariform drug effects
Echothiophate	Topical ocular	1 wk or more	Glaucoma and accommodative esotropia
Malathion	Topical	—	Pediculosis (lice)
Avanafil	Oral	5 h	Erectile dysfunction
Sildenafil	Oral	4–6 h	Erectile dysfunction, pulmonary arterial hypertension
Tadalafil	Oral	36 h	Erectile dysfunction, benign prostatic hyperplasia, pulmonary arterial hypertension
Riociguat	Oral	8 h	Pulmonary arterial hypertension

IM, Intramuscular; *IV,* intravenous.

Edrophonium is also used in the diagnosis of **myasthenia gravis** and in distinguishing between a **myasthenic crisis** and a **cholinergic crisis** in myasthenia patients being treated with a cholinesterase inhibitor such as **pyridostigmine** (see later). Myasthenia gravis is an **autoimmune disease** in which antibodies are directed against nicotinic receptors in skeletal muscle. These antibodies inactivate and destroy the receptors and thereby impair neuromuscular transmission, causing severe fatigue. Myasthenia gravis most often affects the muscles of the face, throat, and neck.

Patients with myasthenia gravis may experience muscle weakness from either undertreatment or overtreatment with a cholinesterase inhibitor drug. In the untreated condition and in patients not receiving adequate doses of the drug, muscle weakness is caused by an acetylcholine deficiency and is called a **myasthenic crisis.** In this situation, a test dose of **edrophonium** will increase acetylcholine levels and muscle strength. In patients who are overtreated with a cholinesterase inhibitor, muscle weakness is caused by an excessive amount of acetylcholine at the neuromuscular junction, causing **depolarization neuromuscular blockade** similar to that produced by **succinylcholine** (see Chapter 7). This condition is called a **cholinergic crisis,** and a test dose of edrophonium will cause muscle weakness to increase. This finding indicates that the patient's dose of cholinesterase inhibitor should be decreased.

Neostigmine, Physostigmine, and Pyridostigmine. Physostigmine is a plant alkaloid that is well absorbed from the gut and penetrates the blood-brain barrier. **Neostigmine** and **pyridostigmine** are synthetic drugs that exist as positively charged compounds at physiologic pH. Hence, they are not as well absorbed from the intestines and do not cross the blood-brain barrier in comparison with physostigmine.

Neostigmine and related drugs are substrates for cholinesterase in a manner similar to that of acetylcholine, except that the drug-enzyme intermediate is slowly hydrolyzed (degraded) by the enzyme (Fig. 6.6). Although the enzyme is occupied by neostigmine or a related drug, it is unable to hydrolyze acetylcholine, whose synaptic concentration is

thereby increased. When used in the long-term treatment of **myasthenia gravis, neostigmine** and **pyridostigmine** improve muscle tone and reduce eyelid and facial ptosis. Although either drug can also reduce diplopia (double vision) and blurred vision, diplopia is often resistant to treatment with tolerated doses of these drugs. If excessive doses are used, muscle weakness can increase as a result of a depolarizing neuromuscular blockade resulting from excessive levels of acetylcholine.

Corticosteroids and other **immunosuppressant drugs** are also used in treating myasthenia in order to reduce the formation of antibodies to the nicotinic receptor. They are often used in combination with cholinesterase inhibitors. Thymectomy is sometimes performed to counteract autoimmune mechanisms in persons with myasthenia gravis.

As with edrophonium, **neostigmine** and **pyridostigmine** are often used during surgery to reverse the effects of **curariform neuromuscular blocking drugs** when muscle relaxation is no longer required (see Chapter 7). Neostigmine has been used in the treatment of postoperative urinary retention and abdominal distention, but other treatments are usually preferred.

Physostigmine has been used to treat glaucoma, but other drugs are employed today. It is available for parenteral administration as an **antidote** to the adverse effects caused by an overdose of atropine or other antimuscarinic drugs, including those contained in certain poisonous plants such as the deadly nightshade and jimson weed.

Quasi-reversible Cholinesterase Inhibitors
The quasi-reversible cholinesterase inhibitors are all **organophosphate compounds.** A few of them, including **echothiophate, isoflurophate,** and **malathion,** have been used as therapeutic agents. Most of them are used as **pesticides,** however, and some of them (such as soman and sarin) were developed as chemical warfare agents (see Chapter 5). Because of the widespread use of organophosphates as pesticides, they are responsible for cases of **accidental** and **intentional poisoning** every year (Box 6.2).

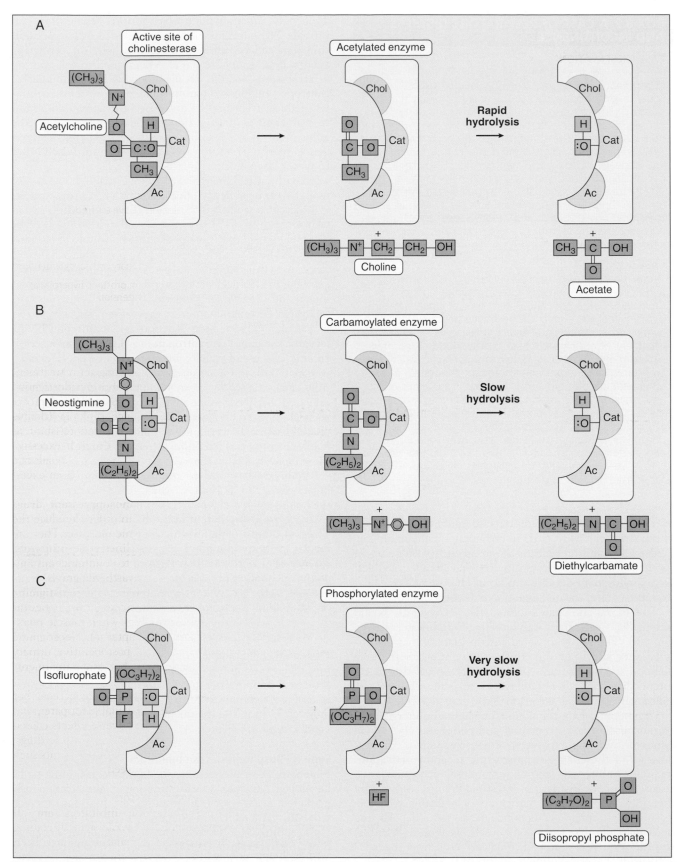

FIG. 6.6 Mechanisms of cholinesterase inhibition. (A) The active site of cholinesterase includes the choline subsite (*Chol*), the catalytic subsite (*Cat*), and the acyl subsite (*Ac*). Acetylcholine binds to these subsites, and the acetate moiety forms a covalent bond with a serine hydroxyl group at the catalytic subsite as choline is released. The acetylated enzyme is then rapidly hydrolyzed to release acetate. (B) Carbamates (e.g., neostigmine) also bind to the active site and form a carbamoylated enzyme that is slowly hydrolyzed by cholinesterase. (C) Organophosphates (e.g., isoflurophate) form a strong covalent bond with the catalytic site of cholinesterase and are very slowly hydrolyzed by the enzyme. *HF*, Hydrofluoric acid.

The quasi-reversible cholinesterase inhibitors are esters of phosphoric acid. Most of these organophosphates are highly lipid-soluble and are effectively absorbed from all sites in the body, including the skin, mucous membranes, and gut. **Organophosphate toxicity** can occur after dermal or ocular exposure or after the oral ingestion of these compounds.

The organophosphates form a tight, covalently bound intermediate with the **catalytic site of cholinesterase** (see Fig. 6.6). The phosphorylated intermediate is then **hydrolyzed very slowly** by the enzyme, accounting for the long duration of action of these compounds. The covalently bound intermediate is further stabilized by a spontaneous process called **aging,** in which a portion of the drug molecule is lost.

Organophosphate compounds **augment cholinergic neurotransmission** at both central and peripheral cholinergic synapses. Systemic exposure to these compounds can produce all of the effects of **muscarinic receptor activation,** including salivation, lacrimation, miosis, accommodative spasm, bronchoconstriction, intestinal cramps, and urinary incontinence. Excessive activation of nicotinic receptors by organophosphate compounds leads to a depolarizing neuromuscular blockade and muscle weakness. **Seizures, respiratory depression,** and **coma** can result from the overactivation of acetylcholine receptors in the CNS.

The clinical use of organophosphates is primarily in the treatment of ocular conditions. **Echothiophate** has been used to treat chronic **glaucoma** that does not respond adequately to more conservative therapy (see Table 6.4). The long duration of action of these drugs can provide 24-hour control of intraocular pressure, a condition that can be difficult to achieve with shorter-acting agents. Echothiophate has also been used to treat a form of **strabismus** (ocular deviation) called **accommodative esotropia.** In affected patients, the cholinesterase inhibitors reduce strabismus by increasing the accommodation-to-convergence ratio. Accommodation refers to the adjustment of the lens for close vision, whereas convergence refers to the rotation of the eyes toward each other to view close objects.

Malathion is primarily used as a pesticide, but it is also used to treat **head lice** (pediculosis capitis). For this purpose, it is administered as a 0.5% lotion (OVIDE) and kills ova as well as adult lice.

Management of Organophosphate Poisoning. Poisoning may result from accidental exposure to organophosphate pesticides used in agricultural and gardening applications or from exposure to chemical warfare agents such as the nerve gases soman and sarin. Management of this toxicity involves the following: decontamination of the patient, support of cardiovascular and respiratory function, use of an acetylcholine receptor antagonist (e.g., **atropine**) to block excessive acetylcholine, and use of pralidoxime to regenerate cholinesterase (see Box 6.2). Atropine effectively counteracts the muscarinic effects caused by organophosphates and other cholinesterase inhibitors. Because of the extremely high levels of acetylcholine at cholinergic synapses during organophosphate exposure, however, the **atropine doses** required in the management of this poisoning are usually **much higher** than those typically used in the treatment of medical conditions.

Pralidoxime is used to regenerate cholinesterase after organophosphate poisoning, which serves to decrease acetylcholine levels and is particularly helpful in reducing nicotinic receptor stimulation and relieving muscle weakness. The high affinity of pralidoxime for phosphorus enables it to break the phosphorus bond with cholinesterase and thereby regenerate the enzyme. It is important to administer pralidoxime as soon as possible after organophosphate exposure because "aging" of the organophosphate reduces the ability of pralidoxime to regenerate cholinesterase.

Centrally Acting, Reversible Cholinesterase Inhibitors
Donepezil, galantamine, and **rivastigmine** are centrally acting, reversible cholinesterase inhibitors that readily cross the blood-brain barrier and act to increase the concentration of acetylcholine at central cholinergic synapses. These drugs are used in the treatment of **Alzheimer's disease** and are discussed in Chapter 24.

Type 5 Phosphodiesterase Inhibitors
Sildenafil was the first phosphodiesterase inhibitor to be developed to treat **erectile dysfunction** in men; it is famously marketed as VIAGRA. Other drugs in this class include **tadalafil, vardenafil,** and **avanafil** (see Table 6.4). Tadalafil is also approved for the treatment of the symptoms of **benign prostatic hyperplasia (BPH),** and both it and sildenafil are also approved for **pulmonary arterial hypertension (PAH;** see later). These drugs potentiate the vasodilation effect of acetylcholine released from parasympathetic neurons originating in the pelvic plexus, increasing penile blood flow and improving **penile erection** during sexual stimulation. Penile

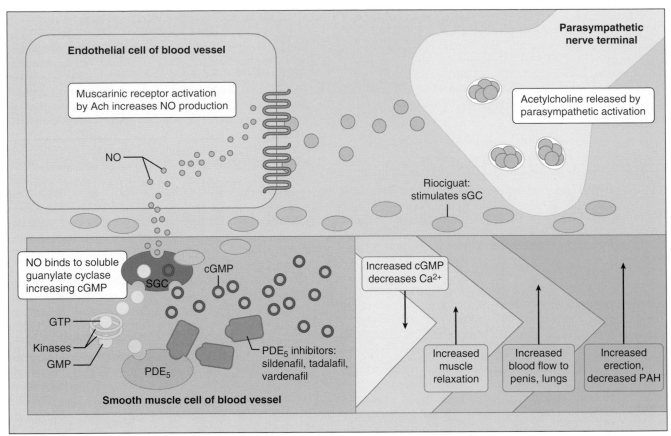

FIG. 6.7 Mechanisms of action of PDE$_5$ inhibitors and Riociguat. The normal erection process begins with the release of acetylcholine from parasympathetic nerves onto acetylcholine receptors on endothelial cells of arterioles supplying the penis. Endothelial cells are stimulated to produce NO (nitric oxide), which diffuses into adjacent smooth muscle cells of the arteriole. NO activates its target receptor, soluble guanylate cyclase (sGC), which increases levels of cGMP. This, in turn, decreases calcium ions and muscle contraction. Increased muscle relaxation equals increased blood flow to the penis (or lung), and this leads to increased blood volume and erection. With age or disease, the erection process fails but can be treated pharmacologically. Sildenafil paved the way for ED treatment by using the mechanism of action of blocking type 5 phosphodiesterase (PDE$_5$), leading to greater cGMP levels. Riociguat, an agent indicated for the treatment of pulmonary arterial hypertension (PAH), facilitates NO binding to sGC and also directly stimulates sGC.

erection occurs when acetylcholine activates muscarinic M$_3$ receptors in vascular endothelial cells, leading to increased production and release of **nitric oxide** (Fig. 6.7). Nitric oxide then diffuses into vascular smooth muscle cells in the corpus cavernosum, binding to **soluble guanylate cyclase** and increasing synthesis of **cGMP,** leading to muscle relaxation and vasodilation. Sildenafil and related drugs inhibit the breakdown of cGMP by **type 5 phosphodiesterase** (5-PDE), leading to elevated levels of cGMP and increased smooth muscle relaxation, which then results in increased blood flow into the penis and erection.

Pharmacokinetics

Sildenafil is rapidly absorbed after oral administration and has an oral bioavailability of about 40%. The absorption of sildenafil is reduced if it is taken with a high-fat meal, whereas the absorption of vardenafil and tadalafil is not affected by food. These drugs have an onset of action 30 to 60 minutes after drug administration. Sildenafil is metabolized by cytochrome P450 3A4 (CYP3A4), and its N-desmethyl metabolite has about half the activity of the parent compound. Whereas **sildenafil and vardenafil have half-lives of about 4 hours** and durations of action of 4 to 6 hours, **tadalafil has a half-life of 17 hours** and a duration of action of 36 hours. For this reason, men should not take more than one dose of tadalafil in a 24-hour period.

Vardenafil is available as a tablet for oral ingestion and as an oral disintegrating tablet that is dissolved on the tongue (STAXYN). The latter formulation provides higher blood levels than the oral tablet (LEVITRA). Both formulations should be taken about 60 minutes before sexual activity. A potential advantage of **avanafil,** the newest member of this class, is its fast onset of action (15–30 minutes) owing to its rapid rate of absorption.

Adverse Effects and Interactions

The adverse effects of sildenafil and related drugs are usually mild and transient and include **headache, nasal congestion,** dyspepsia, myalgia, back pain, and **visual disturbances.**

The 5-PDE inhibitors reduce **supine blood pressure** by about 7 to 8 mm Hg in normal subjects, which ordinarily is not significant. However, these drugs should not be used by men who take nitroglycerin or another **organic nitrate** because the nitrates also increase cGMP formation (see Chapter 11, Fig. 11.3). Concurrent administration of 5-PDE inhibitors and nitroglycerin can cause profound **hypotension,** reflex tachycardia, and worsening of **angina pectoris.** A number of deaths have occurred in men who took both sildenafil and nitroglycerin. The 5-PDE inhibitors can also augment the hypotensive effects of other vasodilators, including α-adrenoceptor antagonists (e.g., doxazosin), used to treat symptoms of urinary obstruction in men with BPH (see Chapter 9).

Sildenafil and related drugs are primarily metabolized by CYP3A4, and inhibitors of this cytochrome P450 isozyme can reduce the clearance and elevate the plasma levels of these drugs. The CYP3A4 inhibitors include cimetidine, erythromycin, ketoconazole, itraconazole, and compounds found in grapefruit juice. The initial dose of sildenafil or related drugs should be reduced by 50% in men who are also taking a CYP3A4 inhibitor.

Indications

In addition to its efficacy in treating erectile dysfunction, **tadalafil** has been shown to significantly improve urinary symptoms of **BPH,** such as sudden urges to urinate, difficulty in starting micturition, a weak urine flow, and frequent urination, including at night. Daily administration of tadalafil was shown to improve both erectile dysfunction and BPH in comparison to a placebo. The mechanisms by which tadalafil improves symptoms of BPH appear to include cGMP-mediated vasodilation in prostate and bladder tissue, as well as relaxation of the prostate and bladder smooth muscle in a way that reduces obstruction to urine outflow.

Sildenafil (as REVATIO) and **tadalafil** (as ADCIRCA) are both approved for the treatment of **PAH.** These drugs were found to improve exercise ability in patients with idiopathic or hereditary PAH as well as those with connective tissue diseases. PAH is partly caused by the impaired release of nitric oxide by vascular endothelial cells, resulting in deficient cGMP levels in pulmonary vascular smooth muscle. Sildenafil and tadalafil increase levels of cGMP by inhibition of type 5 phosphodiesterase, causing relaxation of pulmonary vascular smooth muscle and decreasing pulmonary artery pressure.

Soluble Guanylate Cyclase Stimulators

Riociguat (ADEMPAS) is a first-in-class drug for treating PAH that has a dual mode of action. It sensitizes **soluble cyclic guanylate cyclase** (sGC) to endogenous NO by stabilizing the NO-sGC binding complex. Riociguat also directly stimulates sGC without NO present via a different binding site. The effect of both actions is an increase in intracellular levels of cGMP (see Fig. 6.7). It was approved for the treatment of PAH and pulmonary hypertension after showing improvement in exercise and functional class in clinical trials. Riociguat should not be used with phosphodiesterase-5 inhibitors due to the resulting systemic hypotension. Other treatments for PAH include **epoprostenol** (prostacyclin) and endothelin receptor antagonists such as **bosentan** (see Chapter 26).

SUMMARY OF IMPORTANT POINTS

- The sympathetic and parasympathetic divisions of the autonomic nervous system have opposing effects in many tissues. Drugs that activate one division often have the same effects as drugs that inhibit the other division.
- Acetylcholine is the primary neurotransmitter at parasympathetic and somatic neuroeffector junctions, and norepinephrine is the transmitter at most sympathetic junctions. Nitric oxide is a neurotransmitter that produces vasodilatation in vascular beds and is found in the ENS.
- The ENS also utilizes other nonadrenergic-noncholinergic neurotransmitters, including several peptides and serotonin.

- Most autonomic drugs activate or block receptors for acetylcholine or norepinephrine in smooth muscle, cardiac tissue, and glands. A few drugs affect neurotransmitter synthesis, storage, release, or metabolism. These are called *indirect-acting drugs*.
- The direct-acting acetylcholine receptor agonists include choline esters (e.g., bethanechol) and plant alkaloids (e.g., pilocarpine). Pilocarpine is used to treat glaucoma and dry mouth.
- The cholinesterase inhibitors indirectly activate acetylcholine receptors by increasing the synaptic concentration of acetylcholine. These drugs have both parasympathomimetic and somatic nervous system effects.
- The reversible cholinesterase inhibitors include edrophonium, which is used to diagnose myasthenia gravis, and neostigmine and pyridostigmine, which are used to treat myasthenia gravis.
- The quasi reversible cholinesterase inhibitors are organophosphate compounds that are widely used as pesticides and less commonly used in medical therapy. Echothiophate can be used to treat ocular conditions, whereas malathion is used to treat pediculosis.
- Organophosphate toxicity is treated with atropine and a cholinesterase reactivator called *pralidoxime*.
- Sildenafil and related drugs inhibit the degradation of cGMP by 5-PDE and thereby potentiate the vasodilative action of nitric oxide in the penis and other tissues. These drugs are used to treat male erectile dysfunction, benign prostatic hypertrophy, and pulmonary artery hypertension (PAH).
- Riociguat increases cyclic GMP levels by directly stimulating guanylate cyclase, and it is also used to treat PAH.

Review Questions

1. A woman with facial muscle spasms is treated with an agent that inhibits the release of acetylcholine. Which side effect is most likely to occur in this patient?
   (A) bradycardia
   (B) urinary incontinence
   (C) dry mouth
   (D) diarrhea
   (E) constriction of the pupils
2. A man complains of dry mouth after radiation therapy for throat cancer, and he is treated with cevimeline. Which mechanism produces the therapeutic effect of this drug?
   (A) activation of muscarinic M_2 receptors
   (B) increased formation of IP_3
   (C) increased cAMP levels
   (D) increased cGMP levels
   (E) increased potassium efflux
3. A woman in a smoking cessation program receives a drug that reduces craving and withdrawal effects. Which effect results from receptor activation by this drug?
   (A) sodium influx
   (B) potassium efflux
   (C) increased cAMP
   (D) increased cGMP
   (E) IP_3 formation

4. A man receives a drug that increases cGMP levels. Which adverse effect is most likely to result from this medication?
   (A) constipation
   (B) cough
   (C) dry mouth
   (D) sedation
   (E) headache

5. An agricultural worker is brought to the emergency department after the abrupt onset of bowel and bladder incontinence and muscle weakness while she was working. She is given oxygen and antidotal drug treatments. Which drug mechanism would increase muscle strength in this patient?
   (A) blockade of muscarinic receptors
   (B) activation of nicotinic receptors
   (C) increased neurotransmitter degradation
   (D) induction of drug-metabolizing enzymes
   (E) increased urinary excretion of weak acids

CHAPTER 7

Cholinergic Receptor Antagonists

OVERVIEW

The acetylcholine receptor antagonists are drugs that selectively block one of both types of cholinergic receptors, **either muscarinic** or **nicotinic receptors.** Together, these drugs affect almost every organ system in the body and have a wide range of clinical applications. The muscarinic receptor blockers are used to **relax smooth muscle, decrease gland secretions,** or **increase heart rate.** The nicotinic receptor antagonists primarily consist of neuromuscular blocking agents used to **relax skeletal muscle during surgery.** This chapter focuses on the pharmacologic properties, clinical use, and adverse effects of these drugs.

MUSCARINIC RECEPTOR ANTAGONISTS

Muscarinic receptor antagonists (blockers) compete with acetylcholine for its receptors at **parasympathetic neuroeffector junctions** and thereby inhibit the effects of parasympathetic nerve stimulation. Hence, these drugs are sometimes called **parasympatholytic drugs.**

The muscarinic blockers include the **belladonna alkaloids** obtained from plants as well as a number of semisynthetic and synthetic drugs. These agents have similar effects on target organs, but they differ in their pharmacokinetic properties and clinical uses. Because the sympathetic and parasympathetic nervous systems have opposing effects in many tissues, the effects produced by muscarinic receptor antagonists are often similar to those evoked by adrenoceptor agonists. For this reason, these two classes of drugs are sometimes used in combination in the treatment of obstructive pulmonary disease (see Chapter 27) and other conditions.

Belladonna Alkaloids

The belladonna alkaloids are extracted from various plants found in temperate climates around the world, including *Atropa belladonna* (the deadly nightshade), *Datura stramonium* (jimson weed), and *Hyoscyamus niger*. **Belladonna,** which is an Italian for "beautiful lady," came from the description of courtesans who put belladonna plant extract in their eyes to cause **pupil dilation (mydriasis),** considered a sign of sexual arousal during the Renaissance.

Atropine, scopolamine, and **hyoscyamine** are examples of belladonna alkaloids. The belladonna alkaloids can be highly toxic and are sometimes the cause of accidental or intentional poisonings (Box 7.1). In fact, atropine was named after *Atropos,* one of the gods of Fate in Greek mythology, who killed mortals by "cutting the thread of life."

Atropine and Scopolamine

Chemistry and Pharmacokinetics. **Atropine** and **scopolamine** are nonionized tertiary amines that are well absorbed from the gut and are readily distributed to the central nervous system. After systemic administration, they are excreted in the urine with a half-life of about 2 hours. After **topical ocular administration,** they have longer-lasting effects because they bind to pigments in the iris that slowly release the drugs. People with darker irises bind more atropine and experience a more prolonged effect than do people with lighter irises. The ocular effects gradually subside over several days.

Pharmacologic Effects. The muscarinic blockers inhibit the effects of parasympathetic nerve stimulation and thereby relax smooth muscle, increase heart rate and cardiac conduction, and inhibit exocrine gland secretion. As shown in Fig. 7.1, as the dose of atropine increases, the severity of its effects increases. The signs of **atropine toxicity** are expressed by the mnemonic *"dry as a bone, blind as a bat, and red as a beet,"* referring to the anti-secretory, paralysis of visual accommodation, and vasodilation produced by large doses of atropine.

Ocular Effects. Atropine and related drugs relax the iris sphincter muscle, leading to pupil dilation (mydriasis).

BOX 7.1 A CASE OF DILATED PUPILS AND HALLUCINATIONS

CASE PRESENTATION

A 16-year-old boy was brought to the emergency department by his friends after he became highly agitated and experienced visual hallucinations, claiming that one of his friends had a mailbox for a head. His examination showed dry skin and mucous membranes, absent bowel sounds, and sinus tachycardia. His pupils were dilated, and his vision was blurred. The boy had ingested some seeds from plants growing in a vacant lot, but he denied the use of alcohol or other substances. The plant material was collected and later identified as *Datura stramonium*. His laboratory findings were normal, and his blood alcohol level was zero. Gastric lavage was performed, and activated charcoal was administered to remove any unabsorbed substances. The patient became more agitated and delusional over time, and he was given an intravenous infusion of physostigmine. This treatment was repeated after 20 minutes, and his symptoms gradually subsided. Twelve hours later, the patient was much improved. He continued to improve over the next 36 hours and was discharged from the hospital with normal vital signs and mental status.

CASE DISCUSSION

Jimson weed *(D. stramonium)* is a hallucinogenic plant containing belladonna alkaloids found throughout the United States. Ingestion or inhalation of any part of the plant can result in anticholinergic toxicity with the clinical presentation resembling that seen in cases of atropine poisoning. Some fatalities have occurred from the ingestion of this plant. Treatment is aimed at removing plant material from the gastrointestinal tract, keeping the patient safe, and counteracting severe anticholinergic effects with physostigmine, a cholinesterase inhibitor. Physostigmine increases levels of acetylcholine in peripheral tissues and the brain and thereby counteracts manifestations of atropine toxicity. Physostigmine may cause adverse effects such as bronchospasm, and should be reserved for persons with serious cardiovascular toxicity (such as severe tachycardia) or central nervous system toxicity (severe delirium or agitation, hallucinations, or seizures).

Muscarinic blockers also relax the ciliary muscle, thereby increasing the tension on the suspensory ligaments attached to the lens and causing the lens to flatten so that it is focused on distant objects. This prevents the lens from increasing its refractive power to focus on near objects (accommodation), a condition called *cycloplegia* (paralysis of accommodation). These drugs also inhibit lacrimal gland secretion and can cause dry eyes.

Cardiac Effects. Standard doses of atropine and related drugs increase the heart rate and atrioventricular conduction velocity by blocking the effects of the vagus nerve on the sinoatrial and atrioventricular nodes. When intravenous administration of atropine is begun, however, the low dose of the drug causes a paradoxical slowing of the heart rate. This effect probably results from stimulation of the vagal motor nucleus in the brainstem. After the full dose has been administered, an increase in heart rate is observed.

Respiratory Tract Effects. In addition to producing bronchial smooth muscle relaxation and bronchodilation, atropine and other muscarinic receptor antagonists act as potent inhibitors of secretions in the upper and lower respiratory tract.

Gastrointestinal and Urinary Tract Effects. Atropine reduces lower esophageal muscle tone and can cause gastroesophageal reflux. Muscarinic receptor blockers relax gastrointestinal muscle, except sphincters, and reduce intestinal motility, thereby increasing gastric emptying time and intestinal transit time. They also inhibit gastric acid secretion. Sufficient doses of these drugs can cause constipation. Atropine relaxes the detrusor muscle of the urinary bladder and can cause urinary retention.

Central Nervous System Effects. Atropine and scopolamine are distributed to the central nervous system, where they can block muscarinic receptors and produce **both sedation and excitement.** Scopolamine is more sedating than atropine and has been used as an adjunct to anesthesia. Standard doses of atropine typically cause mild stimulation, followed by a slower and longer-lasting sedative effect. With

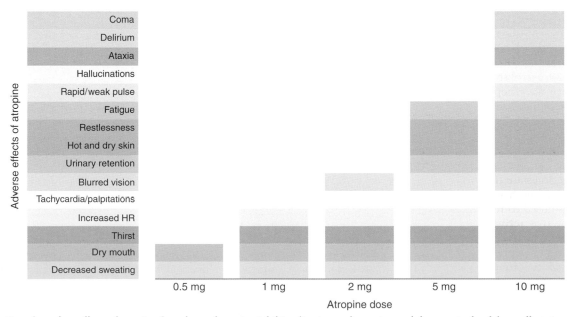

Fig. 7.1 Dose-dependent effects of atropine. Low doses of atropine inhibit salivation and sweating, and the magnitude of these effects increases as the dosage increases. Higher doses produce tachycardia, urinary retention, and central nervous system effects.

higher doses of atropine, patients can experience an acute confusional state known as *delirium*. Higher doses of muscarinic antagonists sometimes cause **hallucinations.** Other drugs in high doses, such as the antihistamine **diphenhydramine** obtained from abuse of over-the-counter cold and cough medicines, can also interact with muscarinic receptors and produce delirium and hallucinations (see Chapter 25).

Other Effects. The muscarinic receptor antagonists **inhibit sweating,** which can reduce heat loss and lead to hyperthermia, especially in children. The increased body temperature can cause cutaneous vasodilation, and the skin can become **hot, dry,** and **flushed.**

Ocular Indications. To obtain a relatively localized effect on ocular tissues, muscarinic receptor blockers are administered via topical instillation of a solution or ointment. These drugs are typically used to produce mydriasis and facilitate ophthalmoscopic examination of the peripheral retina. They can also be used to produce cycloplegia and permit the accurate determination of refractive errors, especially in younger patients with strong accommodation. Because muscarinic receptor blockers can **reduce muscle spasms and pain** caused by inflammation, they are useful in the treatment of iritis and cyclitis (inflammation of the iris and ciliary muscles) associated with infection, trauma, or surgery.

Cardiac Indications. Atropine can be used to treat sinus bradycardia in cases in which the slow sinus rhythm reduces the cardiac output and blood pressure and produces symptoms of hypotension or ischemia. This type of symptomatic bradycardia sometimes occurs after a myocardial infarction. **Atropine** is usually given intravenously for this purpose, but it can be injected endotracheally if a vein is not accessible. In patients with symptomatic atrioventricular block, **atropine** or **glycopyrrolate** can be used to increase the atrioventricular conduction velocity.

Respiratory Tract Indications. Because of its bronchodilating effects, atropine was once used to treat asthma and other obstructive lung diseases. It is no longer used for this purpose, however, because of its many adverse effects. For example, it impairs ciliary activity, thereby reducing the clearance of mucus from the lungs and causing the accumulation of viscid material in the airways. As discussed later in this chapter, **ipratropium** is now used instead of atropine to treat obstructive lung diseases. **Atropine** and other muscarinic receptor blockers are used to reduce salivary and respiratory secretions and thereby prevent airway obstruction in patients who are receiving general anesthetics. **Glycopyrrolate** is often used for this purpose today (see the section on other indications).

Gastrointestinal and Urinary Tract Indications. Atropine and related drugs are used to relieve **intestinal spasms** and **pain** associated with several gastrointestinal disorders, and they are also used to relieve urinary bladder spasms in persons with an **overactive bladder.**

Atropine was once used to reduce gastric acid secretion in patients with peptic ulcer, but the large doses required for this purpose often produced intolerable side effects, and these drugs are seldom used for this purpose today. As discussed later, a selective muscarinic M_1 receptor blocker, **pirenzepine,** is available in some countries to treat peptic ulcer disease.

Central Nervous System Indications. A **transdermal formulation of scopolamine** can be used to prevent motion sickness. The skin patch slowly releases scopolamine over a period of 3 days and is thought to work by blocking acetylcholine neurotransmission from the vestibular apparatus to the vomiting center in the brainstem. As discussed in Chapter 24, muscarinic receptor blockers are also used in the treatment of Parkinson's disease.

Other Indications. Atropine and glycopyrrolate (see later) are used in two other clinical contexts. First, they are used to prevent muscarinic side effects when cholinesterase inhibitors are given to patients with **myasthenia gravis.** Second, as discussed in Chapter 6, they are used to reverse the muscarinic effects of **cholinesterase inhibitor overdose.** In this setting, supranormal doses may be required to counteract the large concentrations of acetylcholine that have accumulated at acetylcholine synapses, and the atropine dosage must be titrated to the patient's response. Atropine and glycopyrrolate will not counteract the effects of nicotinic receptor activation caused by cholinesterase inhibition. The muscle weakness resulting from nicotinic receptor stimulation can be attenuated by adding pralidoxime to the treatment regimen.

Hyoscyamine

Hyoscyamine, the levorotatory stereoisomer of racemic atropine, is the natural form of the alkaloid that occurs in plants. It is primarily responsible for the pharmacologic effects of atropine. Formulations of hyoscyamine for oral or sublingual administration are used to treat **intestinal spasms** and other gastrointestinal symptoms (see Chapter 28).

Semisynthetic and Synthetic Muscarinic Receptor Antagonists

In the search for a more selective muscarinic receptor antagonist, investigators have developed a large number of semisynthetic and synthetic blocking agents. Although the pharmacologic effects of these agents are **similar to those of atropine,** their unique pharmacokinetic properties are advantageous in specific situations.

Ipratropium and Tiotropium

Ipratropium (ATROVENT) and **tiotropium** (SPIRIVA), quaternary amine derivatives of atropine, are administered by inhalation to patients with **obstructive lung diseases.** Because these drugs are not well absorbed from the lungs into the systemic circulation, they produce few adverse effects. For example, unlike atropine, they do not impair the ciliary clearance of secretions from the airways. This makes them particularly useful in treating patients with **asthma, emphysema,** and **chronic bronchitis.** The respiratory effects and uses of these compounds are discussed more thoroughly in Chapter 27.

Dicyclomine, Oxybutynin, Solifenacin, and Related Drugs

Dicyclomine is a synthetic amine used to relax intestinal smooth muscle and thereby **relieve irritable bowel symptoms,** such as intestinal cramping. **Oxybutynin, tolterodine, darifenacin, solifenacin,** and **trospium** are used to reduce the four major symptoms of an **overactive bladder:** daytime urinary frequency, nocturia (frequent urination at night), urgency, and incontinence. Oxybutynin is now available in both oral and topical (gel) formulations. Compared with other muscarinic receptor antagonists, darifenacin, solifenacin, tolterodine, and trospium appear to have a more selective action on the urinary bladder and may cause fewer adverse effects such as dry mouth and blurred vision. These *uroselective* blockers are administered once or twice daily.

Glycopyrrolate

Glycopyrrolate blocks muscarinic receptors throughout the body. Low doses preferentially inhibit secretions, and the drug is administered preoperatively to inhibit excessive salivary and respiratory tract secretions. It is also used during anesthesia to inhibit the secretory and vagal effects of cholinesterase inhibitors (e.g., **neostigmine**) that are used to reverse nondepolarizing neuromuscular blockade induced by curariform drugs (e.g., **vecuronium**). A new formulation of **glycopyrrolate** (Cuvposa) was recently approved to reduce chronic **severe drooling** in patients aged 3 to 16 years with neurologic conditions such as cerebral palsy.

Tropicamide

Tropicamide is a synthetic drug developed for topical ocular administration as a mydriatic agent (pupil dilator). It is given just before ophthalmoscopy to facilitate **examination of the peripheral retina.** It has a short duration of action (about 1 hour) and is often preferable to atropine and scopolamine for short-term mydriasis.

Pirenzepine

Pirenzepine, a muscarinic receptor antagonist that is selective for M_1 receptors, was developed to reduce vagally-stimulated gastric acid secretion in patients with **peptic ulcers.** It blocks M_1 receptors on paracrine cells and inhibits the release of histamine, a potent gastric acid stimulant. Pirenzepine is available in Canada and Europe but not in the United States. It is currently under investigation for slowing myopia progression in children.

NICOTINIC RECEPTOR ANTAGONISTS

The acetylcholine nicotinic receptor antagonists include **ganglionic blocking agents** and **neuromuscular blocking agents** (Fig. 7.2).

Ganglionic Blocking Agents

Drugs that block autonomic ganglia were among the first drugs to be developed for reducing the excessive activity of the sympathetic or parasympathetic nervous system and indicated for the treatment of severe essential hypertension and malignant hypertension. However, their lack of selectivity for sympathetic or parasympathetic ganglia and numerous adverse effects gradually led to their obsolescence as more selective drugs were discovered. Only **mecamylamine** remains on the market as a ganglionic blocker for treating hypertension.

Neuromuscular Blocking Agents

The **neuromuscular blocking agents** (also referred to as **paralytics** or **muscle relaxants**) bind to the muscle type of nicotinic acetylcholine receptor and inhibit neurotransmission at skeletal neuromuscular junctions, causing muscle weakness and paralysis. These agents can be divided into two groups, one consisting of **nondepolarizing blockers,** which are competitive antagonists at the neuromuscular junction, and the other consisting of the **depolarizing blocker** succinylcholine. The neuromuscular blocking agents are extremely dangerous compounds because they can produce complete respiratory failure in a patient lacking external ventilatory support. The neuromuscular blockers are primarily responsible for the rare occurrence of "anesthesia awareness" during surgery because they can render a patient immobile without affecting mental status.

Nondepolarizing Neuromuscular Blocking Agents

General Properties. The nondepolarizing neuromuscular blocking agents, also known as **curariform drugs,** include **atracurium, cisatracurium, pancuronium, rocuronium,** and **vecuronium.** One of the original drugs, tubocurarine, was extracted from plants used by native South Americans as arrow poisons for hunting wild game. **Curare** is another name for the arrow poisons and their chemical derivatives. The curariform drugs are not well absorbed from the gut and do not cross the blood-brain barrier. Hence, they do not cause poisoning when meat containing these substances is ingested.

Chemistry and Pharmacokinetics. The pharmacologic properties of curariform drugs are listed in Table 7.1. These drugs are positively charged quaternary amines having an amino-steroid structure (pancuronium, rocuronium, and vecuronium) or a benzylisoquinoline structure (atracurium, cisatracurium). The nondepolarizing neuromuscular blocking agents are administered **only by the intravenous route.**

Whereas most nondepolarizing paralytic agents are eliminated by renal and biliary excretion of the unchanged compounds and hepatic metabolites, most of the isomers of **atracurium** are hydrolyzed by plasma esterases. However, the specific isomer known as **cisatracurium** spontaneously decomposes by nonenzymatic chemical (Hoffman) degradation. Hence, **cisatracurium** is the **preferred paralytic agent** for critically ill patients with impaired hepatic and renal function. In patients with normal renal and hepatic function, atracurium and cisatracurium have an intermediate duration of action comparable to that of vecuronium and rocuronium.

Mechanisms and Effects. The curariform drugs act as **competitive antagonists of acetylcholine at nicotinic receptors** in skeletal muscle, and this accounts for their muscle-relaxing effects. After a curariform drug is administered, it first paralyzes the small and rapidly moving muscles of the eyes and face and then paralyzes the larger muscles of the limbs and trunk. Finally, it paralyzes the intercostal muscles and diaphragm, causing respiration to cease. This sequence of paralysis is fortunate in that it enables the relaxation of abdominal muscles for surgical procedures without producing apnea. Respiratory function should always be closely monitored in patients receiving a neuromuscular blocking agent, however.

Curariform drugs **stimulate the release of histamine from mast cells,** and they block autonomic ganglia and muscarinic receptors (see Table 7.1). These actions can cause **bronchospasm, hypotension,** and **tachycardia.** Newer drugs, such as cisatracurium, rocuronium, and vecuronium, tend to cause less histamine release and fewer autonomic side effects than does pancuronium.

Interactions. The muscle-relaxing effects of curariform drugs are **potentiated by volatile inhalational anesthetic**

Sites of action of cholinergic antagonists

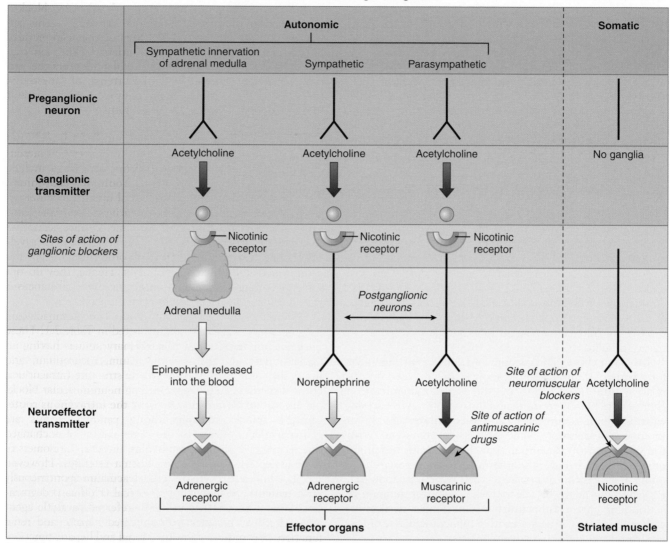

Fig. 7.2 Sites of action of cholinergic antagonists. Autonomic and somatic pathways are shown, and three types of cholinergic antagonists are portrayed. Ganglionic blockers block the first half of both the sympathetic and parasympathetic pathways, and the sympathetic innervation of the adrenal medulla. Antimuscarinic agents block the second half of the parasympathetic pathway only. The site of action of the neuromuscular blockers is only on the nicotinic receptors of the somatic nervous system, which blocks muscle contraction (paralysis).

TABLE 7.1 Properties of Neuromuscular Blocking Agents

DRUG	DEPOLARIZING AGENT	HISTAMINE RELEASE[a]	GANGLIONIC BLOCKADE[b]	EFFECTS REVERSED BY CHOLINESTERASE INHIBITORS	DURATION OF ACTION (MINUTES)	ROUTES OF ELIMINATION
Succinylcholine[c]	Yes	Minimal	None	No	Short (5–10)	Plasma (butyryl) cholinesterase
Atracurium	No	Varies[d]	Low	Yes	Intermediate (30–60)	Plasma esterase
Cisatracurium	No	None	Low	Yes	Intermediate (30–60)	Spontaneous chemical degradation
Pancuronium	No	None	Medium	Yes	Long (60–120)	Renal excretion
Rocuronium	No	None	Low	Yes	Intermediate (30–60)	Biliary and renal excretion
Vecuronium	No	None	Low	Yes	Intermediate (30–60)	Biliary and renal excretion and hepatic metabolism

[a]May cause bronchospasm, hypotension, and excessive salivary and bronchial secretions.
[b]May cause hypotension and tachycardia.
[c]May cause bradycardia by stimulating parasympathetic (vagal) ganglia, or may cause tachycardia and hypertension by stimulating sympathetic ganglia.
[d]At higher doses (e.g., for tracheal intubation), histamine release becomes clinically significant.

agents (e.g., **sevoflurane**) and by the aminoglycoside antibiotics, tetracycline antibiotics, and calcium channel blockers. The effects of paralytic agents are also more pronounced in patients who have neuromuscular disorders such as myasthenia gravis.

The muscle-relaxing effects of curariform drugs can be reversed by administering a **cholinesterase inhibitor** (e.g., **neostigmine**), which acts by increasing acetylcholine levels at the neuromuscular junction and counteracting the neuromuscular blockade. Neostigmine reversal should not be attempted until patients have demonstrated partial recovery of neuromuscular function as measured using a nerve stimulator.

Indications. The neuromuscular blockers are primarily used to induce muscle relaxation during surgery and thereby facilitate surgical manipulations. These drugs are sometimes used as an adjunct to electroconvulsive therapy to prevent injuries that might be caused by involuntary muscle contractions. They are also used to facilitate **intubation** of the respiratory tract to enable ventilation and endoscopic procedures (e.g., bronchoscopy). During the clinical use of neuromuscular blocking agents, the degree of neuromuscular blockade can be determined by monitoring the contraction of a small limb muscle in response to nerve stimulation.

Drug Selection. The selection of a nondepolarizing agent for a particular clinical application is usually based on the relative **duration of action** and the degree of drug-induced changes in blood pressure and heart rate. **Atracurium, cisatracurium, rocuronium,** and **vecuronium** provide an intermediate duration of action (30–60 minutes). With the exception of atracurium, which can cause histamine release at higher doses, the intermediate-acting drugs have minimal effects on cardiovascular and respiratory function. Pancuronium might be selected when a longer duration of action is required. **Tubocurarine is no longer used clinically** because it is associated with a higher incidence of histamine release and other adverse effects.

Pancuronium and rocuronium are used in a number of **state lethal injection protocols.** For example, in the three-drug protocol used in many states, a barbiturate (or less-effectively, a benzodiazepine) is used as the first drug to anesthetize (or sedate with benzodiazepine) the condemned inmate, followed by pancuronium to paralyze the inmate's muscles, and finally potassium chloride infusion to cause death by cardiac arrest. Neuromuscular blockers used in this situation are controversial as if the first drug is not effective or properly administered, the second drug paralyzes the inmate so no response can be made.

Depolarizing Neuromuscular Blocking Agents

Succinylcholine, the only depolarizing agent available for clinical use today, is composed of two covalently linked molecules of acetylcholine. Succinylcholine binds to nicotinic receptors in skeletal muscle and causes **persistent depolarization** of the motor end plate. When the drug is first administered, it produces transient muscle contractions called **fasciculations.** The fasciculations are quickly followed by a **sustained muscle paralysis.** Succinylcholine is not hydrolyzed as rapidly by cholinesterase as is acetylcholine, and this appears to partly account for the persistent depolarization and muscle paralysis.

Table 7.1 compares the properties of succinylcholine with those of the curariform drugs. Succinylcholine has a **short duration of action** (5–10 minutes) owing to its hydrolysis by plasma cholinesterase. The sequence of muscle paralysis produced by succinylcholine is similar to that produced by curariform drugs. The effects of succinylcholine, however, are **not reversed by cholinesterase inhibitors,** and no pharmacologic antidote exists to reverse an overdose of succinylcholine.

Succinylcholine is used to produce muscle relaxation before and during surgery and to facilitate **intubation of the airway.** Because of its shorter duration of action, succinylcholine offers the best chance for resumption of spontaneous breathing if endotracheal intubation proves difficult; thus, it is the preferred neuromuscular blocker for adults with emergency airway situations. Before the drug is administered in a nonemergent situation, patients should be interviewed to screen for personal or family history suggestive of **atypical cholinesterase.** Individuals with this inherited disorder cannot metabolize succinylcholine at normal rates and are susceptible to prolonged neuromuscular paralysis and apnea after receiving the usual doses of the drug.

When possible, a serum potassium level should be obtained before administering succinylcholine. Succinylcholine can cause **hyperkalemia** sufficient to cause cardiac arrest in persons with unhealed skeletal muscle injury such as follows **third-degree burns,** and it should not be used in these individuals until the injury heals. Many conditions involving muscle weakness, such as paralysis caused by spinal cord injury, also present an increased risk of hyperkalemia owing to the upregulation of acetylcholine receptors at the neuromuscular junction. Children are more susceptible to the consequences of hyperkalemia, and succinylcholine is therefore used **less frequently in pediatric patients.** Succinylcholine can also cause postoperative myalgia, particularly in the muscles of the neck, back, and abdomen. This effect probably results from the muscle fasciculations produced by the drug. Finally, succinylcholine has been associated with a rare complication known as **malignant hyperthermia,** which is also associated with inhalation anesthetics (see Chapter 21).

Neuromuscular Blockade Reversal Agent

A drug called **sugammadex** is now available to rapidly reverse the effects of steroidal neuromuscular blocking agents. It is a modified *gamma* (γ)-cyclodextrin compound that forms a tight inactive complex with **rocuronium** and vecuronium that is rapidly excreted in the urine. Sugammadex produces a faster recovery of neuromuscular function than neostigmine and reduces the risk of postoperative respiratory dysfunction. In contrast to cholinesterase inhibitors, sugammadex is effective in subjects demonstrating complete paralysis when tested with a nerve stimulator. Sugammadex appears to be safe and well tolerated.

SUMMARY OF IMPORTANT POINTS

- Muscarinic acetylcholine receptor antagonists relax smooth muscle, increase heart rate and cardiac conduction, and inhibit exocrine gland secretion. They include belladonna alkaloids (e.g., atropine and scopolamine) and semisynthetic and synthetic drugs (e.g., ipratropium).

- Muscarinic blockers are used to treat bradycardia, obstructive lung diseases, intestinal spasms, and overactive urinary bladder. They are also used to reduce salivary and respiratory secretions and to produce mydriasis and cycloplegia.
- Atropine toxicity can cause dryness of the mouth and skin, blurred vision, tachycardia, palpitations, urinary retention, delirium, and hallucinations.
- Nicotinic acetylcholine receptor antagonists include nondepolarizing neuromuscular blocking agents known as *curariform drugs*, such as pancuronium, rocuronium, and cisatracurium. These drugs are used to produce muscle relaxation during surgery.
- Curariform drugs competitively block nicotinic receptors in skeletal muscle. They do not cause muscle fasciculations, and their effects can be reversed by cholinesterase inhibitors.
- Succinylcholine is a depolarizing neuromuscular blocking agent with a short duration of action. It produces muscle fasciculations followed by muscle paralysis. Its effects are not reversed by cholinesterase inhibitors.
- Sugammadex is available to rapidly reverse the effects of steroidal (non-depolarizing) neuromuscular blocking agents.

Review Questions

1. Which drug produces transient muscle fasciculations followed by muscle paralysis that is not reversed by neostigmine?
   (A) rocuronium
   (B) hyoscyamine
   (C) cisatracurium
   (D) succinylcholine
   (E) pancuronium

2. Toxic doses of scopolamine would be expected to cause all of the following effects EXCEPT
   (A) hallucinations.
   (B) bronchospasm.
   (C) hyperthermia.
   (D) urinary retention.
   (E) blurred vision.

3. Topical ocular administration of tropicamide will cause
   (A) contraction of the ciliary muscle.
   (B) vasoconstriction.
   (C) miosis.
   (D) relaxation of the iris sphincter muscle.
   (E) lacrimation.

4. The therapeutic use of darifenacin is based on its ability to
   (A) relax bronchial smooth muscle.
   (B) relax urinary bladder smooth muscle.
   (C) relax uterine smooth muscle.
   (D) inhibit salivary secretions.
   (E) relax gastrointestinal muscle.

5. Sugammadex, used to reverse an overdose with neuromuscular blockers, has a unique mechanism of action best described as which one of the following?
   (A) agonist at cholinergic acetylcholine receptors.
   (B) antagonist at cholinergic acetylcholine receptors.
   (C) antagonist at muscarinic acetylcholine receptors.
   (D) forms an inactive drug complex.
   (E) inhibits acetylcholinesterase.

CHAPTER 8

Sympathetic Neuropharmacology and Adrenergic Agonists

CLASSIFICATION OF ADRENOCEPTOR AGONISTS

Direct-Acting Adrenoceptor Agonists

Catecholamines
- Norepinephrine
- Epinephrine
- Dopamine
- Dobutamine
- Isoproterenol (ISUPREL)

Noncatecholamines
- Phenylephrine (VAZCULEP)
- Midodrine (ORVATEN)
- Albuterol (PROVENTIL, VENTOLIN)
- Salmeterol (SEREVENT)[a]
- Oxymetazoline[b]
- Apraclonidine (IOPIDONE)[c]
- Clonidine (CATAPRES)[d]
- Mirabegron (MYRBETRIQ)

Indirect-Acting Adrenoceptor Agonists
- Cocaine
- Amphetamine
- Solriamfetol (SUNOSI)

Mixed-Acting Adrenoceptor Agonists
- Ephedrine
- Pseudoephedrine (SUDAFED)

Other Drugs
- Metyrosine (DEMSER)
- Droxidopa (NORTHERA)
- Angiotensin II (GIAPREZA)

[a]Also terbutaline (Brethine), fenoterol (Berotec), formoterol (Foradil), arformoterol (Brovana), and levalbuterol (Xopenex).
[b]Also available as oxymetazoline with the local anesthetic, tetracaine, in a nasal spray for dentistry (Kovanaze).
[c]Also brimonidine (Alphagan P).
[d]Also dexmedetomidine (Precedex), tizanidine (Zanaflex), and lofexidine (Lucemyra).

OVERVIEW

Sympathetic Neurotransmission

The sequence of events involved in sympathetic neurotransmission and sites of drug action are illustrated in Fig. 8.1. **Norepinephrine** is synthesized from the amino acid **tyrosine,** which is converted to *dopa* (dihydroxyphenylalanine) by the rate-limiting enzyme in the pathway, tyrosine hydroxylase. *Dopa* is then converted to **dopamine** by dopa decarboxylase, and dopamine is stored in neuronal vesicles and then converted to **norepinephrine** by dopamine β-hydroxylase.

Norepinephrine is released into the synapse by **calcium-mediated exocytosis** in response to nerve stimulation. Once in the synapse, norepinephrine activates postsynaptic *alpha* (α-) and *beta* (β-)adrenoceptors as well as presynaptic autoreceptors that exert negative feedback and inhibit further release of norepinephrine.

Norepinephrine is removed from the synapse primarily by neuronal reuptake via a transport protein known as the *catecholamine transporter* located in the neuronal membrane. The reuptake of norepinephrine limits the duration of presynaptic and postsynaptic receptor activation and enables the neurotransmitter to be used again for neurotransmission. Once inside the neuron, norepinephrine is sequestered in storage vesicles. The catecholamine transporter can also sequester epinephrine and related drugs.

The enzymes **catechol-O-methyltransferase (COMT)** and **monoamine oxidase (MAO)** primarily serve to inactivate norepinephrine not taken up by presynaptic neurons. These enzymes are found in many tissues, including the liver and gut. MAO is also located inside neuronal mitochondria and degrades cytoplasmic norepinephrine not accumulated by storage vesicles.

DRUGS AFFECTING ADRENERGIC NEUROTRANSMISSION

Fig. 8.1 also shows the sites of action of drug that affect adrenergic neurotransmission, including the neuronal blocking agents, such as reserpine and bretylium, used in pharmacology research but no longer have any clinical use.

The synthesis of norepinephrine is inhibited by **metyrosine,** which is a competitive inhibitor of tyrosine hydroxylase. Metyrosine is used to inhibit norepinephrine and epinephrine synthesis in persons with **pheochromocytoma,** an adrenal medullary tumor that secretes large amounts of these substances and causes severe hypertension (see Chapter 10).

The most important drugs used clinically to reduce excessive sympathetic stimulation of various organs are the **adrenoceptor antagonists.** These include **phentolamine,** which selectively blocks α-adrenoceptors; **propranolol,** which selectively blocks β-adrenoceptors; and **labetalol,** which blocks both receptor types. These drugs are described in Chapter 9.

Drugs that bind and activate α- or β-adrenoceptors are known as **direct-acting adrenoceptor agonists,** whereas **indirect-acting agonists** such as cocaine increase the synaptic concentration of norepinephrine as shown in Fig. 8.1. Other drugs inhibit the breakdown of norepinephrine by COMT or MAO. As discussed in Chapters 22 and 24, these inhibitors also exert effects on the central nervous system.

ADRENERGIC NEUROTRANSMISSION

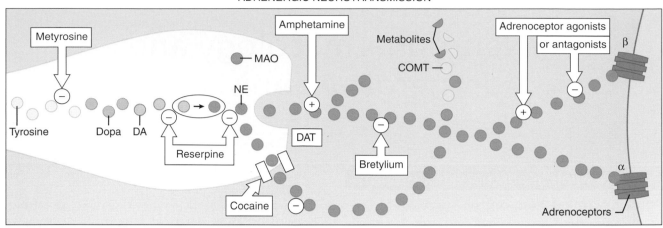

FIG. 8.1 Sympathetic neurotransmission and sites of drug action. Norepinephrine *(NE)* is synthesized from tyrosine in a three-step reaction: tyrosine to dopa (dihydroxyphenylalanine), dopa to dopamine *(DA)*, and dopamine to NE. The conversion of tyrosine to dopa is inhibited by metyrosine. The vesicular storage of DA and NE is blocked by reserpine, and the release of NE in response to nerve stimulation is blocked by bretylium. After activating post-synaptic receptors, NE is sequestered by neuronal reuptake—a process blocked by cocaine. Amphetamine indirectly increases the transport of NE into the synapse. Postsynaptic adrenoceptors are activated or blocked by adrenoceptor agonists or antagonists, respectively. *α*, *α*-adrenoceptors; *β*, *β*-adrenoceptors; *COMT*, catechol-O-methyltransferase; *DAT*, dopamine transponder; *MAO*, monoamine oxidase; (−), inhibits; (+), stimulates.

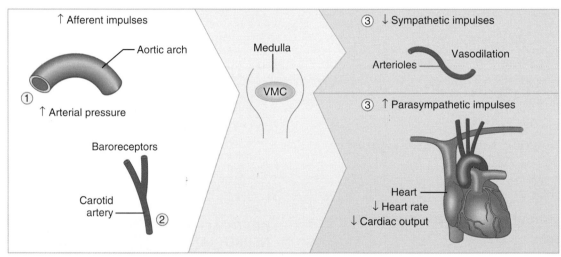

FIG. 8.2 The baroreceptor reflex. (1) Increased arterial pressure activates stretch receptors in the aortic arch and carotid sinus. (2) Receptor activation initiates afferent impulses to the brainstem vasomotor center (VMC). (3) Via solitary tract fibers, the VMC activates the vagal motor nucleus, which increases vagal (parasympathetic) outflow and slows the heart. At the same time, the VMC reduces stimulation of spinal intermediolateral neurons that activate sympathetic preganglionic fibers, and this decreases sympathetic stimulation of the heart and blood vessels. By this mechanism, drugs that increase blood pressure produce reflex bradycardia. Drugs that reduce blood pressure attenuate this response and cause reflex tachycardia.

Drugs Modulating the Baroreceptor Reflex

In addition to exerting their primary pharmacologic actions, a number of adrenoceptor agonists and antagonists modulate the **baroreceptor reflex**, as illustrated in Fig. 8.2.

When a drug or a physiologic action increases blood pressure, this activates stretch receptors (mechanoreceptors) located in the aortic arch and in the carotid sinus at the bifurcation of the carotid artery. Receptor activation initiates impulses that travel via afferent nerves to the brainstem vasomotor center. Stimulation of the vagal motor nucleus (via nerves from the solitary tract nucleus) leads to an increase in vagal (parasympathetic) outflow, a decrease in heart rate, and a decrease in the sympathetic nerve outflow from the vasomotor center. The effect on the heart rate is called **reflex bradycardia.**

If a drug lowers the blood pressure sufficiently, it may reduce the baroreceptor tone and thereby produce an acceleration of the heart rate and activation of sympathetic vasoconstriction. In this case, the effect on the heart rate is called **reflex tachycardia.**

ADRENOCEPTOR AGONISTS

The adrenoceptor agonists are a large group of drugs whose diverse effects make them valuable in the treatment of a number of clinical conditions, ranging from cardiovascular emergencies to the common cold. Although some of these drugs exert their effects on multiple organ systems, others target a specific organ. The spectrum of effects produced by a particular adrenoceptor agonist depends on its affinity for different types of adrenoceptors.

Adrenoceptors

Adrenoceptors were originally classified as **α-adrenoceptors** or **β-adrenoceptors** based on the relative potency of

TABLE 8.1   Properties of Adrenergic, Dopamine, and Imidazoline Receptors

TYPE OF RECEPTOR	MECHANISM OF SIGNAL TRANSDUCTION	EFFECTS
Adrenoceptors		
α_1	Phospholipase C activation, increased IP_3 and release of calcium	Contraction of smooth muscles, exocrine gland secretion, neuronal excitation
α_2	Inhibition of adenylyl cyclase and decreased cAMP	Inhibition of norepinephrine release, decrease in secretion of aqueous humor, decrease in secretion of insulin, platelet aggregation, and central nervous system effects
β_1	Adenylyl cyclase activation, increased cAMP, protein kinase activation	Increase in secretion of renin and increase in heart rate, contractility, and conduction
β_2	Adenylyl cyclase activation, increased cAMP, protein kinase activation	Glycogenolysis, relaxation of smooth muscles, and uptake of potassium in skeletal muscles
β_3	Adenylyl cyclase activation, increased cAMP, protein kinase activation	Lipolysis, thermogenesis in skeletal muscle, uterine relaxation, and other effects
Dopamine receptors		
D_1	Increased cAMP	Relaxation of vascular smooth muscles
D_2	Decreased cAMP, increased potassium currents, and decreased calcium influx	Modulation of neurotransmission in the sympathetic and central nervous systems
Imidazoline receptors	Uncertain; receptors not fully characterized.	Natriuresis and decrease of sympathetic outflow from the central nervous system

cAMP, Cyclic adenosine monophosphate; *IP₃,* inositol triphosphate.

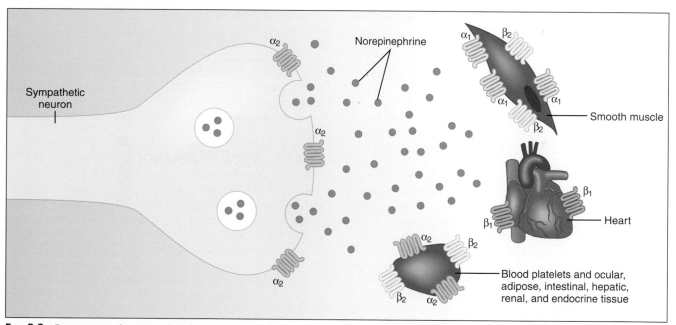

FIG. 8.3   Primary tissue locations of α-adrenoceptors and β-adrenoceptors. Whereas α_1- and β_2-adrenoceptors are primarily located in smooth muscle, β_1-adrenoceptors are predominantly found in cardiac tissue. Some α_2-adrenoceptors are located on sympathetic (and parasympathetic) neurons, where they inhibit neurotransmitter release. Other α_2- and β_2-adrenoceptors are located in blood platelets and a variety of organ tissues. The α- and β-adrenoceptors are also found in the central nervous system.

adrenoceptor agonists in different tissues. For example, epinephrine and norepinephrine are more potent than isoproterenol at adrenoceptors in smooth muscle, and these were designated α-adrenoceptors, whereas isoproterenol is more potent than epinephrine and norepinephrine at adrenoceptors in cardiac tissue, and these receptors were called β-adrenoceptors.

As shown in Table 8.1 and Fig. 8.3, subtypes of α- and β-adrenoceptors have been identified on the basis of several criteria, including differences in signal transduction and physiologic effects and differences in agonist affinity for

different receptors. The receptor subtypes have been cloned and their molecular structures determined.

α-Adrenoceptors

The α-adrenoceptors can be differentiated on the basis of their location and function. The **α_1-adrenoceptors** are primarily located in smooth muscle at sympathetic neuroeffector junctions, but these receptors are also found in exocrine glands and in the central nervous system. Three main subtypes of α_1-adrenoceptors have been identified (α_{1A}, α_{1B}, and α_{1D}), but the functional roles of these receptors have not been clearly established. The α_2-adrenoceptors are widely distributed in presynaptic neurons, various tissues, and blood platelets (see Fig. 8.3)—and subtypes of these receptors have also been identified.

The α_1-adrenoceptors mediate **contraction** of vascular smooth muscle, the iris dilator muscle, and smooth muscle in the lower urinary tract (bladder, urethra, and prostate) and other tissues. The α_2-adrenoceptors located on sympathetic postganglionic neurons serve as **autoreceptors,** whose activation leads to feedback inhibition of norepinephrine release from nerve terminals. The α_2-receptors are also found in blood platelets and in ocular, adipose, intestinal, hepatic, renal, and endocrine tissue. In blood platelets, α_2-receptors mediate platelet aggregation. In the pancreas, α_2-receptors mediate the inhibition of insulin secretion that occurs when the sympathetic nervous system is activated.

β-Adrenoceptors
Table 8.1 summarizes the effects of three subtypes of β-adrenoceptors.

Activation of $\boldsymbol{\beta_1}$**-adrenoceptors** produces cardiac stimulation, leading to a positive **chronotropic effect** (increased heart rate), a positive **inotropic effect** (increased contractility), and a positive **dromotropic effect** (increased cardiac impulse conduction velocity). Activation of β_1-receptors also increases **renin secretion** from renal juxtaglomerular cells.

The $\boldsymbol{\beta_2}$**-adrenoceptors** mediate **relaxation** of bronchial, uterine, and vascular smooth muscle (see Fig. 11.3). In skeletal muscle, β_2-receptors mediate potassium uptake. In the liver, they mediate **glycogenolysis** (breakdown of glycogen and release of glucose), which increases the glucose concentration in the blood. Whereas epinephrine and norepinephrine are equally potent at β_1-receptors in cardiac tissue, epinephrine is more potent than norepinephrine at β_2-receptors in smooth muscle.

A third subtype of the β-adrenoceptor are $\boldsymbol{\beta_3}$**-adrenoceptors.** These receptors mediate **lipolysis** (breakdown of triglycerides in adipose tissue), **thermogenesis** in skeletal muscle, **smooth muscle relaxation,** and other effects. The first selective **agonist** for the β_3-adrenoceptor approved by the US Food and Drug Administration (FDA) was an extended-release formulation of **mirabegron** (see the following section).

Dopamine Receptors
Dopamine receptors are activated by dopamine but not by other adrenoceptor agonists. The subtypes of dopamine receptors include $\mathbf{D_1}$**-receptors,** which mediate vascular smooth muscle relaxation, and $\mathbf{D_2}$**-receptors,** which modulate neurotransmitter release. **Fenoldopam** is a D_1-receptor agonist used in treating acute severe hypertension (see Chapter 10).

Imidazoline Receptors
Imidazoline receptors are activated by adrenoceptor agonists that possess an imidazoline structure. These receptors, which are not cloned or fully characterized, are found in the central nervous system and in several peripheral tissues. The antihypertensive effect of **clonidine** appears to result from activation of both α_2-adrenoceptors and imidazoline receptors in the central nervous system, leading to a reduced

sympathetic outflow to the heart and vascular smooth muscle. The pharmacologic properties of clonidine and related drugs are discussed in Chapter 10.

SIGNAL TRANSDUCTION
The adrenergic and dopamine receptors are guanine nucleotide binding protein–coupled receptors (GPCRs) located in cell membranes of target tissues.

Activation of $\boldsymbol{\alpha_1}$**-adrenoceptors** is coupled with activation of **phospholipase C,** which catalyzes the release of **inositol triphosphate (IP3)** from membrane phospholipids. In smooth muscle, IP_3 stimulates the **release of calcium** from the sarcoplasmic reticulum, leading to muscle contraction. By this action, α_1-adrenoceptor agonists cause vasoconstriction and increase blood pressure. In exocrine glands, formation of IP_3 leads to calcium release and gland secretion.

Activation of $\boldsymbol{\alpha_2}$**-adrenoceptors** leads to **inhibition of adenylyl cyclase** and decreased levels of cyclic adenosine monophosphate (cAMP) in sympathetic neurons and other tissues. This action reduces aqueous humor secretion in the eye and elicits the other effects of α_2-adrenoceptor agonists. Activation of D_2-receptors also **reduces cAMP formation.**

Activation of $\boldsymbol{\beta}$**-adrenoceptors** and D_1-receptors leads to **stimulation of adenylyl cyclase** and an increase in the levels of cAMP in cardiac tissue and smooth muscle. cAMP activates **protein kinase A,** which phosphorylates other proteins and enzymes. The cellular response depends on the specific proteins that are phosphorylated in each tissue. In cardiac tissue, calcium channels are phosphorylated, thereby augmenting calcium influx and cardiac contractility. In smooth muscle, cAMP produces muscle relaxation via effects on multiple targets, including potassium channels, calcium channels, and myosin light chain kinase (see Fig. 11.3).

CLASSIFICATION OF ADRENOCEPTOR AGONISTS
The adrenoceptor agonists mimic the effect of sympathetic nervous system stimulation and are sometimes called **sympathomimetic drugs.** These drugs are divided into three groups based on their mode of action. The **direct-acting agonists** bind and activate adrenoceptors. As shown in Fig. 8.4, the **indirect-acting agonists** increase the stimulation of adrenoceptors by increasing the concentration of norepinephrine at sympathetic neuroeffector junctions in one of two ways. Cocaine inhibits the **catecholamine transporter** located in the plasma membrane of the presynaptic sympathetic neuron and thereby decreases the neuronal reuptake of norepinephrine and increases its synaptic concentration (see Chapter 25). **Amphetamine** and related drugs are transported into the sympathetic nerve terminal by the catecholamine transporter. Once inside the sympathetic neuron, amphetamines inhibit the storage of norepinephrine by neuronal vesicles. This increases the cytoplasmic concentration of norepinephrine, leading to reverse transport of norepinephrine into the synapse by the catecholamine transporter. The **mixed-acting agonists** (e.g., pseudoephedrine) have both direct and indirect actions.

Direct-Acting Adrenoceptor Agonists
The direct-acting agonists include several catecholamines and various noncatecholamine drugs.

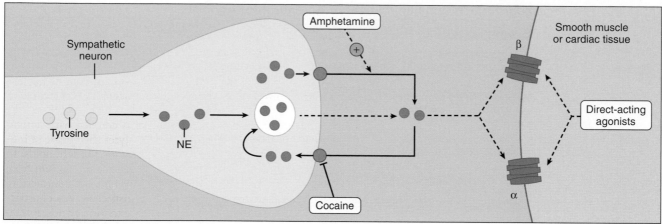

FIG. 8.4 Mechanisms of indirect-acting and direct-acting adrenoceptor agonists. Cocaine blocks norepinephrine reuptake by the catecholamine transporter. Amphetamine inhibits the storage of norepinephrine by neuronal vesicles, leading to reverse transport of norepinephrine into the synapse by the catecholamine transporter. Direct-acting agonists bind to and activate adrenoceptors. α, α-Adrenoceptor; β, β-adrenoceptor; *NE*, norepinephrine.

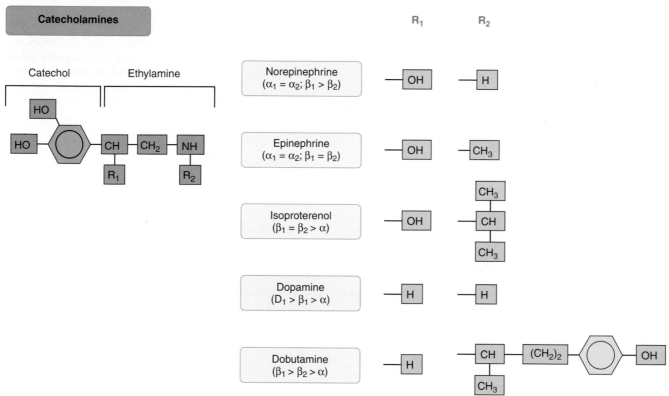

FIG. 8.5 Structures of selected adrenoceptor agonists. Catecholamines contain the catechol moiety and an ethylamine side chain. The amine nitrogen substitution (R_2) determines the relative affinity for α- and β-adrenoceptors, with larger substitutions (e.g., in isoproterenol and dobutamine) decreasing the affinity for α-adrenoceptors and increasing the affinity for β-adrenoceptors. Note that dopamine has an even higher affinity for dopamine D_1 receptors than for adrenoceptors.

Catecholamines

The naturally occurring catecholamines include **norepinephrine,** an endogenous sympathetic neurotransmitter; **epinephrine,** the principal hormone of the adrenal medulla; and **dopamine,** a neurotransmitter and the precursor to norepinephrine and epinephrine. Synthetic catecholamines include **isoproterenol** and **dobutamine.**

Chemistry and Pharmacokinetics. Each catecholamine consists of the catechol moiety and an ethylamine side chain (Fig. 8.5). The catecholamines are rapidly inactivated by MAO and COMT. For this reason, these drugs have low oral bioavailabilities and short plasma half-lives, and they

must be administered parenterally when a systemic action is required (such as in the treatment of anaphylactic shock).

Mechanisms and Effects. As shown in Fig. 8.5 and Table 8.2, the various catecholamines differ in their affinities and specificities for receptors. The size of the alkyl substitution on the amine nitrogen (R_2) determines the relative affinity for α- and β-adrenoceptors. Drugs with a large alkyl group (e.g., isoproterenol) have greater affinity for β-adrenoceptors than do drugs with a small alkyl group (e.g., epinephrine). **Epinephrine** is a potent agonist at all α- and β-adrenoceptors. Norepinephrine differs from epinephrine only in that it has greater affinity for β_1-adrenoceptors than

TABLE 8.2   Pharmacologic Effects and Clinical Uses of Adrenoceptor Agonists

DRUG	PHARMACOLOGIC EFFECT (AND RECEPTOR)	CLINICAL USE
Direct-acting catecholamines		
Dobutamine	Cardiac stimulation (β_1) and vasodilation (β_2)	Cardiogenic shock, acute heart failure, and cardiac stimulation during heart surgery
Dopamine[a]	Renal vasodilation (D_1), cardiac stimulation (β_1), and increased blood pressure (β_1 and α_1)	Cardiogenic shock, septic shock, heart failure, and hypotension; adjunct to fluid administration in hypovolemic shock
Epinephrine	Vasoconstriction (α_1) and cardiac stimulation (β_1) to increase blood pressure; bronchodilation (β_2)	Anaphylaxis, cardiac arrest, ventricular fibrillation; reduction in bleeding during surgery, and prolongation of the action of local anesthetics
Isoproterenol	Cardiac stimulation (β_1) and bronchodilation (β_2)	Atrioventricular block and bradycardia
Norepinephrine	Vasoconstriction and increased blood pressure (α_1)	Hypotension and shock
Direct-acting noncatecholamines		
Albuterol	Bronchodilation (β_2)	Asthma
Brimonidine	Decreased aqueous humor formation (α_2)	Postoperative control of intraocular pressure; open-angle glaucoma and ocular hypertension
Apraclonidine	Decreased aqueous humor formation (α_2)	Short-term presurgical and postoperative control of intraocular pressure
Clonidine	Decreased sympathetic outflow from central nervous system (α_2 and imidazoline)	Hypertension, opioid dependence
Dexmedetomidine	Sedation (α_2)	Adjunct to anesthesia
Midodrine	Vasoconstriction (α_1)	Orthostatic hypotension
Oxymetazoline	Vasoconstriction (α_1)	Nasal and ocular decongestion
Phenylephrine	Vasoconstriction, increased blood pressure, and mydriasis (α_1)	Nasal and ocular decongestion, mydriasis, maintenance of blood pressure, and treatment of shock
Terbutaline	Bronchodilation (β_2)	Asthma, premature labor
Indirect-acting agents		
Amphetamine	Increase in norepinephrine release, central nervous system stimulation	Narcolepsy, attention-deficit disorder
Cocaine	Inhibition of norepinephrine uptake	Local anesthesia
Mixed-acting agents		
Ephedrine	Vasoconstriction (α_1)	Nasal decongestion, bronchodilation, and hypotension
Pseudoephedrine	Vasoconstriction (α_1)	Nasal decongestion

[a]Dopamine is a catecholamine with both direct and indirect actions.

for β_2-adrenoceptors. Because of this difference, norepinephrine constricts all blood vessels, whereas epinephrine constricts some blood vessels but dilates others. **Isoproterenol** is a selective β_1- and β_2-adrenoceptor agonist because it has little affinity for α-receptors. **Dobutamine** primarily stimulates β_1-receptors, with smaller effects on β_2- and α-receptors. **Dopamine** activates D_1-receptors, β_1-receptors, and α-receptors. Unlike the other catecholamines, dopamine also stimulates the release of norepinephrine from sympathetic neurons. For this reason, dopamine is both a direct-acting and an indirect-acting receptor agonist.

Cardiovascular Effects. Fig. 8.6 compares the cardiovascular effects when norepinephrine, epinephrine, isoproterenol, and dopamine are given by intravenous infusion.

The cardiovascular effects of **norepinephrine** primarily result from activation of α_1-adrenoceptors. Activation produces vasoconstriction and increases peripheral resistance, which in turn increases the systolic and diastolic blood pressure. Norepinephrine can cause reflex bradycardia if blood pressure increases sufficiently to activate the baroreceptor reflex.

Epinephrine increases the systolic blood pressure but can increase or decrease the diastolic blood pressure. The increased systolic pressure results partly from an increased heart rate and cardiac output. The effect on diastolic pressure depends on the relative stimulation of α_1- and β_2-adrenoceptors, which mediate vasoconstriction and vasodilation, respectively. Lower doses of epinephrine produce greater stimulation of β_2-receptors than α_1-receptors, especially in the vascular beds of skeletal muscle, thereby causing vasodilation and decreasing diastolic blood pressure. Higher doses produce more vasoconstriction throughout the body and can increase both diastolic and systolic pressure.

Isoproterenol activates β_1- and β_2-adrenoceptors and produces vasodilation and cardiac stimulation. It usually lowers the diastolic and mean arterial pressure, but it can increase the systolic pressure by increasing the heart rate and contractility. Its potent chronotropic effect can cause tachycardia and cardiac arrhythmias. For this reason, an alternative drug (e.g., dobutamine) is usually administered to increase cardiac output in cases of heart failure.

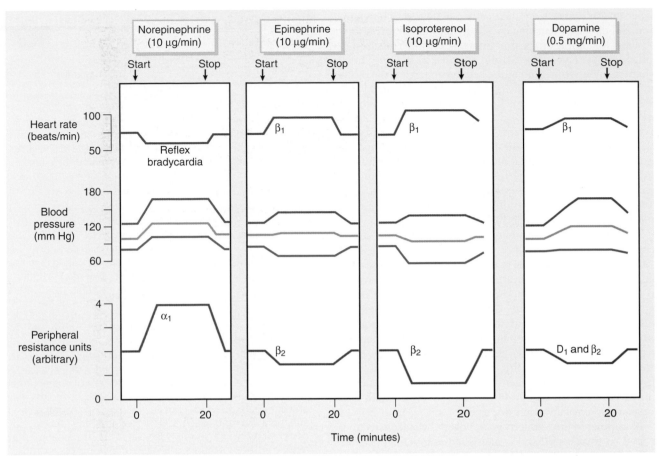

FIG. 8.6 Comparison of the cardiovascular effects of four catecholamines when a low dose of each drug is given by intravenous infusion. *Arrows* indicate when the infusion was started and stopped. The blood pressure recordings show systolic, diastolic, and mean arterial pressure. Peripheral resistance is expressed on an arbitrary scale, ranging from 0 to 4 units. The reflex mechanism, adrenoceptors (α_1, β_1, and β_2), or dopamine (D_1) receptors responsible for changes in the heart rate and peripheral resistance are illustrated. Norepinephrine increases peripheral resistance and blood pressure, and this leads to reflex bradycardia. Epinephrine increases heart rate while reducing peripheral resistance, and the mean arterial blood pressure increases slightly. Isoproterenol increases heart rate but significantly lowers peripheral resistance, and the mean arterial pressure declines. Dopamine increases heart rate (and increases cardiac output) while lowering vascular resistance, and the mean arterial pressure increases.

Dobutamine selectively increases myocardial contractility and stroke volume while producing a smaller increase in heart rate. These actions can increase cardiac output in persons with acute heart failure. Dobutamine also reduces vascular resistance by activating β_2-adrenoceptors, thereby reducing the impedance to ventricular ejection. In patients with heart failure, this effect contributes to an increased stroke volume and cardiac output (see Chapter 12).

When given in low doses, **dopamine** selectively activates D_1-receptors in renal and other vascular beds, thereby causing vasodilation and an increase in renal blood flow. At slightly higher doses, dopamine activates β_1-adrenoceptors in the heart, thereby stimulating cardiac contractility and increasing cardiac output and tissue perfusion. At even higher doses, dopamine activates α_1-adrenoceptors and causes vasoconstriction.

Respiratory Tract Effects. Epinephrine and isoproterenol are potent bronchodilators. Although they have been used in the treatment of asthma, more selective β_2-adrenoceptor agonists are usually employed for this purpose today.

Adverse Effects. Catecholamines can cause excessive **vasoconstriction,** leading to tissue ischemia and necrosis. Localized tissue ischemia can result from extravasation of an intravenous drug infusion or from the accidental injection of epinephrine into a finger, such as when a patient is self-injecting epinephrine to stop an acute allergic reaction. The administration of excessive doses of catecholamines can reduce blood flow to vital organs, such as the kidneys, or cause **excessive cardiac stimulation** that leads tachycardia and other cardiac dysrhythmias. The β-adrenoceptor agonists can cause **hyperglycemia** secondary to glycogenolysis, and this is usually undesirable in patients with diabetes.

Specific Drugs

Catecholamines are used to treat several types of **shock.** Shock is a condition in which the circulation to vital organs is profoundly reduced as a result of inadequate blood volume **(hypovolemic shock),** inadequate cardiac function **(cardiogenic shock),** or inadequate vasomotor tone **(neurogenic shock and septic shock).** Septic shock is associated with massive vasodilation secondary to the production of toxins by pathogenic microorganisms. It is sometimes called "warm shock" to distinguish it from hypovolemic and cardiogenic shock in which the patient's extremities are usually cold because of inadequate blood flow. Some cases of septic shock, however, may also cause hypoperfusion and cold extremities. **Anaphylactic shock,** resulting from severe immediate hypersensitivity reactions, is usually manifested by hypotension and difficult breathing caused by bronchoconstriction.

Catecholamine drugs that increase blood pressure are called **vasopressors.** These drugs are used in treating shock when organ function is impaired because mean arterial blood pressure is less than 60 mm Hg. **Hypovolemia** should always be corrected by intravenous fluid administration before the use of vasopressors because vasopressors will not be effective if hypovolemia is present. In cases of cardiogenic shock, mechanical devices (e.g., the intraaortic balloon pump) are usually superior to pharmacologic agents in their ability to improve coronary artery perfusion and cardiac performance while reducing myocardial ischemia and cardiac work. Such devices are often used in conjunction with vasopressor drugs in the treatment of this condition.

Dopamine is used to treat **septic** or **cardiogenic shock** when patients remain hypotensive despite adequate fluid administration. Dopamine is usually started at a dose of 2 mg/kg body weight per minute, and then the dose is titrated to achieve the desired blood pressure. Although low doses of dopamine can increase urine output by augmenting renal blood flow in normal subjects, ample evidence indicates that low doses of dopamine are usually not effective in preventing and treating **acute renal failure.** The most effective means of protecting the kidneys in patients with shock appears to be the maintenance of mean arterial pressure of greater than 60 mm Hg with intravenous fluids and adequate doses of a vasopressor agent.

Norepinephrine, which is a **potent vasoconstrictor,** is used to treat septic shock and is often given to persons with cardiogenic shock when the response to dopamine is inadequate or is accompanied by marked tachycardia. Norepinephrine is also used to treat hypotension caused by decreased peripheral resistance that can occur in persons who have received excessive doses of a vasodilator drug. **Phenylephrine** is also used for this purpose, as described later in this chapter.

In cases of **anaphylaxis, epinephrine** is the treatment of choice (Box 8.1). By producing bronchodilation and increasing blood pressure, epinephrine counteracts the effects of histamine and other mediators that are released from mast cells and basophils during immediate hypersensitivity reactions. Epinephrine is used as a vasoconstrictor to **reduce bleeding** during surgery and to **prolong the action of local anesthetics** by retarding their absorption into the general circulation. Epinephrine is also used as a cardiac stimulant in the treatment of **cardiac arrest** and **ventricular fibrillation.** Isoproterenol is used to treat refractory **bradycardia** and **atrioventricular block** when other measures have not been successful. Although it has been used to treat **asthma,** a selective β_2-adrenoceptor agonist is usually preferred for this indication because it does not increase the heart rate as much as isoproterenol.

Dobutamine is a cardiac stimulant (inotropic agent) that also produces vasodilation. It is used as a **cardiac stimulant during heart surgery** and in the short-term management of **acute heart failure** and **cardiogenic shock.** Dobutamine is not routinely used in treating septic shock, however, because its vasodilator effect can further reduce vascular resistance and blood pressure. Its utility in hypotensive patients is limited to situations in which hypotension is caused by bradycardia.

BOX 8.1 A CASE OF AIRWAY OBSTRUCTION

CASE PRESENTATION
A 6-year-old boy sustained a bee sting on the tongue. He developed edema of the face, lips, eyelids, tongue, and throat and experienced breathing difficulties. Paramedics administered epinephrine intramuscularly and transported the patient to the hospital, where he received oxygen and intravenous dexamethasone (a corticosteroid). The child previously had an allergic reaction to a bee sting that did not require hospitalization. Because of his respiratory distress, he was intubated and mechanically ventilated for 24 hours. The edema subsided, and the boy was extubated and discharged in good condition.

CASE DISCUSSION
Insect stings are common and can result in immediate hypersensitivity reactions that range from localized pain and rash to more severe reactions involving laryngeal edema, bronchospasm, and hypotension. Stings in the oropharyngeal area have a greater potential to cause airway obstruction and may require intubation and more aggressive treatment than stings in other areas of the body. Hypersensitivity reactions are mediated by immunoglobulin E, which cross-links antigens on mast cells and basophils, leading to the release of histamine and other chemical mediators that cause edema and laryngospasm. The primary treatment of severe hypersensitivity reactions (anaphylaxis) is the immediate intramuscular administration of epinephrine. Some patients require oxygen, and corticosteroids may prevent delayed bronchoconstriction by counteracting inflammation and edema. Hypotension and shock may occur in the most severe cases, and these reactions may require intravenous fluids, oxygen, and vasopressor drugs.

Noncatecholamines

These drugs do not contain a catechol moiety, and they are not substrates for COMT. Some of the noncatecholamines are also resistant to degradation by MAO. For this reason, noncatecholamines are effective after oral administration and have a longer duration of action than do catecholamines.

Phenylephrine

Pharmacokinetics. Phenylephrine is adequately absorbed after oral or topical administration and can also be administered parenterally. The drug is partly metabolized by MAO in the intestine and liver.

Mechanisms and Effects. Phenylephrine activates α_1-adrenoceptors and causes **smooth muscle contraction.** This produces vasoconstriction and increases vascular resistance and blood pressure. Ocular administration of phenylephrine leads to contraction of the iris dilator muscle and dilation of the pupil **(mydriasis).**

Indications. Phenylephrine is used as a **nasal decongestant** in patients with **viral rhinitis,** an infection that can be caused by more than a hundred serotypes of rhinovirus, as well as other viruses, and is referred to as the "common cold." Phenylephrine is also used by patients with **allergic rhinitis,** an inflammation of the nasal mucosa caused by histamine released from mast cells during allergic reactions. The drug's vasoconstrictive effect on the nasal mucosa reduces vascular congestion and mucus secretion to open the nasal passages and facilitate breathing. Both topical and oral preparations are available for this purpose.

In patients with **allergic conjunctivitis**, an inflammation of the eyes associated with hay fever or other allergies, phenylephrine can be used as a topical **ocular decongestant**. The ocular preparation of phenylephrine is also used to induce **mydriasis** and thereby facilitate ophthalmoscopic examination of the retina. In contrast to the muscarinic receptor antagonists used for this purpose (e.g., **tropicamide**), phenylephrine does not relax the ciliary muscle to prevent accommodation for near vision.

Phenylephrine can be administered intravenously to treat forms of **hypotension** and **shock** caused by decreased peripheral vascular resistance. These include hypotension caused by excessive doses of vasodilator drugs, drug-induced shock, septic shock, and neurogenic shock such as resulting from spinal cord injury. Phenylephrine is also used to **maintain blood pressure during surgery** (e.g., when hypotension is induced by anesthetic agents).

Midodrine

Midodrine forms an active metabolite that selectively **activates α_1-adrenoceptors** in the arteriolar and venous circulation, leading to increased systolic and diastolic blood pressure in the standing, sitting, and supine positions. The drug is rapidly absorbed after oral administration and is used to treat postural (orthostatic) hypotension in persons who are considerably impaired by this condition (e.g., those with severe diabetic autonomic neuropathy). It is also used to treat hypotension caused by infections in infants or induced by psychotropic agents and hypotension in persons undergoing renal dialysis. The primary adverse effect of midodrine is **hypertension** when persons are supine.

Albuterol, Salmeterol, Terbutaline, and Related Drugs

Chemistry and Pharmacokinetics. Albuterol, salmeterol, and terbutaline are examples of selective β_2-adrenoceptor agonists that can be given by inhalation. Albuterol and terbutaline can also be given orally, and terbutaline is available for injection. The oral bioavailability of these drugs is 30% to 50% because of their incomplete absorption and first-pass metabolism. They are partly metabolized to inactive compounds before undergoing renal excretion. About 50% of albuterol is converted to an inactive sulfate conjugate. These drugs are often administered by inhalation in the treatment of respiratory diseases. Their duration of action is about 4 to 6 hours after inhalation or oral administration.

Mechanisms, Effects, and Indications. The β_2-adrenoceptor agonists cause smooth muscle relaxation in several tissues. These drugs produce bronchodilation and are beneficial in the treatment of **asthma** and chronic obstructive lung diseases (e.g., **COPD**). Several other β_2-adrenoceptor agonists have been introduced to treat asthma, including **fenoterol**, **formoterol**, **arformoterol**, **levalbuterol**, and **salmeterol**, known collectively as *long-acting β-agonists* (LABAs). The properties and use of these drugs are described in Chapter 27.

Terbutaline is also used off label in the short-term management of **preterm (premature) labor**, which is defined as labor that begins before the 37th week of gestation. The drug relaxes the uterus and maintains pregnancy for 24 to 48 hours in the majority of cases, which is called **tocolysis**. Although the tocolytic effect is of limited duration and value, the treatment may delay delivery long enough to enable corticosteroids to be given to prevent neonatal respiratory distress syndrome. The FDA has recently added a warning to injectable terbutaline products stating that the drug **should not be used in pregnant women** for prevention or prolonged treatment (beyond 48–72 hours) of preterm labor because of the risk of serious and potentially fatal maternal heart problems.

The adverse effects of albuterol and other selective β_2-adrenoceptor agonists include **tachycardia, muscle tremor,** and **nervousness** caused by activation of β_2-adrenoceptors in the heart, skeletal muscle, and central nervous system.

Imidazoline Drugs

Chemistry and Pharmacokinetics. The imidazoline compounds activate α-adrenergic and imidazoline receptors. Some imidazolines are administered by topical ocular or nasal administration, whereas others are administered by systemic routes. After systemic administration, these drugs are partly metabolized and then excreted in the urine and have a duration of action lasting several hours.

Mechanisms, Effects, and Indications. Based on their clinical use, the imidazolines can be divided into three groups. The first group consists of **oxymetazoline** and similar drugs that selectively activate α_1-adrenoceptors and cause vasoconstriction. These drugs are used as topical **nasal** and **ocular decongestants**. Oxymetazoline is available as a nasal spray and ophthalmic solution without prescription. Because it may increase blood pressure, it should not be used by persons with hypertension or heart disease without consulting a health care provider. Topical nasal decongestants should never be used for more than 3 to 5 days to avoid **rebound congestion** that results from excessive vasoconstriction and tissue ischemia. Oxymetazoline and similar decongestants can also cause central nervous system and cardiovascular depression if they are absorbed into the systemic circulation and distributed to the brain. For this reason, these drugs should be used with caution in children under 6 years of age and in the elderly.

Both **epinephrine** and **oxymetazoline** are used as vasoconstrictors in local anesthetic formulations. The coadministration of a vasoconstrictor with a local anesthetic limits the systemic absorption of the local anesthetic. This increases the duration of action and decreases adverse effects (see Chapter 21).

The second group of imidazoline compounds includes **apraclonidine** and **brimonidine**. After topical ocular administration, these agents activate ocular α_2-adrenoceptors in the ciliary body and thereby reduce aqueous humor secretion (see Box 6.1). Apraclonidine and brimonidine are both used to prevent short-term elevations of intraocular pressure after **cataract surgery** and other types of ocular surgery. The utility of these drugs as single agents in treating chronic open-angle glaucoma is limited by the development of tolerance within several months of starting therapy. However, a fixed combination of brimonidine and the carbonic anhydrase inhibitor brinzolamide (see Chapter 13) has been found to be an effective treatment for open-angle glaucoma and ocular hypertension and may be particularly useful in patients unable to tolerate β-adrenoceptor antagonists such as timolol.

The third group of imidazoline agents consists of **clonidine, dexmedetomidine,** and **tizanidine,** which selectively activate α_2-adrenoceptors in the central nervous system. In fact, clonidine has a 200-fold greater affinity for α_2- than for α_1-adrenoceptors. Activation of α_2-adrenoceptors leads to a reduction in sympathetic outflow from the vasomotor center in the medulla, and clonidine is used to treat **hypertension** (see Chapter 10). The activation of α_2-adrenoceptors in the central nervous system is also responsible for the sedative and analgesic effects of clonidine and dexmedetomidine. Clonidine has been used to for sedation during pediatric procedures and to reduce anxiety and anesthetic requirements in pediatric surgery. It has also been used to treat attention deficit/hyperactivity disorder (ADHD) in children and adolescents by reducing the firing rate of neurons releasing norepinephrine in the prefrontal cortex, and thereby reducing impulsivity and hyperactivity. Clonidine is also used for treating insomnia in ADHD patients, and it has been used in persons being treated for **drug dependence** (see Chapter 25), where it facilitates withdrawal and abstinence from opioids, benzodiazepines, alcohol, and cocaine. The newest clonidine-like drug is **lofexidine** and the first such agent specifically indicated for **reduction of opioid withdrawal symptoms** to ease abrupt opioid discontinuation in adults.

Dexmedetomidine is indicated for sedation of intubated and mechanically ventilated patients during treatment in an intensive care setting. It has also been used as an **adjunct to anesthesia** during surgical procedures because of its ability to facilitate sedation and analgesia and to prevent delirium during emergence from anesthesia. Dexmedetomidine has the advantage of not causing respiratory depression in these settings.

Tizanidine (ZANAFLEX) also activates α_2-adrenoceptors in the central nervous system and produces muscle relaxation from a central action. It is used to treat conditions with **muscle spasticity** arising from spinal cord injury or multiple sclerosis and other neurodegenerative diseases (see Chapter 24).

Mirabegron

Preclinical studies using cell lines transfected with human adrenoceptors showed that **mirabegron** is a selective agonist of the β_3-adrenoceptor. Mirabegron relaxes the detrusor smooth muscle which increases urinary bladder capacity. Mirabegron is indicated for the treatment of overactive bladder with symptoms urge urinary incontinence, urgency, and urinary frequency. The commonly listed but rare adverse effect of **angioedema** is noted (see Chapter 4). There is also a warning that mirabegron can **increase in blood pressure,** negating its use in patients with uncontrolled hypertension. There are also mirabegron-drug interactions for many drugs that share **metabolism at the CYP2D6** hepatic enzyme as mirabegron inhibits the activity of this enzyme.

Droxidopa

Droxidopa is a recently approved drug for treatment of orthotension with a nonreceptor medicated mechanism of action. Droxidopa is a **precursor to norepinephrine** in its biosynthetic pathway and effectively increases the amount of norepinephrine produced and released. Norepinephrine then acts as per usual on α_1-receptors in the blood vessels to constrict vascular smooth muscle and raise blood pressure.

Recently, the human kidney hormone **angiotensin II** was approved and marketed under the brand name of GIAPREZA. It is indicated for the treatment of **hypotension in septic shock.** Further discussion of the angiotensin pathway and use of angiotensin receptor blockers to treat hypertension is presented in Chapter 10.

Indirect-Acting Adrenoceptor Agonists
Amphetamine and Tyramine

Amphetamine and related compounds have high lipid solubility and increase synaptic concentrations of norepinephrine in the central and peripheral nervous systems by mechanisms previously described, causing vasoconstriction, cardiac stimulation, increased blood pressure, and central nervous system stimulation. The **central nervous system effects** are discussed in greater detail in Chapters 22 and 25.

Tyramine is a naturally occurring amine found in a number of foods, including bananas. Under normal conditions, tyramine is rapidly degraded by MAO in the gut and liver. In patients receiving **MAO inhibitors** for the treatment of depression, however, tyramine can be absorbed from foods in an amount sufficient to exert a sympathomimetic effect and increase blood pressure markedly. The interaction between foods containing tyramine and MAO inhibitors is discussed in Chapter 22. Tyramine is not available for clinical use.

Cocaine

Cocaine, a naturally occurring alkaloid, acts as a **local anesthetic** and also stimulates the sympathetic nervous system by blocking the neuronal reuptake of norepinephrine at both peripheral and central synapses. The sympathomimetic effects of cocaine are similar to those of amphetamine. Cocaine produces both vasoconstriction and cardiac stimulation and elevates blood pressure. The vasoconstrictive effect can cause ischemia and necrosis of the nasal mucosa in people who abuse cocaine. The sympathomimetic effects of cocaine also appear to be responsible for the severe hypertension and cardiac damage that may occur in people who abuse cocaine. The **local anesthetic** and **central nervous system effects** of cocaine are discussed further in Chapter 21. Cocaine also **blocks the reuptake of dopamine,** leading to its rewarding effects and drug abuse, as discussed in Chapter 25.

Solriamfetol was recently approved by the FDA with an **orphan drug** designation (see Chapter 4). It is a dopamine and norepinephrine reuptake inhibitor (DNRI) approved to increase wakefulness in adult patients who experience excessive daytime sleepiness due to narcolepsy or obstructive sleep apnea (OSA). By blocking the reuptake of dopamine and norepinephrine, wakefulness is promoted by increased availability of those neurotransmitters in the brain.

Mixed-Acting Adrenoceptor Agonists

A few drugs activate adrenoceptors by both direct and indirect mechanisms, including **dopamine** (see earlier), **ephedrine,** and **pseudoephedrine.** These agents indirectly increase synaptic concentrations of norepinephrine in a manner similar to that of amphetamine.

Ephedrine and Pseudoephedrine

Pharmacokinetics. Ephedrine is a naturally occurring alkaloid obtained from plants of the genus *Ephedra*, which is also called *ma huang*. **Pseudoephedrine,** an isomer of ephedrine, is used as a nasal decongestant in the treatment of colds and allergies. It is well absorbed from the gut and has sufficient lipid solubility to enter the central nervous system. Pseudoephedrine is relatively resistant to metabolism by MAO and COMT, contributing to a duration of action of several hours.

Mechanism, Effects, and Indications. Ephedrine and pseudoephedrine **activate α- and β-adrenoceptors** by direct and indirect mechanisms. Via the activation of α_1-adrenoceptors, these drugs produce vasoconstriction, making them useful as **nasal decongestants** in the treatment of **viral** and **allergic rhinitis.** Because of the risks of adverse effects and limited evidence of effectiveness, the FDA recommends that **cough and cold medications,** including those containing pseudoephedrine and phenylephrine, should not be used in children under 6 years of age. These products often contain combinations of decongestants, antihistamines, and cough suppressants.

By activating β-adrenoceptors, ephedrine and pseudoephedrine produce **bronchodilation,** and ephedrine preparations were historically used in the treatment of asthma, but selective β_2-adrenoceptor agonists are considered more safe and effective for this purpose.

The adverse effects of ephedrine and pseudoephedrine include **tachycardia** and **increased blood pressure.** Urinary retention may result from α_1-adrenoceptor activation and contraction of the sphincter muscle of the bladder, especially in men with prostatic hypertrophy. These drugs also cause central nervous system stimulation and insomnia.

Availability and Legal Status. The availability of ephedrine and pseudoephedrine is now restricted in the United States by the **Combat Methamphetamine Epidemic Act** and by various state acts because the drugs have been used illegally to synthesize methamphetamine. These acts provide that only limited quantities of single-ingredient pseudoephedrine preparations can be purchased without a prescription and stipulate several record-keeping requirements. Some states have implemented tracking systems to prevent multiple purchases at different locations, and the quantity and dosage of ephedrine and pseudoephedrine products available for purchase without a prescription is now limited in most US states. Herbal preparations containing *Ephedra* were formerly used to suppress appetite as an aid to losing weight, but the FDA has banned the sale of such products because **fatalities** have resulted from excessive cardiovascular stimulation following their use.

SUMMARY OF IMPORTANT POINTS

- Norepinephrine is synthesized from tyrosine in sympathetic nerve terminals. The conversion of tyrosine to dopa is inhibited by metyrosine, a drug used in treating pheochromocytoma.
- Direct-acting adrenoceptor agonists bind and activate α- and β-adrenoceptors, whereas indirect-acting agonists, such as cocaine, increase the synaptic concentration of norepinephrine.
- Activation of α_1-adrenoceptors mediates smooth muscle contraction, leading to vasoconstriction, dilation of the pupils, and contraction of the bladder sphincter muscle. Phenylephrine and pseudoephedrine cause α_1-receptor-mediated vasoconstriction and are used as nasal decongestants.

- Activation of α_2-adrenoceptors inhibits the release of norepinephrine from sympathetic neurons, decreases the secretion of aqueous humor, and decreases the secretion of insulin. Selective α_2-adrenoceptor agonists are used to reduce intraocular pressure (apraclonidine and brimonidine), reduce systemic blood pressure (clonidine), produce sedation (dexmedetomidine), and facilitate drug abstinence (clonidine, lofexidine).
- Activation of β_1-adrenoceptors produces cardiac stimulation and increases the secretion of renin, whereas activation of β_2-adrenoceptors mediates smooth muscle relaxation. The β_1-adrenoceptor agonists—such as dobutamine—are used to increase cardiac output and blood pressure, whereas the β_2-adrenoceptor agonists—such as albuterol—are employed as bronchodilators in treating asthma.
- The catecholamines include norepinephrine, epinephrine, isoproterenol, dopamine, and dobutamine. These drugs are rapidly metabolized, must be administered parenterally, and are used primarily to treat cardiac disorders and various types of shock.
- In addition to activating adrenoceptors, dopamine activates D_1-receptors and thereby increases renal blood flow.
- Noncatecholamines (e.g., phenylephrine, albuterol, pseudoephedrine) are resistant to degradation by COMT and have a longer duration of action than catecholamines.

Review Questions

1. Which property is characteristic of the sympathetic nervous system?
   - (A) discrete activation of specific organs
   - (B) long preganglionic neurons
   - (C) action terminated by cholinesterase
   - (D) inhibits the enteric nervous system
   - (E) activated by increased arterial blood pressure
2. A man is given a drug that inhibits the synthesis of norepinephrine. Which response would result from this treatment?
   - (A) diarrhea
   - (B) bronchodilation
   - (C) renin secretion
   - (D) decreased heart rate
   - (E) salivation
3. A man with diabetic autonomic neuropathy complains of dizziness and fainting when arising from bed in the morning. Which drug would be most beneficial to this patient?
   - (A) dobutamine
   - (B) albuterol
   - (C) midodrine
   - (D) clonidine
   - (E) isoproterenol
4. A woman is given topical ocular apraclonidine after cataract surgery. Which mechanism is responsible for the desired effect?
   - (A) inhibition of adenylyl cyclase
   - (B) activation of adenylyl cyclase
   - (C) activation of phospholipase C
   - (D) inhibition of phospholipase C
   - (E) release of calcium from the sarcoplasmic reticulum

5. A child with asthma is being treated with albuterol to prevent bronchospasm. Which side effect is typically associated with this drug?
   (A) sedation
   (B) rapid heart rate
   (C) muscle weakness
   (D) low blood pressure
   (E) blurred vision

6. After being stung by a bee, a child is given an intramuscular injection of epinephrine. Which action would lead to bronchodilation?
   (A) increased cAMP levels
   (B) increased cyclic guanosine monophosphate (cGMP) levels
   (C) increased IP3 levels
   (D) calcium influx
   (E) sequestration of calcium

CHAPTER 9

Adrenergic Receptor Antagonists

OVERVIEW

Excessive sympathetic nervous system activity contributes to a number of diseases, including common cardiovascular disorders, such as **hypertension, angina pectoris, and cardiac dysrhythmias.** Drugs that reduce sympathetic stimulation, **sympatholytic drugs,** are used in the management of cardiovascular diseases and other diseases such as glaucoma, migraine headache, and urinary obstruction. The adrenoceptor antagonists are the most important group of sympatholytic drugs used today. The sympathetic neuronal blocking agents (reserpine, guanethidine) discussed in Chapter 6 also have a sympatholytic effect but are no longer used clinically.

The **adrenoceptor antagonists** include drugs that block α-adrenoceptors, β-adrenoceptors, or both. Their **therapeutic effects** are almost entirely caused by blockade of α_1- and β_1-adrenoceptors. Blockade of α_1-adrenoceptors relaxes vascular and other smooth muscles in tissues innervated by the sympathetic nervous system, whereas blockade of β_1-adrenoceptors reduces sympathetic stimulation of the heart. Blockade of α_2- or β_2-adrenoceptors is responsible for many of the adverse effects of these drugs, and drugs that selectively block either α_1- or β_1-adrenoceptors have been developed in an effort to avoid these adverse effects.

α-ADRENOCEPTOR ANTAGONISTS

The α-adrenoceptor antagonists, or **α-blockers,** can be distinguished on the basis of their selectivity for adrenoceptor subtypes and by their noncompetitive or competitive blockade of these receptors.

Nonselective α-Blockers

Agents that block both α_1- and α_2-adrenoceptors are called **nonselective α-blockers.** Phenoxybenzamine and phentolamine are examples. Phenoxybenzamine is a **noncompetitive antagonist,** and phentolamine is a **competitive antagonist.**

Phenoxybenzamine

Pharmacokinetics and Mechanism of Action. Phenoxybenzamine is administered orally and undergoes nonenzymatic chemical transformation to an active metabolite that forms a long-lasting covalent bond with α-adrenoceptors, resulting in noncompetitive receptor blockade (Fig. 9.1). The drug exhibits a slow onset of action owing to the time required to form its active metabolite, but it has a long duration of action of 3 to 4 days because of its stable drug-receptor binding.

Effects and Indications. Phenoxybenzamine decreases vascular resistance and lowers both supine and standing blood pressure. As shown in Table 9.1, phenoxybenzamine is used to treat **hypertensive episodes** in patients with **pheochromocytoma,** which is a tumor of the adrenal medulla that secretes huge amounts of catecholamines, causing extremely high blood pressure. In this setting, phenoxybenzamine is used to control hypertension until surgery can be performed to remove the tumor (Box 9.1).

Phentolamine

Chemistry and Pharmacokinetics. Phentolamine is an imidazoline compound that is structurally related to oxymetazoline and other agents in the imidazoline class of adrenoceptor agonists (see Chapter 8). After intravenous administration, the onset of action is almost immediate, and the duration of action is 10 to 15 minutes. After intramuscular or subcutaneous administration, the onset of action is 15 to 20 minutes, and the duration is 3 to 4 hours. The drug is metabolized chiefly in the liver before excretion in the urine.

Mechanisms, Effects, and Indications. Phentolamine is a competitive adrenoceptor antagonist (see Fig. 9.1) that produces vasodilation, decreases peripheral vascular resistance, and decreases blood pressure. It is used in the treatment of **acute hypertensive episodes** caused by

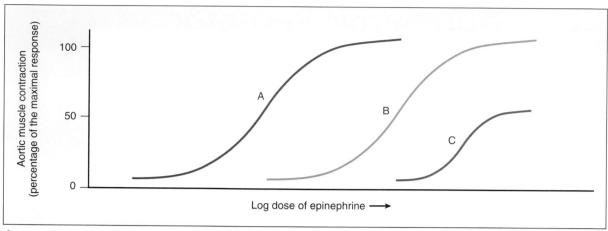

FIG. 9.1 Competitive and noncompetitive blockade of epinephrine-induced aortic smooth muscle contraction by phentolamine and phenoxybenzamine. Three dose-response curves are compared. (A) is the curve of epinephrine alone, and (B) is the curve of epinephrine in the presence of phentolamine. Because phentolamine is a competitive α-adrenoceptor antagonist, epinephrine can surmount its effect. (C) is the curve of epinephrine in the presence of phenoxybenzamine. Because phenoxybenzamine is a noncompetitive antagonist, it reduces the maximal effect of epinephrine.

TABLE 9.1   Mechanism, Effects, and Clinical Use of Adrenoceptor Antagonists

DRUG	MECHANISM OF ACTION	PHARMACOLOGIC EFFECTS	CLINICAL USE
α-blockers			
Alfuzosin, tamsulosin	Competitive α_1-blocker	Relax bladder, urethral, and prostate smooth muscle	Urinary symptoms caused by benign prostatic hyperplasia
Doxazosin, prazosin, terazosin	Competitive α_1-blocker	Cause vasodilation and decrease blood pressure; relax bladder, urethral, and prostate smooth muscle	Hypertension; urinary symptoms caused by benign prostatic hyperplasia
Phenoxybenzamine	Noncompetitive α_1- and α_2-blocker	Causes vasodilation; decreases blood pressure	Hypertension in pheochromocytoma
Phentolamine	Competitive α_1- and α_2-blocker	Causes vasodilation; decreases vascular resistance and blood pressure	Hypertension in pheochromocytoma; treat necrosis and ischemia after injection of an α-adrenoceptor agonist
β-blockers			
Acebutolol	β_1-blocker with ISA and MSA	Decreases cardiac rate, output, O_2 demand, AV node conduction, and blood pressure	Hypertension; cardiac dysrhythmias
Atenolol	β_1-blocker	Same as acebutolol	Hypertension; angina pectoris; acute myocardial infarction
Betaxolol	β_1-blocker	Same as acebutolol; decreases intraocular pressure	Glaucoma
Bisoprolol	β_1-blocker	Same as acebutolol	Hypertension
Esmolol	β_1-blocker	Same as acebutolol	Acute supraventricular tachycardia and hypertension
Metoprolol	β_1-blocker with MSA	Same as acebutolol	Hypertension; angina pectoris; acute myocardial infarction
Nadolol	β_1- and β_2-blocker	Same as acebutolol	Hypertension; angina pectoris; migraine headache
Nebivolol	β_1-blocker	Same as acebutolol	Hypertension
Pindolol	β_1- and β_2-blocker with ISA and MSA	Same as acebutolol	Hypertension
Propranolol	β_1- and β_2-blocker with MSA	Same as acebutolol	Hypertension; angina pectoris; cardiac dysrhythmias; hypertrophic subaortic stenosis; essential tremor; migraine headache; acute thyrotoxicosis; acute myocardial infarction; pheochromocytoma

TABLE 9.1 Mechanism, Effects, and Clinical Use of Adrenoceptor Antagonists—Cont'd

DRUG	MECHANISM OF ACTION	PHARMACOLOGIC EFFECTS	CLINICAL USE
Timolol	β_1- and β_2-blocker	Same as acebutolol; also decreases intraocular pressure	Hypertension; acute myocardial infarction; migraine headache; glaucoma
α- and β-blockers			
Carvedilol	β_1- and β_2-blocker; α_1-blocker	Causes vasodilation; decreases heart rate and blood pressure in patients with hypertension; increases cardiac output in patients with heart failure	Hypertension; heart failure
Labetalol	β_1- and β_2-blocker with MSA; α_1-blocker	Causes vasodilation; decreases heart rate and blood pressure	Hypertension

AV, Atrioventricular; *ISA,* intrinsic sympathomimetic activity (partial agonist activity); *MSA,* membrane-stabilizing activity (local anesthetic activity).

BOX 9.1 A CASE OF HEADACHE, ANXIETY, AND A RACING HEART

CASE PRESENTATION
A 38-year-old man complains of the recent onset of episodes of headache, nervousness, sweating, a racing heart, and rapid breathing. The episodes last from a few minutes to over an hour and occur several times a day. On physical examination, his pulse is 86 beats/min, his respiration rate is 24/min, and his blood pressure is 210/110 mm Hg. The patient has no history of hypertension and is taking no medications. He is given oxygen and intravenous labetalol to gradually reduce heart rate and blood pressure. His 24-hour urinary vanillylmandelic acid concentration is 10.8 mg (normal <7 mg/24 h), his epinephrine is elevated at 186 mcg (normal <22 mcg/24 h), and norepinephrine is 135 mcg (normal 12–85 mcg/24 h). A computed tomography image shows a 1.7 × 2.1 cm soft tissue density in the left suprarenal area but no other abnormalities, and he is placed on metoprolol to control high blood pressure until surgery, and phenoxybenzamine and metyrosine right before surgery. His blood pressure is gradually reduced to 118/65 mm Hg, and he is started on a high-salt diet to maintain plasma volume. A week later, he undergoes laparoscopic left adrenalectomy, and his medications are gradually withdrawn. His blood pressure stabilizes at 120/70 mm Hg, and he is discharged after an uneventful recovery with no discharge medication required.

CASE DISCUSSION
Pheochromocytoma is a rare tumor of the adrenal medulla that secretes huge quantities of epinephrine and norepinephrine. The peak age of onset is 40 years. Symptoms may be intermittent or continuous and include headache, anxiety, sweating, rapid breathing, and tachycardia. The diagnosis is established by abdominal imaging and measurement of urinary catecholamines and vanillylmandelic acid. If the tumor has not metastasized, it can be surgically removed with no sequelae. Blood pressure should be controlled until surgery with adrenoceptor antagonists, and phenoxybenzamine is often used for this purpose along with a β-blocker to reduce cardiac stimulation and prevent dysrhythmias and cardiac ischemia. Alternatively, metyrosine (see Chapters 8 and 10) can be used with phenoxybenzamine to control blood pressure preoperatively, and the drug is useful in managing patients when surgery is contraindicated or when the tumor has metastasized. Patients are usually given a high-sodium diet (>5000 mg daily) to counteract catecholamine-induced volume contraction and the orthostatic hypotension caused by α-receptor blockade. If the tumor is unilateral, replacement of corticosteroids is not necessary after adrenalectomy.

α-adrenoceptor agonists. It is also used to counteract **localized ischemia** caused by accidental injection or extravasation (leakage from an intravenous infusion) of epinephrine or other vasopressor amines. Accidental injection of a finger with an epinephrine auto-injector may result in localized vasoconstriction, ischemia, and necrosis. This condition can be treated by injecting the finger with phentolamine. In this setting, phentolamine competes with epinephrine for vascular α-adrenoceptors, leading to vasodilation and a return of blood flow to the affected digit.

Phentolamine and other nonselective α-blockers are **not useful in treating chronic hypertension,** because they evoke reflex tachycardia and may cause dizziness, headache, and nasal congestion.

Selective α_1-Antagonists
Agents that selectively antagonize α_1-adrenoceptors include **alfuzosin, doxazosin, prazosin, silodosin, tamsulosin,** and **terazosin.** Prazosin, the original drug in this class, was developed to treat hypertension. These drugs are primarily used to treat urinary symptoms in men with benign prostatic hyperplasia.

General Properties
Pharmacokinetics. The selective α_1-adrenoceptor antagonists are administered orally and undergo varying amounts of first-pass and systemic metabolism. The drugs are highly bound to plasma proteins, and they are excreted in the bile, urine, and feces.

Mechanisms, Effects, and Indications. The selective α_1-blockers **relax vascular and other smooth muscles,** including those of the urinary bladder, urethra, and prostate. Because they produce vasodilation and decrease blood pressure, they are used to treat essential (primary) hypertension. The cardiovascular effects of α- and β-blockers in patients with hypertension are depicted in Fig. 9.2.

The selective α_1-blockers do not cause as much reflex tachycardia as do phentolamine and other agents that nonselectively block both α_1- and α_2-adrenoceptors. This is because blockade of α_2-adrenoceptors on sympathetic

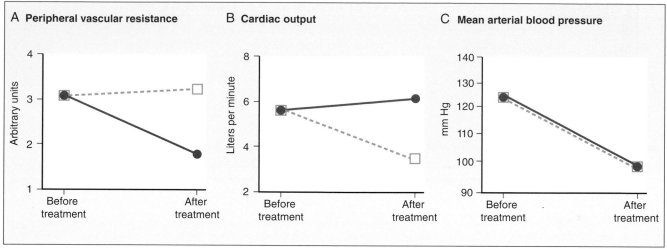

FIG. 9.2 Cardiovascular effects of α_1-adrenoceptor antagonists (*solid line*) and β_1-adrenoceptor antagonists (*dotted line*) in patients with hypertension. (A) The α_1-blockers reduce peripheral vascular resistance, whereas β_1-blockers can cause a slight increase in peripheral resistance as a result of reflex vasoconstriction. (B) The β_1-blockers reduce cardiac output, whereas the α_1-blockers can increase cardiac output by decreasing cardiac afterload and aortic impedance to ventricular ejection of blood. (C) Both α_1-blockers and β_1-blockers reduce mean arterial blood pressure.

neurons prevents feedback inhibition of norepinephrine release and thereby leads to increased activation of cardiac β_1-adrenoceptors and tachycardia (Fig. 9.3). The use of selective α_1-blockers to treat hypertension is discussed in greater detail in Chapter 10.

The selective α_1-blockers are quite helpful in treating **lower urinary tract symptoms** associated with **benign prostatic hyperplasia** and other conditions. Men with these conditions complain of urinary frequency, urgency, and nocturia (need to urinate more frequently at night). Prostatic enlargement may obstruct urinary outflow, and there is good evidence that activation of α_1-adrenoceptors in the bladder, the urethra, and the nervous system contributes to urinary tract obstruction in these men (Fig. 9.4). Blockade of α_1-receptors relaxes smooth muscles in these tissues and relieves urinary tract symptoms. These drugs can be used in combination with **finasteride** or **dutasteride** (see Chapter 34) for relief of urinary symptoms. **Tadalafil,** a type 5 phosphodiesterase inhibitor, has also been approved for treating symptoms of benign prostatic hyperplasia (see Chapter 6).

The most common adverse effects of α_1-blockers include **hypotension, dizziness,** and **sedation,** which are attributed to excessive vasodilation and to the central nervous system effects of these drugs. Doxazosin and terazosin appear to be associated with a higher incidence of these adverse effects than tamsulosin and alfuzosin. A small percentage of men experience abnormal ejaculation when taking α_1-blockers.

Specific Drugs

Prazosin, whose half-life is shorter than the half-lives of other α_1-antagonists, has a duration of action of about six hours. It undergoes considerable first-pass and systemic metabolism before renal and biliary excretion.

Doxazosin and **terazosin** are longer-acting α_1-blockers that are usually administered once a day to treat **hypertension** or to relieve lower urinary tract symptoms. Their duration of action ranges from about 20 hours (terazosin) to about 30 hours (doxazosin).

Alfuzosin, silodosin, and **tamsulosin** selectively block the α_{1A}-**adrenoceptor,** which is the α_1-receptor subtype that

mediates contraction of the ureter and urinary bladder. The relative affinity of these agents for the α_{1A}- to α_{1B}-receptors ranges from 4:1 for tamsulosin to 162:1 for silodosin. These more **uroselective** α_{1A}-blockers relieve **lower urinary tract symptoms** without causing as much hypotension, dizziness, and sedation as nonselective α_1-blockers. In fact, their side effect profiles are similar to those of placebo. Alfuzosin, silodosin, and tamsulosin are only indicated for treating symptoms of urinary outflow obstruction in men with prostatic hyperplasia and are not used to treat hypertension.

β-ADRENOCEPTOR ANTAGONISTS
Classification

The β-adrenoceptor antagonists, or **β-blockers,** include (1) nonselective drugs that block β_1- and β_2-receptors, (2) drugs that selectively block β_1-receptors, and (3) drugs that block α_1-, β_1-, and β_2-receptors. These drugs are listed with their pharmacologic properties in Table 9.2 (see also Table 9.1). The first of these drugs to be developed for clinical use were the nonselective blockers. In addition to blocking β_1-adrenoceptors in the heart and other tissues, they block β_2-adrenoceptors in blood vessels, lungs, and the liver. **Nadolol, pindolol, propranolol,** and **timolol** are examples of nonselective β blockers The selective β_1-blockers were developed later to avoid the adverse effects of β_2-blockade, such as bronchoconstriction, prolongation of hypoglycemia after excessive insulin administration, decreased peripheral blood flow during exercise, and a risk of cold extremities. These effects result from blockade of β_2-receptors in the lungs, liver, and vascular smooth muscle. The selective β_1-blockers include **atenolol, esmolol,** and **metoprolol.** There is no clear rationale for choosing a nonselective β-blocker in treating cardiovascular conditions, as the clinical benefits are derived from β_1-blockade, and the same can be said for most of the other indications for β-blockers.

General Properties
Pharmacokinetic Properties

Most of the β-blockers can be administered orally, whereas esmolol is given parenterally, and propranolol can be given

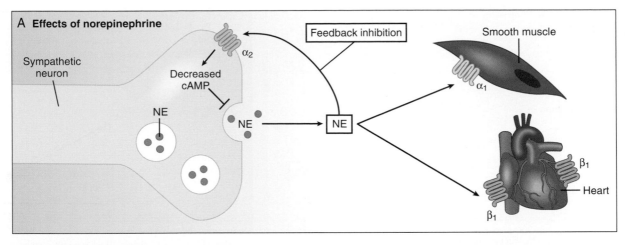

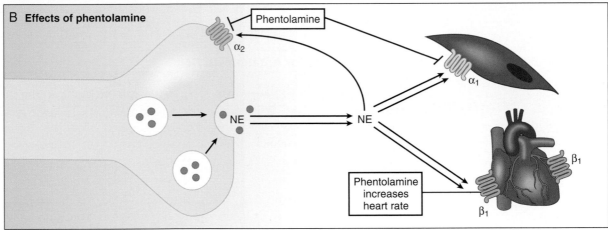

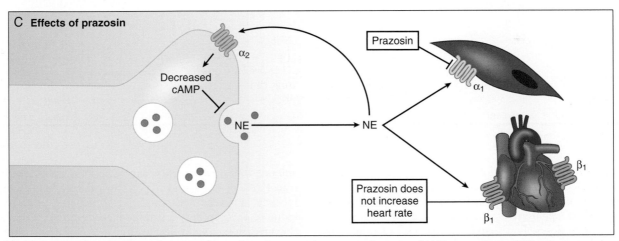

Fig. 9.3 A comparison of the effects of norepinephrine, phentolamine, and prazosin on heart rate. (A) Norepinephrine (*NE*) activates presynaptic α_2-adrenoceptors (α_2), and this inhibits the formation of cyclic adenosine monophosphate (*cAMP*) and decreases the release of NE. (B) Phentolamine blocks α_2-adrenoceptor–mediated inhibition of NE release. This increases the stimulation of cardiac β_1-adrenoceptors (β_1) and results in tachycardia. (C) Prazosin, a selective α_1-blocker, does not block α_2-adrenoceptor–mediated inhibition of norepinephrine release. Therefore, prazosin causes less tachycardia than does phentolamine. α_1, α_1-adrenoceptors.

orally or parenterally. In addition, timolol, carteolol, and betaxolol are administered as eye drops for the treatment of glaucoma (see Chapter 6). β-blockers differ in their hydrophilicity and ability to cross the blood-brain barrier. Hydrophilic β-blockers, such as atenolol (brain:blood ratio of 0.1:1), are less likely to cause central nervous system side effects compared with lipophilic propranolol and metoprolol, with brain:blood ratios of 17:1 and 14:1, respectively. At

the same time, the lipophilicity of propranolol enables it to enter the brain and be used for the prophylaxis of migraine headache.

Mechanisms and Effects

The β-blockers competitively block the activation of β-adrenoceptors by epinephrine, norepinephrine, and adrenoceptor agonists. The selective β_1-blockers have greater

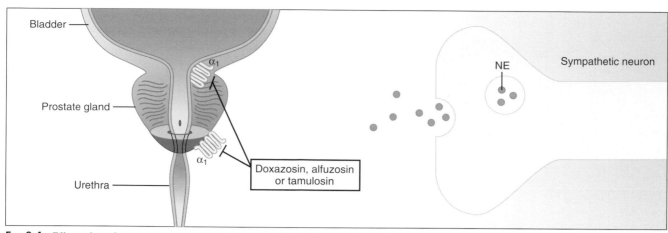

FIG. 9.4 Effects of α_1-adrenoceptor antagonists on the urinary bladder. Prostatic hyperplasia leads to obstruction of urine outflow from the bladder through the urethra. An α_1-blocker (e.g., doxazosin, alfuzosin, or tamsulosin) will relax smooth muscle in the bladder, urethra, and prostate and, thereby, facilitate micturition in patients with prostatic hyperplasia. α_1, α_1-adrenoceptors; *NE*, norepinephrine.

TABLE 9.2   Pharmacologic Properties of β-Adrenoceptor Antagonists

DRUG	LIPID SOLUBILITY	ORAL BIOAVAILABILITY	ELIMINATION HALF-LIFE	INTRINSIC SYMPATHOMIMETIC ACTIVITY	MEMBRANE-STABILIZING ACTIVITY
Nonselective β-blockers					
Nadolol	Low	35%	15–20 h	None	None
Pindolol	Medium	75%	3–4 h	Medium	Low
Propranolol	High	25%	4–6 h	None	High
Timolol	Medium	50%	4–6 h	None	None
Selective β-blockers					
Acebutolol	Medium	40%	10–12 h[a]	Low	Medium
Atenolol	Low	50%	6–7 h	None	None
Esmolol	Low	—	10 min	None	None
Metoprolol	Medium	40%	3–4 h	None	Low
α- and β-blockers					
Carvedilol	Not known	30%	6–8 h	None	None
Labetalol	Medium	20%	6–8 h	None	Low

[a]Includes half-life of active metabolite.

affinity for β_1- than for β_2-adrenoceptors and are also known as **cardioselective β-blockers** because the heart predominantly contains β_1-receptors. The β_1-selectivity of these drugs is most apparent at low doses and is progressively lost at higher doses. Fortunately, lower doses of β-blockers are usually sufficient to produce the desired clinical effect while avoiding many side effects. In addition to producing β-receptor blockade, some drugs exhibit **membrane-stabilizing (local anesthetic)** and a low degree of **intrinsic sympathomimetic (partial agonist) activity,** as outlined in Table 9.2. The therapeutic relevance of these properties has never been clearly established, and the clinical effectiveness of β-blockers is mostly, if not entirely, due to antagonism of β_1-adrenoceptors. The local anesthetic effect of β-blockers, such as propranolol, has little clinical importance except that it precludes topical ocular administration that might anesthetize the cornea.

Blockade of **cardiac β_1-adrenoceptors** reduces heart rate, cardiac contractility, and atrioventricular conduction velocity. β-blockers reduce cardiac output and blood pressure (see Fig. 9.2), and all of the orally administered β-blockers are used to treat arterial hypertension. In the kidneys, β_1-receptor blockade reduces **renin secretion** from the juxtaglomerular cells, leading to reduced synthesis of angiotensin, and thereby contributing to a reduction in blood pressure. β-blockers reduce cardiac oxygen demand and many of the drugs are used to treat angina pectoris. A few, including acebutolol, are used to treat cardiac dysrhythmias (see Table 9.1).

As mentioned previously, many of the adverse effects of β-blockers result from **blockade of β_2-adrenoceptors.** In the lungs, antagonism of β_2-adrenoceptors can cause **bronchoconstriction** in patients with asthma, and nonselective β-blockers should be avoided in these persons. If a β-blocker is required to treat an asthmatic patient, a selective β_1-blocker should be used. In the liver, β_2-adrenoceptor blockade inhibits epinephrine-stimulated **glycogenolysis** and can reduce hepatic glucose output during hypoglycemia caused by excessive insulin administration. The β-blockers can also block some of the early signs of hypoglycemia (e.g., tachycardia), which would otherwise alert a diabetic patient to this problem. For these reasons, β-blockers should be used cautiously in patients with diabetes and particularly in those who have insulin-dependent diabetes and are susceptible to hypoglycemic episodes caused by excessive insulin administration.

Specific Drug Properties

Atenolol is administered orally or parenterally and is primarily used to treat **hypertension, angina pectoris,** and **acute myocardial infarction.** It shows less variability in its oral absorption than other β-blockers and is mostly excreted unchanged in the urine. Its low lipid solubility is believed responsible for its lower incidence of central nervous system side effects (e.g., vivid dreams, tiredness, and depression).

Esmolol has a much shorter half-life than other β-blockers and is administered intravenously to treat **hypertension** and **supraventricular tachycardia** when these occur during surgery and in other acute situations. Esmolol is rapidly metabolized to inactive compounds by plasma esterase enzymes.

Metoprolol is used to treat **hypertension, angina pectoris,** and **acute myocardial infarction.** It can be administered orally or parenterally, and it is extensively metabolized by cytochrome P450 enzymes before undergoing renal excretion.

Pindolol is the only β-blocker with noticeable **intrinsic sympathomimetic activity** (ISA), whereby it exerts a weak agonist effect on β-adrenoceptors. This effect can be observed when a treated patient is resting and sympathetic tone is low, and the drug's ISA results in a smaller reduction in heart rate than caused by other β-blockers. Pindolol is only approved for the treatment of hypertension.

Propranolol has many clinical uses, partly because it was the first of the currently available β-blockers to be developed. It is used to treat **hypertension, angina pectoris,** and **cardiac dysrhythmias** (conditions discussed in the chapters of Section III); **hypertrophic subaortic stenosis**—a form of hypertrophic cardiomyopathy that impedes the ejection of blood from the ventricles; and **essential tremor**—a benign condition characterized by involuntary trembling of the hands. **Propranolol** is also used to prevent **migraine headache** and as adjunctive therapy in the treatment of **acute thyrotoxicosis, acute myocardial infarction,** and **pheochromocytoma.** Patients with thyrotoxicosis often experience tachycardia and palpitations because thyroid hormones increase the effects of sympathetic stimulation of the heart. Propranolol is used to reduce these symptoms until the underlying thyroid disorder can be treated. Propranolol and other β-blockers are frequently administered to patients with **acute myocardial infarction** because clinical trials have shown that β-blockers reduce the incidence of sudden death and mortality in these patients. In patients with **pheochromocytoma,** propranolol is used to reduce cardiac stimulation caused by circulating catecholamines released from this adrenal medullary tumor. Propranolol, acebutolol, and pindolol exhibit varying degrees of **membrane-stabilizing activity.** Hence, these agents are not employed as eye drops in the treatment of glaucoma.

Timolol was the first β-blocker to be used to treat **glaucoma** and is available as an ophthalmic solution for topical ocular administration. The drug is absorbed through the cornea and penetrates to the ciliary body where it reduces aqueous humor secretion and intraocular pressure. **Carteolol** and **betaxolol** have similar effects and use. Timolol is also given orally to treat hypertension.

α- AND β-ADRENOCEPTOR ANTAGONISTS

Carvedilol and **labetalol** are agents that block α_1-, β_1-, and β_2-adrenoceptors. Their effects, uses, and properties are shown in Tables 9.1 and 9.2. Carvedilol also possesses antioxidant activity. All of these actions contribute to its cardioprotective effects in persons with cardiovascular disorders. The **antioxidant effects** of carvedilol include (1) inhibition of lipid peroxidation in myocardial membranes, (2) scavenging of free radicals, and (3) inhibition of neutrophil release of O_2. In addition, carvedilol has **antiapoptotic properties** that can prevent myocyte death and reduce infarct size in persons with myocardial ischemia. For these reasons, carvedilol has been called a "**third-generation β-blocker**" and neurohumoral antagonist," and its value in treating myocardial infarction has been established in clinical trials. Carvedilol has also been used in the treatment of hypertension. As discussed further in Chapter 12, it also decreases cardiac afterload, increases cardiac output, and reduces mortality in patients with heart failure.

Labetalol is primarily used in the treatment of hypertension. It is 5 to 10 times more potent as a β-blocker than as an α-blocker, but both actions are believed to contribute to its antihypertensive effect. Labetalol decreases heart rate and cardiac output as a result of blocking β_1-adrenoceptors, and it decreases peripheral vascular resistance as a result of α_1-receptor blockade.

SUMMARY OF IMPORTANT POINTS

- The α-adrenoceptor antagonists relax smooth muscle and decrease vascular resistance, whereas the β-adrenoceptor antagonists reduce heart rate and cardiac output. Both α- and β-blockers reduce blood pressure.
- The nonselective α-blockers include phenoxybenzamine (a noncompetitive blocker) and phentolamine (a competitive blocker). These drugs block both α_1- and α_2-adrenoceptors and are primarily used to treat hypertensive episodes caused by pheochromocytoma.
- The selective α_1-blockers include alfuzosin, doxazosin, prazosin, tamsulosin, and terazosin. These drugs are used to treat urinary obstruction caused by benign prostatic hyperplasia, high blood pressure, and other conditions.
- The nonselective β-blockers, which antagonize both β_1- and β_2-adrenoceptors, include nadolol, pindolol, propranolol, and timolol. Pindolol possesses intrinsic sympathomimetic (partial agonist) activity, and propranolol exerts membrane-stabilizing (local anesthetic) activity.
- The selective β_1-blockers include acebutolol, atenolol, esmolol, and metoprolol. These drugs cause less bronchoconstriction than nonselective β-blockers and have other advantages over nonselective blockers.
- The β-blockers have a variety of clinical applications, including the prevention of migraine headache and the treatment of hypertension, angina pectoris, cardiac dysrhythmias, and glaucoma.

- Carvedilol blocks α- and β-adrenoceptors and exerts cardioprotective effects that make it particularly useful in the treatment of myocardial infarction and heart failure.

Review Questions

For Questions 1 to 4, for each patient described, select the most appropriate drug therapy from the following lettered choices:

(A) alfuzosin
(B) carvedilol
(C) betaxolol
(D) phenoxybenzamine
(E) phentolamine

1. A woman experiences pain and ischemia in her finger after accidentally injecting it with epinephrine that she carries for emergency treatment of severe allergic reactions.

2. A man complains of urinary urgency, frequency, and nocturia and is found to have enlargement of the prostate gland.

3. A patient with essential hypertension requires a drug that reduces both cardiac output and peripheral resistance.

4. A man with episodic severe hypertension is found to have markedly elevated levels of epinephrine and norepinephrine metabolites in his urine and needs a long-acting drug to lower blood pressure before surgery.

5. Which drug is most likely to slow recovery from hypoglycemia in a diabetic patient who has taken an excessive dose of insulin?

(A) metoprolol
(B) doxazosin
(C) propranolol
(D) phenoxybenzamine
(E) atenolol

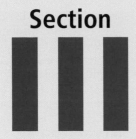

Section

III

CARDIOVASCULAR, RENAL, AND HEMATOLOGIC PHARMACOLOGY

CHAPTER 10 Antihypertensive Drugs

OVERVIEW

An estimated 950 million people around the world have **hypertension** (high blood pressure), which is defined as a sustained systolic blood pressure of 140 mm Hg or higher or a sustained diastolic blood pressure of 90 mm Hg or higher. Numerous studies have shown that untreated high blood pressure damages blood vessels, accelerates **atherosclerosis,** and produces **left ventricular hypertrophy.** These abnormalities contribute to the development **of ischemic heart disease, stroke, heart failure,** and **renal failure,** which are among the most common causes of death worldwide.

Hypertension

Over the past several decades, health professionals and public officials have increased efforts to educate the public about the hazards of untreated hypertension, and this has led to a significant increase in the number of hypertensive individuals who are aware of their condition and treat it effectively with lifestyle changes and drug therapy. The effective treatment of high blood pressure appears to be one of the factors that has contributed to a nearly 60% reduction

in the incidence of stroke and at least a 50% reduction in the mortality rate from coronary artery disease since 1970.

About 95% of the cases of hypertension are considered to be **primary hypertension** that cannot be attributed to a specific cause. The other 5% of cases are classified as **secondary hypertension,** which results from an identifiable cause such as chronic kidney disease or hyperaldosteronism. In some cases, secondary hypertension can be corrected by medication or surgery.

Although the cause of primary hypertension in any specific patient is usually unknown, numerous genetic and lifestyle factors are associated with it. These include obesity, lack of exercise, the so-called *metabolic syndrome* (abdominal obesity, hyperlipidemia, and insulin resistance), elevated dietary sodium intake, and excessive consumption of alcohol.

Vascular **endothelial cell dysfunction** also contributes to the development of hypertension. The endothelium regulates vascular smooth muscle tone through the synthesis and release of relaxing factors such as **nitric oxide** and **prostacyclin** and vasoconstricting factors such as **angiotensin II** and

TABLE 10.1　Classification of Blood Pressure for Adults and Follow-Up Recommendations

BLOOD PRESSURE CLASSIFICATION	SBP (MMHG)	DBP (MMHG)	FOLLOW-UP RECOMMENDATIONS
Normal	<120	and <80	Check again in 2 years
Prehypertension	120–139	or 80–90	Check again in 1 year
Stage 1 hypertension	140–159	or 90–99	Confirm within 2 months
Stage 2 hypertension	>160	or >100	Evaluate within 1 week to 1 month[a]

DBP, Diastolic blood pressure; *SBP,* systolic blood pressure.
[a]Based on blood pressure level and clinical situation.

endothelin-1. Angiotensin II may cause vascular injury by activating growth factors that cause vascular smooth muscle proliferation and hypertrophy as well as fibrotic changes in the vascular wall. Oxidative stress increases vasoconstrictive factors but decreases relaxing factors, thereby contributing to the development of hypertension. Several antihypertensive drugs, including carvedilol and angiotensin inhibitors, appear to counteract endothelial cell dysfunction and reduce some of the adverse consequences of hypertensive disease.

Classification of Blood Pressure

Blood pressure is classified as shown in Table 10.1. This classification uses the term **prehypertension** for those with blood pressures ranging from 120 to 139 mm Hg systolic, 80 to 89 mm Hg diastolic blood pressure, or both. This designation helps identify persons in whom early adoption of **lifestyle changes** that decrease blood pressure could prevent the progression of blood pressure to hypertensive levels (see later). These persons are not candidates for drug therapy unless they have **diabetes,** and a trial of lifestyle changes fails to reduce their blood pressure to the desired level of 130/80 mm Hg or less for diabetics.

The classification includes two stages of hypertension that confer differences in follow-up recommendations and management. In addition to providing information about lifestyle modifications, stage 1 hypertension should be confirmed within 2 months and then treated appropriately. Stage 2 hypertension should be treated immediately if blood pressure is greater than 180/110 mm Hg. For lower blood pressures, stage 2 hypertension should be evaluated and treated within 1 month.

Regulation of Blood Pressure

From a systemic hemodynamic perspective, blood pressure is regulated primarily by the **sympathetic nervous system** and the **kidneys** through their influence on cardiac output and peripheral vascular resistance (PVR). Vasoactive and other substances produced within the blood vessel wall also have a substantial role in the regulation of blood pressure and in the pathophysiology of hypertension.

Cardiac output, which is the product of stroke volume and heart rate, is increased by sympathetic stimulation via activation of β_1-adrenoceptors in the heart, and it is influenced by the kidneys through their regulation of blood volume, which is one of the factors determining the cardiac filling pressure and stroke volume.

PVR is chiefly determined by the resistance to blood flow through the arterioles, whose cross-sectional area depends on arteriolar smooth muscle tone in the various vascular beds.

Via activation of α_1-adrenoceptors, the sympathetic nervous system stimulates arteriolar smooth muscle contraction, and this leads to vasoconstriction. Blood-borne substances such as vasopressin and angiotensin II also cause vasoconstriction, whereas locally released adenosine, serotonin, endothelin, and prostaglandins also affect arteriolar smooth muscle tone. These substances serve to regulate blood flow through the tissues and influence arterial pressure.

The sympathetic nervous system provides **short-term control** of blood pressure through the **baroreceptor reflex.** This reflex modulates sympathetic stimulation of cardiac output and PVR and adjusts blood pressure in response to postural changes and altered physical activity. The kidneys are responsible for the **long-term control** of blood pressure via the regulation of plasma volume and the **renin-angiotensin-aldosterone axis.** By these mechanisms, the sympathetic system and kidneys maintain arterial blood pressure within a fairly narrow range when a person is at rest, and they adjust blood pressure appropriately in response to postural changes and physical activity.

In normotensive individuals, an increase in blood pressure leads to a proportional increase in sodium and water excretion by the kidneys so that blood volume is reduced and blood pressure returns to its normal *set point.* In hypertensive patients, the set point at which blood pressure is controlled is higher than normal, the regulation of blood pressure is defective, and an increase in blood pressure is not followed by a proportional increase in sodium and water excretion by the kidneys. Although studies have shown that PVR is elevated in most hypertensive patients, it is not clear whether this is the cause or the result of hypertension.

Sites and Effects of Antihypertensive Drug Action

The four major categories of antihypertensive drugs are diuretics, sympatholytic drugs, angiotensin inhibitors, and other vasodilators. These drugs lower blood pressure through actions exerted at one or more of the following sites: kidneys, sympathetic nervous system, renin-angiotensin-aldosterone axis, or vascular smooth muscle (Fig. 10.1).

Antihypertensive drugs can be characterized in terms of their cardiovascular effects (Table 10.2) and their effects on serum potassium and cholesterol measurements (Table 10.3). They can also be characterized in terms of the **compensatory mechanisms** invoked by their hypotensive effect. Compensatory reactions serve to return blood pressure to the pretreatment level and include reflex tachycardia, fluid retention by the kidneys, and activation of the renin-angiotensin-aldosterone axis. Whereas most antihypertensive drugs are taken orally on a long-term basis, some are administered parenterally for the management of **hypertensive**

Physiological control of blood pressure and sites of drug action

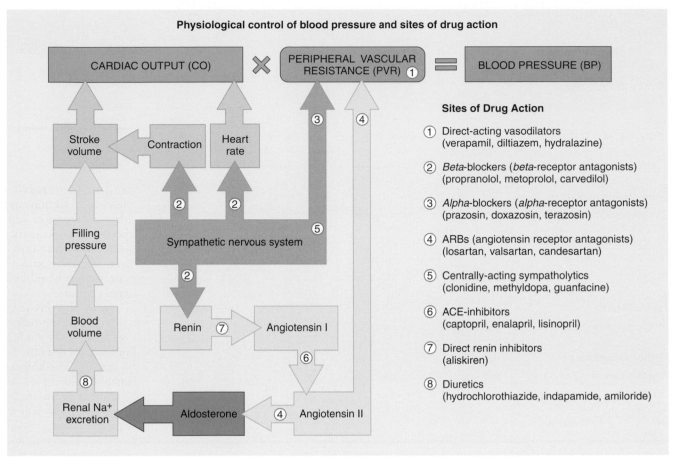

FIG. 10.1 Physiologic control of blood pressure and sites of drug action. Blood pressure is the product of cardiac output and peripheral vascular resistance (PVR). These parameters are regulated on a systemic level by the sympathetic nervous system and the kidneys. Antihypertensive drugs act to suppress excessive sympathetic activity and modify renal function to counteract the mechanisms responsible for hypertension. Sites of action of the following drugs are shown: *1,* vasodilators; *2,* β-adrenoceptor antagonists (β-blockers); *3,* α-adrenoceptor antagonists (α-blockers); *4,* angiotensin receptor antagonists; *5,* centrally acting sympatholytics; *6,* angiotensin-converting enzyme (ACE) inhibitors; *7,* direct renin inhibitors; and *8,* diuretics. The vasodilators, sympatholytic drugs, and angiotensin inhibitors reduce PVR; β-adrenoceptor blockers primarily reduce cardiac output; and diuretics promote sodium excretion and reduce blood volume.

emergencies. The treatment of this condition is discussed at the end of the chapter.

DIURETICS

Chapter 13 provides detailed information about the various classes of diuretics and their uses, mechanisms of action, and pharmacologic properties. The discussion here focuses on the diuretics most commonly used to treat hypertension: the thiazide and related diuretics, and the potassium-sparing diuretics.

Diuretics increase renal sodium excretion, and this **natriuretic effect** appears to be responsible for their antihypertensive activity. The thiazide diuretics have a moderate natriuretic effect and are the diuretics used most frequently in the treatment of hypertension. The loop diuretics may cause more natriuresis than do thiazides but are usually less effective in treating hypertension than are thiazide diuretics and have a greater potential to cause hyponatremia. Loop diuretics can be used to treat hypertension when a thiazide diuretic is not effective or is contraindicated. The potassium-sparing diuretics have a relatively low natriuretic effect and are primarily used in combination with a thiazide or loop diuretic to reduce potassium excretion and prevent hypokalemia.

Thiazide and Related Diuretics

Thiazide diuretics reduce blood pressure by two mechanisms, both stemming from their ability to increase sodium and water excretion. When they are first administered to a patient, the drugs decrease blood volume and thereby decrease cardiac output (Fig. 10.2; see Table 10.2). With continued administration over weeks and months, they also decrease PVR, and this appears to account for much of their long-term antihypertensive effect. The decreased PVR may result from a reduction in the sodium content of arteriolar smooth muscle cells, which decreases muscle contraction in response to vasopressor agents such as norepinephrine and angiotensin. This relationship is supported by the finding that the effect of a thiazide on PVR is reduced if patients ingest enough dietary sodium to counteract the natriuretic effect of the drug. The use of a thiazide typically reduces blood pressure by 10 to 15 mm Hg.

Hydrochlorothiazide is the thiazide diuretic often used to treat hypertension. **Indapamide** and **chlorthalidone** have similar efficacy, and indapamide has the additional benefit of causing **vasodilation** via calcium channel blockade. Recent clinical trials have shown that the combination of indapamide and an angiotensin inhibitor effectively controls blood pressure while reducing the risk of stroke

TABLE 10.2 Cardiovascular Effects of Antihypertensive Drugs

DRUG CLASSIFICATION	PERIPHERAL VASCULAR RESISTANCE	CARDIAC OUTPUT	BLOOD VOLUME	PLASMA RENIN ACTIVITY	LEFT VENTRICULAR HYPERTROPHY
Diuretics					
Thiazide and loop diuretics	Decrease	Decrease	Decrease	Increase	No change or decrease
Potassium-sparing diuretics	Decrease	Decrease	Decrease	Increase	No change or decrease
Sympatholytic drugs					
α-adrenoceptor antagonists	Decrease	No change or increase	No change or increase	No change or decrease	Decrease
β-adrenoceptor antagonists	No change or decrease	Decrease	No change or decrease	Decrease	Decrease
Centrally acting drugs	Decrease	No change or decrease	Increase[a]	Decrease	Decrease
Angiotensin inhibitors					
Angiotensin-converting enzyme inhibitors	Decrease	No change or increase	No change	Increase	Decrease
Angiotensin receptor antagonists	Decrease	No change or increase	No change or increase	Increase	Decrease
Aliskiren	Decrease	No change or increase	No change or increase	Decrease	Decrease
Vasodilators					
Calcium channel blockers	Decrease	No change or increase[b]	No change	No change or increase	Decrease
Other vasodilators					
Hydralazine	Decrease	Increase	Increase	Increase	Increase
Minoxidil	Decrease	Increase	Increase	Increase	Increase
Nitroprusside	Decrease	Increase	Increase	Increase	No change or increase
Fenoldopam	Decrease	Increase	No change	Increase	No change

[a]An exception is guanfacine, which may cause no change in blood volume or decrease it slightly.
[b]An exception is verapamil, which may increase or decrease cardiac output.

TABLE 10.3 Pharmacologic Effects of Antihypertensive Drugs on Serum Potassium and Cholesterol Measurements

DRUG CLASSIFICATION	SERUM POTASSIUM	TOTAL CHOLESTEROL	LOW-DENSITY LIPOPROTEINS	HIGH-DENSITY LIPOPROTEINS	TRIGLYCERIDES
Diuretics					
Thiazide and loop diuretics	Decrease	Increase	Increase	No change or decrease	Increase
Potassium-sparing diuretics	Increase	Unknown	Unknown	Unknown	Unknown
Sympatholytic drugs					
α-adrenoceptor antagonists	No change	Decrease	Decrease	Increase	Decrease
β-adrenoceptor antagonists	Slight increase	No change or increase	No change or increase	Variable	No change or increase
Centrally acting drugs	No change	No change	No change	No change	No change
Angiotensin inhibitors					
Angiotensin-converting enzyme inhibitors	Increase	No change	No change	No change	No change
Angiotensin receptor antagonists	Increase	No change	No change	No change	No change
Aliskiren	Increase	No change	No change	No change	No change
Vasodilators					
Calcium channel blockers	No change	No change	No change	No change	No change
Other vasodilators					
Hydralazine	No change	No change	No change	No change	No change
Minoxidil	No change	No change	No change	No change	No change
Nitroprusside	No change	Not applicable[a]	Not applicable[a]	Not applicable[a]	Not applicable[a]
Fenoldopam	Decrease	No change	No change	No change	No change

[a]Nitroprusside is used only for short-term management of hypertension.

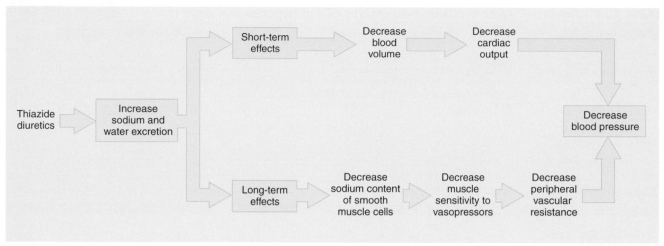

FIG. 10.2 Antihypertensive actions of thiazide diuretics. Initially, thiazide diuretics decrease blood volume and thereby decrease cardiac output. Over time, the drugs decrease peripheral vascular resistance (PVR), an action that may be secondary to a reduction in the sodium content of smooth muscle cells.

and myocardial infarction in hypertensive patients. Some clinical trials have demonstrated superior reductions in the incidence of stroke and cardiac events with chlorthalidone *versus* hydrochlorothiazide, which is possibly related to the longer duration of action of chlorthalidone.

Hydrochlorothiazide has often been used for the initial treatment of persons with mild to moderate hypertension, though recent clinical trials suggest that an angiotensin inhibitor or calcium channel blocker (CCB) may be preferable because of the superior ability of these agents to control blood pressure for the entire day and because they tend to cause fewer adverse effects. Thiazide diuretics are also used in combination with other types of antihypertensive agents. Drugs from different classes often have additive or synergistic effects on blood pressure, and a diuretic may prevent the compensatory fluid retention evoked by another agent.

The common adverse effects and interactions of thiazide diuretics and other antihypertensive agents are summarized in Table 10.4. Thiazides may cause **hypokalemia,** which may contribute to cardiac arrhythmias and muscle weakness. Using a low dosage of a thiazide diuretic (e.g., 12.5–50 mg of hydrochlorothiazide per day) usually produces a maximal antihypertensive effect with minimal hypokalemia. Using a higher dosage causes more hypokalemia but does not have a greater effect on blood pressure. Thiazides elevate plasma levels of **glucose, uric acid,** and **lipids** in some patients. Less commonly, they cause **hematologic toxicity** and aggravate hepatic disease. They can also evoke a compensatory increase in **renin secretion,** which is one reason why using the drug in combination with an angiotensin inhibitor is effective. Nevertheless, numerous clinical trials have shown that thiazide diuretics are effective and relatively safe when serum potassium, glucose, uric acid, and lipid levels are monitored appropriately. In addition, thiazides are among the least expensive agents available for treating hypertension.

One other advantage of taking thiazide diuretics is that they appear to offer protection against **osteoporosis,** a condition in which bone demineralization and loss of bone mass make patients more susceptible to fractures. Thiazides are probably beneficial in this condition because they decrease the urinary excretion of calcium.

Loop Diuretics

Despite the greater natriuretic effect of loop diuretics, they are usually **less effective** than thiazide diuretics in the treatment of hypertensive patients with normal renal function. For this reason, loop diuretics are usually reserved for use in hypertensive patients who have poor renal function and a serum creatinine level greater than 2.3 mg/dL.

Potassium-Sparing Diuretics

Examples of potassium-sparing diuretics are **amiloride, spironolactone,** and **triamterene.** These agents have a mild natriuretic effect, and they reduce renal potassium excretion and thereby **prevent hypokalemia** caused by thiazide and loop-acting diuretics.

Spironolactone and eplerenone are **mineralocorticoid receptor antagonists** that have an impressive ability to lower blood pressure when combined with other drugs; they are used in treating hypertension that cannot be controlled with combinations of three or more other agents. **Eplerenone** is similar to spironolactone but has fewer endocrine side effects. Eplerenone has been found to cause regression of left ventricular hypertrophy in hypertensive patients and regression of microalbuminuria in patients with type 2 diabetes.

SYMPATHOLYTIC DRUGS

The sympatholytic drugs used in the treatment of hypertension include adrenoceptor antagonists and the **centrally acting α_2-adrenoceptor agonists.** The pharmacologic effects of these drugs are summarized in Tables 10.2 and 10.3, and their common adverse effects and drug interactions are listed in Table 10.4.

Adrenoceptor Antagonists
α-Adrenoceptor Antagonists
Selective α_1-blockers, such as **doxazosin, prazosin,** and **terazosin,** are not recommended for the initial treatment of high blood pressure but can be added to other drugs when blood pressure is not adequately controlled. Although they effectively inhibit sympathetic stimulation of arteriolar contraction, leading to vasodilation and decreased vascular resistance, these drugs have several disadvantages. The

TABLE 10.4 Adverse Effects and Drug Interactions of Antihypertensive Agents

DRUG CLASSIFICATION	COMMON ADVERSE EFFECTS	COMMON DRUG INTERACTIONS
Diuretics		
Thiazide and loop diuretics	Blood cell deficiencies, hyperlipidemia, hyperuricemia, hypokalemia, and other electrolyte changes; aggravation of diabetes	Increase serum levels of lithium. Hypotensive effect decreased by NSAIDs and augmented by ACE inhibitors.
Potassium-sparing diuretics	Hyperkalemia	Hyperkalemic effect increased by ACE inhibitors and potassium supplements.
Sympatholytic drugs		
α-adrenoceptor antagonists	Dizziness, first dose syncope, fluid retention, and orthostatic hypotension	Hypotensive effect increased by β-adrenoceptor antagonists and diuretics.
β-adrenoceptor antagonists	Bradycardia, bronchoconstriction, depression, fatigue, impaired glycogenolysis, and vivid dreams	Cardiac depression increased by diltiazem and verapamil. Hypotensive effect decreased by NSAIDs.
Centrally acting drugs		
Clonidine	Dry mouth, fatigue, rebound hypertension, and sedation	Hypotensive effect decreased by tricyclic antidepressants. Sedative effect increased by CNS depressants.
Guanfacine	Same as clonidine but milder	Same as clonidine.
Methyldopa	Autoimmune hemolytic anemia, hepatitis, and lupus-like syndrome; others same as clonidine	Hypotensive effect increased by levodopa. Other interactions same as those of clonidine.
Angiotensin inhibitors		
ACE inhibitors	Acute renal failure, angioedema, cough, hyperkalemia, metallic taste, neutropenia, and rash	Increase serum levels of lithium. Hyperkalemic effect increased by potassium-sparing diuretics and potassium supplements. Hypotensive effect decreased by NSAIDs.
Angiotensin receptor antagonists	Hyperkalemia	Serum levels of drug increased by cimetidine and decreased by phenobarbital.
Aliskiren	Hyperkalemia	Aliskiren reduces serum levels of furosemide. Cyclosporine increases levels of aliskiren.
Vasodilators		
Calcium channel blockers		
Dihydropyridine drugs[a]	Dizziness, edema, gingival hyperplasia, headache, and tachycardia	Serum levels of drug increased by azole antifungal agents, cimetidine, and grapefruit juice.
Diltiazem	Atrioventricular block, bradycardia, constipation, dizziness, edema, gingival hyperplasia, headache, and heart failure	Increases serum levels of carbamazepine, digoxin, and theophylline. Decreases serum levels of lithium.
Verapamil	Same as diltiazem	Same as diltiazem.
Other vasodilators		
Hydralazine	Angina, dizziness, fluid retention, headache, lupus-like syndrome, and tachycardia	Hypotensive effect decreased by NSAIDs.
Minoxidil	Angina, dizziness, fluid retention, headache, hypertrichosis, pericardial effusion, and tachycardia	Hypotensive effect decreased by NSAIDs.
Nitroprusside	Dizziness, headache, increased intracranial pressure, methemoglobinemia, and thiocyanate and cyanide toxicity	None.
Fenoldopam	Headache and nausea	None identified.

ACE, Angiotensin-converting enzyme; *CNS,* central nervous system; *NSAIDs,* nonsteroidal anti-inflammatory drugs.
[a]The dihydropyridine drugs include amlodipine, felodipine, isradipine, nicardipine, and nifedipine.

α_1-blockers may evoke **reflex activation** of the sympathetic nervous system and can increase the heart rate, contractile force, and circulating norepinephrine levels and thereby increase myocardial oxygen requirements. Because they activate the renin-angiotensin-aldosterone system and cause fluid retention, α_1-blockers are often given with a diuretic.

The α_1-blockers can also cause **orthostatic hypotension,** and the initial administration of an α_1-blocker may cause **"first dose" syncope** in some patients, particularly patients taking a diuretic. This can be prevented by beginning treatment with a low dose of the blocker at bedtime and withholding the diuretic for a day until the body adjusts to the lowered blood pressure. The pharmacokinetic properties of α-blockers are covered in Chapter 9.

β-Adrenoceptor Antagonists

The β-blockers lower blood pressure by blocking β_1-adrenoceptors in the heart and other tissues. Blockade of cardiac β_1-receptors reduces cardiac output by **decreasing the heart rate and contractility.** Blockade of β_1-receptors in renal juxtaglomerular cells **inhibits renin secretion,** which in turn reduces the formation of angiotensin II and the subsequent release of aldosterone. The drugs also appear to reduce sympathetic outflow from the central nervous system. Hence, β-blockers have actions at several sites affecting blood pressure.

Clinical trials have shown that β-blockers have beneficial effects in hypertensive persons with other cardiovascular diseases. In persons with **coronary heart disease,** β-blockers reduce myocardial ischemia and lower the risk of myocardial infarction (see Chapter 11). In persons who have had a **myocardial infarction,** β-blockers are **cardioprotective** and prevent sudden death, primarily by reducing the heart rate and decreasing the risk of ventricular arrhythmias. In persons with **heart failure,** β-blockers improve symptoms and survival (see Chapter 12). Hence, β-blockers are sometimes useful in treating hypertension in patients with other cardiovascular diseases, and they are often combined with angiotensin inhibitors in treating patients with heart failure.

The β-blockers are no longer recommended for the initial treatment of hypertension in persons without another cardiovascular disease. Recent meta-analyses of clinical trial data suggest that β-blockers such as **atenolol** are less likely to prevent stroke, myocardial infarction, and death in patients without coronary heart disease in comparison with the calcium channel blockers, renin-angiotensin system inhibitors, and diuretics. Clinical guidelines now recommend an angiotensin inhibitor, CCB, or diuretic for the initial treatment of hypertensive patients without a preexisting heart disease.

The β-blockers are usually **well tolerated** and are unlikely to cause orthostatic hypotension or to produce hepatic, renal, or hematopoietic toxicity. However, β-blockers may cause fatigue, depression, vivid dreams, and reduced exercise capacity.

Nonselective β-blockers are contraindicated in persons with **asthma** or chronic obstructive pulmonary disease because these drugs may cause bronchospasm owing to β_2-blockade. In **diabetics,** nonselective β-blockers may delay recovery from hypoglycemia by blocking β_2-receptor-mediated glycogenolysis and hepatic glucose production, and they may mask symptoms of hypoglycemia. Chapter 9 describes the pharmacologic properties of β-blockers. **Labetalol,** which blocks α- and β-receptors, is used to treat chronic hypertension and hypertensive emergencies. Because of its α-adrenoceptor-blocking activity, it can cause orthostatic hypotension. **Esmolol** is an intravenously administered, ultrashort-acting β_1-blocker used to treat hypertension in surgical patients and in persons with hypertensive emergencies. **Carvedilol** is a third-generation α- and β-blocker with antioxidant properties that can protect the vascular wall from free radicals that damage blood vessels. **Nebivolol** is a selective β_1-blocker with antioxidant properties, and it also increases the release of endothelial **nitric oxide** and exerts vasodilation. Nebivolol provides another option for treating hypertension in patients with heart failure.

Centrally Acting Drugs

The centrally acting sympatholytic drugs include **clonidine, guanfacine,** and **methyldopa.** These drugs reduce sympathetic outflow from the central vasomotor center to the circulation primarily through activation of $\alpha 2$-adrenoceptors in the brainstem medulla. In the case of methyldopa, it must first be converted to an active metabolite (methyl-norepinephrine) by central neurons, which then activates α_2-receptors. The centrally acting drugs lower the blood pressure primarily by reducing vascular resistance while having little effect on heart rate and cardiac output.

Clonidine and related drugs cause more side effects than other antihypertensive drugs and are not recommended for chronic treatment of most patients with high blood pressure. Clonidine is occasionally used for the treatment of **hypertensive urgencies** in the outpatient setting because it slowly reduces blood pressure to a safe level after a single oral dose. It is also used to reduce the sympathetic nervous system symptoms of alcohol, opioid, or nicotine withdrawal (see Chapter 25). **Methyldopa** has been used to treat hypertension in pregnant women because extensive experience has shown that it does not harm the fetus.

The side effects of centrally acting drugs include **sedation, dry mouth, and impaired mental acuity.** Severe **rebound hypertension** can occur if they are discontinued abruptly, and the dosage should be tapered gradually over 1 to 2 weeks if treatment is to be stopped. **Methyldopa** is well known for its ability to cause immunologic effects, including a Coombs-positive **hemolytic anemia,** autoimmune hepatitis, and other organ dysfunction. Because tricyclic antidepressant drugs can block the effects of centrally acting sympatholytic drugs, the two classes of drugs should not be used concurrently.

ANGIOTENSIN INHIBITORS

The angiotensin system inhibitors include the **angiotensin-converting enzyme (ACE) inhibitors,** the **angiotensin receptor blockers (ARBs),** and a direct renin inhibitor called **aliskiren.** The ACE inhibitors and ARBs are effective and well tolerated and are among the preferred drugs for the initial treatment of most hypertensive patients. ACE inhibitors and ARBs have been shown to reduce the risk of stroke, and they are particularly useful in persons with diabetes or heart failure. The pharmacologic properties of these drugs are summarized in Tables 10.2 and 10.3, and their adverse effects and drug interactions are listed in Table 10.4.

The actions of drugs affecting the **renin-angiotensin-aldosterone axis** are shown in Fig. 10.3. The primary stimuli to renin secretion are (1) a reduction in arterial pressure in renal afferent arterioles, (2) a fall in sodium chloride concentration in the distal renal tubule, and (3) sympathetic nervous system activation of β_1-adrenoceptors on renal juxtaglomerular cells. When blood pressure falls and renin is released, a cascade of events serves to return blood pressure to the preexisting level. Renin is a protease that converts circulating angiotensinogen to angiotensin I. ACE is a protease primarily located in the pulmonary vasculature that converts the physiologically inactive angiotensin I to the active angiotensin II. Angiotensin II activates two types of **angiotensin receptors,** called AT_1 and AT_2. The AT_1 receptors are coupled with enzymes that increase the formation of inositol triphosphate and various arachidonic acid metabolites and decrease the formation of cyclic adenosine monophosphate. The effects resulting from activation of AT_1 receptors include (1) contraction of vascular smooth muscle

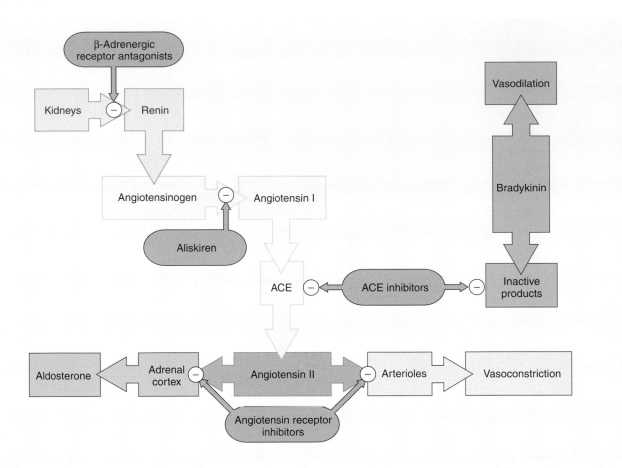

FIG. 10.3 Actions of antihypertensive drugs on the renin-angiotensin-aldosterone axis. β-adrenoceptor antagonists inhibit sympathetic stimulation of renin secretion. Aliskiren directly inhibits renin and the formation of angiotensin I. ACE inhibitors block the formation of angiotensin II and inhibit the breakdown of bradykinin, a vasodilator. Angiotensin receptor antagonists (e.g., losartan) block angiotensin II AT$_1$-receptors in smooth muscle and adrenal cortex. *ACE,* Angiotensin-converting enzyme.

leading to generalized vasoconstriction, (2) secretion of aldosterone from the adrenal cortex, (3) increased reabsorption of sodium from the proximal tubule, (4) increased release of norepinephrine from sympathetic nerves, and (5) stimulation of cell growth in the arteries and heart. AT$_2$ receptors appear to have roles in cardiovascular and metabolic functions.

Angiotensin-Converting Enzyme Inhibitors
Mechanism of Action
ACE inhibitors act by binding to the zinc atom at the enzyme's active site and prevent the catalysis of angiotensin I to angiotensin II. Reducing circulating angiotensin II lowers blood pressure primarily by **reducing vascular resistance.** ACE inhibitors have little effect on cardiac output or blood volume in otherwise healthy persons (see Table 10.2). ACE inhibitors decrease both arterial pressure and venous pressure, and this in turn reduces cardiac afterload and cardiac preload, respectively. By reducing angiotensin-stimulated aldosterone secretion, ACE inhibitors prevent the compensatory increase in sodium retention and plasma volume that can occur with some other antihypertensive drugs. In patients treated with ACE inhibitors, renal sodium retention is decreased, renal potassium retention is increased, and serum potassium levels typically increase by about 0.5 mEq/L. Because ACE also catalyzes **bradykinin,** a

vasodilator, ACE inhibitors may act partly by inhibiting its degradation.

The ACE protease that converts angiotensin I to angiotensin II is formally known as ACE$_1$, a membrane bound protein that is expressed mainly in the lungs. **ACE2** is a distinct soluble enzyme that is found on the epithelial surface of the lung, intestine, and heart and is the target of the pandemic coronavirus **SARS-CoV-2 spike protein** (see Chapter 43). ACE inhibitors used to treat hypertension do not appear to act at the ACE$_2$ protease.

Pharmacokinetics
ACE inhibitors undergo varying degrees of first-pass hepatic inactivation after oral administration, and several of the ACE inhibitors have **active metabolites.** Except for **captopril,** the duration of action of most ACE inhibitors is about 24 hours, and the drugs are administered once or twice daily to treat hypertension and other disorders (Table 10.5).

Adverse Effects
ACE inhibitors can cause **fetal and neonatal injury and death** when administered to pregnant women, especially during the second and third trimesters. Therefore, use of these drugs should be discontinued when pregnancy is detected. ACE inhibitors can also cause renal failure in patients who have a rare condition known as **bilateral renal**

TABLE 10.5   Pharmacokinetic Properties of Selected Angiotensin Inhibitors

DRUG	ORAL BIOAVAILABILITY	ABSORPTION REDUCED BY FOOD	ACTIVE METABOLITE	DURATION OF ACTION (HOURS)
Angiotensin-converting enzyme inhibitors				
Benazepril	37%	No	Benazeprilat	24
Captopril	75%	30%–40%	None	6–12
Enalapril	60%	No	Enalaprilat[a]	24
Fosinopril	36%	No	Fosinoprilat	24
Lisinopril	25%	No	None	24
Quinapril	60%	25%–30%	Quinaprilat	24
Ramipril	55%	No	Ramiprilat	24
Angiotensin receptor antagonists				
Candesartan	15%	No	None	24
Losartan	33%	10%	Carboxylic acid metabolite	24
Valsartan	25%	40%	None	24
Direct renin inhibitor				
Aliskiren	2.5%	Yes (high fat)	None	24

[a]Enalaprilat is available as a separate drug for intravenous administration.

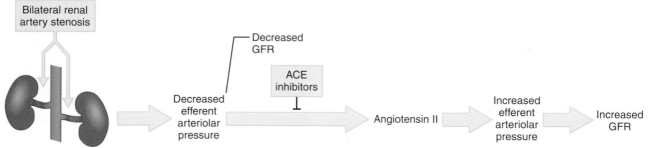

Fig. 10.4   Effects of ACE inhibitors in patients with bilateral renal artery stenosis. Renal blood flow is reduced in the presence of bilateral renal artery stenosis. In affected patients, glomerular filtration is maintained by elevating efferent arteriolar pressure via vasoconstriction produced by angiotensin II. By blocking the formation of angiotensin II, ACE inhibitors can severely impair glomerular filtration and lead to renal failure. *ACE,* Angiotensin-converting enzyme; *GFR,* glomerular filtration rate.

artery stenosis because these persons depend on angiotensin II to maintain renal blood flow and glomerular filtration, as illustrated in Fig. 10.4.

The ACE inhibitors are usually well tolerated and do not adversely affect the lifestyle of most hypertensive patients. The most common side effect is a **dry cough** that is probably caused by increased bradykinin levels. Less commonly, bradykinin accumulation may contribute to the development of **angioedema,** manifested as painful swelling of the lips, face, and throat. Rash and an **abnormal taste sensation** may occur in persons receiving captopril due to the presence of a sulfhydryl group as the drug's zinc-binding moiety.

Interactions

The antihypertensive action of ACE inhibitors is **augmented** by diuretics and CCBs, and combination products containing an ACE inhibitor and one of these drugs are available. ACE inhibitors can interact with potassium-sparing diuretics and potassium supplements to increase serum potassium levels and cause **hyperkalemia.** They can also increase serum lithium levels and provoke **lithium toxicity** in patients receiving lithium compounds for the treatment of a bipolar disorder. Nonsteroidal anti-inflammatory drugs,

such as **ibuprofen,** can impede the effects of ACE inhibitors as well as other antihypertensive agents.

Indications

Because they have excellent antihypertensive action and few bothersome side effects, ACE inhibitors are used in the management of **mild to severe hypertension** in patients with a wide variety of traits and concomitant diseases, as outlined in Table 10.6. These drugs protect against stroke and myocardial infarction and are of particular value in treating hypertensive patients with coexisting heart failure, myocardial infarction, chronic kidney disease, or diabetes mellitus.

Studies have also shown that ACE inhibitors increase cardiac output and survival in patients with **heart failure** (see Chapter 12). These agents also reduce the incidence of overt heart failure and increase survival in persons with myocardial infarction and significant left ventricular dysfunction (a cardiac ejection fraction of less than 40%). The ejection fraction is the percentage of blood ejected from the left ventricle during each systole.

In **diabetic patients** who exhibit early signs of renal impairment (e.g., albuminuria and increased serum creatinine levels), ACE inhibitors exert a **renoprotective effect.**

TABLE 10.6　Selection of Antihypertensive Drugs for Patients With Specific Traits or Concurrent Diseases

PATIENT CHARACTERISTIC	MOST PREFERRED DRUGS	LEAST PREFERRED DRUGS
Age over 65 years	ARB, ACEI, CCB, thiazide diuretic	Clonidine, β-blocker
African heritage	Thiazide diuretic, CCB	β-blocker
Pregnant	Methyldopa, labetalol	ACEI, ARB, aliskiren
Angina pectoris	β-blocker, CCB	Hydralazine, minoxidil
Myocardial infarction	ACEI, ARB, β-blocker, aldosterone antagonist	Hydralazine, minoxidil
Congestive heart failure	ACEI, ARB, β-blocker, thiazide or loop diuretic	Verapamil
Stroke prevention	ARB, ACEI, CCB, thiazide diuretic	
Kidney disease	ACEI or ARB	
Diabetes	ACEI, ARB, CCB, thiazide diuretic	
Asthma	CCB, ACEI, ARB, thiazide diuretic	β-blocker
Benign prostatic hyperplasia	α-blocker	
Migraine headache	β-blocker, CCB	
Osteoporosis	Thiazide diuretic	

ACEI, Angiotensin-converting enzyme inhibitor; *ARB,* angiotensin receptor blocker; *CCB,* calcium channel blocker.

Studies indicate that ACE inhibitors reduce the progression of renal failure and the subsequent need for renal dialysis in these patients. Moreover, if an ACE inhibitor is withdrawn, the progression of nephropathy resumes. Based on these findings, experts now recommend that an ACE inhibitor be given to **diabetic patients** with albuminuria or increased serum creatinine levels, regardless of whether they have hypertension.

Blood pressure is the most important determinant of the risk of **stroke,** and ACE inhibitors are among the agents that reduce the incidence of both primary and secondary stroke. The renin-angiotensin system appears to be involved in the development and progression of cerebrovascular disease, and clinical trials suggest that ACE inhibitors and ARBs have a cerebroprotective effect beyond their blood pressure-lowering ability.

Specific Drugs

Three classes of ACE inhibitors have been developed. In each class, a different chemical group binds the zinc ion in ACE. The only sulfhydryl compound is **captopril;** the phosphoryl agents include **fosinopril;** and the carboxyl derivatives include **benazepril, enalapril, lisinopril, quinapril,** and **ramipril.** All of these drugs, except **captopril** and **lisinopril,** are enzymatically transformed into active metabolites. **Enalaprilat,** the active metabolite of enalapril, is available for intravenous administration; the other ACE inhibitors are administered orally. **Perindopril** is a **prodrug** and is converted to perindoprilat, the biologically active metabolite, by ester hydrolysis.

The orally administered ACE inhibitors undergo considerable first-pass inactivation, and their oral bioavailability ranges from 25% to 75% (see Table 10.5). In comparison with other ACE inhibitors, which are administered one or two times a day, captopril has a shorter half-life and must be administered two or three times a day.

Angiotensin Receptor Blockers

These drugs selectively block **angiotensin AT1 receptors** in various tissues and thereby reduce vasoconstriction, aldosterone secretion, sodium reabsorption by the proximal tubule, and norepinephrine release from sympathetic nerve terminals. ARBs are often effective when used alone, and they can be combined with a diuretic, CCB, or other antihypertensive agent when greater blood pressure reduction is needed. Some studies show a benefit of combining an ACE inhibitor with an ARB in high-risk patients with diabetic nephropathy and other conditions.

Many orally effective ARBs are now available, including **candesartan, irbesartan, losartan, telmisartan, valsartan,** and others. In the treatment of hypertension, these drugs are as effective as the ACE inhibitors but only rarely cause the dry cough that occurs with ACE inhibitors. Recent clinical trials have found that the ARBs can reduce the risk of the cardiovascular consequences of hypertension. In these studies, losartan produced a greater reduction of **left ventricular hypertrophy** and the risk of **stroke** and new-onset **diabetes** than did atenolol, despite having similar blood pressure-lowering effects. With regard to diabetes, ARBs such as **telmisartan** have been shown to increase insulin sensitivity by activating the peroxisome proliferator-activated receptor-γ (see Chapter 35). Moreover, **telmisartan** was shown to be as effective as **ramipril** in protecting a broad range of patients at increased risk of cardiovascular and other diseases, and telmisartan had a more powerful blood pressure-lowering ability than ramipril.

The ARBs do not increase serum glucose, uric acid, or cholesterol levels but may cause **hyperkalemia, neutropenia,** and elevated serum levels of hepatic aminotransferase enzymes. As with the ACE inhibitors, the ARBs can cause **fetal injury and death** and should not be used during pregnancy.

Direct Renin Inhibitor

Aliskiren is the first orally effective direct renin inhibitor to be approved for treatment of hypertension. It binds to the active site of renin, preventing cleavage of angiotensinogen and formation of angiotensin I. Thus, aliskiren lowers **plasma renin activity** and levels of angiotensin I and angiotensin II. Hence, aliskiren can protect against compensatory increases in angiotensin II evoked by other drugs. Aliskiren has equal or superior blood pressure-lowering ability compared with other drugs and a placebo-like side effect profile. It is available as a single-ingredient preparation and in preparations containing hydrochlorothiazide, amlodipine, or valsartan. Aliskiren appears to be a safe and effective option for the treatment of high blood pressure.

VASODILATORS

The vasodilators include the CCBs and other agents such as **hydralazine, minoxidil,** and **nitroprusside.** The pharmacologic effects, adverse effects, and drug interactions of these agents are summarized in Tables 10.2, 10.3, and 10.4.

Calcium Channel Blockers

CCBs are used to treat **hypertension, angina pectoris, peripheral vascular disorders,** and **cardiac arrhythmias.** Chapter 11 discusses the pharmacologic properties of these drugs in more detail, whereas this chapter focuses on their antihypertensive actions.

By blocking calcium ion channels in the plasma membranes of smooth muscle, the CCBs **relax vascular smooth muscle** and cause **vasodilation.** CCBs have a greater effect on arteriolar smooth muscle than on venous smooth muscle, and their effect on blood pressure is primarily caused by a reduction in PVR, with relatively little effect on venous capacitance, cardiac filling pressure, and cardiac output.

Whereas all of the CCBs relax vascular smooth muscle, **diltiazem** and **verapamil** also have significant effects on cardiac tissue and can reduce the heart rate and cardiac output. Most CCBs, including **amlodipine, felodipine, isradipine, nicardipine,** and **nifedipine,** belong to the dihydropyridine class. The dihydropyridine drugs have little direct effect on cardiac tissue at usual therapeutic levels; however, they can evoke **reflex tachycardia.**

The CCBs are among the most widely recommended drugs for the initial treatment of high blood pressure, and they are often combined with diuretics or angiotensin system inhibitors. CCBs protect against stroke, coronary heart disease, and kidney disease. In fact, **verapamil** and **diltiazem** reduce protein excretion in patients with **kidney disease** and may be used with an ACE inhibitor or ARB for this purpose. The CCBs are relatively free of adverse effects and do not alter levels of serum glucose, lipids, uric acid, or electrolytes. Occasionally, dihydropyridine CCBs cause gingival hyperplasia in persons with poor dental care. They are particularly useful in treating hypertensive patients who have asthma or are of **African heritage** (see Table 10.6). Because of the need to obtain 24-hour blood pressure control in hypertensive patients, a long-acting CCB such as amlodipine or a sustained-release formulation such as the nifedipine gastrointestinal system should be employed.

Other Vasodilators
Hydralazine and Minoxidil

Hydralazine and minoxidil are powerful orally effective vasodilators primarily used in combination with other antihypertensive drugs to treat **moderate to very severe hypertension.** When used alone, they often evoke **reflex tachycardia** and cause **fluid retention,** and they can precipitate angina in susceptible patients. To prevent these problems, hydralazine or minoxidil is usually given in combination with two other drugs: a diuretic plus either a β-adrenoceptor antagonist or another sympatholytic agent. Hydralazine has been associated with a **lupus-like syndrome,** whereas minoxidil

can cause **hypertrichosis** (excessive hair growth), particularly in women. In fact, minoxidil is marketed as a topical formulation for the treatment of several forms of **alopecia** (baldness) in men and women. For many reasons, hydralazine and minoxidil are reserved for treating hypertension resistant to other drugs.

Nitroprusside

Sodium nitroprusside is one of several drugs used in the management of **hypertensive emergencies.** The drug is administered by intravenous infusion and has a short half-life. Nitroprusside is rapidly metabolized to **cyanide** in erythrocytes and other tissues. Cyanide is then converted to **thiocyanate** in the presence of a sulfur donor. Both thiocyanate and cyanide gradually accumulate during nitroprusside infusion. For this reason, the duration of therapy with this drug is usually limited to a few days. During drug administration, the patient's blood pressure should be monitored frequently, and thiocyanate levels should be checked every 72 hours to detect potential toxicity.

Fenoldopam

Fenoldopam is a rapid-acting, intravenously administered vasodilator used to treat **hypertensive emergencies** (see later). It activates vascular **dopamine D1-receptors** and produces vasodilation in systemic vascular beds, including coronary, renal, and mesenteric vessels. In the kidney, fenoldopam dilates both afferent and efferent arterioles, thereby increasing renal blood flow. The drug is rapidly converted to inactive conjugates with an elimination half-life of about 5 minutes. Fenoldopam can reduce serum potassium levels, which should be monitored at 6-hour intervals during drug infusion.

THE MANAGEMENT OF HYPERTENSION

The Eighth Joint National Committee on Hypertension (JNC 8) published its guidelines for treatment in 2014. As with earlier JNC reports, JNC 8 stresses the importance of lifestyle modifications and recommends starting drug therapy with a **thiazide diuretic, ACE inhibitor, angiotensin receptor blocker,** or **calcium channel blocker** for most patients.

Lifestyle Modifications

Patients with hypertension should be encouraged to pursue **lifestyle changes** that can improve general health and lower their blood pressure. Effective strategies include exercise and weight loss, moderation of alcohol intake, and a diet that is rich in fruits, vegetables, and nuts and low in sodium, such as the DASH (Dietary Approaches to Stop Hypertension) or American Heart Association diet. Unless hypertension is severe, patients should try lifestyle modifications for several months before instituting drug therapy.

Selection of Drug Therapy

The JNC 8 recommends three methods for initiating and modifying drug therapy. These methods represent different approaches to drug selection and titration. As a general rule, a single drug is recommended for starting therapy if blood pressure is less 160/100 mm Hg, and a 2-drug combination is suggested for those with higher pressures. Doses of each drug are then increased until blood pressure is controlled or the maximum effective dose is reached and alternative drugs are considered.

Clinical experience has shown that many patients with high blood pressure require more than one drug to achieve target blood pressure levels. Studies have found that therapy with more than one drug increases the likelihood of achieving a desired blood pressure, and drug combinations often achieve blood pressure reduction with lower doses of the component drugs, thereby reducing the incidence of adverse effects. A number of **combination drug products** are now available that can be taken once or twice daily. These products can be less expensive and more convenient to use than two single-drug products, and they enhance patient adherence to the treatment regimen. The combinations include those with a CCB and an angiotensin inhibitor, such as **amlodipine** and **valsartan** (EXFORGE). Other combinations contain a thiazide diuretic with an ACE inhibitor or a CCB. Recently, a combination of **nebivolol** and **valsartan** was approved (BYVALSON). Unless intolerable side effects occur or hypertension is severe, drugs should be given a trial of several weeks before their effectiveness is evaluated or medications are changed.

Patients with Specific Traits or Diseases

Table 10.6 summarizes the most preferred and least preferred drugs for hypertensive patients with specific traits or concurrent diseases. These recommendations are only guidelines, and individual patient characteristics should always be considered when selecting drug therapy. For example, patients with **chronic kidney disease** (CKD) and proteinuria should receive an ACE inhibitor or angiotensin receptor blocker. For most blacks, a thiazide diuretic or CCB are first-line choices.

For patients with **diabetes mellitus,** guidelines recommend that blood pressure be controlled to the level of 130/80 mm Hg or lower (Box 10.1). This is because rigorous control of blood pressure is essential for reducing the progression of **diabetic nephropathy** to end-stage renal disease. Clinical trials found that ACE inhibitors, ARBs, and CCBs have demonstrated benefits in patients with both type 1 and type 2 diabetes. The ACE inhibitors and ARBs are important components of antihypertensive regimens for patients with diabetes because of their ability to reduce the progression of diabetic nephropathy. Recommendations for persons with other traits and conditions are shown in Table 10.6.

Hypertensive Emergencies and Urgencies

Hypertensive emergencies are characterized by **severe elevations in blood pressure** (>180/120 mm Hg) complicated by target organ dysfunction (e.g., encephalopathy or intracranial hemorrhage). These situations require an immediate reduction in blood pressure to limit organ damage. **Hypertensive urgencies** are situations with severe elevations of blood pressure without target organ dysfunction, such as with persons who have upper levels of stage 2 hypertension associated with severe headache, shortness of breath, or severe anxiety.

The initial goal of treatment of hypertensive emergencies is to reduce blood pressure by no more than 25% within the first hour and then to 160/100 mm Hg within the next 2 to 6 hours. If this level of blood pressure is well tolerated, gradual reductions to normal blood pressure can be implemented in the next 24 to 48 hours. Excessive reductions in blood pressure can precipitate renal, cerebral, or coronary ischemia and should be avoided. For this reason,

---

BOX 10.1 A CASE OF INCREASING BLOOD PRESSURE AND PROTEINURIA

CASE PRESENTATION

An overweight 46-year-old African American woman with an 8-year history of type 2 diabetes and a 5-year history of hypertension has been seen regularly by her health care providers. Her diabetes has been treated with dietary restrictions and metformin, although her target glycosylated hemoglobin A_{1c} level (<7%) has not been achieved. Her blood pressure had been controlled with a thiazide diuretic, but over the past 2 years, her blood pressure readings have increased and now average 138/86 mm Hg. Her latest test results showed microalbuminuria (proteinuria) of 50 m/min over 24 hours. Valsartan, amlodipine, and glipizide were added to her treatment regimen, and the thiazide diuretic was discontinued. She was scheduled to see a dietitian and exercise counselor.

CASE DISCUSSION

The prevalence of both type 2 diabetes and hypertension is higher in black patients than in other populations, and both diseases increase the risk of proteinuria and chronic kidney disease. A greater proportion of black hypertensive patients exhibit microalbuminuria (>30 m/min) compared with white patients. For these reasons, it is important that patients achieve target A_{1c} and blood pressure levels (<130/80 mm Hg) to slow the progression of kidney disease. Several types of drugs can be combined with metformin to help patients control blood glucose and A_{1c} levels, including glipizide and incretin mimetics such as sitagliptin (see Chapter 35). Because a thiazide diuretic can decrease insulin sensitivity, it was decided to replace this patient's diuretic with valsartan and amlodipine to achieve the target blood pressure level and slow the progression of nephropathy. Although diuretics and calcium channel blockers are often preferred for the initial treatment of black patients with hypertension, angiotensin inhibitors can be effective when combined with other drugs. Lifestyle changes can help the patient achieve target A_{1c} and blood pressure levels while controlling body weight.

---

short-acting nifedipine is no longer an acceptable treatment for hypertensive emergencies or urgencies.

A number of drugs can be used to treat hypertensive emergencies and urgencies, and therapy should be guided by clinical judgment and the consideration of individual patient characteristics. Parenterally administered drugs are usually used, although oral **clonidine** can be used for less-severe hypertensive urgencies because it slowly reduces blood pressure to a safe level. The drugs most often used in treating most types of hypertensive emergencies include **fenoldopam, nicardipine, labetalol,** and **sodium nitroprusside. Nitroglycerin** is useful for hypertensive emergencies in persons with **acute coronary ischemia,** and **enalaprilat** may be of value in patients with acute **left ventricular failure** (but not acute myocardial infarction). **Esmolol** is useful in persons with **aortic dissection** and **perioperative** hypertension.

Pheochromocytomas are nonmalignant, catecholamine-releasing tumors located in the medulla of the adrenal gland. They occur in 1 of every 1000 patients with hypertension. These tumors are highly vascularized and contain high concentrations of norepinephrine and epinephrine, which is released in a continuous or paroxysmal fashion, the latter causing a **hypertensive crisis.** Treatment is by surgical removal, and patients are pretreated by the administration of **phenoxybenzamine** to induce a long-lasting α-adrenoceptor blockade and β-blockers. **Metyrosine** is also often used as it inhibits tyrosine hydroxylase and subsequent biosynthesis of catecholamines.

SUMMARY OF IMPORTANT POINTS

- The four major classes of antihypertensive drugs are the diuretics, sympatholytic drugs, angiotensin inhibitors, and vasodilators.
- Thiazide diuretics initially reduce blood volume and cardiac output, but their long-term effect on blood pressure is primarily caused by decreased PVR.
- Sympatholytic drugs used in the treatment of hypertension include α-adrenoceptor antagonists, β-adrenoceptor antagonists, and centrally acting drugs. Except for the β-blockers, which reduce cardiac output, the sympatholytics reduce blood pressure primarily by decreasing PVR.
- The angiotensin inhibitors include ACE inhibitors (e.g., lisinopril), ARBs (e.g., losartan), and direct renin inhibitor, aliskiren. These drugs reduce PVR and aldosterone levels, with little effect on blood volume or cardiac output in patients who do not have heart failure.
- The vasodilators include the CCBs, hydralazine, minoxidil, and nitroprusside. These drugs reduce PVR, and some of them (hydralazine and minoxidil) provoke reflex tachycardia and fluid retention.
- The management of high blood pressure begins with lifestyle modifications and then proceeds to the use of an angiotensin inhibitor or CCB for many patients without comorbid conditions. Thiazide diuretics are often combined with other drugs. Patients with heart disease often benefit from the use of a β-blocker and an angiotensin system inhibitor. Angiotensin system inhibitors are particularly useful in preventing kidney disease. ARBs appear to protect against stroke more than other drugs.

Review Questions

1. A patient with type 2 diabetes and hypertension has recently developed proteinuria. Which drug would be most likely to slow the progression of renal disease in this patient beyond its ability to lower blood pressure?
   (A) metoprolol
   (B) enalapril
   (C) nifedipine
   (D) lisinopril
   (E) diltiazem

2. A man with a history of poor dental hygiene and high blood pressure complains of tender and swollen gums during an appointment with his dentist. Which antihypertensive drug might be contributing to this condition?
   (A) irbesartan
   (B) metoprolol
   (C) nifedipine
   (D) hydrochlorothiazide
   (E) doxazosin

3. Which drug binds to renin and inhibits its activity?
   (A) aliskiren
   (B) atenolol
   (C) enalapril
   (D) hydrochlorothiazide
   (E) valsartan

4. What is the mechanism by which irbesartan lowers blood pressure?
   (A) inhibiting renin
   (B) blocking angiotensin AT1 receptors
   (C) decreasing calcium entry into smooth muscle
   (D) inhibiting formation of angiotensin II
   (E) antagonizing aldosterone

5. Which drug blocks α- and β-adrenoceptors, and also has antioxidant and other beneficial effects?
   (A) carvedilol
   (B) amlodipine
   (C) propranolol
   (D) hydrochlorothiazide
   (E) doxazosin

CHAPTER 11 Antianginal Drugs

OVERVIEW
Coronary Heart Disease

The spectrum of coronary heart disease (CHD), a subset of cardiovascular disease, includes **chronic angina pectoris** (stable angina) and a group of acute coronary syndromes consisting of **unstable angina** and **myocardial infarction** (MI) (Fig. 11.1). Two forms of MI can be distinguished by the presence or lack of ST-segment elevation on the electrocardiogram, as described more fully in Chapter 16. All of these conditions are caused by myocardial hypoxia due to coronary artery ischemia (inadequate blood flow) resulting from atherosclerosis, formation of thrombi (blood clots), or coronary vasospasm.

Typical angina results from the formation of atherosclerotic plaques in vessel walls that limit coronary blood flow and the supply of oxygen to the myocardium. The symptoms of angina, often described as resembling a heavy weight or pressure on the chest, occur when the oxygen supply is insufficient to meet the demand imposed by increased physical exertion. The condition is called **stable angina** if angina attacks have similar characteristics and occur in similar circumstances each time. It is known as **unstable angina** if the frequency and severity of attacks increase over time. Unstable angina, which may be caused by occlusion

of a coronary vessel by small platelet thrombi and ruptured atheromatous plaque, is often the forerunner of MI. **Variant angina (Prinzmetal angina)** is caused by acute coronary **vasospasm** and may occur at rest or during sleep.

Table 11.1 lists five classes of drugs and compares their efficacy in treating different forms of CHD. This chapter focuses on the anti-ischemic agents: **organic nitrites and nitrates, calcium channel blockers** (CCBs), and **β-adrenoceptor antagonists** (β-blockers), which are the primary agents used to treat angina symptoms. Chapter 15 discusses drugs for hyperlipidemia, and Chapter 16 covers antithrombotic drugs (e.g., aspirin). The latter two groups of drugs have been shown to reduce the risk of MI and death in persons with CHD.

Mechanisms and Effects of Antianginal Drugs

The antiischemic agents used in treating angina serve to prevent or counteract myocardial ischemia and thereby increase exercise tolerance and reduce the frequency of anginal attacks. This is accomplished by restoring the balance between myocardial oxygen supply and demand by either increasing oxygen supply or decreasing oxygen demand. The factors that determine supply and demand are illustrated in Fig. 11.2.

Myocardial oxygen supply is primarily determined by **coronary blood flow** and **regional flow distribution** but is also influenced by **oxygen extraction.** In patients with coronary artery disease, the subendocardial tissue is more likely to be affected by ischemia because it is not as well perfused as the subepicardial tissue. The use of nitrates or CCBs (vasodilator drugs) can reduce ischemia by increasing total coronary flow and the distribution of coronary flow to ischemic subendocardial tissue. The drugs increase perfusion of subendocardial tissue by dilating collateral vessels and by decreasing intraventricular pressure and resistance to perfusion. The β-blockers improve the distribution of coronary flow by reducing intraventricular pressure. Cardiac tissue extracts a higher percentage of oxygen from the blood than does any other tissue, and this factor is not affected by drugs.

Myocardial oxygen demand is determined by the amount of energy required to support the work of the heart. The factors that influence cardiac work include **heart rate, cardiac contractility,** and **myocardial wall tension.** Contractility is directly related to the amount of cytosolic calcium available to stimulate the shortening of myocardial fibers. As contractility increases, the velocity of fiber shortening and peak systolic muscle tension also increase. Myocardial wall tension is equal to the product of ventricular volume (radius) and pressure, divided by wall thickness. Ventricular wall tension is primarily determined by arterial and venous blood pressure.

Antianginal drugs act by several mechanisms to **reduce myocardial oxygen demand.** The β-blockers and ivabradine

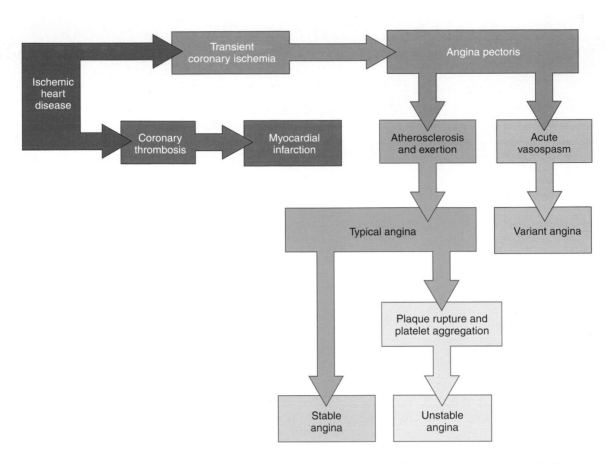

Fɪɢ. 11.1   Classification and pathophysiology of ischemic heart disease. Variant angina, also called *Prinzmetal angina*, is considered a form of unstable angina if the angina attacks occur with increasing severity or frequency.

TABLE 11.1   Efficacy of Drugs Used in the Treatment of Coronary Heart Disease[a]

DRUG CLASS	TYPICAL ANGINA PECTORIS		VARIANT ANGINA	MYOCARDIAL INFARCTION
	STABLE ANGINA	UNSTABLE ANGINA		
Organic nitrites and nitrates	++	++	++	++
Calcium channel blockers	++	0 to ++	+++	0
β-adrenoceptor antagonists	++	++	0	+++
Ranolazine	++	Uncertain	0	Uncertain
ACE inhibitors	0 to ++	0 to ++	0 to ++	+++
Antithrombotic drugs (e.g., aspirin)[b]	+++	+++	0 to ++	+++
Cholesterol-lowering agents	+++	+++	0 to ++	+++

ACE, Angiotensin-converting enzyme.
[a]Ratings range from 0 (not efficacious) to +++ (highly efficacious).
[b]Includes antiplatelet, anticoagulant, and fibrinolytic drugs.

both decrease heart rate, while β-blockers also decrease cardiac contractility. The organic nitrates, CCBs, and ranolazine reduce ventricular wall tension and oxygen demand via their effects on ventricular volume and pressure. Dilation of veins decreases venous pressure, cardiac filling pressure, and ventricular diastolic pressure (preload). Dilation of arteries decreases arterial and aortic pressure and thereby reduces ventricular systolic pressure (afterload) and the impedance to the ventricular ejection of blood. The organic nitrates act primarily on venous tissue and predominantly affect preload, whereas the CCBs act mostly on arteriolar muscle

to reduce afterload. Ranolazine (see later) appears to work throughout the cardiac cycle.

In **typical angina,** which is caused by increased oxygen demand in the face of a limited oxygen supply, vasodilators, β-blockers, and other drugs act primarily by decreasing oxygen demand through the mechanisms described previously. They can also increase the perfusion of ischemic subendocardial tissue. In **variant angina,** chest pain usually occurs at rest (when oxygen demand is relatively low), and ischemia results in a reduction in oxygen supply secondary to coronary artery spasm. Under these conditions, vasodilators

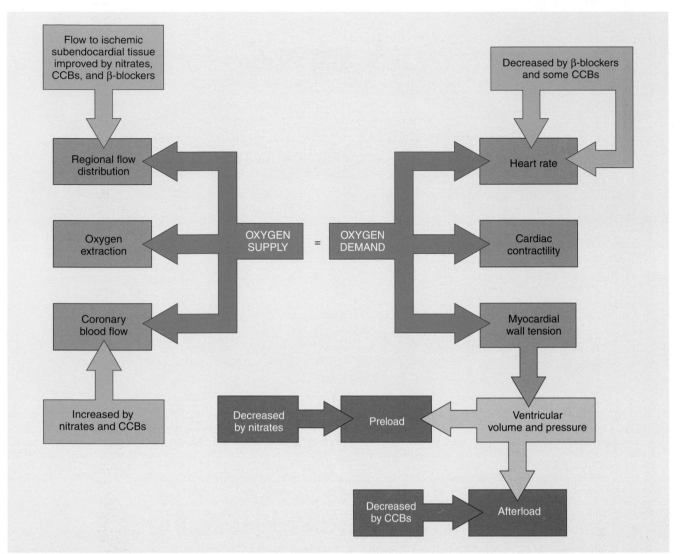

Fig. 11.2 Effects of organic nitrites and nitrates, calcium channel blockers, and β-adrenoceptor antagonists (β-blockers) on myocardial oxygen supply and demand.

increase oxygen supply by relaxing coronary smooth muscle and restoring normal coronary flow. The β-blockers are not effective in variant angina because they do not counteract vasospasm and increase coronary blood flow. The β-blockers may actually reduce coronary blood flow by blocking the vasodilation effect of epinephrine, an effect that is mediated by β_2-adrenoceptors in coronary smooth muscle.

VASODILATORS

Two classes of vasodilators are used in the management of angina pectoris. The first consists of organic nitrites and nitrates, and the second consists of CCBs.

Organic Nitrites and Nitrates

The organic nitrites and nitrates are esters of nitrous acid and nitric acid, respectively. **Amyl nitrite,** the only nitrite compound used to treat angina, is administered by inhalation. **Nitroglycerin** (glyceryl trinitrate), isosorbide dinitrate, and isosorbide mononitrate are compounds with sufficient solubility in water and lipids to enable rapid dissolution and absorption after sublingual, oral, or transdermal administration. The onset and duration of action

of these drugs vary with their physical properties, route of administration, and rate of biotransformation. Amyl nitrite has the **most rapid onset** and the shortest duration of action, whereas isosorbide compounds have the slowest onset and the longest duration. Nitroglycerin has an intermediate onset and duration. All of these compounds are extensively metabolized in the liver.

Amyl Nitrite

Amyl nitrite is a volatile liquid that can be inhaled and absorbed through the lungs. Its action is rapid in onset (within 30 seconds) and brief in duration (3–5 minutes). Amyl nitrite is effective in the **treatment of acute angina attacks,** as well as in the **initial management of cyanide poisoning.** In patients with cyanide poisoning, amyl nitrite is used until intravenous **sodium nitrite** and **sodium thiosulfate** can be administered. The nitrites oxidize hemoglobin to methemoglobin. In comparison with hemoglobin, methemoglobin has a greater affinity for cyanide, and this allows it to trap the compound in the form of cyanmethemoglobin. Thiosulfate is then administered to convert cyanide to inactive thiocyanate.

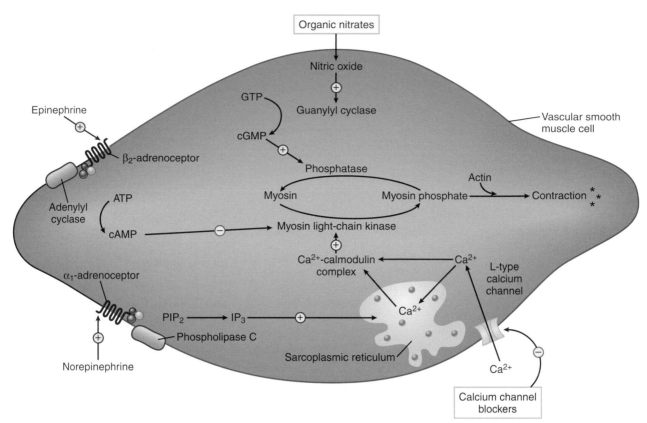

Fig. 11.3 Regulation of vascular smooth muscle contraction. Vascular smooth muscle contraction occurs when calcium (Ca^{2+}) enters smooth muscle via L-type calcium channels, binds to calmodulin, and activates myosin light-chain kinase. This leads to the formation of myosin phosphate, which interacts with actin to cause muscle contraction. Calcium influx is inhibited by CCBs, leading to muscle relaxation. Organic nitrates release nitric oxide, which activates guanylyl cyclase and increases the formation of cyclic guanosine monophosphate (cGMP). Investigators believe that cGMP causes smooth muscle relaxation by activating kinases that increase myosin phosphatase activity and decrease myosin phosphate levels. α_1-adrenoceptor agonists activate phospholipase C, which increases the formation of inositol triphosphate (IP3) from phosphatidylinositol bisphosphate (PIP2), leading to increased release of calcium from the sarcoplasmic reticulum. β_2-adrenoceptor agonists increase the formation of cyclic adenosine monophosphate (cAMP), which activates kinases that inhibit myosin light-chain kinase.

Amyl nitrite and other similar agents are sometimes abused and used recreationally, called **"poppers."** They became popular with gay males in urban settings; now, they are abused among a variety of persons associated with the club scene. Like other inhalant drugs of abuse (see Chapter 25), amyl nitrite can produce **euphoria** and **increase sexual libido.** They also relax involuntary smooth muscles found in the vagina and anus. A number of significant health problems arise from the misuse of poppers, including immune system suppression, red blood cell dysfunction, and overdose.

Nitroglycerin, Isosorbide Dinitrate, and Isosorbide Mononitrate

Pharmacokinetics. Nitroglycerin and isosorbide preparations are used to **prevent and treat angina attacks. Nitroglycerin** is available in formulations for sublingual, transdermal, topical, oral, and intravenous administration. The drug's solubility in water and lipids permits its rapid dissolution and absorption after **sublingual** or buccal administration for the treatment of acute angina attacks. Its high lipid solubility and low dosage have enabled the formulation of skin patches known as films for transdermal administration. The patches slowly release the drug for absorption through the skin into the circulation and are used in the **prevention of angina attacks.** In ointment form, nitroglycerin is absorbed through the skin over a period of several hours. The ointment is primarily used in hospitalized patients with **angina** or **MI.** Nitroglycerin is administered orally in the form of sustained-release capsules used to prevent angina attacks. The drug is well absorbed from the gut but undergoes considerable first-pass inactivation, thereby necessitating the use of larger doses when administered orally. Nitroglycerin is also available as an intravenous solution used chiefly to reduce preload but also to reduce afterload in patients who have **acute heart failure** associated with MI and other conditions.

Isosorbide dinitrate can be administered sublingually or orally and is used for both the prevention and the treatment of angina attacks. Isosorbide dinitrate produces the same pharmacologic effects as nitroglycerin, but it has a slightly slower onset of action and a greater duration of action. It is converted to an active compound, **isosorbide mononitrate,** which is now available as a drug preparation itself.

Mechanisms and Pharmacologic Effects. The organic nitrates appear to act by releasing **nitric oxide** in vascular smooth muscle cells (Fig. 11.3). The mechanisms by which nitroglycerin and other organic nitrates release nitric oxide are uncertain. Some evidence suggests the involvement of thiol (-SH) compounds in this process. Recent evidence supports the involvement of **aldehyde dehydrogenase** in the release of nitric oxide as well as in the development of **nitrate tolerance** (see next section).

TABLE 11.2 Pharmacokinetic Properties of Calcium Channel Blockers Used in the Treatment of Coronary Heart Disease[a]

DRUG	ORAL BIOAVAILABILITY	EXCRETED UNCHANGED IN URINE	ELIMINATION HALF-LIFE (HOURS)
Dihydropyridine drugs			
Amlodipine	75%	10%	40
Felodipine	20%	1%	14
Nicardipine	35%	1%	3
Nifedipine	60%	1%	3
Nimodipine	13%	<1%	1.5
Other calcium channel blockers			
Diltiazem	55%	3%	5
Verapamil	25%	3%	5

[a]Values shown are the mean of values reported in the literature.

Nitric oxide is a gas that **activates guanylyl cyclase,** forming cyclic guanosine monophosphate (cGMP). Cyclic GMP activates cGMP-dependent kinases that appear to cause **relaxation of vascular smooth muscle** by phosphorylating proteins that decrease intracellular calcium mobilization and decrease phosphorylation of myosin light chains by increasing activity of myosin light-chain phosphatase (an enzyme that removes phosphate; see Fig. 11.3).

The organic nitrates **preferentially relax venous smooth muscle** and have a relatively smaller effect on arteriolar smooth muscle. This leads to venous pooling of blood, a decrease in the venous blood return to the heart, and a decrease in ventricular volume, pressure, and wall tension. By these mechanisms, the nitrates reduce cardiac work and oxygen demand and thereby relieve or prevent angina pectoris. By reducing **cardiac preload,** nitrates also reduce cardiac output and thereby contribute to a reduction in blood pressure. If blood pressure falls sufficiently, reflex tachycardia can be invoked. The nitrates do not have any direct effects on myocardial tissue.

Tolerance. Continuous administration of nitroglycerin and other organic nitrates often leads to pharmacodynamic tolerance to their vasodilation effects. It has been demonstrated to occur with intravenous, transdermal, and oral administration of the nitrates, including sustained-release preparations of them. To **prevent nitrate tolerance** and loss of therapeutic effect, skin patches should be removed for at least 10 hours each day, and long-acting oral medications should be administered only once or twice a day.

Several mechanisms have been proposed to explain nitrate tolerance, but none has been proved conclusively. Studies suggest that **oxygen free radicals** (O_2^-) are formed during the release of nitric oxide from organic nitrates by mitochondrial **aldehyde dehydrogenase,** and it is proposed that these radicals inactivate aldehyde dehydrogenase and thereby decrease nitric oxide formation and lead to tolerance.

Adverse Effects and Interactions. The most common adverse effects of organic nitrates are caused by excessive vasodilation, including **headache, hypotension, dizziness,** and **reflex tachycardia.** Tachycardia increases oxygen demand and can counteract the beneficial effects of nitrates, so patients should be cautioned to avoid excessive doses of these drugs. To prevent reflex tachycardia,

a β-blocker can be used together with an organic nitrate or other types of vasodilators. The hypotensive effect of organic nitrates is potentiated by **sildenafil** and other 5-phosphodiesterase inhibitors used in treating **erectile dysfunction** (see Chapter 6). Both classes of drugs increase cGMP levels and cause vasodilation. Profound hypotension leading to reflex tachycardia and angina may occur if these drugs are used concurrently, and some episodes have been fatal.

Calcium Channel Blockers

The CCBs include several subgroups. **Amlodipine, felodipine, isradipine, nicardipine, nifedipine,** and **nimodipine** belong to the dihydropyridine class and have similar pharmacologic properties. **Diltiazem** and **verapamil** are unique members of other classes.

All of the CCBs, **except nimodipine,** are indicated for the treatment of **hypertension** (see Chapter 10). Diltiazem and verapamil are also used to treat certain types of **cardiac arrhythmias** (see Chapter 14). Nimodipine is indicated for the treatment of **subarachnoid hemorrhage,** and its use is described later. The CCBs used in the management of **angina pectoris** include several dihydropyridine drugs (amlodipine, felodipine, nicardipine, and nifedipine) and the nondihydropyridine drugs diltiazem and verapamil.

Pharmacokinetics

The pharmacokinetic properties of the seven antianginal CCBs are summarized in Table 11.2. These CCBs are well absorbed after oral administration, but most of them undergo significant first-pass metabolism. Diltiazem, nicardipine, nifedipine, and verapamil have relatively **short half-lives** and are available in sustained-release preparations that are administered once or twice daily. Amlodipine and felodipine have **longer half-lives,** and their immediate-release formulations are administered once or twice a day.

Mechanisms and Pharmacologic Effects

The **calcium ion channels** are located in the plasma membrane of smooth muscle and cardiac tissues. The influx of calcium through these channels leads to membrane depolarization and initiates or strengthens muscle contraction. CCBs bind to these channels and alter their conformation in a way that **prevents the entry of calcium** into cells (see

TABLE 11.3 **Cardiovascular Effects of Calcium Channel Blockers Used in the Treatment of Angina**

DRUG	CORONARY BLOOD FLOW	HEART RATE AND CONTRACTILITY	AV CONDUCTION VELOCITY
Amlodipine, nicardipine, nifedipine, felodipine	↑↑	→ or ↑ (reflex)	→ or ↑ (reflex)
Diltiazem	↑↑	↓	↓
Verapamil	↑↑	↓ or ↓↓	↓ or ↓↓

AV, Atrioventricular.

Fig. 11.3). By this mechanism, CCBs produce smooth muscle relaxation and suppress cardiac activity.

Calcium channels are classified on the basis of their electrophysiologic properties. The two main types of voltage-activated calcium channels are the L (long) type and the T (transient) type. **L-type calcium channels** are high-voltage channels that are slowly inactivated, and their calcium influx has a relatively long duration. **T-type calcium channels** are low-voltage channels that are rapidly inactivated, and their calcium influx is more transient. Both L-type and T-type channels are found in vascular smooth muscle and in the sinoatrial (SA) and atrioventricular (AV) nodes. Only L-type channels, however, are found in the muscle cells of the heart. CCBs differ in their affinity for the different types of calcium channels. All of the currently available CCBs selectively bind to L-type channels.

Whereas all CCBs cause vascular smooth muscle to relax, they differ markedly in their effects on cardiac tissue (Table 11.3). The dihydropyridine drugs, which are potent vasodilators, can reduce blood pressure sufficiently to evoke reflex tachycardia. At therapeutic doses, the dihydropyridine drugs do not suppress cardiac function as much as the other CCBs. **Diltiazem** and **verapamil** decrease SA node automaticity, cardiac contractility, and AV node conduction velocity to a greater degree than the other CCBs and can significantly reduce cardiac output in patients with heart failure.

Adverse Effects

The most common side effects of CCBs are **fatigue, headache, dizziness, flushing, peripheral edema,** and other manifestations of vasodilation and hypotension. CCBs can also cause **constipation** by relaxing gastrointestinal smooth muscle and reducing peristalsis. In retrospective case-control studies, investigators found a higher incidence of MI, congestive heart failure, and deaths from CHD in the group of patients who took immediate-release forms of **nifedipine** and other short-acting CCBs than in the control group. Authorities now recommend that a long-acting CCB or a **sustained-release formulation** of nifedipine or felodipine be used for treating chronic cardiovascular disorders. The CCBs occasionally cause **gingival hyperplasia** (gingival overgrowth) in persons with poor dental hygiene or care. This condition is amenable to dental treatment. Unlike diltiazem and verapamil, dihydropyridine CCBs do not affect digoxin serum levels significantly.

Specific Drugs

Amlodipine, felodipine, nicardipine, and **nifedipine** are the dihydropyridine CCBs approved for the treatment of angina. Amlodipine has a long elimination half-life and is administered once a day. **Felodipine** and **nifedipine** are available in sustained-release formulations given once daily.

Nimodipine is used for the purpose of reducing the neurologic complications of **subarachnoid hemorrhage,** which is one of the causes of stroke (as an oral solution in NYMALIZE). The drug dilates small cerebral vessels and increases collateral circulation to the affected areas of the brain. It also reduces neuronal damage caused by the excessive release of calcium that is evoked by cerebral ischemia. Nimodipine should be given only by mouth or feeding tube and never by intravenous administration, a method that has caused **severe hypotension, cardiac arrest,** and **fatalities.**

Diltiazem and verapamil are effective treatments for **typical** and **variant angina.** Because these drugs can suppress cardiac contractility, caution should be exercised when administering them to patients with heart failure, especially verapamil. In patients who have typical angina without heart failure, the drugs have the advantage of reducing the heart rate and contractility in addition to their effects on myocardial wall tension. Both verapamil and diltiazem reduce the clearance of digoxin and can thereby increase serum digoxin levels and precipitate digoxin toxicity. Digoxin doses should be reduced in patients receiving these drugs.

BETA-ADRENOCEPTOR ANTAGONISTS

The pharmacologic properties of β-adrenoceptor antagonists, or β-blockers, are discussed in Chapter 9, and their use in the treatment of hypertension and arrhythmias is discussed in Chapters 10 and 14, respectively.

Among the β-blockers used in the management of angina are **atenolol, metoprolol, nadolol,** and **propranolol.** These β-blockers are often used in **typical angina pectoris** and **acute MI,** but they are not used in the management of vasospastic angina or acute anginal attacks. In typical angina, they prevent ischemic episodes because of their ability to prevent exercise-induced tachycardia and increased myocardial oxygen demand. They can also prevent reflex tachycardia induced by either organic nitrates or dihydropyridine CCBs. In the post-MI setting, β-blockers decrease the risk of recurrence and **improve survival.**

The β-blockers have a **negative inotropic effect** that can be hazardous to patients with heart failure if large doses are given. Because the combination of verapamil and a β-blocker may significantly reduce cardiac output, it should usually be avoided. The combination of a β-blocker and diltiazem is less hazardous.

OTHER ANTIANGINAL AGENTS
Ivabradine

Ivabradine is a novel **heart rate–lowering drug** that has been approved for the treatment of chronic angina and heart failure. The drug reduces the heart rate by blocking the **If current** (the so-called "funny current") in the **SA node,** which is a mixed Na^+-K^+ inward current activated by hyperpolarization, modulated by the autonomic nervous system, and responsible for diastolic depolarization and cardiac impulse initiation. Clinical trials have reported mixed results with ivabradine in the treatment of chronic angina. Some trials found that ivabradine reduced the frequency of angina attacks and improved total exercise duration, while other trials did not. Adverse effects forced discontinuation of the drug in 13% of patients in one study due to headache, visual disturbances, bradycardia, atrial fibrillation, and atrioventricular block. In a study of patients with heart failure, ivabradine reduced the worsening of **heart failure,** need for hospitalization, and mortality in these subjects. It has been suggested the drug may be most useful in patients with both angina and heart failure. Ivabradine is metabolized by CYP3A4, and strong inhibitors of this isozyme should not be given concurrently.

Agents That Alter Metabolism

For many years, the pharmacotherapy of angina has been dependent on vasodilators and drugs that decrease heart rate and contractility. A new group of drugs has emerged that reduce angina episodes by improving myocardial metabolism without altering heart rate or blood pressure. These agents include **ranolazine** and **trimetazidine.**

Ranolazine has been approved as a first-line agent for **chronic stable** angina and is particularly useful for patients with a heart rate less than 70/min or low blood pressure. The drug's primary mechanism is to block excessive prolongation of the **late inward sodium current** (I_{Na-L}) in myocardial cells. This abnormal current leads to increased sodium-calcium exchange, intracellular calcium accumulation, and increased left ventricular wall tension. By blocking I_{Na-L}, ranolazine decreases diastolic wall tension, improves diastolic subendocardial perfusion, and reduces oxygen consumption. Unlike other antianginal drugs, ranolazine has no effect on heart rate or blood pressure.

In clinical trials, ranolazine **increased exercise capacity** and **reduced anginal frequency,** the need for nitroglycerin, and the incidence of atrial fibrillation while improving quality of life. The drug seems to be an attractive alternative or supplement to conventional antianginal agents and can be used with β-blockers and nitrates. The most common side effects of ranolazine are mild **dizziness, headache, nausea,** and **constipation.** The drug increases the QTc interval of the electrocardiogram and is contraindicated in persons with QT prolongation and in those taking QT-prolonging drugs (see Chapter 14) or those with hepatic impairment (because the drug is metabolized in the liver). Because of its short half-life, a sustained-release preparation of the drug is available.

The heart uses glucose, fatty acids, and lactate as sources of energy. Although fatty acids are the major fuel for the heart, glucose is metabolized more efficiently and generates more energy per unit of oxygen used. **Trimetazidine** inhibits ketoacyl coenzyme-A thiolase, a key enzyme in the β-**oxidation pathway of fatty acid metabolism.** The resulting decrease in fatty acid oxidation evokes a compensatory increase in glucose metabolism and reduces oxygen consumption by about 20%. Clinical studies show that the drug decreases the number of anginal episodes and increases the duration of exercise before a 1-mm ST-segment depression appears on the electrocardiogram (ECG). **Trimetazidine**

BOX 11.1 A CASE OF CHEST PAIN ON EXERTION

CASE PRESENTATION

A 57-year-old construction foreman who is a heavy smoker complained to his physician of a pressure-like discomfort in the retrosternal area. The problem began about a month before and occurred two or three times a week. The discomfort occurred only when he was working, disappeared when he rested, and never lasted for more than 15 minutes. Except for a blood pressure of 150/100 mm Hg, his physical examination findings and electrocardiogram were normal. Blood samples were obtained for chemical analysis, including a complete lipid profile.

After ruling out other causes of the patient's chest discomfort, the physician made a provisional diagnosis of typical angina pectoris and prescribed sublingual nitroglycerin for the relief of acute chest discomfort. The patient was started on an amlodipine-losartan drug combination and a low dose of aspirin. He was also encouraged to monitor his blood pressure regularly and to enroll in a smoking cessation program. He was scheduled to see his physician again in 3 weeks.

CASE DISCUSSION

The risk factors for coronary heart disease (CHD) include hypertension and smoking. Whereas β-blockers have often been preferred for treating hypertension in persons with CHD, recent clinical trials have indicated that long-acting CCBs are as effective as β-blockers for the prevention of death and MI in angina patients. Moreover, CCBs may be more effective than β-blockers for the prevention of stroke. Amlodipine is a long-acting dihydropyridine CCB that is suitable for the control of blood pressure and the prevention of angina symptoms. Studies have shown that amlodipine reduces hospitalization and the need for revascularization in patients with angina. Combining amlodipine with an angiotensin receptor blocker will also enable the patient to achieve normal blood pressure in a shorter amount of time using lower doses of each drug.

Aspirin can prevent the formation of platelet thrombi and reduce the risk of MI and death in persons with angina. Patients with CHD should be evaluated for hyperlipidemia and treated appropriately with dietary restrictions and drug therapy to retard the progression of atherosclerosis. These patients should also be considered for angiographic evaluation of their coronary arteries to determine whether angioplasty or coronary artery bypass grafting would be beneficial.

---

has also been found to increase ejection fraction in persons with left ventricular dysfunction. However, long-term safety and efficacy data are needed. The drug has been approved in many countries but not in the United States.

MANAGEMENT OF ANGINA PECTORIS

In patients with angina pectoris, the primary objectives of drug therapy are to relieve acute symptoms, prevent ischemic attacks, improve the quality of life, and reduce the risks of MI and other potential cardiovascular problems, as illustrated in Box 11.1. Treatment of concurrent hypertension, hyperlipidemia, diabetes, and obesity can slow coronary artery disease progression, whereas antithrombotic agents (e.g., aspirin) reduce the risk of coronary thrombosis and MI. In fact, **aspirin** has been shown to prolong the life of persons with stable angina.

If a patient has only an occasional angina episode, **sublingual nitroglycerin** can be used as needed to relieve acute symptoms. If episodes occur predictably with exertion, sublingual nitroglycerin or isosorbide dinitrate can be taken as a prophylactic measure just before exertion. If the severity of angina requires regular use of sublingual nitroglycerin, however, prophylactic therapy should be considered. In some cases, angiography should be performed to determine whether percutaneous coronary intervention (angioplasty) or coronary artery bypass grafting is appropriate.

For patients who might benefit from **prophylactic therapy,** a β-blocker, a long-acting nitrate, or a CCB might be chosen for initial therapy, whereas **ranolazine** offers an attractive alternative or adjunct to traditional drugs for angina. Studies show that β-blockers lower the risk of MI and possibly improve survival in patients with stable angina, and a meta-analysis of clinical studies found that β-blockers reduced anginal episodes more than did CCBs. However, rates of cardiac death and MI were similar in patients receiving β-blockers and CCBs.

Patients with **unstable angina** have a high risk of MI and should receive aspirin or other antithrombotic drugs to prevent platelet aggregation and thrombus formation. These patients should be considered for coronary revascularization and stent insertion. CCBs are less suitable than β-blockers for patients with unstable angina or a recent MI because the dihydropyridine CCBs have the potential to cause reflex tachycardia and because verapamil and diltiazem have the potential to suppress cardiac contractility and can increase the frequency of heart failure in persons with ventricular systolic dysfunction.

The β-blockers are **ineffective in treating variant angina,** which is caused by coronary vasospasm. This condition is usually treated with a CCB.

In patients who have angina and concomitant asthma, a CCB is usually preferred because β-blockers may cause bronchoconstriction, whereas CCBs may relax bronchial smooth muscle. In angina patients with diabetes, a CCB is often used, but a $β_1$-adrenoceptor blocker or a third-generation β-blocker such as **carvedilol** may be advantageous in some patients. In patients with heart failure, a long-acting nitrate may be required for angina prophylaxis because the low doses of β-blockers typically used in heart failure may not prevent angina symptoms (see Chapter 12).

SUMMARY OF IMPORTANT POINTS

- In patients with coronary artery disease, lifestyle changes and drugs that lower cholesterol levels (e.g., statins) may slow the progression of atherosclerosis. Aspirin and statins decrease coronary events and mortality in persons with CHD.
- In patients with typical angina, antianginal drugs act by decreasing myocardial oxygen demand. The organic nitrites and nitrates, CCBs, and ranolazine decrease myocardial wall tension, whereas the β-adrenoceptor antagonists (β-blockers) and nondihydropyridine CCBs decrease the heart rate and contractility, and ivabradine decreases heart rate.
- Nitrates and dihydropyridine CCBs have the potential to cause reflex tachycardia, but this effect can be prevented by concurrent administration of a β-blocker.

- Continuous exposure to nitrates leads to tolerance. Nitrate tolerance may be caused by the inactivation of aldehyde dehydrogenase and decreased release of nitric oxide.
- All CCBs have similar vasodilation activity. Verapamil and diltiazem also produce significant cardiac depression, and verapamil has a greater effect than diltiazem on cardiac contractility. Verapamil and diltiazem can increase serum digoxin levels and cause digitalis toxicity.
- In patients with a history of MI, the β-blockers have been found to reduce the incidence of ventricular arrhythmias that cause sudden death.
- Calcium channel blockers and organic nitrates are effective in the treatment of vasospastic angina, whereas the β-blockers are not.
- Ranolazine is a novel agent that reduces ischemic symptoms in patients with angina by preventing myocardial sodium and calcium overload.

Review Questions

1. Which mechanism is responsible for the vasodilation effect of verapamil?
   - (A) increased levels of cGMP
   - (B) decreased binding of calcium to calmodulin
   - (C) decreased formation of IP_3
   - (D) increased myosin light-chain kinase activity
   - (E) increased metabolic efficiency
2. Which effect is caused by both atenolol and diltiazem?
   - (A) decreased cAMP levels
   - (B) increased cGMP levels
   - (C) decreased heart rate
   - (D) relaxation of arterial smooth muscle
   - (E) inhibition of sodium influx
3. What is the mechanism by which isosorbide dinitrate increases cyclic GMP levels?
   - (A) inhibition of phosphodiesterase
   - (B) inactivation of aldehyde dehydrogenase
   - (C) blockade of β-adrenoceptors
   - (D) release of nitric oxide
   - (E) blockade of calcium channels
4. A man with obstructive pulmonary disease requires therapy to prevent anginal attacks. Which drug should be avoided in this patient?
   - (A) verapamil
   - (B) felodipine
   - (C) isosorbide mononitrate
   - (D) diltiazem
   - (E) propranolol
5. Which agent prevents myocardial cell calcium overload and thereby decreases ventricular wall tension?
   - (A) ranolazine
   - (B) nitroglycerin
   - (C) amlodipine
   - (D) ivabradine
   - (E) trimetazidine

CHAPTER 12

Drugs for the Treatment of Heart Failure

OVERVIEW

In the United States, **heart failure** affects nearly 5 million individuals, is the primary cause of more than 40,000 deaths per year, and is a contributing factor in an additional 220,000 deaths. The overall mortality rate in patients with heart failure is about eight times as high as that in the normal population, and the 5-year mortality rate for patients with heart failure approaches 50%.

Pathophysiology of Heart Failure

Heart failure is the end stage of a number of cardiovascular disorders that ultimately impair the ability of the ventricle to fill with blood or to eject blood into the circulation. **Ischemic heart disease** is the most common cause of heart failure. Other important causes of heart failure include hypertension, valvular disorders, arrhythmias, viral and congenital cardiomyopathy, and constrictive pericarditis. Less commonly, heart failure results from severe anemia, thiamine deficiency, or the use of certain anticancer drugs, such as **doxorubicin** (see Chapter 45). Over time, these disorders produce molecular and cellular changes in cardiac myocytes and connective tissue that lead to a series of structural and functional alterations in the ventricular wall. This process, known as **cardiac** or **ventricular remodeling,** is characterized by cardiac dilatation, ventricular wall thinning, interstitial fibrosis, and wall stiffness. These changes impair the ability of the heart to relax or contract.

Cardiac remodeling is believed to result primarily from the activation of neuroendocrine systems in response to myocardial ischemia, the excessive stretch of muscle fibers, or other pathologic stimuli. The neuroendocrine systems implicated in this process include the **renin-angiotensin-aldosterone** axis, the **sympathetic nervous system, various inflammatory cytokines,** and local mediators such as endothelin. These mediators activate biochemical pathways that induce myocyte hypertrophy, apoptosis, collagen production, fibrosis, and other effects that lead to cardiac remodeling and loss of ventricular function. For example, angiotensin II, which is formed locally in the myocardium in response to mechanical stretch and other stimuli, can induce collagen production and proliferation of fibroblasts. Chronic sympathetic nervous system stimulation of the injured myocardium produces myocyte hypertrophy, increases the production of myocardial cytokines (e.g., tumor necrosis factor *alpha*), and ultimately leads to myocyte death via activation of apoptotic pathways.

The hallmark of heart failure is a **reduction in stroke volume and cardiac output** at any given diastolic muscle fiber length, as determined by measuring the ventricular end-diastolic pressure (preload). The reduced stroke volume can be caused by **diastolic dysfunction** or **systolic dysfunction** and is manifested as an inability of the ventricles either to fill properly or to empty properly, respectively. Systolic dysfunction can result from decreased cardiac contractility secondary to a dilated or ischemic myocardium. Diastolic dysfunction can result from decreased compliance (increased stiffness) of ventricular tissue secondary to left ventricular hypertrophy or fibrosis. Hence, both systolic and diastolic heart failure can be caused or exacerbated by the process of cardiac remodeling.

In cases of **left ventricular failure (left-sided heart failure),** the left ventricle does not adequately pump blood forward, so the pressure in the pulmonary circulation increases. When the increased pressure forces fluid into the lung interstitium, this causes **congestion** and edema (Fig. 12.1). **Pulmonary edema** reduces the diffusion of oxygen and carbon dioxide between alveoli and the pulmonary capillaries.

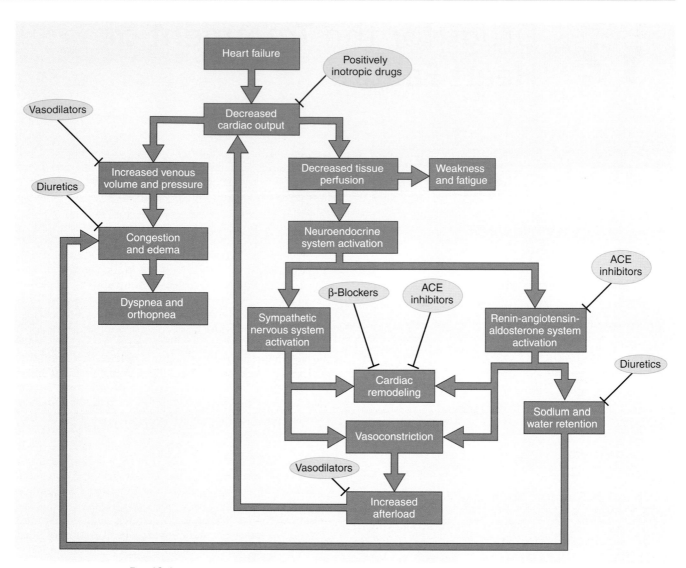

Fig. 12.1 Pathophysiology and treatment of heart failure. ACE, Angiotensin-converting enzyme.

This causes **hypoxemia** (deficient oxygenation of the blood) and can lead to **dyspnea** (difficulty in breathing), including **exertional dyspnea** (dyspnea provoked by exercise), **orthopnea** (intensified dyspnea when lying flat), and **paroxysmal nocturnal dyspnea** (edema-induced bronchoconstriction when sleeping).

The combination of edema-related hypoxemia and the heart's failure to pump sufficient blood to adequately perfuse the tissues can lead to generalized tissue hypoxia and organ dysfunction. For this reason, patients with heart failure often experience symptoms of weakness and fatigue and have reduced exercise capacity.

In cases of **right ventricular failure (right-sided heart failure)**, congestion in the peripheral veins leads to **ankle edema** in the ambulatory patient and to **sacral edema** in the bedridden patient. It also leads to **hepatojugular reflux,** characterized by an increase in jugular vein distention when pressure is applied over the liver. Ultimately, right-sided failure can lead to left-sided failure as the left ventricle is forced to work harder in an attempt to maintain cardiac output.

The reduction in cardiac output that occurs in heart failure triggers a cascade of **compensatory neuroendocrine**

responses. Although these responses attempt to restore cardiac output via the Frank-Starling mechanism (see Fig. 12.1), they are often maladaptive and counterproductive. The reduction in tissue perfusion activates both the sympathetic nervous system and the renin-angiotensin-aldosterone system, both of which in turn stimulate vasoconstriction. Arterial vasoconstriction increases aortic impedance to left ventricular ejection and thereby decreases cardiac output, especially in patients with a weak, dilated heart. When angiotensin II stimulates the secretion of aldosterone and antidiuretic hormone, this increases the amount of sodium and water retention, the plasma volume, and the venous pressure. In addition, angiotensin II and sympathetic activation lead to cardiac remodeling and ventricular wall thinning or fibrosis, which often reduce systolic and diastolic function. Hence, the net result of the neuroendocrine responses is often a further reduction in cardiac output and an increase in circulatory congestion.

Mechanisms and Effects of Drugs for Heart Failure
The primary goals of drug therapy for heart failure are to **improve symptoms,** slow or **reverse deterioration** in

TABLE 12.1 Cardiovascular Effects of Drugs Used in the Treatment of Heart Failure[a]

DRUG	CARDIAC CONTRACTILITY	HEART RATE	PRELOAD REDUCTION	AFTERLOAD REDUCTION	RISK OF ARRHYTHMIA	OTHER EFFECTS
Digoxin	+	−	++	0 to +	++	Increases parasympathetic tone and decreases sympathetic tone
Dobutamine	++	+ to ++	0 to +	+ to ++	+ to ++	Increases blood pressure
Milrinone	+	0 to ++	++	++	++	
ACE inhibitors	0	0	++	++	0	Reduces blood pressure
Hydralazine	0	+ (R)	0	++	+	Reduces blood pressure
Isosorbide dinitrate	0	+ (R)	++	+	0	Reduces pulmonary congestion
Nesiritide	0	0 to + (R)	++	++	0	Reduces venous and arterial blood pressure
Loop-acting diuretics (furosemide and others)	0	0	+	0	0	Reduces edema and congestion
Carvedilol	0	0 to −	0	+	0	Blocks *alpha-* and *beta-* adrenoceptors

ACE, Angiotensin-converting enzyme.
[a]Effects are indicated as follows: decrease (−); no change or variable (0); increase ranging from small (+) to large (++); and reflex (R).

myocardial function, and **prolong survival.** Drugs can also be used to treat underlying conditions, control arrhythmias, prevent thrombosis, and treat anemia.

The pharmacologic agents used to **treat heart failure** include drugs that (1) increase cardiac output, (2) reduce pulmonary and systemic congestion, and (3) slow or reverse cardiac remodeling. Cardiac output can be increased by positively inotropic drugs that increase cardiac contractility and by vasodilators that reduce cardiac afterload and the impedance to left ventricular ejection. Vasodilators also reduce venous pressure, circulatory congestion, and edema. Diuretics are used to mobilize edematous fluid and reduce plasma volume, thereby decreasing circulatory congestion. Angiotensin and sympathetic inhibitors have been shown to favorably influence **cardiac remodeling** and increase survival in persons with heart failure.

Table 12.1 compares the cardiovascular effects of drugs discussed in this chapter. Each of these drugs partly counteracts the loss of myocardial function and the maladaptive responses that occur during heart failure; however, none of the current therapies, either alone or in combination, has been completely satisfactory. Because heart failure has such a high incidence and poor prognosis, a much greater effort has been expended in the search for better means to treat it. The most significant development in recent decades has been the use of angiotensin inhibitors, *beta*-adrenoceptor blockers, and other agents that attenuate cardiac remodeling and reduce the mortality rate in patients with heart failure. Ultimately, however, the successful treatment of patients with heart failure may require the development of drugs that activate genes capable of repairing or replacing myocardial tissue.

POSITIVELY INOTROPIC DRUGS

Derived from the Greek words for "fiber" (*inos*) and "turning" or "to turn" (*tropikos*), the term *inotropic* refers to a change in muscle (fiber) contractility. Drugs that increase

cardiac contractility are said to have a **positive inotropic effect** and are commonly referred to as *inotropic drugs* or *agents.* The inotropic agents most often used in the treatment of heart failure are the digitalis glycoside called **digoxin,** the *beta*-adrenoceptor agonist known as **dobutamine,** and a phosphodiesterase inhibitor named **milrinone.** These drugs increase cardiac contractility by increasing calcium levels in cardiac myocytes. Dobutamine and milrinone increase calcium influx by increasing intracellular cyclic adenosine monophosphate (cAMP) levels, either by stimulating cAMP formation by adenylyl cyclase (dobutamine) or by inhibiting cAMP breakdown by phosphodiesterase (milrinone).

Digoxin
Despite the fact that the **digitalis glycosides** such as digoxin have been used to treat heart failure for more than 200 years, their effectiveness and place in therapy have been difficult to establish. Recent clinical trials indicate that digoxin provides a definite, yet limited, benefit to patients with heart failure caused by systolic dysfunction.

Drug Properties
A large number of **digitalis glycosides** have been isolated from the leaves of *Digitalis* (foxglove) plants, as well as from toad secretions. Digoxin is the only glycoside that is extensively used today.

Chemistry and Pharmacokinetics. Digoxin is composed of a steroid, a lactone ring, and three sugars linked by glycosidic bonds. The steroid nucleus of digoxin is different from that of human steroids, and it lacks most of the effects produced by gonadal or adrenal steroids.

As shown in Table 12.2, digoxin is adequately absorbed from the gut and has a **long half-life** of about 36 hours. It is primarily eliminated by renal excretion of the parent compound. The **P-glycoprotein** located in the luminal membrane of proximal tubule cells pumps digoxin into the urine.

TABLE 12.2 Pharmacokinetic Properties of Positively Inotropic Drugs[a]

DRUG	ORAL BIOAVAILABILITY	ONSET OF ACTION	DURATION OF ACTION	ELIMINATION HALF-LIFE	EXCRETED UNCHANGED IN URINE	THERAPEUTIC SERUM LEVEL
Digoxin	75%	1 h	24 h	36 h	60%	0.5–2 ng/mL
Dobutamine	NA	1 min	<10 min	2 min	0%	NA
Milrinone	NA	3 min	Variable	4 h	60%	NA

NA, Not applicable.
[a]Values shown are the mean of values reported in the literature.

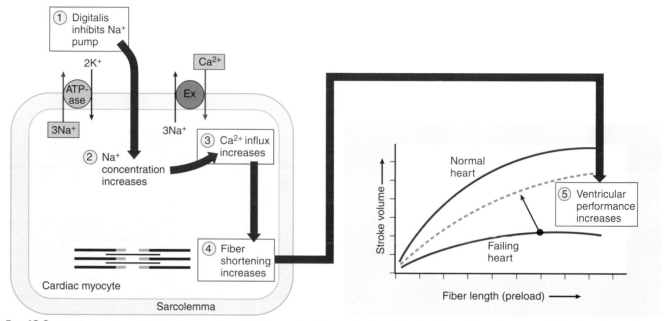

FIG. 12.2 Mechanisms by which digoxin exerts its positive inotropic effect on the heart. Digoxin inhibits the sodium pump (*ATPase*) in the sarcolemma and increases the concentration of intracellular sodium. The high sodium concentration increases the activity of the sodium-calcium exchanger (*Ex*), thereby causing more calcium to enter or remain inside the cardiac myocyte. Calcium activates muscle fiber shortening and increases cardiac contractility, which in turn increases stroke volume at any given fiber length (preload).

Because digoxin has a low therapeutic index, serum concentrations are useful in assessing the adequacy of the dosage and evaluating potential toxicity and should be in the range of 0.5 to 2 ng/mL.

Mechanisms and Pharmacologic Effects. Digoxin produces a unique constellation of effects on the cardiovascular system. It has a **positive inotropic effect** (an increase in the force of contraction), a **negative chronotropic effect** (a decrease in the heart rate), and a **negative dromotropic effect** (a decrease in conduction velocity). Digoxin is unique in its ability to strengthen cardiac contraction while decreasing heart rate.

Positive Inotropic Effect. Digoxin produces a modest positive inotropic effect by **increasing intracellular calcium** as a result of inhibiting the sodium pump (Na+, K+-ATPase) in the plasma membrane (sarcolemma). When the sodium pump is inhibited, the concentration of intracellular sodium is increased, thereby increasing the activity of the sodium-calcium exchanger and causing more calcium to enter the cardiac myocyte (Fig. 12.2). The increase in cytoplasmic calcium stimulates the release of additional calcium from the sarcoplasmic reticulum and increases the rate of myofibril shortening (muscle contraction) and the peak systolic muscle tension. These actions increase stroke volume and cardiac output as shown in Fig. 12.3. The stroke volume

is the amount of blood pumped by the ventricle during each systole, and the cardiac output is the amount of blood ejected from either ventricle of the heart per minute.

Electrophysiologic and Electrocardiographic Effects. Digoxin increases parasympathetic nervous system activity while decreasing sympathetic activity. These actions decrease heart rate and atrioventricular (AV) node conduction velocity while increasing AV node refractory period (Fig. 12.4).

Digoxin also has potential adverse effects on the heart, including an ability to increase abnormal impulse formation by evoking spontaneous **afterdepolarizations** (see Fig. 12.4). These abnormal depolarizations occur during or after cardiac repolarization and lead to **extrasystoles** (premature or coupled beats) and **tachycardia** (rapid beating of the heart). The afterdepolarizations appear to be caused by excessive calcium influx into cardiac cells, and they are more likely to occur after higher doses of digoxin have been given.

Digoxin has several electrocardiographic effects (see Fig. 12.4). It shortens the ventricular action potential duration by accelerating repolarization, and this **decreases the QT interval.** It reduces the AV node conduction velocity and thereby increases the PR interval. Finally, it causes ST segment depression, which gives rise to the so-called "**hockey stick** configuration" of the ST segment.

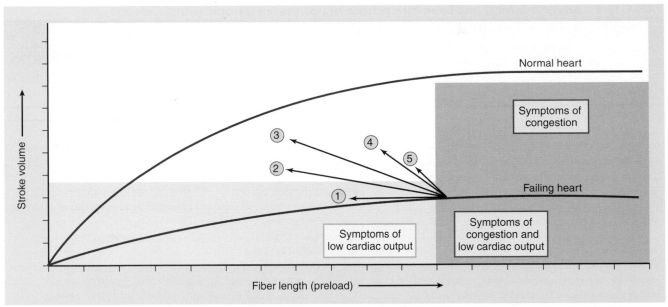

Fig. 12.3 Effect of drug treatment on ventricular performance. Effects of the following drugs or drug combinations are shown: *1*, a diuretic or a nitrate; *2*, nitroprusside or an angiotensin-converting enzyme (ACE) inhibitor; *3*, a positively inotropic drug plus a vasodilator; *4*, dobutamine; and *5*, digoxin. The positively inotropic drugs increase stroke volume at any given fiber length and thereby decrease venous pressure and preload. Some vasodilators (e.g., ACE inhibitors) decrease afterload and thereby increase stroke volume. Vasodilators can also decrease preload.

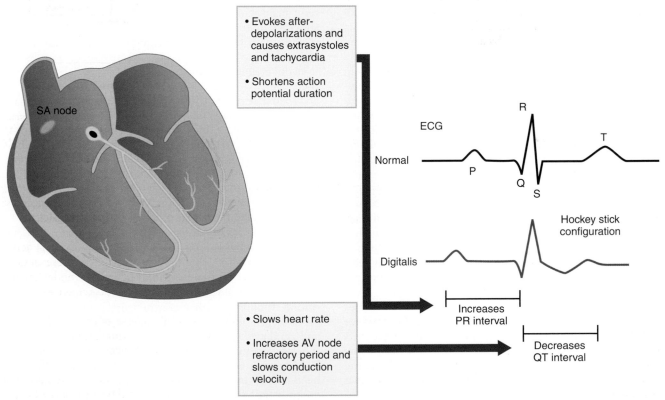

Fig. 12.4 Electrophysiologic and electrocardiographic effects of digoxin. Digoxin causes an increase in parasympathetic (vagal) tone and a decrease in sympathetic tone. These actions slow the heart rate by decreasing sinoatrial (SA) node automaticity. The increased vagal tone and decreased sympathetic tone also slow the atrioventricular (AV) node conduction velocity while increasing the AV node refractory period. The reduced AV conduction velocity increases the PR interval on the electrocardiogram. In ventricular tissue, digoxin shortens the action potential duration, and this decreases the QT interval. Toxic concentrations of digoxin may evoke afterdepolarizations throughout the heart and thereby cause extrasystoles and tachycardia. Digoxin also causes ST-segment depression, which gives rise to the so-called "hockey stick configuration" on the electrocardiogram.

Adverse Effects. The most common adverse effects of digoxin are **gastrointestinal, cardiac,** and **neurologic** reactions. Frequently, the earliest signs of toxicity are anorexia, nausea, and vomiting. These reactions are often associated with elevated serum concentrations and may forewarn more serious toxicity.

Arrhythmias, usually the most serious manifestation of digoxin toxicity, can include AV block and various

TABLE 12.3 Adverse Effects and Drug Interactions of Positively Inotropic Drugs

DRUG	COMMON ADVERSE EFFECTS	COMMON DRUG INTERACTIONS
Digoxin	Anorexia, nausea, and vomiting; arrhythmias; blurred vision; chromatopsia; gynecomastia; and seizures	Antacids, cholestyramine, diltiazem, quinidine, and verapamil
Dobutamine	Excessive vasoconstriction and tachyarrhythmias	Adrenoceptor agonists and antagonists
Milrinone	Arrhythmias, hypotension, and thrombocytopenia	Unknown

tachyarrhythmias. **Atrial tachycardia** with AV block is one of the most common types of digitalis-induced arrhythmia, but digoxin can also cause ventricular arrhythmias. **Hypokalemia** can precipitate arrhythmias in patients receiving digoxin, and the serum potassium level should be determined immediately if arrhythmias occur in these patients.

The neurologic effects of digoxin toxicity are usually caused by excessive plasma levels of the drug and include **blurred vision** and yellow, green, or blue **chromatopsia** (a condition in which objects appear unnaturally colored). Severe digoxin toxicity can precipitate seizures.

Because digoxin has some estrogenic activity, it occasionally causes **gynecomastia** (excessive growth of male mammary glands).

Interactions. Several drugs can interact with digoxin (Table 12.3). Because **antacids** and **cholestyramine** can reduce the absorption of digoxin and decrease its therapeutic effects, their administration should be separated from the administration of digoxin by at least 2 hours. **Diltiazem, quinidine,** and **verapamil** reduce digoxin clearance and increase serum digoxin levels by inhibiting P-glycoprotein mediated renal excretion, thereby contributing to digitalis toxicity. When digoxin is used concurrently with these drugs, only 50% of the usual dose of digoxin should be given, and serum digoxin levels should be monitored. Loop-acting and thiazide diuretics can cause **hypokalemia** and precipitate digitalis toxicity because the reduced serum potassium concentration increases digitalis binding to the sodium pump.

Indications. The improvement produced by digoxin in patients with systolic heart failure probably results from a combination of a modest inotropic effect and attenuation of the neuroendocrine consequences of heart failure, such as increased heart rate and vasoconstriction. Digoxin is generally not used to treat diastolic heart failure because contractility is usually not impaired in this disorder.

Clinical trials have shown that although digoxin does not prolong survival, it reduces symptoms and the need for hospitalization and improves the quality of life of patients with heart failure. Moreover, patients who have been withdrawn from digoxin have experienced a greater worsening of heart failure compared to those who weren't withdrawn from digoxin.

Digoxin has also been used to slow the ventricular rate in patients with **atrial fibrillation** (AF). By slowing AV node conduction velocity and increasing AV node refractory period, digoxin reduces the number of ectopic impulses that are transmitted to the ventricles. However, a recent clinical trial (ROCKET AF) found that digoxin use in patients with AF was associated with increased cardiovascular and all-cause mortality. Ventricular rate control in AF is usually accomplished with a non-dihydropyridine calcium channel blocker or a beta-adrenoceptor blocker.

Digoxin Immune Fab

An **antidote** for severe digoxin toxicity is available in the form of **digoxin immune Fab.** It is made from immunoglobulin fragments taken from sheep previously immunized with a digoxin derivative. This antibody preparation is administered intravenously and can rapidly reverse digoxin toxicity by binding to digoxin.

Dobutamine

Dobutamine is the *beta*-adrenoceptor agonist most frequently used in treating heart failure, partly because it selectively stimulates cardiac contractility and usually causes less tachycardia than other *beta*-agonists. Dobutamine also activates *beta*$_2$-adrenoceptors in vascular smooth muscle, decreasing vascular resistance and cardiac afterload, and thereby augmenting cardiac output. The drug is administered by continuous intravenous infusion in the short-term management of **acute heart failure** and **cardiogenic shock.** Symptomatic improvement has been documented in patients with heart failure receiving a continuous infusion of dobutamine for 3 to 5 days, and some patients may benefit from dobutamine administration for up to 30 days. However, there is no evidence that such treatments improve survival, and high doses may increase mortality. For this reason, many authorities believe dobutamine and other intravenous inotropes should be limited to the short-term management of patients with severe heart failure.

The properties and effects of dobutamine are summarized in Tables 12.1 to 12.3 and are described in greater detail in Chapter 8.

Milrinone

Milrinone is occasionally used in treating acute heart failure and other conditions **requiring myocardial stimulation.** The drug inhibits **type 3 phosphodiesterase,** an enzyme that converts cAMP to inactive 5'-AMP. By increasing the concentration of cAMP in myocytes, milrinone stimulates cardiac contractility, as described previously. It also increases cAMP in vascular smooth muscle and produces vasodilation (see Fig. 11.3), so it is sometimes called an **inodilator.**

Milrinone is used for the short-term management of heart failure in patients who are not responsive to other drugs. It has also been used for inotropic support of infants and children awaiting **cardiac transplantation** and for other conditions requiring myocardial stimulation. Intravenous administration of milrinone can provide both hemodynamic and symptomatic improvement in persons with advanced heart failure. However, long-term use can cause thrombocytopenia and ventricular arrhythmias and is associated with increased mortality in patients with severe heart failure (Table 12.4). Despite these limitations, **infants awaiting cardiac transplantation** have received the drug for up to 6 months without serious adverse effects.

TABLE 12.4 Important Findings in Studies of Drugs in the Treatment of Heart Failure

DRUG OR DRUG CLASS	SUMMARY OF FINDINGS
Digoxin	Digoxin decreased rate of hospitalization for worsening heart failure but did not decrease mortality. Clinical worsening of heart failure occurred with digoxin withdrawal.
Milrinone	Milrinone increased mortality rate in patients with severe heart failure and caused more arrhythmias than digoxin.
ACE inhibitors	ACE inhibitors decreased mortality rate in mild, moderate, and severe heart failure, and decreased risk of heart failure in post-myocardial infarction patients and in asymptomatic patients with left ventricular dysfunction.
ACE inhibitor plus candesartan	Addition of candesartan to ACE inhibitor reduced mortality in heart failure patients.
Enalapril versus nitrate plus hydralazine	In chronic heart failure, the overall risk of sudden death was decreased by enalapril more than by nitrate plus hydralazine, though black patients benefitted more from hydralazine plus nitrate.
Carvedilol	Carvedilol increased exercise tolerance, improved ejection fractions, and decreased hospital admissions and mortality in patients with heart failure.
Nesiritide	Nesiritide reduced venous pressure, vascular congestion, and dyspnea in patients with decompensated heart failure.
Spironolactone	Spironolactone decreased mortality in severe heart failure at 24 months.

ACE, Angiotensin-converting enzyme.

VASODILATORS

The vasodilators used in treating heart failure include the **angiotensin inhibitors,** the combination of **hydralazine** and **isosorbide dinitrate, sacubitril,** and **nesiritide.** The angiotensin inhibitors include angiotensin-converting enzyme (ACE) inhibitors and angiotensin receptor blockers. Vasodilators are useful in the treatment of heart failure because of their ability to reduce venous and arterial pressure. The reduction in venous pressure decreases edema, whereas the dilation of arteries reduces cardiac afterload and increases cardiac output. In addition, the angiotensin inhibitors slow or reverse **cardiac remodeling,** which may be responsible for their beneficial effect on the survival of patients with heart failure.

Angiotensin-Converting Enzyme Inhibitors

The ACE inhibitors reduce the formation of angiotensin II and are used in the treatment of **diabetic nephropathy, hypertension,** and **heart failure.** The pharmacologic properties of these drugs are described in Chapter 10.

Angiotensin II has several actions that contribute to the pathogenesis of heart failure, including vasoconstriction and increased secretion of aldosterone and antidiuretic hormone. **Ramipril, enalapril, lisinopril,** and other ACE inhibitors prevent these effects and reduce plasma volume, venous pressure, and edema while increasing cardiac output by reducing arterial resistance and cardiac afterload.

In addition, ACE inhibitors counteract the adverse effects of angiotensin that contribute to cardiac remodeling in patients with heart failure.

ACE inhibitors have been shown to decrease mortality in patients with heart failure and to prevent the transition from asymptomatic to overt heart failure, thus supporting the early use of an ACE inhibitor in patients with **asymptomatic heart failure.**

In patients with **acute myocardial infarction,** treatment with an ACE inhibitor has been found to improve survival when it is administered within 24 hours of the onset of symptoms. Investigators believe that this benefit is partly caused by the inhibition of angiotensin II–induced cardiac remodeling, which would otherwise lead to cardiac dilatation, wall thinning, and expansion of the infarct zone in these patients.

Angiotensin Receptor Blockers

Angiotensin II receptor blockers (ARBs), such as **valsartan** and **candesartan,** prevent the binding of angiotensin II to AT_1 receptors and have pharmacologic and clinical effects that are similar to those of the ACE inhibitors. Unlike ACE inhibitors, ARBs do not inhibit bradykinin degradation and are not prone to induce chronic cough, an effect that occurs in 3% to 20% of persons treated with ACE inhibitors.

Clinical trials have found that ARBs reduce mortality and hospitalization in persons with heart failure and appear to be as effective as ACE inhibitors in treating heart failure. ARBs are particularly indicated in patients who cannot tolerate an ACE inhibitor.

Natriuretic Peptide

Natriuretic peptides include **atrial natriuretic peptide** (ANP) and **B-type natriuretic peptide** produced and released by cardiac ventricles in response to excessive stretching. **Nesiritide** (NATRECOR) is a form of human B-type natriuretic peptide obtained from *Escherichia coli* using recombinant DNA technology. It is approved for the treatment of patients with **acutely decompensated heart failure** who have shortness of breath (dyspnea) at rest or with minimal activity.

Nesiritide binds to a **guanylate cyclase receptor** in vascular smooth muscle and endothelial cells, leading to increased intracellular concentrations of cyclic guanosine monophosphate (cGMP). cGMP acts as a second messenger to dilate venous and arterial smooth muscle, thereby leading to reductions in venous and arterial pressure in patients with heart failure. Clinical trials show that nesiritide **reduced pulmonary capillary wedge pressure,** a clinical measure of venous pressure and cardiac preload, and thereby decreased vascular congestion and dyspnea in decompensated patients with heart failure. The most common adverse effect of nesiritide is hypotension, although most cases were not symptomatic. Because nesiritide is a peptide drug, it must be given intravenously, and it is eliminated by intracellular proteolysis. The drug can be used alone or with other standard therapies for heart failure.

Neprilysin inhibitor

Neprilysin is an endogenous **endopeptidase** enzyme that degrades vasoactive peptides such as bradykinin and **natriuretic peptides.** Inhibition of neprilysin raises the levels of these peptides, leading to decreased cardiac remodeling, decreased vasoconstriction, and reduced sodium retention. Because neprilysin also degrades angiotensin II to inactive products, neprilysin inhibition must be combined with an inhibitor of the renin-angiotensin-aldosterone system. **Sacubitril** is a neprilysin inhibitor that is available in a 1:1 molecular ratio combination with **valsartan** (ENTRESTO). Sacubitril is a prodrug that is rapidly converted to its active metabolite sacubitrilat by plasma esterases.

The sacubitril-valsartan combination is touted as the first new drug in over a decade to **decrease death rates** in patients with systolic heart failure. In a large phase 3 clinical trial (PARADIGM-HF), sacubitril-valsartan decreased cardiovascular death and hospitalization due to heart failure by 20% more than did enalapril alone in patients with heart failure and a low ventricular ejection fraction. Clinical trials have also found sacubitril to be effective in combination with an ACE inhibitor, and combinations of sacubitril and an angiotensin inhibitor are also effective in the treatment of hypertension. Sacubitril-valsartan caused few adverse effects in clinical trials, and only a low percentage of patients discontinued the drug.

Hydralazine and Nitrates

Isosorbide dinitrate primarily relaxes **venous** smooth muscle, whereas **hydralazine** preferentially relaxes **arterial** smooth muscle. The combined use of these two drugs reduces cardiac preload and afterload, leading to reduced venous pressure and edema and to increased cardiac output, respectively. Hence, the effects of isosorbide dinitrate plus hydralazine are similar to those produced by the angiotensin inhibitors. It was found that this drug combination decreased mortality more than placebo but less than **enalapril.** For this reason, the hydralazine-isosorbide dinitrate combination is sometimes used to treat patients with heart failure who cannot tolerate an angiotensin inhibitor.

Clinical trials also found that black patients with heart failure had a lesser benefit from ACE inhibitors than did whites, whereas the effect of hydralazine plus isosorbide dinitrate was greater in black patients. The African American Heart Failure Trial provided further evidence of the beneficial effects of hydralazine plus isosorbide dinitrate on the **survival of black patients** with heart failure.

BETA-ADRENOCEPTOR ANTAGONISTS

Once contraindicated in heart failure because of their negative inotropic effect, the *beta*-adrenoceptor antagonists (*beta*-blockers) have emerged as one of the primary treatments for this cardiac condition. This practice resulted from advances in the understanding of the role of the sympathetic nervous system in cardiac remodeling and the progression of heart failure.

Excessive sympathetic nervous system activity contributes to **cardiac remodeling** in several ways. Sympathetic activation of cardiac *beta*-receptors produces tachycardia and increased oxygen demand, thereby increasing infarct size and the propensity for cardiac remodeling in persons with myocardial infarction. Sympathetic activation also increases activation of the renin-angiotensin-aldosterone system, whose role in cardiac remodeling was described earlier. In addition, chronic stimulation of cardiac *beta*-receptors leads to both **myocyte hypertrophy and**

apoptosis in a manner that contributes to cardiac dilatation and ventricular wall thinning. Finally, activation of the sympathetic system increases the production of **cardiac cytokines,** including tumor necrosis factor (TNF)-*alpha* and interleukins. These cytokines also induce myocyte hypertrophy and apoptosis and produce alterations in the intracellular matrix that contribute to fibrosis and ventricular wall stiffness.

The benefits of therapy with *beta*-blockers are caused by the ability of these drugs to reduce excessive sympathetic stimulation of the heart and circulation in patients with heart failure. Several clinical trials have shown that some *beta*-blockers, particularly **carvedilol, metoprolol,** and **bisoprolol,** benefit patients with mild to severe heart failure caused by left ventricular systolic dysfunction.

Carvedilol is a *beta*$_1$- and *beta*$_2$-blocker that also produces vasodilation via *alpha*$_1$-receptor blockade. Carvedilol and its metabolites also have antioxidant properties (described in Chapter 9), and it exhibits anti-inflammatory and anti-apoptotic properties that may contribute to its beneficial effects in heart failure.

In several clinical trials, carvedilol has been found to increase left ventricular ejection fraction, improve symptoms, and slow disease progression. These studies show that carvedilol reduces both hospitalization and mortality in persons with heart failure when it is added to a standard treatment regimen. Carvedilol is currently recommended for patients with symptomatic heart failure who do not have hypotension, pulmonary congestion, or AV block. Patients should be monitored for the adverse effects of carvedilol, which include bradycardia, worsening heart failure, and dizziness or light-headedness caused by vasodilation and decreased blood pressure. **Metoprolol** and **bisoprolol** have also been shown to produce beneficial effects in patients with heart failure.

Because the beneficial effects of *beta*-blockers in heart failure have a delayed onset of action, whereas potential adverse cardiac effects can occur immediately, patients are started on low doses of a *beta*-blocker, and the dose is then gradually increased every 2 to 3 weeks until the target dose is achieved over a period of several months. Patients should be regularly monitored because *beta*-blockers can increase symptoms for 4 to 10 weeks before improvement is noted.

ALDOSTERONE ANTAGONISTS

Spironolactone and **eplerenone** are mineralocorticoid receptor antagonists that compete with aldosterone for the mineralocorticoid receptor in renal tubules and other tissues. These drugs act on the kidneys to increase sodium excretion, decrease potassium excretion, and exert a moderate diuretic effect. Hence, spironolactone is classified as a potassium-sparing diuretic, and its pharmacologic properties and use are described in Chapter 13.

The Randomized Aldactone Evaluation Study (RALES) found that spironolactone reduced mortality in persons with **severe heart failure.** This benefit has been attributed to the prevention of the adverse effects of excessive aldosterone levels on the heart and to an elevation of the serum potassium level. The survival benefits of these drugs were in addition to those provided by angiotensin inhibitors and *beta*-blockers. After the RALES study, many physicians began using aldosterone antagonists in patients with mild to moderate heart failure. The increased use of these drugs in elderly patients who may have renal insufficiency was initially associated with a large increase in the incidence of hospitalization and death caused by **hyperkalemia.** Hence, patients taking an aldosterone antagonist should be monitored closely.

Aldosterone can produce **endocrine side effects** resulting from its binding to androgen and progesterone receptors, leading to gynecomastia and impotence in some male patients. **Eplerenone** is a newer aldosterone antagonist that produces fewer endocrine side effects than **spironolactone** (1% versus 10% in clinical trials). Eplerenone is more expensive, however, and it seems reasonable to begin with spironolactone and switch to eplerenone if endocrine side effects develop.

DIURETICS

In patients with heart failure, diuretics are used to reduce plasma volume and edema and thereby relieve the symptoms of volume overload, such as shortness of breath (dyspnea).

Loop diuretics (e.g., **bumetanide, furosemide,** and **torsemide**) have greater natriuretic activity than other diuretics and are preferred for reducing plasma volume in heart failure. However, they must be used carefully to avoid dehydration, hyponatremia, and hypokalemia. **Hypokalemia increases the risk of digoxin toxicity,** and patients with heart failure should be closely monitored for this condition. Thiazide diuretics can be used when a lesser degree of diuresis is required in the treatment of heart failure, and they can be combined with loop diuretics in patients with volume overload despite significant doses of loop diuretics. The pharmacologic properties of diuretics are described in greater detail in Chapter 13.

MANAGEMENT OF HEART FAILURE

In patients with heart failure, the goals of therapy are to relieve symptoms, improve quality of life, and prolong survival. Acute heart failure may require hospitalization and the administration of intravenous vasodilators (such as nitrates and nesiritide), diuretics, inotropic agents, and oxygen. Once stabilized, patients can often be managed with oral medications, dietary restrictions, and exercise guidelines (Box 12.1). Although bed rest may relieve symptoms of heart failure during the early course of therapy, many patients benefit from an incremental exercise program after their condition has improved.

The management of chronic heart failure depends on the underlying cause, the degree of cardiac dysfunction, and the particular signs and symptoms exhibited by the patient. Although some drugs prolong survival, heart failure continues to have a high mortality rate. Drug therapy for heart failure caused by systolic dysfunction typically includes a diuretic, an angiotensin inhibitor, possibly in combination with sacubitril, and a *beta*-adrenoceptor blocker. An aldosterone antagonist (spironolactone or eplerenone) can be added when indicated. Some patients benefit from the addition of digoxin or the combination of hydralazine and an organic nitrate. Anticoagulant and antiplatelet drugs may be needed by some patients. Other classes of drugs are being developed, and the treatment of heart failure will continue to evolve as new drugs are developed.

SUMMARY OF IMPORTANT POINTS

- Heart failure is a common manifestation of coronary heart disease, chronic hypertension, valvular disorders, and other cardiovascular conditions.
- Angiotensin inhibitors and *beta*-adrenoceptor blockers attenuate cardiac remodeling and disease progression while increasing cardiac output and survival in persons with heart failure.
- In patients with heart failure, digoxin increases cardiac contractility and cardiac output and reduces symptoms of weakness and fatigue and the need for hospitalization.
- Digoxin augments parasympathetic tone and thereby slows the AV node conduction velocity and increases the AV node refractory period. These actions slow the ventricular rate in patients with atrial fibrillation.
- Digoxin is primarily eliminated by renal excretion and has a relatively long half-life.
- The adverse gastrointestinal, cardiac, and neurologic effects of digoxin include anorexia, nausea, vomiting, arrhythmias, blurred vision, chromatopsia, and seizures.

- Digoxin immune Fab can be used to treat life-threatening digoxin toxicity.
- Loop-acting diuretics are used to mobilize edematous fluid in patients with heart failure.
- Positively inotropic drugs (e.g., dobutamine) and vasodilators (e.g., nesiritide, a recombinant human B-type natriuretic peptide) are used in the treatment of acute decompensated heart failure.

Review Questions

1. Inhibition of neprilysin leads to increased levels of which endogenous substance?
   - (A) angiotensin II
   - (B) natriuretic peptide
   - (C) both angiotensin II and natriuretic peptide
   - (D) neither angiotensin II or natriuretic peptide
   - (E) nitric oxide
2. A man is brought to the emergency department complaining of nausea and vomiting, blurred and abnormally colored vision, and palpitations. Which drug is most likely responsible for these effects?
   - (A) dobutamine
   - (B) lisinopril
   - (C) digoxin
   - (D) milrinone
   - (E) furosemide
3. Which drug has been demonstrated to increase survival in persons with heart failure?
   - (A) furosemide
   - (B) carvedilol
   - (C) milrinone
   - (D) digoxin
   - (E) hydralazine-isosorbide dinitrate
4. Which mechanism is responsible for the cardiovascular effects of nesiritide?
   - (A) inhibition of adenylyl cyclase
   - (B) stimulation of adenylyl cyclase
   - (C) inhibition of guanylyl cyclase
   - (D) stimulation of guanylyl cyclase
   - (E) inhibition of phosphodiesterase
5. Which drug blocks alpha-1, beta-1, and beta-2 adrenoceptors?
   - (A) carvedilol
   - (B) metoprolol
   - (C) propranolol
   - (D) dobutamine
   - (E) phentolamine

Diuretic Drugs

OVERVIEW

Diuretics are used in the **management of edema** associated with cardiovascular, renal, and endocrine abnormalities, as well as in the treatment of hypertension, glaucoma, and several other clinical disorders (Table 13.1). The drugs act at various sites in the nephron to cause **diuresis** (an increase in urine production). Most diuretics inhibit the reabsorption of sodium from the nephron into the circulation and thereby increase **natriuresis** (the excretion of sodium in the urine). Several types of diuretics also increase **kaliuresis** (the excretion of potassium in the urine) and affect the excretion of magnesium, calcium, chloride, and bicarbonate ions.

NEPHRON FUNCTION AND SITES OF DRUG ACTION

Sodium and other electrolytes are reabsorbed into the circulation at various sites throughout the nephron by active and passive processes that involve **ion channels, transport proteins,** and the **sodium pump** (Na^+,K^+-ATPase). Ion channels are unique membrane proteins through which a specific ion moves across the cell membrane in the direction determined by the electrochemical gradient for the ion. The transport proteins include **symporters,** which transport two or more ions in the same direction, and **antiporters,** which transport ions in opposite directions across cell membranes. Most diuretics block a specific ion channel or transporter in the tubular epithelial cells. The sites and mechanisms by which diuretics affect ion reabsorption and secretion in the nephron are illustrated in Box 13.1.

Glomerular Filtration

Urine formation begins with glomerular filtration, a process in which an ultrafiltrate of blood is forced out of the glomerular capillaries and into the nephron lumen by the hydrostatic pressure in these capillaries. In healthy individuals, this filtrate is essentially free of blood cells and plasma proteins. **Digitalis glycosides** and other cardiac stimulants can indirectly cause diuresis by increasing cardiac output, renal blood flow, and the glomerular filtration rate. These drugs are described in greater detail in Chapter 12. The diuretic drugs described in this chapter do not increase the glomerular filtration rate, and some of them may indirectly reduce it by decreasing plasma volume and renal blood flow.

Proximal Tubule

The proximal tubule is an important site of tubular reabsorption and secretion. Essentially, all of the filtered glucose, amino acids, and other organic solutes are reabsorbed in the early portion of the proximal tubule. About 85% of filtered sodium bicarbonate is reabsorbed in the proximal tubule, and this reabsorption is inhibited by a class of diuretics known as **carbonic anhydrase (CA) inhibitors.** For reasons described later in this chapter, these drugs are relatively weak diuretics and are seldom used for this purpose, although their actions are useful in the treatment of glaucoma and other conditions.

About 40% of filtered sodium chloride is reabsorbed in the proximal tubule. This is a relatively unimportant site of diuretic action, however, because inhibition of sodium chloride reabsorption in the proximal tubule leads to greater sodium chloride reabsorption in more distal segments of the nephron.

The proximal tubule is the major site of the active tubular secretion of organic acids and bases into the nephron lumen, including both endogenous compounds (e.g., uric acid) and drugs (e.g., penicillins). The **loop diuretics** and **thiazide diuretics** are also secreted by proximal tubular cells into the tubular lumen.

Loop of Henle

The loop of Henle is responsible for the reabsorption of about 35% of the filtered sodium chloride. This segment is also where calcium and magnesium are reabsorbed. The loop also enables the urine to be concentrated by transporting sodium chloride into the surrounding interstitium where a hypertonic interstitial fluid is formed. This fluid attracts water from the adjacent collecting duct under the influence of antidiuretic hormone and thereby increases the urine concentration. The reabsorption of sodium from the thick ascending limb is inhibited by **loop diuretics,** which can produce a greater diuresis than any other class of diuretics.

Distal Tubule

The early distal tubule is responsible for the reabsorption of 5% to 10% of the filtered sodium chloride, and this reabsorption is inhibited by **thiazide and related diuretics.** Because of the smaller amount of sodium reabsorbed in the distal tubule, the diuretic effect of thiazides is less than that of the loop diuretics.

Collecting Duct

The collecting duct serves to adjust the final composition and volume of urine to regulate extracellular fluid composition and pH and thereby maintain physiologic homeostasis. The collecting duct is the site of action of **aldosterone** and **antidiuretic hormone.** Aldosterone is a mineralocorticoid that increases sodium reabsorption, thereby promoting sodium retention by the body. Antidiuretic hormone increases the reabsorption of water from the collecting duct, which conserves body water and concentrates the urine. The actions of these hormones are partly responsible for maintaining plasma volume and osmolality in the normal range.

The collecting duct is responsible for the reabsorption of about 3% of the filtered sodium chloride. This reabsorption is coupled with potassium and hydrogen excretion. The **potassium-sparing diuretics** inhibit these processes and are primarily used to reduce potassium excretion and prevent hypokalemia.

TABLE 13.1 Usefulness of Diuretics in the Management of Various Clinical Disorders[a]

DISORDER	THIAZIDE AND RELATED DIURETICS	LOOP DIURETICS	POTASSIUM-SPARING DIURETICS	OSMOTIC DIURETICS	CARBONIC ANHYDRASE INHIBITORS
Cerebral edema	0	0	0	+	0
Cirrhosis	+	++	+	0	0
Congestive heart failure	+	++	+	0	0
Diabetes insipidus	++	0	0	0	0
Epilepsy	0	0	0	0	+
Glaucoma	0	0	0	+	++
High-altitude sickness	0	0	0	0	++
Hyperaldosteronism	0	0	+	0	0
Hypercalcemia	0	++	0	0	0
Hypertension	++	+	+	0	0
Hypokalemia	0	0	++	0	0
Nephrolithiasis	++	0	0	0	0
Nephrotic syndrome	+	++	+	0	0
Pulmonary edema	+	++	+	0	0
Renal impairment	+	++	0	+	0

[a]Ratings range from 0 (not useful) to ++ (highly useful).

BOX 13.1 SITES AND MECHANISMS OF ACTION OF DIURETICS

In the proximal tubule (A), carbonic anhydrase catalyzes the reversible conversion of hydrogen ion and bicarbonate to carbon dioxide and water, thereby enabling the reabsorption of sodium bicarbonate. This process is inhibited by carbonic anhydrase inhibitors, such as acetazolamide.

In the thick ascending limb of the loop of Henle (B), the $Na^+,K^+,2Cl^-$ symporter transports sodium, potassium, and chloride ions into the tubular cells, and then sodium is transferred to the interstitial fluid by the sodium pump. Potassium back-diffuses into the lumen and contributes to the positive transepithelial potential that drives paracellular calcium and magnesium reabsorption. By inhibiting the symporter, the loop diuretics reduce the back-diffusion of potassium and increase the excretion of calcium and magnesium.

In the distal tubule (C), sodium is transported into tubular epithelial cells by the Na^+,Cl^- symporter and then is transferred to interstitial fluid by the sodium pump. The Na^+,Cl^- symporter is inhibited by thiazide and related diuretics.

In the collecting duct (D), sodium enters the principal cells through sodium channels. Sodium is then transferred into the interstitial fluid by the sodium pump, while potassium is pumped in the opposite direction and then moves through potassium channels into the tubular fluid. Aldosterone stimulates these processes by increasing the synthesis of messenger RNA that encodes for sodium channel and sodium pump proteins. The potassium-sparing diuretics exert their effects via two mechanisms: amiloride and triamterene inhibit the entrance of sodium into the principal cells, whereas spironolactone blocks the mineralocorticoid receptor and thereby inhibits sodium reabsorption and potassium secretion.

BOX 13.1 SITES AND MECHANISMS OF ACTION OF DIURETICS—cont'd

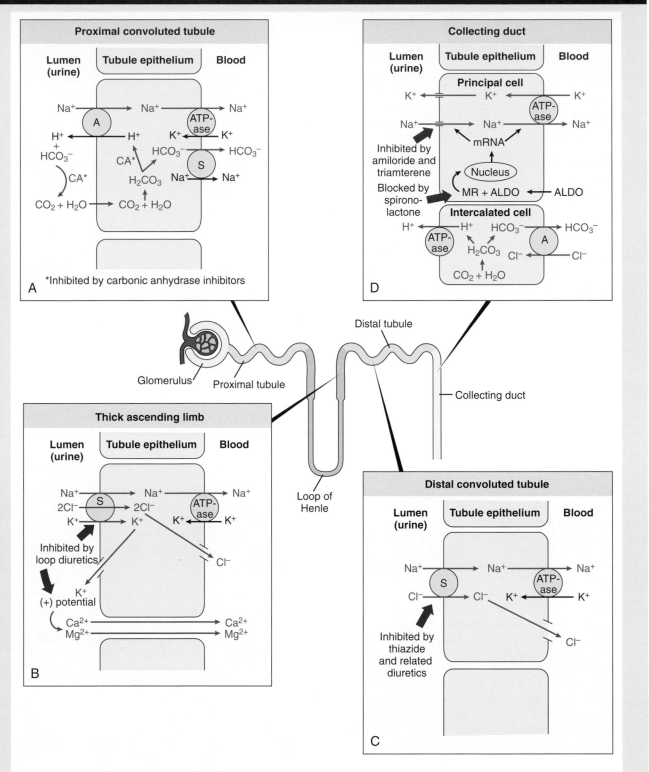

A, Antiporter; *ALDO*, aldosterone; *CA*, carbonic anhydrase; *MR*, mineralocorticoid receptor; *mRNA*, messenger RNA; *S*, symporter.

TABLE 13.2   Pharmacokinetic Properties of Diuretics[a]

DRUG	ORAL BIOAVAILABILITY	ELIMINATION HALF-LIFE (HOURS)	ROUTE OF ELIMINATION	DURATION OF ACTION (HOURS)
Thiazide and related diuretics				
Hydrochlorothiazide	70%	5	60% R and 40% M	12 for oral
Indapamide	90%	16	70% R and 30% M	30 for oral
Metolazone	65%	8	80% R and 20% M	18 for oral
Loop diuretics				
Bumetanide	85%	1.25	65% R and 35% M	5 for oral 1 for IV
Ethacrynic acid	100%	1	65% R and 35% M	7 for oral 2 for IV
Furosemide	60%	2	60% R and 40% M	7 for oral 2 for IV
Torsemide	80%	3.5	30% R and 70% M	7 for oral 7 for IV
Potassium-sparing diuretics				
Amiloride	20%	8	R	24 for oral
Spironolactone	65%	1.5	M	60 for oral
Triamterene	50%	4	M	14 for oral
Osmotic Diuretics				
Glycerol	95%	0.07	M	1 for oral
Mannitol	NA	1	R	7 for IV
Carbonic anhydrase inhibitors				
Acetazolamide	70%	7.5	R	10 for oral
Dorzolamide	NA	Biphasic[b]	R and M	8 for topical

IV, Intravenous; *M*, metabolism; *NA*, not applicable (not administered orally); *R*, renal.
[a]Values shown are the mean of values reported in the literature.
[b]Dorzolamide is eliminated in a biphasic manner with a rapid decline in serum levels followed by a much slower release from erythrocytes and has a half-life of 4 months.

DIURETIC AGENTS

Thiazide and Related Diuretics

The thiazides and related diuretics are the most commonly used diuretics. They are orally efficacious, have a moderate natriuretic effect, and have few adverse effects in most patients.

Drug Properties

Chemistry and Pharmacokinetics. Thiazides are sulfonamide compounds and were the first orally administered diuretics to be widely used for the treatment of hypertension and edema. Thiazides exhibit good oral bioavailability and are actively secreted into the nephron by proximal tubular cells, and they travel through the nephron lumen to reach their site of action in the distal tubule. Some of the thiazides are partially metabolized before excretion in the urine (Table 13.2).

Mechanisms and Pharmacologic Effects. Thiazide diuretics act on the early portion of the **distal tubule** to inhibit the **Na+, Cl− symporter** that participates in the reabsorption of sodium and chloride from this segment of the nephron (see Box 13.1). This action leads to the delivery of a greater volume of sodium chloride-enriched tubular fluid to the late distal tubule and collecting duct, which in turn stimulates the exchange of sodium and potassium at these sites. In the process, a small amount of sodium is reabsorbed as potassium is secreted into urine in the tubules. By this mechanism, thiazides have a kaliuretic effect that leads to **hypokalemia** in some patients.

As shown in Table 13.3, thiazides increase magnesium excretion, but—unlike many diuretics—they decrease **calcium excretion** in the urine. The reduced calcium excretion appears to result from decreased expression of calcium transport proteins, including the epithelial calcium channel, calbindin, and the sodium-calcium exchanger protein, in renal tubules after thiazide administration. The ability of thiazides to reduce calcium excretion is the basis for their use in the treatment of kidney stones caused by excessive calcium in the urine.

Adverse Effects and Interactions. Table 13.4 lists the common adverse effects and interactions of thiazides and other diuretics. Thiazide diuretics sometimes cause hypokalemia, particularly in patients whose dietary potassium intake is inadequate. Hypokalemia can eventually lead to **hypokalemic metabolic alkalosis** (Fig. 13.1). In this disorder, hydrogen ions enter body cells as potassium leaves these cells in an attempt to correct the plasma potassium deficiency. As the plasma potassium level falls, more hydrogen ions are secreted into urine in the tubules in exchange for sodium, and this further contributes to the development of metabolic alkalosis. In cases of hypokalemic metabolic alkalosis, potassium chloride is administered intravenously and orally. Correction of the serum potassium level then leads to correction of the acid-base disturbance as potassium

TABLE 13.3   Effects of Diuretics on Plasma pH and Urinary Excretion of Electrolytes[a]

| DRUG | PLASMA pH | ELECTROLYTES EXCRETED | | | | |
		Ca^{2+}	HCO$_3^-$	K$^+$	Mg^{2+}	Na$^+$
Thiazide and related diuretics	0 or ↑	−	0 or +	++	++	++
Loop diuretics	0 or ↑	++	0	++	++	+++
Potassium-sparing diuretics	0 or ↓	−	0	−	−	+
Osmotic diuretics	0	+	+	+	++	+++
Carbonic anhydrase inhibitors	↓	0 or +	+++	+	−	+

[a]Acute effects are shown and are indicated as follows: decrease (−); no change or variable (0); and increase ranging from small (+) to large (+++).

TABLE 13.4   Adverse Effects and Drug Interactions of Diuretics

DRUG	COMMON ADVERSE EFFECTS	COMMON DRUG INTERACTIONS
Thiazide and related diuretics		
Hydrochlorothiazide	Blood cell deficiencies; electrolyte imbalances; and increased blood cholesterol, glucose, or uric acid levels	Potentiates the diuretic effect of loop diuretics.
Indapamide	Electrolyte imbalances and increased blood cholesterol, glucose, or uric acid levels	Same as hydrochlorothiazide.
Metolazone	Blood cell deficiencies, electrolyte imbalances, and increased blood cholesterol or glucose levels	Same as hydrochlorothiazide.
Loop diuretics		
Bumetanide	Blood cell deficiencies, electrolyte imbalances, hearing impairment, and hypersensitivity reactions	Diuretic effect decreased by NSAIDs. Administration with ACE inhibitors may cause excessive hypotension.
Ethacrynic acid	Blood cell deficiencies, electrolyte imbalances, hearing impairment, and rash	Diuretic effect decreased by NSAIDs.
Furosemide	Blood cell deficiencies; electrolyte imbalances; hearing impairment; hypersensitivity reactions; increased blood cholesterol, glucose, or uric acid levels; and photosensitivity	Same as bumetanide.
Torsemide	Electrolyte imbalances and increased blood cholesterol, glucose, or uric acid levels	Same as bumetanide.
Potassium-sparing diuretics		
Amiloride	Blood cell deficiencies, gastrointestinal distress, and hyperkalemia	Administration with ACE inhibitors or potassium supplements may cause hyperkalemia. Administration with NSAIDs may cause renal failure.
Spironolactone	Gynecomastia, hyperkalemia, and impotence	Administration with ACE inhibitors or potassium supplements may cause hyperkalemia.
Triamterene	Same as amiloride	Same as amiloride.
Osmotic diuretics		
Glycerol	Heart failure; nausea and vomiting; and pulmonary congestion and edema	Potentiates effects of other diuretics.
Mannitol	Same as glycerol	Same as glycerol.
Carbonic anhydrase inhibitors		
Acetazolamide	Blood cell deficiencies, drowsiness, hepatic insufficiency, hyperglycemia, hypokalemia, metabolic acidosis, paresthesia, and uremia	Serum levels of weak bases, such as amphetamine, ephedrine, and quinidine, are increased by CA inhibitors. Serum levels of CA inhibitors are increased by salicylates.
Dorzolamide	Bitter taste, blurred vision, ocular discomfort, allergic reactions	Unknown.

ACE, Angiotensin-converting enzyme; *CA,* carbonic anhydrase; *NSAIDs,* nonsteroidal anti-inflammatory drugs.

displaces hydrogen ions from body cells and fewer hydrogen ions are secreted by the collecting duct.

In addition to causing electrolyte and acid-base disturbances, the thiazides can cause several metabolic abnormalities, including **elevated blood glucose, uric acid,** and **lipid levels.** Thiazides appear to decrease insulin sensitivity and thereby contribute to the development of diabetes in some patients. In addition, thiazide-induced hypokalemia can decrease insulin secretion (see Fig. 13.1). Hyperuricemia, which is caused by inhibition of uric acid secretion from

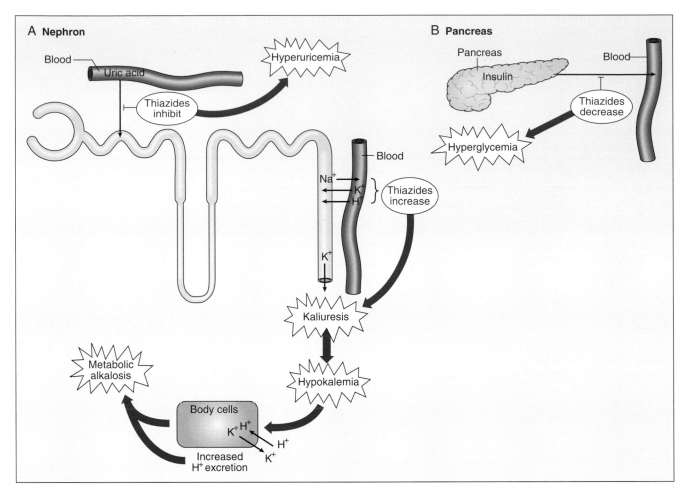

Fig. 13.1   Adverse effects of thiazide diuretics. (A) Inhibition of uric acid secretion in the proximal tubule can lead to hyperuricemia and gout. Increased potassium secretion in the collecting duct can cause hypokalemia. Hypokalemia can lead to metabolic alkalosis by promoting the exchange of intracellular potassium for hydrogen ions and by increasing the excretion of hydrogen ions. The increased excretion is caused by lack of availability of potassium for exchange with sodium in the collecting duct. (B) In the presence of hypokalemia, the amount of insulin secreted by the pancreas can be reduced, thereby leading to hyperglycemia. Other mechanisms can also be involved in the development of hyperglycemia.

the proximal tubule, can lead to the development of gout. The effects of thiazide diuretics on serum lipid levels are discussed in greater detail in Chapter 10.

Indications. Thiazide diuretics are widely used in the management of cardiovascular and renal diseases (see Table 13.1). They are often prescribed for **hypertension** and can be used to treat **edema** associated with **heart failure, cirrhosis, corticosteroid therapy, estrogen therapy,** and **renal disorders,** such as **nephrotic syndrome.** Because thiazides reduce calcium excretion and decrease urinary calcium levels, they are helpful in treating patients with **nephrolithiasis** (kidney stones) associated with **hypercalciuria.**

Thiazides are also used to treat nephrogenic **diabetes insipidus.** In this disorder, the kidneys are not responsive to circulating antidiuretic hormone, and patients may excrete from 10 L to 20 L of urine per day. Thiazides exert a paradoxical antidiuretic effect in these patients and reduce the excessive urine volume dramatically. In cases of diabetes insipidus, the effectiveness of thiazides is believed to stem from a reduction in plasma volume caused by these drugs. The reduced plasma volume serves to increase sodium and water reabsorption from the proximal tubule, so that less water is delivered to the diluting segments of the nephron. As a result, the urine output falls.

Hydrochlorothiazide

The several thiazide compounds that are available have almost identical actions but differ in their potency and pharmacokinetic properties. Hydrochlorothiazide is the most frequently prescribed thiazide diuretic.

Thiazide-Like Diuretics

Thiazide-like diuretics have a different chemical structure, but their actions and uses are similar to those of the thiazides. These drugs include **chlorthalidone, indapamide,** and **metolazone.** Indapamide has both diuretic and vasodilator actions and is indicated for the treatment of **hypertension** and **heart failure.**

Loop Diuretics

Drug Properties

Chemistry and Pharmacokinetics. As with the thiazides, most of the loop-acting diuretics have a sulfonamide structure. The pharmacokinetic properties of loop diuretics are summarized in Table 13.2.

Mechanisms and Pharmacologic Effects. Loop diuretics **inhibit the Na$^+$,K$^+$,2Cl$^-$ symporter** in the ascending limb of the loop of Henle and thereby exert a powerful natriuretic effect. In comparison with other diuretics, loop diuretics can

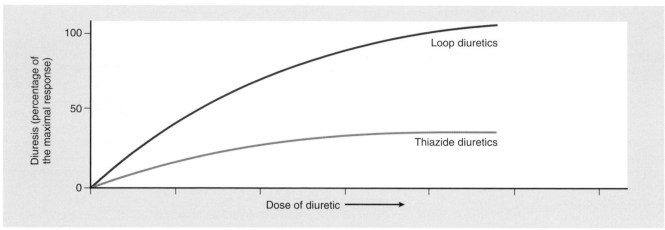

Fig. 13.2 Dose-response curves of loop and thiazide diuretics. Loop diuretics produce dose-dependent diuresis throughout their therapeutic dosage range, whereas thiazide diuretics have a relatively flat dose-response curve and a limited maximal response.

inhibit the reabsorption of a greater percentage of filtered sodium. Loop diuretics are sometimes called **high-ceiling diuretics** because they produce a dose-dependent diuresis throughout their clinical dosage range. This property can be contrasted with the rather flat dose-response curve and limited diuretic capability of thiazides and other diuretic drugs (Fig. 13.2).

In addition to their natriuretic effect, the loop diuretics produce kaliuresis by increasing the exchange of sodium and potassium in the late distal tubule and collecting duct via the same mechanisms as those described for the thiazide diuretics. Loop diuretics also increase **magnesium and calcium excretion** by reducing the reabsorption of these ions in the ascending limb (see Box 13.1). This action results from inhibition of the Na+,K+,2Cl− symporter, which reduces the back-diffusion of potassium into the nephron lumen. The reduction of potassium back-diffusion decreases the transepithelial electrical potential that normally drives the paracellular reabsorption of magnesium and calcium. Inhibition of this process thereby increases magnesium and calcium excretion.

Adverse Effects and Interactions. Loop diuretics can produce a variety of **electrolyte abnormalities,** including hypokalemia, hypocalcemia, hypomagnesemia, and metabolic alkalosis. These diuretics can also increase blood glucose and uric acid levels in the same manner as the thiazide diuretics. In some patients, use of loop diuretics causes **ototoxicity** with manifestations such as tinnitus, ear pain, vertigo, and hearing deficits. In most cases, the hearing loss is reversible. Other adverse effects and drug interactions are listed in Table 13.4.

Indications. Loop diuretics are used when intensive diuresis is required and cannot be achieved with other diuretics. Loop diuretics are highly effective in the treatment of **pulmonary edema,** partly because of the vasodilation that occurs when they are administered intravenously. They are the preferred diuretics in the treatment of persons with renal impairment because—unlike thiazide and other diuretics—they are effective in patients whose creatinine clearance drops below 30 mL/min. Loop diuretics are often the drugs of choice for patients with edema caused by heart failure, cirrhosis, and other disorders. Although they are prescribed for patients with hypertension, the thiazide diuretics

are usually preferred for this condition. Loop diuretics can be used to treat **hypercalcemia,** whereas the thiazide diuretics can increase serum calcium levels slightly.

Bumetanide, Furosemide, and Torsemide
Bumetanide, furosemide, and **torsemide** are sulfonamide derivatives with similar pharmacologic actions and effects. These drugs can be administered orally or intravenously. In comparison with other loop diuretics, **torsemide** has a somewhat longer half-life and a significantly longer duration of action after intravenous administration (see Table 13.2). All three of the drugs are partly metabolized before they are excreted in the urine.

Ethacrynic Acid
Ethacrynic acid is the only loop diuretic that is not a sulfonamide derivative, and it is occasionally used when patients are allergic or intolerant to the sulfonamide drugs in this class. Otherwise, it is seldom used because it tends to produce more **ototoxicity** than do other loop diuretics.

Potassium-Sparing Diuretics
Two types of potassium-sparing diuretics exist: the epithelial **sodium channel blockers** and the **aldosterone receptor antagonists**.

Amiloride and Triamterene
Amiloride and triamterene are epithelial **sodium channel blockers.** By blocking the entry of sodium into the principal tubular cells of the late distal tubule and collecting duct (see Box 13.1), these drugs prevent sodium reabsorption at this site and indirectly reduce the secretion of potassium into the tubular filtrate and urine. Through these actions, the potassium-sparing diuretics produce a modest amount of natriuresis but decrease kaliuresis. Amiloride and triamterene are primarily used to prevent and treat **hypokalemia** induced by thiazide and loop diuretics. The properties, effects, and uses of amiloride, triamterene, and other potassium-sparing diuretics are outlined in Tables 13.1 to 13.4.

The most characteristic adverse effect of the potassium-sparing diuretics is **hyperkalemia,** but this is unlikely to occur unless the patient also ingests potassium supplements or other drugs that increase serum potassium levels (e.g., angiotensin antagonists) or unless the patient has a renal disorder that predisposes to hyperkalemia.

Treatment of hyperkalemia is the sole indication for **patiromer** (VELTASSA), a new drug with the novel mechanisms of binding up potassium in the gastrointestinal (GI) tract. Patiromer is not absorbed, and the binding of potassium reduces the concentration of free potassium in the GI lumen, resulting in a reduction of serum potassium levels.

Spironolactone

Spironolactone is a structural analog of aldosterone that competitively **blocks aldosterone binding** to the **mineralocorticoid receptor** in epithelial cells of the late distal tubule and collecting duct. When activated, the mineralocorticoid receptor interacts with DNA to promote expression of genes for sodium channels and the sodium pump that enable sodium reabsorption and potassium secretion. By blocking these actions, spironolactone reduces sodium reabsorption and the accompanying secretion of potassium.

Spironolactone is adequately absorbed from the gut and has a **long duration of action** despite its short elimination half-life, indicating that its cellular actions persist longer than circulating drug levels (see Table 13.2). Spironolactone is used to prevent hypokalemia in the same manner as amiloride and triamterene, and it has a special role in the treatment of primary **hyperaldosteronism**. Clinical trials have shown that spironolactone reduces mortality in persons with heart failure, as described in Chapter 12. Its use in this condition, however, has been associated with an increased incidence of hyperkalemia. Because of its **antiandrogenic effect**, spironolactone is also used in the treatment of polycystic ovary disease and hirsutism in women.

The adverse effects of spironolactone include **gynecomastia** and **impotence** in men (caused by the drug's antiandrogenic effects) and hyperkalemia. **Eplerenone** is a newer aldosterone antagonist that produces fewer endocrine side effects than does spironolactone. Eplerenone is used to counteract the effects of excessive aldosterone in persons with heart failure (see Chapter 12).

Osmotic Diuretics

Glycerol and **mannitol** are examples of osmotic diuretics. These diuretics increase the osmotic pressure of the plasma and thereby attract water from interstitial and transcellular fluids. Because of this action, mannitol is used to treat **cerebral edema** and reduce intracranial pressure. Glycerol and mannitol are both used in the treatment of **acute glaucoma**. By attracting water from ocular fluids into the circulation, the drugs reduce intraocular volume and pressure. Glycerol is administered orally for this purpose, whereas mannitol is administered intravenously.

Mannitol is also used as a diuretic. After intravenous administration, it is filtered at the glomerulus but is not reabsorbed from the renal tubules. It osmotically attracts and retains water as it moves through the nephron and into the urine. This action reduces the tubular sodium concentration and the concentration gradient between the tubular fluid and cells and thereby retards the reabsorption of sodium. Hence, mannitol has both direct and indirect actions that promote diuresis. The diuretic effect of mannitol has been used to improve renal function in the oliguric phase of **acute renal failure**. Evidence for a renoprotective effect of mannitol has been obtained in studies of persons having renal transplantation.

Mannitol has also been administered along with intravenous fluids to **maintain renal function** and reduce the renal toxicity of **antineoplastic platinum compounds** (e.g., cisplatin), and mannitol is used to promote the renal excretion of toxic substances in cases of drug overdose or poisoning.

The primary adverse effect of mannitol is **excessive plasma volume expansion**, which is most likely to occur if the drug is administered too rapidly or with too large a volume of intravenous fluid. Excessive plasma volume can lead to heart failure and pulmonary congestion and edema in susceptible patients.

Carbonic Anhydrase Inhibitors
Drug Properties

The **CA inhibitors** were the first sulfonamide derivatives to be used as diuretics, and their discovery eventually led to the development of the thiazide and loop diuretics. **Acetazolamide, dorzolamide,** and other CA inhibitors are relatively **weak diuretics** and are seldom used for this purpose today. Instead, their ability to inhibit CA has led to their use in the treatment of disorders, such as **high-altitude sickness** and **glaucoma.**

Pharmacokinetics. **Acetazolamide** is one of several orally administered CA inhibitors, whereas **dorzolamide** is used as an ophthalmic solution to treat glaucoma. Dorzolamide is partly absorbed from the eye into the circulation and undergoes some metabolic transformation before it is excreted in the urine. The drug is eliminated in a biphasic manner, with a rapid decline in serum levels followed by a much slower release from erythrocytes, and it has a half-life of 4 months. The pharmacokinetic properties of acetazolamide and dorzolamide are outlined in Table 13.2.

Mechanisms, Pharmacologic Effects, and Indications. Acetazolamide and other drugs in this class inhibit CA throughout the body. This enzyme catalyzes the conversion of carbon dioxide and water to carbonic acid, which spontaneously decomposes to bicarbonate and hydrogen ions.

When the ciliary process forms aqueous humor, CA participates by catalyzing the formation of bicarbonate, which is secreted into the posterior chamber of the eye, along with water and other substances that make up the aqueous humor. In patients with **glaucoma**, inhibition of CA reduces **aqueous humor secretion** and intraocular pressure. The CA inhibitors are used in the treatment of both the acute and chronic form of glaucoma, although they must be combined with other drugs to treat the acute form. Traditionally, the CA inhibitors have been administered orally to patients with glaucoma. Now, some of these drugs—including dorzolamide—are available for topical ocular administration. Dorzolamide is administered every 8 hours in the treatment of chronic ocular hypertension and open-angle glaucoma.

CA is also required for the **reabsorption of sodium bicarbonate from the proximal tubule** and for the secretion of hydrogen ions in the collecting duct. In the reabsorption of sodium bicarbonate, bicarbonate must be converted to carbon dioxide and water by CA because the apical cell membrane of the tubular epithelial cells is impermeable to bicarbonate. The carbon dioxide and water can diffuse into the tubular cells, where CA converts them back to bicarbonate, which is then transported into the interstitial fluid for diffusion into the circulation (see Box 13.1). Inhibition of this process by acetazolamide and other CA inhibitors causes a marked reduction in the reabsorption of sodium bicarbonate and a corresponding increase in its renal excretion. This leads to alkalinization of the urine and produces a mild form of **hyperchloremic metabolic acidosis.** The hyperchloremia results from the increased reabsorption of chloride as a compensation for reduced bicarbonate reabsorption.

CA inhibitors are seldom used as **diuretics,** although they are used occasionally to **alkalinize the urine.** They are effective in the prevention and treatment of **high-altitude sickness (mountain sickness),** in part because the metabolic acidosis produced by the drugs counteracts the respiratory alkalosis that can result from hyperventilation in this condition. By counteracting respiratory alkalosis, the drugs enhance ventilation acclimatization and maintain oxygenation during sleep at a high altitude. The drugs also counteract fluid retention and cause a decrease in cerebral spinal fluid (CSF) pressure, which can be elevated with acute high-altitude sickness. At the same time, CA inhibitors prevent the fall in CSF pH that occurs in this disorder.

Inhibition of CA in the central nervous system elevates the seizure threshold. For this reason, CA inhibitors have been used occasionally for the treatment of **epilepsy.**

Adverse Effects and Interactions. Acetazolamide and other orally administered CA inhibitors can cause **drowsiness, paresthesia,** and other **central nervous system effects** as well as hypokalemia and hyperglycemia. Less commonly, they are associated with various hypersensitivity reactions and blood cell deficiencies. By increasing the pH of the renal tubular fluid and alkalinizing the urine, the CA inhibitors **decrease the excretion of weak bases**—such as amphetamine, pseudoephedrine, and quinidine—and thereby increase their serum levels and cause drug toxicity.

Antidiuretic Hormone Antagonists

Conivaptan and **tolvaptan** are nonpeptide antagonists of antidiuretic hormone (arginine vasopressin). **Conivaptan** blocks both V_{1A} and V_2 receptors, whereas **tolvaptan** is V_2 selective. The V_2 receptors are coupled with insertion of aquaporin channels in the apical membranes of the renal collecting ducts, leading to reabsorption of water (antidiuretic effect). By activating these receptors, antidiuretic hormone helps maintain plasma osmolality in the normal range. Antagonism of V_2 receptors by conivaptan and tolvaptan causes **free water excretion** or aquaresis, and the drugs have been called **aquaretics.**

Conivaptan and **tolvaptan** are approved for treating **euvolemic** and **hypervolemic hyponatremia** (low serum sodium concentration) in hospitalized patients, but they are contraindicated in hypovolemic hyponatremia. Conivaptan is given as an intravenous infusion, usually for 4 days, and typically increases free water clearance by 3,800 mL and serum sodium concentration by 6.5 mEq/L. Almost 70% of patients achieve a normal serum sodium concentration of 135 mEq/L after 4 days of conivaptan therapy. Tolvaptan is an orally administered drug congener of conivaptan indicated for treating hyponatremia (Box 13.2).

Conivaptan and tolvaptan are extensively metabolized by CYP3A4 and should not be given with potent 3A4

BOX 13.2 A CASE OF LETHARGY, FATIGUE, AND CONFUSION

CASE PRESENTATION

A 58-year-old woman was taken to the emergency department after becoming weak and confused and falling down. Two years ago, she was diagnosed with moderately severe hyponatremia due to the syndrome of inappropriate antidiuretic hormone secretion (SIADH) after complaining of chronic lethargy and fatigue. She was managed at that time with fluid restriction that maintained the serum sodium values in the range of 126 mmol/L to 132 mmol/L (normal 135 mmol/L to 145 mmol/L). After the current admission, the serum sodium was 118 mmol/L. Despite fluid restriction, the sodium level did not improve significantly, and she was placed on alternate day tolvaptan to avoid increasing the sodium level too rapidly. She exhibited profound diuresis, and the serum sodium increased to 130 mmol/L after two doses of tolvaptan. Her symptoms improved dramatically, and she was discharged with a serum sodium of 138 mmol/L and prescribed fluid restrictions. She will be monitored and evaluated for continued tolvaptan therapy.

CASE DISCUSSION

Hyponatremia is the most common electrolyte abnormality in older adults. It can be classified as hypervolemic, euvolemic, or hypovolemic. SIADH typically results in a euvolemic hyponatremia that is often managed by fluid restriction, though this treatment is difficult to maintain over a period of time. Vasopressin (antidiuretic hormone) antagonists, such as conivaptan and tolvaptan, can be used to treat hyponatremia if fluid restriction is not effective. These agents can elicit a profound diuresis in patients with SIADH and must be used cautiously to avoid excessive or too rapid correction of serum sodium levels. Occasionally, these agents can be given chronically, such as once weekly, to manage hyponatremia in patients who cannot be managed with fluid restriction alone, but patients must be closely monitored to avoid hypernatremia and other treatment complications.

inhibitors. Conivaptan and tolvaptan may increase serum levels of **midazolam, simvastatin,** and other drugs metabolized by 3A4. The most common adverse reactions reported with conivaptan are infusion site reactions. Both agents can cause hypernatremia if excessive doses are given.

MANAGEMENT OF EDEMA

Edema is a condition in which fluid accumulates in the interstitial space and body cavities, either because of increased hydrostatic pressure in the capillary beds or because of inadequate colloid osmotic pressure in the plasma. The plasma osmotic pressure is primarily influenced by the osmotic attraction of water by sodium and plasma proteins. Conditions that cause edema as a result of increased hydrostatic pressure include **heart failure** and **certain renal diseases,** all of which cause sodium and water retention. Conditions that cause edema as a result of inadequate colloid osmotic pressure include severe dietary protein deficiency and hepatic diseases (e.g., cirrhosis). In conditions such as cirrhosis, the liver is unable to synthesize adequate albumin and other plasma proteins to maintain plasma osmotic pressure. Hepatic cirrhosis can lead to ascites (accumulation of fluid within the peritoneal cavity) and portal hypertension. This disorder can be managed with dietary salt restriction and the use of diuretics (e.g., spirono-lactone and furosemide).

Nephrotic syndrome, a renal disease that leads to excessive protein excretion in the urine (proteinuria), can cause edema by this mechanism. Infection, neoplasms, and thromboembolism can also cause edema by various mechanisms that include inflammation, increased capillary fluid permeability, and increased hydrostatic pressure caused by obstruction of blood vessels.

The primary treatment of edema is to **correct the underlying disorder** and restore plasma osmotic pressure and hydrostatic pressure to normal values. In acute life-threatening situations (e.g., cerebral edema and pulmonary edema), **diuretics** and other drugs must be administered immediately to prevent tissue hypoxia, injury, and death. In milder forms of edema, diuretics can be used as short-term adjunct treatments that serve to mobilize edematous fluid while an attempt is made to correct the underlying cause. Most cases of mild peripheral edema, however, can be managed without pharmacologic therapy by correcting the underlying disorder or discontinuing a causative drug.

SUMMARY OF IMPORTANT POINTS

- Diuretics are drugs that increase urine production. Most diuretics inhibit the reabsorption of sodium from various sites in the nephron.
- Thiazide diuretics inhibit sodium chloride reabsorption from the distal tubule. They cause natriuresis and kaliuresis, but they decrease calcium excretion. They are primarily used to treat hypertension, edema, hypercalciuria, and nephrogenic diabetes insipidus.
- Loop diuretics inhibit the $Na^+,K^+,2Cl^-$ symporter in the ascending limb and thereby increase sodium, potassium, calcium, and magnesium excretion. They are chiefly used to treat heart failure, renal failure, pulmonary edema, and hypercalcemia.
- Thiazide and loop diuretics can cause hypokalemia and other electrolyte disturbances, as well as hyperglycemia and hyperuricemia.
- Potassium-sparing diuretics, which inhibit potassium secretion in the collecting duct, are primarily used to prevent hypokalemia, which can be caused by thiazide and loop diuretics. Spironolactone is used to treat severe heart failure and hyperaldosteronism.
- Osmotic diuretics increase the osmotic pressure of plasma and retain water in the nephron. They are used to treat cerebral edema, glaucoma, and the oliguria of acute renal failure.
- Carbonic anhydrase inhibitors, which are weak diuretics that inhibit sodium bicarbonate reabsorption from the proximal tubule, can cause a mild form of metabolic acidosis. They reduce aqueous humor secretion and are primarily used to treat glaucoma.
- Conivaptan and tolvaptan are antidiuretic hormone receptor antagonists that increase free water excretion and are used to treat euvolemic or hypervolemic hyponatremia.

Review Questions

For each drug description (1–4), select the correct drug from the following choices:

   (A) spironolactone
   (B) furosemide
   (C) hydrochlorothiazide
   (D) acetazolamide
   (E) mannitol

1. Large intravenous doses of this drug may cause tinnitus, vertigo, and hearing loss.
2. Administration of this drug to persons with renal insufficiency can cause hyperkalemia.
3. This drug can be used to increase the renal excretion of weakly acidic drugs, such as amphetamine.
4. This drug can be used to increase calcium excretion in persons with hypercalcemia.
5. Which diuretic is used in the treatment of high altitude (mountain) sickness?
   (A) mannitol
   (B) hydrochlorothiazide
   (C) acetazolamide
   (D) amiloride
   (E) torsemide

CHAPTER 14

Drugs for Cardiac Dysrhythmia

CLASSIFICATION OF ANTIDYSRHYTHMIC DRUGS

Sodium Channel Blockers

- Disopyramide (NORPACE)[a]
- Lidocaine[b]
- Propafenone (RYTHMOL)[c]

Beta-Adrenoceptor Blockers

- Metoprolol (LOPRESSOR)[d]

Potassium Channel Blockers

- Amiodarone (CORDARONE)
- Dronedarone (MULTAQ)
- Ibutilide (CORVERT)
- Dofetilide (TIKOSYN)
- Sotalol (BETAPACE)

Calcium Channel Blockers

- Diltiazem (CARDIZEM)
- Verapamil (CALAN)

Miscellaneous Drugs

- Adenosine (ADENOCARD)
- Digoxin (LANOXIN)
- Magnesium sulfate
- Ivabradine (CORLANOR)
- Ranolazine (RANEXA)

[a] Also quinidine and procainamide. Quinidine is also combined with dextromethorphan in NEUDEXTA.
[b] Also mexiletine.
[c] Also flecainide.
[d] Also esmolol (BREVIBLOC), propranolol (INDERAL), and acebutolol (SECTRAL).

OVERVEIW

Cardiac arrhythmia literally means cardiac arrest, but cardiac dysrhythmias occur when the origin, rhythm, or rate of heartbeats are abnormal. Dysrhythmias often result from ischemic or structural heart disease and are a major cause of cardiovascular dysfunction and death. Cardiac dysrhythmias occur primarily because of disturbances in cardiac impulse formation or conduction, and they can originate in any part of the heart. Those arising in the atria or atrioventricular (AV) node are called **supraventricular dysrhythmias**, whereas those arising in the ventricles are called **ventricular dysrhythmias**. Those in which the heart rate is too rapid are called **tachydysrhythmias**, and those in which the heart rate is too slow are called **bradydysrhythmias**.

Some dysrhythmias are benign and do not necessarily require treatment. Others require treatment because they produce symptoms, reduce cardiac output and blood pressure significantly, or because they can precipitate more serious and even lethal rhythm disturbances. Both **pharmacologic** and **electrical methods**, as well as **surgical ablation**

of focal dysrhythmia-generating tissue, are used to prevent and terminate dysrhythmias. Clinical trials have shown that antidysrhythmic drugs have limited effectiveness while exhibiting considerable potential to cause dysrhythmias themselves or to produce other adverse effects, particularly in patients with ventricular heart disease. For this reason, drugs are often employed as adjuncts to electrical methods, such as pacemakers and implantable defibrillators in treating ventricular dysrhythmias. However, many patients with supraventricular dysrhythmias may benefit from drugs that prevent or reduce the frequency of their dysrhythmia and symptoms of palpitations and tachycardia. This chapter describes the pathophysiology of dysrhythmias and the mechanisms by which **antidysrhythmic drugs** maintain or restore normal sinus rhythm.

Cardiac Action Potentials and Electrocardiographic Findings

In a normal heart, each heartbeat originates in the sinoatrial (SA) node, the rhythm of heartbeats is regular, and the heart rate is about 70 beats/min at rest (normal sinus rhythm). Fig. 14.1 depicts the relationships among ion currents, cardiac action potentials in phases 0 through 4, and findings on the surface electrocardiogram (ECG) in a healthy individual.

The SA node, located in the right atrium, is the site of origin of the normal heartbeat. The SA node spontaneously depolarizes to form an impulse conducted through the atrium to the AV node and then through the bundle of His, bundle branches, and Purkinje fibers to the ventricular muscle.

The **spontaneous depolarization of the SA node** is primarily caused by the influx of sodium and potassium as the efflux of potassium subsides. The depolarizing pacemaker current is known as the **"funny current"** or I_f and is blocked by **ivabradine** (see later and in Chapter 11). When the threshold potential (TP) is reached at about −40 mV, the SA node is more rapidly depolarized by sodium and calcium influx to generate an impulse that can be conducted to the rest of the heart.

As the impulse is conducted to atrial and ventricular muscle cells, these cells are rapidly depolarized by the influx of sodium through the fast sodium channel. As the heart cells depolarize to about −40 mV, the slow calcium channels open. The influx of calcium through these channels during phase 2 serves to activate muscle contraction. Cardiac tissues become repolarized during phase 3 as a result of the efflux of potassium through several types of rectifier potassium channels, an efflux that occurs when the influx of calcium declines.

As shown in Fig. 14.1, the surface ECG is a summation of action potentials generated by the heart during the cardiac cycle. The **P wave** represents atrial depolarization, whereas the **PR interval** corresponds to the time required to conduct the action potential through the atria and the

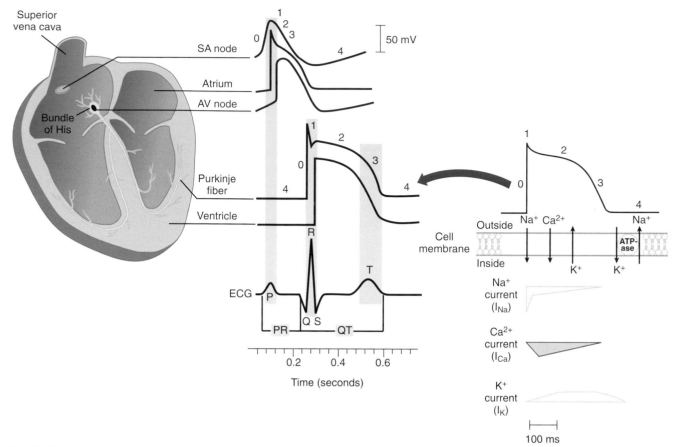

Fig. 14.1   Relationships among ion currents, cardiac action potentials, and the findings on surface electrocardiogram *(ECG)*. The normal heartbeat originates in the sinoatrial *(SA)* node. The impulse is conducted through internodal fibers to the atrioventricular *(AV)* node and then through the bundle of His, bundle branches, and Purkinje fibers to the ventricular muscle. On the ECG, the P wave represents atrial depolarization, the QRS complex represents ventricular depolarization, and the T wave represents ventricular repolarization. The PR interval is primarily related to the conduction time through the AV node, and the QT interval represents the time between ventricular depolarization and repolarization. In phase 0, ventricular depolarization is caused by sodium influx through the fast sodium channel. In phase 1, the membrane is transiently repolarized as a result of potassium efflux. In phase 2, the membrane potential is relatively stable because of the concurrent influx of calcium and efflux of potassium. In phase 3, repolarization is caused by continued potassium efflux as calcium influx declines. In phase 4, the ion balance is returned to normal by the action of the sodium pump (Na$^+$,K$^+$-adenosine triphosphatase [ATPase]). Calcium is removed from the cell by the sodium-calcium exchanger and the calcium ATPase (not shown).

AV node. The **QRS complex** and the **T wave** represent the time intervals of ventricular depolarization and repolarization, respectively. Hence, the **QT interval** represents the duration of the ventricular action potential.

Pathophysiology of Dysrhythmias

Dysrhythmias can be caused by coronary ischemia and tissue hypoxia, structural heart disease, electrolyte disturbances, overstimulation of the sympathetic nervous system, general anesthetics, and other conditions or drugs that perturb cardiac action potentials. Dysrhythmias appear to result from a number of mechanisms, including abnormal impulse formation, impulse conduction, and repolarization. Yet, the mechanisms responsible for specific dysrhythmias have been difficult to define, and it has been concluded that a spectrum of mechanisms contributes to such common dysrhythmias as ventricular tachycardia and atrial fibrillation. Hence, not all patients with these dysrhythmias respond in the same way to a particular therapy, and it is not surprising that most drug treatments have incomplete efficacy for many dysrhythmias.

Reentry is the term applied to a mechanism believed to underlie several supraventricular and ventricular dysrhythmias. The reentry of previously depolarized cardiac tissue

results from different rates of impulse conduction and repolarization (heterogeneity) in a particular part of the heart. For example, heterogeneity in the His-Purkinje conduction pathway and ventricular tissue is thought to contribute to various forms of ventricular tachycardia.

Abnormal Impulse Formation

Abnormal impulse formation can generate extra heartbeats (**extrasystoles**) and result in **tachycardia.** The two mechanisms that are primarily responsible for abnormal impulse formation are increased automaticity and the occurrence of afterdepolarizations. These are shown in Box 14.1.

Increased Automaticity

Spontaneous phase 4 depolarization generates an action potential that can be propagated to other parts of the heart. The SA node is the usual site of spontaneous impulse initiation (**automaticity**), but other cardiac tissues—including the AV node and the His-Purkinje system tissues—are also capable of spontaneous depolarization. Pathologic conditions or drugs can cause these tissues to depolarize more rapidly and thereby generate abnormal impulses. For example, overstimulation of the sympathetic nervous system or use

BOX 14.1 THE ELECTROPHYSIOLOGIC BASIS OF DYSRHYTHMIAS

ABNORMAL IMPULSE FORMATION

The two mechanisms primarily responsible for abnormal impulse formation are increased automaticity and afterdepolarizations.

Increased automaticity can be caused by any change that decreases the time required for depolarization from the maximal diastolic potential (MDP) to the threshold potential (TP). Increased automaticity occurs if the rate of diastolic depolarization (the slope of phase 4) in the SA node or in latent pacemakers is increased. It also occurs if a shift of the TP occurs to a more negative value or if a shift occurs of the MDP to a more positive value.

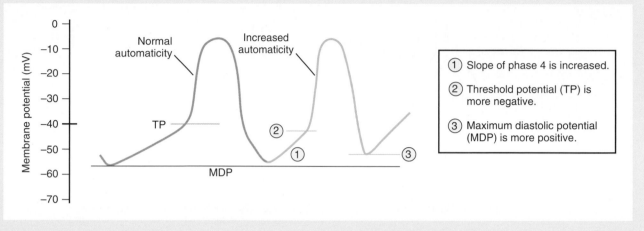

Afterdepolarizations can result from abnormal calcium influx into cardiac cells during or immediately after phase 3 of the ventricular action potential and are sometimes provoked by prolonged ventricular repolarization. Afterdepolarizations can lead to extrasystoles and tachycardia.

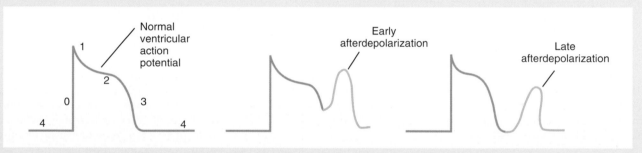

ABNORMAL IMPULSE CONDUCTION

Reentry is the conduction of an impulse into previously depolarized tissue.

In **ventricular tissue,** reentry is believed to result from decreased conduction speed and spread of the impulse (decremental conduction) as the amplitude of the action potential declines due to ischemia or structural abnormalities. This leads to unevenness (heterogeneity) of depolarization and repolarization in adjacent areas of the ventricle, enabling reentry and excitation of previously depolarized ventricular tissue. Ventricular reentry is manifested as tachycardia or fibrillation.

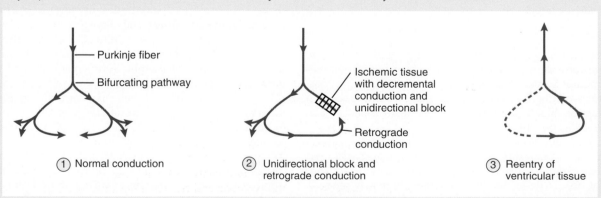

Continued

BOX 14.1 THE ELECTROPHYSIOLOGIC BASIS OF DYSRHYTHMIAS—cont'd

Reentry in the **atrioventricular (AV) node** is the most common electrophysiologic mechanism responsible for paroxysmal supraventricular tachycardia (PSVT). Reentry occurs when a premature atrial depolarization arrives at the AV node and finds that one pathway (β) is still refractory from the previous depolarization. The other pathway (α), however, is able to conduct the impulse to the ventricle. Retrograde conduction of the impulse through pathway β leads to reentry of the atrium and results in tachycardia. In the AV node, the unidirectional block results from the β pathway's longer refractory period, which blocks anterograde conduction but permits retrograde conduction after it has recovered its excitability.

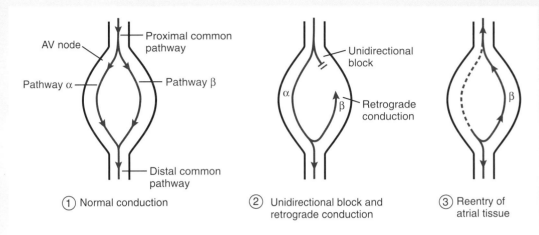

① Normal conduction   ② Unidirectional block and retrograde conduction   ③ Reentry of atrial tissue

of sympathomimetic drugs increases automaticity and can cause **tachydysrhythmia.**

The rate at which action potentials are generated in the SA node and elsewhere in the heart depends on the time required to depolarize the tissue from the maximal diastolic potential (MDP) to the TP. Automaticity is increased if the MDP becomes more positive or if the TP becomes more negative. Serum electrolyte abnormalities, hypoxia, and structural heart defects can affect the MDP or TP in this manner and lead to dysrhythmias.

Afterdepolarizations

Afterdepolarizations result from the spontaneous generation of action potentials during or immediately after phase 3 repolarization. Afterdepolarizations are believed to be triggered by **abnormal calcium influx** and can be provoked by digoxin as well as by other drugs or potassium channel defects that prolong cardiac repolarization and the QT interval (see later).

Reentry

When cardiac impulse conduction and repolarization are not uniform in a particular region of the heart, impulses may reenter previously depolarized tissue causing extra beats and tachycardia. It is sometimes caused by a **unidirectional conduction block** in a bifurcating conduction pathway, as described in Box 14.1.

In ventricular tissue, ischemia and infarction can cause a reduction in the resting membrane potential and a decrease in membrane responsiveness. Under these conditions, cells do not depolarize as rapidly or completely during phase 0, which reduces the rate of conduction and slows the spread of the impulse to surrounding ventricular tissue. This phenomenon, called **decremental conduction**, leads to nonuniformity (heterogeneity) of tissue depolarization and

repolarization in adjacent tissues and enables reentry causing tachycardia or fibrillation.

Reentry in the AV node is the most common mechanism causing paroxysmal supraventricular tachycardia (PSVT). Of the several forms of PSVT, the form that occurs in patients with **Wolff-Parkinson-White syndrome** involves an accessory AV node conduction pathway through the bundle of Kent. However, in the most common form of PSVT, the reentrant circuit is located entirely within the AV node. In this form of PSVT, a premature atrial impulse is blocked in one pathway, is conducted through the AV node via the other pathway, and reenters the atrium by retrograde conduction (see Box 14.1). In AV node reentry, the unidirectional block results from the **difference in the refractory periods** due to heterogeneity of repolarization of the two pathways.

Drug-Induced Dysrhythmias

Drugs can induce dysrhythmias by several mechanisms. **Sympathomimetic drugs and digoxin** can cause tachydysrhythmias by mechanisms described earlier. Other drugs cause dysrhythmias by slowing ventricular repolarization and evoking a form of polymorphic ventricular tachycardia called *torsades de pointes* (French for "fringe of pointed tips"). The prolongation of ventricular repolarization and the QT interval is believed to evoke afterdepolarizations that produce tachycardia. In this disorder, each QRS complex has a configuration that differs from the preceding one. The types of drugs causing *torsades de pointes* include **antidysrhythmic drugs** that block potassium channels (e.g., dofetilide and sotalol) and antipsychotic drugs, such as **thioridazine.**

Mechanisms and Classification of Antidysrhythmic Drugs

Most antidysrhythmic drugs act by blocking specific ion channels in cardiac tissue and thereby suppress abnormal

TABLE 14.1 Electrophysiologic Properties of Selected Antidysrhythmic Drugs[a]

DRUG	ATRIOVENTRICULAR (AV) NODE Ectopic Automaticity	Conduction Velocity	Refractory Period	HIS-PURKINJE SYSTEM AND VENTRICLE Conduction Velocity	Refractory Period	Heart Rate	ELECTROCARDIOGRAM PR Interval	QRS Duration	QT Interval
Class I drugs									
Quinidine	↓	↑ or ↓	→ or ↑	↓↓	↑↑	↑ or ↓	↑ or ↓	↑↑	↑↑
Lidocaine	↓	→	→	→ or ↓	↑ or ↓	→	→	→	→ or ↓
Flecainide	↓	↓	→ or ↑	↓↓	↑	→	↑	↑↑	↑
Class II drugs									
Propranolol	↓	↓↓	↑↑	→	→	↓↓	↑↑	→	→ or ↓
Class III drug									
Amiodarone	↓	↓	↑	↓	↑↑	↓	↑	↑	↑↑
Dofetilide	→	→ or ↓	↑	→	↑↑	→	→	→	↑↑
Sotalol	↓	↓	↑	→	↑↑	↓	↑	→	↑↑
Class IV drugs									
Verapamil, diltiazem	↓	↓↓	↑↑	→	→	↓↓	↑↑	→	→
Other drug									
Adenosine	↓	↓↓	↑↑	→	→	↑	↑↑	→	→

[a]Effects are indicated as follows: decreased (↓); greatly decreased (↓↓); no change (→); increased (↑); greatly increased (↑↑).

impulse formation or conduction or prolong repolarization. Drugs that block sodium or calcium channels can reduce abnormal automaticity and slow conduction of the cardiac impulse. Drugs that block potassium channels prolong repolarization and the action potential duration and increase the refractory period of cardiac tissue. Other drugs block β-adrenoceptors and reduce sympathetic stimulation of cardiac automaticity and conduction velocity that contributes to some dysrhythmias.

On the basis of these mechanisms, Vaughan-Williams divided the antidysrhythmic drugs into four main classes: **Class I,** sodium channel blockers; **Class II,** β-adrenoceptor antagonists (β-blockers); **Class III,** potassium channel blockers; and **Class IV,** calcium channel blockers. Although this classification system is useful, a few drugs (such as **adenosine**) do not fit into any of these categories, while drugs such as amiodarone could fit in several classes. Tables 14.1 and 14.2 compare the electrophysiologic and pharmacokinetic properties of the various groups and subgroups of antidysrhythmic drugs.

SODIUM CHANNEL BLOCKERS

The largest group of antidysrhythmic drugs are the Class I sodium channel blockers. These drugs slow phase 0 depolarization and cardiac conduction, and thereby increase QRS duration. The Class I drugs bind to sodium channels when the channels are in the open and inactivated states and dissociate from the channels during the resting state (Box 14.2). The sodium channel blockers have the most pronounced effect on cardiac tissue that is firing rapidly because sodium channels in this tissue spend more time in the open and inactivated states than in the resting state. This is called **use-dependent blockade.** Because of use-dependent blockade, sodium channel blockers suppress cardiac conduction

in more persons with tachycardia than in persons with a normal heart rate.

The drugs in Class I have been subdivided into three groups (IA, IB, and IC) based on whether they have greater affinity for the open state or the inactivated state and based on their rate of dissociation from sodium channels (rate of recovery). As shown in Box 14.2, **Class IA drugs** have greater affinity for the open state and have a slow recovery; **Class IB drugs** have greater affinity for the inactivated state and have a rapid recovery; and **Class IC drugs** have greater affinity for the open state and a very slow recovery.

Class IA Drugs

Disopyramide, procainamide, and **quinidine** are Class IA drugs. These drugs have similar electrophysiologic effects and clinical indications and efficacy. They differ in pharmacokinetic properties and adverse effects though all of them can be **prodysrhythmic.**

Drug Properties

The Class IA drugs block the **fast sodium channel** and delayed potassium channels. Therefore, they slow phase 0 depolarization and phase 3 repolarization in ventricular tissue (Fig. 14.2). These actions decrease conduction velocity and prolong action potential duration and refractory period (see Table 14.1), which increases QRS duration and the QT interval. Class IA drugs suppress abnormal (ectopic) automaticity but usually do not affect SA node automaticity and the heart rate.

All of the Class IA drugs have some degree of **antimuscarinic** (atropine-like) activity and reduce vagal inhibition of SA depolarization and AV node conduction, thereby increasing heart rate. **Disopyramide** has the greatest antimuscarinic effect, procainamide has the least, and quinidine

TABLE 14.2   Pharmacokinetic Properties of Antidysrhythmic Drugs[a]

DRUG	ORAL BIOAVAILABILITY (%)	ONSET OF ACTION	DURATION OF ACTION	ELIMINATION HALF-LIFE	EXCRETED UNCHANGED IN URINE (%)	THERAPEUTIC SERUM CONCENTRATION
Class IA drugs						
Disopyramide	90	1 h	6 h	7 h	50	2–7 mg/mL
Procainamide	85	1 h	5 h	3.5 h	55	4–8 mg/mL
Quinidine	75	1 h	7 h	6 h	30	2–5 mg/mL
Class IB drugs						
Lidocaine	NA	See text	See text	1.5 h	1	1.5–6 mg/mL
Mexiletine	90	1 h	10 h	11 h	10	0.5–2 mg/mL
Class IC drugs						
Flecainide	75	3 h	21 h	14 h	30	0.2–1 mg/mL
Propafenone	10	3 h	10 h	6 h	<1	0.06–0.1 mg/mL
Class II drugs						
Esmolol	NA	<5 min	20–30 min	0.15 h	<2	0.5–1 mg/mL
Metoprolol	35	1 h	15 h	3.5 h	7	15–25 mg/mL
Propranolol	35	0.5 h	4 h	4 h	<0.5	0.2–1 mg/mL
Class III drugs						
Amiodarone	45	2 weeks	4 weeks	40 days	0	0.5–2.5 mg/mL
Dofetilide	90	1 h	12 h	10 h	80	NA
Ibutilide	NA	5 min	NA	6 h	<10	NA
Sotalol	90	2 h	15 h	12 h	90	1–4 mg/mL
Class IV drugs						
Diltiazem	55	2 h	8 h	5 h	3	0.1–0.2 mg/mL
Verapamil	25	2 h	9 h	5 h	3	0.1–0.3 mg/mL
Miscellaneous drugs						
Adenosine	NA	30 s	1.5 min	<10 s	0	NA
Digoxin	75	1 h	24 h	35 h	60	0.5–2 ng/mL
Magnesium sulfate	NA	<5 min	NA	NA	100	NA

NA, Not applicable (not administered orally).
[a]Values shown are the mean of values reported in the literature.

is intermediate. All of these drugs may promote **(prodysrhythmic effect)** as well as suppress cardiac dysrhythmias and their use has declined for this reason, particularly for the treatment of ventricular dysrhythmias.

Quinidine

Quinidine is an isomer of quinine, an alkaloid used to treat fever and malaria. The pharmacokinetic properties of quinidine and other antidysrhythmic drugs are summarized in Table 14.2. Quinidine is usually administered orally, and it is partly metabolized in the liver and excreted in the urine. The most common adverse effect of quinidine is **diarrhea,** which often necessitates discontinuation of its use. Less commonly, quinidine causes excessive prolongation of the QT interval and **torsades de pointes,** which can cause syncope secondary to a reduction in cardiac output. **Thrombocytopenia** can also occur with quinidine use. Higher doses of quinidine produce a constellation of **neurologic symptoms** called *cinchonism* that include tinnitus, dizziness, and blurred vision.

Quinidine is also formulated in combination with dextromethorphan (Neudexta) for the treatment of emotional lability **(pseudobulbar affect)** in patients with neurodegenerative diseases (see Chapter 24).

Procainamide

Procainamide is a derivative of the local anesthetic procaine. It is well absorbed from the gut and is converted to an active metabolite, *N*-acetylprocainamide, which has Class III antidysrhythmic properties. Long-term use of procainamide often causes a reversible **lupus erythematous–like syndrome**, with arthralgia and a butterfly rash on the face, necessitating drug discontinuation.

Persons who have the slow-acetylator phenotype (see Chapter 2) develop the lupus-like syndrome more often and earlier during treatment than do rapid acetylators. The drug-induced lupus condition can be distinguished from idiopathic lupus using serologic tests for anti-DNA antibodies. Although not a first-line drug for any disrrhythmia, procainamide is occasionally used to terminate the wide QRS complex form of **acute ventricular tachycardia** and to convert atrial fibrillation to sinus rhythm.

BOX 14.2 ELECTROPHYSIOLOGIC PROPERTIES OF SODIUM CHANNEL BLOCKERS

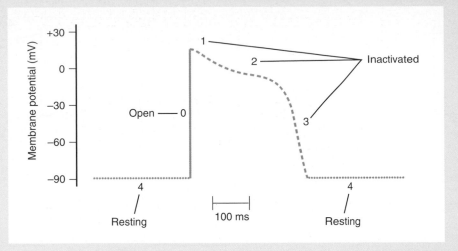

During phase 0 of the ventricular action potential, the sodium channels open to depolarize the cell. The channels are then inactivated and no longer permit sodium entry during phases 1, 2, and 3. The channels must return to the resting state (phase 4) before they can open again during the next action potential.

Drugs dissociate from the sodium channels at different rates (recovery). Drugs with a slow recovery have a greater effect on cardiac conduction velocity.

Drug Class	Example	Sodium Channel Affinity	Rate of Dissociation
Class IA	Quinidine	Open > inactivated	Slow
Class IB	Lidocaine	Inactivated > open	Rapid
Class IC	Flecainide	Open > inactivated	Very slow

Disopyramide

Disopyramide is administered orally to prevent life-threatening **ventricular dysrhythmias,** such as sustained ventricular tachycardia (VT). It should not be used to treat asymptomatic ventricular dysrhythmias because of its potential prodysrhythmic effect. It has negative inotropic and antimuscarinic effects and should be used with caution in patients with heart failure and in elderly patients.

Class IB Drugs

Lidocaine and **mexiletine** are Class IB drugs. Class IB drugs have a greater affinity for inactivated sodium channels than for open channels.

Drug Properties

Chemistry and Pharmacokinetics. Lidocaine is a local anesthetic that also has antidysrhythmic activity. It undergoes extensive first-pass hepatic inactivation after oral administration and is not effective by this route. **Mexiletine** is a lidocaine analog that is not susceptible to first-pass inactivation and is given orally. Lidocaine is rapidly inactivated by hepatic enzymes, whereas mexiletine is more slowly metabolized and has a longer half-life (see Table 14.2).

Mechanisms and Effects. Lidocaine has a more pronounced effect on ischemic tissue than on normal tissue. It has little effect on the normal ECG and is not effective in treating supraventricular dysrhythmias. **Mexiletine** has a greater effect on normal cardiac tissue than does lidocaine.

Adverse Effects. Elevated serum levels of **lidocaine** can cause central nervous system effects such as **nervousness, tremor,** and **paresthesia.** Toxic doses also slow cardiac conduction velocity and can cause cardiac arrest. Because lidocaine is extensively metabolized, concurrent use of drugs that inhibits cytochrome P450 enzymes (e.g., **cimetidine**) can increase the serum levels and lead to adverse effects.

Indications. Lidocaine is no longer used routinely for the treatment of ventricular dysrhythmias (see later), though it is occasionally employed in **refractory ventricular tachycardia** or in cases of ventricular dysrhythmias arising during or after cardiac surgery. The drug is typically administered intravenously as a loading dose followed by a continuous infusion. **Mexiletine** can be administered orally for the suppression of **symptomatic ventricular tachycardia,** sometimes in combination with other drugs.

Class IC Drugs

Flecainide and **propafenone**, which are Class IC drugs, are administered orally. Their properties are outlined in Tables 14.1 and 14.2.

Class IC drugs block both fast sodium channels and the rate of rise of the action potential during phase 0 to a greater extent than do other Class I drugs. By this mechanism, the Class IC drugs markedly slow conduction throughout the heart and especially in the His-Purkinje system. Flecainide and propafenone also inhibit the potassium rectifier current (I_{Kr}) in ventricular tissue and may increase the QT interval, but they rarely cause *torsades de pointes.*

Flecainide

Flecainide is indicated for the treatment of **supraventricular dysrhythmias** and **documented life-threatening ventricular dysrhythmias.** In the past, it was used to suppress

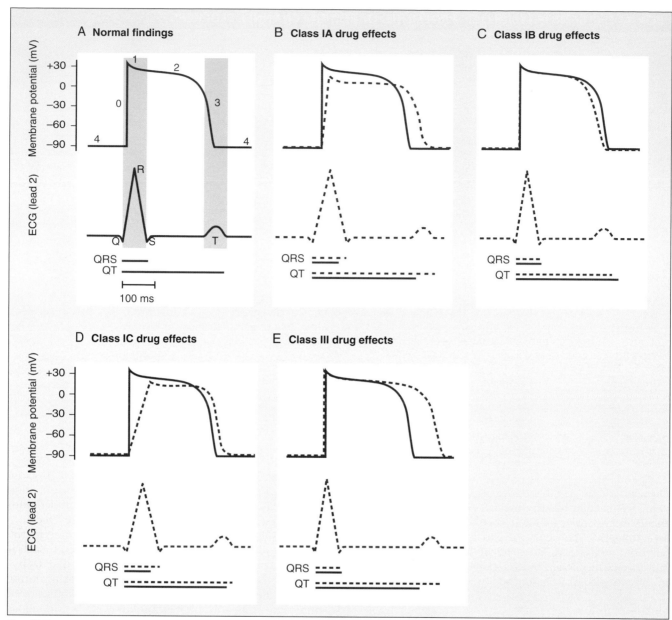

Fig. 14.2 Effects of Class I and Class III antidysrhythmic drugs on the ventricular action potential duration and on the electrocardiogram *(ECG)*. In each panel, the membrane potential scale is in millivolts *(mV)* and the time scale is in milliseconds *(ms)*. *Solid lines and tracings* depict normal findings; *dashed lines and tracings* depict the effects of drug administration. (A) *Lightly shaded vertical bars* show the relationship between the ventricular action potential duration and the findings on ECG in the normally functioning heart. (B) Class IA drugs slow phase 0 depolarization and phase 3 repolarization, thereby increasing the QRS duration and the QT interval. (C) Class IB drugs have little effect on normal cardiac tissue, but they can accelerate phase 3 repolarization and decrease the QT interval slightly. (D) Class IC drugs have the greatest effect on phase 0 depolarization and increase the QRS duration markedly, but they have little effect on phase 3 and the QT interval. (E) Class III drugs have no effect on phase 0, but they markedly prolong phase 3 and increase the QT interval.

nonlife-threatening ventricular dysrhythmias, but this practice was abandoned after the **Cardiac Arrhythmia Suppression Trial (CAST)** showed that flecainide increased mortality in patients who had experienced a myocardial infarction.

Although flecainide does not typically cause afterdepolarizations and *torsades de pointes*, it is capable of increasing the ventricular rate and causing VT by other mechanisms. Other adverse effects of flecainide include bronchospasm, leukopenia, thrombocytopenia, and seizures.

Propafenone

The effect of **propafenone** on fast sodium channels and cardiac conduction is similar to that of flecainide. As with

flecainide, **propafenone prolongs the PR interval and QRS duration**, and can cause some degree of QT prolongation.

Propafenone is administered orally to suppress supraventricular tachycardia and atrial fibrillation. The drug is also used to treat life-threatening forms of ventricular dysrhythmia, such as sustained ventricular tachycardia. Propafenone has the potential to cause ventricular dysrhythmias and **hematologic abnormalities**, including agranulocytosis, anemia, and thrombocytopenia.

Class II Drugs

The Class II antidysrhythmics are β-**adrenoceptor antagonists** (β-blockers) such as **esmolol**, **metoprolol**, and

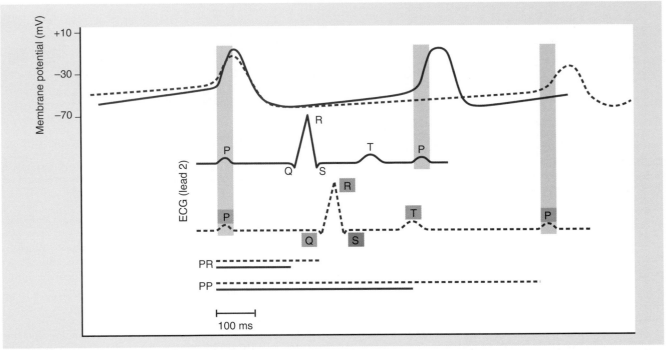

Fig. 14.3 Effects of Class II and Class IV antidysrhythmic drugs on the sinoatrial (SA) node action potential duration and on the electrocardiogram (ECG). The membrane potential scale is in millivolts (mV), and the time scale is in milliseconds (ms). *Solid lines and tracings* depict normal findings; *dashed lines and tracings* depict the effects of drug administration. *Vertical bars* show the relationship between the action potential and the findings on ECG. Class II drugs (β-adrenoceptor antagonists) and Class IV drugs (calcium channel blockers) slow phase 4 depolarization in the SA node and increase the PP interval. They also slow the atrioventricular (AV) node conduction velocity and increase the PR interval.

propranolol. These drugs are used to prevent and treat supraventricular dysrhythmias and to reduce ventricular ectopic depolarizations and sudden death in patients with myocardial infarction.

The β-blockers have antidysrhythmic effects because of their ability to inhibit sympathetic activation of cardiac automaticity and conduction. β-blockers slow the heart rate, decrease the AV node conduction velocity, and increase the AV node refractory period (Fig. 14.3). They have little effect on ventricular conduction and repolarization. The pharmacologic properties of β-blockers are discussed in Chapter 9.

Esmolol

Esmolol, a β-blocker given intravenously, is rapidly metabolized by plasma esterase and has an extremely short half-life. Its pharmacologic properties make it ideally suited for the treatment of **acute supraventricular tachycardia** or **hypertension** during or immediately after surgery, where its short duration of action enables continuous control of the patient's heart rate and blood pressure.

Metoprolol and Propranolol

Metoprolol and propranolol can be administered orally or intravenously to treat and suppress **supraventricular** and **ventricular dysrhythmias**. In patients with **myocardial infarction**, metoprolol is often administered intravenously during the early phase of treatment, followed by oral maintenance therapy that can continue for several months. The β-blockers have been demonstrated to protect the heart against the damage caused by ischemia and free radicals that may be formed during reperfusion of the coronary arteries when fibrinolytic drugs are used.

Class III Drugs

Amiodarone, dofetilide, ibutilide, and **sotalol** are Class III antidysrhythmics that **block potassium currents** that repolarize the heart during phase 3 of the action potential. This causes prolongation of the ventricular action potential duration and refractory period. Except for amiodarone, these agents have little effect on sodium or calcium channels in the heart, and they do not typically slow ventricular conduction or increase QRS duration significantly. The clinical use of Class III agents has increased as the use of Class I agents declined.

Amiodarone

Chemistry and Pharmacokinetics. **Amiodarone** is an organic **iodine compound** that is structurally related to thyroid hormones (Fig. 14.4). It can be administered orally or intravenously and has unusual pharmacokinetic properties. After oral administration, amiodarone is slowly and variably absorbed and is primarily eliminated by biliary excretion. As shown in Table 14.2, the drug's action may not begin for about 2 weeks if loading doses are not given. Hence, oral or intravenous loading doses are used to accelerate the drug's onset of action. The half-life of amiodarone is extremely long (about 40 days with a range of 26–107 days).

Mechanisms and Pharmacologic Effects. Amiodarone is the ultimate multimechanism, all-purpose antidysrhythmic agent, and understanding its actions, indications, and adverse effects is challenging. **Amiodarone** not only blocks potassium channels, but it also blocks sodium channels, calcium channels, and β-adrenoceptors, and it is usually not possible to recognize its mechanism of action in a particular patient or dysrhythmia.

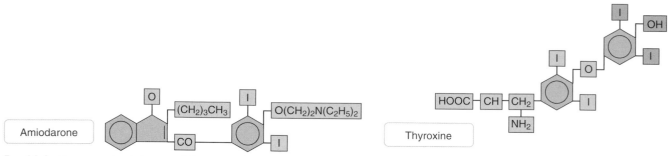

Fig. 14.4 Structures of amiodarone and thyroxine. The structure of amiodarone, which contains two iodine atoms, has some similarity to the structure of thyroid hormones such as thyroxine. Amiodarone can cause hypothyroidism and, less commonly, hyperthyroidism in some persons. The similar parts of the structures of amiodarone and thyroxine are unshaded.

As shown in Table 14.1, **amiodarone** decreases SA node automaticity and AV node conduction velocity, and it prolongs AV node and ventricular refractory periods. It is a powerful inhibitor of ectopic pacemaker automaticity, and it prolongs repolarization and refractory periods throughout the heart. On the ECG, it increases the PR and QT intervals and slightly prolongs QRS duration.

Adverse Effects and Interactions. **Amiodarone** causes a number of adverse effects, most of which are reversible and can be managed by dosage reduction or discontinuation, including **bradycardia**, impaired AV conduction, and QT prolongation leading to *torsades de pointes*. Amiodarone causes **corneal microdeposits** in over 90% of patients, but these are usually benign and do not require intervention. Amiodarone causes **photosensitivity** to ultraviolet light, and patients should avoid sun exposure and use sunscreen. The drug also causes a **blue-gray skin discoloration** that may necessitate dosage reduction or discontinuation. The more serious adverse effects of amiodarone include **hypothyroidism** (6% of patients) or hyperthyroidism (0.9%–2% of patients). Hypothyroidism may be managed with levothyroxine replacement therapy, whereas hyperthyroidism usually necessitates discontinuation of the drug. Tremor, ataxia, and optic or peripheral **neuropathy** may also occur. Hepatic dysfunction should be monitored by determining serum levels of hepatic enzymes every 6 months during treatment.

Pulmonary fibrosis is an uncommon but **potentially fatal reaction** to amiodarone, and patients should have pulmonary function tests and a chest radiograph before starting treatment with a yearly radiograph thereafter. The drug must be discontinued immediately if any sign of pulmonary toxicity occurs.

Amiodarone inhibits the metabolism and excretion of a number of drugs. It can elevate plasma levels of digoxin, flecainide, phenytoin, procainamide, and warfarin, in part by inhibiting P-glycoprotein mediated drug transport. The dosage of these drugs should be decreased in patients receiving concurrent amiodarone therapy. Amiodarone also interacts with inhalational anesthetics and other central nervous system depressants to cause an increased incidence of adverse cardiovascular effects such as **bradycardia**.

Indications. **Amiodarone** is given orally on a long-term basis to **suppress** both **supraventricular** and **ventricular dysrhythmias**, including atrial fibrillation, atrial flutter, supraventricular tachycardia, and VT. Amiodarone is used intravenously to terminate ventricular fibrillation or sustained VT. In this setting, the drug can be given as a loading infusion followed by a maintenance infusion. Amiodarone also appears to be an effective adjunct to implantable cardioverter-defibrillators to reduce the number of shocks required to maintain sinus rhythm.

Dronedarone

Dronedarone is a noniodinated amiodarone analog that has **no effect on thyroid function**. It is indicated for prevention of dysrhythmia in persons with paroxysmal atrial fibrillation or flutter, but "head-to-head" comparisons have found that dronedarone is **less effective** than amiodarone. Moreover, dronedarone has been associated with **liver injury** and life-threatening acute liver failure, and it was found to increase mortality twofold in patients with heart failure. The drug is contraindicated in persons with permanent atrial fibrillation and in those with heart failure, and patients must be monitored every 6 months for the occurrence of these conditions. Dronedarone appears to have a limited role in the treatment of supraventricular dysrhythmias.

Ibutilide and Dofetilide

Ibutilide and **dofetilide** prolong the ventricular action potential duration. Dofetilide selectively blocks the rapidly activating delayed rectifier channel (I_{Kr}) responsible for repolarizing (rectifying) myocardial tissue during phase 3 of the action potential. By inhibiting this outward potassium current, dofetilide prolongs ventricular repolarization and increases refractory periods and the QT interval of the ECG. In contrast to dofetilide, **ibutilide** appears to activate the **slow (late), inward sodium current**, which increases sodium influx and counteracts the outward potassium current so as to slow atrial and ventricular repolarization.

Ibutilide is administered by intravenous infusion. It is rapidly metabolized in the liver, and its metabolites are eliminated in the urine and feces with an average half-life of 6 hours. The drug is indicated for the rapid conversion of **atrial fibrillation** or **flutter** to normal sinus rhythm, though it is more effective for flutter than fibrillation and for recent-onset dysrhythmias. Ibutilide can be used before cardioversion in patients that do not respond to cardioversion alone. The drug does not significantly affect the heart rate, blood pressure, QRS duration, or PR interval. It can induce *torsades de pointes*, and continuous ECG monitoring is required during administration of the drug. Ibutilide should be avoided in patients with a prolonged QT interval (QTc > 440 ms) and those with a history of polymorphic VT.

Dofetilide is administered orally to convert **atrial fibrillation** and for long-term suppression of the dysrhythmia. Because of the drug's potent ability to prolong the QT interval and induce *torsades de pointes*, the ECG must be closely monitored during dosage titration. When therapy is initiated, dosage adjustments are based on the degree of **QT prolongation**. The drug is primarily eliminated by renal excretion, and doses must be reduced in persons with renal insufficiency.

Sotalol

Sotalol is a **nonselective β-adrenoceptor antagonist** that prolongs the cardiac action potential duration and QT interval by blocking the **delayed potassium rectifier current** during phase 3 of the ventricular action potential (see Fig. 14.2). As with other Class II β-blockers, sotalol decreases heart rate, slows the AV node conduction velocity, and increases AV node refractory period without affecting ventricular conduction and QRS duration. Lower doses of sotalol act primarily through β-receptor blockade, whereas higher doses exert more Class III action and prolongation of ventricular repolarization. The drug has a modest negative inotropic effect. The drug is given orally with almost 100% bioavailability. It is excreted unchanged in the urine, and doses should be reduced in persons with elevated serum creatinine levels.

Sotalol is effective in treating a number of supraventricular dysrhythmias and is used for rhythm control in persons with **atrial fibrillation** and **flutter**. However, clinical studies have shown that amiodarone is superior to sotalol for maintaining sinus rhythm in these conditions. Although the drug is not very effective when used alone for prevention of sudden cardiac death in persons with myocardial infarction, it has become a first-line drug as adjunctive therapy in patients with an **implantable cardioverter-defibrillator**. In these persons, sotalol facilitates defibrillation by lowering the defibrillation threshold and reduces the number of shocks required.

Sotalol can cause **bradycardia, bronchospasm, and dyspnea** due to *β*-blockade, and pulmonary edema and heart failure occur in about 3% of patients. A dose-dependent incidence of *torsades de pointes* occurs in about 2% of patients, which is more likely to occur after recent cardioversion.

Class IV Drugs

Diltiazem and **verapamil** are nondihydropyridine **calcium channel blockers** that have significant effects on cardiac tissue. The pharmacologic properties of these drugs are described in Chapter 11. **Diltiazem** and **verapamil** decrease the AV node conduction velocity and increase the AV node refractory period, and they have a smaller effect on the SA node and heart rate. As shown in Table 14.1, they have little effect on the ventricular conduction velocity and refractory period.

Diltiazem and **verapamil** are used for controlling or converting certain **supraventricular dysrhythmias**, but they are not effective in treating ventricular dysrhythmias. They are often used to control the ventricular rate in patients with **atrial fibrillation** or **flutter** and a rapid ventricular response. In this condition, they are more effective than digoxin in controlling ventricular rate. Verapamil can be administered intravenously to terminate PSTV, and it is given orally for chronic treatment of this dysrhythmia.

Calcium channel blockers can exacerbate wide QRS complex VT and should not be given to patients with this dysrhythmia. The dihydropyridine drugs such as nifedipine have less effect on cardiac tissue and no role in the treatment of dysrhythmias.

Miscellaneous Drugs
Adenosine

Adenosine is a naturally occurring nucleoside composed of adenine and ribose. When administered as a rapid intravenous bolus, it has an extremely short half-life of 10 seconds or less. In the body, adenosine is derived from adenosine triphosphate and activates specific G protein–coupled **adenosine receptors**. Stimulation of these receptors leads to activation of acetylcholine-sensitive potassium channels and blockade of calcium influx in the SA node, atrium, and AV node. It thereby causes cell hyperpolarization, slows the AV node conduction velocity, and increases the AV node refractory period. In fact, AV node conduction can be completely blocked for a few seconds, resulting in a brief period of asystole. These actions serve to terminate **supraventricular tachycardia** by preventing the retrograde conduction of reentrant impulses through the AV node. Because of its brief duration of action, adenosine has been termed a pharmacologic counterpart to electrical cardioversion.

Adenosine is primarily used to terminate **acute PSVT**, including the type associated with **Wolff-Parkinson-White syndrome**. It is not indicated for the treatment of atrial fibrillation or flutter. **Dipyridamole**—a vasodilator used to facilitate angiographic studies—inhibits the cellular uptake of adenosine and markedly increases its cardiac effects. Doses of adenosine, therefore, should be reduced in persons who have recently received dipyridamole. Adenosine can cause **bronchospasm** and should be used cautiously in persons with obstructive lung disease.

Digoxin

Digoxin increases vagal tone and thereby slows AV node conduction velocity and increases AV node refractory period. It has been used to slow the ventricular rate in patients with **atrial fibrillation,** though β-blockers and calcium channel blockers are usually preferred for this purpose because of their more rapid onset of action and greater degree of AV nodal blockade. Moreover, a recent clinical trial (ROCKET AF) found that digoxin was associated with increased cardiovascular and all-cause mortality in AF patients.

Magnesium Sulfate

The **magnesium ion**, the second most common **intracellular cation**, has a number of roles in normal cardiac function. Magnesium deficiency can be caused by use of drugs such as loop diuretics or by pathologic states, and this deficiency can contribute to the development of dysrhythmias and congestive heart failure as well as to gastrointestinal and renal disorders.

Magnesium sulfate is administered intravenously to suppress drug-induced *torsades de pointes*, to treat digitalis-induced ventricular **dysrhythmias**, and to treat supraventricular dysrhythmias associated with magnesium deficiency. Magnesium sulfate is also used to treat **pregnant women with severe preeclampsia** (see Chapter 34).

Ivabradine and Ranolazine

Ivabradine and ranolazine are ion channel-blocking agents used in the treatment of angina pectoris. **Ivabradine** blocks the so-called "funny current" responsible for diastolic depolarization in the sinoatrial node, whereas **ranolazine** blocks the late sodium current in ventricular tissue. The pharmacologic properties and clinical use of these drugs are discussed in Chapter 11.

MANAGEMENT OF DYSRHYTHMIAS

Atrial Fibrillation and Flutter

Atrial fibrillation affects millions of people worldwide and is a major cause of morbidity and mortality. The dysrhythmia is probably caused by a disorganized form of reentry in which atrial cells are continuously reexcited by reentrant stimuli as soon as they are repolarized. Under these conditions, the AV node is continuously bombarded with atrial impulses, some of which are conducted to the ventricles, so that the ventricular rate is often rapid and irregular.

There are two general approaches to pharmacologic therapy of atrial fibrillation: rate control and rhythm control. **Ventricular rate control** is essential for all patients to avoid symptoms and development of cardiomyopathy and is the first objective in treating acute atrial fibrillation. Drugs used for this purpose are primarily β-**blockers** and **calcium channel blockers**, which slow AV node conduction velocity and increase its refractory period, so that fewer atrial impulses are transmitted to the ventricles. Although these drugs slow ventricular rate, they do not typically convert atrial fibrillation to normal sinus rhythm (Box 14.3). However, β-blockers can reduce recurrences of atrial fibrillation after conversion to normal sinus rhythm.

After the ventricular rate has been controlled, acute atrial fibrillation can be **converted to normal sinus rhythm** by the use of **direct current cardioversion** (provided the dysrhythmia is of less than 48 hours duration) or by administration of **ibutilide** or **dofetilide**. Many patients whose dysrhythmia is successfully converted will relapse. Several Class I and III drugs are moderately effective (30%–60%) in preventing recurrences and maintaining normal sinus rhythm **(rhythm control)** but at the cost of adverse effects including prodysrhythmia. A recent study found that amiodarone was more effective than sotalol or propafenone for rhythm control, and a meta-analysis indicated that some agents (disopyramide, quinidine, and sotalol) may actually increase mortality.

Because of the modest effectiveness and adverse effects of Class I and III agents, many patients with episodic paroxysmal atrial fibrillation are treated with a β-blocker or calcium channel blocker to control the ventricular rate and with an **anticoagulant** to prevent thromboembolism and stroke (see Chapter 16). **Surgical catheter ablation** of dysrhythmogenic tissue is a treatment option for some patients and is often considered for patients with persistent or paroxysmal dysrhythmias that do not respond well to drug therapy.

Patients who have **Wolff-Parkinson-White syndrome** and develop atrial fibrillation should not be treated with digoxin or verapamil because these drugs can decrease accessory pathway refractoriness and lead to VT. **Atrial flutter** is usually treated in the same manner as atrial fibrillation.

BOX 14.3 A CASE OF SHORTNESS OF BREATH AND PALPITATIONS

CASE PRESENTATION

A 76-year-old man arrives in the emergency department with shortness of breath and chest palpitations for the past 3 hours while at rest. He has a history of hypertension controlled with hydrochlorothiazide and type 2 diabetes controlled with diet and metformin. His electrocardiogram (ECG) shows atrial fibrillation with a rapid and irregular ventricular rate averaging 120 beats/min. He receives diltiazem intravenously, and his ventricular rate becomes more regular with a rate of 85 beats/min, and his symptoms subside. Over the next 24 hours, his ECG continues to show atrial fibrillation with a ventricular rate of 75 beats/min. His serum electrolytes, thyroid function test results, and blood chemistries are within normal limits, and he is placed on heparin and warfarin anticoagulants to prevent thromboembolism and stroke. After discussing treatment options with his physician, he undergoes pharmacologic cardioversion to sinus rhythm with intravenous dofetilide with continuous ECG monitoring, and he is discharged on metformin and lisinopril. He is instructed to call his physician if symptoms of atrial fibrillation resume, and he is scheduled for follow-up evaluations and electrophysiologic studies to determine the most appropriate long-term therapy.

CASE DISCUSSION

Atrial fibrillation is the most common dysrhythmia requiring medical care. Its prevalence increases with age such that 8% of persons over 80 years of age have atrial fibrillation. The dysrhythmia typically causes dyspnea and palpitations and may lead to clot formation on fibrillating atrial leaflets; hence, most patients receive anticoagulants to prevent thromboembolism and stroke. Atrial fibrillation may also cause heart failure because it impairs ventricular filling and emptying. There are two approaches to the long-term management of atrial fibrillation: rate control and rhythm control. In the rate control method, a β-blocker or calcium antagonist is administered to control ventricular rate by slowing AV conduction and increasing the AV refractory period without affecting the underlying atrial fibrillation. In the rhythm control method, electrical or pharmacologic cardioversion is used to restore sinus rhythm, which is then maintained with a Class I or Class III antidysrhythmic drug, such as flecainide or amiodarone. However, many patients will have a recurrence of atrial fibrillation despite treatment, and drugs used for long-term suppression of atrial fibrillation have the potential to cause serious ventricular dysrhythmias. Angiotensin inhibitors appear to lower the relapse rate after cardioversion. A number of new therapies are under development that may overcome some of the limitations of currently available drugs. Some patients benefit from catheter ablation surgery to remove the dysrhythmogenic tissue causing atrial fibrillation.

Supraventricular Tachycardia

PSVT is caused most frequently by a **reentrant circuit in the AV node.** Acute PSVT is often treated with intravenous **adenosine**, which causes AV block and interrupts the reentrant pathway. Alternatively, AV block can be produced by a calcium channel blocker (e.g., **verapamil**) or by a β-blocker (e.g., **esmolol**). **Esmolol** is a short-acting drug whose use is often preferred in perioperative patients. Long-term suppression is usually accomplished by use of a calcium channel blocker, β-blocker, or digitalis glycoside. Surgical ablation of the dysrhythmogenic tissue can also be effective.

Patients with **Wolff-Parkinson-White syndrome** exhibit an **atypical form of PSVT** caused by reentry through an accessory bypass conduction pathway between the atria and ventricles. This form of PSVT can also be terminated with drugs that cause AV block. Long-term treatment may consist of surgical ablation of dysrhythmogenic tissue or use of a sodium or potassium channel blocker to suppress the dysrhythmia.

Ventricular Tachycardia and Fibrillation

Ventricular tachycardia is a dysrhythmia that usually manifests with a monomorphic, regular, wide QRS complex with a rate greater than 100 beats/min. It is often associated with myocardial infarction and is thought to be caused by impaired conduction and reentry in ventricular tissue (see earlier).

Sustained ventricular tachycardia should be treated immediately because of its deleterious effect on cardiac output and myocardial ischemia and because it can lead to **ventricular fibrillation**. If the patient with VT does not have a pulse or is hemodynamically unstable, electric (direct current) cardioversion should be used to terminate the dysrhythmia. If such persons do not respond to three shocks, they should be treated as if they have ventricular fibrillation (see later). In less severe cases of unsustained VT, **amiodarone** may be administered as a series of bolus doses or an intravenous infusion to prevent further episodes and reduce the need for cardioversion. Procainamide is a second-line drug that is occasionally used to treat acute VT. Amiodarone or sotalol can also be used for long-term control of symptomatic dysrhythmias, such as nonsustained VT and frequent premature ventricular beats.

Ventricular fibrillation is the most common cause of **sudden cardiac death**. In ventricular fibrillation, the ECG shows rapid (300–400 per minute), irregular, shapeless depolarizations of variable amplitude and shape. Electrical defibrillation is the treatment of choice for patients with this disorder. If ventricular fibrillation persists after three rapid shocks, intravenous **epinephrine** (or vasopressin) and **amiodarone** are administered, followed by continued attempts at defibrillation. Lidocaine is no longer used routinely for this purpose, but some authorities suggest trying it if other measures fail.

An **implantable cardioverter-defibrillator** is the most effective long-term treatment for patients with **life-threatening sustained VT or ventricular fibrillation**. These patients should also be treated with β-**blockers** and with an ACE inhibitor or angiotensin receptor blocker. β-blockers are the only antidysrhythmic drugs that have been shown to reduce mortality in patients with previous episodes of VT or ventricular fibrillation. **Class I sodium channel blockers** such as quinidine are not often used for treatment of VT or ventricular fibrillation because they increase the risk of sudden cardiac death. **Amiodarone** and **sotalol** are not as effective as an implantable cardioverter-defibrillator for the long-term suppression of ventricular dysrhythmias, but they can be used in conjunction with an implantable cardioverter-defibrillator to reduce the number of shocks required to maintain normal sinus rhythm. **Radiofrequency catheter ablation** of VT foci may benefit some patients with monomorphic VT.

Patients who have taken an overdose of a **tricyclic antidepressant drug** (e.g., **imipramine**) can develop a **wide QRS complex tachycardia** believed to result from the blockade of cardiac sodium channels by the antidepressant. The treatment for this particular form of VT includes the intravenous administration of sodium bicarbonate, which increases dissociation of the antidepressant from sodium channels. **Magnesium sulfate** and β-**blockers** have also been used successfully.

Torsades de Pointes

Torsades de pointes is a polymorphic VT that can be induced by drugs (including **tricyclic antidepressants** and **antipsychotic agents**) or electrolyte abnormalities that prolong the QT interval and predispose cardiac cells to afterdepolarizations. This dysrhythmia can also result from a congenital prolonged QT syndrome. Patients with a drug-induced dysrhythmia can be treated by withdrawal of the causative agent, correction of any electrolyte abnormalities, such as hypokalemia, intravenous administration of **magnesium sulfate**, and cardiac overdrive pacing. These treatments act in part by shortening the QT interval.

SUMMARY OF IMPORTANT POINTS

- Antidysrhythmic drugs suppress the abnormal impulse formation or conduction leading to dysrhythmias or increase the refractoriness of cardiac tissue.
- Antidysrhythmic drugs are divided into four main classes, with Class I consisting of sodium channel blockers, Class II consisting of β-adrenoceptor antagonists (β-blockers), Class III consisting of potassium channel blockers, and Class IV consisting of calcium channel blockers.
- Class IA drugs (e.g., quinidine) slow conduction and prolong refractory periods, thereby increasing the QRS duration and the QT interval. Because of their prodysrhythmic effects, their use has declined in favor of Class III agents.
- Class IB drugs such as lidocaine have little effect on normal cardiac tissue and electrocardiographic findings, but they can decrease the QT interval slightly. Lidocaine is no longer used routinely for acute ventricular dysrhythmias. Mexiletine is an orally effective analog of lidocaine that has been used for prevention of life-threatening or symptomatic ventricular dysrhythmias.
- Class IC drugs have a greater effect than other sodium channel blockers on cardiac conduction but have little effect on the action potential duration. Flecainide and propafenone are used to treat supraventricular dysrhythmias and life-threatening ventricular dysrhythmias.
- Class II drugs (β-blockers), which slow the AV node conduction velocity and prolong the AV node refractory period, are used to treat supraventricular dysrhythmias. They also reduce the incidence of fatal ventricular dysrhythmias in patients with myocardial infarction.
- Class III drugs (e.g., amiodarone, dofetilide, ibutilide, and sotalol) prolong the action potential duration,

refractory periods, and QT interval. Dofetilide blocks the potassium rectifier current while ibutilide activates the delayed inward sodium current.

- Amiodarone is given intravenously in the treatment of ventricular tachycardia and fibrillation and can be given orally for chronic prophylaxis. Ibutilide and dofetilide are used for acute termination and chronic prophylaxis of atrial fibrillation. Sotalol is used for both acute and chronic treatment of supraventricular and ventricular dysrhythmias.
- Class IV drugs (calcium channel blockers) slow the AV node conduction velocity, prolong the AV node refractory period, and thereby terminate the AV node reentry responsible for supraventricular tachycardia. They are also used for rate control in patients with atrial fibrillation.
- Adenosine is administered as a rapid intravenous bolus to terminate acute supraventricular tachycardia.

Review Questions

1. After beginning drug therapy to suppress ventricular tachycardia, a man reports cold intolerance and lethargy, and his thyroid-stimulating hormone level is found to be elevated. Which drug is most likely responsible for this adverse reaction?
   - (A) procainamide
   - (B) dronedarone
   - (C) dofetilide
   - (D) verapamil
   - (E) amiodarone

2. A woman is placed on an antidysrhythmic drug that dissociates very slowly from ventricular sodium channels. Which electrocardiographic finding results from this property?
   - (A) prolonged PR interval
   - (B) shortened PR interval
   - (C) prolonged QRS duration
   - (D) prolonged QT interval
   - (E) sinus bradycardia

3. A man is administered a drug that selectively blocks the rapidly activating delayed rectifier channels. Which electrocardiographic change should guide dosage adjustments with this drug?
   - (A) QT prolongation
   - (B) QRS widening
   - (C) PR prolongation
   - (D) T wave inversion
   - (E) heart rate

4. A woman with supraventricular tachycardia is given an intravenous bolus of adenosine. What is the mechanism by which this drug acts to terminate the dysrhythmia?
   - (A) increased chloride influx
   - (B) increased cyclic guanosine monophosphate
   - (C) increased calcium influx
   - (D) increased potassium efflux
   - (E) decreased sodium influx

5. Which drug should be avoided in persons with asthma?
   - (A) sotalol
   - (B) diltiazem
   - (C) flecainide
   - (D) quinidine
   - (E) lidocaine

CHAPTER 15

Drugs for Hyperlipidemia

OVERVIEW

Lipids are necessary molecules for human life. **Cholesterol** and phospholipids are essential components of cell membranes, and cholesterol is the precursor to steroid compounds that fulfill vital physiologic functions (see Chapters 33 and 34). **Triglycerides,** composed of three **fatty acids** and glycerol, are oxidized to generate energy for muscle contraction and metabolic reactions. Despite the essential roles of these and other lipids, elevated blood levels of cholesterol and triglycerides can lead to coronary artery disease and other disorders.

Hyperlipidemia and **hyperlipoproteinemia** are general terms for elevated levels of lipids and lipoproteins in the blood, whereas **hypercholesterolemia** and **hypertriglyceridemia** refer to high concentrations of cholesterol or triglycerides. Hypercholesterolemia contributes to the development of **atherosclerosis, coronary artery disease,** and other atherosclerotic vascular diseases (Fig. 15.1). Hypertriglyceridemia can lead to **pancreatitis,** but its role in

atherosclerosis and heart disease is uncertain. Clinical trials of drugs that reduce serum triglycerides have not consistently reduced adverse cardiovascular events and have not reduced mortality.

Because **coronary heart disease (CHD)** is a leading cause of premature death in developed countries, it is important to eliminate **modifiable risk factors** contributing to it. In addition to hyperlipidemia, these factors include **hypertension, cigarette smoking,** and a low level of **high-density–lipoprotein (HDL) cholesterol** (<40 mg/dL). **Nonmodifiable risk factors** include **male gender, family history** of premature CHD (CHD in male relatives under 55 years old or female relatives under 65 years old), and **aging** (men over 45 years, women over 55 years). **Diabetes mellitus** and other forms of **atherosclerotic vascular disease** (e.g., aortic aneurysm and carotid artery disease) are considered **CHD risk equivalents** in determining goals for treatment of hyperlipidemia. Persons with these conditions are believed to have the same risk for future occurrences of CHD as persons who already have CHD (e.g., angina pectoris, myocardial infarction).

Women have a lower risk of heart disease until after menopause, which may result from the favorable effect of estrogens on serum lipoprotein levels and production of apoprotein A-I. Estrogens may also have beneficial effects on microcirculation and energy metabolism.

After discussing lipoprotein metabolism and the causes and types of hyperlipoproteinemia, this chapter describes how lifestyle changes and drug therapy can reduce the occurrence of coronary artery disease and save lives. Meta-analyses of clinical trials indicate that CHD mortality decreases 15% for every 10% reduction in the serum cholesterol levels.

Lipoproteins and Lipid Transport

Because lipids are insoluble in plasma water, they are transported in blood in the form of lipoproteins, which have a core of hydrophobic (water-evading) lipids surrounded by a shell of hydrophilic (water-attracting) proteins and phospholipids. Lipoproteins are classified according to their buoyant density and include very-low-density (VLDL), low-density (LDL), intermediate-density (IDL), and high-density lipoproteins (HDL). Each class of lipoproteins is distinguished by its apoprotein and lipid composition, as well as its specific role in lipid transport. The composition and metabolism of lipoproteins are illustrated in Box 15.1.

Chylomicrons

Chylomicrons have the responsibility of transporting dietary lipids from the intestines to adipose tissue and liver. When cholesterol and triglycerides are ingested, they are emulsified in the intestines by the bile acids and other bile secretions, and the emulsified lipids are combined with proteins to form chylomicrons in the gut wall.

A **Normal arterial wall**

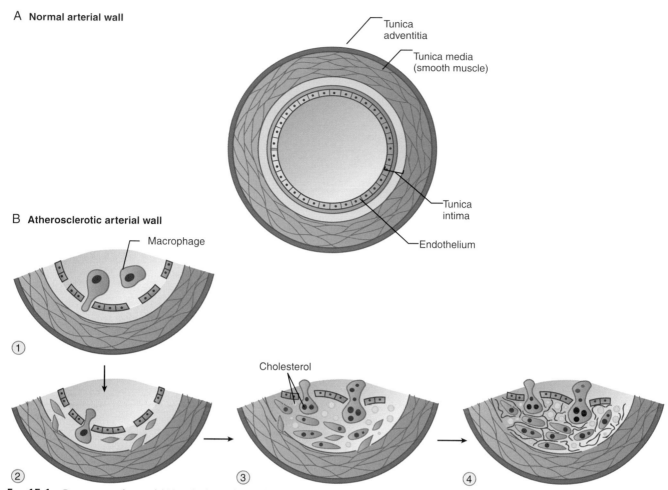

B **Atherosclerotic arterial wall**

FIG. 15.1   Comparison of normal (A) and atherosclerotic (B) arterial walls. Steps in the pathogenesis of atherosclerosis are as follows: (1) Damage to the endothelium is followed by an invasion of macrophages. (2) Endothelial and macrophage growth factors stimulate smooth muscle cells to migrate into the tunica intima and to proliferate. (3) Oxidized cholesterol accumulates in and around macrophages (foam cells) and muscle cells. (4) Collagen and elastic fibers form a connective tissue matrix that results in a fibrous plaque.

After chylomicrons are secreted into the circulation, they deliver triglycerides to adipose tissue via the action of a **lipoprotein lipase** located in the vascular endothelial cells. By this process, chylomicrons are converted to a cholesterol-rich chylomicron remnant that transports cholesterol to the liver.

Very-Low-Density and Low-Density Lipoproteins

VLDL are assembled in the liver from triglycerides, cholesterol, phospholipids, and protein and then secreted into the circulation (see Box 15.1). VLDL delivers triglycerides to adipose tissue in the same manner as chylomicrons. During this process, the VLDLs are transformed into IDL and LDL that contain a higher percentage of cholesterol (Fig. 15.2).

LDL transports cholesterol to peripheral tissues for incorporation into cell membranes, sterols, and steroids. In this process, LDL binds to specific LDL receptors located in the plasma membrane of cells and recognizes apoprotein B-100 on the surface of LDL molecules. After binding to its receptor, LDL undergoes endocytosis and is incorporated into lysosomes for the processing of cholesterol and protein.

LDL can also deliver cholesterol to macrophages in nascent atheromas and thereby contribute to the development of atherosclerosis (see Fig. 15.1). The macrophages are thereby transformed into foam cells as they become filled with oxidized cholesterol.

High-Density Lipoproteins

HDL have several roles in lipid metabolism. As HDL circulates in the blood, it exchanges apoproteins C and E with VLDL so as to enable the delivery of VLDL triglycerides to adipose tissue via lipoprotein lipase. HDL also mediates so-called reverse cholesterol transport believed to protect against the development of atherosclerosis. Moreover, HDL constituents appear to inhibit coagulation, platelet aggregation, and oxidative damage to the vascular endothelium.

The HDLs are small lipoproteins whose high density is caused by their greater protein to lipid ratio. Nascent HDL particles are formed as discs in the liver from apoprotein A-I and phospholipid. In the circulation, HDL acquires cholesterol from tissues and from macrophages in atheromas via **adenosine triphosphate (ATP)–binding cassette transporters,** and then the cholesterol is esterified by **lecithin–cholesterol acyltransferase (LCAT)** and transferred to the HDL core.

HDL delivers cholesterol esters to the liver and other tissues in a process called **reverse cholesterol transport** via direct and indirect pathways. In the direct pathway,

BOX 15.1 LIPOPROTEIN METABOLISM AND ATHEROSCLEROSIS

The liver is the central processing site for lipoprotein metabolism. Cholesterol is derived from three sources: (1) biosynthesis from acetyl-CoA, (2) delivery of dietary cholesterol by chylomicron remnants, and (3) endocytosis of low-density-lipoprotein (LDL) cholesterol by LDL receptors.

Triglycerides are formed in the liver from fatty acids derived from lipolysis of triglycerides in adipose tissue. Triglycerides, cholesterol, cholesterol esters, phospholipids, and apoproteins B100, C-I, and E are assembled by the endoplasmic reticulum (microsomes) and Golgi bodies in the liver to form very-low-density lipoproteins (VLDLs),

which are secreted into the circulation. The microsomal triglyceride transport protein combines lipids with apolipoprotein B-100 to form a nascent VLDL that acquires additional triglycerides before transfer to Golgi bodies, where it is incorporation into vesicles that are secreted from the liver by exocytosis. Once secreted into the circulation, VLDL accepts apoproteins C-II and E from high-density lipoproteins (HDLs) and then returns these apoproteins to HDL as they deliver triglycerides (as fatty acids) to adipose and other tissues via the action of lipoprotein lipase (LL) located in the capillary endothelium.

COMPOSITION OF LIPOPROTEINS

Lipoprotein	Core Lipids[a]	Apoproteins[a]
Chylomicron	Dietary triglycerides and cholesteryl esters	B-48, C, E, and A
VLDL	Endogenous triglycerides and cholesteryl esters	C, B-100, and E
LDL	Cholesteryl esters	B-100
HDL	Cholesteryl esters, phospholipids	A-I, A-II, C-II, E, and D

[a]Listed in order of quantitative importance.

With the removal of apoproteins and triglycerides, VLDLs are transformed into LDLs and intermediate-density lipoproteins. The LDLs deliver cholesterol to various sites in the body, including peripheral tissues and the liver via endocytosis by LDL receptors. LDL cholesterol is also incorporated into atherosclerotic plaques.

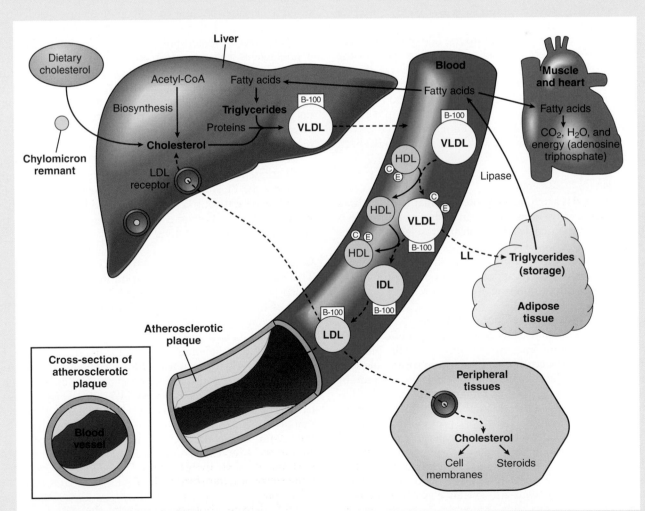

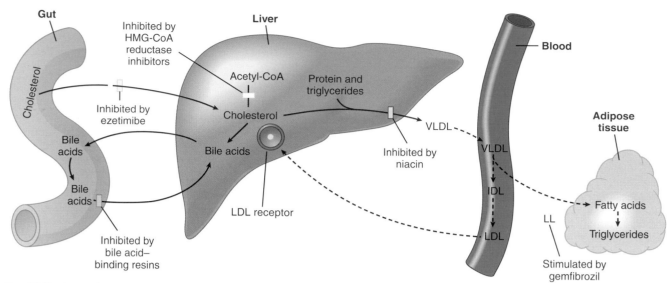

FIG. 15.2 Sites and mechanisms of drugs for hyperlipidemia. Ezetimibe inhibits the absorption of dietary and biliary cholesterol from the intestines. The HMG-CoA reductase inhibitors block the rate-limiting step in cholesterol biosynthesis. The bile acid–binding resins inhibit the reabsorption of bile acids from the gut. Niacin inhibits the secretion of very-low-density lipoproteins (VLDLs) from the liver, and fibrates such as gemfibrozil stimulate lipoprotein lipase to increase the hydrolysis of VLDL triglycerides and the delivery of fatty acids to adipose and other tissues. *IDL*, Intermediate-density lipoprotein; *LL*, lipoprotein lipase.

cholesteryl esters are acquired by the liver and other tissues via so-called scavenger receptors such as scavenger receptor B1 and then are converted to steroids by the adrenal glands, ovaries, and testes, or excreted into the bile or converted to bile acids by the liver. The indirect pathway involves the transfer of cholesterol esters to VLDL or LDL via **cholesterol ester transfer protein** (CETP). The contribution of reverse cholesterol transport to CHD is supported by epidemiologic studies that show an inverse relationship between HDL levels and the risk of disease, but efforts to reduce disease by increasing HDL levels with drug therapy have been disappointing.

Lipoprotein (a)

Lipoprotein (a) is a unique lipoprotein similar to LDL whose physiologic function is unknown and whose occurrence is genetically determined. It is found in atherosclerotic plaques of some individuals, and serum levels of lipoprotein (a) are highly correlated with coronary artery disease as measured on an angiogram. **Niacin** appears to lower lipoprotein (a) levels, but other lipid-lowering drugs do not.

Causes and Types of Hyperlipoproteinemia

Hyperlipoproteinemia occurs as a result of genetic or environmental factors that increase the formation of lipoproteins or reduce the clearance of lipoproteins from the circulation. These factors include biochemical defects in lipoprotein metabolism, excessive dietary intake of lipids, endocrine abnormalities, and use of drugs that perturb lipoprotein formation or catabolism. Table 15.1 provides information about the characteristics and types of hyperlipoproteinemia.

Primary hyperlipoproteinemias are relatively rare disorders, and each of which is caused by a **monogenic defect** (a specific defect at a single gene). In some disorders, LDL-cholesterol (LDL-C) levels are severely elevated because of a deficiency of LDL receptors or a defect in the structure of apoprotein B. In the latter case, LDL receptors do not recognize LDL, so LDL removal from the circulation is markedly

impaired. In other disorders, VLDL and triglyceride levels are severely elevated because of a lipoprotein lipase deficiency that prevents the delivery of triglycerides to adipose tissue.

Most cases of hyperlipoproteinemia do not result from a single gene defect but instead result from the influence of several genes that predispose the patient to milder forms of hyperlipoproteinemia, particularly in the presence of excessive dietary intake of lipids. These milder forms, called **polygenic-environmental hyperlipoproteinemias** are much more common than primary hyperlipoproteinemias and are responsible for most cases of accelerated atherosclerosis.

Secondary hyperlipoproteinemias are commonly caused by the presence of alcoholism, diabetes mellitus, or uremia or by the use of drugs such as β-adrenoceptor antagonists, isotretinoin, oral contraceptives, or thiazide diuretics. They are less commonly caused by hypothyroidism, nephrotic syndrome, or obstructive liver disease.

Guidelines for Management of Hypercholesterolemia

The **National Cholesterol Education Program** (NCEP) has issued periodic evidence-based guidelines for the management of high blood cholesterol and related disorders. The latest recommendations encourage more aggressive reductions in LDL-C in high-risk patients.

The NCEP guidelines (Table 15.2) establish LDL-C goals and levels for initiating **lifestyle changes** and **drug therapy** for persons in different risk categories. For **high-risk** patients (who already have CHD or CHD risk equivalents), the primary goal is to achieve an LDL-C level of less than 100 mg/dL, and lifestyle and drug therapy should be initiated at higher LDL-C levels. The guidelines include an optional LDL-C goal of less than 70 mg/dL for high-risk patients and particularly for those whose LDL-C level is less than 100 mg/dL at baseline. This optional goal is based on clinical trials that show that high-risk patients benefit from LDL-C reduction regardless of their baseline level.

For **moderate-risk** patients (persons with a 10% to 20% risk of developing CHD in 10 years), the guidelines specify

TABLE 15.1 Types and Characteristics of Hyperlipoproteinemia

TYPES	INCIDENCE	TOTAL CHOLESTEROL CONCENTRATION (MG/DL)	TRIGLYCERIDE CONCENTRATION (MG/DL)
Homozygous Familial Hyperlipidemia			
Hypercholesterolemia	Rare	>300	<250
Hypertriglyceridemia	Rare	<250	>300
Mixed hyperlipidemia	Rare	>250	>300
Polygenic-Environmental Hyperlipidemia			
Hypercholesterolemia	Common	200–270	<250
Mixed hyperlipidemia	Less common	>200	>300
Secondary Hyperlipidemia			
Caused by alcoholism, diabetes mellitus, uremia, or use of β-adrenoceptor antagonists,[a] isotretinoin, oral contraceptives, or thiazide diuretics[b]	Common	Normal or increased[b]	Increased
Caused by hypothyroidism, nephrotic syndrome, or obstructive liver disease	Less common	Increased	Normal or slightly increased

[a]Use of β-adrenoceptor antagonist may decrease the high-density–lipoprotein (HDL) cholesterol concentration.
[b]Use of thiazide diuretics may increase the total cholesterol concentration.

TABLE 15.2 Risk Categories and LDL-C Levels for Initiating Lifestyle Changes and Drug Therapy in Adults[a]

RISK CATEGORY	LDL-C GOAL (MG/DL)	LDL-C FOR LIFESTYLE CHANGES (MG/DL)	LDL-C FOR DRUG THERAPY (MG/DL)
HIGH RISK (CHD or equivalents[b]; 10-year risk >20%)	<100 (optional: <70)	≥100 (optional: >70)	≥100 to 130 (optional: >70)
MEDIUM RISK (≥2 risk factors[c]; 10-year risk 10%–20%)	<130	≥130	≥130 to 160
LOW RISK (≤1 risk factor[c]; 10-year risk <10%)	<160	≥160	≥160 to 190

[a]National Cholesterol Education Program Adult Panel III, revised 2004.
[b]Myocardial infarction, angina, myocardial ischemia, noncoronary forms of atherosclerosis, and diabetes mellitus.
[c]Risk factors include cigarette smoking, hypertension, low HDL-C, family history of premature CHD, and age.
CHD, Coronary heart disease; *LDL-C,* low-density lipoprotein cholesterol.

an LDL-C goal of less than 130 mg/dL, with lifestyle and drug therapy initiated if levels are higher than 130 mg/dL. The updated goals recommend that drug therapy be considered for moderate-risk patients with LDL-C levels of 100 to 130 mg/dL. For patients with a **lower risk** of CHD (<10% risk of developing CHD in 10 years), lifestyle and drug therapy is recommended if LDL-C levels are equal to or above 160 mg/dL. There, persons should try to reduce LDL-C with therapeutic lifestyle changes for 6 months before initiating drug therapy.

Secondary causes of hyperlipidemia should be excluded before treatment is considered because abnormal levels of cholesterol or triglycerides can often be corrected by proper management of the underlying condition or by replacing the offending drug with an alternative.

Lifestyle Changes

Therapeutic lifestyle changes embrace **dietary modifications, weight management,** and **physical activity.** These changes are essential in the management of high cholesterol and triglyceride levels and may be effective by themselves in patients with smaller lipid elevations. **Exercise** increases lipoprotein lipase activity and lowers triglyceride levels while increasing HDL levels. The diet of patients with hypercholesterolemia should be low in cholesterol, saturated fat, and calories. **Saturated fat** and **cholesterol** are restricted because each independently increases LDL-C,

and **calories** are restricted to help the patient achieve or maintain an ideal body weight. Restricting dietary fat can reduce LDL cholesterol by 25%.

The guidelines recommend a diet that includes complex carbohydrates, fruits, vegetables, and lean meat for lowering cholesterol and triglyceride levels. Additional reduction in LCL-C can be achieved by including 2 g/day of **plant sterols** and **stanols** (such as β-sitosterol and β-sitostanol) and 10 to 25 g/day of **soluble fiber** in the diet. Stanol and sterol esters (phytosterols) are found in vegetable oils, nuts, seeds, and other dietary sources.

The current diet recommendations specify that cholesterol intake should be under 200 mg/day, and total calories from fat should be limited to 25% to 35% of total calories, with saturated fat limited to less than 7% of total calories, partly because saturated fats downregulate hepatic LDL receptors. Foods containing partially hydrogenated plant oils should be avoided because hydrogenation produces the **trans isomers of fatty acids** that increase LDL-C levels, decrease HDL-C levels, increase systemic inflammation, and reduce the availability of fatty acid precursors to anticoagulant prostaglandins.

Dietary modulations are particularly useful in persons with multiple risk factors or angiographic evidence of coronary artery disease. Studies have shown that diets low in saturated and trans fatty acids and high in linoleic acid and **omega-3 fatty acids (linolenic acid** and those in **fish oils)**

TABLE 15.3 **Effects of Diet and Drug Therapy on Serum Lipid Concentrations**

THERAPY	LDL-C % CHANGE	HDL-C % CHANGE	TRIGLYCERIDES % CHANGE	OTHER EFFECTS
Dietary modifications	↓ 10–25	Typically ↑	↓ 10–25	Decreased weight and blood pressure
Statins	↓ 20–60	↑ 5–10	↓ 10–30	Increase in hepatic LDL receptors
Bile acid sequestrants	↓ 15–30	↑ 3–5	No change	Increase in hepatic LDL receptors
Fibric acid derivatives	↓ 5–20	↑ 5–20	↓ 30–50	Activation of lipoprotein lipase
Ezetimibe	↓ 20	No change	↓ 8	—
Niacin	↓ 10–25	↑ 15–35	↓ 25–30	Decrease in lipolysis and lipoprotein (a)

HDL-C, High-density–lipoprotein cholesterol; *LDL-C,* low-density–lipoprotein cholesterol.

TABLE 15.4 **Pharmacokinetic Properties of Drugs for Hyperlipidemia**

DRUG[A]	ORAL BIOAVAILABILITY (PERCENT)	ELIMINATION HALF-LIFE	ROUTES OF ELIMINATION[B]	OTHER PROPERTIES
HMG-CoA Reductase Inhibitors (Statins)				
Atorvastatin	12	14 h	M and F	Does not cross the blood-brain barrier
Fluvastatin	25	<1 h	M and F	Does not cross the blood-brain barrier
Lovastatin	5	3.5 h	M and F	A prodrug; crosses the blood-brain barrier
Pitavastatin	50	12 h	F > R; M	Not extensively metabolized by P450 enzymes
Pravastatin	17	1.8 h	M and F	Does not cross the blood-brain barrier
Rosuvastatin	20	19 h	M and F	—
Simvastatin	<5	3 h	M and F	A prodrug; crosses the blood-brain barrier
Fibric Acid Derivatives				
Fenofibrate	100	23 h	M	A prodrug
Gemfibrozil	100	2 h	M (98%)	Undergoes enterohepatic cycling
Other Drugs				
Ezetimibe	Variable	22 h	M and F	Localizes in the small intestine
Niacin	100	0.5 h	M and R	—
Lopitamide	7	40 h	M and R	Metabolized by CYP3A4

[a]Bile acid–binding resins (cholestyramine, colestipol, and colesevelam) are not absorbed; they remain in the gastrointestinal tract (0% bioavailability) and are excreted in the feces.
[b]*F,* Fecal; *M,* metabolism; *R,* renal.

improve the ratio of LDL-C to HDL-C. These diets can also reverse the angiographic evidence of coronary atherosclerosis and reduce the mortality rate in patients with CHD. In patients with **hypertriglyceridemia,** supplementing the diet with fish oils that contain **omega-3 fatty acids** often lowers triglyceride levels. A prescription-strength formulation of omega-3-carboxylic acid (EPANOVA) is also available.

DRUGS FOR HYPERCHOLESTEROLEMIA

The most important drugs for treating hypercholesterolemia are the **statins.** Other drugs that can be added to or substituted for statins include the **bile acid–binding resins, ezetimibe,** and **niacin.** Tables 15.3 to 15.5 outline the effects and pharmacokinetic properties of the drugs used to treat hypercholesterolemia and compare them with the effects and properties of other drugs discussed in this chapter.

Statins (HMG-CoA Reductase Inhibitors)

Among the HMG-CoA reductase inhibitors are **atorvastatin, fluvastatin, lovastatin, pitavastatin, pravastatin, rosuvastatin,** and **simvastatin.** The statins are the most

effective drugs for lowering blood cholesterol levels, and clinical trials have shown that they prevent coronary artery disease and reduce mortality. The statins have a relatively good safety record, and their once-daily dosage regimen is highly convenient and fosters patient adherence.

Chemistry and Pharmacokinetics

The **statins** are structurally related to hydroxymethylglutaryl (HMG)-CoA, which is the substrate for HMG-CoA reductase (Fig. 15.3). The drugs have relatively low bioavailability, owing largely to extensive first-pass metabolism. **Lovastatin** and **simvastatin** are inactive **prodrugs** that must be converted to active metabolites in the liver, whereas the other statins are active compounds. All of the drugs, except atorvastatin, have relatively short half-lives (see Table 15.4). Some of the reductase inhibitors are metabolized by cytochrome P450 (CYP) enzymes (see later).

Statins with shorter half-lives are taken in the evening or at bedtime to ensure inhibition of nocturnal cholesterol biosynthesis. **Atorvastatin** and **rosuvastatin** have longer half-lives and can be taken at any time of day. **Lovastatin** should

TABLE 15.5   Common Adverse Effects and Interactions of Drugs for Hyperlipidemia

DRUG	ADVERSE EFFECTS	DRUG INTERACTIONS
Statins	Myopathy, elevated serum hepatic enzyme levels, and hepatitis	Slightly increase warfarin levels; concurrent erythromycin, fibrates, or niacin increase risk of myopathy[a]
Bile acid–binding resins	Constipation, fecal impaction, and rash	Decrease absorption of digoxin, thyroxin, warfarin, and other drugs
Fibrates	Allergic reactions, blood cell deficiencies, and myopathy	Statins or niacin increase the risk of myopathy
Ezetimibe	Headache, myalgia	Cholestyramine decreases absorption
Niacin	Vasodilation, flushing, and pruritus; gastric irritation; glucose intolerance; myopathy	Fibrates or statins increase the risk of myopathy[a]
Lomitapide	Diarrhea, nausea, vomiting, abdominal pain; elevation of serum transaminase levels and hepatotoxicity	Levels increased by CYP3A4 inhibitors; increases levels of statins and warfarin

Statins, HMG-CoA reductase inhibitors; *Fibrates,* fibric acid derivatives; *HMG-CoA,* 3-hydroxy-3-methylglutaryl–coenzyme A.
[a]If niacin must be used in combination with a statin, the safest combination appears to be niacin plus fluvastatin, and the combination that poses the greatest risk is niacin plus lovastatin.

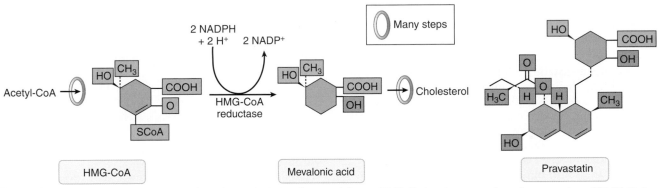

Fig. 15.3   Inhibition of cholesterol biosynthesis by HMG-CoA reductase inhibitors. HMG-CoA reductase catalyzes the conversion of HMG-CoA to mevalonic acid, the rate-limiting enzyme in cholesterol biosynthesis. The reductase inhibitors contain a structure that is similar to the structure of HMG-CoA (the unshaded portions of pravastatin and HMG-CoA), and they compete with the substrate for the catalytic site of the enzyme.

be taken with the evening meal to facilitate its absorption, whereas the other drugs can be taken without regard to food. **Lovastatin** and **simvastatin** cross **the blood-brain barrier** and can cause sleep disturbances in some patients.

Mechanisms and Pharmacologic Effects

HMG-CoA reductase converts HMG-CoA to mevalonic acid and is the rate-limiting enzyme in cholesterol biosynthesis (see Figs. 15.2 and 15.3). By competitively inhibiting this enzyme, statins reduce hepatic **cholesterol biosynthesis** and the amount of cholesterol available for incorporation into VLDL. This leads to a compensatory increase in the number of hepatic **LDL receptors,** which increases the hepatic uptake of LDL-C. Together, these actions cause a substantial reduction in LDL-C. In patients with hypercholesterolemia, statins typically decrease LDL-C levels by 20% to 60%, whereas HDL-C levels are increased by up to 10% (see Table 15.3). The statins also reduce serum triglycerides but are usually not a sufficient treatment for hypertriglyceridemia.

Indications

The statins are used to reduce blood cholesterol levels in persons with **hypercholesterolemia** to achieve the LDL-C goals recommended by the NCEP. The NCEP guidelines recommend using a statin dose that can achieve a 30% to 40% reduction in LDL-C levels. The statins do not have equal potency with respect to reducing LDL-C levels. **Rosuvastatin** is the most potent statin currently available,

followed by **atorvastatin.** Atorvastatin and rosuvastatin also have the greatest effect on triglyceride levels and can be useful in treating patients with **mixed hyperlipidemia.**

Clinical trials of reductase inhibitors have demonstrated that these drugs slow the progression of atherosclerosis, reduce the risk of CHD and other atherosclerotic vascular diseases, and reduce the cardiac mortality rate. A large prospective study of more than 4,000 patients with CHD found that patients treated with **simvastatin** had a lower rate of **death, myocardial infarction, stroke,** and **revascularization procedures.** Some of the benefits produced by statins may result from their ability to improve vascular endothelial function and reduce inflammation. Clinical trials also indicate that statins may also protect against **osteoporosis** and certain forms of **cancer.**

Adverse Effects

The statins are generally well tolerated but may cause serious adverse effects in a small percentage of persons. The most frequent adverse effects are gastrointestinal problems, including abdominal cramps, constipation, diarrhea, and heartburn. Less frequently, statins cause **hepatitis** and elevate serum levels of hepatic enzymes (see Table 15.5). The most serious adverse effect of statins is **rhabdomyolysis,** which is a potentially fatal form of skeletal muscle toxicity **(myopathy).** Only about 0.2% of patients receiving statins develop myopathy, and only a few of these cases progress to rhabdomyolysis.

The precise mechanisms by which statins cause **myopathy** are still being elucidated. The earliest stage of statin-induced myopathy is **myalgia,** which consists of muscle ache or weakness without elevated creatine kinase levels. This stage is reversible on statin withdrawal and resolves in 2 to 3 weeks. Myalgia can be followed by **myositis** or muscle inflammation accompanied by muscle pain, leakage of muscle creatine kinase into the plasma, and elevated creatine kinase levels. Myositis can eventually lead to **rhabdomyolysis** in which muscle cells disintegrate, thereby releasing myoglobin into the circulation. Myoglobin then accumulates in the kidneys and causes acute renal failure. Creatine kinase levels in rhabdomyolysis are often greater than 10 times the upper limit of normal, and persons with this affliction have dark urine resulting from **myoglobinuria.**

Patients taking a statin should be asked to report any sign of unusual, diffuse, or persistent muscle tenderness, pain, or weakness, especially if it is accompanied by malaise, fever, or dark urine. Factors that increase the risk of statin-induced myopathy include **higher doses,** increasing age, female gender, renal or hepatic disease, hypothyroidism, and the use of drugs that inhibit statin metabolism. For example, the highest dose of **simvastatin** (80 mg) has been associated with a much higher incidence of myopathy and rhabdomyolysis than lower doses (10 or 20 mg). The U.S. Food and Drug Administration (FDA) has recommended that patients avoid higher doses of simvastatin and that patients taking CYP3A4 inhibitors (see later), **amiodarone, verapamil,** or **diltiazem** use only the lower doses.

Use of the statin must be discontinued if myopathy is diagnosed or if levels of **creatine kinase** are found to be significantly elevated. No specific treatment exists for rhabdomyolysis except drug withdrawal and fluid administration to maintain renal function. There is anecdotal evidence that **vitamin D** and **coenzyme Q-10** supplements may prevent or improve myopathy in persons taking statins, possibly because these compounds are synthesized in the same pathway as cholesterol, and their production can be reduced by statins.

Clinical trials showing the cardiovascular benefits of statin treatment have also shown a 10% to 25% increase in the incidence of **diabetes** during statin treatment. However, a meta-analysis of trials concluded that statin treatment would prevent five heart attacks for every new case of diabetes. It is currently believed that the benefits of statin therapy outweigh the small increased risk of diabetes.

Interactions

Atorvastatin, lovastatin, and simvastatin are metabolized by CYP3A4, and their plasma concentrations are greatly increased by strong inhibitors of this isozyme, such as **erythromycin, itraconazole,** and **ritonavir. Pitavastatin, pravastatin,** and **rosuvastatin** are mostly excreted unchanged, and their plasma concentrations are not significantly increased by CYP3A4 inhibitors. **Fluvastatin** is metabolized by CYP2C9, and its plasma levels may be increased by inhibitors of this CYP, including some nonsteroidal anti-inflammatory drugs (NSAIDs).

Statins inhibit the metabolism of certain other drugs by CYP enzymes. For example, they **increase warfarin levels** slightly by inhibiting warfarin metabolism. Because statins, fibric acid derivatives, and niacin may cause **myopathies,** the combined use of drugs should be undertaken with great caution using lower doses of each agent employed.

Bile Acid–Binding Resins

Cholestyramine, colestipol, and **colesevelam** are bile acid–binding resins that are moderately effective drugs for hypercholesterolemia and have an excellent safety record. They are especially valuable for patients who cannot tolerate other drugs and for younger patients who may need to have drug therapy for many years.

Chemistry and Pharmacokinetics

The bile acid–binding resins are **high-molecular-weight polymers** containing a chloride ion that can be exchanged for bile acids in the gut. The resins are not absorbed from the gut and are excreted in the feces.

Mechanisms and Pharmacologic Effects

After the resins bind to bile acids, the bile acid–resin complex is excreted. This action prevents the enterohepatic cycling of bile acids and obligates the liver to synthesize replacement bile acids from cholesterol. To obtain more cholesterol for this purpose, the liver increases the number of LDL receptors. Then the levels of LDL-C in the blood are reduced as more cholesterol is delivered to the liver. As shown in Table 15.3, the resins have relatively little effect on HDL-C and triglyceride levels.

Adverse Effects and Interactions

The bile acid–binding resins have few adverse effects. They can cause constipation, fecal impaction, and other gastrointestinal side effects, most of which can be prevented by taking the drugs with a full glass of water and maintaining fluid intake throughout the day. Occasionally, they cause irritation of the perianal area and a skin rash. In the gut, cholestyramine and colestipol can bind to digoxin, thyroxin, warfarin, and other drugs. For this reason, it is best to take the resins 2 hours before or after taking other medications. A newer resin, colesevelam, does not affect the oral bioavailability of digoxin, warfarin, or lovastatin and therefore can be coadministered with most drugs, including HMG-CoA reductase inhibitors.

Indications

The resins are indicated for the treatment of **hypercholesterolemia** and are particularly useful in patients who cannot tolerate other drugs. Although the resins are less effective than the statins, they do not cause hepatitis or myopathy, and they can be given in combination with other drugs to produce an additive effect on serum cholesterol levels. The resins have also been used to treat **chronic diarrhea** due to bile acid malabsorption.

Preparations

Cholestyramine and **colestipol** are available as a powder for mixing with water or juice just before administration, and cholestyramine is also marketed as a chewable bar. To obtain the maximal effect on serum cholesterol levels, these drugs must be taken before each meal and at bedtime. **Colesevelam** is a newer resin available as solid tablets that are usually taken twice daily with meals. It decreases LDL-C to a similar degree as do the other resins and may be more convenient and palatable.

Ezetimibe

Ezetimibe is a unique drug that inhibits the absorption of dietary cholesterol. After oral administration, ezetimibe is absorbed from the intestines and then is metabolized to the pharmacologically **active metabolite ezetimibe-glucuronide.** This active metabolite is distributed by the circulation to the small intestines, where it localizes in the brush border and inhibits the absorption of both biliary and dietary cholesterol. Studies suggest that ezetimibe acts by disrupting a complex of two proteins, annexin-2 and caveolin-1, which mediate cholesterol transport in intestinal brush border cells. The half-lives of ezetimibe and ezetimibe-glucuronide are both 22 hours. The drugs are eliminated in the urine and feces.

Because of its unique mechanism of action, ezetimibe can be used alone or in combination with a statin to treat hypercholesterolemia. A fixed-dose combination of ezetimibe and simvastatin (VYTORIN), and ezetimibe with atorvastatin (LIPTRUZET) are available for this purpose. When administered alone, ezetimibe lowers LDL-C levels 19% to 23%. An incremental reduction of LDL-C levels of about 22% was obtained when ezetimibe was added to statin therapy in one study. Hence, the coadministration of ezetimibe and a statin can achieve reductions in LDL-C similar to that obtained with the highest statin doses. This may permit the use of lower doses of statins to obtain desired LDL-C levels with correspondingly less risk of statin toxicity (Box 15.2). This combination has been found to be effective in treating persons with homozygous familial hypercholesterolemia.

Ezetimibe is generally well tolerated, though it can increase serum hepatic transaminase levels, and some persons experience headaches and myalgia.

Niacin (Nicotinic Acid)

Niacin and the fibric acid derivatives have been used to treat hypertriglyceridemia and to increase HDL-C levels in persons with abnormally low levels of this lipoprotein. The effects and properties of these drugs are shown in Tables 15.3 to 15.5.

Pharmacologic doses of niacin have profound effects on serum lipid levels. The drug has the broadest spectrum of lipid-altering effects of any agent.

Chemistry and Pharmacokinetics

Niacin is also known as *vitamin B_3.* The small amount of niacin that is ingested in food is converted in the body to enzyme cofactors required for oxidative reactions in the metabolism of energy substrates and other substances. These cofactors are nicotinamide adenine dinucleotide (NAD) and its phosphate derivative (NADP). Niacin is well absorbed from the gut and is extensively metabolized before undergoing renal excretion.

Mechanisms and Pharmacologic Effects

The quantity of niacin ingested in food does not have any measurable effect on serum lipid levels. The action of niacin on lipids is a pharmacologic effect that requires the administration of **large doses** (several grams) of the compound each day. Pharmacologic doses of niacin lower LDL-C, lipoprotein (a), and triglyceride levels while raising HDL-C levels.

Niacin acts primarily by inhibiting the formation and secretion of hepatic VLDL, the major carrier of plasma

---

BOX 15.2 A CASE OF WEIGHT GAIN AND DYSLIPIDEMIA

CASE PRESENTATION

A 56-year-old man with a family history of coronary heart disease (CHD) came to his physician to review recent laboratory work. He has battled weight gain over the past several years and now weighs 220 pounds. His waist circumference is 42 inches and his body mass index is 28. He has had hypertension for 4 years that has been treated with lisinopril, and his recent blood pressure readings have averaged 136/84 mm Hg. The patient's laboratory work shows an LDL-C level of 180 mg/dL, an HDL-C level of 40 mg/dL, and a triglyceride level of 175 mg/dL. His other laboratory values are within normal limits. The patient expresses a desire to lose weight and agrees to begin a heart-healthy diet and a structured exercise program. He is placed on atorvastatin to reduce LDL-C levels and is referred to a dietitian and exercise physiologist.

Two months later, the patient returns to his physician for follow-up. He has lost 10 pounds, and his lipid profile now includes an LDL-C of 160 mg/dL, an HDL-C of 44 mg/dL, and a triglyceride level of 155 mg/dL. To further reduce his LDL-C level, colesevelam is added to the patient's treatment regimen, and he is scheduled to see his physician again in 2 months.

CASE DISCUSSION

An estimated 13 million Americans have CHD, which is the leading cause of mortality in the United States. The death rate for CHD has been decreasing steadily for several decades, partly owing to lifestyle changes and improved medical care, but CHD still causes nearly 1 in 5 deaths. The patient in this case has several risk factors for CHD, including advanced age, male gender, hypertension, and an atherogenic dyslipidemia. He also meets several criteria for the so-called *metabolic syndrome.* Hence, it is important to address his modifiable risk factors and prevent progression to symptomatic CHD. The patient has begun lifestyle modifications that may enable him to achieve a normal body weight and triglyceride level. Because of his multiple risk factors for CHD, his LDL-C goal is less than 100 mg/dL, with an optional goal of less than 70 mg/dL. Statins have been shown to reduce LDL-C levels and prevent cardiovascular death, whereas colesevelam may enable the patient to achieve his LDL-C goal more easily and with less risk of adverse effects.

---

triglycerides and the precursor to LDL (see Fig. 15.3). The effect on VLDL secretion is caused partly by **inhibition of lipolysis** in adipose tissue. This action reduces the supply of circulating free fatty acids that the liver uses to synthesize triglycerides for incorporation into VLDL. The inhibition of lipolysis has been attributed to the binding of niacin to a **G protein–coupled receptor** in adipose tissue. Niacin decreases LDL-C levels and particularly the levels of small, dense LDL particles associated with atherosclerosis. At the same time, niacin increases HDL-C levels (see Table 15.3), including the levels of the beneficial HDL_2 component of HDL.

Indications

Because of its favorable effects on serum lipids, niacin is approved to reduce LDL-C and triglyceride levels and to increase HDL-C levels in patients with primary hyperlipidemia and mixed dyslipidemia. The Coronary Drug Project found that niacin reduced the risk of myocardial infarction among men with hypercholesterolemia and atherosclerosis, and it decreased total mortality. Niacin is sometimes combined with a statin or bile acid sequestrant to reduce LDL levels and slow the progression of atherosclerotic disease when a single drug is insufficient, but the benefit of combined therapy on cardiovascular mortality has not been established. Niacin's role in treating **HDL deficiency** remains controversial. A recent clinical trial (AIM-HIGH) was stopped prematurely when it was found that adding extended-release niacin to simvastatin in persons with well-controlled LDL-C levels produced an elevation of HDL levels but did not provide any additional reduction of cardiovascular events. This study confirms the difficulty investigators have had to date in showing a clinical benefit from raising HDL levels with drugs.

Niacin is also used to reduce the risk of pancreatitis in patients with very high triglyceride levels. It is the only antilipemic drug with a consistent ability to reduce **lipoprotein (a)** levels, and it has been used for this purpose.

Adverse Effects and Interactions

The large doses of niacin required to lower serum lipids typically cause vasodilation and flushing of the skin accompanied by pruritus and a feeling of warmth and tingling. This effect can be reduced by pretreatment with aspirin, and some tolerance to this effect develops with continued drug administration. These effects are also reduced with the use of a sustained-release niacin preparation. In a small percentage of patients, niacin can elevate serum transaminase levels and cause hepatitis. It can also cause gastric distress and may aggravate a peptic ulcer. Although niacin can increase blood glucose and aggravate diabetes, clinical trials show it can be used in persons whose diabetes is well controlled with little effect on glucose levels. Finally, niacin may cause hyperuricemia and gout.

Fibric Acid Derivatives
Chemistry and Pharmacokinetics

These drugs are derivatives of a branched-chain carboxylic acid known as fibric acid or **fibrate.** The first drug in this class, clofibrate, is no longer available because of its high incidence of adverse effects. **Gemfibrozil** and **fenofibrate** are currently available in the United States and many other countries.

Mechanisms and Pharmacologic Effects

The fibrates reduce serum levels of triglycerides and LDL-C while raising levels of HDL-C. The fibrates produce these effects by activating a receptor in cell nuclei that regulates gene transcription and is called the **peroxisome proliferator–activated receptor-α** (PPAR-α). In the liver and elsewhere, PPAR-α increases the transcription of certain genes while inhibiting the transcription of others.

The effect of fibrates on serum triglyceride levels is attributed to the PPAR-α–mediated expression of **lipoprotein lipase.** This enzyme is located in the vascular endothelium and catalyzes the hydrolysis and removal of triglycerides from VLDL, thereby lowering serum triglyceride levels (see Fig. 15.2). PPAR-α activation also reduces the expression of an inhibitor of lipoprotein lipase, **apolipoprotein C-III.** Other effects of PPAR-α activation include the expression

of enzymes that oxidize fatty acids. The effects of fibrates on HDL-C are attributed to PPAR-α–mediated expression of apoproteins A-I and A-II, which are important components of HDL. PPAR-α also increases the expression of cholesterol transport proteins (ATP–binding cassette transporters A1 and G1) involved in reverse cholesterol transport (see earlier discussion of HDL).

Fenofibrate reduces serum LDL-C levels by increasing expression of hepatic LDL receptors and by increasing LDL receptor affinity, both via activation of PPAR-α. These actions increase the uptake of LDL-C by the liver and reduce serum LDL-C levels. Fenofibrate causes a greater reduction in LDL-C than does gemfibrozil.

Indications

Gemfibrozil and fenofibrate are indicated for the treatment of **very high triglyceride levels** (higher than 1,500 mg/dL) to prevent pancreatitis when dietary therapy has failed to lower these levels. The benefit of treating moderately elevated triglyceride levels is less clear, and lifestyle changes such as weight loss and exercise can lower such levels in many patients.

The fibrate drugs are also approved for reducing the risk of developing **CHD** in patients who have a triad of elevated LDL-C, low HDL-C, and elevated triglycerides and whose lipidemia has not responded to lifestyle changes or other pharmacologic agents. However, the ability of fibrate drugs to prevent CHD is uncertain. Most clinical trials have found that fibrates do not significantly lower the rates of fatal myocardial infarction or total mortality. The Helsinki Heart Study, which involved 2000 men with hypercholesterolemia, found that gemfibrozil reduced the CHD-related mortality rate, but the overall mortality rate was not affected. In a trial of fenofibrate in patients with type 2 diabetes and mixed dyslipidemia, fenofibrate did not reduce the rates of either fatal or nonfatal myocardial infarction. For this reason, some authorities suggest using niacin, rather than a fibrate, to control dyslipidemia in patients who have not responded to other drugs.

Adverse Effects and Interactions

The fibrates often cause gastrointestinal side effects and, less commonly, blood cell deficiencies and other hypersensitivity reactions. As with the statin drugs, the fibrates can cause myopathy and rhabdomyolysis (see Table 15.5), and the combined administration of statins and fibrates should be avoided or used with great caution. Fibrates can be given with cholestyramine and colestipol, but the doses must be separated by more than 2 hours because the resins reduce fibrate absorption.

DRUGS FOR FAMILIAL HYPERCHOLESTEROLEMIA AND LEPTIN DEFICIENCY

Several drugs are now available to treat patients with familial hypercholesterolemia in combination with dietary restrictions and statins. **Lomitapide** acts to reduce the production of VLDL in the liver and is used to treat **homozygous familial hypercholesterolemia** (HoFH). In the United States, it is only available from physicians and pharmacies certified through an FDA Risk Evaluation and Mitigation Strategy (REMS) because of its potential to cause severe adverse effects.

Lomitapide inhibits the **microsomal triglyceride transfer protein** (MTTP), which is essential for VLDL assembly and secretion in the liver. The drug is used as an adjunct to diet and other lipid-lowering drugs to reduce LDL-C, apolipoprotein B (apo B), and total cholesterol in persons with HoFH. Lomitapide causes gastrointestinal side effects in most patients, and it decreases the absorption of fat-soluble vitamins A, D, and E, and omega-3 fatty acids. These nutrients should be supplemented in patients taking lomitapide. The drug may also cause hepatic toxicity, and serum levels of hepatic enzymes should be monitored. It is also embryotoxic and contraindicated in pregnancy. Lomitapide is metabolized by CYP3A4, and inhibitors of this enzyme must be avoided by those taking the drug. Lomitapide also increases warfarin levels.

Mipomersen is an **antisense oligonucleotide** (complementary strand) that binds to the messenger RNA for **apo B,** preventing the synthesis of apo B required for VLDL production in the liver. Mipomersen is indicated to reduce LDL-C and apo B in persons with HoFH, and it is administered as a weekly injection. The drug may elevate serum hepatic transaminase levels, which must be monitored, and many patients experience injection site reactions, flu-like symptoms, nausea, and headache. Antisense medications are discussed in greater detail in Chapter 46 under *Genetic Pharmacology.*

Evolocumab and alirocumab are monoclonal antibodies to a protease enzyme that destroys LDL receptors in the liver. This enzyme is known as proprotein convertase subtilisin/kexin type 9 (PCSK9). By this mechanism, the hepatic uptake of LDL cholesterol is increased, and the serum cholesterol level falls. These agents are administered subcutaneously every 2 weeks for the treatment of homozygous or heterozygous familial hypercholesterolemia and for patients with demonstrated atherosclerotic cardiovascular disease who are not adequately treated with statins. Their adverse effects include injection site and allergic reactions, and elevated serum levels of hepatic enzymes. Further discussion of these and other monoclonal antibody drugs is presented in Chapter 46.

Bempedoic acid (NEXLETOL) is an adenosine triphosphate-citrate lyase (ACL) inhibitor taken along with dietary changes and maximally tolerated statin therapy for the treatment of adults with heterozygous familial hypercholesterolemia or established atherosclerotic cardiovascular disease who require additional **lowering of LDL-C.**

Leptin Deficiency

Leptin is a peptide hormone released by adipose tissue that transmits information about energy stores to the brain and other organs. In patients with lipodystrophy, the lack of adipose tissue leads to a deficiency of leptin and hypertriglyceridemia with deposition of fat in nonadipose tissue such as the liver and muscle. The lack of leptin signal also leads to excessive calorie intake and further metabolic dysfunction such as insulin resistance. Congenital leptin deficiency may also arise due to mutations in the leptin gene. **Metreleptin** is an analog of human leptin hormone, differing by only one amino acid substitution with methionine, and produced by recombinant biotechnology in *E. coli.* Metreleptin binds to and activates the leptin receptor, leading to an **increase in insulin sensitivity** and **reduced food intake.** It

is administered by a daily subcutaneous injection. Because neutralizing antibodies and a risk of lymphoma can occur after the administration of metreleptin, this new drug is also administered under a specific REMS protocol.

Drug Combinations

Drugs can be used in combination to treat high blood cholesterol in patients who do not respond to a single drug. The most useful combinations are those consisting of a **statin** with **ezetimibe** or a **bile acid–binding resin.** For example, ezetimibe and simvastatin are available in a combination product called VYTORIN, among others. These products enable the use of a lower dose of a statin to achieve target LDL-C levels and reduce the risk of myopathy. Colesevelam is a newer bile acid–binding resin that can be coadministered with statins, and extended-release niacin may be added to a statin when cholesterol levels cannot be controlled with other drugs.

For patients with elevated levels of both cholesterol and triglycerides, a statin can be combined with niacin or a fibrate drug. Niacin is often preferred for this purpose for several reasons: (1) niacin has a greater effect on cholesterol levels than fibrates and may enable the use of lower doses of a statin to control hypercholesterolemia; (2) clinical trials show that niacin lowers cardiovascular and overall mortality; and (3) niacin is less likely than fibrates to cause myopathy and rhabdomyolysis when used in combination with a statin. Niacin and simvastatin are combined in a formulation called SIMCOR for these reasons.

SUMMARY OF IMPORTANT POINTS

- Cholesterol and triglycerides are secreted by the liver in the form of VLDL. After delivering triglycerides to adipose tissue, VLDL becomes LDL. LDL delivers cholesterol to peripheral tissues, the liver, and macrophages in atheromas. HDL transports cholesterol from tissues and atheromas to the liver.
- Hypercholesterolemia is a risk factor for atherosclerosis and coronary artery disease. Hypertriglyceridemia is associated with pancreatitis, and it may have a role in the development of heart disease.
- Patients with high blood cholesterol levels should be managed with lifestyle changes and drug therapy based on the guidelines of the NCEP.
- Ezetimibe inhibits the absorption of dietary and biliary cholesterol from the intestines, thereby causing a reduction in LDL-C levels.
- Atorvastatin and other statins inhibit the rate-limiting enzyme in cholesterol biosynthesis and lead to a secondary increase in hepatic LDL receptors and cholesterol uptake, thereby causing a reduction in serum LDL-C levels.
- Cholestyramine, colestipol, and colesevelam are bile acid–binding resins that prevent the intestinal reabsorption of bile acids and necessitate increased use of cholesterol to replace them, leading to a reduction in LDL-C levels.
- Niacin and the fibric acid derivatives (gemfibrozil and fenofibrate) reduce triglyceride levels and increase HDL-C levels. Niacin inhibits VLDL secretion and reduces triglyceride and LDL-C levels. Fibrates increase

VLDL clearance by increasing lipoprotein lipase activity via activation of PPAR-α.

- Drugs available to treat severe familial hypercholesterolemia in combination with diet and statins include lomitapide and mipomersen. Lomitapide inhibits the microsomal triglyceride transfer protein. Mipomersen in an antisense oligonucleotide to the messenger RNA for apoprotein B.
- Evolocumab and alirocumab are monoclonal antibodies to an enzyme that destroys LDL receptors in the liver and are used to treat familial hypercholesterolemia in patients with atherosclerotic vascular disease.

Review Questions

1. Which drug inhibits the intestinal absorption of cholesterol?
   - (A) colesevelam
   - (B) fenofibrate
   - (C) ezetimibe
   - (D) colestipol
   - (E) niacin

2. A woman taking a drug for high LDL-cholesterol levels experiences muscle tenderness and pain with no apparent cause. Which agent is least likely to cause this adverse effect?
   - (A) atorvastatin
   - (B) niacin
   - (C) fenofibrate
   - (D) colestipol
   - (E) rosuvastatin

3. What is the mechanism by which mipomersen lowers serum cholesterol levels?
   - (A) inhibits microsomal triglyceride transport
   - (B) inhibits cholesterol absorption
   - (C) inhibits cholesterol biosynthesis
   - (D) inhibits apolipoprotein B synthesis
   - (E) increases cholesterol excretion

4. Stimulation of lipoprotein lipase by a fenofibrate results in lowered serum levels of which substance?
   - (A) triglycerides
   - (B) HDL-cholesterol
   - (C) LDL-cholesterol
   - (D) apolipoprotein B
   - (E) phospholipids

5. Which drug increases the utilization of cholesterol to synthesize bile acids?
   - (A) niacin
   - (B) rosuvastatin
   - (C) gemfibrozil
   - (D) ezetimibe
   - (E) colesevelam

CHAPTER 16
Antithrombotic and Thrombolytic Drugs

OVERVIEW

The formation of intravascular thrombi and emboli contributes to the pathogenesis of several important cardiovascular disorders, including myocardial infarction (MI), ischemic stroke, and venous thromboembolism (or deep vein thrombosis [DVT]). This chapter focuses on drugs used in the prevention and treatment of **thromboembolic disorders,** including drugs that inhibit coagulation and platelet aggregation and drugs that lyse thrombi.

Normal Hemostasis

When a small blood vessel is injured, hemorrhage is prevented by **vasoconstriction** followed by formation of a **platelet plug** and a **fibrin clot** (Fig. 16.1). After the vessel is repaired, the clot is removed via the process of **fibrinolysis.**

Vasoconstriction reduces bleeding and blood flow and facilitates platelet aggregation and blood coagulation. Exposure of the blood to extravascular collagen causes adherence of platelets to the injured vessel wall and initiates the sequential activation of numerous **coagulation factors** (blood clotting factors), most of which are serine protease enzymes. In this cascade, the inactive factors are converted to active enzymes by the previous coagulation factor or stimulus. The factors and their synonyms are listed in Table 16.1, and the **coagulation pathways** are illustrated in Fig. 16.2. The **intrinsic pathway** can be activated by surface contact with a foreign body or extravascular tissue, whereas the **extrinsic pathway** is activated by a complex **tissue factor.** The extrinsic pathway is believed to be the most important coagulation pathway for *in vivo* coagulation. The pathways converge with the activation of **factor X,** which is the major rate-limiting step in the coagulation cascade. The activation of factor X leads to the formation of **thrombin;** in turn, thrombin catalyzes the conversion of **fibrinogen** to **fibrin.** The fibrin mesh traps erythrocytes and platelets to complete the formation of a hemostatic thrombus (clot). Thrombin formation and platelet aggregation are mutually supportive, in that platelets release thrombin to promote fibrin formation, and thrombin is a powerful stimulant of platelet aggregation.

Pathologic Thrombus Formation

Arterial thrombi are often overlaid on a disrupted atherosclerotic plaque that exposes blood to plaque material that initiates **platelet aggregation** and **coagulation.** For example, coronary artery atherosclerosis can promote the formation of thrombi that obstruct blood flow and cause **MI.** Formation of thrombi in cerebral arteries can cause an **ischemic stroke.**

Venous thrombi are usually initiated by venous blood pooling and sluggish blood flow that promotes expression of adhesion factors on the surface of venous endothelial cells. Leukocytes can adhere to these cells and release tissue factor that activates coagulation. In leg veins, thrombi can dislodge and travel to the lungs, causing **pulmonary embolism (PE).**

Coagulation has a larger role than platelet aggregation in causing venous thrombi, and anticoagulants are often used to prevent venous thromboembolism. Platelet aggregation is more important in initiating arterial thrombi, although both antiplatelet and anticoagulant drugs are used in prevention and treatment.

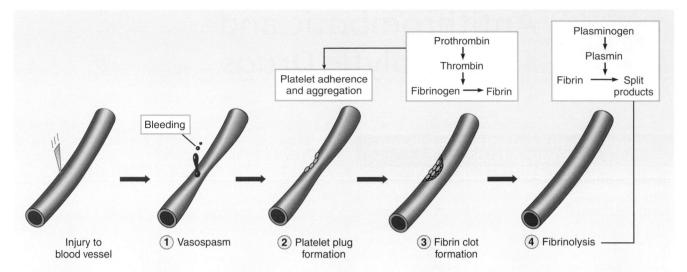

FIG. 16.1   Normal hemostasis. *(1)* When a small blood vessel is injured, vasospasm reduces blood flow and facilitates platelet aggregation and coagulation. *(2)* The platelets, which adhere to extravascular collagen, are activated to release mediators that cause platelet aggregation and the formation of a platelet plug to arrest bleeding. *(3)* Exposure of the blood to tissue factors also activates coagulation and leads to the formation of a fibrin clot, which arrests bleeding until the vessel is repaired. *(4)* After the vessel is repaired, the clot is removed by the process of fibrinolysis.

TABLE 16.1   Coagulation Factors

FACTOR[a]	COMMON SYNONYM	DEPENDENT ON VITAMIN K[b]
I	Fibrinogen	No
II	Prothrombin	Yes
III	Tissue thromboplastin	No
IV	Calcium	No
V	Proaccelerin	No
VII	Proconvertin	Yes
VIII	Antihemophilic factor	No
IX	Plasma thromboplastin component	Yes
X	Stuart factor	Yes
XI	Plasma thromboplastin antecedent	No
XII	Hageman factor	No
XIII	Fibrin stabilizing factor	No

[a]Factor VI is no longer considered to be a coagulation factor.
[b]Proteins C and S, which are endogenous anticoagulants that inactivate factors Va and VIIIa and promote fibrinolysis, are also dependent on vitamin K.

ANTICOAGULANT DRUGS

Anticoagulants are drugs that prevent the formation or expansion of a thrombus. The anticoagulants are classified according to their mechanism of action and include vitamin K antagonists, drugs that potentiate antithrombin III (AT-III), and drugs that directly inhibit thrombin or active factor X. Table 16.2 compares the properties of various anticoagulant drugs.

Warfarin

Chemistry and Mechanisms

Coumarin compounds such as warfarin were originally identified as substances in spoiled clover hay that caused hemorrhagic disease in cattle and were subsequently developed as anticoagulants and rodenticides.

Warfarin and other coumarin derivatives are structurally related to vitamin K. These drugs inhibit the synthesis of coagulation factors whose formation is dependent on vitamin K, **factors II (prothrombin), VII, IX, and X.** As shown in Fig. 16.3, warfarin blocks the reduction of oxidized vitamin K and prevents the posttranslational (following protein synthesis) carboxylation of these coagulation factors. Warfarin also inhibits the synthesis of proteins C and S, which are endogenous anticoagulants that inactivate factors V and VIII and promote fibrinolysis. Inhibition of proteins C and S can cause a transient procoagulant effect when warfarin is first administered. A heparin-type anticoagulant is often administered concurrently until warfarin's anticoagulant effect has developed (see later).

Pharmacokinetic and Pharmacologic Effects

Warfarin is well absorbed from the gut and extensively metabolized before being excreted in the urine. Unlike heparin and related anticoagulants, warfarin crosses the placenta and can cause fetal hemorrhage.

Warfarin has a **delayed onset of action** owing to the time required to deplete the pool of circulating clotting factors after synthesis of new factors is inhibited. The half-life of circulating vitamin K–dependent clotting factors ranges from 6 hours (factor VII) to 50 hours (factor II). Therefore the maximal effect of warfarin is not observed until 3 to 5 days after therapy is started. Patients with acute thromboembolic disorders can be initially treated with a low-molecular-weight heparin (LMWH) plus warfarin, and the LMWH is then withdrawn after warfarin becomes effective. A period of several days is also required for coagulation factor levels to return to normal after warfarin has been discontinued. The recovery of clotting factors can be accelerated by administration of **phytonadione (vitamin K₁),** as described later.

Adverse Effects and Interactions

The most common adverse effect of warfarin is **bleeding** (Table 16.3), which can range in severity from mild nosebleed to life-threatening hemorrhage. Patients should be

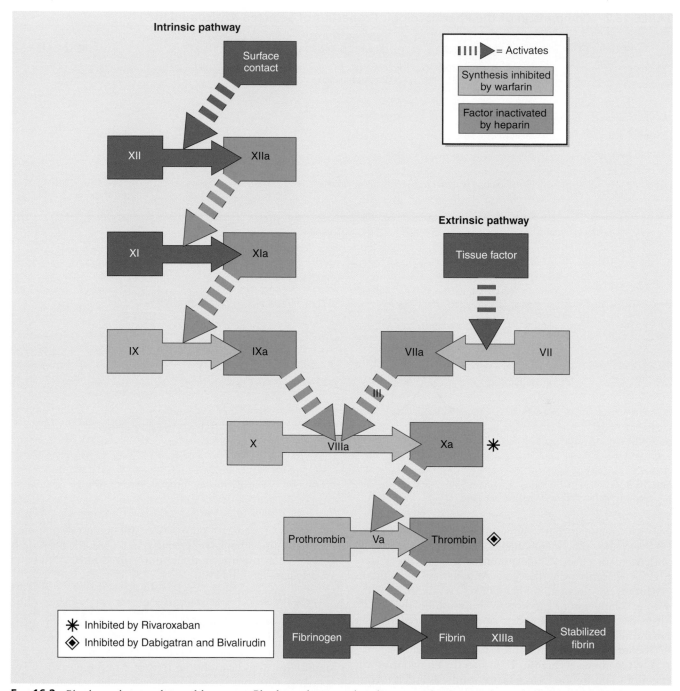

FIG. 16.2 Blood coagulation and sites of drug action. Blood coagulation involves the sequential activation of proteolytic clotting factors. The intrinsic pathway can be activated by surface contact with a foreign body, whereas the extrinsic pathway is activated by tissue factor. The pathways converge with the activation of factor X, which leads to the formation of thrombin and fibrin. Warfarin inhibits the synthesis of the vitamin K–dependent clotting factors. Heparin inactivates various clotting factors. Rivaroxaban inhibits active factor X. Dabigatran and bivalirudin inhibit thrombin.

instructed to report any signs of bleeding, including hematuria and bleeding into the skin **(ecchymoses).**

Warfarin is **contraindicated in pregnancy** because of its potential to cause fetal hemorrhage and various structural malformations referred to as the **fetal warfarin syndrome.** These malformations are partly a result of antagonism of vitamin K–dependent maturation of bone proteins during a process in which these proteins are carboxylated in the same manner as the nascent clotting factors. Warfarin and other vitamin K antagonists block this process and can cause bone deformities and various birth defects that are listed in Table 4.6.

Warfarin interacts with many drugs that either induce or inhibit cytochrome P450 (CYP) enzymes, whereas a few interactions result from antagonism or potentiation of its anticoagulant effect. The most serious interactions are with drugs that **increase the anticoagulant effect** and place the patient at risk of hemorrhage. Because the number of drugs that interact with warfarin is large, patients who are taking this drug should consult a health care provider before starting or discontinuing any other medication.

High doses of **salicylates** reduce prothrombin levels and thereby increase the anticoagulant effect of warfarin. In

TABLE 16.2 Comparison of the Pharmacologic Properties of Selected Anticoagulants

PROPERTY	WARFARIN	HEPARIN AND RELATED DRUGS	DABIGATRAN ETEXILATE	RIVAROXABAN
Mechanism	Vitamin K antagonist	Potentiator of antithrombin III	Direct thrombin inhibitor	Active factor X inhibitor
Active in vitro	No	Yes	No (a prodrug)	Yes
Route of administration	Oral	Parenteral	Oral	Oral
Onset of action	Delayed	Immediate	Immediate	Immediate
Safe to take during pregnancy	No	Yes	Safety not established	Safety not established
Antidote	Phytonadione (vitamin K₁)	Protamine sulfate	Idarucizumab (Praxbind)	Active factor VII or prothrombin complex concentrate

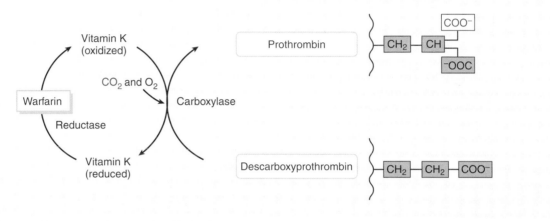

Fig. 16.3 Mechanisms of action of warfarin. Warfarin blocks the reduction of oxidized vitamin K (vitamin K epoxide) and thereby prevents vitamin K–dependent carboxylation of clotting factors.

contrast, treatment with **rifampin** or **barbiturates** induces CYP enzymes that metabolize warfarin and decreases its anticoagulant effect. **Cholestyramine** inhibits the absorption of warfarin from the gut. Amiodarone, cimetidine, erythromycin, fluconazole, gemfibrozil, isoniazid, metronidazole, sulfinpyrazone, and other drugs inhibit the metabolism of warfarin and increase the risk of bleeding. The **prothrombin time** (PT) should be monitored when adding or discontinuing drugs that interact with warfarin.

Phytonadione (vitamin K₁) directly **antagonizes** the effect of warfarin on clotting factor synthesis and is used to treat hemorrhage caused by anticoagulant activity.

Indications

Warfarin is primarily used in the long-term treatment of thromboembolic disorders such as **deep vein thrombosis** (DVT) and for prevention of thrombosis in patients with **atrial fibrillation** or an **artificial heart valve** (Table 16.4). It has also been used with a heparin-type anticoagulant for the treatment of **MI.** The goals of warfarin therapy are to prevent thrombus formation or expansion and to prevent embolization and potentially fatal consequences of thrombosis.

The dosage of warfarin is based on the patient's PT. This measurement is determined by drawing a blood sample, adding a **tissue thromboplastin** preparation to initiate coagulation, and comparing the clotting time of the patient's blood

with that of a control preparation. When an international reference thromboplastin preparation is used, the PT ratio is expressed as the **international normalized ratio** (INR) and is calculated as follows:

$$INR = (PT_{observed}/PT_{control})^{ISI}$$

where the $PT_{observed}$ and $PT_{control}$ are the PTs of the patient and control samples, respectively, and the ISI is the international sensitivity index of the thromboplastin reagent. For most clinical indications, an INR of 2 to 3 is desirable. For patients with mechanical prosthetic heart valves and for those with recurrent systemic embolization, an INR of 3 to 4.5 is recommended.

The patient's PT should be monitored daily during the initiation of warfarin therapy and whenever another drug is added to or withdrawn from the treatment regimen. Concurrent heparin therapy can increase the PT 10% to 20%, and the target INR levels should be increased by the same amount. Once the patient's INR has stabilized, it should be monitored every 4 to 6 weeks.

Treatment of Bleeding

If bleeding occurs, warfarin should be withheld until the bleeding can be evaluated and the patient's INR can be determined. The treatment of bleeding can include a reduction in drug dosage and the administration of **phytonadione (vitamin K₁).** If bleeding is serious or if the INR is markedly

TABLE 16.3   Adverse Effects and Drug Interactions of Antithrombotic Drugs

DRUG	COMMON ADVERSE EFFECTS	COMMON DRUG INTERACTIONS
Anticoagulants		
Warfarin	Birth defects and bleeding	Serum levels altered by drugs that induce or inhibit cytochrome P450, by drugs that inhibit gut absorption, and by drugs that directly increase or decrease the anticoagulant effect.
Rivaroxaban	Bleeding	Serum levels increased by cytochrome P450 3A4 inhibitors and by drugs that inhibit P-glycoprotein (Pgp) drug transport.
Dalteparin, enoxaparin	Bleeding and thrombocytopenia	Risk of bleeding increased by salicylates.
Heparin	Bleeding, hyperkalemia, and thrombocytopenia	Same as dalteparin.
Bivalirudin, dabigatran	Bleeding	Same as dalteparin.
Antiplatelet Drugs		
Abciximab, eptifibatide, tirofiban	Bleeding and thrombocytopenia	Antithrombotic effects increased by anticoagulants and other antiplatelet drugs.
Aspirin	Gastrointestinal irritation and bleeding, hypersensitivity reactions, and tinnitus	Increases hypoglycemic effect of sulfonylureas. Increases risk of gastrointestinal bleeding and ulceration associated with methotrexate, valproate, and other drugs. Inhibits uricosuric effect of probenecid.
Dipyridamole	Gastrointestinal distress, headache, mild and transient dizziness, and rash	Decreases metabolism of adenosine. Increases risk of bradycardia associated with β-adrenergic receptor antagonists.
Clopidogrel	Bleeding, diarrhea, gastrointestinal pain, increased cholesterol and triglyceride levels, nausea, and neutropenia	Increases levels of drugs metabolized by liver microsomal enzymes.
Vorapaxar	Bleeding risk, anemia, and depression	Avoid use with strong CYP3A inhibitors or inducer.
Thrombolytic Drugs		
Alteplase[a]	Bleeding, hypersensitivity reactions, and reperfusion arrhythmias	Increases risk of bleeding associated with anticoagulant and antiplatelet drugs.

aAlso anistreplase, reteplase, streptokinase, and tenecteplase.

TABLE 16.4   Clinical Uses of Antithrombotic Agents

CLINICAL USE	PRIMARY DRUGS
Venous Thromboembolism	
Acute	LMWH, fondaparinux, or direct-acting oral anticoagulant (rivaroxaban, apixaban)
Surgical prophylaxis	LMWH, fondaparinux, or rivaroxaban
Long-term prophylaxis	Warfarin or other oral anticoagulant (rivaroxaban, apixaban, edoxaban, dabigatran)
Pulmonary embolism	Heparin or LMWH, thrombolytic drug, direct-acting oral anticoagulant
Acute Coronary Syndromes	
Unstable angina and non-STE ACS	Aspirin ± clopidogrel or prasugrel; eptifibatide or tirofiban; LMWH or fondaparinux
STEMI	Thrombolytic drug, aspirin, and LMWH
Angioplasty and stent insertion	LMWH or bivalirudin ± abciximab, or eptifibatide; also aspirin, clopidogrel, or prasugrel
Stroke, Thrombotic	
Acute	Heparin or LMWH, thrombolytic drug, aspirin
Prophylaxis, including transient ischemic attacks	Clopidogrel or prasugrel; aspirin plus dipyridamole
Atrial fibrillation	Heparin or LMWH followed by warfarin, dabigatran, or rivaroxaban
Artificial heart valve	Warfarin, aspirin

LMWH, Low-molecular-weight heparin; *non-STE ACS*, non–ST segment elevation acute coronary syndrome; *STEMI*, ST segment elevation myocardial infarction.

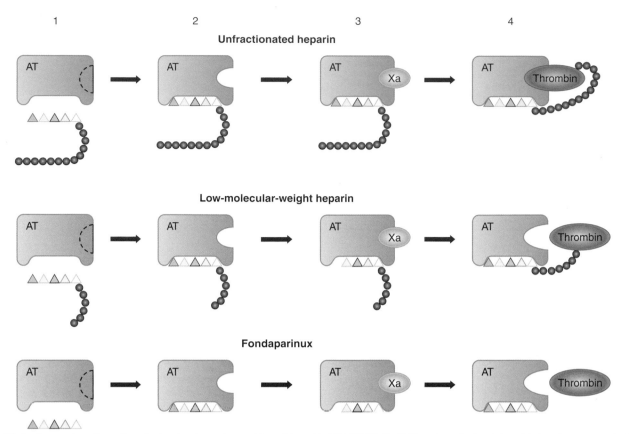

FIG. 16.4 Interaction of heparin and related anticoagulants with antithrombin III (AT-III). (*1, 2*) Heparin and related drugs bind to the pentasaccharide-binding site on AT-III. (*3*) Anticoagulant–AT-III complexes inactivate factor Xa (active Stuart factor). (*4*) Unfractionated heparin–AT-III also inactivates thrombin, whereas low-molecular-weight heparin–AT-III and fondaparinux–AT-III produce little or no inactivation of thrombin, respectively.

elevated (>20), fresh plasma or factor IX concentrate can be administered to rapidly replace clotting factors.

Heparin and Related Drugs

The heparin family of anticoagulants includes unfractionated heparin, LMWHs, and **fondaparinux.** In its natural form, **heparin** contains fractions with high molecular weights ranging from 5000 to 30,000 and fractions with low molecular weights ranging from 2000 to 9000. Enoxaparin and dalteparin are low-molecular-weight fractions that have been developed for clinical use. **Fondaparinux** is a synthetic pentasaccharide whose structure, mechanism, and effects are similar to those of other heparin-type drugs.

Chemistry and Mechanisms

Heparin is a mixture of sulfated mucopolysaccharides found in mast cells, basophils, and the vascular endothelium. For pharmaceutical use, it is obtained from porcine intestine or bovine lung.

As shown in Fig. 16.2, heparin inactivates clotting factors by potentiating the activity of a circulating endogenous anticoagulant called **antithrombin III** (AT-III), which is a powerful inhibitor of active factor II (thrombin) and active factor X (Stuart factor). The activation of AT-III by a heparin-containing pentasaccharide is illustrated in Fig. 16.4.

In contrast to unfractionated heparin, enoxaparin and dalteparin primarily inactivate **active factor X** because the LMWH–AT-III complex has less affinity for thrombin than the heparin–AT-III complex. **Fondaparinux** is an even more selective inhibitor of active factor X (see Fig. 16.4).

Pharmacokinetic and Pharmacologic Effects

Heparin and related anticoagulants are not absorbed from the gut and must be given parenterally. Heparin is usually administered by continuous intravenous infusion. It is removed from the circulation by the reticuloendothelial system, is eliminated from the body by renal and hepatic mechanisms, and has a half-life of approximately 90 minutes. The dosage of heparin is monitored using the **activated partial thromboplastin time** (aPTT) and is considered adequate when the aPTT is 1.5 to 2 times normal.

Enoxaparin and **dalteparin** are administered subcutaneously, and their maximal effect occurs 3 to 5 hours after injection. When these agents are used, the aPTT does not need to be monitored because the anticoagulant activity of LMWH is more predictable than the activity of unfractionated heparin.

Adverse Effects and Interactions

Adverse effects and drug interactions are listed in Table 16.3. The most common adverse effect of fractionated and unfractionated heparin is bleeding due to excessive anticoagulation.

Heparin can also cause two types of **heparin-induced thrombocytopenia** (HIT). Type 1 HIT, which occurs in approximately 25% of patients treated with heparin, is caused by a direct interaction between heparin and platelets, leading to platelet aggregation. Type 1 HIT is usually mild and is reversible within 4 days despite continued heparin treatment. Type 2 HIT is a much less common but more serious condition caused by immunoglobulin-mediated platelet inactivation. This type of HIT has a high risk of thrombotic complications and mortality. Heparin must be discontinued if type 2 HIT occurs.

Heparin occasionally causes **hyperkalemia** because of the suppression of aldosterone secretion.

Indications

Heparin is indicated for the treatment of **acute thromboembolic disorders,** including peripheral and PE, venous thrombosis, and coagulopathies such as disseminated intravascular coagulation. It is used prophylactically to prevent clotting in **arterial and heart surgery,** during **blood transfusions,** and in **renal dialysis** and **blood sample collection.** Heparin is also used to prevent embolization of thrombi that might cause a cerebrovascular event in patients with **acute atrial fibrillation.** Low doses of heparin can be administered subcutaneously to prevent **DVT** and **PE** in high-risk patients.

Enoxaparin and dalteparin are used to prevent **venous thromboembolism** associated with abdominal surgery or knee- or hip-replacement surgery, and in other conditions that place patients at risk for thrombosis. The drugs are administered once before surgery and for 5 to 10 days after surgery. Enoxaparin and dalteparin are also approved to prevent ischemic complications of unstable angina or non–ST segment elevation MI, and they are used in **acute coronary syndrome** (ACS) and **angioplasty.** Enoxaparin is approved for the treatment of DVT and to prevent thromboembolism caused by severely restricted mobility during acute illness.

Fondaparinux is administered subcutaneously for the prophylaxis of DVT in patients having hip fracture or hip-replacement surgery or knee-replacement surgery.

Treatment of Bleeding

The treatment of bleeding caused by unfractionated or LMWH consists of administering **protamine sulfate,** which is a positively charged protein that binds to negatively charged heparin and inactivates it. Protamine sulfate is administered intravenously for this purpose, and the dosage is based on the estimated amount of residual heparin in the body. Measurement of the aPTT 2 to 4 hours after administration is used to guide the need for further protamine treatment. Severe bleeding caused by heparin-type drugs may require the administration of fresh plasma or clotting factors.

Direct Thrombin Inhibitors

The direct thrombin inhibitors include bivalirudin, argatroban, and dabigatran.

Bivalirudin and Argatroban

Bivalirudin is a synthetic derivative of hirudin, a mixture of polypeptides produced in the salivary gland of the medicinal leech, *Hirudo medicinalis.* Because of its peptide structure, bivalirudin is administered intravenously and cannot be given orally because it would be degraded in the gastrointestinal tract. **Bivalirudin binds directly to thrombin** and does not require AT-III as a cofactor, which probably explains why it has a more predictable anticoagulant effect than heparin. Bivalirudin has been used to prevent thrombosis in patients with **unstable angina** and **acute MI,** including those undergoing coronary angioplasty and stent insertion, and clinical trials have established its efficacy and safety. As with other anticoagulants, the most serious adverse effect

of bivalirudin is bleeding. Unlike heparin, it does not cause thrombocytopenia.

Argatroban is a synthetic direct thrombin inhibitor given intravenously for the prophylaxis and treatment of thrombosis in patients with **HIT,** including persons undergoing percutaneous coronary interventions (PCIs) for MI.

Dabigatran

Dabigatran achieved fame as the first new oral anticoagulant to be developed in 50 years, opening the era of orally effective, direct-acting anticoagulants.

Pharmacokinetics. Dabigatran is administered orally as a **prodrug,** dabigatran etexilate, which is converted to dabigatran by esterases in the gut, blood, and liver. It has a half-life of approximately 13 hours and is primarily eliminated by renal excretion of unchanged dabigatran, with approximately 20% excreted after conjugation with glucuronide. Renal impairment prolongs the half-life of the drug, which increases to more than 24 hours if the creatinine clearance decreases to less than 30 mL/min, and doses should be reduced in proportion to the degree of renal dysfunction. Steady-state plasma levels are achieved approximately 3 days after starting therapy.

Mechanism and Effects. Dabigatran is a potent, competitive, reversible inhibitor of **thrombin,** the protease enzyme that converts fibrinogen to fibrin in the final step of blood coagulation. The drug prevents thrombin-activation of platelets, as well as the cross-linking of fibrin monomers. Dabigatran binds to thrombin's active site and inhibits both fibrin-bound and unbound (free) thrombin. This is an advantage over heparin-type drugs that inhibit only free thrombin. Dabigatran's anticoagulant effect is best measured by the **thrombin clotting time** (TT), which assesses the activity of thrombin in a plasma sample. It has little effect on the PT and INR, which measure the extrinsic coagulation pathway.

Indications. Dabigatran is used to reduce the risk of stroke and PE in patients with **nonvalvular atrial fibrillation.** The Randomized Evaluation of Long-term Anticoagulant Therapy (RE-LY) study found that dabigatran was associated with a lower rate of stroke and intracranial bleeding than was warfarin in patients with this condition. Dabigatran may also be preferred because it does not interact with food and most other drugs and does not require laboratory monitoring. Dabigatran is an alternative to warfarin for patients who have been poorly controlled or not well monitored. It is also indicated for treatment and prevention of **DVT** and **PE** in patients who have been treated with a parenteral anticoagulant for 5 to 10 days and for prevention of DVT in those undergoing **hip-replacement surgery.**

Adverse Effects. As with other antithrombotic agents, dabigatran **increases the risk of bleeding** at several sites in the body, including the gastrointestinal tract. Until recently, the lack of a specific reversal agent for dabigatran has been a persistent concern. Idarucizumab (Praxbind) is now available and approved to reverse dabigatran's anticoagulant effect in cases of life-threatening or uncontrolled bleeding or emergency surgery. **Idarucizumab is a monoclonal antibody drug** (Chapter 46) to dabigatran that immediately inactivates it after intravenous administration. Patients should also receive activated charcoal orally and an antifibrinolytic agent such as aminocaproic acid (see later).

Dabigatran also causes **gastrointestinal complaints** such as dyspepsia and gastritis, which may be minimized by taking the drug with food or a histamine H_2 blocker such as famotidine (see Chapter 28).

Interactions. **Dabigatran** etexilate is a substrate for the **P-glycoprotein (Pgp)** transporter (see Chapter 2) in the gut and kidneys, and it should not be coadministered with rifampin and other inducers of Pgp. Dabigatran etexilate can be given to patients taking **Pgp inhibitors** such as verapamil, amiodarone, quinidine, and clarithromycin, but these drugs should be given 2 or more hours before or after dabigatran.

Active Factor X Inhibitors

Apixaban, edoxaban, and **rivaroxaban** are orally administered inhibitors of active factor X (Xa). In the coagulation pathway, Xa is formed at the convergence of the extrinsic and intrinsic pathways, where Xa combines with factor Va to form a prothrombinase complex that converts prothrombin to thrombin (see Fig. 16.2). The drugs bind to the active catalytic site of Xa, inhibiting the activity of both free Xa and that of the prothrombinase complex. Unfortunately, clotting time tests such as the PT are not useful in monitoring the anticoagulant effects of these drugs.

The active factor X inhibitors are used to reduce the risk of **stroke** and **systemic embolization** in persons with **nonvalvular atrial fibrillation,** as well as for prevention of **DVT** and **PE** in persons undergoing **knee- or hip-replacement surgery.** They are also approved for treatment of DVT and PE and to decrease the risk of recurrences of DVT and PE in persons with previous episodes. For the treatment of PE, the drugs are usually given after 5 to 10 days of parenteral anticoagulant therapy. Apixaban and rivaroxaban have been used alone for the initial treatment of DVT.

A meta-analysis of clinical studies concluded that active factor X inhibitors were as effective as warfarin in the prevention and treatment of DVT and PE, while causing significantly fewer episodes of bleeding. Factor Xa inhibitors have a rapid onset of action and do not require laboratory monitoring and individual dose adjustments as is the case with warfarin. In other studies, knee- and hip-replacement patients taking rivaroxaban had fewer episodes of DVT than those taking enoxaparin.

Bleeding is the most common adverse effect of apixaban, edoxaban, and rivaroxaban, and there are no reversal agents available for these agents. Experts suggest administering coagulation factor preparations such as prothrombin complex concentrate, activated prothrombin complex concentrate, or recombinant factor VIIa in cases of severe hemorrhage caused by factor Xa inhibitors, although clinical evidence of effectiveness is not yet available. A **universal antidote** for factor Xa inhibitors called **r-Antidote** is currently under development. It consists of recombinant proteins with a similar structure to factor Xa that bind and rapidly inactivate factor Xa inhibitors but lack enzymatic activity.

Specific Agents

Rivaroxaban is well absorbed after oral administration with a bioavailability of 80% to 100%. It is largely metabolized by P450 isozymes, particularly 3A4, before renal excretion, and dosage adjustments should be considered in patients taking strong 3A4 inhibitors. For prophylaxis of DVT, rivaroxaban is given once a day for 12 days after knee-replacement surgery or 35 days after hip-replacement surgery. When switching patients from warfarin, rivaroxaban should be started when the INR decreases to less than 3.

Apixaban has an oral bioavailability greater than 50%, with a plasma half-life of 8 to 14 hours. It is taken orally twice a day and is eliminated by several routes, including oxidative metabolism and renal and intestinal excretion. Potent inhibitors of CYP3A4 and Pgp are contraindicated with apixaban because they increase plasma drug concentrations. **Edoxaban** is given once daily and has an oral bioavailability of 60%. It is eliminated primarily by renal excretion of the unchanged drug, and it does not inhibit or induce P450 enzymes or Pgp. Edoxaban should not be used in patients with nonvalvular atrial fibrillation whose creatinine clearance is greater than 95 mL/min, because clinical studies have shown an increased risk of ischemic stroke in these patients compared with those taking warfarin. The newest addition to the family of –aban active factor X inhibitors is **betrizaban**. Patients taking betrizaban showed a significant reduction in the incidence of DVT compared with those taking enoxaparin.

ANTIPLATELET DRUGS

The process of platelet aggregation and the sites of antiplatelet drug action are depicted in Fig. 16.5. Platelets bind to the damaged vascular endothelium by the adhesion of platelet **glycoprotein (GP) 1a receptors** to exposed collagen, and adhesion of **platelet GP-1b** receptors via von Willebrand factor, to the injured vascular endothelium. The adherence of platelets to vascular endothelium leads to the synthesis and release of several mediators of platelet aggregation, including **thromboxane A2** (TXA$_2$), **adenosine diphosphate** (ADP), and **5-hydroxytryptamine (serotonin).** These mediators evoke intracellular calcium release that triggers the calcium-dependent association of **GP-2b** and **GP-3a receptors,** enabling the GP-2b/3a complex to bind fibrinogen and cause platelet aggregation. **Aspirin** and **clopidogrel** inhibit the synthesis or release of specific mediators of platelet aggregation, whereas **abciximab, tirofiban,** and **eptifibatide** directly bind and inactivate GP-2b/3a receptors. A new agent called **vorapaxar** blocks PAR-1 receptors to prevent thrombin action on the platelet (see Fig. 16.5).

Aspirin

Aspirin is a **nonsteroidal antiinflammatory drug (NSAID)** that has analgesic, antipyretic, and antiinflammatory effects (see Chapter 30). It also inhibits platelet aggregation and is used to prevent and treat arterial thromboembolic disorders.

Mechanisms and Pharmacologic Effects

Aspirin and other NSAIDs inhibit the synthesis of prostaglandins from arachidonic acid. The most important prostaglandins affecting platelet aggregation are **prostacyclin** (also called *prostaglandin I$_2$* [PGI$_2$]) and **TXA2. Prostacyclin** is synthesized by vascular endothelial cells and inhibits platelet aggregation, whereas **TXA2** is synthesized by platelets and promotes platelet aggregation. Under normal conditions, prostacyclin serves to prevent platelet aggregation and thrombosis, whereas TXA$_2$ becomes predominant during thrombus formation.

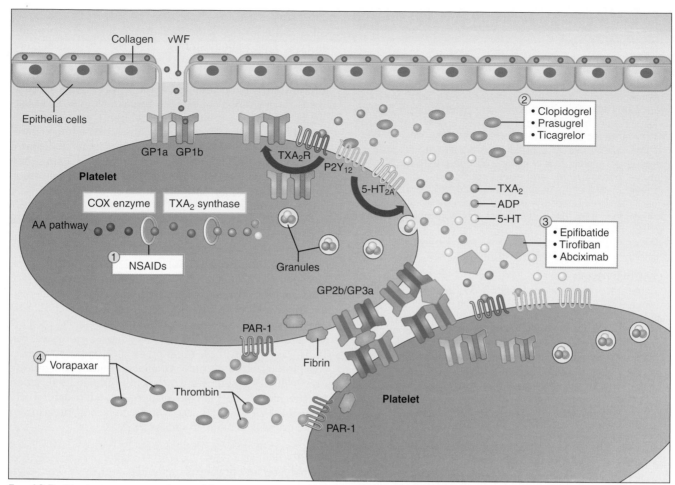

Fig. 16.5 Platelet aggregation and sites of drug action. Platelets adhere to damaged endothelium via linkage of glycoprotein (GP)-1a receptors with exposed collagen and via linkage of GP-1b receptors with von Willebrand factor. This activates the platelets and leads to the synthesis and release (degranulation) of various mediators of platelet aggregation, including thromboxane A_2, adenosine diphosphate (ADP), and 5-hydroxytryptamine (or serotonin), which interact at their target receptors on the platelets. These mediators increase the expression of GP receptors and promote platelet aggregation via the binding of fibrinogen to GP-2b/3a receptors. (1) Nonsteroidal antiinflammatory drugs inhibit the synthesis of thromboxane A_2 by blocking cyclooxygenase. (2) Clopidogrel, prasugrel, ticagrelor, and others block the target of ADP, the purine $2Y_{12}$ receptor. (3) Epifibatide, tirofiban, abciximab, and other agents bind to GP-2b/GP3a proteins and prevent fibrinogen cross-linking of platelets. (4) Vorapaxar is an antagonist at protease-activated receptor-1, which is the target of thrombin on platelets. Not shown are dipyridamole, which inhibits the reuptake of adenosine, increasing adenosine A_2 receptors that are positively coupled to adenylate cyclase, increasing cyclic adenosine monophosphate (cAMP) and phosphate, reducing calcium, and decreasing platelet aggregation. Also not shown is the mechanism of cilostazol, which inhibits type 3 phosphodiesterase and increases cAMP levels.

Low doses of aspirin have been found to selectively **inhibit the synthesis of TXA2** without having as much effect on prostacyclin, whereas higher doses inhibit the synthesis of both prostaglandins. Hence the dosage of aspirin used to inhibit platelet aggregation is usually lower than that used for other pharmacologic effects. Unlike other NSAIDs, aspirin **irreversibly inhibits cyclooxygenase,** the enzyme that catalyzes an early step in TXA_2 synthesis. For this reason, aspirin inhibits platelet aggregation for the life of the platelet and effectively reduces platelet aggregation when administered once a day or every other day.

Indications

Aspirin is often used to prevent arterial thrombosis in patients with ischemic heart disease and stroke, but it has many other indications as well. In patients with a previous **MI** or **stroke,** it has been shown to significantly reduce the risk of a second heart attack or stroke (secondary prevention). Aspirin has also been shown to prevent MI in persons with **coronary artery disease.** However, the evidence for its value in preventing a first stroke or MI (primary prevention) in healthy individuals is less compelling. Some authorities recommend that aspirin be used for primary prevention only in men older than 45 years of age and women older than 55 years of age who have other risk factors for heart disease, because the risk of aspiring-induced bleeding appears to be greater than the benefit obtained. However, many clinicians believe that this risk is justified.

Aspirin is given to patients with acute **MI** (Box 16.1) to prevent enlargement of a coronary thrombus and reduce the severity of cardiac damage. In patients with **transient ischemic attacks,** it can be used to prevent an initial or subsequent stroke. In patients who have **artificial heart valves** or are undergoing **percutaneous coronary angioplasty,** it is used with other drugs to prevent thrombosis. Aspirin is also used to treat persons with peripheral arterial occlusive disease and chronic limb ischemia.

Adverse Effects and Interactions

Aspirin can cause bleeding, especially in the **gastrointestinal tract,** where it inhibits the synthesis of prostaglandins

BOX 16.1 A CASE OF CRUSHING CHEST PAIN

CASE PRESENTATION

A 61-year-old man arrived in the emergency department with crushing chest pain at rest, which had begun an hour previously. He had a history of hypertension treated with hydrochlorothiazide. His vital signs included a blood pressure of 142/92 mm Hg and a heart rate of 88 beats/min. The electrocardiogram showed a 2-mm ST segment elevation in the anterior leads. The man was promptly treated with aspirin and three sublingual doses of nitroglycerin at 5-minute intervals followed by a continuous nitroglycerin intravenous infusion, and metoprolol and morphine by intravenous injection. Because the ST segment elevation and chest pain continued, the patient received clopidogrel and enoxaparin, and then fibrinolysis was accomplished with tenecteplase. He was placed on metoprolol, lisinopril, and clopidogrel and was subsequently transferred to another hospital for angiography and further treatment.

CASE DISCUSSION

There are an estimated 500,000 ST segment elevation myocardial infarction (STEMI) events in the United States annually. The immediate treatment of STEMI includes aspirin to slow progression of coronary thrombosis and nitroglycerin to reduce myocardial oxygen demand, ischemia, and infarct size. The most important objective is restoration of coronary blood flow as soon as possible, and patients with STEMI typically receive thrombolytic therapy or undergo a percutaneous coronary intervention (PCI) (angioplasty with or without stent insertion). For patients who come to hospitals without facilities for PCIs, fibrinolysis with a drug such as tenecteplase is the most viable option. Studies show that clopidogrel and enoxaparin reduce cardiovascular mortality in persons undergoing fibrinolysis or angioplasty. Angiotensin inhibitors may improve left ventricular function in STEMI patients, and β-adrenoceptor antagonists reduce secondary cardiovascular events and mortality.

that promote secretion of bicarbonate and mucus. These substances protect the gastric mucosa from the potentially damaging effects of stomach acid and pepsin. High doses of aspirin and other salicylates may cause **hypoprothrombinemia** and thereby increase the likelihood of bleeding. Other adverse effects of aspirin are discussed in Chapter 30, and interactions are listed in Table 16.3.

Dipyridamole

Dipyridamole is a **coronary vasodilator** and a relatively **weak antiplatelet drug.** It inhibits platelet aggregation by blocking platelet uptake of **adenosine,** leading to increased activation of platelet adenosine A_2 receptors that are positively coupled with adenylate cyclase. This action increases platelet **cyclic adenosine monophosphate (cAMP)** levels, which reduces calcium release and decreases platelet aggregation. The drug has a limited role in the treatment of thromboembolic disorders. A product containing dipyridamole and aspirin (AGGRENOX) has been shown to be more **effective for stroke prevention** than either drug alone, but a study of thousands of patients with ischemic stroke found that AGGRENOX was no more effective than **clopidogrel** for stroke prevention but **caused more major bleeding** episodes.

As a vasodilator, dipyridamole is used during **myocardial perfusion imaging (thallium imaging)** to dilate and evaluate the arteries of patients with coronary artery disease.

Cilostazol

Cilostazol is a vasodilator and antiplatelet drug that **inhibits type 3 phosphodiesterase** (PDE_3) and the breakdown of cAMP, thereby increasing **cAMP levels** in platelets and blood vessels. The drug is indicated for the treatment of **intermittent claudication,** a form of peripheral vascular disease characterized by pain and weakness in a limb leading to limping or lameness. Intermittent claudication is caused by arterial occlusion, and catheter-based procedures to remove arterial blockage are sometimes useful. **Cilostazol can improve blood flow and reduce muscle pain** while increasing walking distance in persons with this disorder. Following oral administration, the drug is metabolized by CYP3A4, and inhibitors of this enzyme such as erythromycin may increase its effects. Headache is the most common side effect of cilostazol.

Adenosine Diphosphate Inhibitors

Mechanism and Effects

Clopidogrel and related drugs block endogenous **adenosine diphosphate (ADP)** from binding to platelet **P2Y12 receptors,** which inhibits activation of GP-2b/3a receptors and prevents ADP-induced platelet aggregation (see Fig. 16.5). As a result, these drugs prevent thrombus formation and prolong bleeding time. **Clopidogrel** and **prasugrel** are irreversible $P2Y_{12}$ antagonists that inhibit platelet function for the life of the platelet. **Cangrelor** and **ticagrelor** are reversible $P2Y_{12}$ antagonists, which can be advantageous in patients about to undergo surgery or PCIs.

Pharmacokinetics

Clopidogrel and **prasugrel** are orally administered prodrugs metabolized to active antiplatelet metabolites by P450 enzymes. **Ticagrelor** does not require activation and has a more rapid onset of action. **Prasugrel** has a more rapid onset of action than clopidogrel because of faster conversion to its active metabolite, and it produces a higher and more consistent level of platelet inhibition than clopidogrel.

Indications

Clopidogrel, prasugrel, and ticagrelor are used for **prevention of thrombosis and MI** in persons with ACSs, including those with unstable angina. For ACSs, drug selection and use are based on the severity of the patient's condition and whether the patient is being managed with pharmacotherapy alone, or with angioplasty and stent insertion as well. In general, the risk of drug-induced bleeding has been found to increase in proportion to drug effectiveness in preventing thrombosis.

Clopidogrel and other ADP-blocking drugs have been shown to reduce **thrombosis and MI** in persons with ACS who are undergoing angioplasty and coronary artery stent insertion. Drug treatment is usually continued for at least 4 weeks after implantation of a bare metal stent and for 1 year in those with a drug-eluting stent. ADP-blocking drugs are sometimes **combined with aspirin** for long-term prevention in persons with ACS, including those with unstable angina. Clinical trials have revealed some differences in the effectiveness and risk of bleeding of specific drugs, and the latest **guidelines should always be reviewed** when selecting drug therapy. For example, studies indicate that ticagrelor is superior to clopidogrel for prevention of stent thrombosis in patients with ACS. Parenteral antiplatelet drug therapy is also used during angioplasty and stent insertion, as described later.

Clopidogrel is also indicated for secondary **stroke prevention,** alone or in combination with aspirin, although combination therapy may not be more effective and increases the risk of bleeding. Clopidogrel is also used to prevent thrombosis in patients with intermittent claudication, chronic arterial occlusion, atrioventricular shunts or fistulas, and open heart surgery.

Ticlopidine is similar to the previously mentioned PY12 receptor blockers. **Cangrelor** is used as an adjunct to PCI to reduce the risk of thrombotic events during and after these procedures. It is given **intravenously** to patients who have not previously received a P2Y$_{12}$ blocker and who are not being given a GP-2b/3a inhibitor during PCI.

Adverse Effects and Interactions

As with aspirin, all the ADP blockers increase the risk of bleeding. In addition, ticagrelor may cause dyspnea. Because it can cause severe neutropenia, ticlopidine is rarely used nowadays.

The activation of clopidogrel by CYP2C19 is inhibited by **proton pump inhibitors (PPIs),** particularly omeprazole, that are used in treating peptic ulcer (see Chapter 28). It has been concluded that clopidogrel and PPIs may be used concurrently without significantly increasing the risk of thrombotic events, but it seems advisable to avoid omeprazole and use dexlansoprazole or another PPI in these patients. Prasugrel is activated primarily by CYP3A4 and CYP2B6 and is not significantly affected by PPIs.

Glycoprotein-2b/3a Antagonists

The final common pathway in platelet aggregation is the **cross-linking of platelets by fibrinogen,** which binds to an activated GP-2b/3a complex on the platelet surface (see Fig. 16.5). The GP-2b/3a complex is a type of **integrin.** Integrins are cell surface transmembrane glycoproteins that function as adhesion receptors to structurally link the cell surface to the cytoskeleton. Antiplatelet effects can be exerted by direct binding of the GP-2b/3a receptors, as shown by the next drugs.

Abciximab

Abciximab was the first platelet GP-2b/3a antagonist to be developed. It consists of the Fab fragment of a chimeric human-murine **monoclonal antibody that binds tightly to platelet GP-2b/3a receptors, preventing fibrinogen binding** and cross-linking of platelets. Abciximab infusion should be stopped 12 hours before surgery because it takes this long for receptor occupancy to decline by 50%.

Abciximab is used to **prevent platelet aggregation** and **thrombosis** in patients undergoing **PCIs,** including coronary angioplasty and stent placement. In this setting, it is administered in combination with aspirin and heparin or LMWH. Abciximab has been shown to **significantly prevent vessel restenosis, reinfarction, and death.** It has also been used as an adjunct to thrombolysis with alteplase and similar drugs (see the discussion of thrombolytic drugs).

The most common adverse effect of abciximab is **bleeding.** Other adverse reactions include **thrombocytopenia** in 5% of patients, as well as hypotension and bradycardia.

Tirofiban and Eptifibatide

Tirofiban and **eptifibatide** also prevent platelet aggregation by preventing fibrinogen cross-linking of platelets. Eptifibatide is a cyclic heptapeptide from rattlesnake venom, whereas tirofiban is a derivative of the amino acid tyrosine. These drugs are **competitive, reversible antagonists** of GP-2/3a receptors and bind receptors less strongly than abciximab. Hence they need to be discontinued only 2 hours before surgery. As with abciximab, these agents are given as an intravenous loading dose followed by a maintenance infusion.

Tirofiban and **eptifibatide** are used in two ways in persons with **unstable angina** and **MI:** (1) to prevent coronary thrombosis in persons with unstable angina or non–ST segment elevation (non–Q wave) MI and (2) to prevent thrombosis in persons having coronary angioplasty or stent placement for ST segment elevation MI. They are often combined with an LMWH in these settings, as well as oral antiplatelet agents.

Bleeding is the major adverse effect of tirofiban and eptifibatide. The incidence of intracranial bleeding and gastrointestinal or genitourinary bleeding caused by tirofiban in one study was 0.1% and 0.2%, respectively. These drugs cause less thrombocytopenia than does abciximab.

Vorapaxar

Vorapaxar is a new drug with a new mechanism of action in preventing platelet aggregation. It is a **protease-activated receptor-1 (PAR-1) antagonist** approved for patients with a history of MI or with peripheral arterial disease (PAD). By occupying the PAR-1 receptor, vorapaxar competitively **inhibits thrombin** access to its target receptor and prevents thrombin-mediated platelet aggregation. In clinical trials, vorapaxar **reduced thrombotic cardiovascular events** and **mortality.**

Thrombolytic Drugs

The breakdown of blood clots begins with the degradation of fibrin by the protease enzyme called plasmin. In this process, circulating **plasminogen** binds to fibrin in clots and is converted to **plasmin** by **tissue plasminogen activator (t-PA),** which is a protease enzyme found on vascular endothelial cells. Plasmin degrades both fibrin and fibrinogen and leads to clot dissolution as blood cells are released and recycled.

Pharmacologic Effects

The **thrombolytic drugs** include recombinant forms of human t-PA named **alteplase, reteplase,** and **tenecteplase,** as well as **streptokinase,** a protein obtained from streptococci, and **anistreplase,** a complex of streptokinase and plasminogen (Fig. 16.6). The recombinant forms of t-PA are active enzymes that convert plasminogen to plasmin and cause fibrinolysis. Streptokinase lacks protease activity and must form an activator complex with plasminogen that converts other plasminogen to plasmin. This complex is available for clinical use as a preparation called anistreplase. The recombinant forms of t-PA are moderately selective for fibrin-bound plasminogen, whereas streptokinase has low fibrin specificity and causes greater degradation of systemic fibrinogen. The properties of thrombolytic agents are listed in Table 16.5.

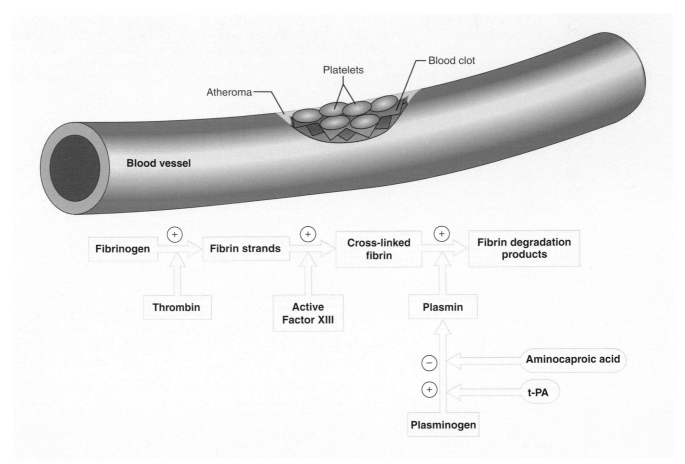

FIG. 16.6 Fibrin formation and fibrinolysis. Platelets adhere to an atheroma, and platelet-bound thrombin converts fibrinogen to fibrin strands, which are then cross-linked by factor XIII to form a stable clot with enmeshed platelets and erythrocytes. Fibrinolysis is catalyzed by plasmin, a proteolytic enzyme formed from plasminogen by tissue plasminogen activator. Plasmin is inhibited by aminocaproic acid and tranexamic acid. *Active factor XIII, fibrin stabilizing factor.*

TABLE 16.5 Properties of Thrombolytic Drugs

	STREPTOKINASE	ALTEPLASE	RETEPLASE	TENECTEPLASE
Administration	Infusion	Infusion	Bolus	Bolus
Allergic reactions	Yes	No	No	No
Systemic fibrinogen depletion	Marked	Mild	Moderate	Minimal
Fibrin specificity[a]	−	++	+	+++
TIMI coronary flow grade 2 out of 3[b]	55%	75%	83%	83%

TIMI, Thrombolysis in myocardial infarction trial.
[a]Fibrin specificity ranges from − (none) to +++ (very high).
[b]Percentage of patients in TIMI trial with a 2 out of 3 coronary blood flow grade after fibrinolysis.

Clinical Use

Thrombolytic drugs are usually administered by intravenous infusion to degrade thrombi in patients with **MI, thrombotic stroke,** or **PE,** and they are used to open thrombosed renal dialysis and central venous catheters. They have also been used in treating **venous thromboembolism,** such as in cases of extensive iliofemoral vein thrombosis, where catheter-directed thrombolysis is used as an adjunct to anticoagulants. For patients with ST segment elevation MI, thrombolytic drugs are used to restore coronary blood flow when patients are not eligible for angioplasty. Thrombolytic agents should be administered as soon as possible and preferably within 6 hours of symptom onset (see Box 16.1). PCIs such as angioplasty and stent insertion are generally preferred over thrombolytic therapy when they are available. A meta-analysis of clinical trials concluded that there is an overall benefit of PCI compared with thrombolytic treatment.

In patients with **acute ischemic stroke,** thrombolytic drugs such as alteplase reduce the incidence of neurologic sequelae and improve outcomes, but treatment must be initiated within 4.5 hours, and preferably within 3 hours, of symptom onset. Combined intravenous and catheter-based intra-arterial administration may be superior to intravenous therapy alone, and mechanical devices to produce embolectomy may provide additional benefits. Thrombolytic drugs are **contraindicated in hemorrhagic stroke** and in patients with any other form of major bleeding or a high risk of bleeding, including those with recent surgery or trauma.

The benefit of thrombolytic therapy for **PE** is uncertain, and treatment is usually reserved for patients who are hemodynamically unstable or whose thrombus does not resolve with anticoagulant therapy.

Adverse Effects and Interactions

Table 16.3 lists adverse effects and drug interactions of thrombolytic drugs. The most common adverse effect is bleeding, and it is important to recognize that these drugs can lyse both normal and pathologic thrombi. Because t-PA selectively activates plasminogen bound to fibrin, the recombinant forms of t-PA cause less bleeding than streptokinase. Arrhythmias (e.g., bradycardia and tachycardia) may occur in MI patients treated with thrombolytic drugs and are probably caused by free radicals generated during the reperfusion of the coronary artery after thrombolysis. Streptokinase can cause various types of hypersensitivity reactions, including fatal anaphylactic shock, and it should not be used repeatedly in the same patient.

Treatment of Bleeding

Aminocaproic acid and tranexamic acid are derivatives of the amino acid lysine. In the circulation, these drugs occupy lysine binding sites on plasmin and thereby prevent it from degrading fibrin. **Aminocaproic acid** is used to stop the bleeding caused by thrombolytic drugs, and it is also used to prevent bleeding in patients who have hemophilia or are recovering from gastrointestinal or prostate surgery. Aminocaproic acid can be administered orally or intravenously and is excreted by the kidneys. Its potential adverse effects include thrombosis, hypotension, and arrhythmias.

Tranexamic acid (LYSTEDA) is taken orally for the treatment of cyclic **heavy menstrual bleeding.** The major adverse effect of tranexamic acid is **thrombosis,** which is increased when hormonal contraceptives are used, especially in women who are obese and smoke cigarettes. Tranexamic acid is also available for injection (CYKLOKAPRON) in patients with hemophilia who need short-term treatment to prevent hemorrhage during and after tooth extraction.

SUMMARY OF IMPORTANT POINTS

- When a small blood vessel is injured, hemorrhage is prevented by the processes involved in normal hemostasis: vasospasm, platelet plug formation, and fibrin clot formation. After the vessel is repaired, the clot is removed via the process of fibrinolysis.
- Orally administered warfarin inhibits vitamin K–dependent synthesis of clotting factors II, VII, IX, and X.
- Heparin-type drugs potentiate inactivation of clotting factors by AT-III. Unfractionated heparin inactivates thrombin and active factor X, whereas LMWHs and fondaparinux primarily inactivate factor X. These drugs are used to prevent and treat venous thromboembolism.
- Bivalirudin is an intravenously administered direct thrombin inhibitor used in persons having coronary angioplasty.

- Dabigatran is an orally administered direct thrombin inhibitor indicated for preventing thromboembolism and stroke in patients with atrial fibrillation.
- Rivaroxaban, apixaban, and edoxaban are given orally to inhibit active factor X for prevention of DVT and PE in patients undergoing knee or hip surgery, and rivaroxaban is used for treatment of DVT.
- Oral antiplatelet drugs act by interfering with the synthesis or activity of mediators of platelet aggregation. Aspirin inhibits TXA_2 synthesis, whereas clopidogrel, prasugrel, and ticagrelor block ADP at $P2Y_{12}$ receptors. Abciximab, tirofiban, and eptifibatide are parenteral antiplatelet drugs that prevent the binding of fibrinogen to GP-2b/3a receptors and are used to prevent thrombosis in persons with ACSs.
- Thrombolytic drugs (e.g., alteplase, reteplase, and tenecteplase) convert plasminogen to plasmin and lead to fibrin degradation. These drugs are used to lyse clots in patients with MI, thrombotic stroke, or PE.
- All of the anticoagulant, antiplatelet, or thrombolytic drugs can cause bleeding. Phytonadione (vitamin K_1) is used to counteract bleeding caused by warfarin. Protamine sulfate is used to neutralize heparins, and aminocaproic acid is used to inhibit fibrinolysis. Idarucizumab (PRAXBIND) is used to treat bleeding caused by dabigatran.

Review Questions

For each drug description (1–4), select the correct drug from the following choices:

    (A) eptifibatide
    (B) prasugrel
    (C) dabigatran
    (D) rivaroxaban
    (E) enoxaparin

1. An orally administered drug that directly inhibits thrombin
2. This drug produces irreversible blockade of platelet adenosine diphosphate P2Y receptors
3. This orally administered inhibitor of active factor X (Stuart factor) is used to prevent and treat DVT
4. This drug is a reversible fibrinogen antagonist at GP-2b/3a receptors
5. Which antithrombotic drug is most likely to cause thrombocytopenia?
    (A) argatroban
    (B) heparin
    (C) tirofiban
    (D) bivalirudin
    (E) rivaroxaban
6. Idarucizumab is used to reverse the activity of which antithrombotic drug in cases of bleeding?
    (A) alteplase
    (B) warfarin
    (C) dalteparin
    (D) dabigatran
    (E) apixaban

CHAPTER 17

Hematopoietic Drugs

CLASSIFICATION OF HEMATOPOIETIC DRUGS

Minerals

- Ferrous sulfate[a]
- Iron dextran (PROFERDEX)[b]

Vitamins

- Folic acid
- Cyanocobalamin (vitamin B$_{12}$, NASCOBAL)
- Hydroxocobalamin (vitamin B$_{12}$, CYANOKIT)

Hematopoietic Growth Factors

Erythropoiesis-stimulating agents

- Epoetin alfa (EPOGEN, PROCRIT)
- Epoetin β (MIRCERA)
- Darbepoetin alfa (ARANESP)
- Methoxy polyethylene glycol-epoetin β (MIRCERA)
- Luspatercept (REBLOZYL)

Colony-stimulating factors

- Filgrastim (NEUPOGEN)[c]
- Pegfilgrastim (NEULASTA)
- Sargramostim (LEUKINE)

Thrombopoietin receptor agonists

- Romiplostim (NPLATE)
- Avatrombopag (DOPTELET)
- Eltrombopag (PROMACTA)

Interleukins

- Oprelvekin (NEUMEGA)

Drugs for Sickle Cell Disease

- Voxelotor (OXBRYTA)
- Crizanlizumab (Adakveo)
- Hydroxyurea (DROXIA)
- L-glutamine (ENDARI)

[a]Also ferrous fumarate, ferrous gluconate, and ferric maltol (ACCRUFER)
[b]Also iron sucrose (VENOFER) and sodium ferric gluconate (FERRLECIT).
[c]Also biosimilars filgrastim (ZARXIO), and filgrastim (GRANIX).

OVERVIEW

Mature blood cells are continuously formed in the bone marrow and are removed from the circulation by reticuloendothelial cells in the liver and spleen. The process by which blood cells are replaced is called **hematopoiesis.** This process requires minerals and vitamins and is regulated by **hematopoietic growth factors** that promote the differentiation and maturation of marrow stem cells to form leukocytes, erythrocytes, and platelets.

Anemia, a subnormal concentration of erythrocytes or hemoglobin in the blood, can result from inadequate erythropoiesis, blood loss, or accelerated hemolysis. Erythropoiesis can be impaired by a lack of essential nutrients, the myelosuppressive effects of certain drugs, or irradiation. Infection,

cancer, endocrine deficiencies, and chronic inflammation can also cause anemia. **Iron, folic acid,** and **vitamin B$_{12}$ deficiencies** are the most common causes of **nutritional anemia.**

This chapter describes the pharmacologic properties and uses of **minerals, vitamins,** and **hematopoietic growth factors** in the treatment of anemia and other blood cell deficiencies. Additionally, novel drugs for the treatment of **sickle cell disease** are also introduced. Table 17.1 lists selected hematopoietic drugs, their brand names, and their uses.

HEMATOPOIETIC DRUGS

Minerals

Iron, an essential dietary mineral, serves as an important component of hemoglobin, myoglobin, and a number of enzymes. The average dietary intake of iron is 18 to 20 mg/day, but people with normal iron stores absorb only about 10% of this amount. Absorption is enhanced twofold or threefold when stored iron is depleted or when erythropoiesis occurs at an accelerated rate. The absorption of iron is regulated by the amount of iron stored in the intestinal mucosa.

Iron is absorbed from the intestines into the circulation where it is bound to **transferrin** and transported to various tissues, including the bone marrow and liver. In these tissues, iron is stored as **ferritin** (Fig. 17.1). In the marrow, iron is incorporated into hemoglobin and packaged into reticulocytes, which enter the circulation and mature into new erythrocytes. The erythrocytes circulate in the blood for about 120 days and then are taken up and degraded by reticuloendothelial cells. These cells later return most of the iron to the plasma so that it can be used again in erythropoiesis. Iron is highly conserved by the body, and only small amounts of it are excreted via the intestinal tract.

The dietary iron requirement per kilogram of body weight is highest in infants and pregnant women, somewhat lower in children and nonpregnant women, and lowest in men. Pregnant women have the greatest need for routine **iron supplementation** because their dietary iron often cannot meet the requirements for maternal and fetal erythropoiesis. Most multivitamin supplements contain iron, and many processed foods, including bread, are supplemented with iron.

If dietary iron intake is inadequate to support sufficient erythropoiesis and maintain a normal hemoglobin concentration in the blood, the body will use stored iron to maintain erythropoiesis until the stores are depleted. When iron stores are significantly depleted, the plasma iron level begins to fall and erythropoiesis is reduced. Over time, these changes lead to **hypochromic microcytic anemia,** a form of anemia in which the mean corpuscular hemoglobin concentration and the mean corpuscular volume are decreased (Box 17.1). The iron preparations described in this chapter are used to prevent and treat **iron-deficiency anemia.**

TABLE 17.1   Selected Hematopoietic Drugs, Brand Names, and Use

DRUG/CLASS	BRAND NAME	USE
Minerals		
Ferrous sulfate	*None*	Iron-deficiency anemia
Iron dextran	Proferdex	Iron-deficiency anemia
Vitamins		
Folic acid	*None*	Megaloblastic anemia, pregnancy
Cyanocobalamin	Nascobal	Pernicious anemia
Erythropoiesis-stimulating agents		
Epoetin alfa	Procrit	Anemia due to chronic kidney disease, AZT use in HIV treatment
Luspatercept	Reblozyl	Anemia due to thalassemia and myelodysplastic syndromes
Colony-stimulating factors		
Filgrastim	Neupogen	Myelosuppressive chemotherapy, bone marrow transplantation
Pegfilgrastim	Neulasta	Chemotherapy-induced neutropenia
Thrombopoietin receptor agonists		
Romiplostim	Nplate	Thrombocytopenia
Avatrombopag	Doptelet	Thrombocytopenia
Interleukins		
Oprelvekin	Neumega	Thrombocytopenia from myelosuppressive chemotherapy

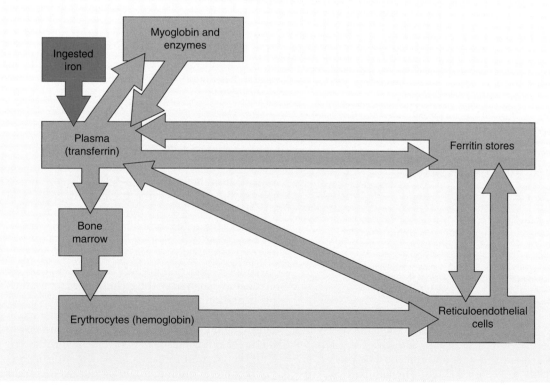

Fig. 17.1 Iron metabolism. Ingested iron is absorbed from the intestinal mucosa into the circulation, where it is bound to transferrin. Iron is distributed to tissues for incorporation into hemoglobin, myoglobin, and enzymes, or it is stored as ferritin. After about 120 days, erythrocytes are degraded by reticulo-endothelial cells, and the iron is returned to the plasma or stored.

Oral Iron Preparations

Iron is administered orally in the form of **ferrous salts,** including **ferrous sulfate, ferrous gluconate,** and **ferrous fumarate.** Iron contained in these preparations is absorbed in the same manner as is dietary iron. In patients with iron deficiency, the amount of iron absorbed increases progressively with larger doses, but the percentage absorbed decreases as the dosage increases. Food can retard iron

BOX 17.1 A CASE OF FATIGUE, SLEEPLESSNESS, AND ICED DRINKS

CASE PRESENTATION

A 25-year-old journalist complained to her health care provider of fatigue, weakness, and sleeplessness due to aching and restless legs. She had a history of heavy menstrual bleeding (menorrhagia), and she reported a recurring desire to chew on ice and consume iced drinks (pagophagia). Laboratory studies showed a hemoglobin (Hb) level of 10.7 (normal 12–15 g/dL), a mean corpuscular volume (MCV) of 75 (normal 80–100 fL/cell), a transferrin saturation (TSAT) of 8% (normal 12%–45%), and a ferritin level of 10 (normal >12 ng/mL). Oral ferrous sulfate was prescribed as 325 mg tablets taken twice daily, and she was also prescribed an estrogen-progestin contraceptive to control menorrhagia. She was also instructed to take psyllium fiber tablets with 8 ounces of water up to four times a day to prevent constipation and to take the iron tablets with a meal if they irritated her stomach. Vitamin C was also recommended to improve iron absorption. Six months later, her symptoms and pagophagia were much improved, and the Hb was 12, MCV 84, TSAT 20%, and ferritin 22.

CASE DISCUSSION

Young women are predisposed to developing iron-deficiency (ID) anemia because of menstruation, and they often have inadequate iron intake to support sufficient erythropoiesis to maintain normal hemoglobin levels. The signs and symptoms of this disorder include weakness and fatigue, cold hands and feet, difficulty sleeping, and pallor. Laboratory values typically show low TSAT and ferritin levels and a low MCV. Pagophagia, a form of pica (the desire to consume nonnutritive substances) is also associated with ID and usually responds to iron supplementation. Her laboratory values showed a deficit in plasma iron availability and iron storage, consistent with a hypochromic, microcytic anemia. She was correctly treated with oral iron supplementation, but ferrous sulfate can be irritating to the stomach, and it often causes constipation. Patients taking this medication should be instructed to increase dietary fiber and fluid intake to prevent constipation and to take the drug with food if they develop gastric irritation, even though this may reduce iron absorption. Vitamin C (ascorbic acid) increases iron absorption and may partly offset the effect of taking iron with food. It can take up to 6 months to normalize iron reserves and hemoglobin levels after beginning iron therapy. Patients who do not respond to oral iron supplementation may be treated with parenteral iron dextran injections.

absorption by 40% to 60%, but the gastric distress caused by iron often necessitates administering iron preparations with food. The percentage of iron absorbed from sustained-release preparations is lower than that absorbed from immediate-release preparations. This is because iron is primarily absorbed from the duodenum, and some of the sustained-release iron is transported to the lower intestinal tract before it is released for absorption.

In iron-deficiency states, oral iron preparations are usually administered three times a day in doses that provide a total of 100 to 200 mg of elemental iron daily. The various iron salts contain different percentages of elemental iron. Ferrous sulfate contains about 20%, so that a 300-mg tablet contains approximately 60 mg of elemental iron. The duration of iron therapy depends on the cause and severity of the iron deficiency. In general, a course of about 4 to 6 months

of oral iron therapy is required to reverse uncomplicated iron-deficiency anemia.

At therapeutic doses, iron salts have **few adverse effects,** but they sometimes cause epigastric pain, nausea, vomiting, diarrhea or constipation, and black stools. Liquid iron preparations can also stain the teeth. Bile acid–binding resins (e.g., cholestyramine) reduce the absorption of iron, whereas ascorbic acid increases iron absorption by maintaining iron in the reduced ferrous state because ferrous iron is better absorbed than is ferric iron. Iron can reduce the absorption of **tetracyclines, fluoroquinolones, levothyroxine,** and **vitamin E.** The administration of these drugs should be separated from iron administration by at least 2 hours. The ingestion of large quantities of iron can cause serious and **potentially lethal toxicity.** Hence, iron preparations should be kept out of the reach of children.

Parenteral Iron Preparations

Iron preparations for parenteral therapy include **iron dextran, iron sucrose,** and **sodium ferric gluconate.** Iron dextran is a mixture of ferric hydroxide and dextran. Both low-molecular-weight and high-molecular-weight iron dextran preparations have been used, but the low-molecular-weight preparations cause fewer adverse effects. Iron dextran is intended for intramuscular or intravenous treatment of iron-deficiency anemia in patients who cannot tolerate oral iron preparations or fail to respond to oral iron therapy. After administration, the iron dextran complex is removed from the circulation by the reticuloendothelial system, and the iron is transferred to the plasma for distribution to the bone marrow and other tissues.

The dosage required for each patient is calculated on the basis of the observed hemoglobin concentration and body weight.

Intravenous administration of **iron dextran** can cause peripheral flushing and hypotensive reactions. Intramuscular administration of iron dextran can cause **injection site reactions,** including pain, inflammation, sterile abscesses, and brown discoloration of skin. For this reason, the preparation must be given by deep intramuscular injection into the outer quadrant of the buttock. A Z-track technique, in which the skin is displaced laterally before injection, is used to avoid leakage into the subcutaneous tissue. Iron dextran administration has rarely caused fatal anaphylactic reactions.

Iron sucrose is a complex of iron hydroxide in sucrose for intravenous administration in the treatment of anemia in patients with chronic kidney disease. Sodium **ferric gluconate** has a similar indication.

Vitamins

Although many vitamins participate in the formation and function of erythrocytes, **folic acid** and **vitamin B$_{12}$** have a critical role in erythropoiesis, and a deficiency of either of them may cause **megaloblastic anemia.** This macrocytic anemia is characterized by an abnormally large red cell volume resulting from continued cell growth in the absence of DNA synthesis during erythropoiesis. Folic acid and vitamin B$_{12}$ serve as cofactors in biochemical reactions involving the addition of single-carbon units to various substrates, and the administration of one of these vitamins can partially compensate for a deficiency of the other. Therefore,

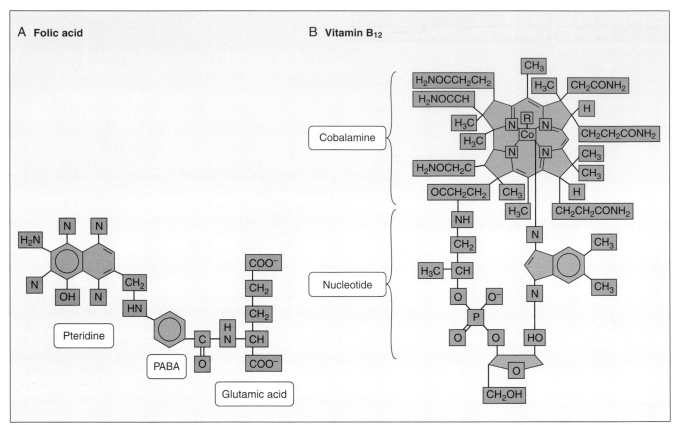

FIG. 17.2 Structures of folic acid and vitamin B$_{12}$. (A) Folic acid consists of pteridine, PABA, and glutamic acid. The unshaded areas represent the bonds that are reduced by folate reductase to form tetrahydrofolic acid. (B) Vitamin B$_{12}$ consists of a porphyrin-like ring with a central cobalt (Co) atom attached to a nucleotide. *PABA*, *p*-Aminobenzoic acid; *R*, CN$^-$ (cyanocobalamin) or OH$^-$ (hydroxocobalamin).

it is critical that the specific vitamin deficiency be correctly identified before therapy is started.

Folic Acid

The structure of folic acid is shown in Fig. 17.2A. Active forms of this vitamin serve as enzyme cofactors that donate single-carbon atoms in the biosynthesis of amino acids and the purine and pyrimidine bases contained in DNA (Fig. 17.3A). Hence, folic acid plays a critical role in **cell proliferation** and **erythropoiesis.**

The requirement for folic acid increases markedly during pregnancy, and inadequate dietary intake of this vitamin can cause **neural tube birth defects,** such as **spina bifida,** and **megaloblastic anemia.** For this reason, folic acid supplementation is especially important before and during pregnancy. The standard US diet provides 50 to 500 mg of absorbable folic acid daily. Women of childbearing age should take an additional 400 mg/day of folic acid, the amount contained in most multivitamin preparations. Since 1998, the US Food and Drug Administration (FDA) requires fortification of enriched cereal grains with 140 mg of folic acid per 100 g of grain. The incidence of neural tube defects in the United States, which had been declining for decades, has fallen at least 25% since the fortification of cereals began.

Folic acid is well absorbed from the jejunum, and oral supplementation is effective both in preventing and in treating megaloblastic anemia associated with **folic acid deficiency.** This disorder often results from insufficient folic acid intake in the diet, but it can also result from impaired folic acid absorption, such as that seen in patients with alcoholism and certain malabsorption syndromes. In

patients with megaloblastic anemia, vitamin B$_{12}$ deficiency must be ruled out before treatment with folic acid is begun. This is because treatment with folic acid may partly correct the anemia caused by a vitamin B$_{12}$ deficiency but will not correct other problems associated with it. Irreversible neurologic damage can occur if a B$_{12}$ deficiency is incorrectly treated with folic acid.

Several drugs can contribute to **folate deficiency.** These include chemotherapeutic **folate reductase inhibitors,** such as trimethoprim, pyrimethamine, and methotrexate (see Chapters 40, 44, and 45). Other drugs inhibit folate absorption, including cholestyramine and certain anticonvulsant drugs (e.g., phenytoin).

Vitamin B12

Vitamin B$_{12}$ consists of a porphyrin-like ring with a central cobalt atom attached to a nucleotide (see Fig. 17.2B). Two synthetic forms of vitamin B$_{12}$, **cyanocobalamin** and **hydroxocobalamin,** are available for the treatment of B$_{12}$ deficiency. In the body, these forms of the vitamin are converted to methylcobalamin or deoxyadenosylcobalamin, which are cofactors for biochemical reactions. Vitamin B$_{12}$ serves as a cofactor for methylation reactions, including the conversion of homocysteine to methionine and the conversion of methylmalonyl coenzyme A (CoA) to succinyl CoA (see Fig. 17.3B).

Vitamin B$_{12}$ is essential for **cell replication and growth, hematopoiesis,** and **myelin synthesis.** It is obtained from dietary meats, dairy products, and eggs, and it is absorbed from the gut in the presence of **intrinsic factor** (a glycoprotein secreted by gastric parietal cells) and calcium. An inadequate secretion of intrinsic factor leads to **vitamin**

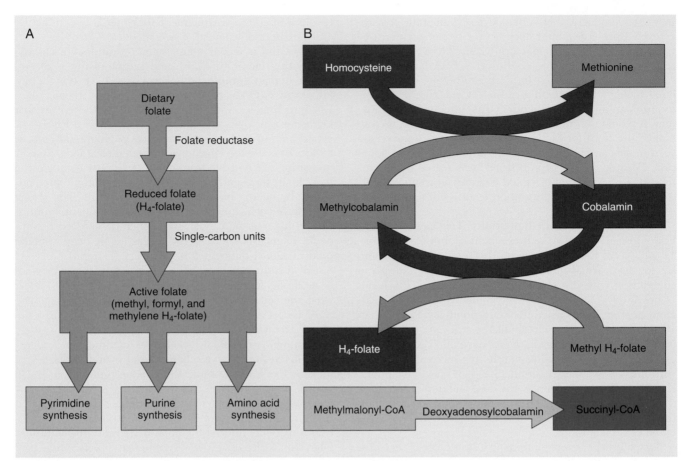

FIG. 17.3 Biochemical reactions involving folic acid and vitamin B_{12}. (A) Dietary folate is reduced by folate reductase to tetrahydrofolate (H_4-folate). Single-carbon units are added to H_4-folate to form active folate, which donates single-carbon units in the synthesis of pyrimidine and purine bases and amino acids. (B) The two active forms of vitamin B_{12} are methylcobalamin and deoxyadenosylcobalamin. These forms are cofactors for methylation reactions, including the conversion of homocysteine to methionine and the conversion of methylmalonyl CoA to succinyl CoA. Methyl H_4-folate donates a methyl group to cobalamin to form methylcobalamin.

B_{12} deficiency and eventually results in so-called **pernicious anemia.** Vitamin B_{12} deficiency is also seen in patients who have malabsorption disorders, in individuals who have had gastrectomy, and in strict vegetarians who have a low dietary intake of the vitamin.

Because vitamin B_{12} is not absorbed from the gut in the absence of an intrinsic factor, the vitamin must be administered intramuscularly in the treatment of pernicious anemia, and treatment must be continued for life. At the start of therapy, injections are given daily for 5 to 10 days. Thereafter, maintenance doses are given once a month. **Nasal spray** formulations of **cyanocobalamin** (NASCOBAL) are available for maintenance therapy after normalization of serum B_{12} concentrations with intramuscular B_{12} injections. In patients with a dietary deficiency of vitamin B_{12}, the vitamin is given orally.

Hydroxocobalamin is also used for out-of-hospital empiric treatment of **cyanide poisoning** resulting from smoke inhalation. In this setting, hydroxocobalamin (CYANOKIT) is administered intravenously, and then it rapidly combines with cyanide to form harmless cyanocobalamin in the blood.

Hematopoietic Growth Factors

Hematopoietic growth factors are a large group of glycoproteins that regulate the production of blood cells and include colony-stimulating factors and cytokines. Growth factors bind to receptors on bone marrow progenitor cells and induce their differentiation and proliferation, leading to the production of erythrocytes, leukocytes, and platelets. Several of these growth factors have been produced by recombinant DNA technology and are now available for the treatment of blood cell deficiencies. These agents are administered by intravenous or subcutaneous injection.

Erythropoiesis-Stimulating Agents

Erythropoietin is secreted primarily by the kidney in adults and binds to erythropoietin receptors on erythroid progenitor cells in the bone marrow, thereby stimulating cell differentiation and proliferation. Several forms of erythropoietin have been developed for treating anemia and are collectively known as **erythropoiesis-stimulating agents (ESAs).** **Epoetin alfa** was the first ESA to be developed and is identical to endogenous human erythropoietin. **Darbepoetin alfa** and **epoetin β** are modified forms of erythropoietin that have longer half-lives than epoetin alfa and are given less frequently. Darbepoetin alfa contains additional polysaccharide molecules, whereas epoetin β contains polyethylene glycol (PEG) molecules attached to the amino acid lysine throughout the erythropoietin structure. Likewise, methoxy polyethylene glycol-epoetin β is a new formulation of epoetin β that produces a more favorable pharmacokinetic profile.

ESAs stimulate erythropoiesis in patients with **anemia caused by chronic renal failure,** as indicated by an increased production of reticulocytes (immature erythrocytes) within 10 days after starting therapy, and an increased hemoglobin level and hematocrit within 2 to 6 weeks as the reticulocytes develop into erythrocytes. ESAs are also used to treat anemia resulting from chemotherapy for nonmyeloid malignancies, anemia caused by zidovudine therapy for **human immunodeficiency virus infection,** and anemia in premature infants. These agents have been used to reduce the need for blood transfusions during surgery and to stimulate erythropoiesis before autologous blood donation. Because the use of iron stores is increased in patients receiving ESAs, patients should be given iron supplements to maintain transferrin saturation levels of at least 20% to support erythropoiesis.

ESAs have significant limitations. The larger doses of ESAs formerly used to achieve hemoglobin levels above 12 g/dL were found to increase the risk of **hypertension, stroke, myocardial infarction, heart failure,** and **death** in comparison with doses used to achieve hemoglobin levels of below 11 g/dL. The FDA recommends that ESA treatment be started only when the hemoglobin level is less than 10 g/dL and that treatment should be reduced or discontinued if levels exceed 10 g/dL. ESAs have also been found to enhance **tumor progression** and shorten survival in patients with breast, non-small cell lung, head and neck, lymphoid, and cervical cancers. Hence, the dose and duration of ESA therapy used in treating anemia caused by cancer chemotherapy should be limited to that required to avoid red blood cell transfusions.

Luspatercept is a recombinant fusion protein that **promotes the maturation of red blood cells** from late-stage erythroid precursors. It is the first and only erythroid maturation drug on the market. **Luspatercept** is indicated for the **treatment of anemia** in adult patients with *beta* thalassemia who require regular red blood cell transfusions and in adult patients with very low- to intermediate-risk myelodysplastic syndromes. Clinical studies show that treatment of patients with thalassemia and myelodysplastic syndromes (MDS) by injection of luspatercept **improved hematology parameters** associated with ineffective erythropoiesis in those disorders.

Erythropoietin Drug Abuse. Erythropoietin and other ESAs are often abused as performance-enhancing drugs in professional sports and in weight rooms. By increasing red blood cells, the oxygen-carrying capacity of the blood is increased, which can increase athletic performance. The premier cyclist Lance Armstrong admitted to erythropoietin use (among other doping agents) and, as a result, lost his seven Tour de France cycling medals and an Olympic bronze medal.

Colony-Stimulating Factors

Neutrophils are the most common type of leukocyte found in the bloodstream and are a type of granulocyte (cells with cytoplasmic granules). Their primary role is to defend against bacterial and fungal infections. The production of neutrophils and other granulocytes is regulated by colony-stimulating factors (CSF) produced by leukocytes, fibroblasts, and endothelial cells. These cytokine factors stimulate the maturation and proliferation of granulocyte progenitor cells by binding to CSF receptors. The CSF cytokine receptors are an example of tyrosine kinase enzyme receptors (see Chapter 3). Recombinant forms of the CSF cytokine have revolutionized the **treatment of leukopenia** (neutropenia) and are essentially devoid of side effects.

Filgrastim is recombinant human **granulocyte colony-stimulating factor** (G-CSF), and **sargramostim** is recombinant human **granulocyte-macrophage CSF** (GM-CSF). Filgrastim is produced in *Escherichia coli* by recombinant DNA techniques and differs from natural G-CSF in that filgrastim is not glycosylated. The addition of a **PEG** moiety to filgrastim (pegylation) creates **pegfilgrastim,** whose molecular size is too large to enable renal clearance, thereby increasing the half-life from about 3.5 hours for filgrastim to 42 hours for pegfilgrastim. Pegfilgrastim is eliminated primarily by neutrophil uptake and metabolism. The longer half-life of pegfilgrastim has enabled less-frequent administration for treating cancer chemotherapy-induced neutropenia. **Filgrastim-sndz** and **tbo-filgrastim** are two biosimilar products given different non-propriety (generic) names to distinguish them in cases where proprietary names may not be used, such as in adverse effect databases. While it is clear what the suffix means in filgrastim-sndz as it is manufactured by Sandoz Pharmaceuticals, the *tbo-* in tbo-filgrastim remains a mystery.

Recombinant G-CSF accelerates granulocyte recovery after **myelosuppressive chemotherapy** and reduces the incidence of infections and shortens hospitalization. It can also be used for prophylaxis of neutropenia in high-risk patients, such as older lymphoma patients treated with curative chemotherapy, and it reduces neutropenia and infection in patients undergoing **bone marrow transplantation.** Filgrastim is also used to mobilize hematopoietic progenitor cells into the peripheral blood when blood is being collected for **leukapheresis,** and patients exposed to lethal **radiation** should receive G-CSF to prevent neutropenia. In patients with HIV infection, G-CSF prevents zidovudine-induced neutropenia. Filgrastim can also be beneficial in the treatment of other forms of congenital or acquired neutropenia, such as aplastic anemia.

Sargramostim (GM-CSF) is used to accelerate myeloid cell (granulocyte) recovery in patients undergoing allogenic **bone marrow transplantation** or chemotherapy for **lymphoma, acute myeloid leukemia,** or **Hodgkin disease.** It has also been used to enhance stem cell mobilization before collection for stem cell transplantation to accelerate myeloid cell recovery after allogenic bone marrow transplantation. Sargramostim can also reduce the incidence of fever and infections in patients with **severe chronic neutropenia.** Although endogenous GM-CSF stimulates the production of several types of cells, sargramostim has little effect on erythrocytes or platelets in deficiency states and serves primarily to accelerate the development of neutrophils.

Filgrastim and **sargramostim** are administered subcutaneously or intravenously once a day for 2 weeks or until the absolute neutrophil count has reached 10,000/μL. Because of its longer half-life, **pegfilgrastim** requires administration only once during each cycle of cancer chemotherapy to manage chemotherapy-induced neutropenia.

Thrombopoietin Receptor Agonists

Thrombopoietin is a glycoprotein hormone manufactured in the liver which stimulates the formation of megakaryocytes in the bone marrow to increase platelet (thrombocyte) production. Although clinical trials with thrombopoietin to treat thrombocytopenia were not successful, recombinant protein analogs that act as thrombopoietin receptor agonists are available.

Romiplostim is a **thrombopoietin receptor agonist** indicated for the treatment of thrombocytopenia in immune thrombocytopenia disorder who did not respond to corticosteroids, immunoglobulins, or splenectomy. Romiplostim is an Fc-peptide fusion protein (peptibody) consisting of human immunoglobulin IgG1 Fc domain, linked to a peptide containing two thrombopoietin receptor-binding domains.

Avatrombopag is a **thrombopoietin receptor agonist** used for the treatment of thrombocytopenia in adult patients with chronic liver disease about to undergo a medical procedure and for patients with chronic immune thrombocytopenia who have had an ineffective response to a previous treatment. **Eltrombopag** is a small molecule agonist at the **thrombopoietin receptor** with the same indications as avatrombopag. Like avatrombopag but not romiplostim which is an injectable, eltrombopag is an oral medication.

Interleukins

Oprelvekin (NEUMEGA) is a recombinant form of **interleukin-11** (IL-11), one of a large number of cytokine growth factors involved in regulating the differentiation and proliferation of blood and immune cells. It is a thrombopoietic growth factor that stimulates the proliferation of megakaryocyte progenitor cells and induces megakaryocyte maturation, resulting in increased platelet production. Oprelvekin is used to prevent severe **thrombocytopenia** and reduce the need for platelet transfusions following myelosuppressive chemotherapy in high-risk patients with nonmyeloid malignancies.

DRUGS FOR SICKLE CELL DISEASE

Sickle cell disease is a group of inherited disorders that acquired its name because red blood cells are distorted from their typical round, doughnut shape to a crescent or sickle shape. Sickle cells die quicker than normal red blood cells, leading to a shortage of oxygen-carrying capacity of the blood, and patients exhibit sickle cell anemia. Because sickle cells are not round and smooth, they often get stuck in blood vessels, causing a painful vaso-occlusive episode (sickle cell crisis). Besides opioid and non-opioid analgesics for the treatment of pain, there are now four FDA-approved medications for the treatment of sickle cell disease.

Voxelotor is a hemoglobin S **polymerization inhibitor** indicated for the treatment of sickle cell disease in adults and pediatric patients 12 years of age and older. This indication is approved under accelerated approval as an orphan drug based on an increase in normal hemoglobin (Hb) in clinical trial participants.

Crizanlizumab is a humanized IgG_2 **monoclonal antibody drug** that binds to P-selectin and blocks interactions with its ligands including P-selectin glycoprotein ligand 1. Binding P-selectin on the surface of the endothelial cells blocks the aggregation between endothelial cells and the platelets, red blood cells, and leukocytes. It is indicated for the treatment of painful vaso-occlusive episodes in sickle cell disease patients. Additional descriptions of monoclonal antibody drugs are provided in Chapter 46.

Hydroxyurea is a DNA synthesis inhibitor used in the treatment of cancer (see Chapter 45) but is also marketed as a treatment to prevent vaso-occlusive episodes in sickle cell patients. Although it is not clear how hydroxyurea benefits patients with sickle cell disease, increased hemoglobin levels in RBCs, decreased neutrophils, increased water content of RBCs, increased plasticity of sickle cells, and decreased adhesion of RBCs to endothelium have been observed.

L-glutamine is the naturally occurring form of the amino acid glutamine. It is thought that L-glutamine increases the availability of reduced glutathione, a free radical scavenger in cells. Because sickle cells are more sensitive to oxidative stress than normal RBCs, a decrease in oxidative stress by increased cell stores of glutathione may be beneficial. It comes as an oral powder to be mixed in milk or juice and given in an amount according to body weight twice a day.

SUMMARY OF IMPORTANT POINTS

- Iron deficiency causes hypochromic microcytic anemia, whereas folic acid or vitamin B_{12} deficiency causes megaloblastic anemia.
- Ferrous sulfate and other ferrous salts are administered orally for several months in the treatment of iron-deficiency anemia.
- Folic acid supplementation is used during pregnancy to prevent anemia and birth defects.
- Folic acid treatment can partly mask the hematologic effect of vitamin B_{12} deficiency but does not prevent irreversible neurologic damage.
- Pernicious anemia is caused by inadequate secretion of intrinsic factor and reduced vitamin B_{12} absorption. It is treated with intramuscular injections of cyanocobalamin or hydroxocobalamin.
- Epoetin alfa, epoetin β, and darbepoetin alfa are recombinant forms of human erythropoietin used to treat anemia caused by chronic renal failure, cancer-related anemia, and anemia caused by other conditions.
- Filgrastim, pegfilgrastim, and sargramostim are recombinant forms of G-CSF or GM-CSF. They are used to treat neutropenia associated with cancer chemotherapy, bone marrow transplantation, and various disease states.
- Oprelvekin is a recombinant form of the cytokine interleukin 11 (IL-11) and is used to prevent severe thrombocytopenia during cancer chemotherapy.
- New drugs for sickle cell disease include voxelotor, a hemoglobin S polymerization inhibitor, and crizanlizumab, a monoclonal antibody drug that prevents platelet-endothelial interactions.

Review Questions

For each numbered patient, select the best treatment from the lettered choices.

    (A) cyanocobalamin
    (B) epoetin
    (C) ferrous fumarate
    (D) filgrastim
    (E) folic acid

1. A 19-year-old woman with lethargy and fatigue is found to have a blood hemoglobin level of 9.8 g/dL (normal range 12–16 g/dL), a low erythrocyte corpuscular volume, and a low erythrocyte hemoglobin concentration.
2. A 47-year-old woman exhibits severe neutropenia after a course of chemotherapy for breast cancer.
3. A 66-year-old man with progressive fatigability and anorexia is found to have a low blood hemoglobin concentration, an elevated mean corpuscular volume, and an elevated serum concentration of methylmalonic acid.

4. A 68-year-old man with diabetic nephropathy and end-stage renal disease exhibits peripheral reticulocytopenia and anemia.
5. Pegylation of a recombinant protein is employed for which purpose?
   (A) increasing oral bioavailability
   (B) decreasing renal excretion rate
   (C) increasing duration of action
   (D) increasing binding to receptors
   (E) reducing adverse effects

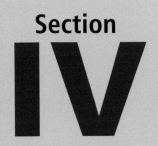
CENTRAL NERVOUS SYSTEM PHARMACOLOGY

CHAPTER 18

Introduction to Central Nervous System Pharmacology

OVERVIEW

The central nervous system (CNS) consists of the brain and spinal cord. Sensory information arrives to the CNS from the special senses and peripheral nerves and is integrated with memories and internal drive states to generate cognitive, emotional, and motor (behavioral) responses. This process occurs because of the complex interplay of **neurotransmitters** and **neuromodulators** acting on their **receptors** to excite or inhibit CNS neurons. In persons with **brain disorders,** structural or functional disturbances of CNS processing produce aberrant cognitive, emotional, or motor responses. Brain disorders are seen in association with a variety of disease processes, including degenerative, ischemic, and psychological disturbances.

Most CNS drugs correct an **imbalance in neurotransmitters or their receptors.** Drugs are used to relieve the symptoms of brain dysfunction, but they usually do not correct the underlying disorder. Although short-term drug treatment may be effective in relieving acute symptoms such as pain and insomnia, drug therapy for many brain disorders is a lifelong process.

After reviewing pertinent concepts of CNS function and neurotransmission, this chapter explains the general mechanisms by which drugs alter CNS activities and processes.

NEUROTRANSMISSION IN THE CENTRAL NERVOUS SYSTEM

Principles of Neurotransmission

In the past century, great debates raged about the nature of neuronal communication in the CNS. The early physiologists believed that neurons communicated by electrical signals directly passing from neuron to neuron in a **hardwired** fashion, much like wires in a telegraph relay. The early pharmacologists argued for chemical transmission, with substances released into the **synapse** between communicating neurons. Modern research shows that both were right to some degree because most neuronal communication occurs by chemical **neurotransmitters** serving as messengers that enable neurons to communicate with one another. However, there is also evidence of direct voltage signaling between neurons at **electrotonic** or **gap junctions.**

The details of chemical neurotransmission undergo constant refinement as new mechanisms and neurotransmitters are discovered. An early statement by Sir Henry Dale, known as **Dale's principle,** suggested that each neuron contained only one type of neurotransmitter. This principle was revised with the finding that neurons may release more than one neurotransmitter, as is the case with cotransmitters (see later). It was also thought that neurotransmitter action was limited to the single synapse where released. The neuroanatomic demonstration of diffuse neuronal systems with fine, widespread projections throughout the CNS, such as norepinephrine and serotonergic fibers arising from brainstem

nuclei, led to the concept of the **chemical soup** or **chemical milieu** model of neurotransmission. Newer methods using *in vitro* brain slice preparations and other techniques show that neurotransmitters can diffuse far from the synapse and affect other neurons at other synapses. Identification of neuroactive substances, both intrinsic and extrinsic to the CNS, that exert generalized effects on neurons strengthened the concept of action at a distance. A **neuromodulator** is a general term for any substance that exerts an effect on neurotransmission among a set of neurons in the brain.

The action of drugs on the CNS is similar to the chemical milieu model of neurotransmission, because drug molecules are widely distributed throughout the brain and can simultaneously interact with receptors on neurons in several different neuronal tracts. This lack of specificity can lead to therapeutic effects and adverse effects at the same time. For this reason, the development of agents that are more selective for specific receptor types and subtypes is a useful approach to improving the therapeutic index of CNS drugs.

Neurotransmitter Synthesis and Metabolism

Neurotransmitters are synthesized in neuronal cell bodies or terminals, and they are stored in neuronal **vesicles** until they are released into a synapse (Fig. 18.1). The release of neurotransmitters is activated by membrane depolarization and calcium influx into the cell. Calcium evokes the interaction of storage vesicle proteins and membrane-docking proteins, leading to **vesicle fusion** with the membrane and **exocytosis** of the neurotransmitter.

After exocytosis, the neurotransmitter may activate presynaptic and postsynaptic receptors. A neurotransmitter's action is then terminated either by its reuptake into the presynaptic neuron or by its degradation to inactive compounds, with degradation catalyzed by enzymes located on presynaptic and postsynaptic neuronal membranes or within the cytoplasm.

Neurotransmitters can also diffuse from the synapse of their origin to affect neurons in the surrounding vicinity. In this way, different neurotransmitters released from different types of neurons form a **chemical milieu,** as described previously. The net influence of the chemical milieu on neurotransmission depends on the concentrations of the excitatory and inhibitory neurotransmitters acting at a particular synapse.

Excitatory and Inhibitory Neurotransmission

CNS neurotransmitters can evoke either an excitatory or an inhibitory synaptic membrane potential and trigger effects at presynaptic and postsynaptic sites on target neurons. If an **excitatory postsynaptic membrane potential** reaches firing threshold, an action potential is conducted along the dendritic and axonal membrane, evoking the release of a neurotransmitter from the nerve terminal.

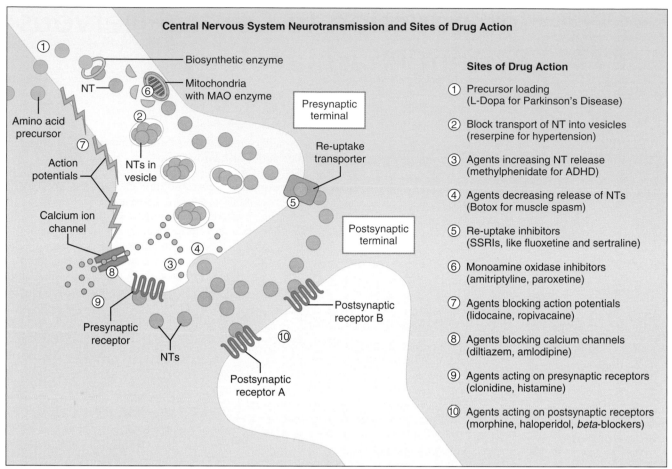

FIG. 18.1   Central nervous system (CNS) neurotransmission and sites of drug action. CNS drugs act primarily by affecting the synthesis, storage, release, reuptake, or degradation of neurotransmitters (NT) or by activating receptors. NTs are synthesized from amino acid precursors accumulated or synthesized in the neurons. The NTs are stored in vesicles whose membranes contain proteins involved in NT. The NTs are released when an action potential–mediated calcium influx initiates interaction of vesicles with the neuronal membrane. This leads to docking and exocytosis. Synaptic NTs activate presynaptic or postsynaptic receptors. The action of NTs is terminated by reuptake into the presynaptic neuron or by enzymatic degradation. Examples of sites of drug action and particular agents are presented in the figure as *1* to *10*.

An **inhibitory postsynaptic membrane potential** hyperpolarizes the neuronal membrane and inhibits the firing of action potentials. Depending on whether a **presynaptic membrane potential** is excitatory or inhibitory, it will increase or decrease the release of a neurotransmitter from the neuron. Presynaptic receptors, also called **autoreceptors,** can also be coupled with **cyclic adenosine monophosphate (cAMP)** or other **second messengers** that modulate neurotransmitter release.

As shown in Box 18.1, the interaction of multiple neurotransmitters at a particular site in a neuronal tract enables the complex interplay of various neuronal systems and contributes to the wide range of functional expression exhibited in the CNS. For example, inhibition of the release of an inhibitory neurotransmitter will actually increase neurotransmission in the target neuron. Similarly, drugs can act in complex ways to affect neurotransmission. **Ethanol** (ethyl alcohol), for instance, can diminish the inhibitory influence of the cerebral cortex on certain human behaviors, thereby increasing drug-induced behaviors, a phenomenon called **behavioral disinhibition.** Ethanol and other CNS depressants, initially or at low doses, exert their effects on the smaller and more numerous inhibitory neurons, creating disinhibition via excitation owing to removal of inhibitory

neurotransmitters. At higher doses, larger excitatory neurons are inhibited, and profound depression of CNS activity can occur.

Fast Versus Slow Signals

Neurotransmitters in the CNS can be characterized as slow or fast, depending on the receptors activated and the persistence of signal transduction pathways. The best examples of **fast neurotransmitters** are *gamma*-aminobutyric acid (GABA) and glutamate acting at **ligand-gated ion channels.** Binding of these amino acid neurotransmitters directly to subunits of the ion channel protein directly initiates ion flow with a signal that lasts for only a few milliseconds. Examples of **slow neurotransmitters** are norepinephrine and serotonin acting at **G protein–coupled receptors.** These activated G protein–coupled receptor proteins initiate a slower, multistep process with alterations in second messengers and membrane effects that can last from many milliseconds to as long as a second. A slow (long-acting) signal can influence the overall tone of a neuron because it can modulate the signals of several other fast neurotransmitters acting on the same neuron. For this reason, slow neurotransmitters can also be called **neuromodulators.**

BOX 18.1 PATTERNS OF NEUROTRANSMISSION IN THE CENTRAL NERVOUS SYSTEM

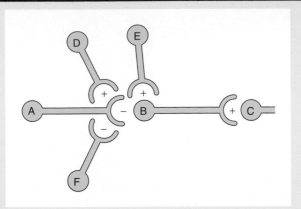

A, B, C, D, E, and F are neurons in a tract that projects from left to right. Neurons B, D, and E release excitatory neurotransmitters (+). Neurons A and F release inhibitory neurotransmitters (−). The net effect of neuronal interactions on neurotransmission from B to C is shown in the accompanying table. Each interaction presupposes that the other neurons are quiescent at that time. Other, more complex interactions are possible.

Interaction	Effect on Neurotransmission (B → C)
A → B	Decreased
D → A → B	Greatly decreased
F → A → B	Increased
E → B	Increased

Neurotransmitters and Receptors

Important neurotransmitters in the CNS include acetylcholine and several amino acids, biogenic amines, and neuropeptides. Table 18.1 lists the names, receptors, mechanisms of signal transduction, and functions of the major neurotransmitters.

The receptors can be divided into two basic groups: **ionotropic receptors,** also called **ligand-gated ion channels,** which are directly associated with ion channels, and **metabotropic receptors,** which are typical **G protein–coupled receptors** (see Chapter 3). Although this terminology is most frequently applied to receptors for amino acid neurotransmitters (e.g., GABA and glutamate), it is equally appropriate for other classes of neurotransmitter receptors.

The **mechanisms of signal transduction** for neurotransmitters in the CNS are similar to those for neurotransmitters in the autonomic nervous system. The activation of ionotropic receptors alters chloride, sodium, potassium, or calcium influx, thereby evoking excitatory or inhibitory membrane potentials. The linkage of metabotropic receptors with G proteins leads to activation or inhibition of adenylyl cyclase and alteration in the levels of intracellular cAMP, or activation of phospholipase C and the formation of inositol triphosphate and diacylglycerol. Metabotropic receptor activity can also modulate ion channel activity via **second messengers** (most notably calcium) that activate protein kinases responsible for the phosphorylation of ion channels. Signal transduction for other receptors in the CNS is discussed in Chapter 3.

Acetylcholine

Acetylcholine, synthesized from acetyl coenzyme A and choline, is degraded to acetate and choline by the enzyme acetylcholinesterase (Fig. 18.2). **Acetylcholine receptors** (also known as **cholinergic receptors**) consist of two main types: **muscarinic receptors** and **nicotinic receptors.** The properties and mechanisms of these receptors are compared in Table 6.2.

Drugs can affect acetylcholine neurotransmission by activating or blocking acetylcholine receptors or by inhibiting cholinesterase. The general pharmacologic properties of acetylcholine receptor agonists and antagonists are described in Chapters 6 and 7, respectively.

In the CNS, acetylcholine acts as an excitatory or inhibitory neurotransmitter in a number of neuronal tracts, including those that innervate the hippocampus, cerebral cortex, and basal ganglia. These tracts participate in memory, sensory processing, and motor coordination, respectively.

Amino Acids

Several amino acids are important neurotransmitters in the brain and spinal cord. Some of them, most notably **GABA** and **glycine,** are inhibitory. Others, such as **glutamate** and **aspartate,** are excitatory.

GABA. The most ubiquitous inhibitory neurotransmitter in the brain and spinal cord is **GABA,** which is biosynthesized from **glutamate,** the most abundant excitatory amino acid (see later). Its receptors are the **ionotropic GABA$_A$ receptors** and the **metabotropic GABA$_B$ receptors.** Most drugs affecting GABA neurotransmission primarily activate or inhibit the GABA$_A$-chloride ion channel complex. This ion channel complex contains receptors for several types of drugs, including the **benzodiazepines** and **barbiturates** (see Chapter 19), **general anesthetics** (see Chapter 21), and **alcohol** (see Chapter 25). Drugs acting at the **GABA$_B$ receptor** are used to control spasticity (see Chapter 24). The functions of GABA include regulation of neuronal excitability throughout the CNS and motor coordination.

Glycine. Glycine is a major inhibitory transmitter in the spinal cord. Its **strychnine-sensitive receptors** are coupled with the chloride ion channel, and activation of these receptors leads to membrane hyperpolarization. The inhibitory actions of glycine are potently antagonized by the alkaloid **strychnine,** a convulsant poison used as a rodenticide. Strychnine poisoning causes disinhibition of motoneurons, leading to convulsions and death through respiratory failure. Glycine also acts as a **coagonist** to the excitatory amino acid glutamate at **N-methyl-d-aspartate (NMDA) receptors** by binding to an allosteric **strychnine-insensitive** site.

Taurine is a sulfur-containing amino acid postulated to act as a neurotransmitter or neuromodulator in the CNS. Taurine is believed to activate both strychnine-sensitive and strychnine-insensitive types of **glycine-binding sites.**

Glutamate and Aspartate. Glutamate and aspartate are acidic amino acids that function as excitatory neurotransmitters throughout the CNS. Their ionotropic receptors consist of three types that differ in their subunit composition and are named for drugs that show the most selectivity for each type: **NMDA, AMPA** (amino-3-hydroxy-5-methyl-4-isoxazole propionate), and **kainate** receptors. These receptors are excitatory because their associated ion channels allow the flow of sodium or calcium ions into neurons, causing

TABLE 18.1   Major Neurotransmitters and Their Receptors in the Central Nervous System

NEUROTRANSMITTER	RECEPTORS	SIGNAL TRANSDUCTION	FUNCTION
Acetylcholine	Muscarinic		
	M_1, M_3, M_5	$\uparrow IP_3$, $\uparrow DAG$, $\uparrow iCa^{2+}$	Excitatory; role in arousal and consciousness, memory consolidation
	M_2, M_4	$\downarrow cAMP$, $\uparrow gK^+$, $\downarrow gCa^{2+}$	Inhibitory; autoreceptor and heteroreceptor, decreases NT release
	Nicotinic	$\uparrow gNa^+$, $\uparrow gCa^{2+}$	Excitatory; increases NT release, role in nicotine dependence
Amino acids			
GABA	$GABA_A$	$\uparrow gCl^-$	Inhibitory (major); ligand-gated ion channel site of action of sedative-hypnotics, alcohol, general anesthetics
	$GABA_B$	$\downarrow cAMP$, $\uparrow gK^+$, $\downarrow gCa^{2+}$	Inhibitory; modulates motor neuron excitability
Glutamate	NMDA, AMPA, KA	$\uparrow gNa^+$, $\uparrow gCa^{2+}$	Excitatory (major); roles in LTP (memory), excitotoxicity of neurons
	$mGlu_1$, $mGlu_5$	$\uparrow IP_3$, $\uparrow DAG$, $\uparrow iCa^{2+}$	Excitatory; memory consolidation, neuronal excitation
	$mGlu_2$-$mGlu_4$, $mGlu_6$-$mGlu_8$	$\downarrow cAMP$, $\uparrow gK^+$, $\downarrow gCa^{2+}$	Inhibitory; role in thalamic sensory processing
Glycine	Strychnine-sensitive	$\uparrow gCl^-$	Inhibitory; highest levels in spinal cord
	Strychnine-insensitive	Coagonist at NMDA receptor	Excitatory; obligate coagonist for function of NMDA receptor
Biogenic amines			
Dopamine	D_1, D_5	$\uparrow cAMP$, $\uparrow PKA$	Excitatory; basal ganglia function, memory and performance
	D_2, D_3, D_4	$\downarrow cAMP$, $\uparrow gK^+$, $\downarrow gCa^{2+}$	Inhibitory; decreases dopamine release, reduces firing of neurons
Norepinephrine	α_1	$\uparrow IP_3$, $\uparrow DAG$, $\uparrow iCa^{2+}$	Excitatory; autonomic nuclei in brainstem
	α_2	$\downarrow cAMP$, $\uparrow gK^+$, $\downarrow gCa^{2+}$	Inhibitory; sympathetic outflow from CNS; decreases pain transmission
	β_1, β_2	$\uparrow cAMP$, $\uparrow PKA$	Excitatory; cortex, limbic system, nucleus accumbens
Serotonin (5-HT)[a]	$5\text{-}HT_1$	$\downarrow cAMP$, $\uparrow gK^+$, $\downarrow gCa^{2+}$	Inhibitory; role in anxiety and depression
	$5\text{-}HT_2$	$\uparrow IP_3$, $\uparrow DAG$, $\uparrow iCa^{2+}$	Excitatory; widespread distribution, role in antipsychotic action
	$5\text{-}HT_3$	$\uparrow gNa^+$, $\uparrow gCa^{2+}$	Excitatory; mediate fast neuronal transmission in neocortex; presynaptic modulation of NT release
	$5\text{-}HT_4$	$\uparrow cAMP$, $\uparrow PKA$	Excitatory; role in cognitive processes, anxiety
Histamine	H_1	$\uparrow IP_3$, $\uparrow DAG$, $\uparrow iCa^{2+}$	Excitatory; increases NT release, role in arousal, anxiety
	H_2	$\uparrow cAMP$, $\uparrow PKA$	Excitatory; located in hippocampus, amygdala, and basal ganglia
	H_3	$\downarrow cAMP$, $\uparrow gK^+$, $\downarrow gCa^{2+}$	Inhibitory; autoreceptor and heteroreceptor, decreases NT release
Neuropeptides			
Opioid peptides	*Mu, delta, kappa*	$\downarrow cAMP$, $\uparrow gK^+$, $\downarrow gCa^{2+}$	Inhibitory, analgesic role in sensory processing, role in drug dependence for opioids and other substances
Tachykinins	NK_1, NK_2, NK_3	$\uparrow IP_3$, $\uparrow DAG$, $\uparrow iCa^{2+}$	Excitatory; role in pain processing, autonomic regulation

AMPA, Amino-3-hydroxy-5-methyl-4-isoxazole propionate; *cAMP,* cyclic adenosine monophosphate; *CNS,* central nervous system; *DAG,* diacylglycerol; *5-HT,* 5-hydroxytryptamine (serotonin); *g,* ion channel conductance; *GABA, gamma*-aminobutyric acid; *i,* intracellular; *IP₃,* inositol triphosphate; *KA,* kainate; *LTP,* long-term potentiation; *NK,* neurokinin; *NMDA,* N-methyl-ᴅ-aspartate; *NT,* neurotransmitter; *PKA,* cAMP-dependent protein kinase.
[a]Over a dozen types of serotonin receptors are cloned; the four given here are the main types.

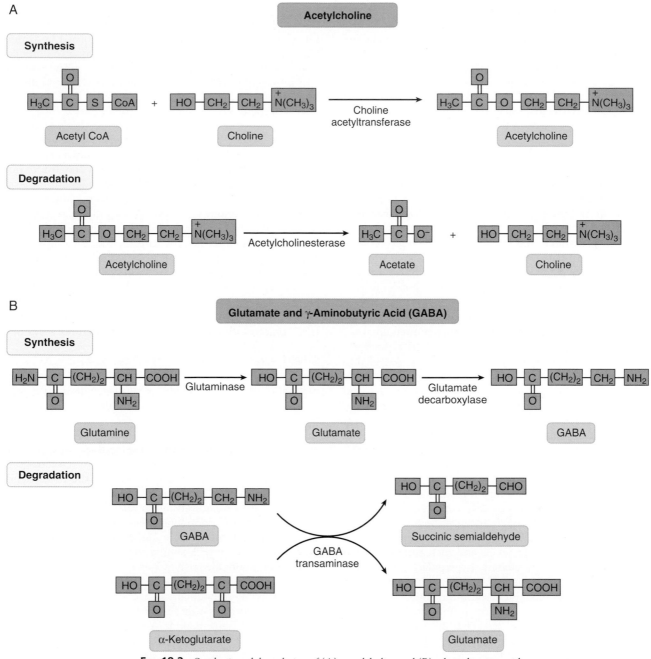

FIG. 18.2 Synthesis and degradation of (A) acetylcholine and (B) selected amino acids.

depolarization and firing of action potentials. Metabotropic glutamate receptors consist of two main classes that are either coupled to phospholipase C and intracellular calcium signaling or are negatively coupled to adenylyl cyclase and decrease cAMP. Glutamate and aspartate participate in the long-term potentiation needed for learning and memory and have a role in neuronal toxicity and apoptosis (cell death) evoked by trauma and ischemia. Antagonists of these excitatory amino acid receptors are used in the treatment of **seizures** (see Chapter 20) and may find use in blocking the overexcitation of neurons that occurs after stroke and in other disorders.

Biogenic Amines

The biogenic amines or monoamines that function as CNS neurotransmitters are the catecholamines dopamine and norepinephrine; serotonin (5-hydroxytryptamine); and histamine. These neurotransmitters, which are formed by decarboxylation of amino acids, are catabolized in part by the enzyme monoamine oxidase.

Dopamine. Dopamine is a major CNS neurotransmitter that binds to five types of dopamine receptors. The D_1 and D_5 receptors activate adenylyl cyclase, thereby increasing cAMP levels. In contrast, the D_2, D_3, and D_4 receptors inhibit adenylyl cyclase and decrease cAMP levels. **Levodopa, clozapine,** and other drugs have effects on various steps in the synthesis and metabolism of dopamine. Dopamine is found in several neuronal tracts originating from the ventral tegmental area, plays a significant role in behavioral and drug reinforcement, and regulates emesis (vomiting), prolactin release, mood states, motor coordination, and olfaction. Its degradation by **monoamine oxidase** results in the formation of homovanillic acid, a metabolite that is subsequently excreted in the urine (Fig. 18.3). Inhibitors of monoamine oxidase increase dopamine levels in the brain and are used for the treatment of parkinsonism.

Norepinephrine. Norepinephrine, which is formed from dopamine, is degraded by **monoamine oxidase** and **catechol-O-methyltransferase** to a number of metabolites. The major metabolite excreted in the urine is **3-methoxy-4-hydroxymandelic acid,** or **vanillylmandelic acid.** The receptors for norepinephrine are α-**adrenoceptors** and β-**adrenoceptors** (also known as α and β-adrenergic receptors), and their classification and properties are described in detail in Chapter 8. Norepinephrine is associated with several neuronal tracts projecting from the **locus ceruleus** in the medulla (brainstem) to the thalamus, cerebral cortex, cerebellum, and spinal cord, and it is found in tracts projecting from the midbrain to the hypothalamus. This ubiquitous neurotransmitter participates in the regulation of anxiety, cerebellar function, learning, memory, mood, sensory processing (including pain), and sleep. Drugs can alter norepinephrine neurotransmission by activating or blocking its receptors or by inhibiting its presynaptic neuronal uptake.

Serotonin. Serotonin, also known as 5-hydroxytryptamine (5-HT), is synthesized from tryptophan, is degraded to **5-hydroxyindoleacetic acid,** and functions as both an excitatory and inhibitory neurotransmitter. Serotonin is found in neuronal tracts projecting from the **raphe nuclei** in the medulla to many other parts of the brain. These tracts are involved in emotional processing and pain processing and have an effect on appetite, mood, sleep, and hallucinations. Serotonin (5-HT) acts on more than a dozen types of receptors; all of them are metabotropic receptors, except for the **5-HT3 receptor,** which is a ligand-gated ion channel protein. The main types and effector mechanisms of 5-HT receptors are outlined in Table 18.1. In most areas of the brain, serotonin has an inhibitory effect mediated by the 5-HT_{1A} receptor, decreasing cAMP levels and increasing potassium conductance, causing membrane hyperpolarization. Drugs can affect serotonergic function by stimulating or blocking 5-HT receptors or by blocking serotonin reuptake.

Histamine. Histamine is a neurotransmitter found in **hypothalamic neurons** that project to all the major parts of the brain, including the cerebral cortex. It is involved in the regulation of the sleep-wake cycle, cardiovascular control, regulation of the hypothalamic-pituitary-adrenal axis, learning, and memory. Histamine acts on two types of receptors in the brain, H_1 and H_3, with action on a third type, H_2, in the periphery. All histamine receptors are metabotropic, with H_1 receptors coupled to the phospholipase C pathway and H_3 receptors negatively coupled to adenylate cyclase. H_3 receptors were originally discovered as autoreceptors on histaminergic neurons but are now known to also inhibit the release of other neurotransmitters. CNS histamine receptors are not currently considered a major site of therapeutic drug action, but antagonism of H_1 receptors is partly responsible for the drowsiness and sedation caused by some **antihistamines.**

Neuropeptides

A number of peptides function as slow neurotransmitters or neuromodulators in the CNS. Unlike other neurotransmitters, **neuropeptides** are synthesized in neuronal cell bodies and are then transported to nerve terminals for release. Once released, they are metabolized by various peptidases, but they do not undergo presynaptic reuptake. Some of the neuropeptides are released as **cotransmitters** with other, nonpeptide neurotransmitters. The cotransmitter neuropeptides usually serve to amplify or prolong the effects of these other neurotransmitters.

A growing number of neuropeptides are known to function as neuromodulators in the CNS. One of the first classes of neuropeptides discovered are the **endogenous opioid peptides (endorphins),** which include **met-enkephalin, dynorphin, and β-endorphin.** The opioid peptides inhibit pain transmission in the spinal cord and midbrain, and, **like morphine, act on opioid receptors.** A second important group consists of **tachykinins,** which include **neurokinins A and B,** and **substance P.** Neurokinins modulate cardiovascular and behavioral responses to stress, and substance P participates in pain processing, emesis, and anxiety.

Other peptides that were originally isolated from peripheral tissues are thought to function as neuromodulators in the CNS. These neuropeptides include **cholecystokinin, gastrin, somatostatin,** and **vasoactive intestinal polypeptide.**

Other Neurotransmitters

Several additional substances, including the gases **nitric oxide** and **carbon monoxide,** appetite-regulating peptides, and purines, also serve as neurotransmitters or neuromodulators in the CNS.

Nitric oxide is a gas formed from arginine by calcium-calmodulin–stimulated nitric oxide synthase in CNS neurons. Evidence suggests that nitric oxide acts as a **retrograde neurotransmitter** in that it is released by the postsynaptic neuron and diffuses to the presynaptic terminal, where it facilitates future neurotransmitter release by elevating levels of cyclic guanosine monophosphate. This action may contribute to long-term potentiation, which is a key process to establishing memory. A similar function is also postulated for **carbon monoxide** in the CNS.

Several recently discovered **appetite-regulating peptides** function as neuromodulators in the CNS. These include **ghrelin,** a peptide synthesized in the stomach and hypothalamus, and **neuropeptide Y** and **orexin,** contained in neurons in the lateral hypothalamus. All three peptides stimulate food intake and increase body weight in animal models. Conversely, **leptin** is a peptide hormone secreted from fat cells that acts on the brain to reduce food intake and increase peripheral energy expenditure. As expected, the pharmaceutical industry has intense interest in developing drug therapies for the treatment of obesity based on these discoveries.

Purines that can serve as neurotransmitters include **adenosine** and **adenosine triphosphate (ATP).** Adenosine activates specific receptors identified as A_1, A_2, and A_3 **receptors.** Activation of A_1 and A_3 receptors increases cAMP formation, whereas activation of A_2 receptors inhibits cAMP formation. The role of adenosine as a central neurotransmitter is not clearly established, but inhibition of A_2 receptors by methylxanthines (e.g., caffeine) causes CNS stimulation. ATP acts on both ionotropic receptors, called **P2X receptors,** and metabotropic **P2Y receptors.** Similarly, the role of ATP in neurotransmission is unclear,

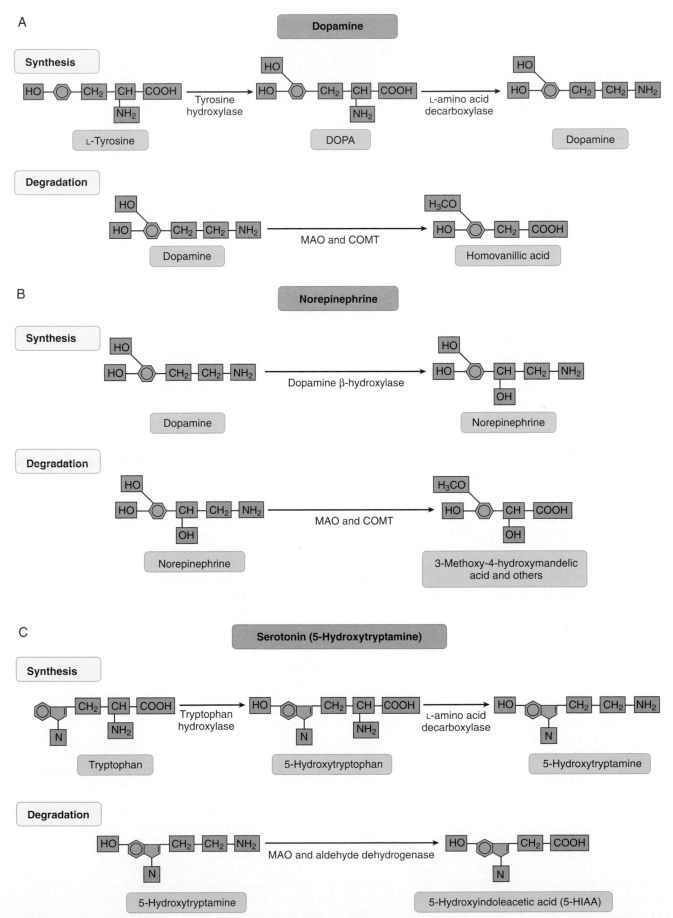

Fig. 18.3 Synthesis and degradation of (A) dopamine, (B) norepinephrine, and (C) serotonin. *COMT*, Catechol-O-methyltransferase; *DOPA*, dihydroxyphenylalanine; *MAO*, monoamine oxidase.

but some evidence indicates that ATP is a cotransmitter that is released with other neurotransmitters in the brain and serves to augment the effects of these neurotransmitters.

MECHANISMS OF DRUG ACTION

Drugs that alter CNS neurotransmitter function generally do so by altering the **synthesis, storage,** or **release** of a neurotransmitter; blocking the **reuptake** of a neurotransmitter; inhibiting the **degradation** of a neurotransmitter; or **activating** or **blocking** neurotransmitter receptors. A few CNS drugs act by directly blocking membrane ion channels or by altering the physiochemical properties of neuronal membranes to inhibit neurotransmission. Although bypassing the membrane receptor and directly modulating second-messenger or signal transduction pathways is an attractive target for novel pharmacologic agents, **lithium** is currently the only CNS drug shown to act by this mechanism.

Neurotransmitter Synthesis, Storage, and Release

Neurotransmitter synthesis can be increased by administering a precursor to a neurotransmitter, such as levodopa. **Levodopa** is taken up by dopamine neurons and is converted to dopamine, thereby increasing the amount of dopamine available for neurotransmission. The vesicular storage of norepinephrine is blocked by **reserpine,** a plant alkaloid first used to treat hypertension. The side effect of severe depression in patients treated with reserpine provided an early clue that neurotransmitter levels may be inadequate in persons with this type of affective disorder (see Chapter 22). Drugs can cause nonexocytotic release of neurotransmitters by interacting with the presynaptic neurotransmitter transporter. For example, **amphetamine** increases the release of norepinephrine by this mechanism and **amantadine** is used therapeutically to increase the release of dopamine in patients with parkinsonism.

Neurotransmitter Reuptake and Degradation

Presynaptic reuptake and enzymatic degradation are the two primary mechanisms for terminating the action of most CNS neurotransmitters, and drugs inhibit both of these processes. **Cocaine** and many antidepressant drugs act by blocking the reuptake of dopamine, norepinephrine, or serotonin. **Donepezil** and **selegiline** are examples of agents that inhibit the degradation of acetylcholine or dopamine and thereby elevate the synaptic concentration of these neurotransmitters.

Receptor Activation or Blockade

Postsynaptic receptors are activated or blocked by several types of CNS drugs. For example, **bromocriptine,** a drug used in the treatment of parkinsonism, acts as an agonist at dopamine receptors, whereas antipsychotic drugs act as antagonists at dopamine and serotonin receptors.

Presynaptic receptors are involved in feedback inhibition of neurotransmitter release. They are called **autoreceptors** when they are activated by the same neurotransmitter that is released by the neuron, and **heteroreceptors** when they are activated by a different neurotransmitter. Activation of presynaptic receptors decreases the concentration of the released neurotransmitter found in synapses, whereas blockade of these receptors increases the concentration. For example, activation of 5-HT_{1D} autoreceptors inhibits the release of serotonin and decreases its concentration in synapses.

Receptor Alterations Caused by Central Nervous System Drug Treatment

As detailed in Chapter 3, receptor proteins not only regulate cell processes but are themselves regulated. Receptors undergo dynamic alteration in response to changes in synaptic neurotransmitter concentrations or in response to long-term drug administration. These alterations can affect the efficiency of receptor coupling to signal transduction pathways (**desensitization** or **sensitization**) or affect the number of receptor proteins expressed by the neuron (**down-regulation** or **up-regulation**). CNS drugs that act on metabotropic or G protein–coupled receptors are particularly noted for their alteration of receptor numbers. Receptor down-regulation may follow a sustained increase in neurotransmitter release, a sustained blockade of neurotransmitter reuptake, or long-term receptor activation by a drug. For example, long-term administration of **morphine** in a patient with chronic pain can cause **down-regulation** of opioid receptors in the brain and spinal cord (Fig. 18.4). Receptor down-regulation is one of the primary mechanisms of pharmacodynamic drug tolerance. Receptor **up-regulation** is a compensatory reaction to a sustained decrease in neurotransmission, a condition that can be caused either by a reduction in neurotransmitter release or by long-term receptor antagonism. For example, daily administration of **haloperidol,** a dopamine receptor antagonist, in a schizophrenic patient can lead to up-regulation of D_2 receptors.

NEURONAL SYSTEMS IN THE CENTRAL NERVOUS SYSTEM

Many CNS diseases and drug treatments affect cognitive processing, memory, motor coordination, and other complex brain functions. It is difficult to attribute these complex functions to specific neuronal tracts because many of the functions are accomplished through the interaction of tracts that communicate with several brain regions and use various neurotransmitters. These six broad areas of functional processing, however, provide an introduction to the neuroanatomy and neuropharmacology of CNS agents.

Cognitive Processing

Cognitive processing occurs in **prefrontal cortical structures,** where sensory information is integrated with past experience and interpreted in a manner that can result in thoughts and behavioral action. The neuronal systems involved in cognitive processing include **association fibers** that arise from areas throughout the brain and converge on the anteromedial frontal, orbital frontal, and cingulate areas of the prefrontal cortex.

Cognitive processing uses memory and is influenced by emotions. At the same time, emotions are largely derived from past experience and cognition. Cognitive processing also encompasses abstract reasoning and forethought, which are processes that do not necessarily result in motor expression but can influence emotional processing and future acts.

Delirium is a general term that refers to disorders of cognitive processing, and one of the manifestations of **schizophrenia** is impaired cognitive processing.

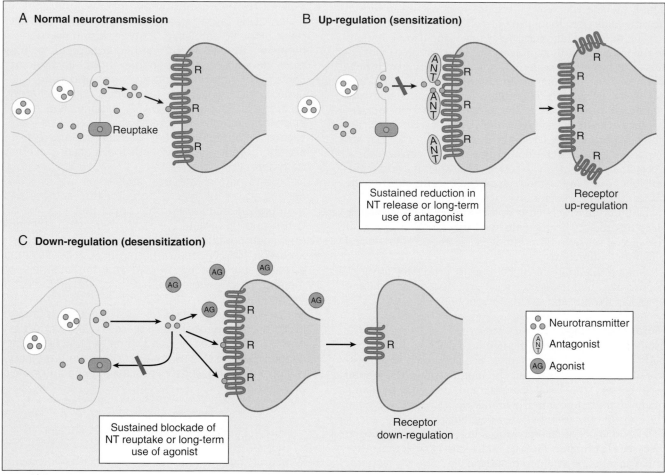

FIG. 18.4 Mechanisms of receptor sensitization and desensitization. (A) Under normal circumstances, the NT activates receptors and is removed from the synapse by neuronal reuptake. (B) The number of receptors can be increased (up-regulated) by a sustained reduction in NT release or by the long-term administration of a receptor ANT. (C) The number of receptors can be decreased (down-regulated) by a sustained blockade of NT reuptake or by the long-term administration of a receptor AG. *AG,* Agonist; *ANT,* antagonist; *NT,* neurotransmitter.

Drugs that affect cognitive processing include antipsychotics, CNS stimulants, hallucinogens, and sedative-hypnotics.

Memory

Memory is the ability to recall events and integrate them into cognitive processing, emotional processing, and ongoing motor activities. One form of memory, called **procedural memory,** is used to recall a set of practiced motor actions (e.g., riding a bicycle or typing on a keyboard), and it involves the interaction of **limbic structures,** the **cerebellum,** and the **basal ganglia.** Another form of memory, called **declarative memory,** involves thoughts and associations that may be used to determine future actions. For example, remembering that touching a hot stove is painful may keep a child from playing near the stove in the future, and remembering that a family member's birthday is approaching may trigger activities such as planning a dinner party. Declarative memory involves neuronal tracts in the **hippocampus, amygdala, thalamus,** and **neocortex.**

Dementia is a term used to describe a number of memory disorders, including **Alzheimer disease.** The involvement of the basal ganglia in procedural memory may explain why some patients with **Parkinson disease** have difficulties with practiced motor actions.

Drugs that affect memory include the **cholinesterase inhibitors** and CNS depressants such as **benzodiazepines.**

Emotional Processing

Emotional processing is responsible for the generation of emotions such as anger, anxiety, fear, happiness, love, and sadness. These emotions represent the conscious perception of neuronal activity originating in the **limbic system,** including the hypothalamus, amygdala, septum, hippocampus, and mammillary bodies, as well as the cingulate and entorhinal portions of the frontal lobe cortex. Emotions contribute to a state of mental preparedness for anticipated future activities. For example, anxiety contributes to a state of heightened vigilance, which may amplify the response to a future stimulus or event.

Disorders in which emotional processing is defective include **anxiety states, mood disorders,** and **schizophrenia.**

Drugs that affect emotional processing in the limbic system include anxiolytic (antianxiety) drugs, antidepressants, antipsychotics, CNS stimulants, opioids, and all drugs that produce drug dependence. Hence, most CNS drugs have some effect on emotional processing.

Sensory Processing

Sensory processing involves neuronal tracts that perceive external stimuli and transmit that information to the brain.

These include the sensory systems responsible for vision, hearing, olfaction, touch, and pain.

The spinothalamic tracts relay touch and pain sensations to the **thalamus,** which projects this information to the **cortex.** The brainstem region known as the **reticular formation** plays a significant role in filtering sensory information before it is relayed to the thalamus and hypothalamus and eventually to the cortex. The reticular formation includes the **locus ceruleus** and **raphe nuclei,** whose neurons release norepinephrine and serotonin, respectively, and play an important role in determining the level of consciousness, sleep, and wakefulness. The cortex of the parietal and occipital lobes and part of the temporal lobe is involved in the recognition and integration of sensory perceptions.

Disorders in which sensory processing is defective include **sleep disorders, chronic pain syndromes,** and **disorders of the special senses** such as blindness, deafness, and taste and olfactory dysfunction.

Among the drugs that affect sensory processing are antidepressants, hallucinogens, local and general anesthetics, opioid analgesics, and sedative-hypnotics.

Motor Processing

Motor processing refers to the neuronal activity that enables body movement. The structures involved in motor processing include the **cerebellum,** the motor strip of the **frontal lobe cortex,** the **basal ganglia,** and the suprasegmental nuclei that are found in the **brainstem** and are involved in the control of posture (e.g., the vestibular nuclei).

Disturbances in motor processing occur in **Parkinson disease, Huntington disease,** and a variety of degenerative and demyelinating neuron disorders.

Drugs that affect motor processing include antiparkinsonian drugs, CNS stimulants, muscle relaxants, antispastic drugs, and sedative-hypnotics.

Autonomic Processing

Autonomic processing involves areas of the brain that integrate the activities of the **peripheral autonomic nervous system** (see Chapter 6). These areas include the **hypothalamus** and portions of the **brainstem,** such as the vasomotor center and the cranial nuclei of parasympathetic nerves.

Disorders of autonomic processing include orthostatic hypotension and postural tachycardia syndrome.

Some CNS drugs alter autonomic processing by affecting the actions of hypothalamic and brainstem nuclei, and others have a direct effect on peripheral autonomic neurotransmission. The drugs that affect autonomic processing include **antidepressants, antiparkinsonian drugs, antipsychotics,** and **drugs used to treat Alzheimer disease.**

SUMMARY OF IMPORTANT POINTS

- CNS drugs act primarily by affecting the synthesis, storage, release, reuptake, or degradation of neurotransmitters or by activating or blocking receptors.
- Long-term administration of drugs sometimes causes up-regulation or down-regulation of receptors. Up-regulation is evoked by receptor antagonists, whereas down-regulation is evoked by receptor agonists or reuptake inhibitors.

- Major CNS neurotransmitters include acetylcholine; amino acids (aspartate, GABA, glutamate, and glycine); biogenic amines (dopamine, histamine, norepinephrine, and serotonin); and neuropeptides such as the endogenous opioid peptides and the tachykinins.
- Some CNS neurotransmitters (e.g., aspartate, glutamate, histamine, and tachykinins) are excitatory; others (e.g., dopamine, GABA, glycine, and opioid peptides) are inhibitory; and still others (e.g., acetylcholine, norepinephrine, and serotonin) are both excitatory and inhibitory, with these actions exerted via different receptors.
- Neurotransmitters can be classified as fast or slow, depending on the type of receptor they activate and the duration of the neuronal signal that they evoke. GABA and glutamate are fast, whereas norepinephrine, neuropeptides, and serotonin are slow.
- Receptors for CNS neurotransmitters can be classified as ionotropic (directly coupled with ion channels) or metabotropic (coupled with G proteins and second messengers).
- Many diseases of the CNS and the corresponding drugs used to treat these diseases have an effect on one or more of the following complex brain functions: cognitive processing, emotional processing, memory, motor processing, sensory processing, and autonomic processing.

Review Questions

1. Which of the following terms best describes a receptor located on a neuronal terminal that binds a neurotransmitter released from another neuron and decreases release of neurotransmitter from the neuronal terminal?
   (A) presynaptic receptor
   (B) heteroreceptor
   (C) postsynaptic receptor
   (D) autoreceptor
   (E) ionotropic receptor

2. Neurotransmitters are made in neurons and released when vesicles fuse with the neuronal membrane. What name is given to this process?
   (A) apoptosis
   (B) phagocytosis
   (C) endocytosis
   (D) pinocytosis
   (E) exocytosis

3. Which one of the following statements best describes the differences between classical neurotransmitters and neuropeptides?
   (A) neuropeptides are synthesized in the cell body
   (B) classical neurotransmitters have a longer duration of action
   (C) neuropeptides undergo rapid reuptake into the presynaptic terminal
   (D) classical neurotransmitters are packaged into vesicles
   (E) neuropeptides are degraded by acetylcholinesterase in the synapse

4. A patient with metastatic lung cancer is treated for chronic pain with daily doses of a long-acting morphine

formulation and oxycodone for breakthrough pain. He complains that the medicines are no longer working. Which one of the following mechanisms may explain the lack of effect of his medicines?

(A) the metabolism of morphine is upregulated
(B) pain intensity has greatly increased
(C) the efficiency of G protein coupling is decreased
(D) opioid receptors are downregulated
(E) the patient is a "drug seeker" and addicted to opioid medications

5. Which one of the following drugs acts by inhibiting neurotransmitter reuptake?

(A) lithium
(B) morphine
(C) fluoxetine
(D) levodopa
(E) donepezil

CHAPTER 19

Sedative-Hypnotic and Anxiolytic Drugs

CLASSIFICATION OF SEDATIVE-HYPNOTIC AND ANXIOLYTIC DRUGS

Benzodiazepines

- Alprazolam (XANAX)
- Chlordiazepoxide (LIBRIUM)
- Clonazepam (KLONOPIN)
- Diazepam (VALIUM)
- Lorazepam (ATIVAN)
- Triazolam (HALCION)[a]
- Midazolam (VERSED)
- Remimazolam (BYFAVO)
- Flumazenil (ROMAZICON)[b]

Barbiturates

- Thiopental (PENTOTHAL)
- Methohexital (BREVITAL)
- Pentobarbital (NEMBUTAL)
- Amobarbital (AMYTAL)
- Phenobarbital (LUMINAL)

Antihistamines

- Diphenhydramine (BENADRYL)
- Doxepin (SILENOR)
- Hydroxyzine (ATARAX)

Anti-Insomnia Agents

- Zolpidem (AMBIEN)[c]
- Zaleplon (SONATA)
- Eszopiclone (LUNESTA)
- Suvorexant (BELSOMRA)[d]
- Ramelteon (ROZEREM)[e]

Nonsedating Anxiolytic Drugs

- Buspirone (BUSPAR)
- Propranolol (INDERAL)

[a] Also estazolam (PROSOM), flurazepam (DALMANE), oxazepam (SERAX), temazepam (RESTORIL), and clorazepate (TRANXENE).
[b] Flumazenil is a competitive antagonist at the benzodiazepine binding site.
[c] Also available as zolpidem tartrate sublingual tablet (INTERMEZZO).
[d] Also lemborexant (DAYVIGO)
[e] Also tasimelteon (HETLIOZ).

OVERVIEW

Sedative-hypnotic drugs are among the most widely used pharmaceutical agents in the world. The **sedative** part of their name refers to the ability of these agents to calm or reduce anxiety, known as an **anxiolytic** effect. The **hypnotic** part of their name describes the ability of these agents to induce drowsiness and promote sleep. This latter action is caused by a greater depression of central nervous system (CNS) activity; most sedative-hypnotic drugs will first cause sedation, then at higher doses produce *hypnosis,* the medical term for sleep. A few agents, however, exert anxiolytic effects without causing sedation or hypnosis.

This chapter describes the pharmacologic properties of benzodiazepines, barbiturates, and other sedative-hypnotic and anxiolytic drugs used in the treatment of anxiety and sleep disorders. Because of their greater safety, fewer adverse effects, and the availability of an antagonist, benzodiazepines have largely replaced the older barbiturates for these indications. Although ethanol (alcohol) has sedative-hypnotic effects, it is not used therapeutically for these purposes; its pharmacologic effects are described in Chapter 25.

ANXIETY DISORDERS

Anxiety is normally an **adaptive response** that prepares a person to react to the challenges of life. Anxiety is characterized by changes in mood (apprehension and fear), sympathetic nervous system arousal, and hypervigilance. When anxiety becomes chronic, it can impair a person's ability to perform the activities of daily living. Moreover, chronic anxiety often leads to visceral organ dysfunction and unpleasant symptoms. For example, patients with chronic anxiety may develop gastrointestinal, cardiovascular, and neurologic problems, including diarrhea, tachycardia, sweating, tremors, and dizziness. Ultimately, anxiety can contribute to heart disease and other disorders, including self-medication, which may lead to substance abuse.

Neurologic Basis of Anxiety

The neuronal pathways involved in anxiety disorders include the **sensory, cognitive, behavioral, motor,** and **autonomic pathways.** Sensory systems, cortical processing, and memory are involved in interpreting a stimulus to be dangerous and creating a state of heightened arousal. Motor systems and autonomic processing participate in the exaggerated responses to an anxiety state.

Growing evidence indicates that the **amygdala,** an almond-shaped structure in the temporal lobe, plays a central role in mediating most of the manifestations of anxiety, including the **conditioned avoidance reaction** (conditioned fear reaction) that underlies anxiety states. In experimental protocols, this reaction can be induced in animals by teaching them that a cue (e.g., a flashing light) will be followed by a noxious stimulus (e.g., a shock to the foot). During the anticipatory period, the animals conditioned in this manner will exhibit signs of anxiety, such as autonomic and behavioral arousal. Electrical stimulation of the amygdala induces signs of anxiety, whereas lesioning the amygdala or the administration of anxiolytic drugs prevents the behavioral and physiologic manifestations of anxiety during the anticipatory period. It is believed that **long-term potentiation** in amygdala neurons establishes the memory of adverse events underlying anticipatory anxiety.

Classification and Treatment of Anxiety Disorders

The appropriate management of anxiety disorders requires an accurate diagnosis, and treatment may involve the use of pharmacologic agents, psychotherapy, or both.

Acute Anxiety

Acute anxiety may develop in response to various factors, such as illness, separation from loved ones, or the anticipation of stressful events. Acute anxiety is often self-limiting and may resolve in a few weeks to a few months without drug treatment. A **benzodiazepine** might provide short-term relief from more severe acute anxiety conditions.

Panic Disorder

Panic disorder is characterized by acute episodes of severe anxiety with marked psychological and physiologic symptoms. During a panic attack, an individual may feel an impending sense of doom that is often accompanied by sweating, tachycardia, tremor, and other visceral symptoms. Patients with panic disorder often respond to drug therapy with a **benzodiazepine** or an **antidepressant drug,** such as a **selective serotonin reuptake inhibitor (SSRI;** see Chapter 22). Benzodiazepines may provide immediate relief from panic attacks during the early phase of therapy, and **alprazolam** and **clonazepam** are benzodiazepines that have been particularly useful in this regard. For long-term treatment, an SSRI antidepressant, such as **fluoxetine,** is often prescribed.

Phobic Disorders

Phobic disorders can be grouped into specific phobia, social anxiety disorder (social phobia), or agoraphobia. Phobias are conditions in which an individual is overly fearful about a particular situation or condition, such as a fear of spiders or traveling in an airplane. Panic disorder can coexist with **agoraphobia,** an intense fear of being in a public place from which it might be difficult or embarrassing to cope with a panic attack. Patients with panic disorder and agoraphobia often show the best outcomes when treated with a combination of psychotherapy and drug therapy. As with panic disorder, phobic disorders are treated with a **benzodiazepine** or an **antidepressant drug.** Benzodiazepines provide acute relief of symptoms and enable patients to more easily benefit from psychotherapy, whereas antidepressants are usually the most effective long-term drug therapy for agoraphobia and social phobia. **Propranolol** is useful in the prevention of **stage fright,** or **acute situational** or **performance anxiety.**

Obsessive-Compulsive Disorder

Obsessive-compulsive disorder (OCD) is characterized by **obsessions,** which are recurring or persistent thoughts and impulses, and **compulsions,** defined as repetitive behaviors in response to obsessions. OCD can be treated effectively with an **antidepressant drug** (see Chapter 22) and psychotherapy.

Generalized Anxiety Disorder

Generalized anxiety disorder (GAD) is characterized by chronic worry and apprehension concerning future events. Short-term therapy with a **benzodiazepine** may relieve acute symptoms and provide a useful bridge to psychotherapy. The severity of the disorder often fluctuates over time, and benzodiazepines may be effectively used on an intermittent basis to help patients deal with exacerbations of the disorder. **Buspirone, a nonsedating anxiolytic,** provides a useful alternative to benzodiazepines for the treatment of chronic anxiety states because it produces little sedation and is not associated with tolerance or dependence. It must be taken for 3 or 4 weeks, however, before its anxiolytic effects are felt. SSRIs, such as **paroxetine,** and the serotonin and norepinephrine reuptake inhibitors (SNRIs) **venlafaxine** and **duloxetine** (see Chapter 22) are also used in the treatment of GAD.

Posttraumatic Stress Disorder

Posttraumatic stress disorder (PTSD) may develop after exposure to a traumatic event, such as sexual assault or military combat. SSRIs are used in the treatment of PTSD. Other medications, such as benzodiazepines, may also be used to treat associated symptoms, such as an exaggerated **startle response** and **flashbacks.**

SLEEP DISORDERS

Sleep is a reversible state of reduced consciousness accompanied by characteristic changes in the electroencephalogram (EEG). Five distinct patterns of brainwave activity occur during sleep, grouped into the four stages of **nonrapid eye movement (NREM) sleep,** and a pattern characterized by paralysis of voluntary muscles and quick, saccadic movement of the eye called **rapid eye movement (REM) sleep.**

As an individual falls asleep, the high-frequency and low-amplitude activity of the alert state gradually diminishes during stages 1 and 2 and is replaced by the low-frequency and high-amplitude activity of **slow-wave sleep** (stages 3 and 4). Over time, the individual returns to stage 1 and eventually to the REM stage. REM sleep is also known as **paradoxical sleep** because the EEG pattern is similar to that in the awake state. A normal adult cycles through the sleep stages about every 90 minutes (Box 19.1).

Sleep patterns change with age and are altered by sedative-hypnotic and other CNS drugs.

Neurologic Basis of Sleep

The neuronal systems involved in sleep include the **basal forebrain nuclei** and the **reticular formation.** Projecting from the basal forebrain to the cortex are cholinergic fibers that are believed to be involved in the induction of sleep. The basal forebrain is the only region of the brain that is active during slow-wave sleep and quiescent at other stages. The reticular formation facilitates the flow of sensory information from the thalamus to the cortex. When reticular nuclei are quiescent, the thalamus does not transfer information to the cortex, and this facilitates the onset of sleep.

Classification and Treatment of Sleep Disorders

Insomnia

Some patients with insomnia find it difficult to go to sleep or to stay asleep during the night, whereas others awaken too early in the morning. In general, the management of insomnia depends on whether the sleep disorder is caused by physiologic, psychologic, or medical conditions. As shown in Box 19.1, the patterns of sleep stages in patients with insomnia are irregular and include longer latency to fall asleep and frequent awakenings.

BOX 19.1 EFFECT OF SEDATIVE-HYPNOTIC DRUGS ON SLEEP ARCHITECTURE TERMINOLOGY

Patterns on the electroencephalogram (EEG) vary with the stage of sleep. When a person falls asleep, the high-frequency and low-amplitude pattern of the **awake state** is gradually replaced by the progressively lower-frequency and higher-amplitude patterns of stages 1 through 4, which collectively are called **non–rapid eye movement sleep (NREM sleep).** Stages 3 and 4 are called **slow-wave sleep.** Another stage, called **rapid eye movement sleep (REM sleep),** is characterized by rapid, jerky eye movements. REM sleep is also called **paradoxical sleep** because it is during

this stage that the pattern on the EEG returns to the pattern seen during the awake state.

NORMAL AND ABNORMAL SLEEP PATTERNS

The normal sleep pattern in adults consists of about five cycles, each of which lasts approximately 90 min. During each cycle, an individual progresses from stage 1 to stage 4 and then returns to stage 1, followed by a period of REM sleep. As the cycles progress through the night, they become shorter, and the amount of slow-wave sleep decreases.

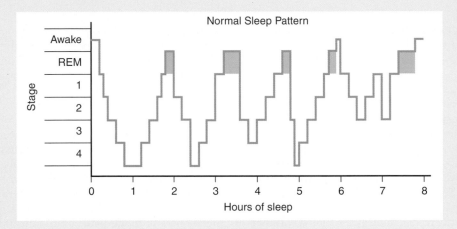

EFFECTS OF DRUGS ON SLEEP ARCHITECTURE

The sleep patterns of patients with insomnia vary widely but are often characterized by reduced amounts of slow-wave sleep and by one or more awakenings during the night. The time required to fall asleep (sleep latency) is usually

prolonged, and the total sleep time is decreased in most patients with insomnia. Elderly adults often have a similar sleep pattern.

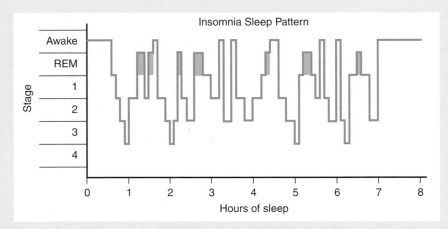

Benzodiazepines and most other hypnotics suppress stage 3 and REM sleep. In contrast, zolpidem, zaleplon, eszopiclone, suvorexant, lemborexant, ramelteon, and

tasimelteon have little effect on sleep architecture. Therefore, the use of these newer agents may better restore the sleep pattern to normal.

Occasional sleeplessness caused by acute stress or a minor illness is usually self-limiting and may not require treatment. More severe insomnia caused by medical conditions whose symptoms interfere with sleep is effectively treated with **benzodiazepines** or other **sedative-hypnotic drugs,** such as **zolpidem** and **zaleplon,** whereas insomnia related to psychological and psychiatric disturbances is best managed with a combination of psychotherapy

and sedative-hypnotic drugs. Benzodiazepines and most other hypnotic drugs **decrease sleep latency** (the time required to go to sleep) and **increase sleep duration.** The newest agents, zolpidem, zaleplon, eszopiclone ('z'-drugs), **orexin receptor antagonists,** and **melatonin agonists,** have the advantages of not significantly affecting sleep architecture and not causing as much tolerance and dependence as the other drugs. For these reasons,

BOX 19.2 DRUG EFFECTS ON SLEEP

State	Rapid Eye Movements	Pattern on EEG	Effect of Benzodiazepines	Effect of Z-Drugs
Awake	No	High-frequency, low-amplitude pattern	Induce sleep	Induces sleep
Stages 1 and 2 sleep	No	Lower-frequency, higher-amplitude pattern than awake state	Increase length of stages	Little change
Stages 3 and 4 sleep	No	Lower-frequency, higher-amplitude pattern than stages 1 and 2	Decrease length of stages	Little change
REM sleep	Yes	High-frequency, low-amplitude pattern	Decrease length of stage	Little change

zolpidem, zaleplon, eszopiclone, suvorexant, lemborexant, ramelteon, and tasimelteon have become the drugs of choice to treat most types of insomnia (Box 19.2).

Other Sleep Disorders

Other sleep disorders include **hypersomnia** (difficulty in awakening), **narcolepsy** (sleep attacks), **enuresis** (bedwetting during sleep), **somnambulism** (sleepwalking), **sleep apnea** (episodes of hypoventilation during sleep), and **nightmares** and **night terrors.** Most of these disorders are managed with a combination of psychotherapy and **antidepressant drugs** or **CNS stimulants. Sodium oxybate** (XYREM), a form of the abused drug *gamma (γ)*-hydroxybutyrate (GHB), was recently approved for the treatment of cataplexy associated with **narcoleptic attacks.** CNS stimulants used to treat narcolepsy and other sleep disorders are discussed in Chapter 22.

SEDATIVE-HYPNOTIC DRUGS

The sedative-hypnotic drugs include **benzodiazepines, barbiturates, antihistamines,** and nonbenzodiazepine agents, such as the **'z'-drugs, orexin receptor antagonists, and melatonin agonists.** The properties of these drugs are summarized in Table 19.1.

Because benzodiazepines have fewer adverse reactions and drug interactions and are safer in cases of overdose, they have largely replaced the barbiturates and other older drugs. Nevertheless, barbiturates are still used when benzodiazepines are ineffective or contraindicated. The sedating antihistamines are occasionally used to treat mild insomnia and anxiety and have less potential for abuse than benzodiazepines and barbiturates. Many over-the-counter (OTC; nonprescription) sleep aids contain antihistamines as their effective ingredient.

Benzodiazepines

The benzodiazepines are a large group of drugs that have similar pharmacologic effects. They are so named because they share the common chemical structure of a benzene ring *(benzo)* joined to a seven-member ring containing two nitrogen molecules *(diazepine)*. The particular use of specific drugs is largely determined by their pharmacokinetic properties and route of administration. Some benzodiazepines were developed and approved to treat anxiety, whereas others are approved for the management of insomnia or for other purposes.

Drug Properties

Pharmacokinetics. The pharmacokinetic properties of various benzodiazepines are compared in Table 19.1. The benzodiazepines are absorbed from the gut and distributed to the brain at rates proportional to their **lipid solubility,** which varies 50-fold among individual drugs in the class. As the plasma concentration of a benzodiazepine declines, the drug is redistributed from the brain to the blood, and this mechanism contributes significantly to the termination of its effects on the CNS.

All benzodiazepines are **extensively metabolized** in the liver. Most benzodiazepines are converted to **active metabolites** in phase I oxidative reactions catalyzed by cytochrome P450 enzymes. The active metabolites of chlordiazepoxide, diazepam, and flurazepam are long acting and contribute to the long duration of action of these agents. The active metabolites of alprazolam, estazolam, midazolam, and triazolam are shorter acting. Each of these active metabolites is eventually conjugated with glucuronate to form an inactive polar metabolite excreted in the urine. Other drugs, namely **oxazepam, temazepam, clonazepam,** and **lorazepam,** bypass phase I oxidation and are metabolized only by phase II conjugation (Fig. 19.1). These drugs may be safer for use by elderly patients, because the capacity to conjugate drugs does not decline with age as much as the capacity for oxidative biotransformation does. Therefore, active metabolites of these four drugs are less likely to accumulate to toxic levels in elderly patients.

Benzodiazepines also undergo some degree of **enterohepatic cycling** that prolongs their duration of action. In fact, some patients who are taking a drug such as diazepam may notice an increased sedative effect after eating a high-fat meal. The fatty meal causes the gallbladder to empty, thereby delivering bile containing diazepam to the intestines for reabsorption into the circulation.

Mechanism of Action. The **benzodiazepines** and **barbiturates** exert their effects on sleep and consciousness by facilitating the activity of the neurotransmitter *gamma-*aminobutyric acid (GABA) at various sites in the brain. GABA, the most ubiquitous inhibitory neurotransmitter in the CNS, regulates the excitability of neurons in almost every neuronal tract. As shown in Fig. 19.2, the $GABA_A$ **receptor–chloride ion channel** has binding sites for benzodiazepines and barbiturates, as well as alcohols, steroids, and inhalational anesthetics. This receptor-ion channel complex is made up of five subunits, with the major form of the complex containing *alpha (α), beta (β),* and *gamma (γ)* subunits. However, there are at least 16 types of these protein subunits (e.g., α_1, α_2, β_1, β_2), and it is not entirely clear which types of subunits make up the $GABA_A$ receptors that mediate the clinical and adverse effects of drugs that bind to them.

TABLE 19.1   Pharmacokinetic Properties and Clinical Uses of Sedative-Hypnotic and Anxiolytic Drugs

DRUG	ONSET OF ACTION[a]	DURATION OF ACTION[a]	ACTIVE METABOLITES	MAJOR CLINICAL USES
Benzodiazepines				
Alprazolam	Fast	Medium	Yes	Anxiety, including panic disorder
Chlordiazepoxide	Fast; very fast (IV)	Long	Yes	Alcohol detoxification; anxiety
Clonazepam	Fast	Medium	No	Anxiety, including panic disorder; seizure disorders
Diazepam	Fast; very fast (IV)	Long	Yes	Alcohol detoxification; anxiety; muscle spasm; seizure disorders; spasticity
Lorazepam	Fast; very fast (IV)	Medium	No	Anxiety; seizure disorders
Midazolam	Very fast (IV)	Short (IV)	Yes	Anesthesia induction; conscious Sedation
Remimazolam	Very fast (IV)	Short (IV)	Yes	Anesthesia induction; conscious Sedation
Triazolam	Fast	Short	Yes	Insomnia
Barbiturates				
Thiopental	Very fast (IV)	Short (IV)	No	Induction of anesthesia
Pentobarbital	Fast	Short	No	Insomnia
Phenobarbital	Slow	Long	No	Seizure disorders
Amobarbital	Fast	Medium	No	Insomnia
Antihistamines				
Diphenhydramine	Fast	Medium	No	Insomnia
Hydroxyzine	Fast	Long	No	Anxiety; sedation
Anti-insomnia agents				
Zolpidem	Fast	Short	No	Insomnia
Zaleplon	Fast	Very short	No	Insomnia; midsleep awakenings
Eszopiclone	Fast	Short	No	Insomnia
Suvorexant	Fast	Medium	No	Insomnia
Ramelteon	Slow	Short	Yes	Sleep-onset insomnia
Nonsedating anxiolytic drugs				
Buspirone	Very slow	Long	No	Chronic anxiety
Propranolol	Fast	Medium	Yes	Situational or performance anxiety

[a]Unless onset and duration of action are specifically indicated for intravenous (IV) administration, they are for oral administration. Very fast, <15 min; fast, 15–59 min; slow, 1–4 h; very slow, 3–4 weeks; short, 1–6 h; medium, 7–12 h; and long, >12 h.

The **benzodiazepine binding site** is located at the interface between α and γ subunits at a site different from the binding site of GABA. Benzodiazepines bind to this site and increase the affinity of GABA for its binding site on the GABA_A receptor–chloride ion channel complex. This is an example of an **allosteric binding site.** Benzodiazepines bind to receptors made up of both α_1 and α_2 subunits, whereas the newer nonbenzodiazepine agents ('z' drugs, see later) are selective for receptors containing α_1 subunits.

Benzodiazepines increase the **frequency** with which the channel opens, whereas barbiturates increase the **length of time** that the channel remains open. By increasing chloride conductance, these drugs cause neuronal membrane **hyperpolarization,** and this in turn counteracts the depolarizing effect of excitatory neurotransmitters. Barbiturates increase chloride conductance **independent** of the presence of GABA, which is why they are capable of causing greater CNS depression and toxicity than the benzodiazepines.

In addition to their effects on GABA, benzodiazepines also inhibit the neuronal reuptake of **adenosine.** This action

increases the inhibitory effect of adenosine on neurons that release acetylcholine from the reticular formation, which is a brainstem structure mediating arousal. The effect of benzodiazepines on adenosine may also explain why these drugs dilate coronary arteries and decrease total peripheral resistance.

Pharmacologic Effects. The benzodiazepines produce a dose-dependent but **limited depression of the CNS.** Lower doses have a sedative and anxiolytic effect, whereas higher doses produce hypnosis (sleep) and moderate sedation, but **not reaching the depth of general anesthesia** needed for loss of reaction to painful stimulus (Fig. 19.3). Benzodiazepines can relieve anxiety at doses that produce relatively little sedation. In contrast to barbiturates, the orally administered benzodiazepines do not produce significant respiratory depression, coma, or death unless they are administered with another CNS depressant (e.g., opioids or alcohol). Because benzodiazepines **work only in the presence of GABA** released by neurons, the depth of CNS depression is limited. Therefore, the **benzodiazepines exhibit a ceiling effect** whereby greater doses do not produce significantly

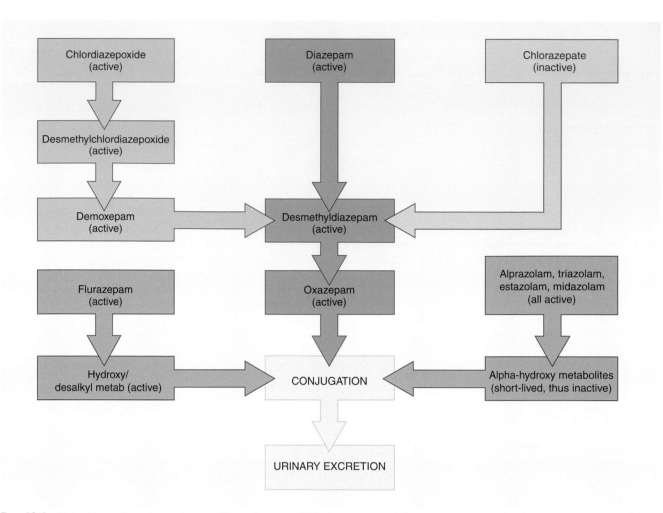

FIG. 19.1 Major biotransformation pathways of benzodiazepines. Chlordiazepoxide and diazepam are converted to long-acting active metabolites. Alprazolam, midazolam, and triazolam are converted to a short-acting active metabolite. Clorazepate is a prodrug and inactive until metabolized. All benzodiazepines, including those with no active metabolites, are eventually converted to glucuronide compounds that are pharmacologically inactive and are excreted in the urine. The benzodiazepines that do not undergo phase 1 metabolism and are directly conjugated include oxazepam, temazepam, lorazepam, and clonazepam ("out the liver cleared"), and these may be the safest benzodiazepines to use in treating elderly patients.

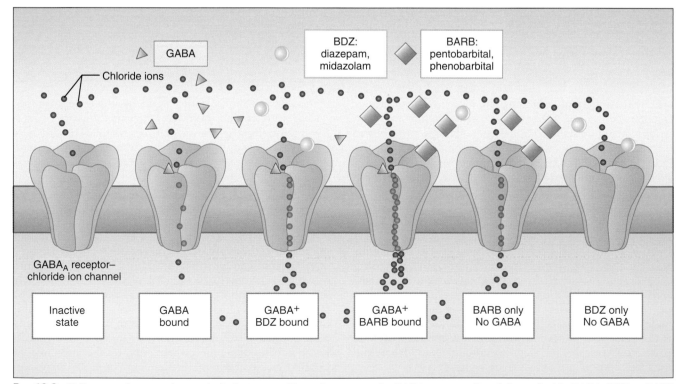

FIG. 19.2 Different mechanisms of action for barbiturates and benzodiazepines at the GABA_A receptor. From left to right: No GABA, BDZ, or BARB present, inactive receptor. GABA bound, receptor activated, Cl⁻ ions enter neuron which inhibits excitation. GABA + BDZ bound, receptor activated more than when only GABA bound. GABA + BARB bound, receptor activated maximally. BARB only no GABA, receptor activated. BDZ only no GABA, no receptor activation.

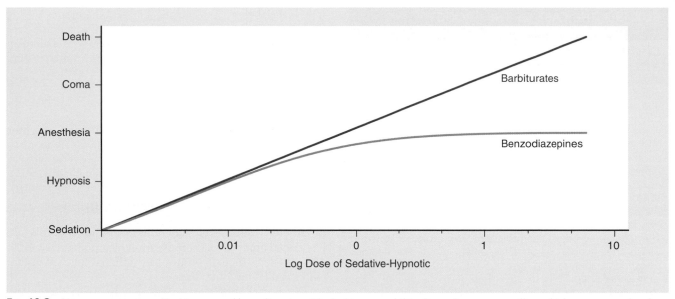

Fig. 19.3 Dose-response curves of barbiturates and benzodiazepines. The barbiturates exhibit a linear dose-response effect, which progresses at low doses from sedation to hypnosis, anesthesia, coma, and death at high doses. Due to a different mechanism of action, benzodiazepines produce sedation and hypnosis but cannot produce anesthesia, coma, or death at high doses. Because of this, benzodiazepines exhibit a ceiling effect. Intravenous administration of benzodiazepines at clinical doses does not produce significant respiratory depression, except when other CNS depressants are co-administered. Benzodiazepines are given intravenously to induce anesthesia but cannot maintain anesthesia as sole agents.

greater effects and do not depress the brain to the point of anesthesia and death. **Barbiturates do not exhibit this ceiling effect** and can produce severe respiratory depression and death after administration of a large dose.

In addition to producing sedative-hypnotic and anxiolytic effects, benzodiazepines can produce **anterograde amnesia,** which means that an individual will not remember what happens from the time that the drug is administered to the time that the drug effects dissipate. This is in contrast to **retrograde amnesia,** in which a person cannot remember what happened before a certain point in time (drug administration). The benzodiazepines produce anterograde amnesia because they interfere with the formation of new memory; they do not affect the ability to recall past events. The amnesic property of benzodiazepines is often useful when patients are undergoing stressful procedures, such as endoscopy or outpatient surgery. When these drugs are used on a long-term basis, such as in treating anxiety, the amnesic properties can have an adverse effect on the patient's ability to function. **Triazolam,** a widely used hypnotic, has been associated with problems caused by its amnesic effect.

Benzodiazepines have anticonvulsant effects and are used in the treatment of seizure disorders (see Chapter 20). Although benzodiazepines cause muscle relaxation only at doses that produce considerable sedation, they are occasionally used to treat muscle spasm and spasticity. The muscle-relaxing effects of benzodiazepines are caused by the fact that these drugs potentiate the effects of GABA in the spinal cord.

Adverse Effects. The adverse effects of benzodiazepines are largely caused by CNS depression. The drugs frequently cause motor incoordination, dizziness, and excessive drowsiness. They impair cognitive processing and can affect concentration, judgment, and planning. They can also interfere with **driving** and other **psychomotor skills.** When longer-acting benzodiazepines (e.g., diazepam) are used to treat

insomnia, they can cause drowsiness and a drug hangover the next day. If this occurs, a shorter-acting drug (e.g., zolpidem or zaleplon) should be substituted for the longer-acting drug. See case in Box 19.3.

Intravenous (IV) administration of benzodiazepines produces greater CNS depression than does oral administration, although IV administration of a benzodiazepine by itself rarely causes respiratory depression. Specific warnings of respiratory depression were issued by the U.S. Food and Drug Administration (FDA) for **midazolam,** an agent formulated solely for intravenous administration. The FDA warning stressed that midazolam should be used cautiously with other CNS depressant agents.

Benzodiazepines have a mild euphoric effect and can reduce behavioral inhibitions in a manner similar to the **disinhibitory** effect of alcohol. The behavioral reinforcement produced by these drugs may contribute to their recreational abuse by polydrug abusers and to their inappropriate long-term use by patients. It appears that the reinforcing effects of benzodiazepines are less than the reinforcing effects of barbiturates but greater than the reinforcing effects of sedating antihistamines and possibly **zolpidem, zaleplon,** and **eszopiclone.** The newest melatonin agonist drugs, **ramelteon** and **tasimelteon,** are unscheduled prescription sedative-hypnotic agents due to lack of reinforcing effects from activation of **melatonin receptors.**

Long-term use of the benzodiazepines can produce **physical dependence,** the severity of which is proportional to the dosage and duration of administration. After several months of continued use, most patients develop some degree of physical dependence. If their medication is abruptly discontinued, they will experience a withdrawal syndrome characterized by rebound anxiety, insomnia, headache, irritability, and muscle twitches. The withdrawal syndrome is usually mild and not life-threatening. Abrupt withdrawal from **alprazolam** has been associated

BOX 19.3 THE CASE OF THE GROGGY GRANDMOTHER

CASE PRESENTATION

A 68-year-old woman was prescribed 5 mg of diazepam for anxiety by her primary care physician after her husband died. She was told to take one in the morning with her breakfast and was advised to increase her activities to "take her mind off her worries." After following the prescribed regimen for a week, she found that she had problems going to sleep, and without consulting her physician, she began to take another diazepam pill at night. She continued taking one diazepam pill in the morning and one pill at night for the next few days. Her friends noted that she was not coming out of her room at the assisted living center as much as she used to, and they knocked on her door to check up on her. They found her still in her nightgown and disorientated. They convinced her to call her doctor, who told her to stop taking the second pill of diazepam at night; the doctor prescribed zolpidem, at a dose of 5 mg, to be taken at night to help her sleep. Over the next few days, the patient was more alert during the day and resumed her activities.

CASE DISCUSSION

The use of benzodiazepines for anxiety disorders has largely replaced any other type of sedative-hypnotic agent, such as barbiturates, for this indication because of their increased safety and effectiveness. However, benzodiazepines are metabolized into many active metabolites, some that have longer durations of actions than their parent drug. Phase 1 or oxidative drug biotransformation (metabolism) in the elderly is reduced, and this patient population is especially sensitive to the buildup of active metabolites of many benzodiazepines, including diazepam. Three agents are better suited in elderly patients; oxazepam, temazepam, and lorazepam do not undergo phase 1 metabolism but are directly conjugated to inactive metabolites. Phase 2 metabolic reactions, such as conjugation, are less affected with aging. The use of zolpidem, a nonbenzodiazepine drug used for insomnia, has a short elimination half-life and leads to little hangover effect the next day, allowing for resumption of normal daytime activities for the elderly patient.

with seizures. To prevent the occurrence of seizures, the dosage of benzodiazepines should be gradually tapered over a period of several weeks. Because the various drugs in the benzodiazepine class exhibit cross-tolerance, any of them can be substituted for another one to prevent or counteract the withdrawal reaction.

Pharmacodynamic tolerance also occurs during long-term use of benzodiazepines. Unlike barbiturates, however, benzodiazepines do not induce their own metabolism or cause pharmacokinetic tolerance.

Although the overall safety of the benzodiazepines is high, in rare cases, their use has been associated with hypotension, arrhythmia (tachycardia or bradycardia), and a number of other, less-common effects. A massive overdose of a benzodiazepines is only fatal when preexisting respiratory conditions exist or the benzodiazepine is taken with other CNS depressants. Benzodiazepine overdose is successfully treated due to the availability of the selective benzodiazepine antagonist **flumazenil.**

The incidence of fetal malformations in the offspring of women who take benzodiazepines during pregnancy is very low. Nevertheless, chronic use of benzodiazepines during pregnancy is not recommended, and benzodiazepines are included in pregnancy category D by the FDA. **Zolpidem** and **zaleplon** appear to be safer in pregnancy and are listed as pregnancy category B.

Interactions and Treatment of Adverse Effects. Several drugs, including flumazenil and β-carboline derivatives, interact with benzodiazepine receptors.

Flumazenil is a competitive **benzodiazepine receptor antagonist.** In addition to blocking the effects of agonists, such as diazepam, it also blocks the effects of inverse agonists (see later) at the benzodiazepine receptor. Flumazenil can be used to counteract the adverse effects of benzodiazepines, such as respiratory depression resulting from intravenous administration of these drugs or in the case of accidental or intentional overdose. Flumazenil is given intravenously and has a rapid onset and a short duration of action. Its potential adverse effects include seizures, arrhythmias, blurred vision, emotional lability, and dizziness.

The β-carboline derivatives act as inverse agonists. An inverse agonist is a drug that decreases the response of an effector system below the basal level (see Chapter 3). The β-carboline drugs act to decrease chloride conductance by the $GABA_A$ receptor–chloride ion channel, and this can cause anxiety and seizures. Some experimental inverse agonists enhance cognitive function ("smart drugs") and are being studied for the treatment of Alzheimer disease.

Indications. Benzodiazepines are effective in the treatment of anxiety disorders, insomnia, muscle spasm, seizure disorders, and spasticity. They are also used for the treatment of alcohol withdrawal. When possible, the use of benzodiazepines should be limited to the short-term treatment of these conditions. If long-term use is medically justified, the physician should carefully monitor drug use to prevent dosage escalation.

Specific Agents

Alprazolam is converted to a short-acting α-hydroxyl metabolite before undergoing glucuronide formation. Alprazolam has a medium duration of action and is used primarily in the management of **anxiety.** Although it has special utility in the treatment of **panic disorder,** the larger doses usually required for controlling panic attacks can cause considerable sedation and contribute to drug dependence. Therefore, for many patients, the panic disorder can be treated instead with antidepressants and behavioral therapy. Alprazolam is useful as a short-term measure to relieve acute symptoms while other therapies are instituted.

Chlordiazepoxide and **diazepam** are converted to long-acting metabolites, including desmethyldiazepam (also called nordiazepam). Desmethyldiazepam is converted to **oxazepam,** which is excreted as a polar glucuronate conjugate (see Fig. 19.1). Chlordiazepoxide and diazepam are effective in the treatment of **anxiety.** In patients undergoing **alcohol detoxification,** these drugs can be used to prevent seizures and other acute withdrawal reactions. The drug dosage is gradually tapered over several weeks.

Diazepam is also used to terminate **acute recurrent seizures** (see Chapter 20), to treat **severe muscle spasm,** and to treat **spasticity** associated with degenerative and demyelinating neurologic disorders.

Oxazepam, temazepam, clonazepam, and lorazepam do not form long-acting metabolites, so they have a short or medium duration of action. They are biotransformed to inactive glucuronide compounds. As mentioned, they may be preferable in the treatment of elderly patients because glucuronide conjugation does not decline significantly with aging. Lorazepam can be administered orally or intravenously and is used to treat **anxiety** and to control **seizures.** Oxazepam is a short-acting drug that is administered to patients with **anxiety.** Temazepam is used primarily to treat **insomnia.**

Estazolam, flurazepam, and triazolam have active metabolites with varying durations of action. Estazolam has a medium duration of action, whereas flurazepam has a longer one, and triazolam has a shorter one. All three drugs are used to treat **insomnia.** A short- or medium-acting drug may be preferred for patients whose primary problem is getting to sleep, whereas a medium- or long-acting drug may be preferred for patients who report waking up too early. The short-acting triazolam is more likely to cause rebound insomnia when it is discontinued. The long-acting flurazepam is less likely to cause rebound insomnia but is more likely to cause daytime drowsiness. Triazolam has been associated with a higher incidence of amnesia, confusion, and delirium, especially in elderly patients. The dose of triazolam in formulations marketed in the United States has been reduced by the FDA, and triazolam has been banned in the United Kingdom.

Recently, label revisions for all of the previously mentioned sedative-hypnotic agents indicated for sleep disorders were made to include warnings regarding the risk of **hypersensitivity reactions,** including anaphylaxis (severe allergic reaction) and angioedema (severe facial swelling), which can occur as early as the first time the sedative-hypnotic agents are taken. In addition, warnings were included for the risk of **complex sleep-related behaviors,** which may include driving, making phone calls, having sex, and preparing and eating food, all while still asleep and with no memory of the behaviors having occurred.

Other Benzodiazepines

Clonazepam is also used for the treatment of **panic disorder** and **other anxiety disorders,** as well as for the treatment of **seizure disorders** (see Chapter 20). As mentioned above, unlike most benzodiazepines, clonazepam does not have active metabolites.

Midazolam is used intravenously as an **induction agent** for patients undergoing surgery or to produce **conscious sedation** for endoscopy, minor outpatient surgery, and other diagnostic procedures. Midazolam is also a benzodiazepine drug that was used recently for **lethal injection** after the barbiturate thiopental was no longer available. After several "botched executions" with midazolam, attorneys on behalf of condemned inmates filed suit against the jailers arguing that midazolam use violated the "cruel and unusual punishment" clause of the 8th Amendment. The case was appealed all the way to the Supreme Court and, in a 5 to 4 vote, the use of midazolam instead of thiopental for lethal injection was upheld. It was the first instance that the Supreme Court considered a basic pharmacology question concerning the differences between barbiturates and benzodiazepines; a question they failed to answer correctly.

Remimazolam is the newest benzodiazepine to join the sedative-hypnotic class. Using the same strategy as the ultra-short opioid remifentanil (see Chapter 23) of rapid metabolism by tissue esterases, the structure of midazolam was modified with an ester linkage to make remimazolam. **Remimazolam** is given by IV injection and indicated for the **induction and maintenance of conscious sedation** for procedures lasting 30 minutes or less.

Barbiturates

The barbiturates include **amobarbital, pentobarbital, phenobarbital,** and **thiopental.** The properties of these drugs are outlined in Table 19.1.

Drug Properties

Pharmacokinetics. The onset and duration of action of barbiturates are determined by their lipid solubility and rate of metabolic inactivation. Highly lipid-soluble drugs (e.g., **amobarbital, pentobarbital,** and **thiopental**) are well absorbed from the gut, rapidly redistributed from the brain to peripheral tissues as plasma concentrations fall, and extensively metabolized to inactive compounds before they are excreted in the urine. Phenobarbital, a more polar drug, is slowly absorbed from the gut and more slowly redistributed from the brain, and this contributes to its longer duration of action. **Phenobarbital** is partly converted to inactive metabolites, but a significant fraction of the parent compound is excreted unchanged in the urine.

Mechanism of Action. Barbiturates bind to an **allosteric site** on the $GABA_A$ receptor–chloride ion channel that is distinct from the allosteric site to which benzodiazepines bind. The barbiturates **increase the affinity** of the receptor for GABA and **the duration of time** that the chloride channel remains open. In contrast to benzodiazepines, barbiturates also act to directly increase chloride influx **in the absence of GABA** (see Fig. 19.2). For this reason, barbiturates **do not exhibit a ceiling effect.** As shown in Fig. 19.3, they have a linear dose-response curve with no ceiling effect. Higher doses of barbiturates increasingly depress the neuronal activity of the CNS, causing anesthesia, coma, and death from cardiorespiratory depression. This is why barbiturates exhibit greater toxicity and a smaller therapeutic index than benzodiazepines.

Pharmacologic Effects. Unlike the anxiolytic effect of benzodiazepines, that of barbiturates is associated with considerable sedation. When used to treat insomnia, barbiturates can cause hangover and daytime sedation. As with benzodiazepines, barbiturates suppress slow-wave and REM sleep. Barbiturates can also cause tolerance and physical dependence during continuous use, and a withdrawal syndrome occurs if the drugs are abruptly discontinued. Short-acting barbiturates (e.g., **pentobarbital**) have been extensively abused.

Interactions. Barbiturates induce cytochrome P450 enzymes in the liver and thereby accelerate their own metabolism, as well as that of other drugs metabolized by these enzymes. Maximal enzyme induction is obtained by the daily administration of phenobarbital, a long-acting agent. Barbiturates also induce the rate-limiting enzyme in porphyrin biosynthesis, α-aminolevulinate synthase, and may thereby exacerbate **porphyria,** a condition in which a hereditary defect causes excessive porphyrin synthesis and excretion, with attendant neurologic and cutaneous manifestations.

Indications. The barbiturates were extensively used to treat anxiety disorders and insomnia before the development of benzodiazepines, but they are seldom used for these purposes today. Unlike benzodiazepines, barbiturates do not produce significant muscle relaxation and are not used in treating muscle spasm or spasticity disorders. They are indicated for the treatment of seizure disorders (see Chapter 20) and for the induction and maintenance of general anesthesia.

Specific Agents

Pentobarbital and **amobarbital** and have been used primarily to treat **insomnia**. **Phenobarbital** is used occasionally to treat **seizure disorders,** and **thiopental** was administered intravenously to induce **anesthesia.** Thiopental is extremely lipid soluble and has a very fast onset of action; it is the only barbiturate available that is classified as an **ultra-short-acting barbiturate.** It is also rapidly redistributed from the brain to other tissues (muscle and fat), which accounts for its ultra-short duration of action. It is no longer available in the United States.

Antihistamines

Some of the **histamine antagonists** (antihistamines) cross the blood-brain barrier and produce varying degrees of sedation, and these drugs have been used to treat **mild insomnia** and **anxiety disorders.** For example, **diphenhydramine** is the active ingredient in several nonprescription sleep preparations, and **hydroxyzine** has been used in the treatment of mild anxiety and is sometimes used as a **sedative** before surgery. **Doxepin** was also recently approved for the treatment of insomnia and has a high affinity for H$_1$ receptors. The sedative action of these drugs is caused by their ability to bind to H$_1$ receptors and reduce acetylcholine released by neurons in the reticular nuclei (reticular activating system).

Drugs that block acetylcholine release, including **antihistamines,** induce drowsiness and sleep via their effects on the cholinergic projections of the reticular nuclei. In contrast, **caffeine** and related **methylxanthines** can increase arousal by blocking presynaptic adenosine receptors, thereby increasing cholinergic activity in the reticular nuclei.

Some tolerance can occur during the long-term use of antihistamines, but these drugs are not associated with physical dependence or significant drug abuse. The pharmacologic properties of antihistamines are discussed in detail in Chapter 26.

Anti-Insomnia Agents
Zolpidem, Zaleplon, and Eszopiclone

The newer agents **zolpidem, zaleplon,** and **eszopiclone** (known as 'z' drugs) have largely replaced older benzodiazepines for the treatment of insomnia. These agents are popular because they cause fewer adverse effects than the older benzodiazepine agents—for example, they have a relative lack of effect on REM or slow-wave sleep—and have less potential for tolerance and dependence. Their shorter duration of action usually precludes daytime sedation and hangover effects. There is evidence that this is a result of greater selectivity at targeting only GABA$_A$ receptors composed of particular subunit combinations, in particular those receptors composed of α$_1$ subunits. (This site of action was previously classified as the "omega$_1$ site.") The older benzodiazepines are less selective and bind to a more widespread distribution of receptor, producing a greater degree of adverse effects on sleep, cognitive performance, and memory. In addition, the elimination half-life of these newer agents is shorter than that of the older benzodiazepine agents, which accounts for a weaker hangover effect. **Zaleplon** has the advantage that its elimination half-life is the shortest at about 1 hour; it can be taken by patients who awaken in the middle of the night and have difficulty going back to sleep. **Zolpidem** is also available in a quick-acting sublingual tablet called EDLUAR.

Orexin Receptor Antagonists

Orexin is a neuropeptide produced in the hypothalamus and promotes wakefulness through interaction with orexin receptors. A role for orexin in wakefulness was confirmed when it was discovered that some people with **narcolepsy** (a dysfunction in sleep causing chronic sleepiness and episodes of falling asleep during the day) have a **loss of orexin-producing neurons** in the brain.

Suvorexant is a first in class drug that works as a **competitive receptor antagonist** at **orexin receptors.** Suvorexant has good oral bioavailability and reaches maximum concentration in the blood after about 2 hours. It has a long elimination half-life of 12 hours after steady-state is reached in nightly users, so caution for next-day sleepiness is warranted. More recently, a second **orexin receptor antagonist** was approved for the treatment of insomnia, called **lemborexant. Lemborexant** has similar bioavailability and time to peak absorption after oral administration as suvorexant but with a longer elimination half-life.

Melatonin and Related Drugs

Melatonin is a neuroendocrine hormone synthesized in the pineal gland. The hormone interacts with specific receptors in the CNS and elsewhere, and it is believed to be the principal mediator of the biologic clock that determines circadian, seasonal, and reproductive rhythms in animal species. In humans, melatonin is released before the onset of sleep and produces drowsiness that facilitates sleep. Studies show that melatonin produces drowsiness even if administered during the daytime.

Melatonin is available without prescription and may be effective in the treatment of **jet lag** in individuals who have rapidly traveled across several time zones and in the treatment of **insomnia in shift-change workers.** If melatonin is taken at bedtime for a few nights, it may accelerate the resetting of the biologic clock in these persons. Melatonin may also be effective in treating **insomnia in elderly patients** who do not secrete adequate melatonin, and it appears to be effective in treating **delayed sleep-phase syndrome** and **non–24-hour sleep-wake disorder.** It should be noted that melatonin is not an FDA-approved drug but is available OTC at health food or supplement stores.

Ramelteon is a new drug that acts selectively at **melatonin receptors** and is approved to treat **sleep-onset insomnia.** Ramelteon does not produce dependence and has little potential for abuse, so it is not a controlled substance. Compared with benzodiazepine drugs, there is no evidence for **rebound**

insomnia after cessation of ramelteon. It should not be used with fluvoxamine, as this SSRI antidepressant is a strong CYP1A2 inhibitor, and concurrent use with ramelteon increases the peak plasma concentration of ramelteon 70-fold.

Tasimelteon is another melatonin agonist recently approved for the **treatment of insomnia for non-24-hour sleep-wake disorder** (Non-24). Non-24 is a serious, chronic sleep disorder marked by disruption of the circadian rhythm. Non-24 affects up to 70% of people who are totally blind, whether **blind from birth or acquired blindness.** Tasimelteon was stealthily marketed by TV commercials that did not mention tasimelteon, but educated the public about the Non-24 disorder in blind persons and gave a website for further information.

Chloral Hydrate

Chloral hydrate is an older hypnotic that is largely obsolete today. It is a prodrug that is converted to its active metabolite, trichloroethanol, by liver enzymes. Its effects are potentiated by alcohol, and the combination of alcohol and chloral hydrate gained fame under the monikers of "Mickey Finn" and "knock-out drops." Chloral hydrate is occasionally used for **preanesthetic sedation** in pediatric patients.

Nonsedating Anxiolytic Drugs
Buspirone

Buspirone is a unique anxiolytic agent that does not share structural similarity with the other agents. The drug is used in the treatment of **chronic anxiety** and produces an anxiolytic effect without causing marked sedation, amnesia, tolerance, dependence, or muscle relaxation. In some patients, it can cause headache, dizziness, and nervousness, but these side effects are usually mild and temporary.

Buspirone is a **partial agonist** at serotonin 5-HT$_{1A}$ receptors and may exert its anxiolytic effect by activating feedback inhibition of serotonin release. By this action, it can cause up-regulation of postsynaptic serotonin receptors. This effect takes time to develop and is consistent with the 3- to 4-week delay in the onset of the anxiolytic effect of buspirone. Buspirone and other drugs affecting serotonin are discussed further in Chapter 26.

Propranolol

Propranolol, a β-adrenoceptor antagonist (β-blocker), is sometimes used to prevent the physiologic manifestations of **stage fright, acute situational,** or **performance anxiety.** When taken an hour before the anticipated anxiety-provoking event, propranolol prevents tachycardia and other signs and symptoms of acute anxiety caused by sympathetic stimulation. The mechanisms and properties of β-blockers are discussed in detail in Chapter 9.

SUMMARY OF IMPORTANT POINTS

- Benzodiazepines, the most widely used sedative-hypnotic drugs, are indicated for the treatment of anxiety disorders, insomnia, muscle spasm, seizure disorders, and spasticity.
- Benzodiazepines bind to an allosteric receptor site on the GABA$_A$ receptor–chloride ion channel and thereby facilitate the binding of GABA and increase

the frequency with which the chloride channel opens. Because benzodiazepines need GABA present to work, the magnitude of CNS depression produced by these drugs is limited and show a ceiling effect.

- Some benzodiazepines (e.g., chlordiazepoxide and diazepam) have long-acting active metabolites. Others (e.g., alprazolam, midazolam, and triazolam) have shorter-acting active metabolites. All benzodiazepines, including those with no active metabolites, are eventually converted to inactive glucuronide compounds. The benzodiazepines that have no active metabolites (e.g., oxazepam, temazepam, lorazepam, clonazepam) may be the safest ones to use in the treatment of elderly patients.
- Benzodiazepines and other hypnotic drugs reduce the time required to fall asleep (sleep latency), reduce early awakenings, and increase total sleep time. Benzodiazepines and barbiturates reduce slow-wave sleep and decrease REM sleep.
- Pentobarbital, phenobarbital, and other barbiturates bind to the GABA$_A$ receptor–chloride ion channel but do not exhibit a ceiling effect and can cause respiratory depression, coma, and death.
- Unlike benzodiazepines, barbiturates induce their own metabolism, as well as that of many other drugs metabolized by cytochrome P450 enzymes.
- Long-term administration of benzodiazepines and barbiturates can lead to tolerance and physical dependence, and abrupt discontinuation of their use will cause symptoms of withdrawal.
- Zolpidem, zaleplon, and eszopiclone are effective, short-acting sedative-hypnotic agents that have little effect on normal sleep architecture and produce few adverse effects.
- Orexin receptor antagonists are the newest class of sedative-hypnotic agents. Drugs in this class are suvorexant and lemborexant.
- Ramelteon is the first prescription drug that acts on melatonin receptors to treat insomnia. A second melatonin agonist approved for the treatment of insomnia is tasimelteon.
- Sedating antihistamines (e.g., diphenhydramine and hydroxyzine) have been used to treat mild insomnia and anxiety. Older hypnotics (e.g., chloral hydrate) are largely obsolete but are occasionally used for preanesthetic sedation.
- Propranolol and other β-adrenoceptor antagonists can be used to prevent the physiologic manifestations of situational or performance anxiety, including tachycardia.
- Flumazenil is a benzodiazepine receptor antagonist that can be used to counteract respiratory depression and other reactions that are usually caused by excessive doses of intravenously administered benzodiazepines.

Review Questions

1. Which of the following molecular processes best describes the mechanism of action of benzodiazepines?
   (A) potentiating the effect of GABA at chloride ion channels

    (B)   blocking glutamate excitation
    (C)   blocking the inactivation of sodium ion channels
    (D)   binding to opioid receptors to produce sedation
    (E)   potentiating the action of the inhibitory amino acid, glycine

2. Benzodiazepines are noted for altering which one of the following aspects of sleep?
    (A)   increasing the time to sleep onset
    (B)   decreasing stage 2 NREM sleep
    (C)   increasing slow-wave sleep
    (D)   decreasing the REM stage of sleep
    (e)   increasing sleep awakenings

3. Which one of the following statements best describes flumazenil?
    (A)   does not produce withdrawal seizures
    (B)   has the longest elimination half-life
    (C)   is not metabolized into an active agent
    (D)   is also used for the treatment of epilepsy
    (E)   is a selective benzodiazepine antagonist

4. Zaleplon differs from zolpidem in which one of the following ways?
    (A)   produces withdrawal seizures
    (B)   has a shorter elimination half-life
    (C)   has a different chemical structure than benzodiazepines
    (D)   shows less tolerance to sedative effects
    (E)   produces greater morning sedation

5. Which one of the following anxiolytic drugs is noted for its lack of sedation?
    (A)   hydroxyzine
    (B)   diazepam
    (C)   oxazepam
    (D)   alprazolam
    (E)   buspirone

CHAPTER 20 Antiepileptic Drugs

CLASSIFICATION OF ANTIEPILEPTIC DRUGS[a]

Drugs for Partial Seizures and Generalized Tonic-Clonic Seizures

- Carbamazepine (TEGRETOL)[b]
- Phenytoin (DILANTIN)
- Phenobarbital (LUMINAL)
- Primidone (MYSOLINE)
- Cenobamate (XCOPRI)
- Valproic acid (DEPAKENE)[c]

Adjunct Drugs for Partial Seizures

- Clorazepate (TRANXENE)
- Felbamate (FELBATOL)
- Gabapentin (NEURONTIN)
- Pregabalin (LYRICA)
- Lamotrigine (LAMICTAL)
- Zonisamide (ZONEGRAN)
- Topiramate (TOPAMAX)[d]

Drugs for Generalized Absence, Myoclonic, or Atonic Seizures

- Clonazepam (KLONOPIN)
- Ethosuximide (ZARONTIN)
- Lamotrigine (LAMICTAL)
- Valproic acid (DEPAKENE)

Drugs for Status Epilepticus

- Diazepam (Valium)
- Lorazepam (Ativan)
- Phenobarbital (Luminal)
- Fosphenytoin (Cerebyx)

Cannabinoid Drugs for Atypical Seizures
- Cannabidiol (EPIDIOLEX)

[a]Note that some drugs are listed more than once.
[b]Also oxcarbazepine (TRILEPTAL) and an extended-release formulation of oxcarbazepine called OXTELLAR XR.
[c]Also available in a delayed release formulation (STAVZOR) and as divalproex sodium (DEPAKOTE, DEPAKOTE ER, DEPAKOTE SPRINKLE CAPSULE).
[d]Also tiagabine (GABITRIL), levetiracetam (KEPPRA), brivaracetam (BRIVIACT), vigabatrin (SABRIL), lacosamide (VIMPAT), ezogabine (POTIGA), eslicarbazepine (APTIOM), rufinamide (BANZEL), clobazam (ONFI), and perampanel (FYCOMPA). Topiramate XR (extended-release) is also now available (QUDEXY, TROKENDI XR) as well as a sprinkle capsule designed to be opened and applied to soft foods (TOPAMAX SPRINKLE).

OVERVIEW

Seizures are episodes of abnormal electrical activity in the brain that cause involuntary movements, sensations, or thoughts. Seizures can result from head trauma, stroke, brain tumors, hypoxia, hypoglycemia, fever, chronic alcohol withdrawal, and other conditions that alter neuronal function. Recurrent seizures that cannot be attributed to any proximal cause are seen in patients with epilepsy. In some patients, epilepsy appears to have a genetic basis. Environmental perturbations (e.g., intrauterine or neonatal complications) have also been implicated in the development of epilepsy. In the United States, epilepsy affects 1% to 2% of the population and is the second most common neurologic disease after stroke.

Classification of Seizures

The two main categories of seizures are partial (focal) seizures and generalized seizures (Table 20.1). A partial seizure originates in one cerebral hemisphere, and the patient does not lose consciousness during the seizure. A generalized seizure arises in both cerebral hemispheres and involves loss of consciousness. Seizures are accompanied by characteristic changes in the electroencephalogram (EEG), as shown in Fig. 20.1. Most seizures are self-limited and last from about 10 seconds to 5 minutes. Some seizures are preceded by an aura, which is a sensation or mood that may help identify the anatomic location of the seizure focus.

About 60% of epileptic seizures are partial seizures. Electroencephalographic abnormalities are seen in one or more lobes of a cerebral hemisphere, and the patient may exhibit motor, sensory, and autonomic symptoms. In **simple partial seizures,** consciousness is not altered. In **complex partial seizures,** however, patients have an altered consciousness and exhibit repetitive behaviors (automatisms). Complex partial seizures often originate in the temporal lobe, in which case the disorder is called either **temporal lobe epilepsy** or **psychomotor epilepsy.** Some partial seizures progress along anatomic lines as the electrical discharges spread across the cortex. For example, a seizure may first involve the fingers, then the hand, and finally the entire arm. This is characteristic of **jacksonian epilepsy,** or **"jacksonian march."** Partial seizures can also evolve into generalized seizures.

The two main types of generalized seizures are tonic-clonic seizures and absence seizures. Generalized tonic-clonic seizures, which were formerly called **grand mal seizures,** begin with a brief tonic phase followed by a clonic phase with muscle spasms lasting 3 to 5 minutes, and they conclude with a postictal period of drowsiness, confusion, and a glazed look in the eyes. **Status epilepticus** is a condition in which patients experience recurrent episodes of tonic-clonic seizures without regaining consciousness or normal muscle movement between episodes. Generalized **absence seizures,** or **petit mal seizures,** are characterized by abrupt loss of consciousness and decreased muscle tone, and they can include a mild clonic component, automatisms, and autonomic effects. On the EEG, generalized absence seizures exhibit a synchronous 3-Hz (three cycles per second) spike-and-dome pattern that usually lasts 10 to 15 seconds.

Less-common types of generalized seizures include **myoclonic seizures** and **atonic seizures** (see Table 20.1).

Neurobiology of Seizures

Epileptic seizures are caused by synchronous neuronal discharges within a particular group of neurons, or **seizure focus,** which is often located in the cerebral cortex but can be found in other areas of the brain. Once initiated, the abnormal discharges spread to other parts of the brain and produce abnormal movements, sensations, or thoughts. The neuronal mechanisms that initiate a seizure are not fully understood, but growing

TABLE 20.1 International Classification of Partial and Generalized Seizures

CLASSIFICATION	CHARACTERIZATION
Partial (focal) seizures	Arise in one cerebral hemisphere
Simple partial seizure	No alteration of consciousness
Complex partial seizure	Altered consciousness, automatisms, and behavioral changes
Secondarily generalized seizure	Focal seizure becomes generalized and is accompanied by loss of consciousness
Generalized seizures	Arise in both cerebral hemispheres and are accompanied by loss of consciousness
Tonic-clonic (grand mal) seizure	Increased muscle tone followed by spasms of muscle contraction and relaxation
Tonic seizure	Increased muscle tone
Clonic seizure	Spasms of muscle contraction and relaxation
Myoclonic seizure	Rhythmic, jerking spasms
Atonic seizure	Sudden loss of all muscle tone
Absence (petit mal) seizure	Brief loss of consciousness with minor muscle twitches and eye blinking

evidence indicates the involvement of excessive excitatory neurotransmission mediated by **glutamate** (Fig. 20.2). Investigators believe that excessive activation by glutamate of N-methyl-D-aspartate (NMDA) receptors displaces Mg^{2+} ions from the **NMDA receptor–calcium ion channel** and thereby facilitates calcium entry into neurons. Calcium contributes to the long-term potentiation of excitatory glutamate neurotransmission by activating the synthesis of **nitric oxide.**

Nitric oxide is a gas that can diffuse backward to the presynaptic neuron, where it facilitates glutamate release via stimulation of a G protein that activates the synthesis of cyclic guanosine monophosphate. These actions further increase NMDA receptor activation and calcium influx, which are believed to contribute to the **depolarization shift** observed in seizure foci. The depolarization shift consists of abnormally prolonged action potentials (depolarizations) that have spikelets. The shift recruits and synchronizes depolarizations by surrounding neurons and thereby initiates a seizure.

Several other mechanisms can be involved in seizures. One is the suppression of inhibitory neurotransmission **of gamma (γ)-aminobutyric acid (GABA),** and another is an increase in calcium influx via T-type calcium channels in thalamic neurons.

Mechanisms of Antiepileptic Drugs

Antiepileptic drugs (AEDs) are believed to suppress the formation or spread of abnormal electrical discharges in the brain. As shown in Table 20.2, the classic AEDs accomplish these actions via three mechanisms: (1) inhibition of the sodium or calcium influx responsible for neuronal depolarization, (2) augmentation of inhibitory GABA neurotransmission, and (3) inhibition of excitatory glutamate neurotransmission. The mechanisms of action of classic and new AEDs are shown in Fig. 20.3.

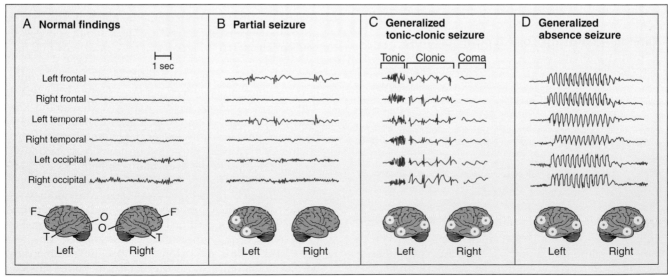

Fig. 20.1 Patterns on electroencephalogram (EEG) in the normal state and during seizures. The locations of seizure foci are shown as *shaded areas* on the cerebral hemispheres. (A) In the normal state, the EEG shows asynchronous alpha (8–12 Hz) and beta (12–30 Hz) rhythms originating in the cortex of the frontal (*F*), temporal (*T*), and occipital (*O*) lobes. (B) During a partial seizure, synchronous discharges are observed in various areas of the brain. In this example, they are seen in the left frontal and left temporal lobes, but they are not seen in other lobes. (C) During a generalized tonic-clonic seizure, the tonic phase is characterized by low-frequency and high-amplitude waves, whereas the clonic phase shows synchronous oscillations. (D) During a generalized absence seizure, a synchronous 3-Hz spike-and-wave pattern is seen throughout the cortex.

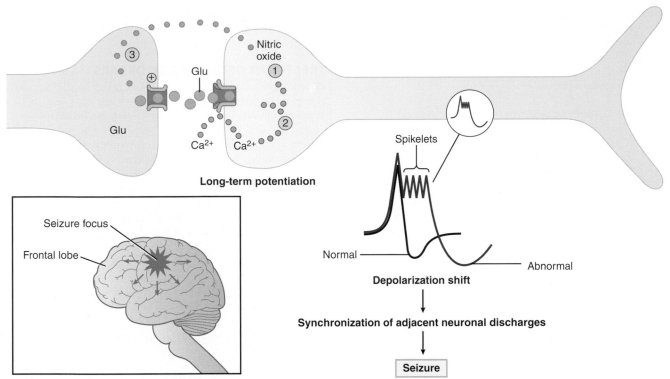

Fig. 20.2 Neuronal mechanisms underlying seizures. In this example, a seizure is caused by the synchronous discharge of a group of neurons (focus) in the cortex. Activation of N-methyl-D-aspartate *(NMDA)* receptors increases calcium influx *(1)* and nitric oxide synthesis *(2)*. Nitric oxide then diffuses to the presynaptic neuron and increases the release of glutamate via formation of cyclic guanosine monophosphate *(3)*. Increased excitatory glutamate neurotransmission leads to long-term potentiation. Long-term potentiation is believed to facilitate a depolarization shift, characterized by prolonged depolarizations with spikelets. The depolarization shift can cause adjacent neurons to discharge synchronously and thereby precipitate a seizure.

TABLE 20.2 Mechanisms of Selected Antiepileptic Drugs

DRUG	EFFECTS ON ION FLUX	EFFECTS ON GABA	EFFECTS ON GLUTAMATE
Carbamazepine	Blocks voltage-sensitive sodium channels	—	—
Phenytoin	Blocks voltage-sensitive sodium channels	—	—
Phenobarbital	—	Enhances GABA-mediated chloride flux	—
Cenobamate	Blocks voltage-sensitive sodium channels	Enhances GABA-mediated chloride flux	—
Valproate	Blocks voltage-sensitive sodium channels and T-type calcium channels	Increases GABA synthesis and inhibits GABA degradation	Decreases glutamate synthesis
Clorazepate	—	Enhances GABA-mediated chloride flux	—
Ethosuximide	Blocks T-type calcium channels	—	—
Gabapentin	—	Increases GABA release	—
Lamotrigine	Blocks voltage-sensitive sodium channels	—	—
Topiramate	Blocks voltage-sensitive sodium channels	Increases GABA activation of GABA$_A$ receptors	Blocks kainate and AMPA receptors

AMPA, α-Amino-3-hydroxy-5-methyl-4-isoxazole propionate acid; *GABA,* γ-aminobutyric acid; *NMDA,* N-methyl-D-aspartate; —, no effect.

Effects on Ion Channels

Under normal circumstances, **voltage-sensitive (voltage-gated) sodium channels** are rapidly opened when the neuronal membrane potential (voltage) reaches its threshold. This causes rapid depolarization of the membrane and the conduction of an action potential along the neuronal axon. When the action potential reaches the nerve terminal, it evokes the release of a neurotransmitter. After the neuronal membrane is depolarized, the sodium channel is inactivated by the closure of the channel's inactivation gate. The inactivation gate must be opened before the next action potential can occur.

Many AEDs, including **carbamazepine, lamotrigine, phenytoin,** and **topiramate,** prolong the time that the sodium channel's inactivation gate remains closed, and this delays the formation of the next action potential. These drugs bind to the channel when it is opened. Because rapidly firing neurons are opened a greater percentage of the time than are slowly firing neurons, the drugs exhibit **use-dependent blockade.** For this reason, the drugs suppress abnormal repetitive depolarizations in a seizure focus more than they suppress normal neuronal activity. By these actions, carbamazepine and other drugs prevent the spread of abnormal discharges in a seizure focus to other neurons.

A few drugs, such as **ethosuximide** and **valproate,** block **T-type (low-threshold) calcium channels** located in thalamic neurons and participate in the initiation of generalized absence seizures.

Effects on GABAergic Systems

AEDs facilitate GABA neurotransmission by various means. Benzodiazepines, such as clonazepam, and barbiturates, such as phenobarbital, enhance GABA activation of the **GABA$_A$ receptor–chloride ion channel** (see Chapter 19). Topiramate also activates the GABA$_A$ receptor. **Gabapentin** increases GABA release, whereas **vigabatrin** inhibits GABA degradation. Drugs that augment GABA may serve to counteract the excessive excitatory neurotransmission responsible for initiating and spreading abnormal electrical discharges.

Effects on Glutaminergic Systems

A few AEDs, including **felbamate, topiramate,** and **valproate,** inhibit glutamate neurotransmission, and other drugs that work via this mechanism are under development. This

is an attractive mechanism of action because it may affect the formation of a seizure focus and thereby terminate a seizure at an early stage of its development.

TREATMENT OF SEIZURE DISORDERS

As indicated in the box at the beginning of this chapter, some of the listed drugs are active against only one or two types of seizures. In contrast, valproate has a broad spectrum of activity and is active against most types of seizures. The newer agents, such as **lamotrigine, topiramate, tiagabine, levetiracetam, zonisamide, pregabalin, lacosamide,** and **ezogabine,** are considered adjunct agents and are primarily used in combination with older drugs for the treatment of partial seizures. These newer agents are particularly useful because complex partial seizures are more resistant to treatment than are other types of seizures.

The pharmacologic properties of AEDs are described in the following sections, whereas the mechanisms of action, adverse effects, contraindications, and drug interactions are given in Table 20.3 (see also Table 20.2). With regard to adverse effects, the results of recent US Food and Drug Administration (FDA) studies showed an **increased risk of suicidal thoughts and behavior** with all antiepileptic agents.

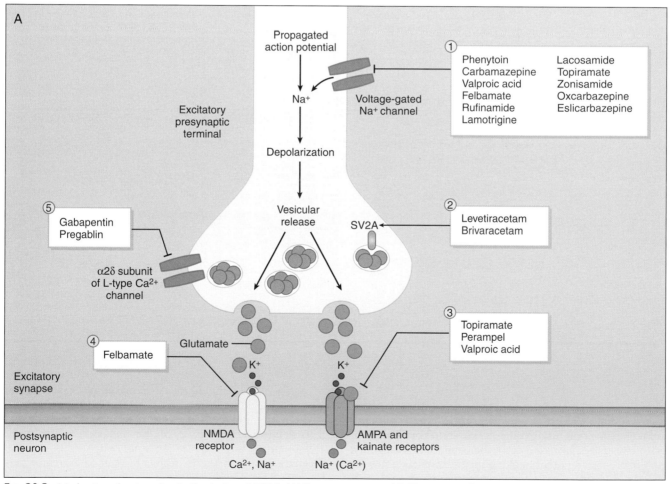

FIG. 20.3 Mechanism of action of antiepileptic drugs (AEDs). (A) Excitatory synapse. (*1*) Phenytoin, carbamazepine, valproic acid, and others inhibit voltage-gated Na$^+$ channels, thereby inhibiting action potentials at excitatory synapse. (*2*) Levetiracetam and brivaracetam bind to the vesicle transporter SV2A, decreasing amount of NT in vesicles. (*3*) Topiramate, perampanel, and valproic acid inhibit the activation of AMPA and kainate glutamate receptors, decreasing excitation. Topiramate and valproic have other actions as well. (*4*) Felbamate inhibits activation of NMDA glutamate receptors, decreasing excitation. (*5*) Pregabalin and gabapentin inhibit the L-type Ca^{+2} channel, decreasing Ca^{+2} inflow and exocytosis of vesicles and NT release.

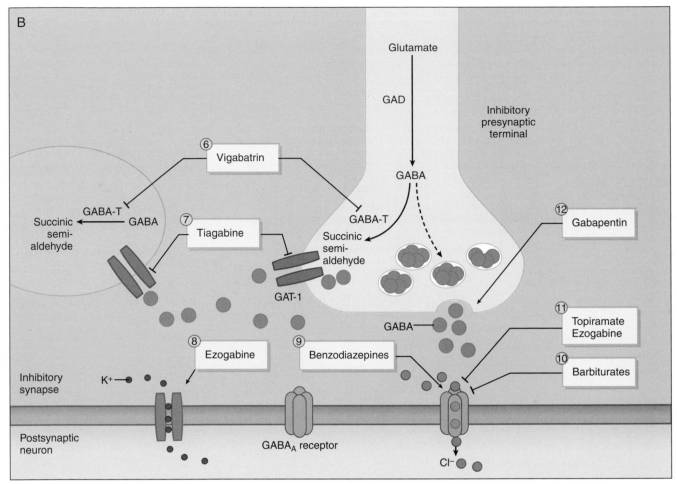

Fig. 20.3, cont'd (B) Inhibitory synapse. *(6)* Vigabatrin is an irreversible inhibitor of GABA transaminase (GABA-T), the enzyme responsible for the breakdown of GABA, increasing levels of GABA. *(7)* Tiagabine binds to the GABA reuptake transporter (GAT-1), permitting greater levels of GABA in the synapse and more neuronal inhibition. *(8)* Ezogabine activates K⁺ ion channels, leading to inward flow of ions and hyperpolarization of neurons. *(9)* Diazepam, clobazam, and other benzodiazepines coactivate GABA$_A$ receptors with GABA, leading to inhibition of neuronal activity. *(10)* Barbiturates like phenobarbital activate GABA$_A$ receptors and increase inhibition. *(11)* Topiramate, ezogabine, and cenobamate augment the activation of the GABA$_A$ receptor by GABA. *(12)* Gabapentin increases the release of GABA from inhibitory neurons. Not shown is the mechanism of action of ethosuximide and valproate, which block T-type (low-threshold) calcium channels that are located in thalamic neurons and underlie the propagation of generalized absence seizures.

Drugs for Partial and Generalized Tonic-Clonic Seizures

The first-line drugs for partial seizures and generalized tonic-clonic seizures are **carbamazepine, phenytoin,** and **valproate. Carbamazepine** and **phenytoin** have a similar mechanism of action and clinical effectiveness, but both drugs induce cytochrome P450 enzymes and increase drug metabolism. **Valproate** acts by a different mechanism and inhibits cytochrome P450 enzymes. Two other drugs that are effective against partial seizures, as well as generalized tonic-clonic seizures, are **phenobarbital** and **primidone.** Very recently, **cenobamate** was approved to treat partial seizures.

Carbamazepine and Oxcarbazepine

Pharmacokinetics. Carbamazepine is adequately absorbed after oral administration and has an active metabolite, **carbamazepine epoxide.** Almost all of the drug is excreted as metabolites in the urine and feces. **Oxcarbazepine** is considered a prodrug in that its activity is attributed to its monohydroxy metabolite. Oxcarbazepine mechanisms and effects, interactions, and indications for treating seizure disorders are the same as those of carbamazepine.

Mechanisms and Effects. Carbamazepine blocks **voltage-sensitive sodium channels** in neuronal cell membranes. As described, blockade of these channels inhibits the spread of abnormal electrical discharges from the seizure focus to other neurons by preventing the release of excitatory neurotransmitters from nerve terminals. Carbamazepine has additional mechanisms of action, but its contributions to its antiepileptic effects are unknown. For example, carbamazepine blocks adenosine receptors in a way that leads to up-regulation of these receptors, and it blocks norepinephrine reuptake in the same way that tricyclic antidepressants block it. The latter action is probably responsible for the mood-elevating effect of carbamazepine.

Carbamazepine can cause drowsiness, ataxia, and other symptoms of central nervous system (CNS) depression, as well as gastrointestinal reactions. Rarely, its use has been associated with **aplastic anemia.** In general, carbamazepine usually produces fewer adverse effects than does phenytoin.

Interactions. Carbamazepine is a **potent inducer** of cytochrome P450 enzymes that metabolize a wide range of drugs. Carbamazepine accelerates its own metabolism as well as

TABLE 20.3   Adverse Effects, Contraindications, and Pregnancy Risk for Select Antiepileptic Drugs

DRUG	MAJOR ADVERSE EFFECTS	CONTRAINDICATIONS	RISK CATEGORY AND EFFECTS OF USE DURING PREGNANCY[A]
Carbamazepine	Aplastic anemia (rare); ataxia, drowsiness, and other symptoms of central nervous system (CNS) depression; gastrointestinal reactions; and nausea	Hypersensitivity	Category C; increased risk of birth defects, abnormal facial features, neural tube defects such as spina bifida, reduced head size, and other anomalies
Phenytoin	Cerebellar symptoms, gastrointestinal disturbances, gingival hyperplasia, hirsutism, megaloblastic anemia and other blood cell deficiencies, osteomalacia, and psychiatric changes	Bradycardia, hypersensitivity, and severe atrioventricular block or sinoatrial dysfunction; Asians with polymorphism in human leukocyte antigen (HLA) allele at higher risk for skin reactions.	Category D; may reduce folate levels, two to three times increased risk of birth defects, fetal hydantoin syndrome
Phenobarbital	Ataxia, cognitive impairment, dizziness, drowsiness, drug dependence, rash, and respiratory depression	Hypersensitivity, porphyria, respiratory depression, and severe liver disease	Category D; bleeding at birth, minor congenital defects
Cenobamate	Somnolence, dizziness, fatigue, headache, nausea, and vomiting.	Hypersensitivity, Familial Short QT syndrome	Co-administration increases phenytoin plasma levels two-fold
Valproate	Drowsiness, gastrointestinal disturbances, hepatic toxicity (rare), pancreatitis (rare), nausea, and weight gain	Hepatic disease and hypersensitivity	Category D; may reduce folate levels; teratogenic during the first trimester; neural tube defects such as spina bifida; decreased cognitive development
Clorazepate	Confusion, drowsiness, drug tolerance, and lethargy	Hypersensitivity	Category D; increased risk of birth defects
Ethosuximide	Dizziness, drowsiness, gastric distress, lethargy, and nausea	Hypersensitivity	Category C
Gabapentin	Ataxia, dizziness, drowsiness, nystagmus, and tremor	Hypersensitivity	Category C
Lamotrigine	Ataxia, diplopia, dizziness, drowsiness, headache, nausea, rash, and Stevens-Johnson syndrome Risk of aseptic meningitis	Hypersensitivity; use cautiously in patients who are taking valproate or have hepatic or renal disease.	Category C; may reduce folate levels
Topiramate	Ataxia, dizziness, drowsiness, nystagmus, paresthesia, and psychomotor impairment	Hypersensitivity; use cautiously during pregnancy, during lactation, or in the presence of hepatic or renal disease.	Category D; recent data showed increased incidence of cleft palate
Zonisamide	Somnolence, anorexia, dizziness, headache, nausea, and agitation or irritability; metabolic acidosis in younger patients	Hypersensitivity	Category C; teratogenic in mice, rats, and dogs and C in monkeys when administered during the period of organogenesis at zonisamide dosage and maternal plasma levels similar to or lower than therapeutic levels in humans

[a]Pregnancy risk categories are defined by the US Food and Drug Administration (FDA) as follows: A, controlled studies show no risk; B, no evidence of risk in humans; C, risk cannot be ruled out; D, positive evidence of risk; and X, contraindicated in pregnancy.

that of many other drugs, including lamotrigine, phenytoin, topiramate, and valproate. For this reason, it decreases the serum level and effects of these drugs. Carbamazepine can also increase lithium toxicity.

Indications. In addition to its use in treating **partial seizures** and generalized tonic-clonic seizures, carbamazepine is the drug of choice for **trigeminal neuralgia** (tic douloureux), a condition that can cause chronic and intense pain on one or both sides of the face. Carbamazepine is also effective as an alternative to lithium in the treatment of **bipolar disease,** a mood disorder discussed in Chapter 22.

Eslicarbazepine

Eslicarbazepine is a recently approved AED closely related to carbamazepine. It shares the same mechanism of action of **blocking voltage-sensitive sodium channels** in neuronal cell membranes. Like carbamazepine, eslicarbazepine can cause drowsiness, ataxia, and other symptoms of CNS

depression. It is approved for the treatment of partial-onset seizures as a sole agent (monotherapy) or as an adjunct to other AEDs.

Phenytoin and Fosphenytoin

Pharmacokinetics. Phenytoin is a hydantoin derivative formerly called *diphenylhydantoin.* It is poorly soluble in water, and different pharmaceutical formulations of it may have different bioavailability. Hence, it is prudent to avoid switching from one formulation to another. If a switch must be made, serum drug levels should be monitored. A new formulation, called **fosphenytoin,** has become available for parenteral administration. Fosphenytoin is more soluble in water, and this prevents precipitation of the drug after intramuscular or intravenous administration.

Phenytoin is converted to an inactive hydroxylated metabolite by cytochrome P450 enzymes. The drug exhibits **dose-dependent kinetics,** whereby lower concentrations are eliminated by a **first-order** process, but higher concentrations saturate biotransformation enzymes and exhibit **zero-order** kinetics. Phenytoin hydroxylation also exhibits genetic **polymorphism.** These factors are responsible for the considerable patient variation in the plasma drug concentrations produced by a given dose. Because of this variation, serum drug levels should be monitored at the start of therapy and whenever toxicity or therapeutic failure occurs.

Mechanisms and Effects. As with carbamazepine, phenytoin **blocks voltage-sensitive sodium channels** by prolonging the inactivation state of these channels. This enables phenytoin to inhibit the repetitive firing of neurons in a seizure focus.

Phenytoin can cause a number of adverse effects. The drug interferes with **folate metabolism,** and this can lead to **megaloblastic anemia.** Folate antagonism can also contribute to birth defects such as those seen in **fetal hydantoin syndrome.** This syndrome is characterized by cardiac defects; malformation of ears, lips, palate, mouth, and nasal bridge; mental retardation; and microcephaly. By impairing cerebellar function, phenytoin can cause ataxia, diplopia, nystagmus, and slurred speech. By interfering with vitamin D metabolism and decreasing calcium absorption from the gut, phenytoin sometimes causes osteomalacia. Phenytoin adversely affects collagen metabolism and thereby contributes to **gingival hyperplasia,** a condition in which the gums can extend down over the teeth if good dental hygiene is not practiced. It can also cause excessive hair growth, known as **hirsutism.** Because of these adverse effects, phenytoin use in children should generally be avoided.

Serious skin reactions, including **Stevens-Johnson syndrome** and **toxic epidermal necrosis,** have been observed in Asian patients administered phenytoin or fosphenytoin. This has been linked to a polymorphism in the human leukocyte antigen (HLA) allele that is more likely to be present in these ethnic populations.

Interactions. Phenytoin induces the **CYP3A4** isozyme and **accelerates the metabolism** of other antiepileptic agents, including felbamate, lamotrigine, topiramate, and valproate. It can also reduce levels of digoxin, steroids, vitamin K, and other drugs. In patients who are being treated with phenytoin, vitamin K supplements are given to prevent hypoprothrombinemia and bleeding. Carbamazepine induces the metabolism of phenytoin and decreases its serum levels, whereas cimetidine and other drugs inhibit the metabolism of phenytoin and increase its serum levels.

Indications. Despite its many adverse effects and drug interactions, phenytoin is widely used in the treatment of **partial seizures** and **generalized tonic-clonic seizures.** As with carbamazepine, it can worsen absence seizures and should not be used in patients with this type of seizure.

Phenobarbital and Primidone

Phenobarbital and **primidone** are both second-line drugs for **partial seizures** and **generalized tonic-clonic seizures.** Phenobarbital, a barbiturate, is the oldest of the currently used AEDs. Its pharmacologic properties are discussed in Chapter 19. Primidone has two active metabolites, phenobarbital and phenylethylmalonamide (PEMA), and the parent drug and its active metabolites probably all contribute to its antiepileptic effects.

Phenobarbital enhances the GABA-mediated chloride flux that causes membrane hyperpolarization. Primidone probably acts primarily by blocking sodium channels and preventing membrane depolarization. It can also **potentiate GABA** via the formation of phenobarbital. Both primidone and phenobarbital are well absorbed from the gut, but primidone has a shorter half-life and therefore reaches steady-state levels more rapidly. Both drugs can cause ataxia, dizziness, drowsiness, and cognitive impairment. In excessive doses, they can depress respiration. **Hypersensitivity** to these drugs develops in a few patients and most frequently manifests as a rash.

Valproate

Pharmacokinetics. Several valproate formulations are available, including the free acid form (**valproic acid),** the sodium salt of valproic acid (**valproate sodium),** and a 1:1 mixture of valproic acid and valproate sodium (**divalproex sodium).** Divalproex sodium is absorbed more slowly than the other formulations, and it usually causes fewer adverse gastrointestinal and CNS side effects. Valproate is well absorbed from the gut and is metabolized to active metabolites and inactive conjugates before it is excreted.

Mechanisms and Effects. Valproic acid (valproate) has **several mechanisms of action** that probably contribute to its broad spectrum of antiepileptic effects. It inhibits voltage-sensitive sodium channels and T-type calcium channels, increases GABA synthesis and decreases GABA degradation, and may decrease glutamate synthesis. By these actions, valproate inhibits the repetitive firing of neurons and the spread of epileptic seizures.

Valproate produces relatively little sedation or drowsiness, but it occasionally causes nausea, gastrointestinal complaints, and weight gain. Mild hepatic toxicity sometimes occurs and is usually reversible. Rarely, the drug has been associated with **fatal hepatic toxicity.** To prevent liver damage, the hepatic function of patients should be monitored when they begin therapy with valproate. Children under 2 years of age are at the greatest risk of liver failure.

Valproate has been associated with an increased incidence of **spina bifida** and other birth defects in the offspring of women treated with the drug during pregnancy. In addition, recent epidemiologic studies showed **impaired cognitive development** in the offspring of women who took valproate during pregnancy compared with those who took another antiepileptic medication.

Interactions. Valproate inhibits the metabolism of other drugs and can increase the serum levels of lamotrigine, phenobarbital, and primidone. It can either increase or decrease the levels of carbamazepine and phenytoin, whereas these drugs decrease the levels of valproate. Because of these interactions, serum levels should always be monitored when another drug is added to or removed from the treatment regimen of a patient with seizure disorders. Patients should be warned that salicylates can increase the serum levels of valproate.

Indications. Of the various AEDs, valproate has the broadest spectrum of activity. It is effective in the treatment of partial seizures and all forms of generalized seizures, and it can be given in combination with other drugs when a single drug does not adequately control seizures (see later). Valproate is also used as an alternative to lithium to treat the manic phase of bipolar disorder (see Chapter 22) and for the prophylaxis of migraines (see Chapter 29).

Cenobamate

Cenobamate was very recently approved for the treatment of partial-onset seizures in adult patients. Cenobamate works like carbamazepine and phenytoin by blocking voltage-gated sodium ion channels but also potentiates the action of GABA at its receptors like a benzodiazepine. It is well-tolerated and has the adverse effects expected from this type of agent, including CNS depression, as noted by somnolence and fatigue, as well as diplopia and headache.

Adjunct Drugs for Partial Seizures

The most difficult seizures to control with drug therapy are partial seizures and, especially, complex partial seizures. Efforts, therefore, have focused on developing new drugs for these seizures. Unlike clorazepate, the following drugs were recently introduced after a resurgence in the development of AEDs. The last two agents are approved as adjunct drugs specifically for the treatment of seizures in children and adults with Lennox-Gastaut syndrome (LGS).

Clorazepate

Clorazepate is a **prodrug** that is converted to an active metabolite of **diazepam** in the liver. Although it primarily has been used to treat patients with **anxiety disorders,** it also has been found useful as an adjunct drug for the treatment of **partial seizures.** It can cause drowsiness and lethargy, and tolerance can occur during long-term use of the drug.

Felbamate

Felbamate was a promising new drug for the treatment of partial seizures and other types of seizures until cases of **fatal aplastic anemia** and **acute hepatic failure** were reported. Since 1994, felbamate has been limited to the treatment of **partial seizures that are refractory** to other drugs. Felbamate has a unique mechanism of action in that it **blocks glycine coactivation of NMDA receptors** and thereby can inhibit processes responsible for the initiation of seizures. Efforts are underway to develop other drugs that act via this mechanism but exhibit less toxicity than felbamate.

Gabapentin

Gabapentin is a GABA analog that appears to act by **increasing the release of GABA** from central neurons. It has no direct effect on the GABA$_A$ receptor–chloride ion channel itself. Gabapentin also inhibits the L-type Ca^{+2} channel like pregabalin (see later). The absorption of gabapentin from the gut is inversely related to the dose. Because the drug has a relatively short half-life, it must be given several times a day. Gabapentin is effective when used in combination with other drugs to treat **all forms of partial seizures,** and studies indicate that, for many patients, it is also effective when used alone. Its adverse effects are minimal at usual therapeutic doses, but it can cause ataxia, dizziness, drowsiness, nystagmus, and tremor. An extended-release form of gabapentin (GRALISE) was recently approved for the treatment of **postherpetic neuralgia;** an additional prodrug formulation, **gabapentin enacarbil** (HORIZANT), was approved for **restless legs syndrome.**

Lamotrigine

Lamotrigine blocks voltage-sensitive sodium channels and thereby interferes with neuronal membrane conduction and the release of excitatory neurotransmitters such as glutamate. It is one of the more effective adjunct drugs for treating **partial seizures** in adults and children. It is also useful in the treatment of **generalized tonic-clonic, atonic,** and **absence seizures** and in the treatment of **LGS,** a syndrome characterized by multiple types of seizures in patients with mental retardation and other neurologic abnormalities. Lamotrigine is also indicated for the treatment of the **manic phase of bipolar disorder.**

Lamotrigine has excellent oral bioavailability. It is mostly conjugated with glucuronate in the liver and excreted by the kidneys. Serum levels of lamotrigine are decreased by carbamazepine and phenytoin and are increased by valproate. Serum levels of valproate are decreased by lamotrigine.

The primary side effects of lamotrigine include **cerebellar dysfunction, drowsiness, and rash.** Patients should be advised to report early signs of skin changes because the rash can progress to **Stevens-Johnson syndrome.** This potentially fatal syndrome, a severe form of erythema multiforme, is characterized by mucocutaneous and systemic lesions. The syndrome is more common in patients who are being treated with the **combination** of lamotrigine and valproate, possibly because valproate increases the serum level of lamotrigine. If children are treated with both drugs, the dosage of lamotrigine should be lower than that used in other patients. Dosage guidelines are provided in the prescription inserts.

The FDA also recently noted the occurrence of **aseptic meningitis** in more than 40 patients receiving lamotrigine in the past 15 years, and an additional warning is now in place in the prescribing information.

Topiramate

Topiramate is a monosaccharide derivative that has several **mechanisms of action,** including blockade of **voltage-sensitive sodium channels, augmentation of GABA** activation of GABA$_A$ receptors, and **blockade** of two types of excitatory glutamate receptors, namely, **kainate receptors** and amino-3-hydroxy-5-methyl-4-isoxazole propionate acid **(AMPA) receptors.**

Clinical studies indicate that about half of patients who have intractable partial seizures experience a 50% reduction in seizure frequency when topiramate is added to their treatment regimen. Therefore, topiramate is approved for adjunct use in the treatment of **partial seizures.** Because it has also demonstrated effectiveness as single-drug therapy (monotherapy) for partial seizures and as an adjunct in the treatment of generalized seizures, it may receive approval for these indications in the future.

Topiramate is adequately absorbed from the gut, is partly metabolized before excretion in the urine, and has a half-life of about 21 hours. Carbamazepine and phenytoin may induce the metabolism of topiramate and decrease its serum level. Topiramate may reduce the serum level of oral contraceptives. The side effects of topiramate include ataxia, dizziness, drowsiness, and other CNS effects listed in Table 20.3. Because of an increased occurrence of **cleft palate** in children born of mothers taking topiramate, it has been recently placed into pregnancy category D.

Perampanel

Perampanel is a recently approved antiseizure medication that acts as a noncompetitive antagonist of the ionotropic **AMPA glutamate receptor** on postsynaptic neurons. It is indicated as adjunctive therapy for the treatment of partial-onset seizures with or without secondarily generalized seizures and for the treatment of primary generalized tonic-clonic seizures in patients 12 years of age and older.

Tiagabine

Tiagabine binds to recognition sites associated with the GABA reuptake transport protein. By this action, tiagabine **blocks GABA reuptake** into presynaptic neurons, permitting greater levels of GABA in the synapse.

Levetiracetam and Brivaracetam

The mechanism of action for **levetiracetam** is not clearly delineated. However, the drug binds to a **synaptic vesicle protein (SV2A),** reducing vesicular packaging of GABA and impeding neurotransmission across synapses. This leads to a decrease in neuronal burst firing present in seizure disorders. Levetiracetam shows effective results as an adjunct drug in treating **partial seizures** in children. **Brivaracetam** also has a high and selective affinity for SV2A and was recently approved as an adjunct drug for treating partial seizures.

Zonisamide

Zonisamide acts at **sodium channels** and voltage-dependent, transient inward currents of **calcium channels** (low-threshold, T-type Ca^{2+} currents). Zonisamide blocks Na^+ channels in the inactivated state and reduces the ion flow in Ca^{2+} channel proteins. With regard to adverse effects, recent data suggest an increased risk of **metabolic acidosis,** especially in younger patients. Health care providers should obtain serum bicarbonate levels before and during treatment, even in the absence of symptoms.

Pregabalin

Pregabalin binds to the *alpha* $(\alpha)_2$-*delta* site on an auxiliary subunit of voltage-gated calcium channels and **reduces the calcium current.** This action may be responsible for its antiseizure effects, as well as analgesic effects, as it is also indicated for **neuropathic pain** associated with **diabetes** and **postherpetic neuralgia.** It was also the first drug approved specifically for **fibromyalgia.** It is also approved for the treatment of **neuropathic pain after spinal cord injury.**

Vigabatrin

Vigabatrin is an **irreversible inhibitor** of GABA transaminase **(GABA-T),** the enzyme responsible for the breakdown of GABA in the brain. The inhibition of the GABA-T enzyme leads to increased levels of the inhibitory neurotransmitter GABA.

Lacosamide

The exact mechanism for the action of **lacosamide** is not entirely known. However, electrophysiologic studies have shown that lacosamide selectively enhances the inactivation of voltage-gated **sodium channels,** resulting in stabilization of hyperexcitable neuronal membranes and inhibition of repetitive neuronal firing.

Ezogabine

Ezogabine has a unique mechanism of action among antiepileptic agents in that it acts at **potassium channels** to increase K^+ ion flow. In this way, ezogabine hyperpolarizes neurons and decreases their firing potential. It has also been shown to **enhance GABA-mediated chloride ion** currents.

Rufinamide

Rufinamide is an antiepileptic agent approved solely for the adjunct **treatment of seizures in children and adults** with **LGS,** a syndrome characterized by multiple types of seizures in patients with mental retardation and other neurologic abnormalities. Rufinamide modulates the activity of sodium channels and, in particular, prolongs the inactive state of the channel.

Clobazam

Clobazam is a benzodiazepine that increases the inhibition by GABA at $GABA_A$ receptors, as do all the other benzodiazepines. Like rufinamide, it is approved solely for the adjunct **treatment of seizures in children and adults with LGS.** It has been granted an orphan drug designation because it is intended to treat a condition that affects fewer than 200,000 people.

Drugs for Generalized Absence, Myoclonic, or Atonic Seizures

Ethosuximide

Pharmacokinetics. Ethosuximide is the most effective and least toxic of the several succinimide derivatives that have been used to treat epilepsy over the past 50 years. It is well absorbed from the gut, widely distributed to tissues, and metabolized to inactive compounds before it is excreted in the urine. Ethosuximide has a long half-life of about 30 hours in children and 55 hours in adults.

Mechanisms and Effects. Ethosuximide inhibits T-type calcium channels in thalamic neurons. These low-threshold channels are believed to be responsible for the pacemaker current that generates the synchronous 3-Hz (three cycles per second) spike-and-dome depolarizations observed on the EEG during absence seizures (see Fig. 20.1). Ethosuximide produces little toxicity, but it can cause dizziness, drowsiness, gastric distress, and nausea, which can usually be minimized by starting treatment with lower doses and then gradually increasing doses to the desired level. See Box 20.1 for a case example.

Interactions. Valproate inhibits the metabolism of ethosuximide and increases its serum levels. Haloperidol, a high-potency antipsychotic drug, can alter the seizure pattern in patients treated with ethosuximide. No other important interactions have been identified.

Indications. Ethosuximide is safe and highly effective in the treatment of generalized absence seizures in children and is the drug of choice for this particular group of patients. Ethosuximide is not very effective, however, in the treatment of adults with absence seizures or of patients with other types of seizures, so valproate (discussed earlier) is often used instead.

Clonazepam and Other Drugs

Clonazepam is a benzodiazepine used to treat **absence, myoclonic,** and **atonic seizures.** It often produces more sedation than other AEDs when used at doses that suppress seizures.

BOX 20.1 THE CASE OF SPACY SUZY

CASE PRESENTATION

Suzy B., a 7-year-old girl in good health with normal development and intelligence, is having problems keeping up with her classroom activities at school. Her parents are called to the school to meet her teacher and are told that Suzy is not paying attention and at times seems to be "spacing out" with a blank stare and is unresponsive to the teacher's questions. The teacher says that at times Suzy "blanks out" from 10 to 15 s at a time, sometimes with repetitive blinking. She states that after these episodes, Suzy seems fine and behaves as if nothing happened and reports that on some days, Suzy may have five or more of these episodes. The concerned parents take Suzy to a neurologist who obtains an electroencephalogram (EEG) tracing while Suzy is having one of these episodes. He notes a characteristic 3-Hz spike-and-dome pattern and tells the parents that Suzy has absence seizures. He starts Suzy on a course of ethosuximide at 250 mg twice a day. Suzy returns to school, and her teacher calls the concerned parents in a few days to report that Suzy is no longer having episodes.

CASE DISCUSSION

Absence seizures (also called *petit mal seizures*) usually last less than 10 s, but they can last as long as 20 s. The seizures begin and end suddenly, and during the seizure, awareness and responsiveness are impaired. Children who have a seizure are not usually aware that they have had one and are completely alert immediately afterward. Simple absence seizures are just "stares." Many absence seizures are complex absence seizures, meaning that muscle activity, such as blinking, occurs. Absence seizures usually begin at age 4 to 12 and occur in children with normal development and intelligence. The most effective medications for absence seizures include ethosuximide, valproic acid, and lamotrigine. Most children take the medicine for 2 years and then, if no episodes have occurred, can usually discontinue antiseizure medications with a good prognosis. In about 75% of cases, absence seizures stop by the age of 18. Children who develop absence seizures before age 9 have a better prognosis for spontaneous remission than children whose absence seizures start after age 10.

Because the efficacy of valproate is equal to or greater than that of clonazepam, it is frequently used instead to treat patients with absence, myoclonic, and atonic seizures.

Lamotrigine is sometimes used as an adjunct for the treatment of absence and atonic seizures.

The pharmacologic properties of valproate and lamotrigine are discussed earlier in this chapter, and those of clonazepam are discussed in Chapter 19.

Drugs for Status Epilepticus

Status epilepticus is a life-threatening emergency. Patients with this condition have recurrent episodes of tonic-clonic seizures without regaining consciousness or normal muscle movement between episodes. If their seizures are not controlled, prolonged hypoxia can lead to **severe brain damage.** Immediate attention must be given to cardiopulmonary support and to the administration of drugs that rapidly terminate the seizures. In fact, published reports indicate that seizures must be controlled within 60 minutes of the onset of an episode in order for a favorable prognosis to be achieved.

The drug of choice for status epilepticus is **diazepam** or **lorazepam.** Either drug is administered as a slow intravenous injection given every 10 to 15 minutes until seizures are controlled or a maximal dose has been administered. The pharmacologic properties of these drugs are described in Chapter 19.

After diazepam or lorazepam has been administered, **phenytoin** (or the newer form, **fosphenytoin**) is often administered intravenously to provide a longer duration of seizure control than is provided by a benzodiazepine. Large doses of **phenobarbital** may be effective if a benzodiazepine or phenytoin fails to control the seizures. In highly resistant cases, general anesthesia can be used to control the seizures.

Cannabinoid Drugs for Atypical Seizures

Cannabidiol (CBD) is the **first in class cannabinoid drug** to be FDA-approved and is marketed as EPIDIOLEX. CBD is labeled for the treatment of seizures associated with **Lennox-Gastaut syndrome** and **Dravet syndrome** in patients 1 year of age and older. Both neurological syndromes are linked to genetic mutations, affect intellectual abilities, and produce seizures that can change in type and frequency as an affected child grows up. CBD is a main ingredient in the marijuana plant but is not psychoactive like tetrahydrocannabinol (THC) and does not directly activate cannabinoid receptors (see Chapter 25). In clinical trials, CBD decreased the frequency and severity of seizures in patients with Lennox-Gastaut and Dravet syndrome. The exact mechanism of action that CBD uses to suppress seizures is not known.

THE MANAGEMENT OF SEIZURE DISORDERS

The effective management of patients with epilepsy requires an accurate diagnosis of the type of seizures that occur and also requires the rational selection and use of drugs.

First-Line Drugs

For **partial seizures** and **generalized tonic-clonic seizures,** carbamazepine, phenytoin, and valproate are first-line drugs, and phenobarbital and primidone are second-line drugs. Carbamazepine generally causes fewer adverse effects than phenytoin, although phenytoin can be slightly less sedating than carbamazepine at equally effective doses. Of the several drugs that have been recently developed as adjunct medications for partial seizures, lamotrigine and topiramate appear particularly attractive at this time. The relative safety and efficacy of these drugs are still being evaluated.

For **generalized absence seizures,** ethosuximide is clearly the first choice in treating children with this condition, which usually has its onset during childhood and often remits during adolescence. Valproate is generally more effective in treating adults with absence seizures and in treating patients with multiple types of seizures.

For **generalized myoclonic and atonic seizures,** valproate is the drug of choice.

For status epilepticus, intravenous treatment with diazepam or lorazepam can be followed by intravenous treatment with fosphenytoin or phenobarbital.

Principles of Drug Use

In most cases, an attempt should be made to control seizures with single-drug therapy (monotherapy) because this will minimize side effects, reduce costs, and increase patient compliance.

Unless the patient is experiencing frequent seizures, it is usually best to start with a single drug and give it in a low dose (one-fourth to one-third of the therapeutic dose). The dose can be gradually increased until effective serum concentrations are achieved or intolerable adverse effects occur. Starting with a low dose enables the patient to develop tolerance to the CNS side effects of AEDs and improves compliance.

If a single drug has significantly reduced the occurrence of seizures but has not eliminated them, it is usually prudent to add another drug to the regimen rather than switch to a new drug. Two drugs acting by different mechanisms may control seizures when a single drug is not adequate. The second drug should be given initially in a low dose, and the dosage should be gradually increased until therapeutic concentrations are reached or adverse effects occur. Because of interactions between AEDs, the doses that are both safe and effective for combination therapy may differ from the doses that are safe and effective for monotherapy. For example, lamotrigine causes a much higher incidence of serious **dermatologic toxicity in children** who are concurrently taking valproate, and lamotrigine should be started at much lower doses in these patients.

Once a satisfactory drug regimen has been achieved, the patient should be monitored periodically for drug toxicity and efficacy. Serum drug levels should be determined whether there is evidence or suspicion of adverse effects, therapeutic failure, or patient noncompliance.

The appropriate duration of AED therapy is a topic of considerable controversy. If a patient undergoing drug therapy has not had a seizure for several years, it seems prudent to consider slowly withdrawing the medication because this will minimize long-term side effects and offer lifestyle benefits and cost savings. About 25% of patients who withdraw from medication will relapse within 1 year, however. Factors that increase the likelihood of relapse include the onset of seizures during adolescence, the occurrence of complex partial seizures or generalized seizures, and abnormal interictal findings on EEGs. If antiepileptic medication is to be discontinued, the dosage should be tapered slowly over several weeks because abrupt withdrawal from medication is associated with a higher incidence of **rebound seizures.**

A number of the antiseizure agents are currently in clinical trials for various other indications, including **bipolar disorder** (see Chapter 22), **trigeminal neuralgia, fibromyalgia,** and other **neuropathic pain states** (see Chapter 23). They are also being used off-label for these disorders and others. Significantly, in 2008 the FDA issued a **warning letter** regarding increased risk of suicidal thoughts and behaviors **(suicidality)** in patients who take these drugs, which may limit the expansion of these agents for wider indications.

SUMMARY OF IMPORTANT POINTS

- Seizures are caused by episodic, synchronous neuronal discharges in the cerebral cortex or elsewhere in the brain. They are classified as partial or generalized seizures on the basis of their clinical characteristics and electroencephalographic pattern.
- Some antiepileptic drugs work by blocking voltage-sensitive sodium channels or T-type calcium channels.

Others augment inhibitory GABA neurotransmission or block excitatory glutamate neurotransmission.
- Carbamazepine, phenytoin, and valproate are the first-line drugs for partial seizures and generalized tonic-clonic seizures.
- Ethosuximide is the drug of choice for generalized absence seizures in children. Valproate and clonazepam are effective in absence, myoclonic, and atonic seizures.
- Gabapentin, lamotrigine, topiramate, and several other new drugs are used as adjuncts in the treatment of partial seizures, and some of these agents have activity against other types of seizures.
- Status epilepticus is a medical emergency that requires intravenous administration of diazepam or lorazepam, sometimes followed by intravenous use of phenytoin (fosphenytoin) or phenobarbital.
- Many antiepileptic drugs interact with other medications. Carbamazepine and phenytoin induce cytochrome P450 enzymes and decrease serum levels of the drugs with which they interact, whereas valproate inhibits the metabolism of the drugs with which it interacts.
- Antiepileptic drugs frequently produce CNS and gastrointestinal side effects, and some drugs cause infrequent but severe hematologic or hepatic toxicity. Valproate and phenytoin are known to cause birth defects, and both of these drugs can reduce folate levels.
- Except in urgent situations, antiepileptic therapy should begin with a low dose of a single drug, and the dosage should be increased until the desired serum concentration or full dosage is achieved. If a single drug is not effective, another drug can be added to the regimen or substituted. Drug use should be discontinued slowly. Serum levels should be monitored to verify adequate dosage and whenever toxicity, therapeutic failure, or noncompliance occurs or is suspected.

Review Questions

1. The molecular mechanism underlying the antiepileptic effects of carbamazepine and phenytoin is best described by which one of the following statements?
   (A) inhibiting low-threshold Ca^{2+} ion channels
   (B) prolonging the inactivation of the Na^+ ion channel
   (C) potentiating the release of GABA by inhibiting GABA reuptake
   (D) increasing the release of GABA by vesicular fusion
   (E) blocking glutamate receptor excitation
2. Which antiepileptic agent gained wider therapeutic use also to treat trigeminal neuralgia and the manic phase of bipolar disorder?
   (A) ethosuximide
   (B) zonisamide
   (C) levetiracetam
   (D) carbamazepine
   (E) phenytoin
3. Which one of the following agents is considered the drug of choice for initial treatment of generalized absence seizure (petit mal) in children?
   (A) ethosuximide
   (B) zonisamide

(C) levetiracetam
(D) carbamazepine
(E) phenytoin
4. Topiramate has which set of three mechanisms of action?
   (A) increases Na⁺ channel inactivation, increases GABA, blocks glutamate
   (B) decreases Na⁺ channel inactivation, decreases GABA, blocks glutamate
   (C) increases Ca²⁺ channel inactivation, increases GABA, blocks glutamate
   (D) decreases Ca²⁺ channel inactivation, increases GABA, blocks glutamate
   (E) decreases Ca²⁺ channel flow, increases GABA, blocks glutamate

5. Gabapentin has which mechanism of action?
   (A) inhibits monoamine oxidase
   (B) has an agonist effect at dopamine receptors
   (C) increases Na⁺ channel inactivation
   (D) blocks reuptake of neurotransmitters
   (E) increases release of neurotransmitters.

CHAPTER
21 Local and General Anesthetics

CLASSIFICATION OF LOCAL AND GENERAL ANESTHETICS

Local Anesthetics

Ester-type drugs
- Cocaine
- Benzocaine (AMERICAINE)
- Chloroprocaine (NESACAINE)[a]

Amide-type drugs
- Lidocaine (XYLOCAINE)
- Bupivacaine (MARCAINE)[b]
- Etidocaine (DURANEST)
- Prilocaine (CITANEST)
- Ropivacaine (NAROPIN)[c]

General Anesthetics

Inhalational anesthetics
- Nitrous oxide
- Halothane (FLUOTHANE)
- Desflurane (SUPRANE)
- Isoflurane (FORANE)
- Sevoflurane (ULTANE)[d]

Parenteral anesthetics
- Pentobarbital (NEMBUTAL)[e]
- Midazolam (VERSED)[f]
- Ketamine (KETALAR)
- Propofol (DIPRIVAN) also Fospropofol (LUSEDRA)
- Etomidate (AMIDATE)
- Fentanyl (SUBLIMAZE)[g]

Other Agents
- Dantrolene (DANTRIUM)[h]

---

[a] Also tetracaine (PONTOCAINE) and proparacaine (OPHTHAINE). The first ester local anesthetic, procaine (NOVOCAIN), is no longer available.
[b] Also available as bupivacaine liposome injectable suspension (EXPAREL).
[c] Also levobupivacaine (CHIROCAINE), mepivacaine (CARBOCAINE), and dibucaine (NUPERCAINAL).
[d] Also enflurane (ETHRANE).
[e] Also methohexital (BREVITAL) and previously, thiopental (PENTOTHAL).
[f] Also remimazolam (BYFAVO).
[g] Also sufentanil (SUFENTA), alfentanil (ALFENTA), and remifentanil (ULTIVA).
[h] Dantrolene is not an anesthetic but is used to treat malignant hyperthermia after general anesthetic or antipsychotic use.

OVERVIEW

Anesthesia is the loss of all sensation, whereas analgesia is the selective loss of pain sensation. Local anesthetics block the conduction of nerve impulses in the peripheral nerves or spinal cord. General anesthetics block cortical neuronal activity underlying consciousness and all sensation.

Local anesthetics, which are used to anesthetize a particular part or region of the body, are given to patients undergoing surgery on the skin and subcutaneous tissues, ears, eyes, joints, or pelvis. They are also used for anesthesia during labor and delivery and for diagnostic procedures

such as gastrointestinal endoscopy. Occasionally, local anesthetics are used to relieve pain associated with pathologic conditions.

General anesthetics are used to prevent consciousness during major surgical procedures. Unlike local anesthetics, general anesthetics produce loss of consciousness and amnesia and thereby prevent the anesthetized patient from recalling the surgical procedure.

LOCAL ANESTHETICS
Drug Properties
Chemistry and Pharmacokinetics

Based on their chemical structure, local anesthetics can be divided into **ester-type** drugs and **amide-type** drugs. Each local anesthetic has a lipophilic (hydrophobic) portion and a hydrophilic portion (Fig. 21.1). The hydrophilic portion, an amine that is a weak base, exists in both ionized and nonionized forms. The ionized, protonated form predominates at lower pH levels, and the nonionized, unprotonated form predominates at higher pH levels. Only the nonionized form can **penetrate neuronal membranes** to reach binding sites on the internal surface of sodium channels. Inflammation and acidosis decrease the pH of tissues, thereby increasing the ionization of local anesthetics. For this reason, local anesthetics are less effective in the presence of these conditions, necessitating larger doses.

Local anesthetics are formulated as hydrochloride salts with a pH less than 7, as the ionized molecule is more soluble and stable than the free base. Once injected, the local anesthetic solution is quickly buffered to the pH of the tissue.

The duration of action of local anesthetics can be **short, medium,** or **long** (Table 21.1). Because local anesthetics act directly at the site of administration, their duration of action is determined primarily by the rate of diffusion and absorption away from the site of administration. Diffusion and absorption, in turn, depend on the chemical properties of the anesthetics and on such factors as local pH and blood flow. In some formulations, **epinephrine** is added to prolong a local anesthetic's duration of action by producing vasoconstriction and slowing its rate of absorption. Because of the risk of ischemia and necrosis, however, local anesthetics with epinephrine are not used to anesthetize tissues with end arteries, such as tissues of the fingers, toes, ears, nose, and penis.

After systemic absorption, **ester-type local anesthetics** are metabolized in the plasma by cholinesterases to p-aminobenzoic acid (PABA) derivatives. **Amide-type local anesthetics** undergo metabolism by hepatic P450 enzymes to yield polar metabolites. In both cases, the metabolites are excreted in the urine.

Mechanism of Action

Local anesthetics cause a reversible inhibition of action potential conduction by **binding to the sodium channel** and decreasing the nerve membrane permeability to sodium.

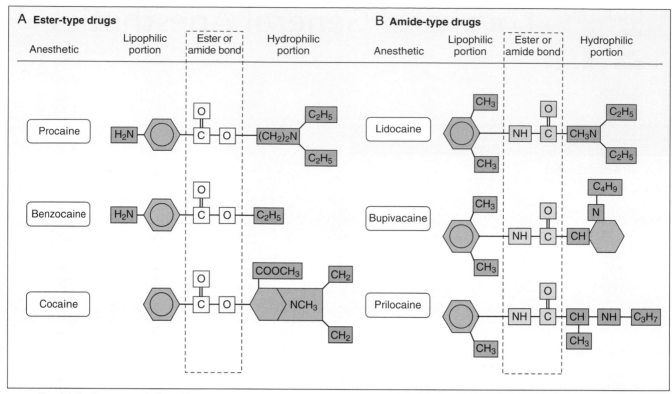

Fig. 21.1 Structures of selected local anesthetics. Note the ester or amide bond that determines the subclass of the local anesthetic agent.

TABLE 21.1 Properties of Selected Local Anesthetics

DRUG	POTENCY	DURATION OF ACTION[a]	PARENTERAL USES	TOPICAL USES
Ester-Type Drugs				
Procaine[b]	Low	Short	Infiltration, nerve block, and spinal anesthesia	None
Benzocaine	Low	Medium	None	Dermal, laryngeal, and oral
Chloroprocaine	Low	Short	Epidural, infiltration, and nerve block anesthesia	None
Cocaine	Low	Medium	None	Laryngeal, nasal, and urogenital
Amide-Type Drugs				
Lidocaine	Intermediate	Short	Epidural, infiltration, nerve block, and spinal anesthesia	Dermal, laryngeal, and oral
Bupivacaine	High	Medium	Epidural, infiltration, nerve block, and spinal anesthesia	None
Etidocaine	Intermediate	Long	Infiltration and nerve block anesthesia	None
Mepivacaine	Intermediate	Short	Epidural, infiltration, nerve block, and spinal anesthesia	None
Prilocaine	Intermediate	Short	Infiltration anesthesia	Dermal
Ropivacaine	High	Long	Epidural, infiltration, and nerve block anesthesia	None

[a]The duration varies with the dose and route of administration. Short, 0.25–1.5 h; medium, >1.5–5 h; and long, >5 h.
[b]Procaine is no longer available in the United States but is included here because it was used for many years and because of the popularity of its trade name (Novocain).

The nonpolar, lipophilic form of the anesthetic molecule passes through the neuronal membrane and switches to the polar, hydrophilic form in the cytoplasm of the neuron. This cationic form of the anesthetic binds to the cytoplasmic side of the sodium channel protein and **prolongs the inactivation state** of the sodium channel (Fig. 21.2). With sodium channels blocked, action potentials cannot propagate along the neuronal fiber, and sensory input is lost.

Pharmacologic Effects

Local anesthetics have a greater affinity for sodium channels that are in the depolarized (open) configuration than

A

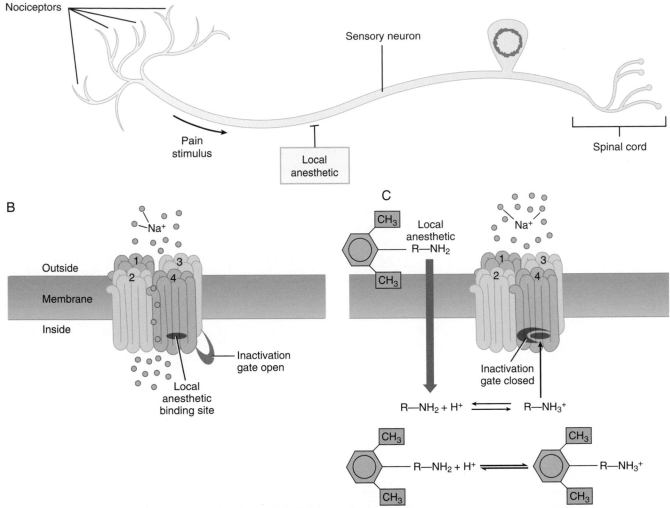

FIG. 21.2 Mechanisms of action of local anesthetics. (A) The local anesthetic binds to sodium channels and blocks the generation and conduction of action potentials in peripheral neurons. (B) The sodium channel includes four large transmembrane domains, each with six transmembrane spanning regions. The inactivation gate is a short, intracellular loop between domains 3 and 4. The local anesthetic binds to amino acid residues located on domain 4. (C) The nonionized form of the local anesthetic (R-NH₂) penetrates the axonal membrane and is then converted to the ionized form (R-NH₃⁺). The ionized form binds to the sodium channel in the open state, and this prolongs the sodium channel inactivation state. Sodium entry is blocked during the inactivation state.

for channels that are closed. Nerve fibers that are firing, therefore, are more susceptible to sodium channel blockade. This **use-dependent blockade** causes selective inhibition of nerve fibers that are stimulated by the surgical procedure, such as pain fibers during suturing. **Size-dependent blockade** refers to the finding that small-diameter fibers are blocked more easily than are larger fibers. Small **unmyelinated C** and **lightly myelinated Aδ** pain fibers, therefore, are more easily anesthetized than are large, myelinated touch fibers. Autonomic and sensory nerves are blocked more easily than are motor nerves. Nerves recover from blockade in the reverse order.

Adverse Effects and Interactions
The adverse effects of local anesthetics are primarily caused by their absorption into the systemic circulation and subsequent alteration of the **central nervous system (CNS)**, **cardiovascular,** and other organ system functions.

Local anesthetics often produce **CNS stimulation** (restlessness, tremor, and euphoria) followed by **inhibition** (drowsiness and sedation). Other symptoms of local anesthetic toxicity include headache, paresthesias, and nausea. Higher concentrations can cause seizures followed by coma. Death is usually caused by respiratory failure.

Adverse cardiovascular effects include **hypotension** and **cardiac depression.** Most local anesthetics are vasodilators, and they also block vasoconstriction induced by the sympathetic nervous system. Most local anesthetics have **antidysrhythmic activity,** but toxic levels of local anesthetics suppress cardiac conduction and can cause tachyarrhythmia characterized by a wide QRS complex.

Local anesthetic **blockade of autonomic ganglia** and **neuromuscular transmission** can lead to loss of visceral and skeletal muscle tone. For this reason, local anesthetics potentiate the effect of neuromuscular blocking drugs (e.g., pancuronium) and must be used with great caution in patients with **myasthenia gravis.**

Allergic reactions to local anesthetics are fairly common. Patients who have repeated applications of topical anesthetics are particularly susceptible to sensitization. The ester-type anesthetics cause **hypersensitivity reactions** more frequently than do the amide-type anesthetics. This is because ester-type anesthetics (e.g., chloroprocaine) are metabolized to PABA. PABA causes allergic reactions in a small percentage of individuals. Patients who are allergic to an ester-type anesthetic will usually tolerate an amide-type anesthetic.

Recently a greater appreciation of the dangers of even the apparently benign administration of topical local anesthetics has caught the attention of the US Food and Drug Administration (FDA). They issued a new warning to highlight the **risk of systemic absorption** and cardiac abnormalities when topical anesthetics are used on large body surfaces or when subsequently covered. This may apply to women undergoing mammography or a number of other medical procedures.

Indications

Local anesthetics are usually administered parenterally but are sometimes applied topically. The route of administration depends on factors such as the site of anesthesia.

Topical Anesthesia. The topical application of local anesthetics is used to anesthetize the skin, mucous membranes, or cornea. A local anesthetic can be applied to the skin to treat pruritus (itching) caused by poison ivy, insect bites, eczema, or cutaneous manifestations of systemic diseases such as chickenpox (varicella). A eutectic mixture of local anesthetics (EMLA) consisting of two or more solid compounds that form a liquid when they are combined is sometimes used to anesthetize the skin before venipuncture or minor surgery. The topical application of a local anesthetic to mucous membranes can relieve pain caused by oral, nasal, laryngeal, or rectal disorders or surgery. For example, an anesthetic ointment is used to relieve the discomfort of hemorrhoids. The topical ocular administration of local anesthetics is used to anesthetize the cornea before diagnostic or surgical procedures (e.g., radial keratotomy), the removal of foreign bodies, and cataract surgery.

Infiltration Anesthesia. Infiltration is probably the most common route used to administer local anesthetics. The process involves injecting an anesthetic directly into subcutaneous tissue just under the skin. Infiltration is used primarily for minor surgical procedures (e.g., suturing a wound) or for the removal of foreign bodies. It is also frequently used for dental procedures. When a local anesthetic is to be administered by infiltration, epinephrine can be added to it to decrease the dose and prolong the duration of action. As mentioned earlier, however, epinephrine should not be used to anesthetize fingers, toes, and other tissues with end arteries.

Iontophoresis. Local anesthetics can also be administered by iontophoresis. This technique uses a small electric current to force molecules of the anesthetic into the tissue. Iontophoresis is used primarily in dentistry. It eliminates the need to inject the anesthetic and is used by some dentists for this reason. A new, needle-free device with the trade name of Zingo delivers powdered lidocaine by rapid gas pressure to reduce the pain of subsequent peripheral injections or blood draws. It is approved for use in children (or adults who act like children).

Nerve Block and Field Block Anesthesia. Nerve block and field block anesthesia are forms of regional anesthesia, the goal of which is to anesthetize an area of the body by blocking the conductivity of sensory nerves from that area. In nerve block anesthesia, a local anesthetic is injected into or adjacent to a peripheral nerve or nerve plexus. For example, a radial nerve block can be used to anesthetize the structures innervated by the radial nerve, including portions of the forearm and hand. An intraorbital block is often used for ocular surgery. Other examples of nerve block anesthesia are brachial plexus and cervical plexus blocks. In field block anesthesia, a local anesthetic is administered in a series of injections to form a wall of anesthesia encircling the operative field.

Spinal Intrathecal Anesthesia. Spinal anesthesia is used to block somatosensory and motor fibers during procedures such as surgery on the lower limb or pelvic structures. A local anesthetic is injected into the subarachnoid, intrathecal space below the level at which the spinal cord terminates. The spread of the anesthetic along the neuraxis is controlled by the horizontal tilt of the patient and by the specific gravity (baricity) of the local anesthetic solution. Hyperbaric solutions of local anesthetics are available for this purpose, and these spread along the neuraxis for about 15 minutes. By this time, they have mixed with cerebrospinal fluid to become isobaric and are said to be "fixed" at a certain level of the spinal cord. Spinal anesthesia can cause headaches associated with cerebrospinal fluid leakage from the lumbar puncture, and respiratory depression can occur if the anesthetic ascends too high up the spinal cord towards respiratory centers in the brainstem. Entry into the CNS by spinal injection also carries a small risk of infection or meningitis.

Epidural Anesthesia. Epidural anesthesia is produced by injecting a local anesthetic into the lumbar or caudal epidural (extradural) space. A local anesthetic, such as bupivacaine, is often administered by this route to provide anesthesia during labor and delivery. After epidural administration, the local anesthetic is absorbed into the systemic circulation. Therefore, doses must be carefully monitored to prevent cardiac depression and neurotoxicity in the mother and neonate.

Specific Agents
Ester-Type Local Anesthetics

Cocaine, a naturally occurring plant alkaloid, was the first local anesthetic to be discovered. It has both local anesthetic and CNS stimulant properties, and it is the only local anesthetic that causes significant vasoconstriction as a result of its **sympathomimetic effect.** Because of its CNS effects and potential for abuse (see Chapter 25), cocaine is seldom used as a local anesthetic. It is occasionally used, however, to anesthetize the internal structures of the nose, where its vasoconstrictive action helps prevent bleeding after nasal surgery. A cocaine solution is applied to gauze and inserted into the nose for this purpose.

Procaine, the first synthetic local anesthetic drug to be prepared after the discovery of cocaine, became the standard of comparison for many years. It is no longer available but is

TABLE 21.2 Properties of Inhalation Anesthetics

DRUG	MINIMUM ALVEOLAR CONCENTRATION (% VOL/VOL)[a]	BLOOD: GAS PARTITION COEFFICIENT	RATE OF INDUCTION	AMOUNT METABOLIZED	AMOUNT OF SKELETAL MUSCLE RELAXATION
Nonhalogenated Drugs					
Nitrous oxide	>100	0.47	Fast	0%	None
Halogenated Drugs					
Desflurane	6.0	0.42	Fast	<2%	Medium
Enflurane	1.7	1.9	Medium	5% (fluoride)	Medium
Halothane	0.75	2.3	Slow	20%	Low
Isoflurane	1.2	1.4	Medium	<2% (fluoride)	Medium
Sevoflurane	1.9	0.63	Fast	<2%	Medium

[a]The minimum alveolar concentration (MAC) is the concentration needed to produce anesthesia in half of the subjects.

included here because of its significance and the popularity of its trade name (NOVOCAIN). Procaine and **chloroprocaine** have a low potency and a relatively short duration of action. They are not effective after topical administration and must be administered parenterally. Both drugs are metabolized to PABA. For this reason, they are more likely to cause **allergic reactions** than amide-type local anesthetics. **Tetracaine** is another ester-type local anesthetic with a longer duration of action than procaine. It is used for infiltration anesthesia. It is also available in a topical spray and gel formulation in combination with **butamben** (butyl aminobenzoate) and **benzocaine** in a preparation called CETACAINE.

Benzocaine, a frequently used topical anesthetic, is available in a number of nonprescription products for the treatment of **sunburn, pruritus,** and other skin conditions. In some patients, the drug causes hypersensitivity reactions, which can exacerbate preexisting dermatitis. Benzocaine is also used to **anesthetize mucous membranes** and is available in cough lozenges and sprays to relieve coughing.

Proparacaine is available in a 0.5% solution for instillation during eye surgery and other ophthalmic procedures.

Amide-Type Local Anesthetics

Lidocaine produces local anesthesia after topical or parenteral administration. The most widely used local anesthetic, it is available in a number of formulations. These include topical solutions and ointments, oral sprays, viscous gels for oral and laryngeal application, and various parenteral formulations. EMLA, a eutectic mixture of the local anesthetics **lidocaine** and **prilocaine,** is available as a cream to anesthetize intact skin to a depth of 5 mm. In pediatric patients, **EMLA cream** has been used for local anesthesia before venipuncture, intravenous cannulation, or circumcision. Lidocaine is also used for infiltration, nerve block, epidural, and spinal anesthesia. Lidocaine is also available as a **transdermal patch** (LIDODERM) approved for postherpetic neuralgia and widely used off-label for conditions such as vertebral fractures.

Etidocaine has properties similar to those of lidocaine, but its duration of action is considerably longer. It is primarily used for infiltration and nerve block anesthesia.

Bupivacaine, mepivacaine, and **ropivacaine** have similar clinical uses but differ in their duration of action, as shown in Table 21.1. **Bupivacaine** has been the most widely used local anesthetic for obstetric anesthesia, but it causes cardiac depression more frequently than do many other local anesthetics. Bupivacaine is also available in a liposome-encapsulated formulation (EXPAREL) for long-acting analgesia in the treatment of postsurgical pain, including C-sections. **Ropivacaine** is a newer drug that may cause fewer cases of cardiac toxicity. **Levobupivacaine** is the isolated $S(-)$-stereoisomer of racemic bupivacaine, which is the active form of the chiral drug mixture. It is used in epidural anesthesia for labor and delivery.

Prilocaine is a congener of lidocaine. It is converted to O-toluidine, a **toxic metabolite** that can cause methemoglobinemia if it is allowed to accumulate. For this reason, prilocaine use is limited to topical and infiltration anesthesia.

Dibucaine is formulated in an ointment used to relieve the pain and itching of hemorrhoids (piles) and other unfortunate problems in the rectal area.

GENERAL ANESTHETICS

The first demonstration of general anesthesia for surgery was performed by William Morton at Massachusetts General Hospital in 1846. The anesthetic that Morton used was **diethyl ether,** and his demonstration had a profound effect on the field of surgery. Before that time, surgery was limited to rapid procedures such as limb amputations with strong men to hold down the patients. General anesthesia and the subsequent development of aseptic techniques permitted the evolution of surgical procedures to the sophisticated level achieved today.

Diethyl ether is no longer used in developed countries because it has a slow rate of induction, causes considerable postoperative nausea and vomiting, and is highly flammable. The use of another anesthetic gas, **cyclopropane,** has also been abandoned because of its explosive nature and its tendency to cause cardiac arrhythmias. A variety of anesthetics are currently available for inhalational use, however. These include **nitrous oxide** and a growing number of halogenated hydrocarbons. The pharmacologic properties of this class of drugs are listed in Table 21.2. A picture showing the mechanism of action for general anesthetics is presented in Fig. 21.3.

Inhalational Anesthetics

Drug Properties

Pharmacokinetics. The inhalational anesthetics are divided into **nonhalogenated** drugs and **halogenated** drugs.

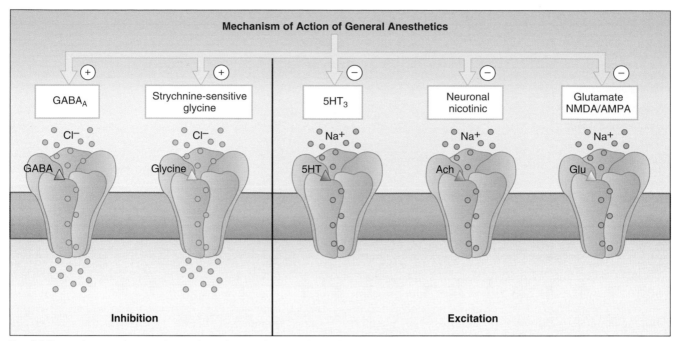

FIG. 21.3 Mechanism of action of general anesthetics. Like antiepileptic drugs, general anesthetics work at a variety of target sites. General anesthetics increase GABA and glycine inhibitory effects and decrease excitatory effects by blocking serotonergic, nicotinic, and glutaminergic neurotransmission.

These anesthetics are either gases or volatile liquids whose gaseous phase can be inhaled.

The **potency** of inhalational anesthetics is expressed in terms of the inspired concentration of the anesthetic required to produce anesthesia in half of the subjects. This is called the **minimal alveolar concentration.** The minimal alveolar concentration value is used to compare potency among different inhalational agents similar to the median effective dose of other drugs.

The pharmacokinetics of inhalational anesthetics differs from that of other drugs because the gaseous anesthetics are absorbed and eliminated through the same organ, the lungs. Moreover, as the activity of inhalational agents is caused by anesthetic molecules in the gas phase, molecules that enter the liquid phase and become soluble in the blood decrease the onset of anesthesia. The movement of anesthetic molecules between the lungs and other tissues is determined by the **partial pressure** of the anesthetic, and as the anesthetic's partial pressure in the blood increases, molecules of the anesthetic move across the blood-brain barrier into the brain and produce anesthesia.

The **induction rate** of anesthesia is determined by three primary factors: (1) the alveolar partial pressure of the anesthetic in the inspired air, (2) the ventilation rate, and (3) the rate at which the anesthetic's partial pressure in the blood increases as the anesthetic is administered. This third factor is largely dependent on the **blood:gas partition coefficient** (Box 21.1).

Because anesthetic molecules move from an area of higher partial pressure to an area of lower partial pressure, both the rate of induction and the depth of anesthesia can be rapidly adjusted by increasing or decreasing the partial pressure of the anesthetic in the patient's inspired air. After the concentration in inspired air is increased or decreased, the concentration in the blood and brain will increase or decrease. The ability to rapidly control the

depth of anesthesia increases the safety of the inhalational anesthetics.

Mechanism of Action. It once was thought that the action of inhalational anesthetics resulted from a nonspecific interaction of anesthetic molecules within the lipid bilayer of neuronal membranes, causing a disruption of ion flow and inhibiting neuronal activity. This hypothesis was supported by the correlation of the anesthetic potency with its lipophilicity, known as the *Meyer-Overton principle* (see oil:gas partition coefficient, Box 21.2).

More recently, the molecular actions of inhalational anesthetics were elucidated. These agents bind to specific amino acid residues in the transmembrane portions of the *gamma*-aminobutyric acid (GABA$_A$) receptor–chloride ion channel. The inhalational anesthetics appear to increase chloride influx and potassium efflux from neurons. Both of these actions cause hyperpolarization of neuronal membranes and reduce membrane excitability. The effect of the anesthetics on chloride flux appears to be caused by a potentiation of the action of GABA at the GABA$_A$ receptor–chloride ion channel. Inhalational anesthetics also reduce sodium and calcium influx, and this prevents nerve firing and the release of neurotransmitters.

Pharmacologic Effects. The induction by general anesthetics is characterized by four stages. **In stage I,** neurons in the spinal cord are prevented from firing, and **analgesia** and **conscious sedation** occur. **In stage II,** inhibition of firing in small inhibitory neurons can cause **paradoxical excitation,** although, with modern balanced anesthesia, this stage is often not observed. **Stage III** is the goal of surgical anesthesia, with **suppression** of the reticular-activating system, **loss of consciousness,** and **inhibition of spinal reflexes.** The latter effect contributes to the muscle relaxation needed for surgery; however, adjunct muscle relaxant agents (see Chapter 7) are commonly used. **Stage IV,** which is to be avoided because it can lead to **cardiovascular collapse,** is

BOX 21.1 PHARMACOKINETICS OF INHALATIONAL ANESTHETICS RATE OF INDUCTION OF ANESTHESIA

The rate of induction of anesthesia is determined by three primary factors: (1) the alveolar concentration, or alveolar partial pressure, of the anesthetic; (2) the ventilation rate; and (3) the rate at which the anesthetic's partial pressure in the blood increases as the anesthetic is administered. This third factor, in turn, is influenced by the blood:gas partition coefficient.

The blood:gas partition coefficient is a measure of the anesthetic's solubility in the blood. In the example shown here, the coefficient of nitrous oxide is 0.47, whereas that of halothane is 2.3.

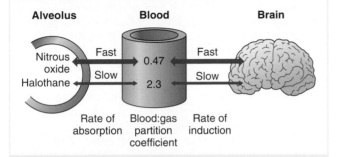

A high blood:gas partition coefficient corresponds with a high degree of solubility in the blood and with a low rate of rise in the anesthetic's partial pressure in the blood during induction. Anesthetics with a low coefficient (e.g., nitrous oxide) have a fast rate of induction because they saturate the blood quickly, and their partial pressure rises quickly. Anesthetics with a higher coefficient (e.g., halothane) have a slow rate of induction because they dissolve slowly in the blood, and it takes a long time for their partial pressure in the blood to rise.

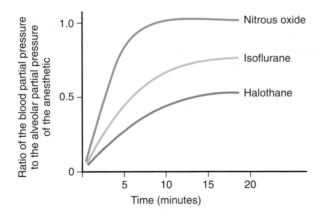

ADJUSTING THE RATE OR DEPTH OF ANESTHESIA

The anesthetic's alveolar concentration and the ventilation rate can be altered by the anesthesiologist to accelerate or slow the rate of induction or recovery, to adjust the depth of anesthesia during surgery, or to maintain tissue oxygenation and eliminate carbon dioxide.

The anesthetic's alveolar concentration after induction is usually about half as high as during induction. In patients having mechanical ventilation, the rate of induction or depth of anesthesia can be adjusted by changing the respiratory rate or tidal volume.

BOX 21.2 MECHANISMS OF ACTION OF INHALATIONAL ANESTHETICS

The potency of an inhalational anesthetic, expressed in terms of the minimal alveolar concentration, is highly correlated with the lipid solubility (oil:gas partition coefficient) of the anesthetic. This correlation suggests that anesthetics interact with a hydrophobic component of neuronal membranes.

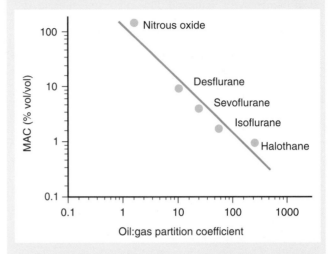

Inhalational anesthetics are believed to bind stereoselectively to hydrophobic regions of neuronal membrane proteins that interface with membrane lipids. The anesthetics potentiate γ-aminobutyric acid (GABA) activity at the $GABA_A$-chloride ionophore and thereby increase chloride flux through the ionophore. They may also inhibit sodium and calcium influx through membrane channels. These actions hyperpolarize the neuronal membrane and inhibit neuron firing and the release of neurotransmitters.

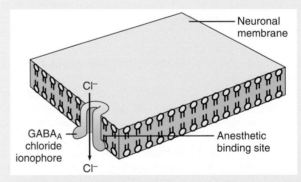

Because of their effects on neuronal membrane proteins, anesthetics disrupt neuronal firing and sensory processing in the thalamus and thereby cause loss of consciousness and analgesia. Anesthetics also inhibit neuronal output from layer V (the internal pyramidal layer) of the cortex, and this reduces motor activity.

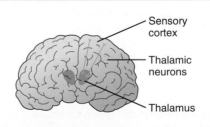

BOX 21.3 THE CASE OF THE ESCALATING APPENDECTOMY

CASE PRESENTATION

A 21-year-old man comes to a small-town hospital with nausea, a low-grade fever, and pain radiating from the lower right quadrant of his abdomen. A history reveals that he was backpacking in the country and was fed some wild berries by his girlfriend. Physical examination reveals tenderness and pain in the lower abdomen, which is worse after the physician presses down and quickly removes his hand. He is diagnosed with acute appendicitis and prepared for emergency surgery. He undergoes general anesthesia with enflurane, and the operation begins. After the surgery, he develops a fever, severe muscle rigidity and contractions, and tachycardia. The anesthesiologist recognizes that he has a case of malignant hyperthermia and administers dantrolene.

CASE DISCUSSION

Appendicitis is inflammation of the appendix, a small pocket off the large intestine commonly thought of as a vestigial organ but recently has been suggested to play a role as a reservoir for intestinal flora and to serve an immune function. When treated promptly by appendectomy, most patients with acute appendicitis recover without difficulty, but if treatment is delayed, the appendix can burst, causing infection and death. Many cases of appendicitis are linked to a blockage in the lumen of the organ and can be caused by impacted feces or even a fruit pit. Malignant hyperthermia is associated with more than 80 genetic defects and appears to be inherited with an autosomal dominant inheritance pattern. Most defects are related to mutations of the ryanodine receptor located on intracellular organelles, such as the sarcoplasmic reticulum, which mediate the release of Ca^{2+} from these intracellular stores. Dantrolene is given by the intravenous route, binds to the ryanodine receptor, and blocks the release of Ca^{2+} and the resultant sequelae that characterize malignant hyperthermia.

noted by depression of the respiratory and vasomotor nuclei in the brainstem.

Adverse Effects. The adverse effects of nonhalogenated and halogenated anesthetics are limited and uncommon and include airway irritation, moderate respiratory depression, and hypotensive effects. Of particular importance with the administration of **halothane** is the toxicity of the liver, called **halothane hepatitis,** which results from a reactive intermediate metabolite that acetylates liver proteins and produces an immune reaction that is fatal in about half of all cases.

Halothane and other halogenated anesthetics can also trigger **malignant hyperthermia,** a rare condition leading to muscle fiber breakdown, rhabdomyolysis (muscle proteins released into the blood), and renal failure (see the case in Box 21.3). Prompt discontinuation of the anesthetic and treatment with **dantrolene,** which prevents Ca^{2+} release from the sarcoplasmic reticulum, are necessary to prevent fatality. Dantrolene is also used in the management of **neuroleptic malignant syndrome** (see Chapter 22).

Specific Agents

Nonhalogenated Drugs. **Nitrous oxide** is the only nonhalogenated anesthetic gas used today. It is the least potent of the inhalational anesthetics, and it does not reduce consciousness to the extent required for major surgical procedures. Nitrous oxide, however, produces more analgesia than do the other inhalational anesthetics, and it is often used for minor surgery and dental procedures that do not require loss of consciousness. Nitrous oxide is frequently used as a component of **balanced anesthesia** in combination with another anesthetic agent and other drugs (see later). The nitrous oxide in balanced anesthesia provides greater analgesia and enables the use of a lower concentration of the other anesthetic agent.

Because nitrous oxide has a low blood:gas partition coefficient, induction and recovery are rapid when it is used. The anesthetic produces virtually no cardiovascular or respiratory depression, and it is generally considered quite safe. It oxidizes the cobalt moiety of vitamin B_{12}, however, and thereby inhibits the methylation of nucleic acids and proteins. Although these effects are minimal during acute exposure, chronic exposure to nitrous oxide can cause **megaloblastic anemia.**

Nitrous oxide, which is also called **"laughing gas,"** often produces mild euphoria when it is administered. For this reason, some recreational use of the drug occurs.

Halogenated Anesthetics. In most areas of the world, halogenated anesthetics replaced older, volatile liquid anesthetics (e.g., **diethyl ether**) because of several advantages. The halogenated drugs have a more **rapid rate** of induction and recovery, cause a much lower incidence of postoperative nausea and vomiting, and are not flammable. However, they produce dose-dependent respiratory and cardiovascular depression. For this reason, respiratory and cardiovascular functions are monitored during the use of halogenated anesthetics, and artificial ventilation and circulatory support are often required. The halogenated anesthetics cause uterine relaxation, which usually limits their use in obstetrics to women having cesarean section. Because halogenated anesthetics produce relatively little analgesia or skeletal muscle relaxation, they are often given in combination with nitrous oxide, opioids, muscle relaxants, and other adjunct drugs in what is called **balanced anesthesia.**

Halothane is the prototypical halogenated anesthetic, and **desflurane, enflurane, isoflurane,** and **sevoflurane** are newer halogenated anesthetics. Halothane is the most potent inhalational agent, but it has several disadvantages. Because of its relatively high blood:gas partition coefficient, its rate of induction and recovery is slower than that of other halogenated anesthetics. Because it sensitizes the heart to catecholamines more than other anesthetics, it places patients at greater risk for **cardiac dysrhythmias.** Hence, the use of epinephrine for hemostasis must be strictly limited in patients receiving halothane. Halothane undergoes appreciable hepatic metabolism and is converted to reactive intermediate metabolites that can produce a hypersensitivity reaction and hepatitis (see earlier). For this reason, a patient who is anesthetized with halothane should not be re-exposed to it for 6 to 12 months. **However, halothane is no longer used in the United States.**

Enflurane and **isoflurane** exhibit more rapid induction and recovery than halothane exhibits. They undergo less metabolic degradation and produce little cardiac arrhythmia. Enflurane and isoflurane produce more **muscle relaxation,** so this reduces the need for muscle relaxants during surgery. They cause more respiratory depression, however,

TABLE 21.3   Properties of Parenteral Anesthetics^a

DRUG	DURATION OF ACTION (MIN)	ANALGESIA	MUSCLE RELAXATION	OTHER EFFECTS
Fentanyl	5–10 for IV; 30–60 for IM	+ + + +	0	Respiratory depression
Remifentanil	As long as infused	+ + + +	0	Respiratory depression, corrected by stopping infusion
Ketamine	5–10 for IV; 12–25 for IM	+ + +	0	Postanesthetic delirium and hallucinations
Midazolam	5–20 for IV; 20–40 for IM	0	+ + +	Amnesia
Etomidate	5–10 for IV	0	0	Little effect on blood pressure
Propofol	5–10 for IV	0	0	Respiratory depression
Pentobarbital	5–10 for IV	0	0	Respiratory depression

IM, Intramuscular administration; *IV,* intravenous administration.
^aValues shown are the mean of values reported in the literature. Ratings range from none (0) to high (+ + + +).

than the other halogenated drugs cause. At high concentrations, enflurane can produce CNS excitation, leading to seizures.

Desflurane and **sevoflurane** have a more rapid rate of induction and recovery than other halogenated anesthetics do, but desflurane is irritating to the respiratory tract, so this limits the concentrations of this agent that can be administered during induction. Sevoflurane is close to an ideal anesthetic. It exhibits a rapid and smooth induction and recovery, and it causes little cardiovascular or other organ system toxicity.

Parenteral Anesthetics

The parenteral anesthetics include barbiturates, benzodiazepines, opioids, and other compounds such as propofol. These drugs are used for a variety of purposes, including preanesthetic sedation, induction of anesthesia, perioperative analgesia, and anesthesia for minor surgical and diagnostic procedures. The properties of parenteral anesthetics are given in Table 21.3.

Pentobarbital is a fast-acting barbiturate used for induction of anesthesia and to produce a medically induced coma in ICU patients. **Thiopental** and **methohexital** are listed as ultra-fast-acting barbiturates; the former is no longer available in the United States, but methohexital is still marketed.

Propofol is a phenol compound that produces a quick and predictable loss of consciousness (induction of anesthesia) and is widely used for procedures such as colonoscopy. Patients recover faster from outpatient surgery when given propofol compared to benzodiazepines or barbiturates. **Fospropofol** is a phosphorylated prodrug of propofol, also for IV administration. These drugs, like the benzodiazepines (below), potentiate GABA activity at the GABA$_A$ receptor–chloride ion channel but are more potent and can work without GABA present. Their use is followed by the administration of an inhalational anesthetic to maintain anesthesia. Both drugs have a rapid onset of action, causing unconsciousness in about 20 seconds. Their duration of action is short (5 to 10 minutes) because they are redistributed from the brain to the peripheral tissues as their blood concentrations fall. **Propofol** has the advantages of being rapidly metabolized and eliminated from the body and causing little drug hangover. **Thiopental** is accumulated in fat and muscle. It is more slowly eliminated from the body, and some hangover can occur. Thiopental is no longer available in the USA. Either drug can depress cardiovascular and

respiratory function. **Methohexital** is also a barbiturate used for rapid induction of anesthesia and has properties similar to those of thiopental.

Etomidate is structurally distinct from the other parenteral anesthetics and is commonly used in the emergency department for rapid induction to induce anesthesia or for conscious sedation. It has a rapid onset of action with low cardiovascular risks and is less likely to cause a significant drop in blood pressure than other induction agents.

Fentanyl is a strong opioid agonist used to treat moderate to severe pain (see Chapter 23). Because of its potent analgesic properties, it is also administered intravenously or by the epidural route in combination with other drugs for surgical or obstetric analgesia and balanced anesthesia. For example, it is used to provide anesthesia during **cardiac surgery** (e.g., coronary artery bypass grafting) because it does not cause cardiovascular toxicity. Fentanyl does not produce amnesia or complete loss of consciousness, so it is often combined with a benzodiazepine (e.g., **midazolam**) to produce amnesia and increased sedation.

Fentanyl has been used in combination with **droperidol,** a member of the antipsychotic class of agents (previously called *neuroleptics*) that produce a condition called **neuroleptanesthesia (twilight sleep).** Droperidol is a butyrophenone compound whose properties are similar to those of the antipsychotic agent, haloperidol (see Chapter 22). The advantage of neuroleptanesthesia is that it provides adequate analgesia and sedation during surgery while maintaining a sufficient level of consciousness to permit the patient to respond to questions during the surgical procedure. The disadvantages of neuroleptanesthesia include **chest wall rigidity,** which is caused by the effects of fentanyl and droperidol on the basal ganglia. Fentanyl has a much shorter half-life than does droperidol, and supplemental doses of fentanyl may be needed during long surgical procedures.

Fentanyl and **sufentanil,** a closely related opioid, are also used with or without a local anesthetic for epidural administration or by the spinal intrathecal route during labor or to provide postoperative analgesia. Other shorter-acting opioids (e.g., **alfentanil** and **remifentanil**) are used intravenously for induction or for ambulatory surgery. **Remifentanil** is unique because it is metabolized extremely rapidly by esterases in the blood and tissues (see opioids in Chapter 23).

Ketamine is chemically and pharmacologically related to **phencyclidine (PCP),** a street drug that is abused because of its pronounced effects on sensory perception (see Chapter 25). Both ketamine and PCP act by blocking the action of excitatory amino acids, primarily glutamate, at *N*-methyl-D-aspartate (NMDA) receptors. By blocking the excitation of neurons, ketamine and PCP depress neuronal activity. Ketamine produces less sensory distortion and euphoria than does PCP and therefore is more suitable for use as an IV anesthetic.

Ketamine produces **dissociative anesthesia,** a mental state in which the individual appears to be dissociated from the environment without complete loss of consciousness. This type of anesthesia is characterized by analgesia, reduced sensory perception, immobility, and amnesia. Unlike many inhalational anesthetics, ketamine usually increases blood pressure, but it has little effect on respiration with typical doses. The main drawback of ketamine is its tendency to cause unpleasant effects during recovery, including delirium, hallucinations, and irrational behavior. Because children are less likely than adults to experience these adverse effects, ketamine is most often used in **pediatric patients** and is given in combination with a benzodiazepine for anesthesia during minor surgical or diagnostic procedures. **Esketamine,** which is the S-enantiomer of racemic ketamine, was very recently approved as a fast-acting antidepressant (see Chapter 22).

Midazolam is a short-acting benzodiazepine used for preoperative sedation as well as for endoscopy and other diagnostic procedures that do not require general anesthesia. Although its onset of action is slower than that of thiopental or propofol, it has the advantage of causing little cardiovascular or respiratory depression. If an overdose of midazolam occurs, the effects of the drug can be reversed by administration of **flumazenil,** a **benzodiazepine antagonist. Remimazolam** is a new IV sedative drug with a shorter elimination half-life than midazolam (see benzodiazepines in Chapter 19) so marketed for short outpatient procedures.

SUMMARY OF IMPORTANT POINTS

- Local anesthetics produce use-dependent blockade of nerve conduction and thereby prevent pain associated with surgical and diagnostic procedures. Autonomic and sensory nerves are blocked more easily than are nerves affecting proprioception, muscle tone, and somatic motor activity.
- Local anesthetics are weak bases. The nonionized form permeates neuronal membranes, and the ionized form binds to the internal surface of sodium channels.
- Ester-type anesthetics (e.g., procaine and chloroprocaine) are converted to PABA and may elicit hypersensitivity reactions.
- Amide-type anesthetics (e.g., lidocaine and mepivacaine) produce fewer allergic reactions than ester-type anesthetics.
- All local anesthetics can cause CNS and cardiac toxicity, including seizures and cardiac arrhythmias.
- General anesthetics include inhalational agents (e.g., nitrous oxide and enflurane) and parenteral agents (e.g., ketamine and propofol).
- The potency of inhalational anesthetics is expressed as the minimal alveolar concentration required to produce anesthesia. The potency is proportional to the oil:gas partition coefficient.
- The rate of induction of inhalational anesthetics is determined in part by the blood:gas partition coefficient. Nitrous oxide has a low coefficient and a rapid rate of induction. Halothane has a higher coefficient and a slower rate of induction.
- All inhalational anesthetics, except nitrous oxide, suppress respiratory function and decrease blood pressure in a dose-dependent manner.
- Parenteral anesthetics are used to induce anesthesia and to provide anesthesia during minor surgical and diagnostic procedures. They are also used in combination with other anesthetics during major surgical procedures.

Review Questions

1. Local anesthetics exert their effects by which one of the following mechanisms?
   (A) increasing K^+ conductance and hyperpolarizing nerves
   (B) blocking the Na^+ channels in nerves
   (C) inactivating the Na^+,K^+-adenosine triphosphatase (ATPase) pump
   (D) blocking excitation at postsynaptic receptors
   (E) blocking by a direct action only at the synapse
2. Epinephrine is sometimes added to commercial local anesthetic solutions for which purpose?
   (A) to decrease the rate of absorption of the local anesthetic
   (B) to decrease the duration of action of the local anesthetic
   (C) to block the metabolism of ester-type local anesthetics
   (D) to enhance the distribution of the local anesthetic
   (E) to act synergistically with the local anesthetic at the nerve ion channel
3. Which of the following characteristics is used to quantitate and compare the potency of gaseous general anesthetics?
   (A) blood:gas partition coefficient
   (B) minimal alveolar concentration
   (C) blood:brain partition coefficient
   (D) rate of uptake and elimination
   (E) relative analgesic potency
4. Which one of the following inhalational anesthetics can provide anesthetic effectiveness only under hyperbaric conditions?
   (A) enflurane
   (B) nitrous oxide
   (C) halothane
   (D) methoxyflurane
   (E) isoflurane
5. Muscle rigidity can be a side effect of which intravenous anesthetic?
   (A) fentanyl
   (B) midazolam
   (C) ketamine
   (D) propofol
   (E) thiopental

CHAPTER 22
Psychotherapeutic Drugs

CLASSIFICATION OF PSYCHOTHERAPEUTIC DRUGS

Antipsychotic Drugs

Typical antipsychotics
- Fluphenazine
- Thioridazine[a]
- Haloperidol (Haldol)

Atypical antipsychotics
- Clozapine (Clozaril)
- Olanzapine (Zyprexa)
- Risperidone (Risperdal)
- Aripiprazole (Abilify)[b]

Antidepressant Drugs

Tricyclic antidepressants
- Amitriptyline (Elavil)[c]
- Imipramine (Tofranil)
- Clomipramine (Anafranil)[d]

Selective serotonin reuptake inhibitors (SSRIs)
- Fluoxetine (Prozac)[e]
- Citalopram (Celexa)
- Sertraline (Zoloft)[f]

Serotonin and norepinephrine reuptake inhibitors (SNRIs)
- Duloxetine (Cymbalta)
- Venlafaxine (Effexor)
- Desvenlafaxine (Pristiq)[g]

Monoamine oxidase inhibitors
- Phenelzine (Nardil)[h]
- Selegiline (Eldepryl)

Atypical Antidepressant drugs
- Bupropion (Wellbutrin, Zyban)[i]
- Trazodone (Oleptro)[j]
- Esketamine (Spravato)[k]

Mood-Stabilizing Drugs
- Lithium (Lithobid)
- Carbamazepine (Tegretol)
- Valproate (Depakote)

Central Nervous System Stimulants
- Amphetamines (Adderall)[l]
- Methylphenidate (Ritalin)[m]
- Modafinil (Provigil)
- Armodafinil (Nuvigil)
- Atomoxetine (Strattera)
- Phentermine (Adipex-P)[n]

---

[a] Also chlorpromazine, trifluoperazine, thiothixene (Navane), perphenazine, and loxapine; also valbenazine (Ingrezza) which is not used as an antipsychotic but the first drug approved for the treatment of tardive dyskinesia produced by antipsychotic agents.

[b] Also quetiapine (Seroquel), brexpiprazole (Rexulti), ziprasidone (Geodon), paliperidone (Invega), lurasidone (Latuda), iloperidone (Fanapt), asenapine (Saphris), pimavanserin (Nuplazid), cariprazine (Vraylar), and lumateperone (Caplyta). Aripiprazole is also available in an extended-release formulation (Aristada).

[c] Also available in a generic combination formulation of amitriptyline with perphenazine.

[d] Also desipramine (Norpramin) and nortriptyline (Pamelor).

[e] Also in combination drug as fluoxetine and olanzapine (Symbyax).

[f] Also escitalopram (Lexapro), fluvoxamine (Luvox), paroxetine (Paxil, Brisdelle), and vortioxetine (Brintellix).

[g] Also milnacipran (Savella), and levomilnacipran (Fetzima).

[h] Also isocarboxazid (Marplan) and tranylcypromine (Parnate).

[i] Also in a combination formulation of bupropion plus naltrexone (Contrave) for weight loss.

[j] Also mirtazapine (Remeron) and vilazodone (Viibryd).

[k] Also brexanolone (Zulresso).

[l] Also dextroamphetamine (Dexedrine), methamphetamine (Desoxyn), and lisdexamfetamine (Vyvanse).

[m] Also dexmethylphenidate (Focalin). Methylphenidate is also formulated in extended-release tablets (Aptensio XR, Concerta), as a transdermal patch (Daytrana), as an oral suspension (Quillivant XR), and chewable tablet (Quillivant ER) for young children.

[n] Also formulated as phentermine plus topiramate, extended release (Qsymia).

OVERVIEW

The major psychiatric disorders include psychoses, such as schizophrenia, and affective disorders, such as depression. Psychoses are disorders in which patients exhibit gross disturbances in their comprehension of reality, as evidenced by false perceptions (hallucinations) and false beliefs (delusions). In contrast, affective disorders are emotional disturbances in which the mood is excessively low (depression) or high (mania). During the past 50 years, tremendous advances have been made in the treatment of these disorders. The newer antipsychotic drugs used to treat schizophrenia and the newer antidepressant and mood-stabilizing drugs used to treat affective disorders cause fewer adverse reactions and are more effective than older psychotherapeutic agents. Treatment-resistant disorders still pose a significant problem to clinicians, but some progress has been made in the treatment of refractory disease. The chapter ends with central nervous system (CNS) stimulants used for attention-deficit/hyperactivity disorder (ADHD), narcolepsy and other sleep disorders, and obesity.

SCHIZOPHRENIA
Clinical Findings

Schizophrenia, the most common form of psychosis, affects about 1% of the world's population. Its hallmarks are delusions, hallucinations, disorganized thinking, and emotional

Positive Symptoms	Negative Symptoms
Agitation	Apathy (avolition)
Delusions	Affective flattening
Disorganized speech	Lack of motivation
Disorganized thinking	Lack of pleasure (anhedonia)
Hallucinations	Poverty of speech (alogia)
Insomnia	Social isolation

abnormalities. Several forms of the disease, including paranoid, disorganized, and catatonic forms, are differentiated on the basis of symptoms.

As shown in Box 22.1, the symptoms of schizophrenia can be divided into two groups. The **positive symptoms,** which include delusions and hallucinations, probably result from excessive neuronal activity in mesolimbic neuronal pathways. These symptoms are usually the primary manifestations of acute psychotic episodes. The **negative symptoms,** which include apathy, withdrawal, and lack of motivation and pleasure, probably result from insufficient activity in mesocortical neuronal pathways. The negative symptoms generally are more difficult to treat, often persist after positive symptoms resolve, and are associated with a poor prognosis.

Dopamine Hypothesis

Many hypotheses exist regarding the biologic basis of schizophrenia. According to the **dopamine hypothesis,** schizophrenia results from abnormalities in dopamine neurotransmission in mesolimbic and mesocortical neuronal pathways (Box 22.2). Much of the evidence supporting this hypothesis is based on the clinical effects of agents that alter dopaminergic transmission.

Several observations support the dopamine hypothesis. First, most antipsychotic drugs block **dopamine D_2 receptors,** and an excellent correlation exists between the clinical potency of these drugs and their *in vitro* binding affinity for these receptors. Second, drugs that act by increasing the neuronal release of dopamine (amantadine) or by blocking the reuptake of dopamine (drugs such as amphetamines and cocaine) can **induce psychotic behavior** that resembles the behavior of schizophrenic patients.

Dopamine turnover in the brain, which reflects the neuronal release of dopamine, can be studied by measuring the concentration of the principal metabolite of dopamine, homovanillic acid, in the cerebrospinal fluid. Although elevated levels of homovanillic acid are not found in patients with chronic schizophrenia, they are found in some schizophrenic patients having acute psychotic episodes. Evidence also exists for a dopamine receptor defect in schizophrenic patients. Positive emission tomography scanning using D_2 receptor ligands has revealed that schizophrenic patients have **decreased D_2 receptor densities** in the prefrontal lobe cortex (but increased D_2 receptor densities in the caudate nucleus). These findings lend overall support to the dopamine hypothesis, although it is clear from the clinical

effectiveness of atypical antipsychotics that 5-hydroxytryptamine ($5\text{-}HT_2$) and other types of dopamine receptors may be involved (Box 22.3).

ANTIPSYCHOTIC DRUGS

Antipsychotic drugs are agents that reduce psychotic symptoms and improve the behavior of schizophrenic patients. Antipsychotic drugs were also called **neuroleptic drugs** because they suppress motor activity and emotional expression. The accidental discovery of the antipsychotic properties of chlorpromazine in the early 1950s began a new era in the treatment of schizophrenia and stimulated research concerning the neurobiology of mental illness and psychopharmacology. Nearly 40 years later, the introduction of **clozapine** had an equally important effect. Clozapine was the first agent to show greater activity against the **negative symptoms** of schizophrenia and to produce a decreased occurrence of **extrapyramidal syndrome (EPS)** than the previous antipsychotic drugs. For this reason, the discovery of clozapine has stimulated the development of new antipsychotic drugs with improved pharmacologic properties.

Mechanism of Action

The antipsychotic drugs interact with multiple neurotransmitter systems. Whereas the therapeutic effects of these drugs are believed to result from a competitive blockade of **dopamine receptors** and **serotonin (5-HT) receptors,** the adverse effects are attributed to the blockade of a variety of receptors (Table 22.1).

Typical antipsychotic drugs have an equal or greater affinity for D_2 receptors than for $5\text{-}HT_2$ receptors. As shown in Fig. 22.1, an excellent correlation exists between the clinical potency of these drugs and their *in vitro* affinity for D_2 receptors. Whereas antagonism of D_2 receptors in mesolimbic pathways is thought to repress the positive symptoms of schizophrenia, blockade of D_2 receptors in the basal ganglia is believed to be responsible for the parkinsonian and other EPS that sometimes occur in patients taking antipsychotic drugs.

Atypical antipsychotic drugs (e.g., **clozapine**) have a greater affinity for 5-HT receptors than for D_2 receptors, and some atypical drugs have increased the affinity for D_3 or D_4 receptors. This is thought to increase their effectiveness in reducing the negative symptoms of schizophrenia (see Box 22.1).

Pharmacologic Effects

The mechanisms by which the blockade of dopamine and serotonin receptors alleviates the symptoms of schizophrenia are not completely understood. Whereas these receptors are blocked immediately when antipsychotic drugs are first administered, the therapeutic effects of the drugs usually require several weeks to fully develop. This is because antipsychotic drugs produce three time-dependent **changes in dopamine neurotransmission.** When first administered, the drugs cause an increase in dopamine synthesis, release, and metabolism. This probably represents a compensatory response to the acute blockade of postsynaptic dopamine receptors produced by antipsychotic drugs. Over time, continued dopamine receptor blockade leads to the inactivation of dopaminergic neurons and produces what has been called **depolarization blockade.** Depolarization blockade results in

BOX 22.2 NEUROBIOLOGY OF SCHIZOPHRENIA AND SITES OF DRUG ACTION

POSTULATED NEURONAL DYSFUNCTION IN SCHIZOPHRENIA

As shown in the accompanying figure, numerous dopamine pathways are found in the brain.

1. **Mesolimbic pathway.** Dopamine travels from the midbrain tegmental area to the nucleus accumbens. Increased activity in this pathway may cause delusions, hallucinations, and other so-called *positive symptoms* of schizophrenia.
2. **Mesocortical pathways.** There are several mesocortical pathways. Decreased activity in the pathway that goes from the midbrain to the prefrontal lobe cortex can cause apathy, withdrawal, lack of motivation and pleasure, and other so-called *negative symptoms* of schizophrenia. Mesocortical dysfunction also disinhibits the mesolimbic pathway.
3. **Nigrostriatal pathway.** The pathway from the substantia nigra to the striatum is involved in the coordination of body movements. Inhibition of this pathway causes the extrapyramidal side effects of antipsychotic drugs.
4. **Tuberoinfundibular pathway.** The pathway from the hypothalamus to the pituitary inhibits the release of prolactin. Inhibition of this pathway leads to elevated serum prolactin levels.

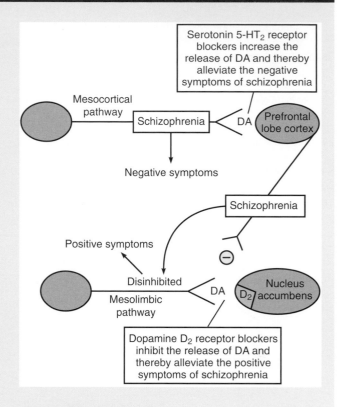

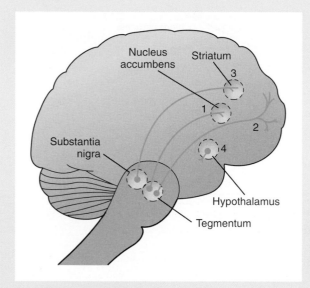

SITES OF DRUG ACTION

Some antipsychotic drugs (e.g., clozapine, olanzapine, and risperidone) block serotonin 5-HT$_2$ receptors in the mesocortical pathway to the prefrontal lobe cortex. This increases the release of dopamine *(DA)* and thereby alleviates the negative symptoms of schizophrenia. Most antipsychotic drugs (including those listed previously) block dopamine D$_2$ receptors in the mesolimbic pathway to the nucleus accumbens, and this alleviates the positive symptoms of schizophrenia.

BOX 22.3 THE CASE OF THE PARANOID POLICEMAN

CASE PRESENTATION

A 24-year-old man employed as a policeman locks himself in an interrogation room, waving his handgun and yelling incoherent statements such as "They aren't going to take me alive!" and "Get out of my head!" His partner tells the police chief that the man has been acting strangely, talking about a conspiracy against him by the other policemen and arriving for work in dirty clothes and unshaven. He was overheard talking and arguing with himself in the locker room that morning, and the partner says they almost got into a fight just minutes ago because the partner wouldn't agree to shoot him when he insisted that he "wouldn't be hurt and was immortal." A medical emergency team arrives on the scene, and at a moment when he is sitting in the corner cowering in fear, they forcibly enter the room, disarm him, and inject haloperidol into his thigh. He is transported to the locked ward of a psychiatric hospital and diagnosed with paranoid schizophrenia.

CASE DISCUSSION

Schizophrenia affects about 1 in 100 males and can be one of the most dangerous of all mental disorders, as it causes those it affects to lose touch with reality. They often show signs of confusion, inability to make decisions, auditory hallucinations, delusions, neglect of personal hygiene, strange statements or behavior, and changes in eating or sleeping habits, energy level, or weight. In the paranoid form of this disorder, schizophrenics develop delusions of persecution or personal grandeur. The first sign of paranoid schizophrenia usually surfaces at ages 15 to 30, and schizophrenia is much more common in males than females. There is no cure, but the disorder can be controlled with antipsychotic medications such as haloperidol. Haloperidol is a good choice for acute psychotic episodes as it is rapidly absorbed and has a high bioavailability after intramuscular injection, with plasma levels reaching their maximum within 20 min after injection.

TABLE 22.1   Mechanisms Responsible for the Therapeutic and Adverse Effects of Antipsychotic Drugs

MECHANISM	THERAPEUTIC EFFECTS	ADVERSE EFFECTS
Blockade of α_1-adrenoceptors	—	Dizziness, orthostatic hypotension, and reflex tachycardia
Blockade of dopamine D_2 receptors	Alleviation of positive symptoms of schizophrenia	Extrapyramidal effects (akathisia, dystonia, and pseudoparkinsonism) and elevated serum prolactin levels
Blockade of dopamine D_4 receptors	Alleviation of negative symptoms of schizophrenia and decrease in the incidence of extrapyramidal side effects	—
Blockade of histamine H_1 receptors	— (Sedation)[a]	Drowsiness and increase in appetite and weight
Blockade of muscarinic receptors	—	Blurred vision, constipation, dry mouth, and urinary retention
Blockade of serotonin 5-HT_2 receptors	Alleviation of negative symptoms of schizophrenia and decrease in the incidence of extrapyramidal side effects	Anxiety and insomnia

[a]Sedation may be considered a therapeutic effect with a typical antipsychotic administered for acute psychosis.

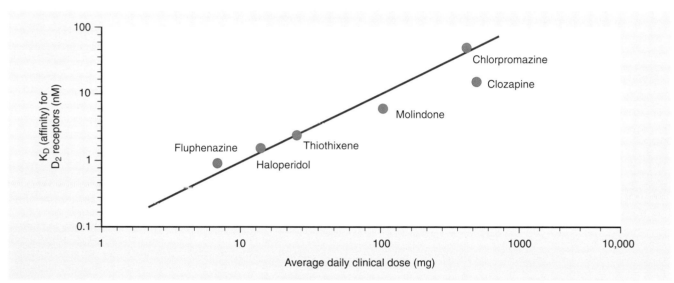

Fig. 22.1   Correlation of antipsychotic drug potency and dopamine D_2 receptor binding. The clinical potency of the typical antipsychotic drugs is highly correlated with their *in vitro* affinity for D_2 (but not D_1) receptors.

reduced dopamine release from mesolimbic and nigrostriatal neurons. This action is believed to alleviate the positive symptoms of schizophrenia while causing EPS. Eventually, the reduction in dopamine release caused by depolarization blockade leads to dopamine receptor up-regulation and supersensitivity to dopamine agonists. This supersensitivity may contribute to the development of a delayed type of EPS called **tardive dyskinesia** (see later).

In mesocortical and nigrostriatal pathways, 5-HT_2 receptors mediate presynaptic inhibition of dopamine release. Blockade of these receptors by atypical antipsychotic drugs may increase dopamine release in these pathways. In the mesocortical pathway, this action may alleviate the negative symptoms of schizophrenia. In the nigrostriatal pathway, increased dopamine release counteracts the EPS caused by D_2 receptor blockade.

Adverse Effects

In the peripheral autonomic nervous system, antipsychotic drugs also block **muscarinic** receptors and **alpha** $(\alpha)_1$-**adrenoceptors,** thereby causing the adverse effects

described in Table 22.2 (see also Table 22.1). Antagonism of α_1-adrenoceptors produces dizziness, orthostatic hypotension, and reflex tachycardia. Muscarinic receptor antagonism produces blurred vision, dry mouth, constipation, and urinary retention. Antagonism of brain H_1 receptors produces drowsiness and weight gain.

The most disturbing adverse effect is the development of **motor abnormalities** after the administration of high-potency, typical antipsychotics. These and other adverse effects specific to particular agents are discussed later.

Neuroleptic malignant syndrome is a severe form of drug toxicity that occurs in 0.5% to 1% of patients treated with antipsychotic drugs. It is a **life-threatening condition** characterized by muscle rigidity, elevated temperature (>38°C), altered consciousness, and autonomic dysfunction (tachycardia, diaphoresis, tachypnea, and urinary and fecal incontinence). The syndrome resembles malignant hyperthermia triggered by halogenated anesthetics in its rapid onset and mortality rate. Neuroleptic malignant syndrome is managed by immediately discontinuing treatment with the offending antipsychotic drug, administering **dantrolene** to prevent

TABLE 22.2   Adverse Effects of Selected Antipsychotic Drugs[a]

DRUG	EXTRAPYRAMIDAL EFFECTS	SEDATION	ANTICHOLINERGIC EFFECTS	ORTHOSTATIC HYPOTENSION	OTHER ADVERSE EFFECTS
Typical Antipsychotics					
Chlorpromazine	+++	++++	+++	++++	Elevated serum prolactin levels and poikilothermy
Fluphenazine	+++++	++	++	++	Same as chlorpromazine
Thioridazine	++	++++	++++	++++	Cardiac arrhythmia, elevated serum prolactin levels, poikilothermy, and retinopathy
Trifluoperazine	++++	++	++	++	Same as chlorpromazine
Thiothixene	++++	++	++	++	Same as chlorpromazine
Haloperidol	+++++	+	+	+	Same as chlorpromazine
Loxapine	++++	+++	++	+++	Same as chlorpromazine
Atypical Antipsychotics					
Clozapine	+	+++++	+++++	++++	Agranulocytosis and cardiac arrhythmia
Olanzapine	+	++	+	+	Weight gain
Risperidone	++	+	+	++	Cardiac arrhythmia and elevated serum prolactin levels

[a]Ratings range from extremely low (+) to extremely high (+++++).

further muscle abnormality (see Chapter 21), and providing supportive care. If future antipsychotic therapy is required in patients who have experienced this syndrome, an atypical drug should be used because the atypical drugs are associated with a lower incidence of neuroleptic malignant syndrome.

Recently, the U.S. Food and Drug Administration (FDA) strengthened warnings against using any type of antipsychotic to treat **dementia-related psychosis in the elderly** after an increased number of deaths attributed to antipsychotic use in this population. In addition, stronger warnings were issued concerning the potential risk for **abnormal motor movements** or **withdrawal effects** in neonates of mothers who took an antipsychotic during their third trimester.

Indications

Antipsychotic agents are primarily used to treat **schizophrenia** and other forms of psychosis, including drug-induced psychosis and psychosis associated with the manic phase of bipolar disorder. They are also used to treat severely agitated patients, including those with dementia and severe mental retardation. Because the older typical antipsychotics have antiemetic activity, some of them are used in the management of nausea and vomiting (see Chapter 28). More recently, some newer antipsychotic agents have been approved as **add-on medications** to those with treatment-resistant depression (see later).

Drug Classification

Antipsychotic drugs were traditionally classified on the basis of their chemical structure, but they are also classified according to whether they display **typical** or **atypical** pharmacologic properties. The **typical antipsychotic drugs** are also considered first-generation antipsychotic agents, and the **atypical antipsychotic drugs** are second-generation antipsychotic agents.

Typical Antipsychotic Agents

Numerous typical antipsychotics are available for the treatment of schizophrenia and related conditions. The four representative examples discussed in detail here are

chlorpromazine, fluphenazine, thioridazine, and **haloperidol.** These drugs have similar therapeutic effects but differ in their relative potency (Table 22.3) and in their side effect profiles (see Table 22.2).

Pharmacokinetics. The typical antipsychotics are adequately absorbed from the gut after oral administration. Several agents are also administered parenterally, including long-acting depot preparations for intramuscular injection. These agents are extensively metabolized to a large number of active and inactive metabolites before they are excreted in the urine, and they have elimination half-lives ranging from 20 to 30 hours (see Table 22.3).

Mechanisms and Pharmacologic Effects. The typical antipsychotic drugs exert their therapeutic effects primarily as a result of D_2 receptor antagonism. After therapy is initiated, the positive symptoms of schizophrenia usually subside in 1 to 3 weeks. Patients become **less agitated** and experience fewer **auditory hallucinations.** Grandiose or paranoid delusions subside and can disappear completely in some patients with continued treatment. At the same time, sleeping and eating patterns become normalized, and behavioral improvement occurs in the form of decreased hostility, combativeness, and aggression. Typical antipsychotic drugs can have some effect on negative symptoms, but it is usually less pronounced than the effect of atypical antipsychotic drugs.

Chlorpromazine and **thioridazine** are considered low-potency agents, **fluphenazine** has a slightly greater potency, and **haloperidol** is a high-potency antipsychotic agent.

Adverse Effects. The most common adverse effects produced by typical antipsychotic drugs are summarized in Table 22.2. Blockade of dopamine receptors in the striatum can cause several forms of EPS, including **akathisia, pseudoparkinsonism,** and **dystonias.** Patients with **akathisia,** or *motor restlessness,* feel compelled to pace, shuffle their feet, or shift positions and are unable to sit quietly. **Pseudoparkinsonism** resembles idiopathic Parkinson disease and is characterized by rigidity, bradykinesia, and tremor. **Dystonia** is a state of abnormal muscle tension that often affects the neck and

TABLE 22.3 Pharmacologic Properties of Selected Antipsychotic Drugs[a]

DRUG	RELATIVE POTENCY[b]	RECEPTOR SELECTIVITY	ROUTE OF ADMINISTRATION	ELIMINATION HALF-LIFE AND ROUTE	MAJOR DRUG INTERACTIONS
Typical Antipsychotics					
Chlorpromazine	Low	$D_2 > 5\text{-HT}_2$	Oral, IM, and IV	30 h (M)	Additive effects with antiadrenergic, anticholinergic, and CNS depressants. Decreases serum levels of lithium. Concurrent use of a β-adrenoceptor antagonist or an antidepressant may increase serum levels of both drugs.
Fluphenazine	High	$D_2 > 5\text{-HT}_2$	Oral and depot IM	20 h (M)	Additive effects with anticholinergic and CNS depressants. Concurrent use of a β-adrenoceptor antagonist or an antidepressant may increase serum levels of both drugs.
Thioridazine	Low	$D_2 > 5\text{-HT}_2$	Oral	30 h (M)	Same as chlorpromazine.
Trifluoperazine	High	$D_2 > 5\text{-HT}_2$	Oral and IM	24 h (M)	Same as chlorpromazine.
Thiothixene	High	$D_2 > 5\text{-HT}_2$	Oral and IM	35 h (M)	Additive effects with anticholinergic and CNS depressants. Concurrent use of a β-adrenoceptor antagonist may increase serum levels of both drugs.
Haloperidol	High	$D_2 > 5\text{-HT}_2$	Oral and depot IM	24 h (M)	Barbiturates and carbamazepine decrease serum levels. Quinidine increases serum levels.
Loxapine	Medium	$D_2 > 5\text{-HT}_2$	Oral and IM	20 h (M)	Concurrent use of an antidepressant may increase serum levels of both drugs.
Atypical Antipsychotics					
Clozapine	Low	$5\text{-HT}_2 = D_4$ and $> D_2$	Oral	24 h (M)	Not established; possible interaction with drugs that induce or inhibit cytochrome P450 isozyme CYP1A2.
Olanzapine	High	$5\text{-HT}_2 > D_2$	Oral	30 h (M)	Same as clozapine.
Molindone	Medium	$D_2 > 5\text{-HT}_2$	Oral	2 h (M)	Additive effects with anticholinergic and CNS depressants. Concurrent use of a β-adrenoceptor antagonist or an antidepressant may increase serum levels of both drugs.
Risperidone	High	$5\text{-HT}_2 > D_2$	Oral	24 h (M)	Not established; possible interaction with drugs that induce or inhibit cytochrome P450 isozyme CYP2D6.

CNS, Central nervous system; D_2, dopamine D_2 receptor; *depot,* long-acting form; *5-HT$_2$,* serotonin 5-HT$_2$ receptor; *IM,* intramuscular; *IV,* intravenous; *M,* metabolized.
[a]Values shown are the mean of values reported in the literature.
[b]Low, 50 to 2,000 mg/day; medium, 20 to 250 mg/day; and high, 1 to 100 mg/day.

facial muscles, including the tongue, pharynx, larynx, and eyes. Patients with dystonia can experience severe reactions, such as oculogyric crisis (a condition in which the eyeballs become fixed in one position, usually upward), glossospasm, tongue protrusion, and torticollis (a contracted state of the cervical muscles, producing twisting of the neck and an unnatural position of the head). Such reactions can be frightening and painful, and pharyngolaryngeal dystonias can be life-threatening. Young males who are given large doses of high-potency drugs are at great risk of developing dystonias.

Although akathisia, pseudoparkinsonism, and dystonias are acute EPS that often occur early in the course of treatment with antipsychotic drugs, **tardive dyskinesia** is a disorder that usually develops after months or years of treatment. The disorder is characterized by abnormal oral and facial movements (e.g., tongue protrusion and lip smacking). In later stages, abnormal limb and truncal movements

may also be observed. Investigators believe that tardive dyskinesia results from supersensitivity to dopamine, which develops during **long-term dopamine receptor antagonism** (see Chapter 18). This hypothesis is supported by the fact that the symptoms of tardive dyskinesia temporarily subside if dopamine receptor blockade is increased by giving larger doses of an antipsychotic drug. This approach, however, eventually leads to further receptor supersensitivity and worsening of the manifestations of tardive dyskinesia.

Typical antipsychotic agents can increase serum **prolactin** levels by blocking dopamine receptors in the tuberoinfundibular pathway (see Box 22.2) and thereby cause **gynecomastia** in men and **menstrual irregularities** in women. Via their effects on the hypothalamus, antipsychotic drugs sometimes impair thermoregulation and cause **poikilothermy,** a condition in which the body temperature tends to approach the ambient temperature. This can lead to hyperthermia (including heat stroke) or hypothermia. In addition, high doses of **thioridazine** can cause **pigmentary retinopathy** and **cardiac toxicity.**

Treatment of Adverse Effects. Acute extrapyramidal effects (akathisia, pseudoparkinsonism, and dystonias) caused by typical antipsychotic drugs can be managed by lowering the drug dosage, changing to an atypical antipsychotic drug, or administering an additional drug to counteract the adverse effects. Drugs that counteract the effects include **benztropine,** an anticholinergic drug; **diphenhydramine,** an antihistamine with significant anticholinergic activity; and **amantadine,** an agent that increases dopamine release in the basal ganglia and can be used in conjunction with an anticholinergic drug.

Tardive dyskinesia is not easily managed and does not necessarily subside if a causative drug is discontinued. Hence, prevention is important. To prevent tardive dyskinesia, antipsychotic drugs should be used in the **lowest doses** for the shortest period of time required to control symptoms of schizophrenia. The drugs should be discontinued periodically to assess the need for continued treatment and possibly to reduce the development of **dopamine supersensitivity.** Patients should be evaluated regularly for early signs of tardive dyskinesia, which are sometimes reversible. Tardive dyskinesia often becomes irreversible if it is not detected early or is allowed to persist.

Once detected, tardive dyskinesia is best managed by reducing the dosage of antipsychotic medication. This results in significant improvement in many patients. Some success has also been reported with the use of **amantadine, dopamine receptor agonists,** and **clozapine.** Other drugs that may be effective include **physostigmine,** an indirect-acting cholinergic agonist, and **benzodiazepines.** However, the first drug for the treatment of antipsychotic-induced tardive dyskinesia was recently approved. **Valbenazine inhibits vesicular monoamine transporter 2 (VMAT2),** preventing the incorporation of monoamines from the synapse back into vesicles in the neuron. Monoamines include dopamine, serotonin (5-HT), and norepinephrine. How exactly this decrease in vesicular store of monoamines translates to decreased symptoms of tardive dyskinesia is not known.

Interactions. The major drug interactions of antipsychotic agents are listed in Table 22.3. The interactions include additive effects on CNS depression when used with other CNS drugs and pharmacokinetic interactions caused by antipsychotics and other drugs existing as substrates for the same cytochrome P450 isozymes.

Specific Agents. Thioridazine and chlorpromazine and are **low-potency** typical antipsychotics with similar properties. Of the two agents, thioridazine produces greater anticholinergic effects, and this probably accounts for its tendency to cause less occurrence of EPS. **Trifluoperazine, thiothixene perphenazine,** and **loxapine** are considered **medium-potency** typical antipsychotics.

Fluphenazine is a relatively **high-potency** typical antipsychotic agent that produces fewer autonomic side effects but more EPS than low-potency antipsychotics. Fluphenazine is available in a long-acting depot preparation intended for intramuscular injection every 1 to 3 weeks and is useful for treating patients who are not compliant with oral medication or are unable to take oral drugs.

The first of the **high-potency** agents and one of the most widely used typical antipsychotic agents is **haloperidol.**

Haloperidol has properties similar to those of fluphenazine and can cause significant EPS (see Tables 22.2 and 22.3). As with fluphenazine, haloperidol is available in a long-acting depot preparation for intramuscular administration. Haloperidol is extensively metabolized in the liver, and its metabolites are excreted in the urine and bile.

In addition to its use in treating psychoses (e.g., **schizophrenia**), haloperidol is used in the treatment of **Tourette syndrome** (*Gilles de la Tourette* syndrome). This syndrome is characterized by facial and vocal tics, coprolalia (compulsive use of obscene words, particularly those related to feces), and echolalia (repetition of another person's words or phrases).

Atypical Antipsychotic Agents

Clozapine, olanzapine, and a number of newer agents are atypical antipsychotics that produce fewer EPS than do older antipsychotic drugs. Besides treatment of schizophrenia, some members of this class are approved for the treatment of acute manic episodes associated with **bipolar disorder,** as either monotherapy or adjunct therapy to lithium or valproate, **treatment-resistant depression, irritability in children with autism,** and for the treatment of **hallucinations and delusion in Parkinson's disease** (see below).

Clozapine. Clozapine has a unique profile of pharmacologic and clinical effects. It was the first of a new generation of **atypical antipsychotic** drugs that cause significantly fewer EPS while exhibiting greater activity against the **negative symptoms** of schizophrenia.

Because clozapine is a potent antagonist of a large number of receptors, it has been difficult to attribute its effects to a particular mechanism of action. It seems likely that its therapeutic effects result from the **blockade of serotonin (5-HT$_2$ receptors) and dopamine D$_4$ receptors.** Both of these actions may contribute to its greater efficacy against the negative symptoms of schizophrenia and to its **lower incidence of EPS.** The use of clozapine is associated with significant sedation and autonomic side effects. Like typical antipsychotics, these adverse effects are caused by antagonism of histamine, muscarinic, and α_1-adrenoceptors. The use of clozapine is also associated with a 1.3% first-year incidence of potentially fatal **agranulocytosis.** Therefore, the FDA requires weekly monitoring of leukocyte counts during the first 6 months of therapy, the period during which the risk of agranulocytosis is greatest. After 6 months, biweekly monitoring of leukocyte counts is required.

Olanzapine. Olanzapine is a chemical analog of clozapine. Its pharmacologic properties are similar to those of clozapine, but **olanzapine causes fewer autonomic side effects** and has not been reported to cause agranulocytosis. As with clozapine, olanzapine causes few EPS. Olanzapine has about twice the affinity for 5-HT$_2$ receptors as it does for D$_2$ receptors, and it can block dopamine D$_3$ and D$_4$ receptors. Although it also blocks histamine, muscarinic, and α_1-adrenoceptors, it does so to a lesser extent than does clozapine leading to fewer adverse autonomic effects.

Clinical trials indicate that olanzapine is as effective as haloperidol in alleviating the **positive symptoms** of schizophrenia, is superior to haloperidol in alleviating the **negative symptoms,** and produces significantly fewer EPS than does haloperidol. The most common adverse reactions to olanzapine are **sedation** and **weight gain.** At higher doses, olanzapine can cause akathisia, pseudoparkinsonism, and dystonias. Olanzapine is also available in combination with the SSRI antidepressant **fluoxetine** (see later) in a formulation (Symbyax) indicated for treatment-resistant depression. **Quetiapine** is a newer olanzapine-type drug indicated for the treatment of schizophrenia and bipolar disorder.

Risperidone. **Risperidone** is a newer atypical antipsychotic drug. Its pharmacologic properties are similar to those of olanzapine, but it appears to cause less sedation, more orthostatic hypotension, and a higher incidence of EPS than olanzapine. Its effects on treating both the positive and negative symptoms of schizophrenia are caused by antagonism at both D_2 and serotonin (5-HT_2) receptors. In some patients, **risperidone elevates levels of serum prolactin.** It also **lengthens the QT interval** seen on the electrocardiogram and can predispose patients to cardiac dysrhythmias, including *torsade de pointes.* **Paliperidone** is the major active metabolite of risperidone and shares its pharmacologic activity as an antagonist at both D_2 and 5-HT_2 receptors. Paliperidone is available in a once-a-day formulation using osmotic drug-release technology to deliver a controlled amount of drug throughout the 24-hour period and in an injectable depot formulation. Other agents sharing the pharmacologic profile of risperidone are **ziprasidone, lurasidone, iloperidone,** and **lumateperone.** A newer agent, **asenapine,** also acts like risperidone but is formulated as a sublingual tablet.

Aripiprazole differs slightly in that it is a **partial agonist** at dopamine and 5-HT_1 receptors but a 5-HT_2 receptor antagonist. Other drugs like aripiprazole include **brexpiprazole** and **cariprazine. Aripiprazole** is also the first drug approved to treat **irritability in autistic children. Pimavanserin** was recently approved for the treatment of hallucinations and delusions associated with Parkinson disease (see Chapter 24).

Treatment Considerations. All typical antipsychotic drugs appear to be equally effective when used in equipotent doses for the treatment of schizophrenia. The highly sedating drugs are no more effective than the less-sedating drugs in calming agitated patients, and the less-sedating drugs are no more effective than the highly sedating drugs in treating withdrawn patients. Hence, the choice of drug is primarily based on the need to minimize autonomic or EPS. Several controlled trials indicate that low-dose regimens are as effective as high-dose regimens and produce fewer side effects.

The **atypical antipsychotic drugs** are an appealing choice for the treatment of schizophrenia, and they may become the drugs of choice for treating most forms of psychosis. In comparison with the typical drugs, the atypical drugs produce a lower incidence of EPS and appear to be more effective against the negative symptoms of schizophrenia. Data on the long-term effectiveness of atypical drugs in patients with chronic schizophrenia, however, have not yet been obtained.

During the first 2 weeks of treatment with an antipsychotic drug, many patients exhibit some alleviation of positive symptoms and an improvement in socialization, mood, and self-care habits. The maximal response to treatment, however, generally requires 6 weeks or longer, at which time it may be possible to reduce the dosage during maintenance therapy. Antipsychotic medication is usually continued for at least 12 months after the remission of acute psychotic symptoms. At that time, a low-dose regimen or gradual withdrawal of medication should be considered in order to reduce the probability of developing **tardive dyskinesia.** Antipsychotic drugs should be tapered slowly before discontinuation because abrupt discontinuation can cause withdrawal symptoms such as insomnia, nightmares, nausea, vomiting, diarrhea, restlessness, salivation, and sweating.

Adjunct Use of Atypical Antipsychotics in Treating Depression. There is increasing use of atypical antipsychotic agents as adjuncts to antidepressant agents in treating depression. These newer antipsychotics are used as "augmentation therapy," or adjunct medications to treat depression that hasn't responded adequately to standard antidepressant treatments. This is known as treatment-resistant depression. The FDA first approved four atypical antipsychotics as adjunct drugs for treatment-resistant depression: **aripiprazole, quetiapine, olanzapine,** and the **combination formulation of olanzapine and fluoxetine.** However, many of the newer atypical antipsychotics often include this indication or are used "off-label" for this purpose.

AFFECTIVE DISORDERS

Affective disorders are also called **mood disorders.** The two most common affective disorders are **major depressive disorder** and **bipolar disorder.** The primary drugs used in their treatment are antidepressant drugs and mood-stabilizing drugs.

Clinical Findings

Major Depressive Disorder

Major depressive disorder (unipolar depression) is characterized by depressed mood, loss of interest or pleasure in life, sleep disturbances, feelings of worthlessness, diminished ability to think or concentrate, and recurrent thoughts of suicide. Depressed patients can also be irritable or anxious.

Bipolar Disorder

Bipolar disorder (previously called **manic-depressive disorder**) is characterized by recurrent fluctuations in mood, energy, and behavior that encompass the extremes of human experience. This disorder differs from major depression in that periods of mania alternate or occur simultaneously with depressive symptoms. The clinical presentation varies widely. The manic phase is characterized by **elevated mood, inflated self-esteem** (grandiosity), increased talking (pressure of speech), racing thoughts (flight of ideas), increased social or work activity, and decreased need for sleep. Manic patients can become hostile and uncooperative. As the manic phase intensifies, some patients experience psychotic symptoms such as delusions.

Typically, the manic phase occurs just before or just after a depressive episode. In many patients, depressive and manic episodes last several weeks or months. In some patients, however, the episodes change within hours or days (rapid cycling bipolar disorder).

Biogenic Amine Hypothesis

According to the **biogenic amine hypothesis,** mood disorders result from abnormalities in serotonin, norepinephrine, or dopamine neurotransmission. Serotonergic fibers projecting from the raphe nuclei in the midbrain to limbic structures are important in regulating mood, among other

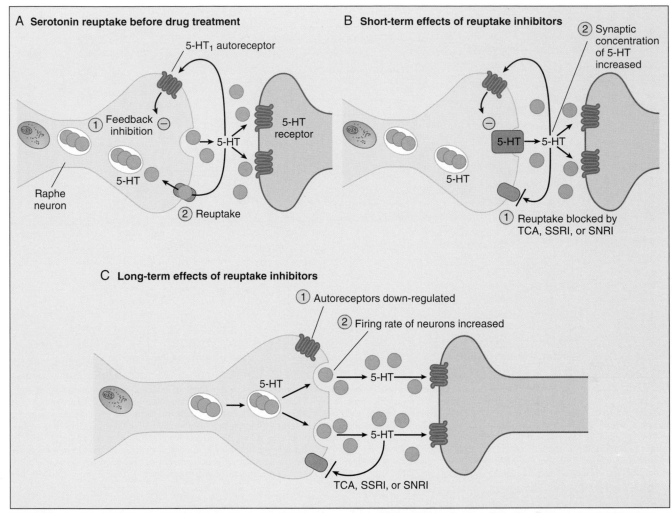

FIG. 22.2 Mechanisms of neuronal reuptake inhibitors. (A) In the absence of a reuptake inhibitor, serotonin (5-hydroxytryptamine [5-HT]) is released from raphe neurons that project to limbic structures. Serotonin activates postsynaptic and presynaptic 5-HT receptors and undergoes reuptake into the presynaptic neuron. (B) When a tricyclic antidepressant (TCA), a selective serotonin reuptake inhibitor (SSRI), or a selective serotonin and norepinephrine reuptake inhibitor (SNRI), the drug blocks the reuptake of 5-HT and increases its synaptic concentration. (C) With continued use of a TCA, an SSRI, or SNRI, increased synaptic concentrations of 5-HT cause the downregulation of presynaptic autoreceptors and an increase in the firing rate of raphe neurons.

functions. The serotonergic system is activated during behavioral arousal and increases cortical awareness of emotional reactions to environmental events. It is believed that impaired serotonin neurotransmission can decrease cortical responsiveness to emotional activation, leading to **affective dysfunction** and **depression.** Noradrenergic fibers that project from the locus ceruleus to the cerebral cortex can also play a role in depression, as can dopaminergic fibers innervating the nucleus accumbens.

Evidence also links depression with abnormal circadian rhythms and melatonin regulation. **Melatonin,** the principal mediator of biologic rhythms, is known to suppress the activity of serotonergic neurons. Investigators postulate that excess melatonin production contributes to the development of depression. This hypothesis is particularly relevant to **seasonal affective disorder,** which usually occurs during the winter months, when daylight is reduced, and melatonin levels are increased. Abnormalities in melatonin and serotonin metabolism can also contribute to the sleep disturbances seen in patients with affective disorders.

The biogenic amine hypothesis is supported by the fact that all antidepressant drugs act to **increase serotonin,** **norepinephrine,** and/or **dopamine neurotransmission** in the brain. Most antidepressant drugs increase the synaptic concentration of serotonin, and this leads to down-regulation of presynaptic autoreceptors. Investigators believe that the downregulation, in turn, increases the firing rate of serotonergic neurons and thereby produces the delayed therapeutic effect of antidepressant drugs. These mechanisms are depicted in Fig. 22.2.

Recent data that antidepressant medications produce an increase in the rate of appearance of new neurons, called **neurogenesis,** in the brain of nonhuman mammals suggest a novel mechanism of antidepressant drug action. Studies have yet to show the correlation between the increased appearance of brain neurons and the clinical effectiveness of antidepressants, but this interesting finding provides another view into the possible causes of depression and its treatment.

ANTIDEPRESSANT DRUGS

Depression can be treated with **tricyclic antidepressants (TCAs), selective serotonin reuptake inhibitors (SSRIs), serotonin and norepinephrine reuptake inhibitors (SNRIs),**

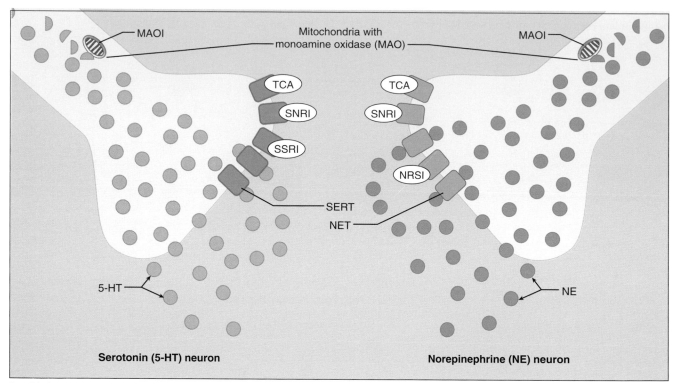

FIG. 22.3 Mechanisms of action for various antidepressant drugs. Two types of neurons are shown, with a serotonergic neuron terminal on the left and a noradrenergic neuron terminal on the right. The serotonin transporter protein (SERT) and the norepinephrine transporter protein (NET) are shown. The tricyclic antidepressants (TCAs) block the reuptake of both serotonin and norepinephrine at the transporter proteins, as shown, but also are nonspecific and promiscuous at other receptor sites not shown (see text). The serotonin and norepinephrine reuptake inhibitors (SNRIs) also block both serotonin and norepinephrine reuptake but do not additionally block a number of other receptors like TCAs. The selective serotonin reuptake inhibitors (SSRIs) inhibit only serotonin reuptake on 5-HT terminals. Both serotonin and norepinephrine are metabolized by monoamine oxidase enzymes in mitochondria. Monoamine oxidase inhibitors (MAOIs) irreversibly to monoamine oxidase and inhibit the degradation of norepinephrine and serotonin (as well as dopamine). Norepinephrine-selective reuptake inhibitors (NSRIs) are not yet developed for the treatment of depression, although some stimulant drugs like atomoxetine are known as NSRIs.

and other antidepressants that have different structures and act by various mechanisms of action. If patients fail to respond to these drugs, **monoamine oxidase inhibitors (MAOIs)** can be used. Fig. 22.3 portrays the molecular mechanisms of action for various antidepressants.

Because depressed patients might attempt suicide, the safety of an antidepressant in overdose is an important consideration when selecting a drug for a particular patient. In addition, all antidepressant medications now contain **boxed warnings** highlighting the risk of increased **suicidal thoughts** and **behavior** in children, adolescents, and adults.

Indications

Antidepressants have been used to treat all forms of **depression** and to treat several other conditions. The antidepressants are also effective in the treatment of certain **anxiety disorders,** such as panic disorder, phobic disorders, and obsessive-compulsive disorder. **Clomipramine** is particularly effective in treating patients with obsessive-compulsive behavior. Some antidepressants are beneficial in the management of certain **sleep disorders,** including somnambulism, night terrors, and enuresis. Antidepressants repress excessive rapid eye movement (REM) sleep and dreaming, which are conditions that contribute to somnambulism and night terrors. In patients with enuresis, antidepressants appear to increase the awareness of the need to urinate and thereby facilitate waking up for this purpose. Other antidepressants also have a role in the treatment of **chronic pain**

syndromes because of their mood-elevating effect and analgesic activity.

The newer SSRIs and SNRIs are used to treat **depression, eating disorders** (e.g., bulimia nervosa and anorexia nervosa), and **anxiety disorders** (e.g., panic disorder, phobic disorders, and obsessive-compulsive disorder). SSRIs and SNRIs may also be effective in the management of other conditions (e.g., **fibromyalgia, autism,** and **premenstrual dysphoric disorder**).

Tricyclic Antidepressants

TCAs include **amitriptyline, imipramine, clomipramine, desipramine,** and **nortriptyline.** These agents are highly effective in the treatment of depression and several other disorders, but they are associated with a high incidence of adverse effects. They also cause severe toxicity when taken in excessive doses, a serious clinical problem when a depressed patient attempts suicide by overdosing on their medication.

Pharmacokinetics

TCAs are incompletely absorbed after oral administration and are extensively metabolized to active and inactive metabolites in the liver. The **tertiary amine** TCAs are deaminated to pharmacologically active **secondary amine** TCAs, and several of these metabolites are available as drugs. For example, **amitriptyline** is converted to **nortriptyline,** and imipramine is metabolized to **desipramine.** The type of amine group determines the selectivity of the pharmacologic action. TCAs and their active metabolites have relatively long half-lives, ranging from 18 to 70 hours.

Mechanism of Action

All TCAs block the neuronal reuptake of norepinephrine and serotonin. They do so by blockade of the reuptake transporter proteins, called the *norepinephrine transporter* [NET] and *serotonin transporter* [SERT], but they do so to differing degrees. The blockade occurs as soon as drug administration begins and causes an immediate increase in the synaptic concentration of serotonin and norepinephrine. The blockade is also believed to trigger a series of adaptive changes in norepinephrine and serotonin neurotransmission.

Pharmacologic Effects

TCAs produce an antidepressant effect that becomes apparent about 2 to 4 weeks after drug therapy is started. Over time, the increased synaptic concentration of serotonin can cause down-regulation of presynaptic autoreceptors and thereby increase the firing rate of serotonergic neurons. The short-term and long-term effects of TCAs and other reuptake inhibitors on serotonin neurotransmission are illustrated in Fig. 22.2.

Adverse Effects

As with many antipsychotic drugs, TCAs produce autonomic side effects by blocking **muscarinic and α-adrenoceptors.** Some of TCAs also produce marked sedation (Table 22.4). In fact, TCAs are often administered at bedtime when their sedative effects can have the added benefit of promoting sleep. TCAs lower the seizure threshold and can induce seizures at therapeutic as well as toxic serum concentrations.

Taking an overdose of a TCA can cause life-threatening **cardiac dysrhythmia,** which frequently manifests as a wide QRS complex tachycardia; marked autonomic effects, including hypotension and sinus tachycardia; excessive sedation; and seizures.

Treatment of Adverse Effects

The type of arrhythmia that occurs with an overdose can be treated by the intravenous administration of **sodium bicarbonate.** Sodium bicarbonate increases the ratio of nonionized TCA to ionized TCA and thereby decreases the binding of the TCA to the sodium channel in cardiac membranes.

Specific Drugs

Nortriptyline and **desipramine** are secondary amines formed by the demethylation of amitriptyline and imipramine, respectively. **Secondary amines block norepinephrine uptake more than they block serotonin reuptake,** and this is especially true of desipramine.

Amitriptyline, clomipramine, and **imipramine** are tertiary amines. They **block serotonin reuptake to a greater extent than do secondary amines.** They also produce more sedation and autonomic side effects than do secondary amines.

Studies have shown that all TCAs are equally effective in relieving depression, although some patients respond better to one drug than to another. The choice of a TCA is based primarily on the relative incidence of adverse effects produced by the different drugs. A drug that causes a higher degree of sedation may be chosen for highly agitated or anxious patients with depression, whereas a drug that causes a lower degree of sedation may be preferred for patients who are more apathetic or withdrawn.

A generic formulation of **amitriptyline** and **perphenazine** (a typical antipsychotic) is available for patients with **depression and moderate to severe agitation and/or anxiety.** With this formulation, patients are sedated by both agents, and depression is also treated with amitriptyline. Additionally, schizophrenic patients with associated depressive symptoms should be considered candidates for pharmacotherapy with perphenazine and amitriptyline tablets.

Selective Serotonin Reuptake Inhibitors

SSRIs are a class of antidepressants that are named by their selective mechanism of action. Commonly recognized SSRIs include **fluoxetine** (Prozac), **citalopram** (Celexa), and **sertraline** (Zoloft). Other SSRIs are **escitalopram, fluvoxamine, paroxetine,** and **vortioxetine.** SSRIs have become the most widely used drugs for the treatment of depression and certain anxiety disorders, such as panic disorder and obsessive-compulsive disorder. They are as effective as TCAs but cause fewer autonomic side effects and less sedation. They are also much safer than TCAs with regard to overdose in that SSRIs seldom cause cardiac arrhythmia and are less likely to induce seizures.

Pharmacokinetics

SSRIs are well absorbed from the gut after oral administration and are extensively metabolized by cytochrome P450 isozymes. **Fluoxetine,** which has a **longer half-life** than the other drugs in this class, is converted to an **active metabolite** that has an even longer half-life. The metabolites of other SSRIs have little or no pharmacologic activity.

Mechanism of Action and Pharmacologic Effects

SSRIs selectively block the neuronal reuptake of serotonin and have much less effect on the reuptake of norepinephrine. Their efficacy in the treatment of depression supports the hypothesis that **serotonin dysfunction** plays a significant role in the pathophysiology of depression. The short-term and long-term effects of serotonin reuptake inhibition are illustrated in Fig. 22.2.

Adverse Effects

SSRIs produce fewer sedative, autonomic, and cardiovascular side effects than TCAs. Unlike TCAs, SSRIs are usually administered in the morning because they tend to increase alertness in patients. Their most common adverse effects are nervousness, dizziness, and insomnia. They occasionally cause **male sexual dysfunction** in the forms of priapism and impotence. Many of the side effects of SSRIs subside with continued use. SSRIs should be used with caution in patients with seizure disorders, hepatic disorders, diabetes, or bipolar disorder.

Specific Drugs

Fluoxetine. Fluoxetine (Prozac) is one of the most popular drugs for the treatment of depression and the first drug approved for the treatment of **bulimia nervosa;** it is also effective in the management of **anorexia nervosa** and **obsessive-compulsive disorder.** The drug is well absorbed

TABLE 22.4 Adverse Effects of Selected Antidepressant Drugs[a]

DRUG	SEDATION	ANTICHOLINERGIC EFFECTS	ORTHOSTATIC HYPOTENSION	CARDIAC CONDUCTION DISTURBANCES
Tricyclic Antidepressants (TCAs)				
Amitriptyline	++++	++++	+++	+++
Clomipramine	++++	++++	++	+++
Desipramine	++	++	++	++
Imipramine	+++	+++	+++	+++
Nortriptyline	++	++	++	++
Selective Serotonin Reuptake Inhibitors (SSRIs)				
Fluoxetine	0	0	0	0
Fluvoxamine	+	0	0	0
Paroxetine	+	+	0	0
Sertraline	0	0	0	0
Serotonin and Norepinephrine Reuptake Inhibitor (SNRI)				
Venlafaxine	+	+	0	+
Monoamine Oxidase Inhibitors (MAOIs)				
Phenelzine	++	++	++	+
Tranylcypromine	+	++	++	+
Other Antidepressant Drugs				
Bupropion	+	+	0	+
Mirtazapine	+	+	++	+
Trazodone	++++	0	+++	+

[a]Ratings range from none (0) to high (++++).

orally and is converted to an active metabolite, **norfluoxetine.** The parent compound has a half-life of 2.5 days, but its active metabolite has a half-life of about 8 days. This long duration of action can be a disadvantage if severe adverse effects occur. It is also available in a once-a-week dosage form called PROZAC WEEKLY.

Fluoxetine causes more drug interactions than other SSRIs. It can impair the regulation of blood glucose levels in diabetic patients. It can also cause a syndrome of **inappropriate antidiuretic hormone secretion,** characterized by persistent hyponatremia and elevated urine osmolality.

Citalopram and Escitalopram. Citalopram has a chemical structure unrelated to that of other SSRIs, TCAs, or other available antidepressant agents. It is a racemic mixture (contains both R and S enantiomers of the drug molecule) and highly selective for serotonin reuptake transporters in preclinical models, owing to the potential to **increase the cardiac QT interval** and the risk of *torsade de pointes*, citalopram was recently restricted to doses no greater than 40 mg/day.

Escitalopram is the pure S-enantiomer (single isomer) of the racemic citalopram drug. Escitalopram (the S-form) is at least 100 times more potent than the R-enantiomer with respect to inhibition of 5-HT reuptake.

Paroxetine and Sertraline. Paroxetine and sertraline have half-lives of 21 and 26 hours, respectively. Paroxetine has a high bioavailability, whereas sertraline undergoes extensive first-pass elimination. Sertraline has relatively little effect on P450 isozymes and causes fewer drug interactions than fluoxetine. Sertraline may be preferred in **elderly**

patients because its elimination is not affected substantially by aging. Paroxetine is somewhat more sedating than either fluoxetine or sertraline. **Low-dose paroxetine** (BRISDELLE) was recently approved for the treatment of vasomotor symptoms ("hot flashes" and night sweats) in perimenopausal women (see Chapter 34).

Fluvoxamine. Fluvoxamine is approved for the treatment of **obsessive-compulsive disorder** but has also been used to treat **depression** and **panic disorder.** Fluvoxamine has a half-life of about 15 hours and can be associated with sedative effects.

Vortioxetine. Vortioxetine is the newest SSRI approved for the treatment of **major depressive disorder (MDD) in adults.** It is a potent, selective inhibitor of serotonin reuptake and has an extremely long elimination half-life of about 66 hours.

Serotonin and Norepinephrine Reuptake Inhibitors

As opposed to older TCA agents that also block both serotonin and norepinephrine reuptake but also interact with many other receptor types to produce adverse effects, new drugs that are selective for both of the reuptake transporters, but not other receptors, are now available. Preclinical studies show that **duloxetine** (CYMBALTA) is a potent and selective inhibitor of **both** neuronal serotonin and norepinephrine reuptake. It is indicated for **major depressive disorder, diabetic peripheral neuropathic pain,** and **generalized anxiety disorder.** Duloxetine was the first approved agent for these disorders in the class of **SNRIs.** Venlafaxine and **desvenlafaxine** are also classified as SNRIs and share the properties and indications of duloxetine. Duloxetine is also indicated for **fibromyalgia.** A newer SNRI, **milnacipran,** is indicated only for the management of pain in patients with **fibromyalgia** (see Chapter 23). Interestingly, the active stereoisomer of milnacipran, called **levomilnacipran,** was recently approved for the treatment of major depression.

Duloxetine and Venlafaxine

Duloxetine and **venlafaxine** are structurally unique antidepressants that strongly inhibit the reuptake of both norepinephrine and serotonin (see Fig. 22.2). Both have a side effect profile similar to that of SSRIs. These agents do not antagonize muscarinic, adrenergic, or histamine receptors and produce few autonomic, sedative, or cardiovascular side effects.

Desvenlafaxine is the major active metabolite of venlafaxine and is approved for the treatment of major depression. It shares the pharmacologic mechanism of action and side effect profile of its parent drug and the other SNRI agents.

Monoamine Oxidase Inhibitors

Because the **MAOIs** have many potentially serious interactions with other drugs and with food, they are not considered drugs of choice in the treatment of depression. They are generally used as alternative therapy when patients have failed to respond adequately to other drugs.

Pharmacokinetics

The first-generation MAOIs, **phenelzine, isocarboxazid,** and **tranylcypromine,** are adequately absorbed from the gut and have relatively short half-lives. They **irreversibly** bind to and inhibit monoamine oxidase, however, and their pharmacologic effects persist for many hours after their serum levels have declined. Phenelzine and tranylcypromine increase serotonin levels more than they do norepinephrine levels in the brain, and their antidepressant effects are probably caused by the downregulation of presynaptic autoreceptors and the subsequent increased firing of serotonergic neurons. As with other antidepressants, the clinical effects of **MAOIs are delayed** for **several weeks** after therapy begins.

Mechanism of Action

The MAOIs bind **irreversibly** to an enzyme, **monoamine oxidase (MAO),** responsible for the degradation of the biogenic amine neurotransmitters, norepinephrine, dopamine, and serotonin. The binding of MAOI prevents the substrate from reaching the active site on the enzyme.

The MAOIs are classified according to their selectivity for the two main types of MAO. MAO-A preferentially oxidizes serotonin but will also metabolize norepinephrine and dopamine. MAO-B preferentially metabolizes dopamine. The inhibition of MAO-A is believed to be responsible for the antidepressant effects of most of the MAOIs, except those with selectivity for MAO-B.

Pharmacologic Effects

MAOIs increase the concentration of dopamine, norepinephrine, and serotonin in storage sites throughout the nervous system. In theory, this increased concentration of monoamines in the brain is the basis for the antidepressant activity of MAOIs.

Adverse Effects

The major adverse effect reported with MAOIs is the occurrence of a **hypertensive crisis,** which is sometimes fatal. Such crises are characterized by some or all of the following symptoms: an occipital headache that may radiate frontally, palpitation, neck stiffness or soreness, nausea or vomiting, sweating, and photophobia. Hypertensive crisis can occur with an MAOI alone or, more commonly, after the administration of sympathomimetic amines or eating food containing **tyramine** (see the discussion of interactions).

Specific Drugs

The first-generation MAOIs for treating depression include **Phenelzine, isocarboxazid,** and **tranylcypromine,** which are irreversible inhibitors of both MAO-A and MAO-B. The second-generation MAOIs include **moclobemide** and are reversible inhibitors of MAO-A (RIMAs). RIMAs are used in many countries to treat depression but are not yet available in the United States. **Selegiline** represents a third type of MAOI, which selectively inhibits MAO-B and is also used in the treatment of Parkinson disease (see Chapter 24). **Selegiline** was recently approved for the treatment of depression in a transdermal patch formulation called EMSAM.

Atypical Antidepressant Drugs

Several other drugs with diverse mechanisms of action are available for the treatment of depression.

Bupropion

The mechanism of action of bupropion is not well understood. It is a relatively weak inhibitor of the neuronal reuptake of dopamine, norepinephrine, and serotonin (at the dopamine transporter [DAT], NET, and SERT). It also acts as a noncompetitive antagonist at nicotinic cholinergic receptors. **Bupropion** produces few anticholinergic side effects, causes very little sedation, and rarely produces cardiovascular effects or sexual dysfunction. It can cause agitation, insomnia, nausea, and weight loss. A new formulation of **bupropion hydrobromide** (APLENZIN) has once-a-day administration. Another formulation of bupropion (ZYBAN) was developed as an adjunct therapy for patients who are attempting to quit smoking cigarettes (see Chapter 25).

Bupropion was recently approved in a **combination pill** with the opioid antagonist, **naltrexone,** called CONTRAVE. It is **indicated for inducing weight loss** in obese patients and as an adjunct to a reduced-calorie diet and increased physical activity. The exact mechanism of action of this bupropion and naltrexone combination is unknown, but preclinical studies suggest an action of both agents on appetite regulation in the hypothalamus and the reward pathways in the mesolimbic dopamine projections.

Trazodone

Trazodone selectively **inhibits the neuronal reuptake of serotonin** and also acts as an **antagonist at the 5-HT$_{2A}$ receptor.** It causes considerable sedation and orthostatic hypotension, but it does not produce anticholinergic side effects and has minimal effects on cardiac conduction.

Mirtazapine

Mirtazapine is a structurally different (tetracyclic) antidepressant than TCAs and has both **antidepressant** and **antianxiety** effects. Mirtazapine blocks presynaptic α_2-adrenergic **autoreceptors** and **heteroreceptors** and thereby increases the neuronal release of norepinephrine and serotonin, respectively. It increases central norepinephrine concentrations to a greater degree than do TCAs, and it is also a potent antagonist of 5-HT$_2$ and 5-HT$_3$ receptors. Mirtazapine is better tolerated and causes fewer adverse reactions than TCAs. It can significantly elevate hepatic enzyme levels, however, and it has been associated with a few cases of **agranulocytosis.**

Vilazodone

The newest antidepressant, **vilazodone,** selectively inhibits the neuronal reuptake of serotonin, like a traditional SSRI, but is also a **partial agonist of the 5-HT$_{1A}$ receptor.** Its mechanism of action is not entirely understood but is thought to be related to its enhancement of serotonergic activity in the CNS. Partial agonism of the 5-HT$_{1A}$ receptor is a relatively novel mechanism of action and is also shared by the anxiolytic **buspirone** (see Chapter 19) and the atypical antipsychotic **aripiprazole** (see earlier).

Esketamine and Brexanolone

Esketamine, the S-enantiomer of racemic **ketamine,** is a **parenteral general anesthetic** (see Chapter 21). **Esketamine is a non-competitive antagonist** of the N-methyl-D-aspartate (NMDA) receptor, a type of **glutamate receptor.** The mechanism by which esketamine exerts its antidepressant effect is unknown, but antagonism of presynaptic NMDA receptors increases glutamate release. It is hypothesized that increased glutamate release activates AMPA glutamate receptors. AMPA receptor activation **increases neurotrophic factors** supporting both fast-acting and long-term antidepressant effects. The major metabolite of esketamine (noresketamine) also demonstrates activity at the same receptor but with less affinity.

Brexanolone is a unique neurosteroid drug and the **first FDA-approved treatment** for **postpartum depression.** It is a **positive allosteric modulator of GABAA receptors,** similar to the action of benzodiazepines (see Chapter 34).

Adverse Interactions of Antidepressant Drugs

The serum levels of TCAs are elevated by concurrent administration of antipsychotic drugs, calcium channel blockers, cimetidine, and SSRIs, which compete with TCA for metabolic enzymes in the liver. Barbiturates, carbamazepine, and phenytoin **decrease the serum levels** of TCAs because of the up-regulation of hepatic metabolic enzymes. As with SSRIs (see later), TCAs should not be used with an MAOI.

Because of their ability to inhibit cytochrome P450 isozymes, SSRIs have significant interactions with a variety of drugs. Among SSRIs, **fluoxetine** has the greatest effect on the **CYP2D isozyme,** and **sertraline** has the least effect. Inhibition of CYP2D can increase the serum levels of antipsychotic drugs, TCAs, and dextromethorphan. Inhibition by SSRIs of CYP2C and CYP3A can increase serum levels of alprazolam, diazepam, carbamazepine, phenytoin, and other drugs. SSRIs can also increase the **hypoprothrombinemic** effect of warfarin.

SSRIs should not be used concurrently with MAOIs because both types of drugs increase the serotonin levels in the brain, and their concurrent use can precipitate **serotonin syndrome.** This syndrome is characterized by agitation, restlessness, confusion, insomnia, seizures, severe hypertension, and gastrointestinal symptoms. At least 2 weeks should elapse between the discontinuation of treatment with either an MAOI or an SSRI and the start of treatment with the other drug. The exception is that 5 weeks must elapse between the discontinuation of fluoxetine and the administration of an MAOI. In addition, **SSRIs** should not be taken concurrently with **triptan** agents used to treat migraine (see Chapter 29). The FDA recently strengthened warnings that the concurrent use of these drugs increases the risk of triggering **serotonin syndrome.**

MAOIs interact with SSRIs, TCAs, and other antidepressant drugs and have the potential to cause severe toxicity when administered with these drugs. Concurrent administration of MAOIs and TCAs or other antidepressants requires dosage reduction and careful monitoring.

MAOIs can cause severe hypertension when administered with sympathomimetic amines or with foods containing **tyramines.** These foods include many types of cheese (especially aged cheeses), beer and some wines (e.g., Chianti), some meats and fish (e.g., canned meat, liver, sardines, and herring), some fruits and vegetables (especially raisins, broad beans, avocados, and canned figs), and some products when consumed in large quantities (chocolate and coffee). The **selegiline patch (Emsam)** at its lowest strength (6 mg) can be used without these dietary restrictions.

Treatment Considerations

Depression is one of the most common mental illnesses. Because it is underdiagnosed, it often goes untreated. The primary treatment for patients with depression is drug therapy, but psychotherapy enhances the response to pharmacologic treatment and increases patient compliance with medication. **Electroconvulsive therapy** is sometimes used as an alternative when antidepressants have been ineffective or are not tolerated. More than 80% of patients respond to treatment with drugs, psychotherapy, electroconvulsive therapy, or a combination of these modalities.

The initial drug used in the treatment of depression is usually either a TCA or an SSRI, depending on clinician preference. A growing body of evidence indicates that SSRIs are better tolerated by patients, produce fewer adverse effects, and are safer in overdose than are TCAs. The disadvantages of SSRIs include their higher cost and the increased tendency of some SSRIs to cause drug interactions. **Sertraline** causes fewer drug interactions than do other SSRIs and may be preferred in the treatment of patients who are taking other drugs that can interact with SSRIs.

If TCAs or SSRIs are not effective or well tolerated, the clinician has a growing choice of SNRIs and atypical antidepressants (e.g., **bupropion, mirtazapine, trazodone,** and **vilazodone**). This class of atypical antidepressants is attractive because of their **low incidence of sedation, autonomic side effects,** and **cardiac toxicity** (see Table 22.4). In comparison with other antidepressants, **vilazodone** has demonstrated a lower incidence of activating side effects, such as nervousness, agitation, and insomnia, and it does not cause sexual dysfunction.

It usually takes 2 to 4 weeks for antidepressants to elevate the mood of depressed patients, and some patients do not respond until after 6 weeks or longer. Some authorities believe that many cases of treatment-resistant depression are caused by inadequate drug dosage, inadequate duration of therapy, or patient noncompliance. Moreover, studies indicate that many patients who failed to respond to treatment in the past will respond to adequate doses of SSRIs, SNRIs, or other new antidepressants.

To prevent relapse, antidepressants are usually continued for 4 to 9 months after remission of depressive symptoms.

MOOD-STABILIZING DRUGS

Indications
Mood-stabilizing drugs act to normalize the swings of affect in **bipolar disorder.** Although the element lithium is the standard agent in this class, a number of other agents are being tested and used for this indication. **Lithium** has been called a mood stabilizer because it reduces both manic and depressive symptoms and thereby tends to normalize the mood in patients with bipolar disorder. Lithium, like other mood stabilizers, however, has greater activity against manic symptoms than it does against depression, and it is primarily used to treat or prevent the **manic phase of bipolar disorder.**

Lithium
Lithium, the lightest of the alkali metal elements, has a single valence electron which it readily loses to form a cation (Li⁺). It was discovered to have a calming effect in patients during the early use of lithium solutions to dissolve urate crystal deposits in patients with gout.

Pharmacokinetics
Lithium, which is administered orally in the form of lithium carbonate or lithium citrate, is available in immediate-release and sustained-release preparations. About 95% to 100% of the administered dose is absorbed from the gut. Lithium is widely distributed throughout the body, with the highest concentrations found in the thyroid gland, bone, and some areas of the brain. The drug is **not metabolized.** It has a half-life of about 24 hours and is excreted in the urine. Lithium is extensively reabsorbed from the renal tubules, and the renal clearance of lithium is about 20% of the glomerular filtration rate. Lithium clearance increases during pregnancy. Sodium competes with lithium for renal tubular reabsorption and thereby can increase the excretion of lithium.

Mechanism of Action
The mechanisms by which lithium produces its mood-stabilizing effects are not well understood. The drug appears to act by suppressing the formation of second messengers involved in neurotransmitter signal transduction, but the relationship between this action and the drug's clinical effect is unclear. Lithium **reduces the formation of inositol triphosphate (IP₃)** by inhibiting two enzymes in the inositol phosphate pathway. These enzymes participate in the regeneration of inositol and the inositol phosphate precursors to IP₃. Lithium also inhibits the uptake of inositol into the cell. By reducing IP₃ formation, lithium reduces the neuronal response to serotonin and norepinephrine, whose effects are partly mediated by IP₃ (see Table 18.1). The mechanisms of action of lithium and other mood-stabilizing agents on the inositol phosphate signaling pathway are shown in Fig. 22.4.

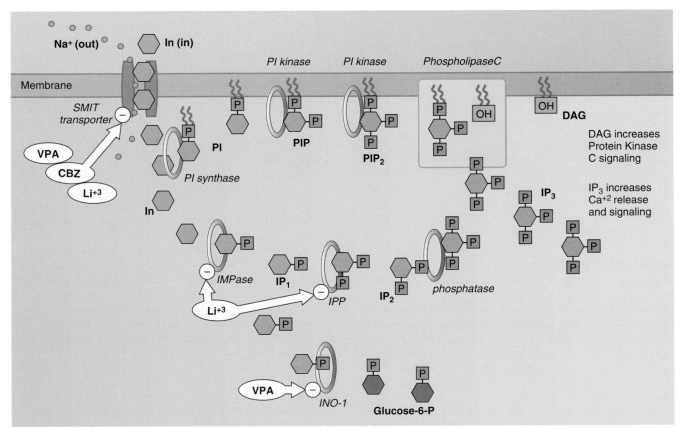

FIG. 22.4 Mechanisms of action of mood-stabilizing agents on the inositol phosphate signaling pathway. Lithium is the standard agent for treating the manic phase of bipolar disorder, but valproic acid (VPA), carbamazepine (CBZ), and others are also used. Neurotransmitter action at GPCRs coupled to Gq activates the IP₃ signaling pathway. Lithium inhibits both the IPP and the IMPase enzymes, which decreases inositol formation. Additionally, lithium, CBZ, and VPA inhibit the uptake of inositol into the cell. VPA has the additional action of inhibiting inositol formation from IP₁ by blocking the enzyme (Ino-1) that converts glucose-6-P into IP₁.

Pharmacologic Effects

Lithium produces a calming effect in manic patients, but the maximal response to lithium often requires several days or weeks of treatment. For this reason, other drugs may need to be used during the early phase of treatment while awaiting the full response to lithium (see later). The serum concentration of lithium should be **monitored** after initiating therapy and at periodic intervals thereafter. Although the concentration should be 0.6 to 1.2 mEq/L, a concentration of 0.8 to 1.0 mEq/L is considered optimal for most patients. Monitoring the concentration serves to verify the adequacy of dosage and may warn of potential toxicity.

Adverse Effects

Lithium has a relatively **low margin of safety** (therapeutic index). Elevated lithium levels can cause neurotoxicity and cardiac toxicity leading to dysrhythmia. Nausea with vomiting can be one of the earliest signs of lithium overdose. It is important for the clinician and patient to distinguish the signs of lithium toxicity from the adverse effects of lithium that often occur with therapeutic serum levels.

Lithium is fairly well tolerated by most patients, but it produces a number of unpleasant side effects that decrease patient compliance. Common side effects include **drowsiness, weight gain,** fine **hand tremor,** and **polyuria.** The hand tremor can usually be controlled by the administration of a *beta* (β)-adrenoceptor antagonist. Lithium causes polyuria because it interferes with the action of antidiuretic hormone and thereby inhibits the kidney's ability to concentrate the urine. In some patients, lithium causes **hypothyroidism** by blocking thyroid hormone synthesis and release.

Interactions

Nonsteroidal anti-inflammatory drugs (NSAIDs) and diuretics **decrease lithium clearance** by about 25% and increase lithium levels. Other drug interactions increase lithium neurotoxicity.

Other Mood-Stabilizing Drugs

Although lithium is the primary drug used to treat and prevent manic symptoms in bipolar disorder, other drugs have been found to have equal or greater efficacy and may be better tolerated by some patients. These include **carbamazepine** and **valproate (valproic acid),** antiepileptic drugs whose pharmacologic properties are described in Chapter 20.

Treatment Considerations

Treatment of bipolar disorder must be individualized on the basis of symptoms, response to drug therapy and other treatment modalities, and the minimization of adverse effects. Drug treatment with **lithium** is often the cornerstone of therapy because lithium can abort an acute manic episode, can prevent future manic episodes, and also appears to exert a mild antidepressive effect. Because of the dynamic nature of the disorder, however, therapy must be frequently reevaluated and modified.

Lithium usually controls an acute manic episode within 1 or 2 weeks after initiation of therapy. Other drugs may be required to control acute symptoms while awaiting the full effect of lithium to develop. **Benzodiazepines** can relieve manic symptoms and promote sleep. An antipsychotic drug may be required to suppress delusions and other psychotic symptoms accompanying mania. **Risperidone, olanzapine, aripiprazole,** and **asenapine** are indicated for the treatment of patients with bipolar disorder and cause fewer adverse effects than do typical antipsychotic drugs (e.g., haloperidol).

Lithium is usually continued for 9 to 12 months after the initial manic episode, and then its use can be slowly tapered, with continued monitoring of symptoms. Many patients experience **hypomanic symptoms** for several days or longer before developing a full manic episode, and lithium therapy can be reinstituted in these patients in an attempt to abort a full manic episode. Long-term prophylactic therapy can be given to patients who have had two or three episodes and to those whose symptoms develop rapidly. Long-term patient compliance with lithium, however, is often poor.

Depression that persists after lithium therapy is instituted may respond to **antidepressant drugs.** The use of antidepressants in patients who have bipolar disorder and are not taking lithium or another mood-stabilizing drug will evoke a manic response **(switch phenomenon)** in many patients.

This growing list of alternatives or adjuncts to lithium for bipolar disorder includes several antiepileptic drugs. **Carbamazepine** exhibits antimanic, antidepressant, and prophylactic effects that are equivalent to those of lithium, and it causes fewer adverse effects in many patients. Moreover, about 60% of manic patients who do not respond to lithium will respond to carbamazepine within the first several days of treatment. Evidence also suggests that lithium and carbamazepine can be synergistic in their antimanic activity in patients with refractory bipolar disorder. **Valproate** is another drug that is approved for the treatment of mania in bipolar disorder. It appears to be especially useful in patients with rapid cycling of manic and depressive episodes and in patients with coexisting substance abuse. Other antiepileptic drugs have demonstrated antimanic activity in clinical studies and may be approved for treating bipolar disorder in the future.

CENTRAL NERVOUS SYSTEM STIMULANTS
Specific Drugs

Amphetamine is the prototypical CNS stimulant, classified as an indirect-acting adrenergic agonist (see Chapter 8). It increases the release of norepinephrine and dopamine from nerve terminals; it enters via the reuptake transporter, reverses the transport mechanism, and inhibits further reuptake of catecholamines. It is available as a **mixture of amphetamine salts** in a formulation called ADDERALL. Other amphetamine derivatives include **dextroamphetamine** (DEXEDRINE), the active isomer of the racemic mixture of amphetamine; **methamphetamine,** the same agent infamous for drug abuse and easy illicit manufacture; and **lisdexamfetamine,** a recently approved prodrug that is converted to dextroamphetamine after absorption.

Methylphenidate (RITALIN), **modafinil** (PROVIGIL), and **armodafinil** (NUVIGIL), the active isomer of modafinil, are also sympathomimetic agents and increase the levels of catecholamines in central and peripheral synapses as amphetamines do but appear primarily to inhibit dopamine reuptake. These stimulants usually cause less irritability, anxiety, and anorexia than does amphetamine. **Atomoxetine** (STRATTERA) is a nonamphetamine drug that has some selectivity as a norepinephrine reuptake inhibitor.

Once-a-day formulations are available for the **amphetamine mixture** (ADDERALL XR), methylphenidate (RITALIN LA, RITALIN-SR, CONCERTA), and dextroamphetamine (DEXEDRINE SPANSULE). **Methylphenidate** is also available in a **transdermal patch** formulation (DAYTRANA).

Indications

ADHD is a neurobehavioral disorder that affects about 5% of children. It is noted by the inability to exercise age-appropriate inhibition of behavior. There are several diagnostic types of ADHD: a predominantly inattentive subtype, a predominantly hyperactive-impulsive subtype, and a combined subtype. ADHD is usually diagnosed and treated in childhood, although there is increasing recognition that the condition can continue into the adult years. It is estimated that more than 2.5 million children in the United States are treated with one of the following stimulants for ADHD on a daily basis. Treatment options include **amphetamine mixture, methylphenidate, dextroamphetamine, methamphetamine,** and **lisdexamfetamine. Atomoxetine** is a unique norepinephrine reuptake inhibitor approved for the treatment of ADHD. **Modafinil** has undergone large, multicenter clinical trials for safety and effectiveness in children; however, as of this writing, it is not approved for the treatment of ADHD. Nevertheless, modafinil appears to be used widely as an off-label drug for ADHD. Two older agents were recently approved for the treatment of ADHD and given new brand names for this indication: **guanfacine extended-release tablets** (INTUNIV) and **clonidine** (KAPVAY). They are both α_2-adrenoceptor agonists used mainly as antihypertensive agents (see Chapter 10).

Narcolepsy is a sleep disorder characterized by excessive daytime sleepiness, even after sufficient nighttime sleep. Other symptoms include cataplexy, sleep paralysis, hypnagogic hallucinations, and automatic behavior; these are often triggered by sudden emotional reactions, such as anger, surprise, or fear, and may last from seconds to minutes. **Amphetamine mixture, dextroamphetamine, methylphenidate, modafinil,** and **armodafinil** are indicated for the treatment of **narcolepsy,** as well as **obstructive sleep apnea/hypopnea syndrome** and **shift work sleep disorder.**

Obesity is commonly defined as having a body weight greater than 20% over one's ideal body weight, but more strict definitions are based on a body mass index greater than 30. In any event, there is no doubt that obesity is a major health concern in developed countries, and **amphetamines** were the first agents available for the treatment of this growing disorder. **Methamphetamine** is still indicated for short-term use in treating exogenous obesity. **Phentermine** is an amphetamine derivative used as an **appetite suppressant (anorectic)** in the treatment of obesity. It acts by stimulating the satiety center in the hypothalamus through sympathomimetic mechanisms. In comparison with amphetamine, phentermine produces less CNS stimulation and has a **lower dependence liability.** Tolerance often develops to the anorectic effects of these drugs after a few weeks to a few months of use. Phentermine is also formulated with the antiseizure agent **topiramate** in an extended-release product (QSYMIA) for the treatment of obesity. **Sibutramine** (MERIDIA) was also widely used as an anorectic but was **recently withdrawn** from the market owing to studies showing a link to increased cardiovascular risk and fatalities.

Adverse Effects

All of the previously described CNS stimulants carry **risks of cardiovascular incidents** ranging from high blood pressure to myocardial infarction. Recent ongoing studies suggest an increased risk of sudden death in children and adolescents being treated for ADHD with stimulants. In young children, their use is also associated with **decreases in growth and weight gain.** They are all controlled substances and, with the exception of **atomoxetine** and other newer drugs to treat ADHD, have a great potential for **drug abuse** (see Chapter 25).

SUMMARY OF IMPORTANT POINTS

- Schizophrenia can result from abnormal function of the dopaminergic pathways in the brain. According to the dopamine hypothesis, this abnormality leads to dysfunctional dopamine neurotransmission in the prefrontal lobe cortex.
- Delusions, hallucinations, and other positive symptoms of schizophrenia can result from excessive dopamine neurotransmission in mesolimbic pathways. Apathy, withdrawal, lack of motivation and pleasure, and other negative symptoms can result from impaired dopamine neurotransmission in mesocortical pathways.
- Typical antipsychotic drugs are believed to act by blocking dopamine D_2 receptors in mesolimbic pathways. Atypical antipsychotic drugs act by blocking serotonin 5-HT$_2$ and D_2 receptors. Both classes of drugs alleviate the positive symptoms of schizophrenia, but the typical drugs cause a higher incidence of EPS (akathisia, pseudoparkinsonism, dystonia, and tardive dyskinesia) and are less effective against the negative symptoms of schizophrenia.
- Low-potency antipsychotics (chlorpromazine and thioridazine) produce more autonomic side effects and sedation than do high-potency drugs (fluphenazine and haloperidol), but the high-potency drugs cause more EPS. Clozapine sometimes causes agranulocytosis, so leukocyte counts must be monitored.
- Depression is believed to result from inadequate serotonergic and noradrenergic neurotransmission in limbic structures and elsewhere in the brain.
- TCAs block serotonin and norepinephrine reuptake. They effectively treat depression, but they have significant autonomic and cardiovascular side effects. When taken in an overdose, they can cause seizures and cardiac arrhythmia.
- SSRIs are antidepressants that have fewer autonomic and cardiovascular side effects and cause less sedation than do TCAs. In comparison with other SSRIs, fluoxetine has a longer half-life and causes more drug interactions. Sertraline causes fewer drug interactions.
- The SNRIs are newer antidepressants that act selectively to block both serotonin and norepinephrine reuptake. As a group, the antidepressants of this class have fewer autonomic and cardiovascular side effects and cause less sedation than do TCAs. Some SNRIs also have additional indications for chronic osteoarthritis pain and fibromyalgia.
- Other antidepressants (e.g., bupropion, mirtazapine, and trazodone) have different pharmacologic profiles that lead to increased biogenic amines in the brain and clinical improvement.

- Nonselective MAOIs (e.g., phenelzine and tranylcypromine) bind to and inhibit MAO type A and type B. These drugs prevent the breakdown of serotonin, norepinephrine, dopamine, sympathomimetic drugs, and amines contained in certain foods. The use of interacting drugs and the consumption of particular foods must be avoided to prevent a hypertensive crisis in patients who are taking MAOIs.
- Lithium is a mood-stabilizing drug that is used primarily to treat and prevent the manic phase of bipolar disorder. It has a narrow therapeutic range, so its serum concentrations must be carefully monitored. Overdose can result in neurotoxicity and cardiac toxicity. Lithium produces many side effects, including tremor, weight gain, and polydipsia. Alternatives to lithium include carbamazepine and valproate.
- Amphetamine, dextroamphetamine, methylphenidate, modafinil, and other amphetamine-like stimulants are indicated for the treatment of ADHD, narcolepsy and other sleep disorders, and obesity. Atomoxetine is a unique non-stimulant agent for ADHD that acts by selective norepinephrine reuptake inhibition.

Review Questions

1. Clinical antipsychotic potency for "typical" antipsychotics correlates with actions at which receptor?
   - (A) dopamine D_2 receptors
   - (A) α_2-adrenergic receptors
   - (C) muscarinic receptors
   - (D) histamine receptors
   - (E) serotonin

2. Which of the following agents is an antipsychotic that can improve both positive and negative symptoms of schizophrenia?
   - (A) chlorpromazine
   - (B) haloperidol
   - (C) thiothixene
   - (D) risperidone
   - (E) thioridazine

3. Which one of the following is not a class of antidepressant medications?
   - (A) SNRIs
   - (B) TCAs
   - (C) MAOIs
   - (D) acetylcholinesterase inhibitors
   - (E) SSRIs

4. The older TCAs share all of the following adverse effects except which one?
   - (A) orthostatic hypotension
   - (B) sedation
   - (C) seizures
   - (D) weight gain
   - (E) sexual dysfunction

5. Foods containing tyramine should be avoided when taken with which class of medications?
   - (A) TCAs
   - (B) MAOIs
   - (C) SSRIs
   - (D) atypical antidepressants
   - (E) antihypertensive medications

CHAPTER 23

Opioid Analgesics and Antagonists

CLASSIFICATION OF OPIOID ANALGESICS AND ANTAGONISTS

Opioid Analgesic
Strong opioid agonists

- Morphine
- Fentanyl (SUBLIMAZE)[a]
- Meperidine (DEMEROL)
- Oxycodone (ROXICODONE)[b]
- Hydromorphone (DILAUDID)[c]
- Methadone

Moderate opioid agonists
- Codeine[d]
- Hydrocodone (ZOHYDRO ER)[e]
- Oliceridine (OLINVYK)

Other opioid agonists
- Dextromethorphan (DM)
- Diphenoxylate (LOMOTIL)
- Loperamide (IMODIUM)[f]
- Tramadol (ULTRAM)[g]

Mixed opioid agonist-antagonists
- Buprenorphine (BUPRENEX)[h]
- Butorphanol (STADOL)[i]

Opioid Antagonists
- Naloxone (NARCAN)[j]
- Naltrexone (REVIA)[k]

[a] Also formulated as a transdermal patch (DURAGESIC), a transmucosal lozenge on a stick (ACTIQ), a buccal film (ONSOLIS), a sublingual tablet (ABSTRAL), a sublingual spray (SUBSYS), and as a nasal spray (LAZANDA). Fentanyl is the most used member of its chemical family; sufentanil (SUFENTA), alfentanil (ALFENTA), and remifentanil (ULTIVA) are others.
[b] Also available as extended-release (OXYCONTIN) and in two abuse-deterrent forms: a crush-proof tablet (OXECTA) and oxycodone with naloxone (TARGINIQ). Oxycodone is also found in many NSAID combinations such as oxycodone with acetaminophen (PERCOCET) or with aspirin (PERCODAN), and the new extended-release formulation of oxycodone with acetaminophen (XARTEMIS XR).
[c] Also formulated as an extended-release tablet (EXALGO).
[d] Available as codeine phosphate or codeine sulfate in numerous generic tablets, also in combination with acetaminophen as TYLENOL #3; in combination with acetaminophen and butalbital (FIORICET); and in combination with phenylephrine and promethazine or chlorpheniramine in numerous cough syrup formulations (PROMETH VC, generics).
[e] Also formulated as hydrocodone bitartate in an extended-release tablet called HYSINGLA; and in many combinations of hydrocodone and an NSAID (with acetaminophen in VICODIN, LORTAB, NORCO; with aspirin in HYCODAN; with ibuprofen in VICOPROFEN), and in cough syrups with phenylephrine (LORTUSS HC), chlorpheniramine (TUSSINEX), or homatropine (HYCODAN); also the prodrug benzhydrocodone is sold in combination with acetaminophen as APADAZ.
[f] Also eluxadoline (VIBERZI), a new opioid drug for diarrhea-predominant IBS in adults.
[g] Also tapentadol (NUCYNTA).
[h] Also formulated as a transdermal patch (BUTRANS), slow-releasing rods for implant (PROBUPHINE), sublingual tablet (SUBUTEX), a buccal film (BELBUCA), a drug-releasing implant (PROBUPHINE), and three combination products containing buprenorphine and naloxone: a sublingual film (SUBOXONE), sublingual tablets (ZUBSOLV), and a buccal transmucosal patch (BUNAVAIL).
[i] Also nalbuphine (NUBAIN) and pentazocine (TALWIN).
[j] Naloxone is also available as a nasal spray for reversing opioid overdose (NARCAN NASAL SPRAY) and in the form of methylnaltrexone bromide as an injection or tablet for opioid-induced constipation (RELISTOR), and in many combination products with buprenorphine (see previous footnote[h]). Other marketed opioid antagonists are naldemedine (SYMPROIC) and naloxegol (MOVANTIK) which are both indicated for opioid-induced constipation.
[k] Also formulated as naltrexone intramuscular depot injection (VIVITROL).

OVERVIEW

The relief of pain by the use of opioid analgesics is an ancient pharmacotherapy still very much in use today. As pain is a symptom associated with many disease states, trauma, and childbirth, this chapter begins with the definition of pain and a review of neural pathways that transmit **nociceptive information** in the central nervous system (CNS), as well as endogenous systems that are activated to suppress pain transmission. General characteristics of opioid analgesics are presented, followed by key features of specific agonists, mixed opioid agonists-antagonists, and pure opioid antagonists. The chapter closes with treatment consideration for various acute and chronic pain states.

PAIN AND ANALGESIC AGENTS

Pain is an unpleasant sensory and emotional experience that serves to alert an individual to actual or potential tissue damage. This damage can be caused by exposure to noxious chemical, mechanical, or thermal stimuli (e.g., acids, pressure, percussion, and extreme heat) or by the presence of a pathologic process (e.g., a tumor, muscle spasm, inflammation, nerve damage, organ distention, or other mechanism that activates nociceptors on sensory neurons). Although pain serves a protective function by alerting a person to the presence of a health problem, its unbridled expression often leads to considerable morbidity and suffering. For this reason, **analgesics** or drugs that relieve pain are used for symptomatic treatment of pain from a wide variety of disease states, ranging from acute and chronic physical injuries to terminal cancer.

Based on their mechanisms of action, analgesics can be classified as **opioid analgesics** or **nonopioid analgesics.** Opioid analgesics act primarily in the spinal cord and brain to **inhibit the neurotransmission of pain.** In contrast, nonopioid analgesics act primarily in peripheral tissues to inhibit the formation of **allogenic** or **pain-producing substances** such as **prostaglandins.** Because most of the nonopioid analgesics also exhibit significant anti-inflammatory activity, they are called **nonsteroidal anti-inflammatory drugs (NSAIDs).** The NSAIDs are described in greater detail in Chapter 30.

261

To facilitate the selection of an appropriate analgesic or anesthetic medication, patients are usually asked to describe their pain in terms of its intensity, duration, and location. In some cases, patients report an **intense, sharp,** or **stinging pain.** In other cases, they describe a **dull, burning,** or **aching pain.** These two types of pain are transmitted by different types of neurons and their primary afferent fibers (Box 23.1). Pain can be further distinguished on the basis of whether it is somatic, visceral, or neuropathic in origin. **Somatic pain** is often well localized to specific dermal, subcutaneous, or musculoskeletal tissue. **Visceral pain** originating in thoracic or abdominal structures is often poorly localized and may be referred to somatic structures. For example, cardiac pain is often referred to the chin, neck, shoulder, or arm. **Neuropathic pain** is usually caused by nerve damage, such as that resulting from nerve compression or inflammation, or from diabetes. Neuropathic pain is characteristic, for example, of **trigeminal neuralgia** (*tic douloureux*), **postherpetic neuralgia,** and **fibromyalgia.**

PAIN PATHWAYS

Exposure to a **noxious stimulus activates nociceptors** on the peripheral free nerve endings of **primary afferent neurons.** The cell bodies of these neurons sit alongside the spinal cord in the dorsal root ganglia and send one axon to the periphery and one to the dorsal horn of the spinal cord. With noxious stimulation, **substance P, glutamate,** and other excitatory neurotransmitters are released from the central terminations of the primary afferent fibers onto neurons of the spinal cord. Many of these terminals synapse directly on **spinothalamic tract neurons** in the dorsal horn, which send long fibers up the contralateral side of the spinal cord to transmit pain impulses via **ascending pain pathways** to the medulla, midbrain, thalamus, limbic structures, and cortex.

As shown in Box 23.1, the primary afferent fibers transmitting **nociceptive** information are **A-δ fibers** and **C fibers,** which are responsible for sharp pain and dull pain, respectively. Spinal reflexes activated by these fibers can lead to withdrawal from a noxious stimulus before pain is perceived by higher structures. Ascending pain pathways consist of two main anatomic-functional projections: the **sensory-discriminative** component to the cerebral cortex, and the **motivational-affective** component to the limbic cortex. Projections to the sensory cortex alert an individual to the presence and anatomic location of pain, whereas projections to limbic structures (e.g., the amygdala) enable the individual to experience discomfort, suffering, and other emotional reactions to pain.

The activation of spinothalamic neurons in the spinal cord is modulated by **descending inhibitory pathways** from the midbrain and by sensory **A-beta (β) fibers** arising in peripheral tissues. These two systems constitute the neurologic basis of the **gate-control hypothesis.** According to this hypothesis, pain transmission by spinothalamic neurons can be modulated, or gated, by the inhibitory activity of other types of large fibers impinging on them. The activation of spinothalamic neurons is also inhibited by peripheral A-β sensory fibers that stimulate the release of **met-enkephalin** from spinal cord interneurons. The A-β fibers are thought to also mediate the analgesic effect produced by several types of tissue stimulation, including **acupuncture** and **transcutaneous electrical nerve stimulation (TENS).** These mechanisms explain the pain relief that may be produced by simply rubbing or massaging a mildly injured tissue.

The **descending inhibitory pathways** arise from **periaqueductal gray (PAG)** in the midbrain, and they project to medullary nuclei that transmit impulses to the spinal cord (see Box 23.1). The medullary neurons include serotonergic nerves arising in the **nucleus magnus raphe (NMR)** and noradrenergic nerves arising in the **locus ceruleus (LC).** When these nerves release **serotonin** and **norepinephrine** in the spinal cord, they inhibit dorsal spinal neurons that transmit pain impulses to supraspinal sites. Nerve fibers from the PAG also activate spinal interneurons that release an endogenous opioid peptide, **met-enkephalin.** The enkephalins act presynaptically to decrease the release of pain transmitters from the central terminations of primary afferent neurons. They also act on postsynaptic receptors on spinothalamic tract neurons in the spinal cord to decrease the rostral transmission of the pain signal. Opioid analgesics **activate the descending PAG, NMR,** and **LC neuronal pathways,** and they also **directly activate opioid receptors** in the spinal cord.

OPIOID PEPTIDES AND RECEPTORS

Since ancient times, **opium,** the raw extract of the poppy plant *Papaver somniferum*, has been used for the treatment of pain and diarrhea. During the 19th century, **morphine** was isolated from opium, and its pharmacologic effects were characterized. Later, specific sites in CNS tissue were discovered that bind morphine and other opioid agonists. The presence of stereoselective receptors for morphine in brain tissue indicated the likelihood of an **endogenous ligand** for these receptors, and this eventually led to the discovery of the three major families of endogenous opioid peptides: **enkephalins, beta (β)-endorphins,** and **dynorphins.**

The opioid peptides are derived from larger precursor proteins that are widely distributed in the brain. Endorphins and dynorphins are large peptides, whereas the two types of enkephalins are small pentapeptides containing Tyr-Gly-Gly-Phe-Met-Leu. Therefore, the two types of enkephalins are called **met-enkephalin** and **leu-enkephalin.**

The **enkephalins are released** from neurons throughout the pain axis, including those in the PAG, medulla, and spinal cord. Enkephalins activate opioid receptors in these areas and thereby block the transmission of pain impulses. The enkephalins appear to act as neuromodulators in that they exert a long-acting inhibitory effect on the release of excitatory neurotransmitters by several neurons.

Opioid agonists mediate their effects at three types of opioid receptors: **mu (μ) opioid receptors, delta (δ) opioid receptors,** and **kappa (κ) opioid receptors.** Most of the clinically useful opioid analgesics, however, have preferential or strong **selectivity for** *mu* **opioid receptors.** Some of the mixed opioid agonist-antagonist agents have *kappa* opioid receptor selectivity, but attempts to develop useful opioid analgesics selective for *delta* opioid receptors have not been successful.

OPIOID DRUGS
Classification

The opioid agents can be classified as full agonists, mixed agonist-antagonists, or pure antagonists.

Based on their maximal clinical effectiveness, the **full agonists** can be characterized as strong or moderate agonists. In experimental pain models, all of the full agonists exert a maximal analgesic effect. In humans, the **strong**

BOX 23.1 PAIN PATHWAYS AND SITES OF DRUG ACTION

Pain activates primary afferent neurons that enter the spinal cord where they synapse with interneurons directly onto spinothalamic tract neurons *(STTs)*. The neospinothalamic tract projects to the primary sensory cortex, which alerts the individual to the presence and location of pain, the **sensory-discriminative** component. The paleospinothalamic tract projects to limbic structures, which mediate the **motivational-affective** response to pain. Descending neuronal tracts from the periaqueductal gray matter activate neurons that release norepinephrine *(NE)*, serotonin (5-hydroxytryptamine, or 5-HT), and enkephalin *(Enk)* in the spinal cord and thereby block ascending pain transmission. Opioid analgesics activate the descending pathways and directly activate opioid receptors on afferent nerve terminals and on STT neurons in the spinal cord. Nonopioid analgesics reduce the activation of primary afferent neurons via inhibition of prostaglandin synthesis. *Glu,* Glutamate; *LC,* locus ceruleus; *NMR,* nucleus magnus raphe; *SP,* substance P.

Primary Afferent Neuron	Ascending Pathway	Projections	Type of Pain	Functions
A-δ (fast)	Neospino-thalamic	Reticular formation, thalamus, and sensory cortex	Intense, sharp, stinging pain	Pain localization and withdrawal reflexes
C (slow)	Paleospino-thalamic	Thalamus, periaqueductal gray matter, and limbic structures	Dull, burning, aching pain	Autonomic reflexes, pain memory, and pain discomfort

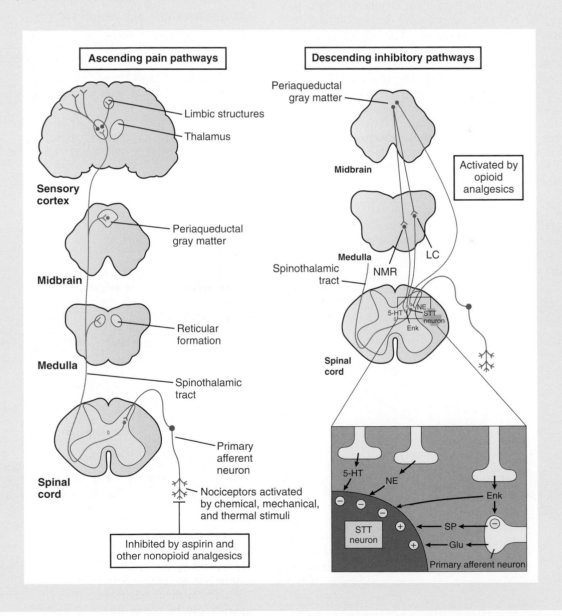

opioid agonists are well tolerated when they are given in a dosage sufficient to relieve severe pain. The **moderate opioid agonists**, however, will cause intolerable adverse effects if they are given in a dosage sufficient to alleviate extremely severe pain. For this reason, the moderate opioid agonists are administered in submaximal doses to treat moderate to mild pain, and they are usually formulated in combination with NSAIDs to enhance their clinical effectiveness.

The **mixed opioid agonist-antagonists** are analgesic drugs that have varying combinations of agonist, partial agonist, and antagonist activity and varying degrees of affinity for the different opioid receptor types.

The **opioid antagonists** have no analgesic effects. They are used to counteract the adverse effects of opioids taken in **overdose** and for the treatment of **drug dependence.**

Drug Properties
Mechanism of Action

The opioid receptors are prominent members of the **G protein–coupled receptor** superfamily. Activation of opioid receptors leads to **inhibition of adenylate cyclase** and a decrease in the concentration of cyclic adenosine monophosphate, an increase in K^+ conductance, and a decrease in Ca^{2+} conductance (Fig. 23.1). The activated $G_{\alpha i}$ subunit of the G protein directly inhibits the adenylate cyclase enzyme, and the $G_{\beta\gamma}$ subunits are thought to mediate the changes at the Ca^{2+} and K^+ channels. These actions cause both **presynaptic inhibition of neurotransmitter release** from the central terminations of small-diameter primary afferent fibers and **postsynaptic inhibition of membrane depolarization** of dorsal horn nociceptive neurons.

Pharmacologic Effects

Central Nervous System. Morphine acts in the CNS to produce analgesia, sedation, euphoria or dysphoria, miosis, nausea, vomiting, respiratory depression, and inhibition of the cough reflex (Box 23.2).

Analgesia is produced by activation of opioid receptors in the spinal cord and at several supraspinal levels, as illustrated in Box 23.1. Effects on midbrain dopaminergic, serotonergic, and noradrenergic nuclei can cause sedation

BOX 23.2 MAJOR PHARMACOLOGIC EFFECTS OF OPIOID AGONISTS

CENTRAL NERVOUS SYSTEM EFFECTS
- Analgesia
- Dysphoria or euphoria
- Inhibition of cough reflex
- Miosis
- Physical dependence
- Respiratory depression
- Sedation

CARDIOVASCULAR EFFECTS
- Decreased myocardial oxygen demand
- Vasodilation and hypotension

GASTROINTESTINAL AND BILIARY EFFECTS
- Constipation (increased intestinal smooth muscle tone)
- Increased biliary sphincter tone and pressure
- Nausea and vomiting (via central nervous system action)

GENITOURINARY EFFECTS
- Increased bladder sphincter tone
- Prolongation of labor
- Urinary retention

NEUROENDOCRINE SYSTEM EFFECTS
- Inhibition of release of luteinizing hormone
- Stimulation of release of antidiuretic hormone and prolactin

IMMUNE SYSTEM EFFECTS
- Suppression of function of natural killer cells

DERMAL EFFECTS
- Flushing
- Pruritus
- Urticaria (hives) or other rash

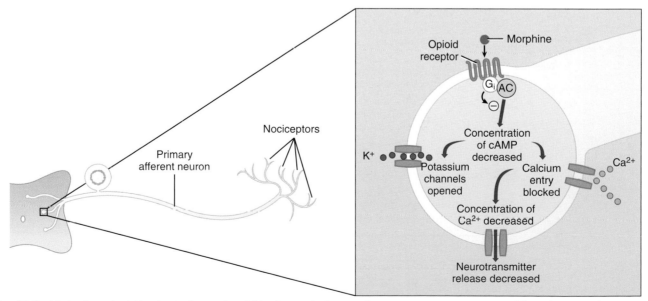

FIG. 23.1 Mechanisms of opioid action in the spinal cord. Morphine and other opioid agonists activate presynaptic mu, *delta,* or *kappa* opioid receptors on primary afferent neurons. These receptors are coupled negatively to adenylate cyclase (*AC*) via G proteins ($G_{\alpha i}$). Inhibition of cyclic adenosine monophosphate (*cAMP*) formation leads to opening of potassium channels and closing of calcium channels. $G_{\beta\gamma}$ subunits may also participate in the modulation of ion channels. Potassium efflux causes membrane hyperpolarization. The closing of calcium channels inhibits the release of neurotransmitters, such as substance P.

and euphoria. Surprisingly, many patients experience **dysphoria** after administration of opioids. **Miosis** (constricted pupils) is produced by the direct stimulation of the Edinger-Westphal nucleus of the oculomotor nerve (cranial nerve III), which activates parasympathetic stimulation of the iris sphincter muscle. Because little or no tolerance develops to miosis, this sign can be **diagnostic of an opioid overdose.**

Codeine and other opioids inhibit the cough reflex at sites in the medulla where this reflex is integrated. The **antitussive actions of opioids** are discussed in greater detail in Chapter 27.

Cardiovascular System. The most prominent cardiovascular effect of morphine and many other opioids is **vasodilation,** which is partly caused by histamine release from mast cells in peripheral tissues. Morphine can cause orthostatic hypotension from decreased peripheral resistance and a reduction in baroreceptor reflex activity. In patients with coronary artery disease, the decreased peripheral resistance leads to a **reduction of cardiac work** and myocardial oxygen demand.

Gastrointestinal, Biliary, and Genitourinary System. Morphine and most other opioids act to **increase smooth muscle tone** in the gastrointestinal, biliary, and genitourinary systems. In the gastrointestinal tract, increased muscle tone leads to inhibition of peristalsis and causes **constipation.** For this reason, the opioids are the oldest and most widely used medication for the treatment of diarrhea (see Chapter 28). Unfortunately, patients with chronic pain do not appear to become tolerant to the constipating effects of opioids, necessitating a continual need for laxatives and other agents.

Morphine and other opioids also **increase the tone of the biliary sphincter** (sphincter of Oddi) and can cause an exacerbation of pain in patients with biliary dysfunction or a gallbladder attack. Opioids also increase the tone of the bladder sphincter and can cause urinary retention in some patients. Because the opioid agonist **meperidine** has **less-pronounced action on smooth muscle,** it is the drug of choice for these patients and for the pain associated with labor.

Other Effects. Opioids have an effect on neuroendocrine and immunologic function. In the hypothalamus, they stimulate the **release of antidiuretic hormone** and **prolactin** and **inhibit** the release of **luteinizing hormone.** Opioids also **suppress** the activity of certain types of lymphocytes, including natural killer cells, and this action may contribute to the high rate of infectious diseases in heroin addicts.

Adverse Effects. The **major adverse effect** of morphine and other opioids is **respiratory depression,** which is usually the cause of death in severe overdoses. Opioids reduce the hypercapnic drive (the stimulation of respiratory centers by increased CO_2 levels) while producing relatively little effect on the hypoxic drive. Opioids reduce the respiratory tidal volume and rate, causing the rate to fall to three or four breaths per minute after an opioid overdose. As the cerebral circulation is exquisitely sensitive to CO_2 levels and responds with an increase in cerebral blood flow leading to **increased intracranial pressure,** opioids should not be used in the case of a **closed-head injury.** The respiratory depressant effects of opioids are rapidly reversed by the intravenous administration of an opioid antagonist such as naloxone (see later).

By stimulating the chemoreceptor trigger zone in the medulla, the opioids also cause **nausea** and **vomiting.** This is seen most often in ambulatory patients because opioids increase the sensitivity of the vestibular organ of the inner ear.

Opioids cause mast cells throughout the body to release histamine, which can cause itching, or **pruritus.** A flushing reaction, noted by redness and a feeling of warmth over the upper torso, may also occur from histamine release.

Allergic reactions to opioid analgesics are not uncommon. In most cases, however, a patient who is allergic to a particular opioid can use an opioid from a different chemical class. For example, someone who is allergic to codeine will probably not be allergic to meperidine or fentanyl.

Tolerance and Physical Dependence

Tolerance is defined as a decrease in initial pharmacologic effect observed after chronic or long-term administration. Repeated administration of an opioid agonist will lead to **pharmacodynamic tolerance** for both the administered opioid and other opioid analgesics. Tolerance primarily results from **down-regulation of opioid receptors.** Interestingly, in animal models, the magnitude of tolerance is inversely proportional to the efficacy of the opioid analgesic. This is because at equianalgesic doses, a more efficacious opioid will occupy a lesser fraction of available opioid receptors than a less-efficacious agent. Tolerance develops to most of the effects of opioids but not to **miosis** and **constipation.** Although considerable tolerance to respiratory depression occurs, a sufficiently high dose of an opioid can still be fatal to highly opioid-tolerant individuals.

Opioid tolerance is usually accompanied by a similar degree of **physical dependence.** Physical dependence is defined as a physiologic state in which a person's continued use of a drug is required for his or her well-being. Tolerance and physical dependence appear with many drug classes and represent the establishment of a new equilibrium between the neuron and its environment (**neuroadaptation),** wherein the neuron becomes less responsive to the drug while requiring continued drug effect to maintain cellular homeostasis. If the chronically used drug is abruptly withdrawn, the equilibrium is disturbed and a **rebound hyperexcitability** occurs owing to the loss of the inhibitory influence of the drug. This produces a withdrawal syndrome, the manifestations of which depend on the particular type of drug (see Chapter 25).

Because opioids demonstrate **cross-tolerance,** one opioid drug can substitute for another opioid drug and prevent symptoms of withdrawal in a physically dependent person. This is the basis for outpatient treatment of opioid dependence by the use of **methadone** or **buprenorphine** (see Chapter 25).

SPECIFIC AGENTS
Strong Opioid Agonists

The strong opioid agonists include naturally occurring drugs, such as **morphine,** and a number of synthetic drugs, including **fentanyl, meperidine,** and **methadone.** These drugs have equivalent analgesic effects but differ in their pharmacokinetic properties (Table 23.1), adverse effects, and uses.

Morphine

Morphine is the principal alkaloid of the opium poppy, *P. somniferum,* and constitutes about 10% of dried opium. Opium also contains **papaverine,** a drug sometimes used

TABLE 23.1 Pharmacokinetic Properties of Selected Opioid Drugs[a]

DRUG	ROUTE OF ADMINISTRATION	DURATION OF ACTION (H)	ELIMINATION HALF-LIFE	ACTIVE METABOLITE
Strong Opioid Agonists				
Fentanyl	Parenteral, transdermal, sublingual, and buccal	1	4 h	No
Meperidine	Oral and parenteral	3	3 h	Yes
Methadone	Oral and parenteral	8	24 h	No
Morphine	Oral and parenteral	4	3 h	Yes
Oxycodone	Oral	4	Unknown	No
Sufentanil	Parenteral	1	2 h	No
Remifentanil	IV infusion only	While infused	4 min	No
Moderate Opioid Agonists				
Codeine	Oral	4	3 h	Yes
Hydrocodone	Oral	4	4 h	No
Other Opioid Agonists				
Dextromethorphan	Oral	6	11 h	No
Diphenoxylate	Oral	6	12 h	Yes
Loperamide	Oral	6	10 h	No
Tramadol	Oral	4	6 h	Yes
Mixed Opioid Agonist-Antagonists				
Buprenorphine	Parenteral	5	5 h	No
Butorphanol	Intranasal and parenteral	3	3 h	No
Nalbuphine	Parenteral	4	5 h	No
Pentazocine	Oral and parenteral	4	4 h	No
Opioid Antagonists				
Naloxone	Parenteral	2	4 h	No
Naltrexone	Oral	24	12 h	Yes

IV, Intravenous.
[a]Values shown are the mean of values reported in the literature.

to relax smooth muscle and treat vasospastic disorders; **noscapine,** used as a cough suppressant; and minor amounts of **codeine.** The diacetic acid ester of morphine is heroin, a drug that is frequently abused (see Chapter 25).

Morphine is well absorbed from the gut, but it undergoes considerable **first-pass metabolism** in the liver, where a significant fraction of the drug is converted to glucuronides. For this reason, larger doses are required when the drug is administered orally than when it is administered parenterally. The principal metabolite of morphine is the 3-glucuronide, which is pharmacologically inactive. A significant amount of the **6-glucuronide** metabolite is also formed; it is **more active than morphine** and has a longer half-life. Hence, the 6-glucuronide metabolite contributes significantly to the analgesic effectiveness of morphine. Morphine is primarily excreted in the urine in the form of glucuronides. A small amount is excreted in the bile and undergoes enterohepatic cycling.

Morphine remains the standard of comparison for opioid analgesic drugs. It is primarily used to treat **severe pain associated with trauma, myocardial infarction,** and **cancer.** In patients with myocardial infarction, it relieves pain and anxiety while also dilating coronary arteries and reducing the myocardial oxygen demand. Morphine is available in both parenteral and oral formulations, including **long-acting oral**

formulations (KADIAN, AVINZA) that are useful in patients with chronic pain. It is also available in a liposome-encapsulated formulation (DEPODUR) for epidural administration for postoperative pain after major surgery.

Fentanyl and Its Derivatives

Fentanyl is a synthetic and highly potent opioid agonist. Fentanyl and its derivatives, including **sufentanil, alfentanil,** and **remifentanil,** are the most potent opioid agonists available. Indeed, tranquilizing darts used to sedate elephants and other large animals in zoos and in the wild are created using a fentanyl derivative called carfentanil (WILDNIL). Because of its high potency and lipid solubility, **fentanyl** has been formulated in a **long-acting transdermal skin patch** (DURAGESIC) to provide continuous pain relief for patients with **severe or chronic pain.** It is also available for breakthrough pain in mucosal, buccal, and nasal spray formulations. It is used by parenteral administration preoperatively and postoperatively and as an **adjunct to general anesthesia.** Fentanyl produces less nausea than morphine but is often associated with truncal rigidity when used as an adjunct to parenteral anesthesia.

Sufentanil, Alfentanil, and **remifentanil** are used as part of anesthesia procedures and are available for intravenous administration. **Remifentanil** is especially useful for short-term procedures and outpatient surgery because it is considered to have an **ultra-rapid onset of action,** reaching blood-brain equilibrium and peak effect within 1 minute after the start of an intravenous infusion. It is also rapidly cleared by nonspecific **esterases** in tissue and blood; therefore, recovery occurs within 5 to 10 minutes after the infusion stops. **Remimazolam,** the newest benzodiazepine on the market, employs the same strategy of rapid plasma and tissue esterase metabolism as the shortest-acting sedative (see Chapter 19).

Meperidine

Meperidine is a synthetic opioid agonist with an unusual profile of pharmacologic properties. It has no antitussive activity and has variable effects on pupil size. Because its effect on gastrointestinal, biliary, and uterine **smooth muscle is less pronounced** than that of morphine, it is less likely than morphine to cause constipation or an increase in biliary pressure. Meperidine **does not prolong labor** as much as morphine does, so it can be used for analgesia in obstetrics.

The parenteral formulation of meperidine is often used as an **obstetric or postsurgical analgesic.** The oral formulation is used to treat **moderate to severe pain** in the outpatient setting. The drug is converted to a toxic metabolite, **normeperidine,** which can cause CNS excitation, convulsions, and tremors when meperidine is administered in large doses or for a prolonged period. Hence, the drug is usually used for the **short-term treatment of acute pain syndromes.**

Oxycodone

Oxycodone is one of several semisynthetic morphine derivatives available as analgesics. Oxycodone is usually administered orally in combination with a nonopioid analgesic (e.g., acetaminophen) to treat **moderate or severe pain.** It is available as a single agent for acute treatment of pain (ROXICODONE) and as **sustained-release oral form of oxycodone** (OXYCONTIN) for long-term treatment of chronic pain syndromes. The OXYCONTIN formulation has been linked to several deaths of opioid abusers after they crushed the pills and dissolved the drug for intravenous administration (see Chapter 25). For this reason, a recently approved crushproof tablet of oxycodone has been made available (OXECTA).

Hydromorphone

Hydromorphone is a semi-synthetic opioid made from morphine. Like all opioids, common adverse effects are dizziness, sedation, constipation, and, at high doses, respiratory depression. It is an older drug and available as generic and brand name in many different formulations by various routes of administration. Hydromorphone formulations are marketed for oral, rectal, transdermal, and IV administration; it is also given intrathecally and by the epidural route.

Methadone

Methadone is a long-acting synthetic opioid agonist. Although it is available in parenteral formulations, it is most often administered orally to ambulatory patients to treat **opioid dependence** or **chronic pain.** Use of the oral formulation by opioid-dependent patients can prevent their craving for heroin or other opioids, but it does not cause significant euphoria or other reinforcing effects. Because of its long duration of action, it can be administered once a day for this purpose. The treatment of opioid-dependent patients in this fashion is called a **methadone maintenance program** (see also Chapter 25).

Moderate Opioid Agonists

The moderate opioid agonists are less potent than the strong opioid agonists. Because they do not produce maximal analgesia at doses that are well tolerated by patients, the moderate agonists are used at submaximal doses, usually in combination with an NSAID analgesic. Fixed-dose combination products containing one of the **moderate opioid agonists** and **acetaminophen, aspirin,** or **ibuprofen** are available for the treatment of moderate pain.

Codeine and Hydrocodone

Codeine is a naturally occurring opioid obtained from the opium poppy. Structurally, it is the 3-O-methyl derivative of morphine. Because codeine contains a methyl group at the 3 position, the principal site of morphine metabolism, codeine undergoes a **lesser degree of first-pass metabolism.** Thus, codeine has greater oral **bioavailability** than morphine.

Codeine is converted to morphine by cytochrome P450 isozyme CYP2D6, and persons with deficient variations of this isozyme obtain little pain relief from the drug. Conversely, pregnant and nursing mothers who are ultra-rapid metabolizers of codeine may pose a risk of lethal morphine exposure to the fetus or nursing infant. A US Food and Drug Administration (FDA) warning in 2007 noted that a published case report of an infant death raised concern that breast-fed babies may be at increased risk of **morphine overdose** if their mothers are taking codeine and are ultra-rapid metabolizers of the drug.

Codeine is a less-potent analgesic than morphine, and the doses required to obtain maximal analgesia produce intolerable side effects, such as constipation. For this reason, codeine is available only in combination with other agents (e.g., NSAIDs) to treat **mild to moderate pain.** Codeine also produces a significant antitussive effect and is included in many cough syrups to **alleviate** or **prevent coughing.**

The uses of **hydrocodone** are similar to those of codeine. Like codeine, it is available only in **combination** medicines, primarily with an NSAID such as aspirin (PERCODAN) or acetaminophen (PERCOCET), and many other formulations. Importantly, the amount of acetaminophen in combination with opioids was recently **limited to 325 mg per dosage unit** to reduce the risk of hepatic toxicity and allergic reactions.

Oliceridine

Oliceridine is the newest opioid on the market and is approved for short-term intravenous use in hospitals or clinics. **Oliceridine** was touted as the first **biased agonist** at the opioid receptor to reach the market. As introduced in Chapter 3, biased agonists all act at the same receptor but activate different signaling pathways; for GPCRs, this means activating G-protein pathways more than *beta*- arrestin 2 pathways. For opioid receptors, a G-protein biased agonist could produce potent analgesia (via G-protein signaling) with **less concurrent respiratory depression and constipation,** effects thought to occur via *beta*- arrestin pathways (Fig 23.2). Interestingly, the FDA label for oliceridine does not mention its role as a G-protein biased opioid agonist.

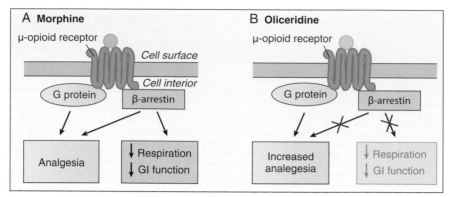

FIG. 23.2 Mechanism of biased opioid agonist. (A) Morphine binds to the μ-opioid receptor and stimulates G-protein (G$_{αi}$) and *beta*-arrestin signaling. G-protein signaling leads to decreased firing of pain neurons and analgesia. *Beta*-arrestin signaling is linked to adverse effects such as respiratory depression and GI constipation. (B) A G-protein biased opioid agonist, perhaps oliceridine, signals primary through the G-protein pathway and produces less adverse effects such as respiratory depression and GI constipation while maintaining analgesic effects.

Other Opioid Agonists

Tramadol is a unique dual-action analgesic. It is an agonist at *mu* **opioid receptors** and inhibits the neuronal **reuptake of serotonin and norepinephrine.** The relationship between neuronal reuptake inhibition and analgesia is not certain. Reuptake inhibition, however, may **potentiate** the inhibitory effects of serotonin and norepinephrine on pain transmission in the spinal cord (see Box 23.1). Tricyclic antidepressants and other neuronal reuptake inhibitors also have analgesic effects, and some **antidepressants** are used to treat **chronic pain** syndromes (Box 23.3). For this reason, investigators believe that neuronal reuptake inhibition by tramadol contributes to the drug's analgesic activity. Thus, the analgesic effect of tramadol is only partly inhibited by opioid antagonists such as naloxone.

Tramadol is administered orally to treat **moderate pain.** It has a definite but limited drug dependence liability. Nevertheless, it has been used successfully in the treatment of **chronic pain syndromes** and produces minimal cardiovascular and respiratory depression. The drug lowers the seizure threshold, and the risk of seizures is increased if tramadol is used concurrently with antidepressants. Like other agents with antidepressant action, the warnings on tramadol have been modified to emphasize the **increased risk of suicidal thought and behaviors** in patients taking this medication. **Tapentadol** is a newer opioid analgesic; like tramadol, it acts at *mu* opioid receptors and reuptake transporters, but it inhibits only norepinephrine reuptake.

Several other opioid agents are available but have little analgesic activity. These include **dextromethorphan,** which has significant antitussive activity and is used in the treatment of **cough** (see Chapter 27) and in combination with **quinidine** for the treatment of **pseudobulbar affect** (emotional lability) often seen in patients with neurodegenerative diseases (see Chapter 24). **Diphenoxylate** and **loperamide,** which activate opioid receptors in gastrointestinal smooth muscle, are used in the treatment of **diarrhea.** **Eluxadoline** is a new opioid drug specifically approved for treatment of **irritable bowel syndrome (IBS) with diarrhea** in adults. This drug binds to several types of opioid receptors, acting as an agonist at *mu* and *kappa* opioid receptors, and an antagonist at *delta* opioid receptors. Activation of *mu* receptors leads to decreased intestinal motility and relief of diarrhea, whereas actions of **eluxadoline** on other opioid

BOX 23.3 THE CASE OF A PAINFUL POX

CASE PRESENTATION
A retired professor visits his primary care physician regarding an itching and painful rash on his abdomen that is distributed like a band across both sides. The physician asks him whether he had chickenpox as a child, to which the professor replies that he did. His physician diagnoses him with shingles and tells him the rash will go away in about a week. Later that same month, the professor returns to the doctor's office regarding pain on his stomach when his clothes rub against it, and sometimes when he is lying in bed. The doctor tells him he has postherpetic neuralgia and prescribes tramadol for the pain.

CASE DISCUSSION
Postherpetic neuralgia is a painful condition that develops after a case of the shingles. Shingles is the name given to a rash that develops from reactivation of chickenpox, the herpes varicella-zoster virus that lay dormant in the cell bodies of the dorsal root ganglia. It is estimated nearly 1 million cases of shingles occur every year in the United States. Shingles affect mostly older persons, with 40% to 50% of cases occurring in people who are 60 years of age and older. Elderly individuals may be more sensitive to shingles due to waning immunologic defenses, or activation of the pox virus by drugs and other disease states. For reasons that are unclear, a number of shingles cases convert to postherpetic neuralgia. Drug treatment for postherpetic neuralgia, a type of neuropathic pain condition, includes antidepressants, opioids, and pregabalin. Tramadol is a unique dual-acting opioid agent; it acts as an agonist at *mu* opioid receptors and inhibits the neuronal reuptake of serotonin and norepinephrine. It has shown effectiveness in a number of neuropathic pain states including postherpetic neuralgia.

receptors reduces the incidence of constipation typically caused by *mu* opioid agonists (see Chapter 28).

Mixed Opioid Agonist-Antagonists and Partial Agonists

The mixed opioid agonist-antagonists are drugs that exhibit partial agonist or antagonist activity at *mu* receptors and show agonist or antagonist activity at *kappa* receptors. Examples are buprenorphine, butorphanol, nalbuphine, and pentazocine.

Pharmacokinetics

The mixed opioid agonist-antagonists have a large chemical group on the nitrogen atom of the morphine molecule, which is responsible for their partial agonist or antagonist activity at opioid receptors. Their pharmacokinetic and pharmacologic properties are shown in Table 23.1. All of the agonist-antagonists can be given parenterally. In addition, pentazocine is available for oral use, and butorphanol is available as a nasal spray. Butorphanol is rapidly absorbed from the nasal mucosa, thereby enabling the use of the drug on an as-needed basis.

Mechanisms and Effects

The most important pharmacologic property of these drugs with respect to their clinical activity is the lack of full agonist effects at *mu* **opioid receptors.** Because of this, the mixed opioid agonist-antagonists produce **less respiratory depression** as the doses are increased than do strong opioid agonists, such as morphine. Hence, the mixed opioid agonist-antagonists are safer to use with regard to respiratory depression and overdose. They also appear to have a lower liability for drug dependence and abuse than do full opioid agonists. The mixed opioids produce less constipation than do most of the full agonists. However, these sometimes cause anxiety, nightmares, and **psychotomimetic effects,** including hallucinations, as a result of the activation of *kappa* **opioid receptors.** They can also **precipitate withdrawal** in a person physically dependent on a full opioid agonist.

Indications

The parenterally administered agonist-antagonist drugs are primarily used for **preoperative** and **postoperative analgesia** and for **obstetric analgesia during labor and delivery.** The orally and nasally administered drugs are used to alleviate **moderate to severe pain.**

Specific Drugs

Buprenorphine, which is a **partial agonist at** *mu* **receptors,** is noted for a slow dissociation from the *mu* opioid receptor after binding. It is somewhat longer acting than most parenterally administered opioid analgesics and can be administered intramuscularly or intravenously. It was recently approved for outpatient treatment of opioid dependence (see Chapter 25) and is available in an oral and sublingual formulation combined with naloxone (as Suboxone) to prevent intravenous abuse and a number of other formulations (see Drug Classification table at beginning of chapter). A transdermal patch formulation was also recently approved (Butrans).

Butorphanol and **nalbuphine** are *kappa* **opioid receptor agonists** and have **partial agonist** or **antagonist** activity at *mu* **opioid receptors.** Both drugs are administered parenterally, and butorphanol is also available as a nasal spray.

Pentazocine is a *kappa* **opioid receptor** agonist with additional activity at *sigma* (σ) **receptors.** σ receptors were once considered a member of the opioid receptor family; it is now known that they are a **distinct class of receptors** mediating the psychotomimetic effects of phencyclidine (PCP) and ketamine (see Chapter 25). Pentazocine is available for parenteral and oral use. The parenteral formulation is primarily used as a preanesthetic medication and as a supplement to surgical anesthesia. The oral formulations are used to treat moderate to severe pain; one formulation contains **naloxone,** a pure opioid antagonist, to discourage parenteral (IV) abuse of the drug. Parenteral use of an oral pentazocine formulation can cause **severe cardiovascular effects,** especially in patients with existing cardiovascular disease. Pentazocine is also available in combination with aspirin or acetaminophen for oral administration.

Opioid Antagonists

Naloxone and **naltrexone** are **competitive opioid receptor antagonists** that can rapidly reverse the effects of morphine and other opioid agonists. These pure opioid antagonists have three primary clinical uses: the treatment of **opioid overdose,** the treatment of **alcohol and opioid dependence,** and decreasing **opioid-induced constipation.**

Naloxone and naltrexone are chemical analogs of morphine, with bulky chemical groups attached to the morphine molecule. This modification allows the molecule to bind to the opioid receptor but prevents the conformation change in the receptor required for agonist activity.

In cases of **opioid overdose,** naloxone is administered intravenously to rapidly terminate respiratory depression and other toxic effects of opioid agonists. Because naloxone has a relatively **short half-life** (see Table 23.1), repeated doses of the drug may be needed to counteract the effects of the longer-lasting opioid agonists. Naloxone is also formulated with opioid agonists in oral medications to prevent crushing of the pill and intravenous abuse. Because naloxone has low bioavailability and is not effective when given orally, it does not block the effects of the oral opioid but would block opioid effects or even precipitate withdrawal if used by the intravenous route.

A nasal spray of naloxone (Narcan Nasal Spray) for reversing opioid overdose is also available and used by many first responders. This life-saving formulation of naloxone is also available in many states to all first responders (including police officers) and family members of chronic pain patients using prescription opioids.

For **opioid maintenance therapy,** naloxone is available in various combinations with the partial opioid agonist **buprenorphine** (discussed in Chapter 25). These combination products contain an opioid partial agonist plus an opioid antagonist and can be prescribed to the opioid-dependent patient by their primary care physician. This is a more palatable treatment option than daily trips to a methadone clinic.

A novel modification of naloxone was produced by the creation of a **PEGylated naloxone.** PEGylation is the pharmaceutical manufacturing process of adding **polyethylene glycol (PEG)** polymers to a drug molecule, which increases drug solubility and generally improves the pharmacokinetic profile. PEGylated naloxone is called **naloxegol** (Movantik) and is indicated for the relief of **opioid-induced constipation.** Opioid analgesics inhibit gastrointestinal (GI) motility, and naloxegol binds to the GI opioid receptors and blocks opioid-induced constipation. Another opioid antagonist with the same indication is **naldemedine.**

Naltrexone, in an oral formulation (ReVia) and in an extended-release injectable suspension (once-a-month, Vivitrol), is also used to treat **alcohol** and **opioid dependence.** In contrast to naloxone, naltrexone has **high oral bioavailability** and can be used on a long-term basis by opioid addicts who have undergone detoxification and are no longer using opioids (see Chapter 25). Like naloxone in **naxologel,** naltrexone comes in a formulation of **methylnaltrexone bromide** (RELISTOR) for the treatment of **opioid-induced constipation.** As methylnaltrexone is restricted from crossing the blood-brain barrier, concurrent opioid agonists still exert their analgesic effects at CNS sites. Its ability to block opioid binding in peripheral tissues decreases opioid-constipating effects (see also Chapter 28). **Methylnaltrexone bromide** comes in a vial and syringe to be self-administered by the patient and was also recently made available in an oral tablet.

THE TREATMENT OF PAIN
Choice of Analgesic
The location, cause, and severity of pain and the risk of producing drug dependence are all factors that influence the way in which pain is managed. As a general rule, patients with acute or chronic pain should be treated with the least potent analgesic that will control their pain. Mild pain usually responds to a nonopioid analgesic, usually an NSAID (see Chapter 30). Moderate to severe pain is often treated with **codeine, hydrocodone,** or **oxycodone** alone or in combination with a nonopioid analgesic. Severe pain usually requires the use of a strong opioid agonist (e.g., **fentanyl, meperidine, methadone,** or **morphine**). Although meperidine can be used for acute postsurgical pain and in other situations in which the duration of treatment is limited to a few days, it should not be used for longer durations because of the possible accumulation of a toxic metabolite (normeperidine).

Acute pain caused by trauma, surgery, or short-term medical conditions can be effectively managed with an analgesic and appropriate treatment of the underlying condition. In patients with acute pain, the risk of producing drug dependence is extremely low. Hence, physicians and other health care professionals should not hesitate to administer adequate doses of a sufficiently strong analgesic to control pain.

Pain associated with **arthritis, neuropathy,** and other **chronic but nonterminal conditions** is more difficult to treat and is often managed with a combination of analgesics, coanalgesics, psychotherapy, physical therapy, and other treatment modalities. Use of opioid analgesics in the treatment of chronic pain is associated with opioid tolerance and a risk of physical dependence, so care must be exercised to prevent dosage escalation, drug dependence, and prescription drug abuse. Strict guidelines for prescription refills should be in place, and a prescription refill flowchart can be used to monitor drug usage and prevent dosage escalation. In some clinics, patients are asked to sign an "opioid contract" in which they agree to procedures that will ensure proper use of opioid drugs, including random drug testing.

Patients with **terminal illnesses,** such as metastatic cancer, should receive sufficient doses of opioid analgesics to control their pain, irrespective of any concerns about the development of tolerance and physical dependence. An example of the **shift in the morphine dose-response curve** in opioid tolerant patients is shown in Fig. 23.3.

Acute Pain
Giving analgesics on an as-needed basis sometimes produces wide swings in pain and sedation during the early phase of treatment. Therefore, in the initial stages of acute pain, analgesics should be given around the clock at regular intervals. The dosage should be titrated to control pain while minimizing sedation and other side effects. As the pain subsides over time and the need for analgesia decreases, the patient can be transferred to an as-needed schedule of medication.

Patient-controlled analgesia is a method of intravenous administration that permits the patient to self-administer preset amounts of an analgesic (e.g., fentanyl) via a syringe pump interfaced with a timing device. The method enables the patient to balance pain control with sedation. Its use depends on the patient's ability to activate the device, so it may not be suitable for elderly patients or for patients immediately after surgery or trauma.

Chronic Pain
Treatment of chronic pain varies greatly with the underlying cause. Although the discussion of specific chronic pain syndromes is beyond the scope of this text, a few general guidelines and comments are offered.

Both **opioid analgesics** and **nonopioid analgesics** are useful in the management of chronic pain syndromes. If pain is associated with inflammation, nonopioid drugs with anti-inflammatory activity can be especially useful. If pain is associated with peripheral nerve or nerve root sensitization, treatment with **transcutaneous nerve stimulation** or a **local anesthetic** may help. In some cases, a cream containing **capsaicin** is effective. Capsaicin activates peripheral nociceptors on primary sensory neurons, thereby leading to increased release of substance P and eventually to the depletion of substance P in the CNS. Capsaicin produces a burning sensation for the first few days of application, but this is gradually replaced by an analgesic effect. Recently, a capsaicin patch formulation (QUTENZA) was approved for treatment of pain caused by **postherpetic neuralgia.**

Chronic pain is frequently seen in association with systemic disorders (e.g., diabetes). When pain has been present for a period of time, the responsiveness of dynamic wide-range nociceptive neurons in the spinal cord increases in a way that increases pain perception and memory. As these neurons become "wound up," their receptive fields increase so that pain is felt over a larger area. These changes appear to contribute to the maintenance of chronic neuropathic pain. Patients with this type of pain may benefit from a combination of nonpharmacologic therapies (e.g., TENS, acupuncture, and physical therapy), analgesic medications, and coanalgesic drugs. The most widely used **coanalgesics** are the **antiepileptic drugs** and the **antidepressant drugs.** These drugs provide pain relief in chronic pain syndromes and may potentiate the effects of opioid and nonopioid analgesics.

Antiepileptic drugs (e.g., **carbamazepine, gabapentin, phenytoin,** and **valproate**) are particularly effective in treating pain syndromes with an intermittent lancinating quality, such as **trigeminal neuralgia** and **postherpetic neuralgia.** They are also useful in syndromes characterized by continuous, burning neuropathic pain. They probably act by inhibiting the conduction of pain impulses in the CNS, but their exact mechanism is unknown. **Pregabalin** (LYRICA) was also one of the first drugs indicated for the pain of **fibromyalgia.** The general properties of these drugs are described in Chapter 20.

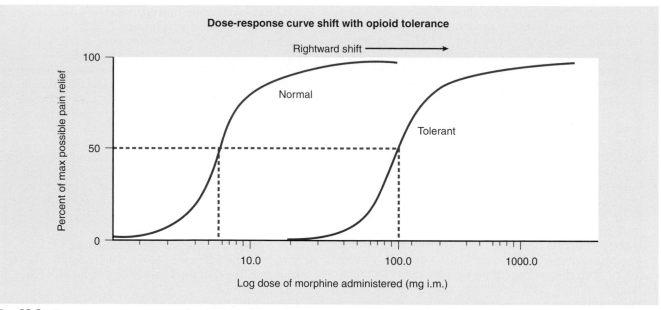

FIG. 23.3 Dose-response curves in normal and opioid-tolerant patients. Percent possible pain relief is plotted on the y-axis (vertical) and dose of morphine on the log x-axis (horizontal). *Dotted lines* represent the ED_{50} dose in these two sample populations. Note that the dose-response curve shifts to the right in the opioid-tolerant group, producing in this example about a 10-fold shift in the ED_{50}. This is the definition of decreased potency in the opioid tolerant dose-response curve. Also note that the efficacy (maximum effect on the y-axis) does not differ between the two curves.

The **tricyclic antidepressants** are the most widely used type of antidepressants for the treatment of chronic pain, as they may be more effective than the selective serotonin reuptake inhibitors in this respect. **Amitriptyline, desipramine,** and other tricyclic antidepressants are particularly effective in the management of postherpetic neuralgia, diabetic neuropathy, migraine headache, and neuropathic pain syndromes. They can also be beneficial in the management of pain associated with chronic fatigue syndrome. Of the newer serotonin-norepinephrine reuptake inhibitor (SNRI) antidepressants, **duloxetine** (CYMBALTA) recently added an indication for treating the pain of **fibromyalgia,** and the newest drug of this class, **milnacipran** (SAVELLA) is indicated only for this type of neuropathic pain. The properties of antidepressant drugs are described in Chapter 22.

Tramadol is a dual-action analgesic that combines opioid receptor activation with inhibition of neuronal reuptake of neurotransmitters in a manner similar to tricyclic antidepressants. As noted previously, tramadol is effective in many neuropathic pain syndromes and causes little constipation, respiratory depression, or drug dependence.

Cancer Pain

Pain is the most common symptom of cancer, and it can be acute, chronic, or intermittent. Cancer-related pain is frequently undertreated. Most patients can be managed with oral medications, including opioid and NSAID analgesics, antidepressant drugs, and antiepileptic drugs. Acupuncture, TENS, and other modalities are also useful. Severe cancer pain usually requires the administration of a strong opioid agonist (e.g., fentanyl, methadone, or morphine). To maintain stable serum drug levels and prevent breakthrough pain, it may be helpful to use a long-acting preparation (e.g., sustained-release morphine tablets or **transdermal fentanyl skin patches**), either alone or in combination with a rapid-acting preparation, such as morphine oral solution.

To help combat the constipation that often occurs with chronic opioid administration in cancer patients, an injectable formulation of **methylnaltrexone bromide** (RELISTOR) was developed. The methyl group on naltrexone, an opioid antagonist, prevents the penetration of the drug into the CNS so that the peripheral actions of opioids on the gut are blocked but not the central actions, such as analgesia. Newer opioid antagonists for the prevention of opioid-induced constipation include **naldemedine** and **naloxegol** (see also Chapter 28).

SUMMARY OF IMPORTANT POINTS

- Pain impulses are transmitted by primary afferent neurons to the spinal cord, where ascending connections from the spinothalamic tract neurons project to limbic structures and the cortex.
- Descending inhibitory fibers from the periaqueductal gray matter activate midbrain and spinal cord neurons that release enkephalins, serotonin, and norepinephrine. Opioids activate these pathways and thereby inhibit ascending pain impulses.
- Opioid drugs include strong and moderate agonists, mixed agonist-antagonists, and pure antagonists.
- In addition to analgesia, opioid agonists can cause sedation, euphoria, miosis, respiratory depression, peripheral vasodilation, constipation, and drug dependence.
- Opioid receptors can be divided into three types: *mu, delta,* and *kappa* opioid receptors. All types mediate analgesia, but *mu* opioid receptors are primarily responsible for analgesic effects, as well as respiratory depression and opioid dependence of most clinical agents.
- The strong opioid agonists include morphine, fentanyl, meperidine, and methadone, which act primarily at

mu opioid receptors. The first three of these agents are used to alleviate severe or moderate pain. Methadone is usually used in the treatment of opioid addiction (methadone maintenance programs).

- The moderate agonists produce maximal analgesia at doses that cannot be tolerated, so they are usually combined with a nonopioid analgesic. The moderate agonists, for example, codeine and hydrocodone, are used to treat moderate or mild pain.
- Other agonists include tramadol, a dual-action analgesic that activates opioid receptors and blocks neuronal reuptake of serotonin and norepinephrine.
- Buprenorphine, butorphanol, nalbuphine, and pentazocine are mixed opioid agonist-antagonists. These drugs exhibit partial agonist or antagonist activity at *mu* opioid receptors and exhibit agonist or antagonist activity at *kappa* opioid receptors. They produce less respiratory depression and are associated with a lower risk of drug dependence than are full opioid agonists.
- Naloxone and naltrexone are opioid antagonists. These antagonists are used to counteract the adverse effects of opioids in overdose or to prevent and treat alcohol and opioid dependence.

Review Questions

1. Most clinically used opioid analgesics are selective for which type of opioid receptor?
   (A) kappa (κ)
   (B) alpha (α)
   (C) beta (β)
   (D) mu (μ)
   (E) delta (δ)

2. Codeine has a greater oral bioavailability compared with morphine because of which reason?
   (A) codeine undergoes less first-pass metabolism
   (B) morphine is conjugated more quickly
   (C) morphine directly passes into systemic circulation
   (D) codeine is available only in liquid formulation
   (E) codeine is metabolized more by hepatic enzymes

3. Which of the following statements best explains the observation that morphine is more likely to cause nausea and vomiting in ambulatory patients?
   (A) morphine inhibits chemoreceptor trigger zone neurons
   (B) morphine sensitizes medulla cough center neurons
   (C) opioids cause sedation, which makes walking more difficult
   (D) patients on opioids eat more
   (E) opioids increase vestibular sensitivity

4. Which of the following opioids is so lipophilic that it is marketed in a skin patch used to treat chronic pain?
   (A) morphine
   (B) naltrexone
   (C) scopolamine
   (D) methadone
   (E) fentanyl

5. In a case of an opioid overdose, naloxone can be given in repeated doses because of which property of naloxone?
   (A) may have a shorter half-life than the opioid agonist
   (B) is effective only at high cumulative doses
   (C) is needed to stimulate the respiratory center
   (D) is safe only in extremely small doses
   (E) is only a partial opioid agonist

CHAPTER 24

Drugs for Neurodegenerative Diseases

CLASSIFICATION OF DRUGS FOR NEURODEGENERATIVE DISEASES

Drugs for Parkinson Disease

Drugs that increase dopamine levels
- Levodopa (LARODOPA)
- Carbidopa (LODOSYN)
- Levodopa and carbidopa (SINEMET)
- Entacapone (COMTAN)[a]
- Tolcapone (TASMAR)[b]
- Selegiline (ELDEPRYL)[c]
- Amantadine[d]

Dopamine receptor agonists
- Bromocriptine (PARLODEL)
- Pramipexole (MIRAPEX)
- Ropinirole (REQUIP)
- Rotigotine (NEUPRO)
- Apomorphine (APOKYN)

Cholinergic receptor antagonists
- Benztropine (COGENTIN)
- Trihexyphenidyl

Adjunct drugs for Parkinsonism
- Istradefylline (NOURIANZ)
- Pimavanserin (NUPLAZID)
- Dextromethorphan and quinidine (NUEDEXTA)

Drugs for Alzheimer Disease

Central acetylcholinesterase inhibitors
- Donepezil (ARICEPT)
- Rivastigmine (EXELON)
- Galantamine (RAZADYNE)

Additional drugs for Alzheimer disease
- Memantine (NAMENDA)[e]
- Caprylidene (AXONA)

Drugs for Huntington Disease
- Diazepam (VALIUM)
- Haloperidol (HALDOL)
- Tetrabenazine (XENAZINE)[f]

Drugs for Multiple Sclerosis
- Interferon *beta* (β)-1b (BETASERON)[g]
- Natalizumab (TYSABRI)[h]
- Mitoxantrone (NOVANTRONE)[i]
- Dalfampridine (AMPYRA)
- Fingolimod (GILENYA)[j]
- Teriflunomide (AUBAGIO)
- Dimethyl fumarate (TECFIDERA)

Drugs for Amyotrophic Lateral Sclerosis
- Gabapentin (NEURONTIN)
- Riluzole (RILUTEK)
- Edaravone (RADICAVA)

Antispastic Drugs[k]
- Baclofen (LIORESAL)
- Cyclobenzaprine (AMRIX)[l]
- Carisoprodol (SOMA)
- Tizanidine (ZANAFLEX)
- Dantrolene (DANTRIUM)
- OnabotulinumtoxinA (BOTOX)[m]

[a] Also in a triple combination of levodopa, carbidopa, and entacapone (STALEVO).
[b] Also opicapone (ONGENTYS).
[c] Also rasagiline (AZILECT) and safinamide (XADAGO).
[d] Also marketed in an extended-release tablet (OSMOLEX ER) or capsule (GOCOVRI).
[e] Also the combination of memantine extended-release and donepezil (NAMZARIC).
[f] Also deutetrabenazine (AUSTEDO)
[g] Also interferon β-1a (AVONEX), peginterferon β-1a (PLEGRIDY).
[h] Newer monoclonal antibody drugs also targeted to specific molecules in MS include daclizumab (ZINBRYTA), and alemtuzumab (LEMTRADA).
[i] Also glatiramer acetate (COPAXONE)
[j] Also siponimod (MAYZENT) and ozanimod (ZEPOSIA).
[k] Note that not all these agents are used uniquely for the treatment of spasticity in neurodegenerative diseases.
[l] Also orphenadrine (NORFLEX) and methocarbamol (ROBAXIN).
[m] Also abobotulinumtoxinA (DYSPORT), incobotulinumtoxinA (XEOMIN), prabotulinumtoxinA (JEUVEAU), and imabotulinumtoxinB (MYOBLOC).

OVERVIEW

Parkinson disease (PD), Huntington disease (HD), Alzheimer disease (AD), multiple sclerosis (MS), and amyotrophic lateral sclerosis (ALS, or Lou Gehrig disease) are **neurodegenerative diseases** characterized by the **progressive loss of neuronal function** in a particular part of the central nervous system (CNS). The signs and symptoms of neurodegenerative diseases do not reflect a normal age-related loss of brain neurons. Instead, these progressive diseases are

the result of an underlying pathologic process. There are a number of important drugs used to treat patients with these devastating neurodegenerative diseases. Spasticity is often a disorder seen along with neurodegenerative diseases; drugs used to treat spasticity close the chapter.

Although the cause of these diseases is unknown, evidence suggests the involvement of heredity, autoimmunity, and environmental factors. Substantial progress has been made in the development of drugs to treat PD and somewhat for AD; however, drug therapy for the other neurodegenerative diseases is limited. New research findings elucidating the pathogenesis of neurodegenerative diseases will enable the development of more successful drugs in the near future.

PARKINSON DISEASE

Parkinson disease (PD), a common neurodegenerative disease, is characterized by a **resting tremor** (involuntary trembling when a limb is at rest), **rigidity** (inability to initiate movements), and **bradykinesia** (slowness of movement). The disease results from the degeneration of **dopaminergic neurons that arise in the substantia nigra** and project to other structures in the basal ganglia.

Etiology and Pathogenesis

The causes of neuron degeneration in PD remain largely unknown. In most cases, heredity appears to have a limited role. Scientists, however, have identified a defective gene responsible for a rare condition called autosomal recessive juvenile parkinsonism, which usually affects people in their teens and 20s.

One of the better-known theories for the cause of PD is called the *oxidative stress theory*. According to this theory, metabolic oxidation of dopamine in the basal ganglia yields highly reactive free radicals that are **toxic to dopaminergic neurons** and lead to their degeneration. Free radicals are molecules that lack an electron in their outer orbits and are capable of extracting an electron from other molecules and thereby cause cell damage. It is not understood, however, why some individuals would be more susceptible to oxidative stress than others.

The basal ganglia are a group of interconnected subcortical nuclei that include the **striatum** (caudate and putamen), **substantia nigra, globus pallidus,** and **subthalamus**. In healthy individuals, the basal ganglia receive input from the cerebral cortex, process this information, and send feedback to the motor area of the cortex in a way that leads to the smooth coordination of body movements. Even simple movements, such as walking, involve a complex sequence of motor acts whose smooth execution requires the continuous interplay of the cortex and basal ganglia. In patients with PD, neuronal degeneration interrupts this interplay. Because the basal ganglia also participate in procedural memory and other cognitive functions, patients with PD may have difficulty remembering how to perform learned motor skills, such as driving a car.

The basal ganglia function via a series of reciprocal innervations among themselves and the cortex (Fig. 24.1). The striatum receives input from the cerebral cortex and substantia nigra and then sends output to the thalamus via the globus pallidus. The thalamus then feeds information back to the motor area of the cortex. Two pathways connect the striatum and the thalamus: a direct pathway—which is excitatory—and an indirect pathway—which is inhibitory. In patients with PD, the degeneration of dopaminergic neurons results in decreased activity in the direct pathway and increased activity in the indirect pathway. As a result, thalamic feedback to the cortex is reduced, and patients exhibit bradykinesia and rigidity.

Excitatory cholinergic neurons also participate in the interconnections between structures in the basal ganglia. In PD, the **degeneration of inhibitory dopaminergic neurons** leads to a relative excess of cholinergic activity in these pathways. For this reason, patients with PD can be treated effectively with drugs that inhibit cholinergic activity or with drugs that increase dopamine levels in the basal ganglia.

Drugs That Increase Dopamine Levels

Dopamine levels in the basal ganglia can be increased by various drugs in different ways. **Levodopa** increases dopamine levels by increasing dopamine synthesis; **selegiline** by inhibiting dopamine breakdown; and **amantadine** by increasing dopamine release from neurons. **Carbidopa** and **entacapone** increase the amount of levodopa that enters the brain and thereby enhance dopamine synthesis. The sites of action of these drugs are illustrated in Fig. 24.2.

Levodopa

Pharmacokinetics. **Levodopa**, also called l-dopa or dihydroxyphenylalanine, is the biosynthetic precursor of dopamine. Levodopa increases the concentration of dopamine in the brain and is the main treatment used to alleviate motor dysfunction in patients with PD. Dopamine itself is not effective in the treatment of PD when administered systemically, because it does not cross the blood-brain barrier to a significant extent.

Levodopa is absorbed from the proximal duodenum by the same process that absorbs large neutral amino acids (see Fig. 24.2). Dietary amino acids compete with levodopa for transport into the circulation, and amino acids can also reduce the transport of levodopa into the brain. For these reasons, the ingestion of high-protein foods can decrease the effectiveness of levodopa, and a protein-restricted diet may improve the response to levodopa in some patients.

Levodopa is metabolized by two enzymes in the periphery. It is converted to **dopamine** by **aromatic amino acid decarboxylase (AAAD)**, and it is metabolized to **methyldopa** by catechol-O-methyltransferase (COMT). A drug that inhibits AAAD (e.g., **carbidopa**) and inhibits COMT (e.g., **entacapone**) are used in combination with levodopa to **prevent breakdown of levodopa in the blood, which increases levodopa in the brain**. AAAD requires vitamin B_6 (**pyridoxine**) as a cofactor. For this reason, vitamin B_6 supplements enhance the peripheral decarboxylation of levodopa and should not be co-administered with levodopa.

Levodopa exhibits a **large first-pass effect**, and about 95% of an administered dose is metabolized in the gut wall and liver before it reaches the systemic circulation. Additional amounts of levodopa are converted to dopamine and methyldopa before the drug enters the CNS. Therefore, only about 1% of the administered dose of levodopa reaches brain tissue.

Mechanisms and Pharmacologic Effects. In the brain, **levodopa** is taken up by dopaminergic neurons in the striatum and **converted to dopamine by AAAD**. This strategy is called **precursor loading**. Levodopa thereby **increases the amount of dopamine** released by these neurons in patients with PD, and it serves as a form of **replacement therapy**. Levodopa can counteract all of the signs of parkinsonism, although the degree and duration of its effectiveness usually are not optimal. As the disease progresses and more dopaminergic neurons are lost, the conversion of levodopa to dopamine declines.

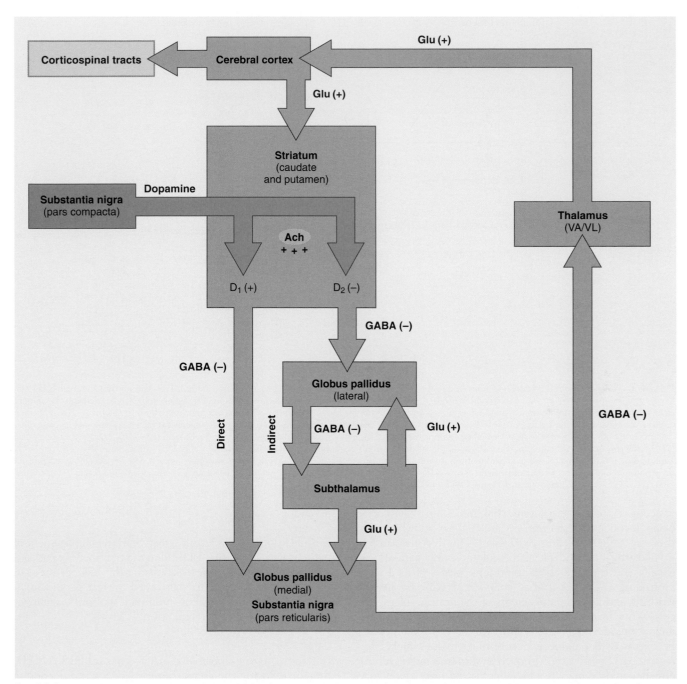

Fig. 24.1 Pathophysiology of Parkinson disease. The striatum receives input from the entire cerebral cortex and the substantia nigra and sends projections to the thalamus via direct and indirect pathways through the globus pallidus, substantia nigra, and subthalamus. Striatal dopamine D_1 receptors excite the direct pathway, whereas D_2 receptors inhibit the indirect pathway. In Parkinson disease, the degeneration of dopaminergic neurons leads to decreased activity in the direct pathway and increased activity in the indirect pathway. As a result of these changes, thalamic input to the motor area of the cortex is reduced, and the patient exhibits rigidity and bradykinesia. *Ach,* acetylcholine; *ACh E,* acetylcholinesterase; *Ach R,* cholinergic receptor; *AMPA R,* glutamate receptor; *APP,* amyloid precursor proteins; *GABA, Gamma*-aminobutyric acid; *Glu,* glutamate; *NSAID,* nonsteroidal anti-inflammatory drug; *PPAR,* peroxisome proliferator-activated receptor; *VA/VL,* ventral anterior and ventral lateral nuclei; (+), excitatory; (−), inhibitory.

About 60% to 70% of **nigrostriatal dopaminergic neurons are lost** before the clinical symptoms of PD are first observed, and the degeneration of these neurons continues throughout the course of the disease. Over time, patients begin to experience two types of fluctuation in the effectiveness of levodopa, both of which are probably related to a reduced concentration of dopamine in the striatum. The first type, a *wearing off* effect, occurs toward the end of a dosage interval. The second type, the *on-off* phenomenon, is characterized by severe motor fluctuations that occur randomly.

Adverse Effects. When levodopa is used alone, **nausea** and **vomiting** occur in about 80% of patients, orthostatic hypotension is reported in 25%, and cardiac dysrhythmias occur in 10%. These effects, which are caused by the action of dopamine on β-adrenoceptors in the case of cardiac arrhythmias, are substantially reduced when **carbidopa** (see later) is administered with levodopa to block the peripheral formation of dopamine.

About 30% of patients who are treated with levodopa on a long-term basis eventually **develop involuntary movements,** or **dyskinesias,** as a result of excessive dopamine

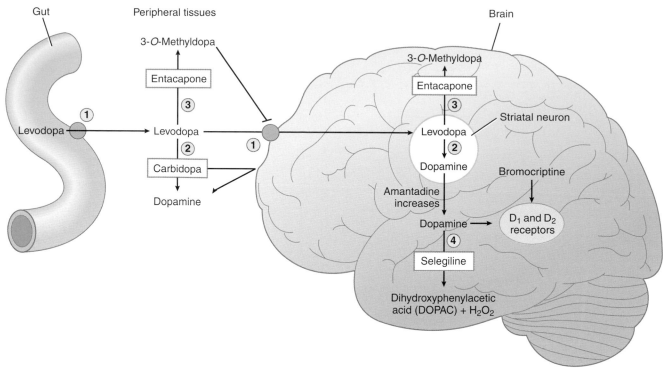

FIG. 24.2 Mechanisms of dopaminergic drugs used in the treatment of Parkinson disease. Levodopa is transported across the gut wall and the blood-brain barrier and is converted to dopamine in striatal neurons. Carbidopa inhibits the peripheral decarboxylation of levodopa and thereby increases the amount of levodopa that enters the brain. Carbidopa does not cross the blood-brain barrier and does not inhibit dopamine synthesis in the brain. Tolcapone and entacapone inhibit the methylation of levodopa in both peripheral tissues and the brain. Tolcapone and entacapone increase levodopa bioavailability and increase brain uptake of levodopa. Selegiline inhibits the degradation of dopamine to dihydroxyphenylacetic acid (*DOPAC*) and hydrogen peroxide (H_2O_2). By this action, selegiline increases dopamine levels in the striatum, and it may reduce the formation of free radicals that are derived from H_2O_2. Amantadine increases the release of dopamine from striatal neurons. Bromocriptine and other dopamine-receptor agonists activate dopamine receptors in the striatum. Numbered structures and enzymes are as follows: (*1*) pump that transports large neutral amino acids; (*2*) aromatic L-amino acid decarboxylase (*AAAD*); (*3*) catechol-O-methyltransferase (*COMT*); (*4*) monoamine oxidase type B (*MAO-B*).

concentrations in the striatum. Dyskinesias most often occur when levodopa concentrations are highest, in which case they are called *peak-dose dyskinesias*. The dyskinesias often involve the oral and facial musculature, and patients can appear as if they are chewing on large pieces of food while protruding their lips. Other common dyskinesias involve writhing and flinging movements of the arms and legs. Less commonly, levodopa causes psychotic effects, including hallucinations and distorted thinking, which are probably caused by excessive dopamine concentrations in mesolimbic and mesocortical pathways. Although **dyskinesias** and **psychotic effects** could be managed by reducing the levodopa dosage, the therapeutic efficacy of the drug would be reduced as well.

Some patients treated with levodopa report sedative effects, agitation, delirium, vivid dreams, or nightmares. Others, however, report a pleasant euphoria after taking the drug.

Interactions. Levodopa has important interactions with a number of medications. Drugs that delay gastric emptying, such as anticholinergic drugs, can slow levodopa absorption and reduce its peak serum concentration. Drugs that promote gastric emptying (e.g., antacids) can increase levodopa bioavailability. Nonselective monoamine oxidase inhibitors (MAOIs)—for example, the antidepressant **phenelzine**—inhibit the breakdown of dopamine and sometimes cause a hypertensive crisis in patients receiving levodopa. Antipsychotic drugs block dopamine receptors and can reduce the effectiveness of levodopa and exacerbate motor dysfunction. Because **clozapine** is much less likely to do this than other antipsychotic drugs, it is often used to manage

psychotic reactions in patients receiving levodopa (see Chapter 22).

Indications. Levodopa is effective in the management of patients with **idiopathic PD** and in the treatment of patients with **postencephalitic parkinsonism**, a disorder portrayed in the movie *Awakenings*. It is also used to treat parkinsonian symptoms caused by carbon monoxide poisoning, manganese intoxication, or cerebral arteriosclerosis.

Carbidopa

Carbidopa, a structural analog of levodopa, **inhibits AAAD**, thereby reducing the conversion of levodopa to dopamine in peripheral tissues and increasing the amount of levodopa that enters the brain (see Fig. 24.2). Carbidopa is highly ionized at physiologic pH, and it does not cross the blood-brain barrier. For this reason, it does not inhibit the formation of dopamine in the CNS.

Carbidopa substantially reduces the gastrointestinal and cardiovascular side effects of levodopa and enables about a 75% reduction in the dosage of levodopa. A **levodopa-carbidopa combination** is available in immediate-release and sustained-release formulations that contain different ratios of the two drugs. The sustained-release formulations are designed to reduce the "wearing off" effect described earlier.

Tolcapone

Tolcapone is a drug used to enhance the effectiveness of levodopa in the treatment of PD. It **inhibits COMT**, the enzyme that metabolizes levodopa to methyldopa in the gut and liver. By this action, tolcapone produces a twofold increase in the oral bioavailability and half-life of levodopa. Because methyldopa competes with levodopa for transport into brain tissue, it may contribute to the *wearing off* and *on-off* effects that occur during long-term levodopa therapy. By inhibiting methyldopa formation, tolcapone may stabilize dopamine levels in the striatum and contribute to a more sustained improvement in motor function.

In clinical studies, **tolcapone** was found to increase the efficacy of levodopa while reducing the dosage requirement. Tolcapone was well tolerated, and most of the side effects were similar in frequency to those reported with use of a placebo. Although tolcapone caused diarrhea and nausea in some patients, these side effects decreased over time. A few reports were made of rare but fatal hepatitis after administration of tolcapone.

Entacapone

Entacapone has the same mechanism of action as tolcapone but is more peripherally restricted in its distribution. It may be safer to use for the treatment of parkinsonism than tolcapone because there are **no reports of hepatic toxicity**. Whereas tolcapone is available only as a single-ingredient product (TASMAR), entacapone is available in combination products with levodopa and carbidopa (STALEVO). The latest catechol-O-methyltransferase (COMT) inhibitor is **opicapone**, which is used in conjunction with levodopa/carbidopa in patients with Parkinson disease experiencing "off" episodes.

Selegiline

Pharmacokinetics. Selegiline, also known as *deprenyl*, is a modified phenylethylamine compound. The drug is well absorbed from the gut and is partly metabolized to amphetamine.

Mechanisms and Pharmacologic Effects. Selegiline **inhibits monoamine oxidase type B** (MAO-B) and thereby prevents the oxidation of dopamine to dihydroxyphenylacetic acid and hydrogen peroxide, as shown in Fig. 24.2. By this action, selegiline **increases dopamine levels** in the basal ganglia and decreases the formation of hydrogen peroxide. In the presence of iron, hydrogen peroxide is converted to hydroxyl and hydroxide free radicals that may participate in the degeneration of nigrostriatal neurons in patients with PD.

There is evidence that selegiline **inhibits the progression of PD** either by inhibiting the formation of free radicals or by inhibiting the formation of an active metabolite of an environmental toxin. However, the ability of selegiline to inhibit disease progression is controversial. It was initially suggested by studies showing that selegiline could prevent a form of parkinsonism induced by 1-methyl-4-phenyl-1,2,3,6-tetrahydropyridine (MPTP). MPTP is a toxic byproduct of the synthesis of *designer* street drugs; in the 1980s, people who took what they thought was a meperidine analog ingested drugs contaminated with MPTP and developed classic signs of parkinsonism. MPTP must be converted to 1-methyl-4-phenylpyridinium by MAO-B before it can damage dopaminergic neurons, and studies have demonstrated that selegiline blocked this reaction. The results of these studies have led some investigators to postulate that idiopathic PD is caused by an **environmental toxin** whose action resembles that of MPTP. Although unfortunate for the drug abusers who were exposed to MPTP, it did lead to an important animal model for parkinsonism and the development of new agents.

Adverse Effects and Interactions. Adverse effects are listed in Table 24.1. Unlike the nonselective MAOIs used in treating mood disorders, **selegiline does not inhibit monoamine oxidase type A** (MAO-A), an enzyme that catalyzes the degradation of catecholamines. For this reason, selegiline is much less likely to cause hypertension when it is administered in combination with sympathomimetic amines or when it is taken with foods that contain tyramine. The drug's selectivity for MAO-B, however, is lost when it is given in higher doses, so the potential for food interaction still exists. Selegiline can cause adverse effects if it is administered with **meperidine** or with selective serotonin reuptake inhibitors (SSRIs; e.g., **fluoxetine**), as noted in Chapter 22.

Indications. Selegiline can be used as a single drug for the treatment of early or mild PD, and it is used as an adjunct with levodopa-carbidopa for advanced disease. Selegiline **reduces the dosage requirement** for levodopa, and it may improve motor function in patients who experience *wearing off* and *on-off* difficulties with levodopa.

The most controversial role of selegiline is its use as a neuroprotective agent. Although some clinical studies have indicated that selegiline slows the progression of PD, others have indicated that it does not.

Recently, a second MAO-B inhibitor, **rasagiline**, was approved as a monotherapy or adjunct medication in the treatment of parkinsonism. It has the same potential adverse effects as selegiline, owing to interactions with tyramine, meperidine, and SSRIs. Most recently, the selective MOA-B inhibitor **safinamide** was approved as an adjunctive treatment to levodopa/carbidopa in patients with PD experiencing "off" episodes.

Amantadine

Amantadine is an **antiviral drug** used in the prevention and treatment of influenza (Chapter 43) but also has a beneficial effect on PD. Amantadine appears to work by **increasing the release of dopamine** from nigrostriatal neurons, but it may also inhibit the reuptake of dopamine by these neurons. Amantadine is generally better tolerated than levodopa or dopamine agonists, but it is also less effective.

Amantadine is used to treat early or mild cases of PD and as an adjunct to levodopa. Its adverse effects include sedation, restlessness, vivid dreams, nausea, dry mouth, and hypotension. It can also cause **livedo reticularis**, which is a reddish-blue mottling of the skin with edema. CNS side effects are more likely to occur in the elderly because of their reduced capacity to excrete the drug via the kidneys. **Amantadine** is also marketed in an extended-release tablet (OSMOLEX ER) or capsule (GOCOVRI). The extended-release capsule has the advantage in that its contents may be sprinkled on soft foods for the PD patient having problems with chewing and swallowing.

Dopamine Receptor Agonists

The dopamine-receptor agonists **directly activate dopamine receptors** in the striatum. Because they do not require a functional dopaminergic neuron to produce their effects, they are sometimes helpful in advanced cases of PD, in which few dopaminergic neurons remain. The drugs work primarily by activating D_2 receptors. As shown in Fig. 24.1, activation of these receptors leads to inhibition of the indirect neuronal pathway from the striatum to the thalamus and increases thalamic stimulation of the motor area of the cortex.

TABLE 24.1 Major Adverse Effects and Major Interactions of Selected Drugs for Neurodegenerative Diseases

DRUG	MAJOR ADVERSE EFFECTS	MAJOR DRUG INTERACTIONS
Drugs for Parkinson Disease		
Drugs that Increase Dopamine Levels		
Amantadine	Dry mouth, hypotension, livedo reticularis, nausea, restlessness, sedation, and vivid dreams.	Benztropine and trihexyphenidyl potentiate CNS side effects.
Levodopa-carbidopa	Agitation; arrhythmias; delirium; distorted thinking, hallucinations, and other psychotic effects; dyskinesias; hypotension; nausea and vomiting; nightmares or vivid dreams; and sedation.	Antacids may increase bioavailability. Anticholinergic drugs may reduce peak serum level. Antipsychotic drugs, such as haloperidol, may decrease effects. Nonselective MAOIs, such as phenelzine, may cause a hypertensive crisis.
Selegiline	Confusion; dyskinesias; hallucinations; hypotension; insomnia; and nausea.	Severe reactions may result if taken with meperidine or with fluoxetine or other SSRIs.
Rasagiline	Same as selegiline.	Same as selegiline.
Tolcapone	Diarrhea and nausea.	Unknown.
Entacapone	Diarrhea and nausea.	Unknown.
Dopamine Receptor Agonists		
Bromocriptine	Confusion, decreased prolactin levels, dry mouth, dyskinesias, hallucinations, nausea, orthostatic hypotension, sedation, and vivid dreams.	Dopamine antagonists may reduce effects.
Pramipexole	Dizziness, hallucinations, insomnia, nausea and vomiting, and sedation.	Cimetidine inhibits renal excretion and increases serum levels.
Ropinirole	Same as pramipexole.	Ciprofloxacin increases serum levels.
Rotigotine	Somnolence, slight BP and HR increase, site irritation.	Sulfite sensitivity; no major drug interactions.
Acetylcholine Receptor Antagonists		
Benztropine	Agitation, confusion, constipation, delirium, dry mouth, memory loss, urinary retention, and tachycardia.	Additive anticholinergic effect with antihistamines and phenothiazines.
Trihexyphenidyl	Same as benztropine.	Same as benztropine.
Drugs for Huntington Disease		
Diazepam	Arrhythmias, CNS depression, drug dependence, hypotension, and mild respiratory depression.	Alcohol and other CNS depressants potentiate effects. Cimetidine increases and rifampin decreases serum levels.
Haloperidol	Extrapyramidal side effects and increased prolactin levels.	Barbiturates and carbamazepine decrease and quinidine increases serum levels.
Drugs for Alzheimer Disease		
Donepezil	Bradycardia, diarrhea, gastrointestinal bleeding, and nausea and vomiting.	Anticholinergic drugs inhibit effects.
Rivastigmine	Risk of bradycardia and AV block; nausea and vomiting, anorexia, weight loss.	Anticholinergic drugs inhibit effects. Nicotine use increases oral clearance.
Galantamine	Risk of bradycardia and AV block; nausea and vomiting	Anticholinergic drugs inhibit effects. Inhibitors of CYP2D6 increase serum levels.
Memantine	Confusion, dizziness, drowsiness, headache, and insomnia.	Carbonic anhydrase inhibitors reduce renal elimination of memantine.
Drugs for Multiple Sclerosis		
Baclofen	Dizziness, fatigue, and weakness	Unknown.
Interferon β-1b	Chills, diarrhea, fever, headache, hypertension, myalgia, pain, and vomiting.	Increases serum levels of zidovudine.
Prednisone	Aggravation of diabetes mellitus, gastrointestinal bleeding, mood changes, pancreatitis, and seizures.	Barbiturates, carbamazepine, phenytoin, and rifampin decrease serum levels.
Drugs for Amyotrophic Lateral Sclerosis		
Baclofen	Dizziness, fatigue, and weakness.	Unknown.
Gabapentin	Ataxia, dizziness, drowsiness, nystagmus, and tremor.	Antacids decrease serum levels.
Riluzole	Asthenia, diarrhea, dizziness, drowsiness, increased hepatic enzyme levels, nausea and vomiting, paresthesias, and vertigo.	Quinolones and theophylline can increase serum levels. Omeprazole, rifampin, and smoking can decrease serum levels.

AV, Atrioventricular; *BP,* blood pressure; *CNS,* central nervous system; *HR,* heart rate; *MAOI,* monoamine oxidase inhibitor; *SSRI,* selective serotonin reuptake inhibitor.

Bromocriptine

Bromocriptine is an **ergot alkaloid** in the same chemical class as the hallucinogen lysergic acid diethylamide (LSD). Other ergot alkaloids used to treat migraine headaches are discussed in Chapter 29. Bromocriptine is a D_2-receptor agonist and a D_1-receptor antagonist. Bromocriptine can serve as a useful adjunct to levodopa in patients who have advanced PD and experience *wearing off* effects and *on-off* motor fluctuations. Interestingly, although the mechanism is not known, **bromocriptine** in a formulation called CYCLOSET was recently approved for the **treatment of type 2 diabetes** (see Chapter 35).

Dopamine-receptor agonists produce **adverse effects that are similar to those of levodopa.** Nausea, which occurs in as many as 50% of patients when they are first treated with a receptor agonist, primarily results from stimulation of dopamine receptors in the vomiting center located in the medulla. Dose-related CNS effects of the receptor agonists include **confusion, dyskinesias, sedation, vivid dreams,** and **hallucinations.** Other adverse effects include orthostatic hypotension, dry mouth, and decreased prolactin levels. Nausea and many other adverse effects subside over time. To enable patients to develop tolerance to the effects, treatment should begin with a low dose, and the dosage should be increased gradually.

Pergolide (PERMAX), is also an ergot alkaloid and direct-acting dopamine agonist, but it was withdrawn from the market in 2007 owing to increased risk of **damage to heart valves**.

Pramipexole and Ropinirole

In contrast to the older dopamine-receptor agonists, **pramipexole** and **ropinirole** are not ergot alkaloids. Both act as selective D_2-receptor agonists. In addition, pramipexole activates D_3-receptors, and this may contribute to its effectiveness in PD. The adverse effects, contraindications, and drug interactions of pramipexole and ropinirole are summarized in Table 24.1.

Clinical studies have shown that pramipexole or ropinirole can **delay the need for levodopa** when used in early stages of PD. In advanced stages, these agents can reduce the "off" period and decrease the levodopa dosage requirement. Thus, although the bromocriptine is primarily used as adjunct therapy in advanced PD, the newer agonists may prove effective as monotherapy in both early and advanced disease.

Pramipexole and ropinirole are also indicated for the **treatment of restless legs syndrome,** a condition characterized by an urge to move the legs at night in bed, often coupled with unpleasant sensations (paresthesias) in the legs that are reduced by movement.

Rotigotine

Rotigotine (NEUPRO) is a newer, nonergot dopamine agonist formulated as a **transdermal patch preparation.** Like pramipexole, rotigotine has selectivity for D_2 over D_1 receptors and additional activity at D_3 receptors, which has been linked to **slowing progression of neurodegenerative diseases.** Like pramipexole and ropinirole discussed previously, the rotigotine patch is also indicated for the treatment of restless legs syndrome.

Apomorphine

Apomorphine, which is chemically related to morphine, does not bind to opioid receptors but rather is a **dopamine receptor agonist.** It is actually an old drug put to a new use and was recently approved for the **treatment of acute, intermittent** hypomobility (*freezing*) episodes associated with advanced PD. It is available for injection only and produces a rapid (within five to 10 minutes) reversal of the hypomobility state.

Cholinergic Receptor Antagonists

Several **centrally acting** anticholinergic drugs are used in the management of PD. Two examples are **benztropine** and **trihexyphenidyl,** which are antagonists at cholinergic muscarinic receptors and also exhibit some antihistamine activity. The anticholinergic drugs are generally less effective than the dopaminergic drugs, but they may be helpful as adjunct therapy in combination with levodopa and other drugs that augment dopaminergic activity. The anticholinergic drugs are **more effective in reducing** tremor than in reducing other manifestations of PD, although they may provide some reduction of bradykinesia and rigidity in patients with mild dysfunction. Benztropine may also inhibit the neuronal reuptake of dopamine by central dopaminergic neurons and thereby prolong the action of dopamine.

In addition to being useful in the treatment of early and advanced PD, the anticholinergic drugs can also reduce parkinsonian symptoms caused by dopamine receptor antagonists, such as **haloperidol** (see Chapter 22).

Adjunct Drugs for Parkinsonism

Istradefylline

Istradefylline is a first in-class adenosine antagonist at the A_2 receptor indicated as adjunctive treatment to levodopa/carbidopa in adult patients with Parkinson disease (PD) experiencing "off" episodes. Although the exact mechanism of the therapeutic effects of istradefylline are unknown, the basal ganglia is rich in A2 receptors and that area in the brain is key to generating movement. **Istradefylline reduced the release of GABA** in the basal ganglia in animal models. It is feasible that less inhibition by GABA increases the motor function of the basal ganglia and reduces "off" episodes in PD patients.

Pimavanserin

Recently, a new atypical antipsychotic agent called **pimavanserin** was approved solely for the treatment of hallucinations and delusions in patients with PD. Antipsychotic agents are discussed further in Chapter 22. Compared to other atypical antipsychotics, **pimavanserin** can be considered the **most selective as a serotonergic receptor antagonist** (at the 5-HT_2 receptors) with little to no affinity for dopamine (including D_2), histamine, muscarinic, or adrenergic receptors.

Dextromethorphan and Quinidine

The combination formulation of **dextromethorphan and quinidine** may be helpful if the PD patient experiences signs of **pseudobulbar affect,** which occurs as sudden outbursts of crying or laughter for no reason. Pseudobulbar affect also occurs with Alzheimer disease (AD), traumatic brain injury, stroke, amyotrophic lateral sclerosis (ALS), and multiple sclerosis (MS). Emotional lability (also called **pseudobulbar affect**) is often seen in patients with neurodegenerative diseases, including AD, MS, and ALS (see later). **Quinidine is an inhibitor of the CYP2D6** metabolic enzyme in the liver. Because **dextromethorphan is metabolized by CYP2D6,** quinidine is added to increase the bioavailability of dextromethorphan. **Dextromethorphan inhibits excitatory glutamate release** by agonist action at *sigma*-1 (σ_1) receptors and is an **antagonist** at **NMDA glutamate receptors**. In this way, the excitatory neurotransmission that underlies emotional lability is reduced.

Treatment Considerations

Optimal management of PD requires that the disabilities of each patient be carefully assessed before drug treatment is recommended. Early disease of mild intensity can be best managed with exercise, nutrition, and education. Speech, occupational, and physical therapies can also be helpful.

For patients whose clinical manifestations are limited to mild tremor and slowness, **anticholinergic drugs** or **amantadine** may be helpful.

For patients with more severe functional disabilities, the **dopaminergic drugs are the most effective treatment**. Combination therapy with **levodopa and carbidopa** is usually prescribed for these patients, but monotherapy with a new dopamine receptor agonist (e.g., pramipexole or ropinirole) may provide an effective alternative for patients who have either early or advanced PD. Clinicians should remember that dopaminergic drugs have a delayed onset of action, so improvement in the patient's condition may not be noted until 2 to 3 weeks after therapy is started.

Tolcapone and **entacapone** inhibit the metabolism of levodopa, and **selegiline** inhibits the metabolism of dopamine, and these agents can be used to enhance the effectiveness of levodopa in patients with early or advanced disease. Some clinicians begin **selegiline** treatment early in the disease in an effort to retard disease progression.

For patients who have more advanced disease and begin to experience the *wearing off* and *on-off* **fluctuations of levodopa-carbidopa,** it is sometimes helpful to change the drug dosage or formulation. For example, the *wearing off* effect can be minimized by increasing the frequency of doses or using a combination of sustained-release and immediate-release formulations. Alternatively, an additional dopaminergic drug can be added to the treatment regimen. The addition of **tolcapone,** for example, may reduce motor fluctuations by increasing and stabilizing levodopa concentrations in the striatum. **Apomorphine,** a nonergot dopamine agonist, may provide quick relief from periods of **hypomobility**.

For PD patients experiencing hallucinations and delusions, **pimavanserin** is available, and for signs of **pseudobulbar affect,** the combination formulation of **dextromethorphan and quinidine** is useful.

ALZHEIMER DISEASE

Etiology and Pathogenesis

Alzheimer disease (AD) is a type of **progressive dementia** for which no cause is known, and no cure has been found. In the United States, AD accounts for about 60% of all cases of dementia in patients over 65 years of age and is associated with more than 100,000 deaths each year. The disease has a tremendous negative effect on patients and their families because of its devastating effects on the **cognitive, emotional,** and **physical function** of the patient with AD (Box 24.1).

AD results from the **destruction of** cholinergic and other neurons in the cortex and limbic structures of the brain, particularly the amygdala, basal forebrain, and hippocampus. Major changes in these structures include cortical atrophy, neurofibrillary tangles, and neuritic plaques containing β-amyloid **protein**. The cholinergic neurons destroyed in AD originate in

the **Meynert nucleus (nucleus basalis)** in the forebrain. These neurons project to the frontal cortex and hippocampus, and they have a critical role in memory and cognition.

Central Acetylcholinesterase Inhibitors

As seen in the treatment of PD above, inhibition of the enzymes that metabolize neurotransmitters is a powerful way to increase neurotransmitter levels. In patients with AD, there is a deficit in cholinergic neurotransmission due to destruction of neurons producing acetylcholine. Treatment with central anticholinesterase inhibitors—such as **donepezil, rivastigmine,** or **galantamine**—is given in an effort to improve cholinergic neurotransmission in the affected areas of the brain. Although these centrally acting cholinesterase inhibitors may slow the deterioration of cognitive function, they do not affect the underlying neurodegenerative process, so the disease is eventually fatal. The adverse effects and drug interactions of donepezil, rivastigmine, or galantamine are outlined Table 24.1.

Donepezil

Studies in patients with AD have demonstrated that those treated with donepezil for 24 weeks had significantly better cognitive function than those treated with a placebo. **Donepezil is a reversible cholinesterase inhibitor** that selectively inhibits cholinesterase in the CNS and increases acetylcholine levels in the cerebral cortex. The drug is well absorbed after oral administration and crosses the blood-brain barrier. Because it has a long half-life of about 70 hours, it is administered once a day. The adverse effects of donepezil include diarrhea, nausea, and vomiting, but these are usually mild and transient. Unlike tacrine (see later), **donepezil is not associated with hepatotoxicity.**

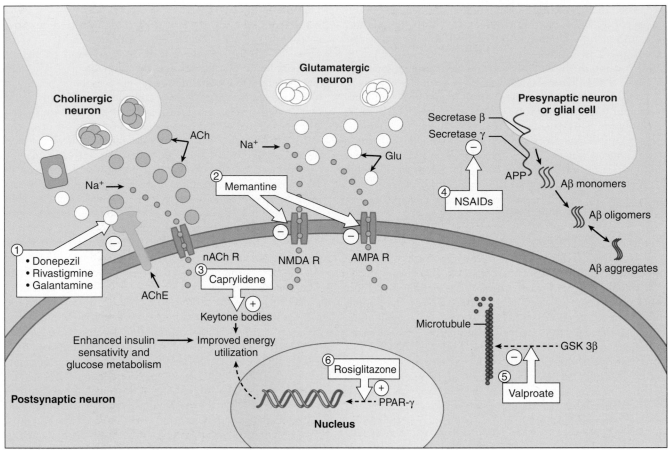

FIG. 24.3 Mechanism of action of drugs for the treatment of Alzheimer disease. *(1)* The central acetylcholinesterase inhibitors—donepezil, rivastigmine, and galantamine—block the acetylcholinesterase enzyme and increase synaptic concentration of acetylcholine. *(2)* Memantine blocks glutamate neurotransmission at NMDA receptors. *(3)* Caprylidene improves energy utilization by neurons in the AD patient. *(4)* NSAIDs such as fluriprofen may decrease formation of aggregates by inhibiting secretase enzymes. *(5)* The antiepileptic drug (AED) valproic acid may block the dissociation of microtubules and by action on GSK-3β. *(6)* The antidiabetic agent—rosiglitazone—increases insulin sensitivity and glucose utilization, which has been shown to improve cognitive function in AD patients. Mechanism and drugs at *(4)*, *(5)*, and *(6)* are not approved yet for treatment of AD but are in clinical trials. *Glu,* glutamate; *GSK-3β,* glycogen synthase kinase 3β; *NMDA,* N-methyl-d-aspartate

Tacrine was the first centrally acting cholinesterase inhibitor approved for the treatment of AD. It has a lower bioavailability and a shorter half-life than donepezil, and it must be administered several times a day. Tacrine, an acridine compound, is associated with a **significant incidence of hepatotoxicity** and with peripheral cholinergic side effects— such as diarrhea, nausea, and urinary incontinence. Because of these adverse effects, few patients can tolerate the higher doses required to demonstrate cognitive improvement in AD, and tacrine (COGNEX) has been withdrawn from the market.

Rivastigmine and Galantamine

Rivastigmine is a newer, centrally acting, reversible cholinesterase inhibitor. Taken in divided doses, it significantly delays the global cognitive impairment associated with AD for at least 6 months in clinical trials. Recently, a **transdermal formulation of rivastigmine** (EXELON PATCH) was introduced; it is applied every 24 hours, increasing patient compliance and simplifying caregiver administration. **Galantamine** is also a newer, centrally acting, reversible cholinesterase inhibitor. It was discovered from the extracts from the bulbs of the daffodil, *Narcissus pseudonarcissus.* Like rivastigmine, it has been shown to slow the progression of AD. The mechanisms of action for these drugs and other agents are shown in Fig. 24.3.

Additional Drugs for Alzheimer Disease

Memantine is a recently approved agent with a new mechanism of action for the treatment of the dementia of AD. Memantine is a low potency, **noncompetitive antagonist at the N-methyl-d-aspartate (NMDA) receptor**. It is hypothesized to work by attenuating the excitotoxic effects of glutamate that may underlie the pathologic process of neuronal loss in AD. It is excreted largely unchanged as the parent molecule. The combination of **memantine extended-release with donepezil** (NAMZARIC) is also available to improve efficacy and compliance.

Using a different approach to treat AD, **caprylidene** was developed as **medical food** that is metabolized into ketone bodies, which the brain can use for energy when the processing of glucose is impaired. Magnetic resonance imaging (MRI) scans of the elderly and those with AD reveal a significantly decreased ability for glucose uptake, the brain's preferred source of energy. Caprylidene replaces depleted glucose levels to treat patients with age-associated memory impairment and AD.

HUNTINGTON DISEASE
Etiology and Pathogenesis

HD, also called Huntington chorea, is an **autosomal dominant hereditary disorder** that is characterized by abnormally expansive or **choreoathetoid movements** (dancelike movements) of the limbs, rhythmic movements of the tongue and face, and mental deterioration that leads to personality disorders, psychosis, and dementia. Patients are usually in their late 30s when the disease begins, and progressive respiratory depression usually causes death in 10 to 15 years.

HD is caused by the **degeneration of *gamma*-aminobutyric acid (GABA) neurons** in the striatum and elsewhere in the brain. This degeneration may be fueled by excessive release of the excitatory amino acid glutamate and glutamate-induced neurotoxicity. The loss of GABA neurons that project from the striatum to the lateral globus pallidus leads to disinhibition of thalamic nuclei and to an increase in thalamic input to the motor area of the cortex (see Fig. 24.1).

Treatment

The symptoms of HD are consistent with **excessive dopaminergic activity** in the basal ganglia. Therefore, **drugs that block dopamine receptors** (e.g., **haloperidol**) and other antipsychotic drugs (see Chapter 22) produce some improvement in motor function and are also helpful in relieving the psychosis that accompanies the disease. **Diazepam** and other benzodiazepine drugs (see Chapter 19) potentiate GABA and can also reduce excess movements in patients with HD. The efficacy of benzodiazepines, however, declines significantly with disease progression.

Tetrabenazine, the first drug approved specifically for the treatment of chorea in HD, was recently approved by the U.S. Food and Drug Administration (FDA). It is a monoamine depletor for oral administration. However, the precise mechanism by which tetrabenazine exerts its antichorea effects is unknown. **Tetrabenazine reversibly inhibits the human vesicular monoamine transporter type 2 (VMAT2)**, resulting in decreased uptake of monoamines into synaptic vesicles and depletion of monoamine stores (e.g., dopamine, serotonin, and norepinephrine), leading to decreased neurotransmitter released from nerve terminals. It is likely that decreased neurotransmission from these neurotransmitters decreases the episodes of chorea. A second VMAT2 inhibitor for treatment of the symptoms of HC is **deutetrabenazine.**

In the future, new treatments may result from identification and gene editing correction (using CRISPR) of the *huntingtin* gene. Drugs that inhibit glutamate neurotoxicity might also prove useful in the treatment of this disease.

MULTIPLE SCLEROSIS
Etiology and Pathogenesis

MS is a chronic disease characterized by the **demyelination of neurons** in the CNS. Although its cause is unknown, the disease is postulated to have an **autoimmune** or **viral** origin. Demyelination leads to disruption of nerve transmission and is accompanied by an inflammatory response and the formation of plaques in the brain and spinal cord. These plaques typically contain decreased numbers of oligodendrocytes (myelin-forming cells). The neurologic symptoms of MS, which depend on the area of the brain that is affected, can include pain, spasticity, weakness, ataxia, fatigue, and problems with speech, vision, gait, and bladder function. Many patients experience **relapses** and **remissions**, but some have a more severe and unremitting progression of disease.

Treatment

Interferon β-1b was the first drug to demonstrate an ability to halt and even reverse the progression of MS in some cases. In clinical studies, the drug was found to **reduce the frequency of relapses** and the number of new lesions detected by MRI in patients who were ambulatory, had a relapsing-remitting type of MS, and had experienced at least two exacerbations during the last 2 years. Interferon β-1b is a synthetic analog of a recombinant interferon-β produced in *Escherichia coli*. Although the drug's exact mechanism of action is unknown, its effects in patients with MS may be caused by its immunomodulating properties. **Interferon β-1b increases the cytotoxicity of natural killer cells** and increases the phagocytic activity of macrophages. In addition, it reduces the amount of interferon-γ secreted by activated lymphocytes. Because interferon-γ has been shown to exacerbate the symptoms of MS, a reduction in its secretion may halt the disease. The pharmacologic effects and uses of various interferons are discussed more thoroughly in Chapter 46.

Recently, another interferon product, **interferon β-1a**, was approved to treat the relapsing forms of MS. Like its predecessor, it works as an immunomodulator and is synthesized by recombinant protein pathways. **Peginterferon β-1a** is a PEGylated (polyethylene glycol) derivative of interferon β-1a, which provides a longer duration of action.

A monoclonal antibody preparation called **natalizumab** works by blocking the molecular pathway involving cell adhesion that draws lymphocytes into the CNS. The presence of lymphocytes around neuronal fibers is implicated in the immune processes that contribute to the pathology of MS. The monoclonal preparation, **daclizumab**, is made up of antibodies to the interleukin-2 (IL-2) receptor. The exact mechanism of action for daclizumab is unknown, but antibody formation with the IL-2 receptor blocks interleukin-mediated activation of lymphocytes.

Alemtuzumab is a CD52-directed cytolytic **monoclonal antibody** (Chapter 46) approved for the treatment of patients with relapsing forms of MS. Because of its potentially **life-threatening adverse effects** of autoimmune, infusion reactions, and increased malignancies, alemtuzumab should only be used in patients who have not responded to two or more other treatments for MS.

Mitoxantrone belongs to the class of antineoplastic agents and was recently approved for the treatment of MS. It acts by **suppressing the activity** of T cells, B cells, and macrophages that are thought to lead the attack on the myelin sheath. **Glatiramer acetate** is a synthetic protein that mimics the structure of myelin basic protein, a component of the myelin covering nerve fibers. This drug blocks myelin-damaging T cells by acting as a **myelin decoy**. In placebo-controlled clinical trials with relapsing-remitting MS, those taking the glatiramer acetate drug had significantly reduced episodes of relapse compared with control subjects.

Two new drugs were recently approved for treatment of MS. The first one, **dalfampridine**, was shown to improve walking in patients with MS. This was demonstrated by an increase in walking speed. It works by **blocking potassium channels** and thereby enhances conduction in damaged nerves. The second new agent, **fingolimod**, is a **sphingosine-1-phosphate receptor modulator** and blocks the egress of lymphocytes from lymph nodes, reducing the number of lymphocytes in peripheral blood. It is indicated for patients with the relapsing form of MS. The exact mechanism by which fingolimod works is unknown but may involve **reduction of lymphocyte migration** into the CNS and decreased immune reactions that destroy nerve myelination. After the success of fingolimod, two other agents of this class were marketed: **siponimod** and **ozanimod**.

Teriflunomide is another new agent used to treat relapsing forms of multiple MS. It is believed to reduce the proliferation of overactive immune cells (including T- and B-cells) that attack and damage the nerves in the CNS by acting as a pyrimidine synthesis inhibitor. The major adverse risk of teriflunomide is **hepatic toxicity**, as this was noted in rheumatoid arthritis patients taking the similar drug **leflunomide** (see Chapter 30).

Dimethyl fumarate is another new agent for the treatment of relapsing forms of MS. Its mechanism of action is unknown, but its main metabolite is monomethyl fumarate (MMF). MMF activates the Nuclear factor (erythroid-derived 2)-like 2 (Nrf2) pathway. The Nrf2 pathway regulates the cellular response to oxidative stress.

Acute exacerbations are treated with **adrenal corticosteroid drugs**, most notably **prednisone**. These drugs have anti-inflammatory activity and are discussed in Chapter 33. In patients with MS, **prednisone shortens the duration of exacerbations** and **ameliorate symptoms**, possibly by decreasing edema. They are administered orally in milder cases and are given parenterally in high doses in more severe cases.

AMYOTROPHIC LATERAL SCLEROSIS
Etiology and Pathogenesis
ALS, also called **Lou Gehrig disease,** is a **progressive disease of the motor neurons**. It is characterized by muscle wasting, weakness, and respiratory failure, leading to death in 2 to 5 years. The cause of ALS is unknown, but evidence suggests a defect in superoxide dismutase, an enzyme that scavenges superoxide radicals.

Treatment
The current treatment for ALS is largely symptomatic. Spasticity can be partly controlled with **baclofen,** a GABA$_B$ receptor agonist whose properties are outlined in Table 24.1 and discussed later. The decline in muscle strength may be slowed by **gabapentin,** an antiepileptic drug discussed in Chapter 20.

Although many drugs have been studied for their potential to reduce the progression of ALS and prolong the length of survival, the first drug specifically approved for use in the treatment of ALS is **riluzole**. This drug has been shown to prolong the time before patients require a tracheotomy and also to prolong life by approximately 3 months. Riluzole is believed to **protect motor neurons from the neurotoxic effects of excitatory amino acids** (e.g., glutamate) and to prevent the anoxia-related death of cortical neurons. Its exact mechanism of action is unclear, but it may inhibit voltage-gated sodium channels that mediate the release of glutamate from neurons. Clinical studies in patients with ALS indicate that riluzole is more effective in those with bulbar-onset disease than in those with limb-onset disease.

Edaravone is touted as a nootropic ("smart drug") and neuroprotective agent used for neurological recovery. It is a **free radical scavenger and reduces neuronal damage** due to oxidative stress. Edaravone was effective in clinical trials with ALS patients and is officially FDA-approved for the treatment of amyotrophic lateral sclerosis.

ANTISPASTIC AGENTS
Antispastic agents are used to treat **skeletal muscle spasms** that may occur from injury or a neurologic disease. The term **antispasmodic agent** is also used; however, this term is more properly applied to **spasmolytic** agents that may be used in the treatment of smooth muscle disorders, such as irritable bowel syndrome (see Chapter 28). Antispastic agents are also known as **muscle relaxants,** and many of the older agents do not have clear mechanisms of action. **Spasticity** is frequently treated with physical therapy, but antispastic drugs such as **baclofen** (see Table 24.1) may be useful in severe cases. It is useful for reducing spasticity resulting from MS, particularly for the relief of flexor spasms and the concurrent pain, clonus, and muscular rigidity.

Baclofen is a GABA$_B$ **receptor agonist,** and these G protein–coupled receptors (GPCRs), when activated, reduce motor neuron excitability. Baclofen is available in oral, injectable, and intrathecal infusion formulations.

Cyclobenzaprine and **orphenadrine** are older agents indicated for the short-term treatment of muscle spasms caused by acute painful, musculoskeletal conditions. They do not appear effective in treating spasticity from CNS diseases such as MS, ALS, or cerebral palsy. Their mechanism of action is not clear but includes centrally mediated effects on catecholamine reuptake, and antimuscarinic and antihistaminergic receptor actions. **Methocarbamol,** a carbamate derivative of **guaifenesin,** is a CNS depressant with sedative and musculoskeletal relaxant properties. It is an older agent, and its exact mechanism of action is not known, except to say **general CNS depression**. It does not directly affect muscle contraction or neurotransmitter action at the muscle end-plate junction.

Carisoprodol is also indicated for the short-term treatment of muscle spasms caused by musculoskeletal conditions. The major metabolite of carisoprodol is **meprobamate,** which is an old barbiturate-like "minor tranquilizer" still available as an anxiolytic, but its use has largely been replaced by the safer benzodiazepines. It is unclear whether carisoprodol has any effects itself or is simply a prodrug for meprobamate.

Tizanidine, a **centrally acting alpha$_2$-adrenoceptor agonist,** is also indicated for the management of spasticity of MS. It is thought to reduce spasticity by blocking nerve impulses through presynaptic inhibition of motor neurons, resulting in decreased spasticity without a reduction in muscle strength.

Dantrolene acts by blocking the release of calcium ions from the sarcoplasmic reticulum in muscle fibers. This decouples the excitation-contraction at the muscle end-plate and directly relaxes skeletal muscle. It is a life-saving drug in cases of **malignant hyperthermia** triggered by halogenated anesthetics (see Chapter 21), is used in **neuroleptic malignant syndrome** seen with high-potency antipsychotics (see Chapter 22), and is also indicated for the management of spasticity from a number of disorders (e.g., after strokes, in paraplegia, in cerebral palsy, or in patients with MS).

Botulinum toxin A, widely known by its trade name, Botox, has recently been approved for a number of medical indications besides the more famous (or infamous) use as a cosmetic agent for removing wrinkles. It is now named **onabotulinumtoxinA** as new preparations of botulinum A needed to each have distinct generic names (see below). OnabotulinumtoxinA is used to treat upper-limb spasticity in stroke patients, for cervical dystonia and other symptoms of PD, for strabismus ("cross-eyed"), and for blepharospasm (spasms of the eyelids). It was also recently approved to treat urinary incontinence resulting from detrusor overactivity in patients with spinal cord injury and MS. **OnabotulinumtoxinA** paralyzes muscles by blocking the release of acetylcholine on the presynaptic side of the muscle end-plate junction (see Chapter 6).

The success of BOTOX spawned the development of additional biologicals obtained from botulinum toxin that are useful in the treatment of spasticity and other disorders. These newer agents include **abobotulinumtoxinA, incobotulinumtoxinA, prabotulinumtoxinA,** and **imabotulinumtoxinB.**

SUMMARY OF IMPORTANT POINTS

- Parkinson disease is a chronic disease caused by degeneration of dopaminergic neurons that arise in the substantia nigra. It is characterized by resting tremor, rigidity, and bradykinesia.
- Parkinson disease is primarily treated with drugs that increase dopamine levels in the basal ganglia or activate dopamine receptors.
- Levodopa is converted to dopamine by AAAD. It is often administered along with carbidopa, which inhibits the peripheral decarboxylation of levodopa and increases its brain uptake.
- Other drugs that increase dopamine levels in the basal ganglia include tolcapone and entacapone—which inhibit methylation of levodopa—and selegiline and rasagiline—which inhibit the breakdown of dopamine catalyzed by MAO-B. Amantadine increases dopamine release and may inhibit its neuronal reuptake.
- Direct-acting dopamine-receptor agonists include bromocriptine, pramipexole, ropinirole, and rotigotine. These drugs are often used as adjuncts to levodopa in the treatment of patients whose response to levodopa is inadequate.
- Levodopa and other dopaminergic drugs can cause significant adverse effects, including nausea, dyskinesias, nightmares, and orthostatic hypotension.
- Cholinergic receptor antagonists can reduce the tremor seen in Parkinson disease, but their effectiveness is limited.
- New drugs are available like pimavanserin and the combination of dextromethorphan and quinidine to treat the psychosis and emotional lability that can occur with neurodegenerative diseases.
- Huntington disease is caused by degeneration of GABA neurons in the striatum and other parts of the brain. Degeneration of neurons leads to excessive dopamine neurotransmission and choreoathetoid movements. Drugs specific for HC include VMAT2 inhibitors, which decrease monoamine neurotransmitters.
- Alzheimer disease is a progressive dementia partly caused by loss of cholinergic neurons in the cortex and limbic structures of the brain. Donepezil, rivastigmine, and galantamine—centrally acting, reversible cholinesterase inhibitors—as well as memantine, an

NMDA antagonist, produce some cognitive improvement in patients with this disease.
- Multiple sclerosis is a demyelinating disease whose exacerbations may be attenuated with corticosteroid drugs. Treatment with interferon β-1b and other immunomodulators retard disease progression in some patients. Dalfampridine, a potassium channel blocker, improves walking ability, whereas fingolimod and others reduce lymphocyte infiltration and autoimmune destruction of oligodendrocytes. Other new agents target patients with relapsing forms of MS.
- Amyotrophic lateral sclerosis is a progressive disease of the motor neurons. Riluzole, the first drug approved for its treatment, has a limited effect on patient survival. The antioxidant edaravone also reduces the progression of ALS.
- Antispastic drugs include baclofen, working at the GABAB receptor, central muscle relaxants, and biologicals derived from botulinum toxins.

Review Questions

1. Which of the following is not a mechanism of action for antiparkinsonism agents?
   (A) Direct dopamine agonist
   (B) Precursor loading
   (C) Dopamine metabolism inhibition
   (D) Cholinergic receptor blocking
   (E) Selective dopamine reuptake inhibition
2. Cardiac arrhythmias after initial doses of levodopa (L-dopa) are occasionally observed. Which of the following most likely explains this occurrence?
   (A) Direct action on cardiac dopamine receptors
   (B) Decreased release of catecholamines
   (C) Direct β-adrenoceptor stimulation
   (D) Increased release of dopamine
   (E) Interaction with vagal cholinergic receptors
3. Anticholinergic agents are useful in the treatment of parkinsonism because of which one of the following mechanisms?
   (A) Decreased levels of acetylcholine from loss of neurons
   (B) Continuing degeneration of dopamine neurons
   (C) Neurotransmitter imbalance in the basal ganglia
   (D) Increased activity of acetylcholinesterase
   (E) Increased release of dopamine in basal ganglia
4. Selegiline, an antidepressant also used for the treatment of Parkinson disease, has which one of the following mechanisms of action?
   (A) It is a selective MAO-B inhibitor
   (B) It blocks the reuptake of dopamine
   (C) It irreversibly binds to COMT
   (D) It increases release of dopamine vesicles
   (E) It blocks muscarinic cholinergic receptors
5. Baclofen is used to treat muscle spasticity because it...
   (A) is a receptor agonist at GABAB receptors.
   (B) blocks acetylcholine receptors.
   (C) enhances the release of GABA vesicles.
   (D) is an antagonist as glutamate receptors.
   (E) increases GABA action at Cl⁻ ion channel.

Drugs of Abuse

CLASSIFICATION OF DRUGS OF ABUSE

Central Nervous System Depressants

Alcohols and glycols
- Ethanol
- Methanol
- Ethylene glycol
- Isopropyl alcohol
- Fomepizole (ANTIZOL)[a]

Barbiturates and benzodiazepines
- Pentobarbital (NEMBUTAL)
- Flunitrazepam (ROHYPNOL)
- *Gamma* (γ)-hydroxybutyrate (GHB)

Opioids
- Heroin
- Fentanyl
- Oxycodone (OXYCONTIN)

Central Nervous System Stimulants

Amphetamine and its derivatives
- Amphetamine
- Methamphetamine
- Methylene-dioxy-methamphetamine (MDMA)

Other stimulants
- Cocaine
- Caffeine
- Nicotine[b]

Other Psychoactive Drugs

Cannabis and its derivatives
- Marijuana
- Dronabinol (MARINOL)[c]
- Nabilone (CESAMET)

Hallucinogens
- Lysergic acid diethylamide (LSD)
- Mescaline
- Psilocybin
- Phencyclidine (PCP)

OTC drugs of abuse
- Dextromethorphan (DM)
- Diphenhydramine (BENADRYL)

Drugs for Treating Drug Dependence
- Disulfiram (ANTABUSE)
- Acamprosate calcium (CAMPRAL)
- Naltrexone (REVIA, DEPADE, VIVITROL)
- Methadone
- Buprenorphine (SUBUTEX)[d]
- Nicotine (NICORETTE, NICODERM)
- Bupropion (ZYBAN)
- Varenicline (CHANTIX)

[a] Used for the treatment of methanol or ethylene glycol poisoning.
[b] Synthetic stimulants such as cathinones are "emerging drugs of abuse" and sold as "bath salts."
[c] Also formulated as dronabinol oral solution (SYNDROS); synthetic cannabinoids sold as "herbal incense" with names like K2 and SPICE are also known as "emerging drugs of abuse."
[d] Also formulated as a buprenorphine transdermal patch (BUTRANS), slow-releasing rods for implant (PROBUPHINE), sublingual tablet (SUBUTEX), and two combination products containing buprenorphine and naloxone: a sublingual tablet (SUBOXONE) and a buccal transmucosal patch (BUNAVAIL).

OVERVIEW

This chapter addresses the grave medical, legal, and social problems of drug abuse, also called *substance abuse*. It begins with a review of general concepts and mechanisms of drug abuse, moves on to specific classes and agents that are likely to be abused, and follows with an update on prescription drugs, steroids, and inhalant abuse. The chapter ends with a discussion of pharmacologic agents used to treat drug dependence and those agents' mechanisms of action.

Drug Abuse

It is human nature that some individuals will experiment with occasional use of or become dependent on **mind-altering substances.** Nearly every society in recorded history has sanctioned the use of certain drugs while banning the use of others. In many Western countries, for example, products containing ethanol, nicotine, or caffeine are socially acceptable or at least tolerated by the majority of the population, whereas the use of cocaine, marijuana, hallucinogens, and

other psychoactive drugs is illegal. In other countries, the use of alcohol is discouraged, but the use of other psychoactive drugs, such as marijuana, is socially acceptable. Hence, what constitutes drug abuse from a social or political perspective is highly dependent on cultural attitudes and legal restrictions.

From a medical and psychological perspective, drug abuse can be defined as the use of a drug in a manner **detrimental** to the health or well-being of the drug user, other individuals, or society as a whole. **Drug abuse is not restricted to the use of illegal drugs,** as the cumulative health and social effects caused by the use of alcoholic beverages and tobacco products in the United States far outweigh the negative effects of all illicit drug use.

Drug Dependence

Drug dependence is a condition in which an individual feels compelled to repeatedly administer a psychoactive drug. When this is done to avoid physical discomfort or withdrawal, it is known as **physical dependence;** when it has a psychological aspect (the need for stimulation or pleasure, or to escape reality), then it is known as **psychological dependence.** Repeated drug use is a learned behavior that is reinforced, both by the pleasurable effects of the drug and by the negative effects of drug abstinence (withdrawal). These effects are the basis of drug craving in drug-dependent individuals. **Psychological dependence** is caused by the positive reinforcement of drug use that results from the activation of neurons located in the nucleus accumbens. **Physical dependence** is a state in which continued drug use is required to prevent an unpleasant **withdrawal syndrome.** Hence, physical dependence leads to negative reinforcement of drug use. Both psychological and physical dependence appear to result from **neuronal adaptation** to the presence of the drug, albeit in different areas of the brain.

Psychological Dependence. The craving for **alcohol, barbiturates, caffeine, cocaine, opioids,** and **tobacco** is remarkably similar, despite the varied behavioral and physiologic effects that these drugs produce. This similarity supports the hypothesis that psychological dependence is mediated by a **common neuronal pathway** that leads to **behavioral reinforcement** of drug use. Psychoactive drugs that evoke behavioral reinforcement of their use appear to sensitize dopaminergic neurons that project from the ventral tegmental area to the **nucleus accumbens.** Other psychoactive drugs that are used for their mind-altering effects, including **lysergic acid diethylamide (LSD),** have a much smaller effect on the dopamine pathway and cause little reinforcement, resulting in less compulsive use of LSD and other such agents.

Much evidence indicates that **dopamine** mediates drug reinforcement by binding to dopamine D_1 receptors in the **nucleus accumbens.** This signal transduction pathway activates adenylyl cyclase, increasing cyclic adenosine monophosphate (cAMP) levels and activating cAMP-dependent kinases. The kinases, in turn, activate other proteins in the signal transduction pathway, including **transcription factors.** In the accumbens, the transcription factor, cAMP-response element-binding protein, increases the synthesis of

G proteins, cAMP-dependent protein kinases, and other cell transduction molecules that **amplify** responses to dopamine. Dopamine release onto accumbens neurons also increases the expression of **glutamate receptors,** which strengthens synaptic pathways for dopamine neurotransmission in a manner much like the molecular mechanisms of learning discovered in the hippocampus. These mechanisms lead to **sensitization** to dopamine, which underlies the behavioral reinforcement of drug use.

The peak of dopamine release in the nucleus accumbens occurs at the time of the drug's **peak effect** on the central nervous system (CNS). The degree of short-term reinforcement of drug use is linked to the **rate of increase of dopamine levels** in the nucleus accumbens. This relationship appears to account for the propensity of some drugs to produce drug dependence. It also appears to explain the difference in reinforcement effects produced by different routes of administration of a particular drug. For example, the oral administration of an opioid or cocaine causes less reinforcement and psychological dependence than does the intravenous administration or inhalation of an equivalent dose of the same drug. The differences in effect are determined by the rate at which the drug is distributed to the brain and the rate at which dopamine levels in the nucleus accumbens are increased. Fig. 25.1 illustrates the neuroanatomy and mechanisms of reinforcement for drugs of abuse.

Physical Dependence. Physical dependence, also called **neuroadaptation,** results from the adaptations of specific neurons or areas of the brain to the continued presence of a drug. **Physical dependence** is observed outwardly only by the development of a drug-specific withdrawal syndrome if the drug is discontinued or blocked, as during **drug abstinence.** For this reason, physical dependence contributes to the continued use of a drug to avoid unwanted symptoms. The negative effects of nicotine withdrawal, for example, are responsible for the high relapse rate in persons trying to stop smoking cigarettes. The withdrawal symptoms are often opposite to the drug's acute effect, unmasking the neuroadaptation that acted to balance the effects of chronic

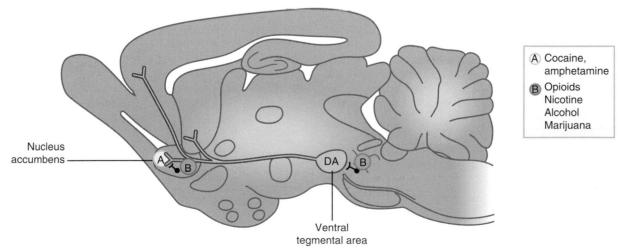

FIG. 25.1 Neural pathways and mechanisms underlying reinforcement of drug abuses. A schematic of a rat brain (midsagittal section) is shown for anatomic reference. Dopamine (*DA*) is present in the cell bodies of neurons in the ventral tegmental area (VTA) that project rostral to the nucleus accumbens and frontal cortex. Dopamine released in the nucleus accumbens is the final common pathway for reinforcing drugs (and addictive behaviors). Cocaine and amphetamines cause an increased release of dopamine directly at the nerve terminals in the nucleus accumbens. Opioids, nicotine, alcohol, and marijuana work via interneurons (GABAergic neurons) in the nucleus accumbens and the VTA to increase the release of dopamine indirectly.

drug administration. For example, opioids inhibit neurons regulating the peristaltic tone of the gastrointestinal tract and cause constipation; diarrhea is a classic sign of opioid withdrawal.

Drug Addiction

Drug addiction usually refers to an extreme pattern of drug abuse in which an individual is continuously preoccupied with drug procurement and use and thus neglects other responsibilities and personal relationships. Addiction is usually associated with a high level of drug dependence. The term *addict* has a pejorative connotation, however, and the modern treatment of substance abuse as a disease state calls for the use of the term *drug-dependent individuals* or *patients*. Such patients are said to have a **substance use disorder (SUD),** as outlined in the *Diagnostic and Statistical Manual of Mental Disorders*, used by psychiatrists.

Classification of Drugs of Abuse

The psychoactive drugs used by some individuals for nonmedicinal purposes can be classified as CNS depressants, CNS stimulants, and miscellaneous agents, with the latter group including marijuana, hallucinogens, and phencyclidine (PCP). In many cases, individuals with a substance abuse disorder are using legal or illegal substances as self-medication for **comorbid disorders** such as anxiety or depression. After describing the pharmacologic effects of these drugs and any clinical use that they may have, this chapter discusses the treatment of substance abuse. Tables 25.1 to 25.3 provide information about the manifestations and treatment of drug intoxication and withdrawal.

CENTRAL NERVOUS SYSTEM DEPRESSANTS
Alcohols and Glycols

In North America, about 12 million individuals have one or more symptoms of alcoholism, making **alcohol abuse** the number one substance abuse problem. In the United States alone, the cost of health care, lost work hours, criminal activity, and other problems related to alcohol use is roughly $90 billion each year.

The alcohols and glycols most commonly ingested are ethanol, methanol, and ethylene glycol. Whereas ethanol selectively produces CNS depression at normal doses, even relatively small doses of methanol and ethylene glycol affect multiple organ systems and can produce severe or life-threatening toxicity, even when ingested in relatively small doses.

Ethanol

Ethanol, or **ethyl alcohol,** is classified as a CNS depressant and has pharmacologic effects similar to those of barbiturates and benzodiazepines.

Pharmacokinetics. Ethanol has sufficient lipid solubility to enable rapid and almost complete absorption from the gut. It is more rapidly absorbed from the duodenum than from the stomach, and food slows its absorption by slowing the rate of gastric emptying. Ethanol is widely distributed throughout the body and has a volume of distribution roughly equivalent to the total body water, or about 38 L/70 kg of body weight.

As shown in Fig. 25.2, ethanol is primarily oxidized by **alcohol dehydrogenase** to form acetaldehyde and is then oxidized by **acetaldehyde dehydrogenase** to form acetate. The acetate derived from ethanol enters the citric acid

TABLE 25.1   Common Signs and Symptoms of Drug Intoxication

DRUG	MOTOR AND SPEECH IMPAIRMENT	EMOTIONAL AND PERCEPTUAL MANIFESTATIONS	CARDIOVASCULAR MANIFESTATIONS	OTHER MANIFESTATIONS
Alcohol	Ataxia, incoordination, loquacity, and slurred speech	Euphoria, impaired attention, irritability, mood changes, and sedation	Flushed face	Nystagmus
Amphetamines	Agitation and loquacity	Decreased fatigue, euphoria, grandiosity, hypervigilance, and paranoia	Hypertension or hypotension and tachycardia	Chills, mydriasis, nausea, nystagmus, sweating, and vomiting
Barbiturates	Same as alcohol	Same as alcohol	Hypotension	Nystagmus
Benzodiazepines	Same as alcohol	Same as alcohol	Hypotension	Nystagmus
Cocaine	Same as amphetamines	Altered tactile sensation ("cocaine bugs"), decreased fatigue, euphoria, grandiosity, hypervigilance, and paranoia	Same as amphetamines	Same as amphetamines
Hallucinogens	Dizziness, incoordination, tremor, and weakness	Depersonalization, derealization, hallucinations, illusions, and synesthesia	Tachycardia	Blurred vision, mydriasis, and sweating
Marijuana	Loquacity and rapid speech	Euphoria, hallucinations (with high doses), jocularity, and sensory intensification	Hypertension and tachycardia	Conjunctivitis, dry mouth, increased appetite, and tightness in chest
Opioids	Motor slowness and slurred speech	Apathy, euphoria or dysphoria, impaired attention, and sedation	None	Miosis
Phencyclidine	Agitation, ataxia, muscle rigidity, and slurred speech	Anxiety, delusions, emotional lability, euphoria, and hallucinations	Hypertension and tachycardia	Hostility, miosis, nystagmus, and violent behavior

TABLE 25.2 Emergency Treatment of Drug Intoxication

DRUG	PHARMACOLOGIC TREATMENT	NONPHARMACOLOGIC TREATMENT
Alcohol	None	Support vital functions
Amphetamines	Lorazepam for agitation and haloperidol for psychosis	Monitor and support cardiac function
Barbiturates	None	Support vital functions
Benzodiazepines	Flumazenil	Support vital functions
Cocaine	Lorazepam for agitation or seizures	Support vital functions
Hallucinogens	Lorazepam for agitation	Give reassurance and support vital functions
Marijuana	Lorazepam for agitation	Give reassurance and support vital functions
Opioids	Naloxone	Support vital functions
Phencyclidine	Lorazepam for agitation and haloperidol for psychosis	Minimize sensory input

TABLE 25.3 Common Signs and Symptoms of Drug Withdrawal

DRUG	CENTRAL NERVOUS SYSTEM MANIFESTATIONS	MUSCULOSKELETAL MANIFESTATIONS	CARDIOVASCULAR MANIFESTATIONS	OTHER MANIFESTATIONS
Alcohol	Altered perceptions, insomnia, irritability, and seizures	Tremor	Hypertension and tachycardia	Delirium tremens, nausea, and sweating
Amphetamines	Depression, drowsiness, dysphoria, fatigue, increased appetite, and sleepiness	None	Bradycardia	None
Barbiturates	Anxiety, insomnia, irritability, and seizures	Muscle twitches	Hypertension and tachycardia	None
Benzodiazepines	Agitation, anxiety, dizziness, and insomnia	Muscle cramps and myoclonic contractions	Hypertension and tachycardia	None
Cocaine	Same as amphetamines	None	Bradycardia	None
Marijuana	Irritability, mild agitation, and sleep disturbances	None	None	Nausea and stomach cramps
Nicotine	Anxiety, dysphoria, hostility, impatience, irritability, and restlessness	None	Decreased heart rate	Increased appetite
Opioids	Anxiety, dysphoria, irritability, restlessness, and sleep disturbances	Muscle aches	Hypertension and tachycardia	Diarrhea, fever, mydriasis, piloerection,[a] sweating, vomiting, and yawning

[a]Because piloerection causes *goosebumps* or *gooseflesh,* patients withdrawing from opioids are sometimes described as "going cold turkey."

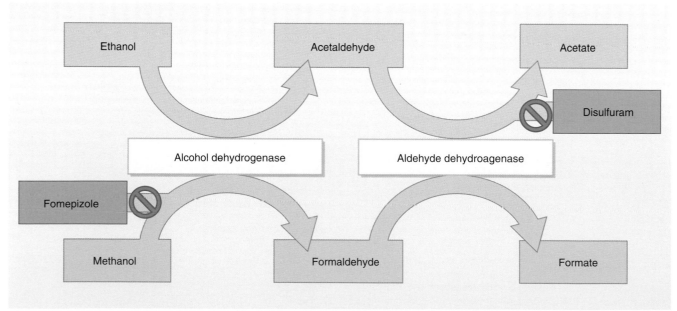

FIG. 25.2 Metabolism of ethanol and methanol. Alcohols are oxidized to aldehydes by alcohol dehydrogenase. The aldehydes are oxidized to acetate or formate by aldehyde dehydrogenase. Disulfiram inhibits aldehyde dehydrogenase and leads to the accumulation of acetaldehyde during ethanol ingestion. Fomepizole inhibits alcohol dehydrogenase and is used in methanol or ethylene glycol poisoning.

cycle for further oxidation to carbon dioxide and water. The oxidation of ethanol uses significant quantities of nicotinamide adenine dinucleotide (NAD), and the depletion of NAD is responsible for some of the metabolic effects of ethanol described later. Ethanol at higher or chronic doses also undergoes oxidation by cytochrome P450 enzymes, namely the **CYP2E1** isozyme. Unlike alcohol dehydrogenase metabolism, CYP2E1 metabolism is induced by long-term alcohol use, contributing to alcohol tolerance in heavy drinkers.

About 2% of ethanol is excreted unchanged by the kidneys and lungs. The concentration of ethanol in alveolar air is about 0.05% of that in the blood, and this relationship is used to estimate the **blood alcohol concentration (BAC)** in exhaled air when the **breathalyzer test** is administered. Because ethanol can markedly impair the psychomotor skills required to safely drive a vehicle, nearly all nations prohibit the operation of motor vehicles while under the influence of alcohol. As of July 2004, the legal limit of blood alcohol is a BAC less than 0.08% (80 mg/dL) in all states and federal territories of the United States.

The capacity of alcohol dehydrogenase to metabolize ethanol is limited because the enzyme is saturated at relatively low ethanol concentrations. Hence, ethanol metabolism exhibits **zero-order kinetics,** except when serum concentrations of ethanol are very low. For this reason, the BAC is largely determined by the rate of ethanol ingestion. An adult weighing 70 kg usually metabolizes only about 10 mL of absolute ethanol per hour, which is roughly equivalent to the amount of ethanol contained in one alcoholic drink. A BAC of 0.08% to 0.10% in most cases is reached after consuming two to four standard drinks in an hour. A standard drink is a 12-ounce serving of beer, a 5-ounce glass of wine, or 1.5-ounces (shot) of 80 proof distilled spirits.

Central Nervous System Effects, Mechanisms, and Interactions. Ethanol potentiates the actions of γ-**aminobutyric acid (GABA)** in a manner similar to that of benzodiazepines and barbiturates (see Chapter 19). It thereby produces sedative-hypnotic, anxiolytic, amnesic, and anticonvulsant effects. However, long-term ethanol use or ethanol withdrawal may lower the seizure threshold and thereby cause seizures. Predictably, ethanol **potentiates** the effects of benzodiazepines and barbiturates, so the combination of any of these drugs with ethanol can produce fatal CNS depression.

Ethanol at low doses produces **disinhibition** and **mild euphoria,** which facilitate social interactions by reducing behavioral inhibitions and self-consciousness. These reinforcing effects are correlated to the rise of the BAC, which probably determines the rate at which **dopamine increases** in the nucleus accumbens. In many individuals, reinforcement leads to the continued consumption of alcoholic beverages and to ethanol intoxication. This problem is exacerbated by the limited rate at which ethanol can be eliminated from the body.

Ethanol inhibits the release of acetylcholine from CNS neurons, and this action may contribute to the sedation and delirium that occur during alcohol intoxication. Ethanol also **inhibits the release of antidiuretic hormone** (vasopressin) from the pituitary gland and thereby produces a diuretic effect. This diuretic effect is augmented by the consumption of large volumes of alcoholic beverages, such as a six-pack of beer.

Ethanol produces vasodilation and increases heat loss from the body, partly by interfering with temperature regulation by the hypothalamus. Hence, alcohol consumption can contribute to **hypothermia** during cold weather.

Other Effects, Mechanisms, and Interactions. In addition to producing CNS effects, ethanol ingestion produces a variety of short-term and long-term **cardiovascular** and **autonomic** effects.

Blood pressure fluctuations are caused by the combination of peripheral vasodilation, depression of regulatory centers in the medulla, and the release of norepinephrine from sympathetic neurons. Consumption of large amounts of ethanol on a long-term basis can eventually lead to alcoholic cardiomyopathy and cardiac arrhythmias.

In alcoholic patients, **thiamine deficiency** secondary to a poor diet is commonly observed, which leads to nerve demyelination. This, in turn, causes peripheral neuropathies, characterized by paresthesias and reduced sensory acuity. Thiamine deficiency can also cause **Wernicke-Korsakoff syndrome,** a behavioral disorder characterized by confusion, severe anterograde and retrograde amnesia, ataxia, nystagmus, and ophthalmoplegia. The administration of thiamine substantially reverses all but the amnesic effects seen in patients with this syndrome.

Alcoholic patients can also develop several metabolic disorders. The depletion of NAD causes several citric acid cycle metabolites and lactate to accumulate and eventually contributes to liver degeneration (**cirrhosis**) and impaired glycogenolysis. The resulting hypoglycemia exacerbates the effects of ethanol on the CNS. A dietary deficiency of folate can lead to megaloblastic anemia, whereas a deficiency of other vitamins and antioxidants contributes to the overall tissue damage observed in alcoholism.

The consumption of significant quantities of ethanol during pregnancy is responsible for the occurrence of **fetal alcohol syndrome,** which is characterized by low birth weight, **microcephaly,** facial abnormalities (flattening), mental retardation, heart defects, and other abnormalities.

Other Alcohols and Glycols

Methanol, also called **methyl alcohol** or **wood alcohol,** is a highly toxic form of alcohol that can cause profound **anion gap metabolic acidosis** and severe damage to the eyes. As shown in Fig. 25.2, methanol is converted to formaldehyde and then to formate. Formate is primarily responsible for **optic nerve damage,** which can result in visual field impairment or permanent blindness. In cases of methanol poisoning, patients are treated with ethanol, which serves to saturate alcohol dehydrogenase and thereby prevent the formation of formaldehyde and formate. Ethanol has a greater affinity for alcohol dehydrogenase than does methanol. Hemodialysis is also used to reduce methanol levels in severe intoxication. **Fomepizole,** an inhibitor of alcohol dehydrogenase, can also be administered; this prevents the formation of toxic metabolites in cases of methanol and ethylene glycol poisoning.

Isopropyl alcohol, which is contained in many formulations of rubbing alcohol, produces more CNS depression than does ethanol or methanol. Isopropyl alcohol is converted to **acetone,** a substance that can be smelled on the breath. The treatment of intoxication is largely supportive.

Ethylene glycol is contained in automobile antifreeze and deicing fluids, and its ingestion can cause anion gap metabolic acidosis and serious toxicity to the kidneys, lungs, and CNS. Owing to its sweet taste and appealing color, children often die of ethylene glycol poisoning from automobile antifreeze left accessible in the garage. Ethylene glycol is metabolized to oxalic acid, and calcium oxalate crystals may be found in the urine of patients after ethylene glycol ingestion. Treatment consists of supporting vital functions, giving **ethanol** or **fomepizole,** managing acidosis, and performing hemodialysis.

Barbiturates and Benzodiazepines

The pharmacologic properties of barbiturates and benzodiazepines are discussed in Chapter 19. These drugs are sedative-hypnotic agents prescribed for the treatment of anxiety disorders, insomnia, and other conditions. They are used recreationally for their euphoric and anxiolytic effects, and some polydrug users use them to reduce the irritability and anxiety associated with cocaine or amphetamine use.

The short-acting barbiturates (e.g., **pentobarbital**) are among the most widely abused sedative-hypnotic drugs. Several benzodiazepines have also been used illicitly, including **flunitrazepam.** Although this drug is not approved for use in the United States, it is used throughout much of the world as an anxiolytic or hypnotic drug. In the United States, it is widely available from street dealers and is sometimes referred to as "**roofies,**" derived from its trade name, ROHYPNOL. Flunitrazepam gained notoriety as a party drug, a club drug, and a drug that contributes to **date rape.** It is an extremely potent benzodiazepine that is tasteless when dissolved in a beverage. Flunitrazepam produces drowsiness, impaired motor skills, and anterograde amnesia. Hence, victims do not recall events that happen while under the influence of the drug.

The long-term use of barbiturate or benzodiazepine drugs can lead to psychological and physical dependence, and their abrupt withdrawal produces symptoms that are similar to those caused by alcohol withdrawal (see Table 25.3).

Gamma (γ)-**hydroxybutyrate (GHB)** usually comes as an odorless liquid, slightly salty to the taste, and is sold in small bottles. It has also been found in powder and capsule form. The use of this club drug has resulted in deaths from CNS depression and from synergistic effects when mixed with alcohol. It is also listed by the Drug Enforcement Administration as a **predatory** or **date-rape drug.** Its exact mechanism of action is unknown, but it has agonist activity at **GABA_B receptors** in the brain.

Opioids

The most commonly abused illicit opioid drug is **heroin.** This drug is prepared from morphine by the addition of acetyl groups, so structurally, it is known as **diacetylmorphine.** Heroin is highly potent and water-soluble and thus can be injected intravenously. Because it rapidly enters the brain after injection, heroin can produce an intense euphoric sensation called a **rush.** Long-term heroin users develop considerable drug tolerance and physical dependence, and they undergo a wide variety of withdrawal symptoms (see Table 25.3) if they abruptly discontinue their use of the drug (Box 25.1).

Fentanyl is a potent opioid that is often sold as 'heroin' and leads to much of the deaths by opioid overdose seen today. It is sold by overseas chemical laboratories and

---

BOX 25.1 THE CASE OF THE OVERDOSED OPIOID ADDICT

CASE PRESENTATION
An 18-year-old man is brought to the emergency room in an unresponsive state with depressed respiration; pinpoint pupils; and cold, clammy skin. His pulse rate is 40 beats/min. There are multiple needle tracks on both his arms. He is administered 2 mg of naloxone in an intravenous bolus and within minutes is sitting up and acting bellicose, complaining to the emergency room staff that they "ruined his high."

CASE DISCUSSION
The needle tracks and the triad of apnea or depressed respiration, miosis (pinpoint pupils), and a comatose state indicate that the patient arrived at the hospital in an opioid overdose condition. Needle tracks in his arms suggest heroin use, although prescription opioids are also increasingly injected intravenously in opioid-dependent individuals. Naloxone is a pure opioid receptor antagonist and can quickly reverse the near-death condition of an opioid overdose, a phenomenon sometimes called the *Lazarus effect,* from the biblical story. As the elimination half-life of naloxone is sometimes shorter than that of the opioid that caused the overdose, patients may be given multiple doses of naloxone and monitored so that a relapse does not occur. It is recommended that patients who receive naloxone be continuously observed for a minimum of 2 hours after the last dose. It is not uncommon that the overdosed individual will be angry at the hospital staff for reversing the opioid effect, and naloxone may precipitate an opioid withdrawal syndrome.

---

shipped to the USA as fentanyl or a closely related fentanyl analog (e.g., methylfentanyl). Other opioids produce effects **similar to those of heroin and fentanyl,** but usually to a lesser degree. These effects vary with the potency and pharmacokinetic properties of the opioid and with the route of administration. Opioids administered orally tend to produce less euphoria and dependence than do opioids administered by intravenous or smoking routes. For this reason, an orally administered drug such as **methadone** (see Chapter 23) can be used to prevent the craving for heroin as well as the opioid withdrawal reaction without causing significant reinforcement or exacerbating drug dependence. **Oxycodone,** in the slow-release formulation marketed as OXYCONTIN, gained notoriety among street users because a dose intended for 24-hour pain relief in patients with chronic pain could be crushed and injected intravenously for a powerful "rush." This has led to an increase in the number of deaths caused by opioid overdose, which started the present **opioid overdose epidemic.** Opioid analgesics are the main class of agents leading to **prescription drug abuse** (see later).

CENTRAL NERVOUS SYSTEM STIMULANTS

The CNS stimulants include **amphetamine, amphetamine derivatives, cocaine, caffeine,** and **nicotine.** The amphetamine compounds and cocaine increase the synaptic concentration of norepinephrine and dopamine and exert sympathomimetic effects. They also induce a **release of dopamine in the nucleus accumbens** because this is the final common pathway for all chronically abused drugs and reinforced behaviors.

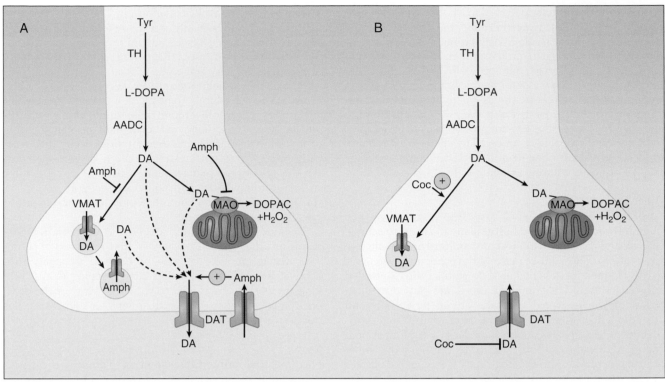

FIG. 25.3 Comparison of the mechanism of action of cocaine and amphetamine in a dopamine neuron. (A) Amphetamine and its derivatives increase synaptic concentration of dopamine (in this example, same for norepinephrine) by gaining entry into the presynaptic terminal through the reuptake transporter protein (*DAT*) to increase the amount of dopamine (*DA*) packaged into vesicles and increase DA vesicular release. Amphetamine additionally facilitates the reverse transport of DA from inside the neuron out through the reuptake transporter into the synapse. At high concentrations, amphetamine, but not all derivatives, also inhibits monoamine oxidase and, by this additional mechanism, can increase the levels of catecholamines. (B) Cocaine has a more limited mechanism of action compared with amphetamines. This natural product blocks dopamine uptake and facilitates the packaging of dopamine into vesicles. *AADC*, aromatic L-amino acid decarboxylase; *Amph*, amphetamine; *Coc*, cocaine; *DOPAC*, dihydroxyphenylacetic acid; *L-DOPA*, levodopa; *MAO*, monoamine oxidase; *TH*, tyrosine hydroxylase; *Tyr*, tyrosine; *VMAT*, vesicular monoamine transporter.

Amphetamine and Its Derivatives

Amphetamine and its derivatives **increase the synaptic concentration** of **norepinephrine** and **dopamine** by gaining entry into the presynaptic terminal through the reuptake transporter protein and increasing the amount of catecholamines packaged into vesicles. It also increases the release of catecholamines from vesicles. Amphetamine additionally facilitates the **reverse transport** of the catecholamines inside the terminal out through the reuptake transporter into the synapse. At high concentrations, amphetamine, but not all derivatives, also **inhibits monoamine oxidase** and, by this additional mechanism, can increase the levels of catecholamines (Fig. 25.3).

The use of amphetamines produces a constellation of central and peripheral effects, including euphoria, insomnia, psychomotor stimulation, anxiety, loss of appetite, increased concentration, decreased fatigue, respiratory stimulation, and hyperthermia. It also produces **sympathomimetic effects** such as mydriasis, tachycardia, and hypertension. Increased dopamine levels in the nucleus accumbens cause euphoria and other reinforcing effects, whereas the jittery and anxious feelings produced by amphetamines primarily result from an enhanced release of norepinephrine in the central and peripheral nervous systems.

The amphetamines, including methamphetamine, have legitimate medical indications such as **attention-deficit/hyperactivity disorder (ADHD), narcolepsy** and other **sleep disorders,** and **obesity** (see Chapter 22).

Methamphetamine

Amphetamine and methamphetamine are closely related sympathomimetic amines, and both are drugs of abuse. Of the two, **methamphetamine** is often preferred by abusers because it causes less norepinephrine to be released and can be more easily pyrolyzed (burned) and smoked. When the methamphetamine-free base is extracted by ether, pyrolyzed, and smoked, it is called **ice** or **crystal meth.** The euphoria produced by smoking "ice" is much greater than that produced by taking methamphetamine orally, presumably because of the faster rate at which dopamine levels are increased by inhaling the drug. The inexpensive cost and relative ease of making methamphetamine from precursor drugs found in non-prescription cold medicines enabled an illicit cottage industry in small-scale meth labs.

Other Amphetamine Derivatives

Several other amphetamine derivatives have been clandestinely synthesized and sold as **designer drugs** on the street. These include **3,4-methylenedioxy-methamphetamine (MDMA),** a drug called **"ecstasy"** or **"X."** MDMA produces both psychostimulant and psychotomimetic effects by increasing dopamine and serotonin levels in the brain.

Users of MDMA report that the drug causes euphoria, increases empathy, enhances pleasure, heightens sexuality, and expands consciousness without loss of control. MDMA, however, causes various unpleasant effects (e.g., nausea, anorexia, and anxiety), and its use can be life-threatening.

A number of deaths have occurred in MDMA users owing to **cardiac arrhythmias, hyperthermia, rhabdomyolysis,** and **disseminated intravascular coagulation.** MDMA is **neurotoxic** to serotonergic neurons, with clear degeneration of serotonergic pathways in animal models. The use of MDMA in humans likely destroys serotonergic brain neurons, which can contribute to some of the associated psychiatric complications, including panic reactions, psychosis, depression, and suicide. These disorders are prevalent in MDMA users today and will probably be observed to a greater extent later in these individuals when neuronal injury is compounded by the loss of neurons during aging.

Other Stimulants

Cocaine

Cocaine produces both psychostimulant and local anesthetic activity and has limited clinical use as a local anesthetic (see Chapter 21). Thus, unlike many of the other drugs discussed in this chapter, it is a Schedule II drug under the Controlled Substances Act. The stimulant effects are caused by **inhibition of the neuronal reuptake** of norepinephrine and dopamine. Cocaine binds to the neurotransmitter transport proteins and causes them to undergo a conformational change that reduces their capacity to transport dopamine or norepinephrine into the neuron. It is a reuptake blocker in the same manner as an antidepressant. Cocaine also increases the uptake of dopamine or norepinephrine into vesicles. By these mechanisms, cocaine increases the synaptic concentration of these neurotransmitters. Fig. 25.3 compares the mechanism of action of cocaine and amphetamine in a dopamine neuron.

Cocaine is an alkaloid derived from the leaves of a plant indigenous to South America, *Erythroxylon coca*. When native South Americans chew the leaves to relieve fatigue, relatively few adverse effects are seen. Use of the purified forms of cocaine, however, is associated with significant drug dependence, as well as cardiovascular, pulmonary, and neural toxicity.

In the past, many cocaine users took powdered cocaine hydrochloride by insufflation (snorting). Cocaine taken in this manner is absorbed across the nasal mucosa and into the circulation. More recently, a cocaine-free base became available in the form of pellets or rocks, called *crack*, because of the cracking sound made during the processing of cocaine powder to the base form. Unlike cocaine powder, crack cocaine can be smoked. Crack cocaine becomes aerosolized when it is heated, and inhaling the substance into the lungs causes it to be rapidly absorbed into the circulation. Inhalation of crack cocaine produces serum levels comparable to those obtained by intravenous administration of the drug. For this reason, crack cocaine produces a euphoric effect that is more intense than that obtained by snorting cocaine. The higher serum levels achieved with crack cocaine use also increase the potential for overdose toxicity, particularly during repeated administration.

The common signs and symptoms of cocaine intoxication are listed in Table 25.1. Unlike other drugs of abuse, cocaine can **alter tactile sensation,** causing its users to feel as if insects were crawling under their skin (**"cocaine bugs"**) and causing them to scratch and produce self-inflicted skin lesions. Cocaine often stimulates respiration at lower doses, and high doses can produce irregular breathing and apnea

known as **Cheyne-Stokes respiration.** The local anesthetic actions of cocaine probably contribute to the drug's **cardiac toxicity** when high doses are administered.

With frank overdoses, the potential for neurotoxicity and cardiac toxicity increases. Cocaine overdose victims often experience delirium and can become aggressive and violent. The pulse can become rapid, weak, and irregular. In some cases, cocaine overdose causes **tonic-clonic seizures** (including status epilepticus), **malignant encephalopathy,** or **myocardial infarction.** When fatalities occur, they typically result from ventricular fibrillation or cardiac arrest. For this reason, the management of cocaine overdose must include cardiovascular and pulmonary support, as well as the administration of a benzodiazepine (e.g., **lorazepam**) to control agitation or seizures.

Cocaine withdrawal produces fatigue, depression, nightmares or other sleep disturbances, and increased appetite. The management of cocaine withdrawal is largely supportive. **Bromocriptine,** a dopamine receptor agonist (see Chapter 24), has been used to reduce craving for the drug, but the effectiveness of this treatment for withdrawal has not been firmly established.

Nicotine

Nicotine, the principal alkaloid of plants of the genus *Nicotiana*, is widely available in the form of various tobacco products that can be chewed or smoked.

Nicotine is a lipid-soluble tertiary amine. It is rapidly absorbed into the circulation from the mouth or the respiratory tract and is then quickly distributed to the brain. The drug's CNS effects are rapidly terminated by redistribution from the brain to the peripheral tissues. Although nicotine has a half-life of about 30 minutes, it is metabolized to the active metabolite, **cotinine,** which has a half-life of about 2 hours. The induction of cytochrome P450 enzymes by tars contained in cigarette smoke accelerates the metabolism of nicotine, and this leads to the development of **pharmacokinetic tolerance** to the drug. Because the use of cigarettes accelerates the metabolism of *beta* (β)-adrenoceptor antagonists, benzodiazepines, opioids, and theophylline, cigarette smokers may require higher doses of these drugs to maintain therapeutic serum levels.

Nicotine activates cholinergic **nicotinic receptors** in the central and peripheral nervous systems and produces a complex constellation of subjective and physiologic effects. The CNS effects of nicotine are similar to those of psychostimulants and include **mild euphoria, increased arousal and concentration, improved memory,** and **appetite suppression.** In addition to activating nicotinic receptors, nicotine **inhibits monoamine oxidase.** The drug's ability to inhibit this enzyme partly explains its ability to activate dopaminergic neurotransmission and its dependence liability. The monoamine oxidase inhibitors used in treating depression, however, do not cause significant drug dependence or the intense drug craving associated with nicotine use. More directly, nicotine increases the release of dopamine in the nucleus accumbens, as with all other addictive drugs and behaviors, and strongly initiates drug dependence.

Electronic vaporizing devices for nicotine self-administration ("E-cigs," "vape") are the latest innovation in the delivery of nicotine. Using a vape is not smoking, as there is **no combustion of nicotine leaves.** Vaping occurs by the rapid heating of a small volume of **nicotine solution,** which is then inhaled. The vaping industry continues to grow at a rapid pace, with a vape shop seemingly occupying a location in every strip mall across the nation. **Nicotine is not regulated by the FDA,** but tobacco is. However, state laws and the FDA are drafting regulations at this moment. The nicotine solution is made up of nicotine and a solvent, such as ethylene glycol. The **long-term effects of smoking ethylene glycol** are not known. There are also cases of children exposed to nicotine solutions, drinking or through the skin, and in need of ER care because of the resultant nicotine toxicity. On the other hand, it is not known if vaping as a substitution for smoking cigarettes leads to decreased cancer rates.

Caffeine

Caffeine citrate is occasionally administered intravenously to treat **apnea in neonates.** It is also available in non-prescription tablets to prevent **fatigue.**

Caffeine is a methylxanthine that produces mild stimulation by **blocking adenosine receptors** on neurons throughout the CNS. Because adenosine inhibits dopamine release, caffeine indirectly enhances dopamine neurotransmission. This action is probably responsible for the drug's stimulant effects and dependence liability.

Caffeine is the most widely ingested drug in the world; it is contained in coffee, cola beverages, teas, and many other products. Caffeine use **combats fatigue; elevates mood;** and **increases alertness, concentration, motivation,** and **talkativeness.** By arousing the sympathetic system, it causes a **mild stimulation** of heart rate and blood pressure. Caffeine also relaxes most smooth muscles and causes diuresis by increasing renal blood flow.

Because caffeine **increases the secretion** of gastric acid and pepsin, it can contribute to gastritis and peptic **ulcers.** High doses of caffeine produce nausea, vomiting, increased muscle tone, and tremors. Although extremely high doses of caffeine can cause delirium, seizures, and even death, these doses are almost impossible to reach by ingesting a caffeinated beverage such as coffee. They can be reached by ingesting caffeine tablets, but abuse of caffeine tablets is limited by the fact that large doses of them produce such unpleasant symptoms.

The manifestations of caffeine withdrawal are **relatively mild;** they include headache, impaired concentration, irritability, depression, anxiety, flu-like symptoms, and blurred vision. The withdrawal symptoms can be lessened by reducing caffeine consumption gradually over a period of several weeks.

Emerging Drugs of Abuse: Synthetic Stimulants

Synthetic cathinones are new drugs chemically related to **cathinone,** a stimulant found in the *khat* plant. *Khat* is a shrub grown in East Africa and southern Arabia, where people chew its leaves for their mild stimulant effects. Synthetic cathinones are commonly sold as "bath salts" and then **smoked to obtain stimulant effects.** The synthetic variants of cathinone are **more potent than the natural product** and have led to numerous ER admissions and, in some cases, death.

OTHER PSYCHOACTIVE DRUGS
Cannabis and Its Derivatives

The best-known form of cannabis is **marijuana,** which consists of the dried flowers and leaves of *Cannabis sativa* and is a popular and illegal drug of abuse. The primary cannabinoid in marijuana is *delta* **(Δ)⁹-tetrahydrocannabinol (THC).** When cannabis is inhaled, about 20% of the THC is absorbed into the circulation. In contrast, when cannabis is ingested orally, only about 6% of the THC is absorbed from the gut, owing to the extensive first-pass metabolism. THC has multiple effects on neuronal function. It binds stereospecifically to membrane **cannabinoid receptors** in neurons, and this action is linked with inhibition of adenylyl cyclase and cAMP production. The recently discovered endogenous ligand for cannabinoid receptors is called **anandamide** (from *ananda*, the Sanskrit word for *bliss*). Anandamide binds to cannabinoid receptors, decreases the level of cAMP via G proteins, and inhibits voltage-gated calcium channels that regulate neurotransmitter release. Through these and other actions, THC appears to modulate the activity of acetylcholine, dopamine, and serotonin.

When marijuana is smoked, pyrolysis releases THC and other substances. The plasma level of THC peaks within several minutes, then it falls rapidly during the first hour, as the drug is redistributed to adipose tissue. Thereafter, it declines slowly, owing to metabolism and excretion in the urine and feces. Because of its **high lipophilicity,** THC is stored in fat, and the drug and its metabolites can be detected in the body for weeks.

Marijuana use initially causes mild stimulation followed by a depressive phase. The stimulant phase is described as a dreamlike **euphoric state** characterized by an **altered sense of time, increased visual acuity, difficulty in concentrating,** and **impaired short-term memory.** The depressive phase is characterized by **drowsiness, lethargy,** and **increased appetite.** The psychoactive effects of marijuana depend somewhat on the environment and the extent of prior use of the drug. For example, first-time users are more likely to experience anxiety than are habitual users. The common **signs and symptoms of marijuana intoxication and withdrawal** are listed in Tables 25.1 and 25.3.

Marijuana has been implicated as a cause of **amotivational syndrome,** characterized by a lack of desire to work or excel in any part of life. It has also been described as a **gateway drug** whose initial use leads to the subsequent use of other drugs (e.g., cocaine or heroin). Little scientific evidence supports either of these claims. Marijuana, however, causes minor **decreases in the levels of testosterone** in men, **low birth weight in neonates,** increased **fetal malformations,** and **decreased ovulation** in females. Studies in humans have consistently demonstrated that **marijuana reduces aggressive behavior,** even though animals injected with THC may show aggression. There is also some evidence linking marijuana use in adolescents to **schizophrenia,** although these data are controversial.

Experimental studies have demonstrated that cannabinoids are effective in the treatment of **asthma, glaucoma,** and **nausea and vomiting.** This is because their use causes bronchodilation, decreased intraocular pressure, and inhibition of nausea. Their use can also cause tachycardia. In the United States, a synthetic cannabis derivative called **dronabinol** (MARINOL) is approved for the **treatment of nausea** caused by cancer chemotherapy and for the **stimulation of appetite** in patients with acquired immunodeficiency syndrome (AIDS) who are experiencing anorexia. The drug is administered orally for these purposes. More recently, nabilone (CESAMET), another cannabinoid agonist, was also approved for the same indications.

Medical and Recreational Use of Marijuana

As of this writing, 34 states in the United States and the District of Columbia have laws legalizing marijuana for medical or recreational use. These states license the operation of **medical marijuana clinics** and **marijuana retail stores** in spite of being in violation of federal law. Proponents of **medical marijuana** maintain that the natural plant is superior to isolated compounds such as dronabinol and nabilone. Research of the medical benefits of marijuana is limited, as most pharmacologists and investigators do not have a Schedule I license. However, clinical studies are emerging that show marijuana could be **helpful in treating a range of medical conditions,** from headache and insomnia to chronic pain and cancer. There may be an additional benefit in legalizing medical marijuana; studies show that states that legalized medical marijuana saw a **decrease in opioid-related fatalities.** At the same time, marijuana does produce **dopamine release in the nucleus accumbens** and can produce **drug dependence.**

There is evidence that marijuana use by adolescents negatively impacts educational attainment and success; however, marijuana use in adolescents has not significantly increased in states that legalized recreational use. More controversially, as noted above, marijuana use has been linked to **triggering psychosis and schizophrenia** in young individuals. Importantly, without rescheduling marijuana from Schedule I to Schedule II or III, research on the long-term effects of marijuana will be slow coming.

Emerging Drugs of Abuse: Synthetic Cannabinoids

Synthetic cannabinoids refer to a growing number of **THC analogs** that were first used in research and later brought to the convenience store market. They are marketed as "safe and legal" alternatives to marijuana and sold under the names of K2 and SPICE as "herbal incense." The packages of synthetic cannabinoids contain dried and shredded plant material that is sprayed with synthetic cannabinoid chemicals. Synthetic cannabinoids are popular among the young but **much more dangerous** and lead to **greater ER admissions** than natural marijuana. Deaths have occurred from the abuse of this new class of abused chemicals.

Hallucinogens

Prescription drugs, fever, and disorders such as schizophrenia are all capable of causing hallucinations, which are false perceptions that result from abnormal sensory processing. Unlike prescription drugs, however, drugs such as **LSD, mescaline,** and **psilocybin** can produce **hallucinations without causing delirium.** LSD is a synthetic ergot derivative, **mescaline** is found in the *Peyote* cactus, and **psilocybin** is found in mushrooms (*Psilocybe coprophila*) that grow on cow excrement. These street drugs are taken orally and usually begin to produce hallucinations within an hour. The effects of LSD can last as long as 12 hours, whereas the effects of mescaline and psilocybin last about 6 hours. The mechanisms responsible for the effects are not completely understood. Some evidence indicates that LSD selectively activates certain subtypes of **serotonin (5-HT) receptors** in the neocortex, limbic system, and brainstem. According

to one hypothesis, the activation of **5-HT$_2$ receptors in the reticular formation** leads to the generalization of sensory stimuli to evoke hallucinations.

Although the use of LSD or mescaline usually causes **visual hallucinations,** it can also cause auditory, tactile, olfactory, gustatory, kinesthetic, and synesthetic hallucinations. Visual hallucinations often follow a temporal pattern in which amorphous bursts of light are followed by geometric forms and then by faces or scenes. Some users also report the occurrence of **synesthesia,** a condition in which one sensory modality assumes the characteristics of another. In a synesthetic hallucination, for example, sounds may be seen or colors may be heard.

The hallucinogens have little effect on cognitive function or arousal. If mood changes occur, they are generally an exaggeration of the predrug mood and are highly context dependent. They are usually pleasant, but they can be terrifying and cause sufficient anxiety to resemble a panic attack. Mood changes are accompanied by somatic signs of sympathetic activation, including increased heart rate, increased blood pressure, and dilated pupils. Nausea and vomiting can occur, particularly with mescaline use.

Overdoses are rarely serious, but the occasional **panic attack ("bad trip")** may require intervention that consists of removing the patient to a quiet room and having someone remain with the patient for reassurance.

Phencyclidine

PCP is a widely used street drug, despite its reputation for causing dangerous side effects and efforts to reduce its supply by limiting the sale of chemicals used in its synthesis. PCP was originally developed as a **dissociative anesthetic** similar to **ketamine,** but the occurrence of a high incidence of post-anesthetic hallucinations and delirium forced its removal from the market.

Sometimes called **"angel dust,"** PCP can be taken via various routes. The drug is incompletely and erratically absorbed from the gut, so it is usually smoked. In some cases, it is sprinkled on tobacco or marijuana and then smoked. In other cases, it is combined with cocaine and heroin before it is used.

The use of PCP produces a unique spectrum of effects that result from the **blockade of glutamate N-methyl-D-aspartate (NMDA) receptors** and action at less characterized receptors called *sigma* (σ) **receptors.** As shown in Table 25.1, these effects include euphoria, hallucinations, and psychotomimetic activity, sometimes accompanied by **hostility** and **violent behavior.** PCP causes little tolerance, physical dependence, or withdrawal effects.

PRESCRIPTION DRUG ABUSE

The **nonmedical use** or **abuse of prescription drugs** is a serious and growing public health problem. It is estimated that 48 million people ages 12 and older have used prescription drugs for nonmedical reasons. This represents about 20% of the U.S. population. Most alarming is the fact that recent government data showed that nearly 20% of young teenagers reported using opioids (VICODIN or OXYCONTIN) without a prescription, making these medications among the most commonly abused drugs by adolescents, second only to marijuana. Drug dealers routinely sell prescription drugs in addition to their illicit wares. **Accessibility** is likely a contributing factor, with a growing number of medications available in the home medicine cabinet and through some **online pharmacies** that dispense medications without prescriptions and identity verification, allowing minors to order the medications easily over the Internet.

Unintentional fatal drug overdoses nearly doubled from 1999 to 2004, mostly from the use and abuse of opioid analgesic drugs. Drug overdose is now the **leading cause of accidental death** in the United States, surpassing deaths from automobile accidents in 2012. For the first time since records were kept, more than half of drug overdose admissions to hospital emergency rooms were a result of an overdose of prescription drugs (mostly opioids), rapidly eclipsing the number of admissions for illicit drug overdose. Educational efforts by governmental agencies, by the media, and by physicians are making an impact, and the pharmaceutical companies are developing formulations that will make overdose on prescription drugs less likely. An example of this is the new formulation of the potent opioid **oxycodone** in a crush-proof tablet (see Chapter 23).

OTC DRUGS OF ABUSE

Over-the-counter (OTC) or **non-prescription drug abuse** is rampant in our society. Non-prescription drug abuse is defined as the use of an OTC drug product in a manner not indicated on the label. OTC drug abuse includes such actions as taking more of a drug than recommended or self-medicating for health problems not indicated on the label. For example, using popular cold and cough remedies every night to get to sleep is OTC drug abuse. The propensity for certain individuals to alter their brains with mind-altering substances is not restricted to adults and, in many individuals, begins with adolescent experimentation. National survey data indicate that about 3.1 million persons aged 12 years and older abuse OTC drugs at least once in their lifetime. An alarming 26% of 9th graders reported abusing OTC cough medicines to get high, which was greater than the 25% of them using marijuana for the same reason. The two most abused OTC drugs are dextromethorphan (DM) and diphenhydramine. Many non-prescription cold and cough remedies contain both DM and diphenhydramine; however, these two drugs will be considered individually.

Dextromethorphan

Dextromethorphan (DM) is a drug that was developed from CIA and Navy-sponsored research in the 1950s. The goal of this classified project was to identify a non-addictive substitute for the use of codeine as a cough suppressant. After trying many chemicals, DM was selected as it suppressed cough but was not addictive to experienced opioid users (see Chapter 27).

OTC remedies containing DM are legal, relatively cheap, and easily available. Many parents would not question the discovery of cough medicine in their kid's bedroom but would be seriously concerned if they found a bag of marijuana. But a drug-to-drug comparison reveals that cough medicines containing DM and other abused OTC drugs send more young adults to the ER than the use of marijuana. In the last decade, there was an increased number of dextromethorphan abuse cases in the ER, which was largely due to increased admissions for adolescents. At high doses consistent with drug abuse, DM acts at other receptors and

in other ways to produce the mind-altering effects sought by abusers.

Diphenhydramine

The second commonly abused OTC drug is diphenhydramine. **Diphenhydramine, an antihistamine at the H₁ receptor,** is the active ingredient in various Benadryl® and other OTC products. Diphenhydramine is mainly found as a sedative-hypnotic agent in OTC sleep aids and 'PM' forms of cold medicine. Diphenhydramine is an old drug and was the first prescription antihistamine approved by the Food and Drug Administration (FDA) in 1946. Diphenhydramine is an example of one of the first drugs approved as a prescription-only medication that later switched to OTC status, although prescription-only, injectable formulations of diphenhydramine still exist. Injectable diphenhydramine is administered alongside epinephrine (from an EpiPen®) for the treatment of anaphylaxis.

Abuse of diphenhydramine is typically carried out by taking higher than recommended oral doses of diphenhydramine-containing allergy or cough and cold medicines. At high doses, diphenhydramine loses its selectivity for blocking histamine receptors and blocks the activity of other neurotransmitter-receptor systems in the brain, most prominently, acetylcholine receptors. The anticholinergic effect of diphenhydramine produces delirium, severe confusion, and hallucinations. The **anticholinergic delirium caused by high doses of diphenhydramine** is often misdiagnosed as schizophrenic psychosis. Epileptic seizures can also occur with high-dose diphenhydramine.

STEROID DRUG ABUSE

Anabolic steroids are synthetic drugs similar to the male hormone **testosterone.** They are available in tablets, in powder, or by intramuscular injection and are abused to improve muscle growth **(bulking),** endurance, and strength (see Chapter 34). They are classified as controlled substances, making it illegal to possess an anabolic steroid without a prescription. In response to a growing clandestine industry manufacturing precursors and designer steroids, the Anabolic Steroid Control Act of 2004 listed an additional 32 steroid agents as Schedule III controlled substances.

Unlike other drugs of abuse, there is no immediate rush or euphoria experienced by the steroid abuser. Abuse of steroids is driven by desires to change one's physical appearance and increase athletic ability. Anabolic steroids can lead to **heart attack, stroke, hepatic toxicity, renal failure, and serious psychiatric problems.** Use in males leads to a reduction of the testes and sperm production. In females, steroid abuse results in the growth of facial hair, menstrual cycle dysfunction, enlargement of the clitoris, and reduced breast size.

There is also evidence that steroid abuse contributes to violent crime owing to **increased aggression** associated with users of anabolic steroids. Most unfortunate, media reports of a number of celebrity athletes exposed as steroid users send a dangerous message to youth who often revere these athletes as role models.

INHALANT ABUSE

Although attention in the drug abuse field is focused on the nonmedical use of prescription drugs, alcohol, tobacco, or illegal drugs, there are increasing numbers of children and adolescents abusing the most easily obtained mind-altering substances: **household solvents, sprays,** and **cleaners.** According to nationwide studies, more than 15% of eighth graders reported using inhalants to "get high." Inhalants are also among the most deadly of abused substances, with even a single session of inhalant abuse able to cause death from **cardiac arrest.** Regular inhalant abuse results in toxicity to the brain, heart, kidneys, and liver.

Products such as nail polish remover, lighter fluid, spray paints, deodorant and hair sprays, pressurized air cleaners, and any type of liquid fuel are soaked in rags or emptied in plastic bags and their concentrated vapors inhaled, a practice called **huffing** or **sniffing.** The latest reports indicate that the organic solvents in these products, such as **toluene,** activate the dopamine system much like any other abused drug, leading to repeated administration and drug dependence.

MANAGEMENT OF DRUG ABUSE
The use of psychoactive drugs can cause several distinct clinical problems, including drug intoxication or overdose, drug withdrawal, and drug dependence. The severity of these problems varies markedly among different classes of drugs and patterns of drug use. A diagnosis of drug intoxication or dependence in a particular individual is based on the individual's history, psychological assessment, physical examination findings, and laboratory findings.

Drug Intoxication and Withdrawal
The initial treatment of drug intoxication or overdose consists of supporting cardiovascular and pulmonary functions. **Naloxone** or **flumazenil** can be administered to counteract the acute CNS depression caused by toxic doses of an opioid or a benzodiazepine, respectively (see Table 25.2). **Lorazepam** can be used to control agitation, and an antipsychotic drug (e.g., **haloperidol**) can be administered for psychosis, which can occur with PCP overdose. Haloperidol should not be used in cases of cocaine overdose, however, because it lowers the seizure threshold and can exacerbate or precipitate seizures.

The next stage of treatment is the management of withdrawal reactions that occur as the drug is eliminated from the body. The pharmacologic treatment of withdrawal consists primarily of substitution therapy and symptomatic relief.

A benzodiazepine (e.g., **lorazepam** or **chlordiazepoxide**) can be administered to suppress the acute manifestations of withdrawal from alcohol, including delusions, hallucinations, a coarse tremor, and agitation (**delirium tremens**). The benzodiazepine is then gradually withdrawn over several weeks.

Methadone is usually used to suppress withdrawal reactions in opioid users because it is long-acting and orally effective. Methadone is also given on a long-term basis in the outpatient treatment of heroin dependence (see later).

Clonidine, an alpha$_2$ (α_2)-adrenoceptor agonist (see Chapter 8), is effective in reducing the sympathetic nervous system symptoms of alcohol, opioid, or nicotine withdrawal, and it may facilitate continued abstinence in persons who are dependent on these drugs. **Lofexidine** is the newest central *alpha$_2$* adrenoceptor agonist specifically approved to treat opioid withdrawal symptoms.

Treatment of Drug Dependence
After treatment of drug intoxication and withdrawal, attention can be directed to the more difficult problem of treating drug dependence. In this endeavor, behavioral therapy and personal motivation are as important as subsequent pharmacologic treatments. Patients are rarely cured, and most clinicians view treatment as a **lifelong process** in which patients are continually recovering. Twelve-step groups, such as Alcoholics Anonymous (AA) and Narcotics Anonymous (NA), have been successful in reducing recidivism, partly because they recognize that the individual is always in a state of remission from drug or alcohol dependence and that an ever-present possibility exists of slipping into drug use again.

Among the pharmacologic agents used for the treatment of alcohol dependence is **disulfiram,** a drug that **inhibits acetaldehyde dehydrogenase.** When disulfiram is taken and ethanol subsequently ingested, the accumulation of acetaldehyde causes nausea, profuse vomiting, sweating, flushing, palpitations, and dyspnea. Because of its ability to cause these extremely unpleasant symptoms, disulfiram is sometimes prescribed to encourage alcoholic patients to abstain from ethanol use. Other drugs that can cause disulfiram-like effects when administered concurrently with ethanol include **metronidazole** (a drug used in the treatment of protozoal infections) and some of the third-generation **cephalosporin** antibiotics.

Recently, a new **dependence medication for alcohol** called **acamprosate calcium** was approved. It is a synthetic compound with a chemical structure similar to that of the endogenous amino acid homotaurine, which is a structural analog of the amino acid neurotransmitter GABA and the amino acid neuromodulator taurine. The mechanism of action of acamprosate in the maintenance of alcohol abstinence is not completely understood. Chronic alcohol exposure is hypothesized to alter the normal balance between neuronal excitation and inhibition. *In vitro* and *in vivo* studies in animals have provided evidence to suggest that acamprosate can interact with glutamate and GABA neurotransmitter systems centrally, and this has led to the hypothesis that **acamprosate restores this balance.**

Methadone maintenance therapy for the treatment of heroin dependence began in the 1960s and has been successful in terms of decreasing crime associated with illicit drug use and transmission of infectious disease from shared needles. However, owing to the decrease in public funding and long patient waiting lists, the need for daily clinic visits and supervised administration, and the stigma attached to the methadone clinic, this method for providing **opioid substitution therapy** for heroin and opioid dependency is insufficient to meet the needs of all patients.

Buprenorphine is approved for physician outpatient **treatment of opioid dependence** to overcome the limitations of visits to a treatment clinic. It is available in a number of new formulations, often in combination with naloxone (e.g., SUBOXONE) to prevent intravenous abuse. A formulation of buprenorphine implant rods (PROBUPHINE) is especially promising.

Naltrexone is available in oral (ReVia, Depade) and extended-release injectable suspension (once a month; Vivitrol) formulations and is used to treat **alcohol and opioid dependence.** For opioid-dependent patients, naltrexone directly blocks opioid receptors and prevents the euphoria associated with opioid abuse. It is effective for the treatment of alcohol dependence because endogenous opioid systems play a key role in the pathway that leads to the reinforcement of alcohol and other drugs. **Clonidine, a centrally acting α2-agonist,** is used to ease withdrawal symptoms from opioid- or nicotine-dependent patients.

Nicotine chewing gum, lozenges, and skin patches have been developed to mitigate nicotine withdrawal reactions in persons who are trying to quit smoking. These methods of nicotine substitution therapy lead to significant smoking cessation, especially when nicotine doses are sufficiently high. Another drug used to treat nicotine dependence is the antidepressant **bupropion** (Zyban), now available in a long-acting formulation for this purpose. The ability of bupropion to block the reuptake of dopamine may contribute to its effectiveness in treating drug dependence. The combined use of bupropion and nicotine patches is currently being investigated.

Recently **varenicline** (Chantix) was approved for smoking cessation and shows a relatively high degree of success. Varenicline is selective for nicotinic receptors containing $\alpha_4\beta_2$ subunits. The efficacy of varenicline is believed to be the result of **partial agonist** activity, with simultaneous prevention of the full agonist nicotine binding to $\alpha_4\beta_2$-receptors. However, in 2009, the U.S. Food and Drug Administration strengthened the warnings for **varenicline** as serious **neuropsychiatric symptoms** have occurred, including agitation, depressed mood, suicidal ideation, and attempted and successful suicide.

Spurred on by both the commercial and medical success of **bupropion** and **varenicline** for smoking cessation, government and industry leaders are awakening to the treatment needs of drug-dependent individuals. Many anti-craving agents and pharmacologic approaches are currently in development. For example, treatment of cocaine dependence by vaccinations to produce **anti-cocaine antibodies** is in clinical trials. Other approved agents (e.g., clonidine and bromocriptine) are being tested in drug-dependent populations. Progress on the prevention and management of drug abuse and drug dependence will soon lead to more effective pharmacotherapy for these difficult but treatable CNS disorders.

SUMMARY OF IMPORTANT POINTS

- Drug dependence is a condition in which an individual feels compelled to repeatedly administer a psychoactive drug. The condition is caused by positive reinforcement (psychological dependence) and negative reinforcement (physical dependence) from continued drug use.
- Reinforcement of drug use results from increased levels of dopamine in the nucleus accumbens and dopamine sensitization of these pathways.
- Physical dependence, which results from neuronal adaptation to the continued presence of a drug, is usually associated with drug tolerance. Physical

dependence results in a characteristic withdrawal syndrome when drug use is discontinued.
- Alcohol and other CNS depressants produce motor and cognitive impairment, sedation, euphoria, and behavioral disinhibition.
- Amphetamines, cocaine, and other CNS stimulants produce euphoria, agitation, hypervigilance, mydriasis, and sympathetic nervous system arousal. Cocaine also produces an altered tactile sensation, and cocaine overdose can cause severe cardiovascular and neural toxicity.
- Marijuana and cannabis derivatives produce mild euphoria, talkativeness, conjunctivitis, and increased appetite.
- LSD and other hallucinogens cause hallucinations without producing delirium.
- Prescription drug abuse, OTC drug abuse, steroid drug abuse, and inhalant abuse are major substance-abuse problems that affect a growing number of children, adolescents, and adults.
- The treatment of drug dependence and withdrawal can include some type of substitution therapy: a benzodiazepine substituted for alcohol, methadone substituted for an opioid, and nicotine chewing gum or skin patches substituted for cigarettes.
- The treatment of alcohol- and opioid-dependent individuals can include long-acting naltrexone formulations. Naltrexone is an opioid antagonist that blocks the opioid receptor link in the dopamine reinforcement pathway in the nucleus accumbens.

Review Questions

1. Disulfiram effectively treats alcohol (ethanol) dependence by which of the following mechanisms?
   (A). increasing plasma ethanol concentration
   (B). preventing the conversion of ethanol to methanol in the liver
   (C). increasing circulating acetaldehyde concentrations
   (D). blocking the action of ethanol at its cell membrane receptor
   (E). stabilizing the cell membrane to prevent ethanol disruption
2. The fact that the degree of reinforcement for morphine is less than that of heroin is best explained by which one of the following statements?
   (A). morphine is a partial agonist
   (B). heroin binds more tightly to opioid receptors
   (C). morphine is metabolized faster than heroin
   (D). morphine is first metabolized to heroin
   (E). heroin is distributed more rapidly to the brain
3. Synesthesia is an acute pharmacologic effect of which drug of abuse?
   (A). marijuana
   (B). LSD
   (C). cocaine
   (D). PCP
   (E). alcohol
4. Which of the following has not been reported as a health hazard of chronic marijuana abuse?
   (A). low birth weight in neonates

(B). decreased testosterone in men

(C). anovulatory cycle in females

(D). increased fetal malformations

(E). increased intraocular pressure

5. Crack cocaine in the 1990s became more problematic than the powder cocaine of the 1980s because of which difference between the two forms of cocaine?

(A). cocaine in crack is more potent than cocaine in powder form

(B). crack cocaine is not metabolized in humans

(C). reinforcement is greater with inhalation *versus* insufflation

(D). powder cocaine reaches the brain more rapidly than crack cocaine

(E). coca plants in the 1990s were bred for greater cocaine content

PHARMACOLOGY OF RESPIRATORY AND OTHER SYSTEMS

CHAPTER 26

Autacoid Drugs That Mimic Endogenous Substances

CLASSIFICATION OF AUTACOID DRUGS

Histamine H₁ Receptor Antagonists

First-generation antihistamines
- Promethazine (PHENERGAN)
- Diphenhydramine (BENADRYL)
- Chlorpheniramine (CHLOR-TRIMETON)
- Dimenhydrinate (DRAMAMINE)
- Hydroxyzine (ATARAX)[a]

Second-generation antihistamines
- Cetirizine (ZYRTEC)
- Desloratadine (CLARINEX)
- Fexofenadine (ALLEGRA)
- Levocetirizine (XYZAL)
- Loratadine (CLARITIN)

Intranasal antihistamines
- Azelastine (ASTELIN)

Ophthalmic antihistamines
- Ketotifen (ZADITOR)
- Levocabastine (LIVOSTIN)[b]

Histamine H3 receptor antagonists
- Pitolisant (WAKIX)

Serotonergic Drugs

Serotonin agonists
- Buspirone (BUSPAR)
- Sumatriptan (IMITREX)[c]
- Tegaserod (ZELNORM)
- Prucalopride (MOTEGRITY)
- Lorcoserin (BELVIQ)
- Flibanserin (ADDYI)

Serotonin antagonists
- Clozapine (CLOZARIL)
- Cyproheptadine (PERIACTIN)
- Ondansetron (ZOFRAN)[d]

Serotonin synthesis inhibitor
- Telotristat ethyl (XERMELO)

Prostaglandin Drugs
- Alprostadil (CAVERJECT, MUSE)
- Carboprost Tromethamine (HEMABATE)
- Dinoprostone (CERVIDIL)
- Misoprostol (CYTOTEC)
- Epoprostenol (FLOLAN)
- Treprostinil (REMODULIN)
- Latanoprost (XALATAN)[e]
- Selexipag (UPTRAVI)

Endothelin-1 antagonists
- Bosentan (TRACLEER)[f]

[a] Also clemastine (TAVIST), doxepin (SILENOR), meclizine (ANTIVERT), and doxylamine with vitamin B₆ (pyridoxine) in DICLEGIS.
[b] Also epinastine (ELESTAT) and olopatadine (PATANOL).
[c] Also zolmitriptan (ZOMIG), rizatriptan (MAXALT), naratriptan (AMERGE), frovatriptan (FROVA), almotriptan (AXERT), and eletriptan (RELPAX).
[d] Also granisetron (KYTRIL), palonosetron (ALOXI), alosetron (LOTRONEX), and dolasetron (ANZEMET).
[e] Also bimatoprost (LUMIGAN), travoprost (TRAVATAN), and tafluprost (ZIOPTAN).
[f] Also ambrisentan (LETAIRIS) and macitentan (OPSUMIT).

OVERVIEW

Autacoids (also spelled *autocoids*) are substances produced by neural and nonneural tissues throughout the body that act locally to modulate the activity of smooth muscles, nerves, glands, platelets, and other tissues (Table 26.1). Several autacoids also serve as neurotransmitters in the central nervous system (CNS) or substances of the **enteric nervous system,** which innervates the gastrointestinal (GI) tract and internal organs.

Autacoids regulate certain aspects of GI, uterine, and renal function, and they are involved in pain, fever, inflammation, allergic reactions, asthma, thromboembolic disorders, and other pathologic conditions. Drugs that inhibit autacoid synthesis or block autacoid receptors are helpful in treating these conditions, whereas drugs that activate autacoid receptors are useful for inducing labor, alleviating migraine headaches, counteracting drug-induced peptic ulcers, and other purposes.

Autacoids include monoamines, such as **histamine and serotonin,** as well as fatty acid derivatives, including **prostaglandins** and **leukotrienes.** Autacoids activate specific membrane receptors in target tissues, mostly of the G protein–coupled receptor (GPCR) type. Their effects are usually restricted to the tissue in which they are formed, but, under pathologic conditions, extraordinarily large amounts of autacoids can be released into the systemic circulation. These disorders include **carcinoid tumor** and **anaphylactic shock,** which cause the release of copious amounts of serotonin and histamine, respectively, and exert systemic effects, including CNS effects. Most autacoids are rapidly metabolized to inactive compounds, as seen with prostaglandins, and some autacoids undergo tissue reuptake, as evidenced by 5-hydroxytryptamine (5-HT) reuptake transporter proteins in neurons and peripheral cells.

This chapter provides basic information about autacoids and reviews the many types of drugs that influence

TABLE 26.1 Effects of Selected Autacoids

AUTACOID	EFFECTS ON VSM	EFFECTS ON NVSM	OTHER EFFECTS
Histamine	Vasodilation and edema	Contraction of bronchial and other NVSMs	Itching, increase in gastric acid secretion
Serotonin	Vasoconstriction in most vascular beds	Contraction of gastrointestinal and other NVSMs	Central nervous system neurotransmission, stimulation of platelet aggregation
Eicosanoids			
Leukotrienes	Vasoconstriction or vasodilation	Contraction of bronchial and other NVSMs	Inflammatory effects, increase in vascular permeability
Prostaglandin E	Vasodilation	Relaxation of bronchial muscle and contraction of uterine muscle	Inhibition of gastric acid secretion
Prostaglandin F	Vasoconstriction in most vascular beds	Contraction of bronchial and uterine muscle	Increase in aqueous humor outflow
Prostaglandin I	Vasodilation	Contraction	Inhibition of platelet aggregation
Thromboxane A_2	Vasoconstriction	Contraction	Stimulation of platelet aggregation

NVSM, Nonvascular smooth muscle; *VSM,* vascular smooth muscle.

their effects. Some autacoid drugs are covered completely here, whereas other chapters provide more details on other agents.

HISTAMINE AND RELATED DRUGS
Histamine Biosynthesis and Release
Histamine is a biogenic amine produced primarily by mast cells and basophils, which are particularly abundant in the skin, gastrointestinal tract, and respiratory tract. Histamine is also produced by paracrine cells in the gastric fundus, where it stimulates acid secretion by parietal cells. Histamine also functions as a neurotransmitter in the CNS (see Chapter 18).

Histamine is formed when the amino acid **histidine** is decarboxylated in a reaction catalyzed by the enzyme L–histidine decarboxylase. Histamine is stored in granules (vesicles) in mast cells and basophils until it is released. It is released from mast cells when membrane-bound **immunoglobulin E (IgE)** interacts with an IgE antigen to cause mast cell degranulation. This process can be blocked by **cromolyn sodium** and related respiratory drugs, as described in Chapter 27. A number of other stimuli can also cause the release of histamine from mast cells (Fig. 26.1). Stimuli that increase cyclic guanosine monophosphate increase histamine release, whereas those that increase cyclic adenosine monophosphate oppose this action.

Mast cell degranulation can also be triggered by bacterial toxins and by drugs such as **morphine** and **tubocurarine.** Some of these stimuli result in the formation of inositol triphosphate (IP_3) and diacylglycerol (DAG). As with neurons, this causes the release of intracellular calcium and the fusion of granule membranes with the plasma membrane, thereby **releasing histamine** and other compounds. The release of histamine that can occur with morphine administration does not appear to be mediated by opioid receptors because the opioid antagonist naloxone does not inhibit morphine-induced histamine release from mast cells.

Histamine is inactivated by methylation and oxidation reactions that are catalyzed by a methyltransferase enzyme and diamine oxidase, respectively.

Histamine Receptors and Effects
Histamine receptors have been classified as H_1, H_2, and H_3. All three types are typical, seven-transmembrane GPCR proteins.

H_1 **receptors** are involved in allergic reactions that cause **dermatitis, rhinitis, conjunctivitis,** and **other forms of allergy.** Activation of H_1 receptors in the skin and mucous membranes causes vasodilation, increases vascular permeability, and leads to erythema (heat and redness), congestion, edema, and inflammation. Stimulation of H_1 receptors on mucocutaneous nerve endings can cause pruritus (itching), and, in the lungs, it initiates the cough reflex. If sufficient histamine is released into the circulation, total peripheral resistance and blood pressure fall, and the individual may progress to **anaphylactic shock.** Activation of H_1 receptors also causes bronchoconstriction and contraction of most gastrointestinal smooth muscles.

H_2 **receptors** are most noted for increasing **gastric acid secretion,** but they are also involved in **allergic reactions.** For this reason, H_2 receptor antagonists are sometimes used in combination with H_1 receptor antagonists in the treatment of allergies. Activation of H_2 receptors in the heart increases the heart rate and contractility, but the cardiac effects of histamine are not prominent under most conditions.

H_3 **receptors** are located in various tissues in the periphery and on nerve terminals. Agonist activation of these presynaptic receptors in the brain inhibits the release of histamine and other neurotransmitters. An antagonist of H_3 receptors would therefore increase brain levels of histamine.

ANTIHISTAMINE DRUGS
Antihistamines, or **histamine receptor antagonists,** have been categorized on the basis of their receptor selectivity as H_1 receptor antagonists or H_2 receptor antagonists. Chapter 28 outlines the properties of H_2 receptor antagonists, which are used primarily to treat peptic ulcer disease. There is a single H_3 receptor antagonist agent very recently approved for the treatment of narcolepsy (see below).

Histamine H₁ Receptor Antagonists
Classification
The following discussion focuses on the properties and uses of four groups of H_1 receptor antagonists. Chlorpheniramine,

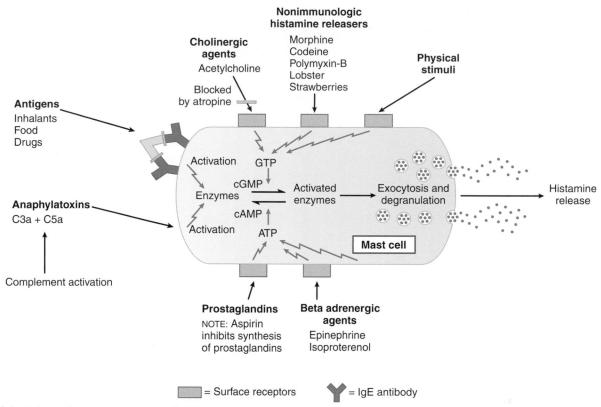

FIG. 26.1 Release of histamine from mast cells. Numerous chemical and physical stimuli activate histamine release from mast cells. Complement activation from serum sickness or bacterial endotoxins produces the anaphylactic peptides C3a and C5a, allergic antigens bind to immunoglobulin E (*IgE*) antibodies, and chemicals and other substances increase guanosine triphosphate (*GTP*) and cyclic guanosine monophosphate (*cGMP*) to activate enzymes causing increased intracellular calcium and release of histamine granules. Beta (*β*)-adrenoceptor agents and some prostaglandins increase adenosine triphosphate (*ATP*) and cyclic adenosine monophosphate (*cAMP*) and reduce activated enzymes.

clemastine, dimenhydrinate, diphenhydramine, hydroxyzine, meclizine, and promethazine are examples of **first-generation** drugs. Cetirizine, fexofenadine, loratadine, and desloratadine are examples of **second-generation** drugs. Drugs in these two groups are administered orally or parenterally. A major difference in the two groups is that the first-generation antihistamines are distributed to the CNS and cause **sedation,** whereas the second-generation antihistamines do not cross the **blood-brain barrier** significantly. Azelastine is an example of an **intranasal antihistamine,** and **levocabastine, ketotifen, epinastine,** and **olopatadine** are used for **ophthalmic** treatment.

Mechanisms and Pharmacokinetics

The H_1 antihistamines contain an alkylamine group that resembles the side chain of histamine and permits them to bind to the H_1 receptor and act as **competitive receptor antagonists.** The drugs can block most of the effects of histamine on vascular smooth muscles and nerves and thereby prevent or counteract allergic reactions.

When antihistamines are administered orally, they are rapidly absorbed and are widely distributed to tissues. Many of them are extensively metabolized in the liver by cytochrome P450 enzymes. Hydroxyzine has an active metabolite that is also available as the drug cetirizine, and this drug is excreted unchanged in the urine and feces.

Azelastine is an H_1 antihistamine marketed as a nasal spray for the treatment of allergic rhinitis. It blocks H_1 receptors and inhibits the release of histamine from mast cells, and it is much more potent than either **sodium cromoglycate** or **theophylline** in its inhibition. The systemic bioavailability of azelastine after intranasal administration is about 40%, and the plasma half-life is about 22 hours. Azelastine is metabolized by cytochrome P450 enzymes to an active metabolite, **desmethylazelastine,** a substance whose plasma concentrations are 20% to 30% of azelastine concentrations. Azelastine and its principal metabolite are both H_1 receptor antagonists. The unchanged drug and its active metabolite are excreted primarily in the feces.

Pharmacologic Effects and Indications

The H_1 antihistamines are all equally effective in treating **allergies,** but they differ markedly in their **sedative, antiemetic,** and **anticholinergic properties** (Table 26.2). The second-generation antihistamines cause little or no sedation, so they are often preferred for the treatment of allergies. Antihistamines are usually more effective when administered before exposure to an allergen than afterward. Hence, individuals with seasonal allergies, such as **allergic rhinitis** (see Chapter 27), should take them on a regular basis throughout the allergy season.

First-Generation Antihistamines

Because the first-generation antihistamines have sedative effects, they are occasionally used to produce **sedation.** They are also used to treat **nausea** and **vomiting,** to prevent **motion sickness** in persons traveling by plane or boat, and

TABLE 26.2   Pharmacologic Properties of Selected Histamine H$_1$ Receptor Antagonists

DRUG	DURATION OF ACTION (H)	SEDATIVE EFFECTS	ANTIEMETIC EFFECTS	ANTICHOLINERGIC EFFECTS
First-Generation Antihistamines				
Chlorpheniramine	6	Medium	None	Medium
Dimenhydrinate	8	High	Medium	High
Diphenhydramine	8	High	Medium	High
Hydroxyzine	6	High	High	Medium
Meclizine	12	Medium	High	Medium
Promethazine	12	High	High	High
Second-Generation Antihistamines				
Cetirizine	24	Low	None	Very low
Fexofenadine	12	Very low	None	Very low
Loratadine	24	Very low	None	Very low
Intranasal Antihistamines				
Azelastine	12	Low	None	Very low

to treat **vertigo** (an illusory sense that the environment or one's own body is revolving).

The most sedating antihistamines are **diphenhydramine, hydroxyzine,** and **promethazine. Doxepin** has antidepressant and anxiolytic effects, but because of its high affinity for blocking central H$_1$ receptors, it was recently approved at low doses for the treatment of insomnia. These drugs are used to induce sleep or for preoperative sedation. Their sedating properties can also be useful in relieving distress caused by the **severe pruritus associated with some allergic reactions.** Persons taking these drugs should be cautioned against driving or operating machinery.

Pheniramine drugs, such as **chlorpheniramine,** are less sedating than other first-generation drugs and are used primarily in the treatment of allergic reactions to pollen, mold spores, and other environmental allergens.

Meclizine, diphenhydramine, hydroxyzine, and **promethazine** have higher **antiemetic activity** than other antihistamines. **Meclizine** is less sedating than diphenhydramine, hydroxyzine, and promethazine, so it is frequently used to prevent **motion sickness** or treat **vertigo. Dimenhydrinate** is a mixture of diphenhydramine and 8-chlorotheophylline and is also used for these purposes. **Promethazine** suppositories are often used to relieve **nausea** and **vomiting** associated with various conditions, and **doxylamine with vitamin B$_6$ (pyridoxine)** is used for the treatment of **morning sickness** in pregnant women (see Chapters 28 and 34).

Second-Generation Antihistamines

The second-generation drugs lack antiemetic activity, so their use is limited to the treatment of **allergies.** None of these drugs cause substantial sedation; however, **cetirizine** is more likely than the other second-generation antihistamines to cause some sedation. Following a common trend in the pharmaceutical industry to market the active enantiomer of racemic drugs already approved, **levocetirizine** is now also available. Because **fexofenadine** has a shorter half-life, it must be taken twice a day, whereas the other second-generation drugs are taken once a day. Fexofenadine and cetirizine are eliminated primarily as the unchanged drug in

the feces and urine, respectively. **Loratadine** and **desloratadine** are metabolized to **active metabolites** that are excreted in the urine and feces.

Intranasal Antihistamines

Azelastine is indicated for the treatment of symptoms of **allergic rhinitis,** including sneezing, nasal itching, and nasal discharge. It is administered as two sprays per nostril twice daily. The drug can cause drowsiness and should be used cautiously when patients are driving or operating machinery.

Ophthalmic Antihistamines

Currently, four antihistamine eyedrop formulations are available. **Levocabastine, epinastine,** and **olopatadine** are selective H$_1$ antagonists for topical ophthalmic use. They are indicated for the temporary relief of the signs and symptoms of seasonal allergic conjunctivitis. **Ketotifen** is a selective, **noncompetitive H$_1$ antagonist** and **mast cell stabilizer.** The action of ketotifen occurs rapidly, with an effect seen within minutes after administration; because of the noncompetitive nature of the H$_1$ receptor antagonism, it has a longer duration of action than the other agents. It is indicated for the temporary prevention of itching of the eye caused by allergic conjunctivitis.

Adverse Effects and Interactions

The H$_1$ antihistamines produce few serious side effects.

First-Generation Antihistamines. Sedation is the most common side effect of the first-generation antihistamines. Paradoxically, however, the drugs can produce **excitement** in infants and children and should be used with caution in these patients.

Diphenhydramine and **promethazine** have the highest **anticholinergic activity** (see Table 26.2), but other first-generation drugs also block cholinergic muscarinic receptors. As a result, the drugs can cause dry mouth, blurred vision, tachycardia, urinary retention, and other atropine-like side effects, including hallucinations. Owing to easy over-the-counter access of some agents (e.g., BENADRYL),

CASE PRESENTATION

A 35-year-old man working as a stockbroker tells his physician that he is constantly sneezing and has a runny nose and itchy, watery eyes whenever he is at his home in the country. He tells his physician that he tried an over-the-counter allergy medicine but that it made him drowsy and feel "like he was living in a fog." His doctor tells him that he has allergic rhinitis, or "hay fever," and prescribes a nasal spray containing azelastine.

CASE DISCUSSION

The most common symptom of seasonal allergies is allergic rhinitis, otherwise known as *hay fever*. Symptoms of allergic rhinitis closely mimic those of the common cold, but with a cold, nasal discharge may be thick and yellow. With allergies, it is generally thin and clear. An allergy is also often accompanied by itchy, watery eyes. Most over-the-counter medications include diphenhydramine, a first-generation antihistamine, but these preparations are known to cause drowsiness. The newer, second-generation antihistamines are fexofenadine and loratadine, which do not cause drowsiness, because they do not readily gain access into the central nervous system. Among the different types of nose sprays are azelastine, an antihistamine, and sprays that contain steroids, such as beclomethasone, fluticasone, or triamcinolone. The drawback to steroid medications is that they may take a week or so to be maximally effective. There is also a nasal spray containing cromolyn sodium, a mast cell stabilizer, available without a prescription.

there is a significant incidence of **drug abuse** and **overdose** with antihistamines.

Anticholinergic toxicity is the principal manifestation of an overdose of first-generation antihistamines. Administration of **physostigmine,** a **cholinesterase inhibitor** that crosses the blood-brain barrier, may be required to counteract the anticholinergic effects of antihistamines in the CNS.

Second-Generation Antihistamines. Astemizole (HISMANAL) also caused prolongation of the QT interval and was removed from the market. **Fexofenadine** is the active metabolite of **terfenadine** (SELDANE). Terfenadine was the first nonsedating H_1 blocker but was withdrawn from the market by the US Food and Drug Administration because it prolonged the QT interval on the electrocardiogram, leading to a type of **cardiac dysrhythmia** called *torsades de pointes*. **Fexofenadine** does not appear to cause cardiac abnormalities. **Cetirizine** and **loratadine** also lack cardiac effects (Box 26.1).

Intranasal Antihistamines. Adverse effects of azelastine are rare and include dizziness, fatigue, headache, nasal irritation, dry mouth, and weight gain.

Ophthalmic Antihistamines. Adverse effects of levocabastine, epinastine, olopatadine, and ketotifen are usually limited to the eyes and include transient stinging and burning. These occur in less than 5% of patients.

Histamine H_3 Receptor Antagonists

Pitolisant is a first-in-class **histamine receptor (H_3) antagonist**/inverse agonist indicated for the treatment of excessive daytime sleepiness (EDS) in adult patients with **narcolepsy.** Unlike standard treatment with amphetamines, **pitolisant** is the first and only treatment for patients with narcolepsy that is **not a controlled substance**. The action of pitolisant in blocking H_3 receptors **increases the synthesis and release of histamine**, a wake-promoting neurotransmitter in the brain.

In the Phase 3 clinical trials conducted in patients with narcolepsy, the **most common adverse effects** that occurred in at least 5% of patients with the use of **pitolisant** were **insomnia** (6%), **nausea** (6%), and **anxiety** (5%). Drug interactions include inhibitors of CYP2D6, drugs that prolong the QT interval, and centrally acting H_1 receptor antagonists.

SEROTONIN AND RELATED DRUGS

Serotonin Biosynthesis and Release

Serotonin, or **5-HT,** is an autacoid and a neurotransmitter produced primarily by platelets, enterochromaffin cells in the gut, and neurons. The greatest concentration of serotonin is in the enterochromaffin cells of the GI tract. As illustrated in Fig. 18.3C, serotonin is synthesized from the amino acid **tryptophan by the action of tryptophan hydroxylase** and is metabolized to **5-hydroxyindoleacetic acid** (5-HIAA) by monoamine oxidase and aldehyde dehydrogenase. 5-HIAA is then excreted in the urine. Serotonin is concentrated in vesicles within the cell and released by calcium-mediated exocytosis like other neurotransmitters.

Serotonin Receptors and Effects

The four main types of **serotonin receptors** are designated as 5-HT_1 through 5-HT_4. The 5-HT_1 and 5-HT_2 receptors have several subtypes that are designated by letters (e.g., 5-HT_{1A} and 5-HT_{1D}). Although most serotonin receptors are GPCRs, the **5-HT_3 receptor** is a ligand-gated ion channel. The mechanisms of signal transduction for serotonin receptors are outlined in Table 18.1.

In the peripheral tissues, the physiologic effects of serotonin include platelet aggregation, stimulation of gastrointestinal motility, and modulation of vascular smooth muscle contraction. Serotonin causes **vasoconstriction** in most vascular beds and contraction of most smooth muscles. In the CNS, serotonin is involved in the regulation of mood, appetite, sleep, emotional processing, and pain processing (see Chapter 18).

Drugs that affect serotonin activity are classified as serotonin agonists, serotonin antagonists, and serotonin reuptake inhibitors. Examples are mentioned later in this chapter and discussed in detail in other chapters.

Serotonin Agonists

Serotonin agonists have been developed for use in the management of several specific disorders (Table 26.3). **Buspirone,** a partial agonist that acts at the 5-HT_{1A} receptor, is used to treat **anxiety** and **depression** (see Chapter 19). **Sumatriptan** and related **triptan** compounds, and some **ergot drugs,** are $5\text{-HT}_{1D/1B}$ receptor agonists used to treat **migraine headaches** (see Chapter 29).

Cisapride was the first 5-HT_4 receptor agonist used for the treatment of **gastroesophageal reflux disease** and **gastrointestinal hypomotility** (see Chapter 28). Activation of 5-HT_4 receptors increases the peristaltic action of the gastrointestinal tract, which is helpful in the treatment of both gastroesophageal reflux disease and gastrointestinal hypomotility.

TABLE 26.3 Serotonin Receptors and Clinical Uses of Serotonin Agonists and Antagonists

DRUG	5-HT RECEPTOR	CLINICAL USE
Serotonin Agonists		
Buspirone	5-HT$_{1A}$	Anxiety, depression
Prucalopride	5-HT$_4$	Irritable bowel syndrome with constipation
Sumatriptan	5-HT$_{1D/1B}$	Migraine headaches
Serotonin Antagonists		
Clozapine	5-HT$_2$	Schizophrenia
Cyproheptadine	5-HT$_2$	Carcinoid syndrome, pruritus, urticaria
Ondansetron	5-HT$_3$	Nausea and vomiting

5-HT, 5-Hydroxytryptamine (serotonin).

However, **cisapride** (PROPULSID) was pulled from the market in the United States in 2000 after post-marketing surveillance revealed a risk of rare but sometimes fatal prolongation of the QT interval on electrocardiogram records (*long QT syndrome*). A newer 5-HT$_4$ agonist, **tegaserod** (ZELNORM), was approved for a narrower indication for women who have **irritable bowel syndrome** with constipation as their main symptom, but it was recently withdrawn from the open market owing to **increased risk of heart attack** or **stroke.** It is still available under an emergency treatment, investigational new drug (IND) protocol for patients who cannot be effectively treated with any other agent. Finally, **prucalopride** was recently approved for the treatment of chronic idiopathic constipation (CIC) in adults (see Chapter 28), and once again there is a 5-HT$_4$ agonist on the market.

Lorcaserin (BELVIQ) is a new antiobesity agent that acts on the serotonin 5-HT$_{2C}$ receptor as an agonist. Lorcaserin is thought to decrease food intake and promote fullness by selectively activating 5-HT$_{2C}$ receptors on proopiomelanocortin (POMC) neurons located in the hypothalamus. The exact mechanism of action is not known. Like other serotonergic agents, lorcaserin carries the risk of serotonin syndrome (see Chapter 22).

Flibanserin (ADDYI) is a new drug indicated for the treatment of premenopausal women with hypoactive sexual desire disorder (HSDD). HSDD is characterized by low sexual desire that causes distress or interpersonal problems and is not due to coexisting medical or psychiatric conditions, the effects of a medication or other drug substance, or problems with the sex partner relationship (see Chapter 34).

Serotonin Antagonists

Examples of serotonin antagonists include clozapine, cyproheptadine, and ondansetron (see Table 26.3).

Clozapine and other drugs are classified as **atypical antipsychotics** that act partly by blocking 5-HT$_2$ receptors in the CNS. They are used in the treatment of **schizophrenia** (see Chapter 22).

Cyproheptadine is a 5-HT$_2$ receptor antagonist that also has H$_1$ antihistamine activity. This makes it useful in managing **urticaria** (hives) and other allergic reactions in which **pruritus** is a prominent feature. Cyproheptadine is administered orally every 8 to 12 hours and can cause slight to moderate drowsiness.

Cyproheptadine is also indicated and useful for the care of patients with **carcinoid tumor.** This tumor can produce huge quantities of serotonin, histamine, and other vasoactive substances that cause a constellation of clinical effects called **carcinoid syndrome.** Affected patients experience malabsorption, violent attacks of watery diarrhea and cramping, and paroxysmal vasomotor attacks characterized by sudden red to purple flushing of the face and neck. The malabsorption and diarrhea can be managed by giving cyproheptadine in combination with opioid antidiarrheal drugs.

Ondansetron was the first selective **5-HT$_3$ receptor antagonist** used as an antiemetic agent in cancer chemotherapy, as well as for treating nausea and vomiting from other causes. It prevents **nausea and vomiting** by blocking the effects of serotonin in the chemoreceptor trigger zone and in vagal afferent nerves in the gastrointestinal tract (see Chapter 28). Closely related gastrointestinal agents sharing the same mechanism of action include **granisetron, alosetron, palonosetron,** and **dolasetron.** Granisetron, like ondansetron, is used to **prevent nausea** and **vomiting** caused by cancer chemotherapy and radiation therapy. **Alosetron** is indicated for treatment of women with irritable bowel syndrome whose predominant bowel symptom is diarrhea. **Palonosetron** is an injectable-only formulation for the prevention of acute or delayed nausea and vomiting associated with initial and repeat courses of emetogenic cancer chemotherapy.

Serotonin Synthesis Inhibitors

Telotristat ethyl is a first-in-class **tryptophan hydroxylase inhibitor indicated for the treatment of carcinoid syndrome** diarrhea in combination with somatostatin analog (e.g., octreotide) therapy in adults inadequately controlled by somatostatin analogues (SSA) therapy. As described in Chapter 18, serotonin is biosynthesized by the conversion of the essential amino acid tryptophan into 5-hydroxytryptophan by tryptophan hydroxylase. 5-hydroxytryptophan is converted to 5-hydroxytryptamine (5-HT, serotonin) by aromatic amino acid decarboxylase (AAD). Inhibition of tryptophan hydroxylase by **telotristat ethyl decreases production of serotonin and reduces the frequency** of carcinoid syndrome diarrhea.

The most common adverse effects of telotristat ethyl were nausea, headache, accumulation of fluid causing swelling (peripheral edema), flatulence, and decreased appetite. It also may cause constipation. The FDA approved telotristat ethyl with a fast-track designation and priority review and classified it as an orphan drug.

Serotonin Reuptake Inhibitors

Serotonin reuptake inhibitors are used in the treatment of **depression** and **other CNS disorders** (see Chapter 22).

EICOSANOIDS AND RELATED DRUGS

Eicosanoids are autacoids derived from **arachidonic acid** (eicosatetraenoic acid) and other 20-carbon fatty acids (*eicos* in Greek means "twenty").

Eicosanoid Biosynthesis and Release

Eicosanoids are made from arachidonic acid and other polyunsaturated fatty acids in the cell membrane. They are freed from their esteric attachment to membrane phospholipids by **phospholipase A$_2$,** an enzyme that is activated by numerous chemical stimuli and by physical stimuli, such as cell damage. The two main groups of eicosanoids are the **prostaglandins** and the **leukotrienes,** whose formation begins with reactions catalyzed by **cyclooxygenase** and **5-lipoxygenase,** respectively. As shown in Fig. 26.2, subsequent reactions convert the products of these reactions to specific prostaglandins and leukotrienes.

Each prostaglandin and leukotriene is assigned a letter and subscript number (e.g., PGE$_2$). The letter refers to the specific ring structure of the substance, and the subscript number indicates the **number of double bonds** in the fatty acid chains.

Eicosanoid end products made in individuals consuming a typical Western diet come primarily from arachidonic acid, containing four carbon double bonds. Because the first

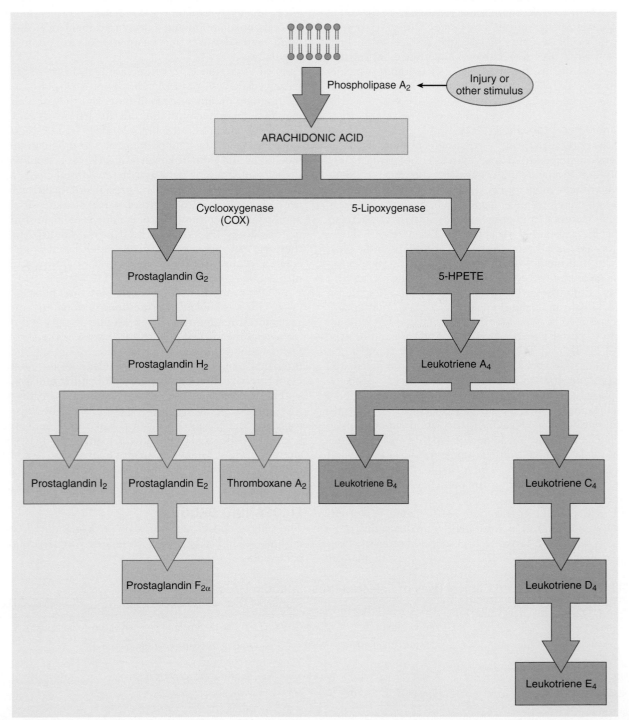

Fig. 26.2 Synthesis of eicosanoids. When phospholipase A$_2$ is activated by an injury or other stimulus, it catalyzes the hydrolysis of arachidonic acid and other 20-carbon fatty acids from cell membrane phospholipids. Arachidonic acid is converted to prostaglandins and leukotrienes by cyclooxygenase and 5-lipoxygenase, respectively. Other enzymes complete the synthesis of specific eicosanoids. *5-HPETE,* 5-Hydroperoxyeicosatetraenoic acid.

double bond is located at the sixth carbon, arachidonic acid is known as an **omega-6 fatty acid.** In diets rich in cold-water fish or plants, cell membranes contain an **omega-3 fatty acid,** eicosapentaenoic acid, with five double bonds starting at the third carbon position. Eicosapentaenoic acid is also a precursor to eicosanoid products, but these products have different biologic activities than eicosanoids generated from arachidonic acid. For example, prostaglandins derived from omega-6 fatty acids have different vasoactive and platelet-aggregating properties than prostaglandins derived from omega-3 fatty acids (see later).

After synthesis, **eicosanoids are released** from the cell to exert local effects on surrounding tissues. Unlike other autacoids, no evidence exists of vesicular storage or calcium-mediated exocytosis for eicosanoid substances within the cell. Because of this, the synthesis of eicosanoids coincides with its release though the cell membrane and into the surrounding tissue.

Eicosanoid Receptors and Effects

All of the naturally released eicosanoids are **short-lived** and locally acting. Eicosanoid drugs exist as either purified preparations of the same naturally occurring substance or closely related synthetic analogs. **Prostaglandins** exert their effects on smooth muscle, platelet aggregation, neurotransmission, glandular secretion, and other biologic activities by activating specific **prostanoid receptors** in target tissues. These receptors are GPCR proteins named according to the prostaglandin that binds with the highest affinity and selectivity; the prostanoid receptor for PGD_2 is DP, the receptor for PGE_2 is EP, and so forth, to identify the ligands for the FP, IP, and TP **(thromboxane)** receptors. To date, four types of EP receptors have been identified, designated EP_1 through EP_4; two types of DP receptors (D_1 and D_2); and one type each of FP, IP, and TP receptors. The signal transduction pathways of prostanoid receptors are diverse and mediated by G proteins that increase or decrease cyclic adenosine monophosphate, or the $DAG-IP_3$ pathway (see Chapter 3). **Thromboxanes,** which are substances derived from prostaglandin synthesis (see Fig. 26.2), also act on smooth muscle and platelet aggregation. Different types of thromboxanes and prostaglandins have different pharmacologic effects and often are opposing effects. The eicosanoid released from a tissue or cell will depend on the particular set of synthetic enzymes contained within the cell.

Whereas **platelet aggregation** is stimulated by **thromboxane A_2 (TXA_2),** it is inhibited by **prostacyclin** (prostaglandin I_2 **[PGI_2]**). Prostacyclin is released primarily from vascular endothelial cells and serves to prevent platelet aggregation under normal conditions. In contrast, TXA_2 is produced and released only when a blood vessel is injured, at which time the adherence of platelets to vascular endothelium activates the platelets and leads to the synthesis and release of TXA_2 (see Chapter 16 and Fig. 16.5).

In some cases, the fatty acid precursor of a prostaglandin or thromboxane has a major effect on its biologic activity. For example, thromboxane A_3 (TXA_3), which is synthesized from eicosapentaenoic acid, an omega-3 fatty acid found in fish oils, produces relatively little platelet aggregation or vasoconstriction in comparison with TXA_2. This difference can largely explain the correlation between **increased fish oil consumption** and a **decreased incidence of thrombotic events** (strokes and heart attacks) in certain native populations.

Both PGE_2 and PGI_2 cause **vasodilation** in several vascular beds. These prostaglandins appear to play a role in maintaining **pulmonary blood flow,** and they also serve to maintain the **patency of the ductus arteriosus** until it is time for its closure. In the kidneys, PGE_2 and PGI_2 produce vasodilation and have important roles in modulating **renal blood flow** and **glomerular filtration.** These actions are particularly important in persons with renal insufficiency and in the elderly. The renal actions of prostaglandin also appear to exert an **antihypertensive effect,** partly by increasing water and sodium excretion. Because **nonsteroidal anti-inflammatory drugs (NSAIDs)** inhibit prostaglandin synthesis, their use can cause or exacerbate renal disorders and may counteract the antihypertensive effect of antihypertensive medications taken concurrently.

Many prostaglandins, including PGE_2 and prostaglandin $F_{2\alpha}$ ($PGF_{2\alpha}$), stimulate **uterine contractions** and increase **gastrointestinal motility.** Their uterine activity is the basis for several therapeutic applications, whereas their gastrointestinal actions can lead to adverse effects (e.g., diarrhea and intestinal cramping). Several prostaglandins also produce a **cytoprotective effect on the gastrointestinal mucosa.**

The **leukotrienes** are produced primarily in inflammatory cells, including mast cells, basophils, eosinophils, macrophages, and polymorphonuclear leukocytes. Leukotrienes C_4 and D_4 (LTC_4 and LTD_4) are the main components of the **slow-reacting substance of anaphylaxis.** These two leukotrienes are secreted in the presence of asthma and anaphylaxis and play a major role in bronchospastic disease.

EICOSANOID DRUGS

The effects and clinical uses of prostaglandin drugs are outlined in Table 26.4 and summarized in the following paragraphs.

TABLE 26.4 Effects and Clinical Uses of Selected Prostaglandin Drugs

DRUG	PG CLASS	EFFECT	CLINICAL USE
Alprostadil	PGE_1	Vasodilation	Erectile dysfunction; patency of the ductus arteriosus
Carboprost tromethamine	$PGF_{2\alpha}$ analog	Contraction of uterine muscle	Abortifacient; postpartum bleeding
Dinoprostone	PGE_2	Contraction of uterine muscle	Abortifacient; cervical ripening
Epoprostenol	PGI_2	Vasodilation	Pulmonary hypertension
Latanoprost	$PGF_{2\alpha}$ analog	Increase in aqueous humor outflow	Glaucoma
Misoprostol	PGE_1 analog	Gastric cytoprotection	Gastric and duodenal ulcers induced by use of NSAIDs

NSAIDs, Nonsteroidal anti-inflammatory drugs; *PG,* prostaglandin.

Eicosanoid Synthesis Inhibitors

Among the groups of drugs that inhibit eicosanoid synthesis are **leukotriene inhibitors** (see Chapter 27), **NSAIDs** (see Chapter 30), and **corticosteroids** (see Chapter 33).

Leukotriene inhibitors act either by inhibiting 5-lipoxygenase or by blocking leukotriene receptors. They are currently used in the management of **asthma,** but other therapeutic applications are being explored.

The **NSAIDs** act by inhibiting cyclooxygenase and are used primarily to alleviate **pain** and **inflammation.**

Corticosteroids block the formation of all eicosanoids, partly by inhibiting phospholipase A_2. They have **antiinflammatory, antiallergic,** and **antineoplastic effects** and are used in the treatment of a wide variety of adrenal diseases and nonadrenal disorders.

Prostaglandin Drugs

Prostaglandin E$_1$ and Prostaglandin E$_1$ Derivatives

Alprostadil is identical to naturally occurring PGE_1 and is available in several formulations for specific clinical uses.

Alprostadil is given by continuous intravenous infusion to maintain the **patency of the ductus arteriosus** in neonates who are awaiting surgery for some types of congenital heart diseases. These include cyanotic heart defects (pulmonary atresia or stenosis, tricuspid atresia, tetralogy of Fallot, and transposition of the great vessels) and acyanotic heart defects (coarctation of the aorta and hypoplastic left ventricle).

Alprostadil is available in injectable, pellet, and cream formulations to treat **erectile dysfunction** in men. For this purpose, the drug is injected into the cavernosa of the penis, or slow-release pellets or drops of cream are inserted into the meatus of the urethra. Adverse effects in men treated with alprostadil include **penile pain,** penile fibrosis, **priapism** (persistent erection), flushing, diarrhea, headache, and fever. Given the rise in the use of oral drugs to treat erectile dysfunction, (for example, **sildenafil** [VIAGRA], **tadalafil** [CIALIS], and **vardenafil** [LEVITRA] [see Chapter 6]) it is likely that alprostadil will be limited to those patients in whom the aforementioned popular drugs are contraindicated.

Misoprostol is a synthetic PGE_1 analog available in an orally administered formulation for the prevention of NSAID-induced **gastric ulcers** and **duodenal ulcers** (see Chapter 28). Misoprostol treatment is particularly useful in patients who take NSAIDs on a long-term basis to alleviate the symptoms of arthritis and other inflammatory conditions. Misoprostol acts locally on the GI mucosa to exert a cytoprotective effect by inhibiting gastric acid secretion and by increasing bicarbonate secretion from mucosal cells. Diarrhea, one of the most common adverse effects of misoprostol use, can be minimized by starting patients on a low dose of the drug and then gradually increasing the dose. In pregnant women, misoprostol is absolutely contraindicated because it can stimulate uterine contractions and cause premature labor.

Misoprostol is also approved for use as an abortifacient in combination with the progesterone receptor antagonist **mifepristone** (RU-486, MIFEPREX). When used in combination, mifepristone and misoprostol are 95% to 97% effective within the first 2 weeks of pregnancy (see Chapter 34).

Prostaglandin E$_2$ and Prostaglandin F$_{2\alpha}$ Derivatives

Dinoprostone and **carboprost tromethamine** are prostaglandin drugs that have oxytocic activity and increase the uterine contractions of pregnant women. Dinoprostone is a formulation of naturally occurring PGE_2, whereas carboprost is a synthetic derivative of $PGF_{2\alpha}$.

Dinoprostone is available as a vaginal insert, gel, or suppository. In pregnant women, the vaginal insert or gel is applied to the vagina or cervix to produce **cervical ripening** before labor induction. The insert may provide more accurate dosing than the gel. The suppository is used to **evacuate the uterine contents** in cases of intrauterine fetal death, benign hydatidiform mole, or second-trimester termination of pregnancy.

Carboprost is administered intramuscularly to **control postpartum bleeding** when other measures have failed and to **terminate pregnancy (abortifacient).** It can cause flushing, diarrhea, vomiting, altered blood pressure, blurred vision, respiratory distress, and other adverse reactions.

Latanoprost was the first prostaglandin drug indicated for the treatment of **glaucoma.** It is administered topically as eyedrops and is used to treat open-angle glaucoma that is resistant to other pharmacologic treatments. Latanoprost is a $PGF_{2\alpha}$ analog that acts on FP receptors to increase aqueous humor outflow via the uveoscleral pathway (see Box 6.1). It can alter the color of the iris and cause a **permanent eye color change** by increasing the amount of melanin in melanocytes. Other synthetic FP receptor agonists developed for the reduction of intraocular pressure in patients with open-angle glaucoma or ocular hypertension are **bimatoprost** and **travoprost,** and **tafluprost.**

Prostaglandin I$_2$ and Prostaglandin I$_2$ Derivatives

Epoprostenol is a formulation of naturally occurring PGI_2 **(prostacyclin)** used to treat **pulmonary arterial hypertension.** Epoprostenol acts on IP receptors to dilate pulmonary blood vessels and increase pulmonary blood flow, thereby counteracting the pathophysiologic consequences of pulmonary hypertension. The drug is administered by continuous intravenous infusion, and the dosage is titrated on the basis of clinical improvement and adverse effects. The most common adverse reactions include flushing, tachycardia, hypotension, diarrhea, nausea, vomiting, and flulike symptoms.

Treprostinil is a stable **analog of prostacyclin** that has a half-life of 2 to 4 hours, and it can be safely administered by a continuous subcutaneous infusion via a self-inserted subcutaneous catheter using a microinfusion pump designed specifically for subcutaneous drug delivery. It is approved to diminish the symptoms (e.g., shortness of breath) associated with physical activity in patients with pulmonary arterial hypertension. **Selexipag** is an orally administered prostacyclin IP receptor agonist indicated for the treatment of pulmonary arterial hypertension. Selexipag is metabolized by esterases to its active metabolite, which is about 40 times more potent than selexipag.

ENDOTHELIN-1 ANTAGONISTS

Endothelin-1 (ET-1) is a peptide autacoid produced by vascular endothelial cells. It activates ET_A and ET_B receptors in vascular smooth muscle and other tissues. The results of ET_A receptor activation are vasoconstriction and cell proliferation, and ET_B receptors mediate vasodilation, antiproliferation, and increased ET-1 clearance. ET-1 may serve physiologically to counteract the vasodilation produced by the endothelin-relaxing factor (nitric oxide), but levels of ET-1 peptide are increased 10-fold in pulmonary arteries of patients with **pulmonary arterial hypertension** (PAH). ET-1 also appears to contribute to cardiac dysfunction during reperfusion after thrombolytic treatment in patients undergoing acute myocardial infarction.

Bosentan (Tracleer) is a **dual ET$_A$ and ET$_B$ receptor antagonist** that is approved for treating PAH. Clinical trials have shown that bosentan significantly improves 6-minute walking distances in persons with class III or IV PAH, while decreasing pulmonary vascular resistance and dyspnea.

Bosentan is administered orally and is generally well tolerated, but 11% of patients have experienced elevated serum aminotransferase levels. For this reason, **liver function tests** should be monitored at baseline and then monthly in persons taking bosentan. Based on animal studies, bosentan is very likely to cause major **birth defects** if used by pregnant women, and it is contraindicated in pregnancy and in women of childbearing age who are not using hormonal contraceptives.

A second ET receptor antagonist, **ambrisentan,** was recently approved for the treatment of PAH. Ambrisentan has much **greater selectivity for ET$_A$ receptors** than for ET$_B$ receptors (>4000-fold), although the clinical effect of such high selectivity is not known. As with bosentan, warnings are made regarding hepatic function and enzyme level monitoring. A third ET receptor antagonist drug indicated for the treatment of PAH, called **macitentan,** is also available.

Although not an endothelin drug, **sildenafil** (Viagra) is now also marketed under a new trade name, Revatio, for the treatment of PAH, along with other PDE$_5$ inhibitors (see Chapter 6). As sildenafil inhibits PDE$_5$, an increase of cyclic guanosine monophosphate within pulmonary vascular smooth muscle cells results in relaxation and vasodilation of the pulmonary vascular bed.

SUMMARY OF IMPORTANT POINTS

- Autacoids include histamine, serotonin, prostaglandins, and leukotrienes. These substances usually act on the same tissue in which they are produced.
- Histamine is the primary mediator of allergic reactions. Stimulation of H$_1$ receptors causes vasodilation, edema, congestion, and pruritus. Stimulation of H$_2$ receptors mediates gastric acid secretion.
- The first-generation H$_1$ receptor antagonists (chlorpheniramine, diphenhydramine, meclizine, promethazine, and others) produce varying degrees of sedation and also have anticholinergic side effects. The second-generation drugs (cetirizine, loratadine, fexofenadine, and desloratadine) are largely devoid of CNS effects.
- The H$_1$ receptor antagonists are used primarily to treat allergies, but meclizine is used to prevent motion sickness, and promethazine is used to treat nausea and vomiting.
- Fexofenadine is the active metabolite of the now-banned terfenadine. Unlike terfenadine, fexofenadine does not prolong the QT interval or cause torsades de pointes. Cetirizine, desloratadine, and loratadine also lack cardiac effects.

- Pitolisant is the first H$_3$ receptor antagonist and is approved for the treatment of narcolepsy.
- Drugs that affect serotonin (5-hydroxytryptamine, or 5-HT) are classified as serotonin agonists, serotonin antagonists, and serotonin reuptake inhibitors.
- Some 5-HT$_1$ receptor agonists can be used to treat migraine headaches, whereas some 5-HT$_2$ receptor antagonists can be used to prevent migraine headaches.
- Cyproheptadine, which is a 5-HT$_2$ receptor antagonist, is used in the management of carcinoid syndrome, which is caused by excessive production of serotonin and other vasoactive substances in patients with carcinoid tumors from enterochromaffin tissue.
- Ondansetron, granisetron, and many other "setron" drugs are 5-HT$_3$ receptor antagonists used in the treatment of nausea and vomiting.
- Eicosanoids are derived from arachidonic acid and other precursor 20-carbon fatty acids. The two main groups of eicosanoids are prostaglandins and leukotrienes. The ratio of omega-6 and omega-3 fatty acids in the diet plays an important role in the activity of eicosanoid end products.
- Alprostadil is PGE$_1$ and misoprostol is a PGE$_1$ derivative. Alprostadil is used to maintain patency of the ductus arteriosus in neonates awaiting surgery for heart defects. It is also used to treat erectile dysfunction in men. Misoprostol is used to prevent gastric and duodenal ulcers in persons taking NSAIDs.
- Dinoprostone, the same as PGE$_2$, is used for cervical ripening before induction of labor and for evacuation of the uterine contents.
- Carboprost and latanoprost are PGF$_{2\alpha}$ derivatives. Carboprost is used to control postpartum bleeding and to terminate pregnancy. Latanoprost and other prostaglandin antiglaucoma drugs that increase the aqueous humor outflow are used to treat glaucoma.
- Epoprostenol is PGI$_2$ (prostacyclin) and treprostinil is a PGI$_2$ derivative; both are used to treat pulmonary arterial hypertension. In addition, bosentan and ambrisentan, endothelin-1 receptor antagonists, and a new formulation of sildenafil are indicated for pulmonary arterial hypertension.

Review Questions

1. Which of the following antihistamines would be best used to treat mild nausea and vomiting caused by motion sickness?
   (A) cetirizine
   (B) fexofenadine
   (C) loratadine
   (D) diphenhydramine
   (E) meclizine
2. Which of the following describes the major difference between a first- and second-generation antihistamine?
   (A) selectivity at H$_1$ receptors
   (B) ability to cross the blood-brain barrier
   (C) effectiveness in treating allergies
   (D) potency at blocking H$_1$ receptors
   (E) indications for use

3. Of the major serotonin (5-HT) receptors identified and used as targets for therapeutic agents, which one is the only one considered a ligand-gated ion channel?
    (A) 5-HT_{1B}
    (B) 5-HT_{1D}
    (C) 5-HT_2
    (D) 5-HT_3
    (E) 5-HT_4
4. Which of the following drugs is the same as PGI_2 (prostacyclin) and is used for the treatment of pulmonary hypertension?
    (A) misoprostol
    (B) alprostadil
    (C) epoprostenol
    (D) treprostinil
    (E) travoprost
5. Latanoprost is an agonist at the PGF_2 receptors and is effective for the treatment of
    (A) cornea abrasions
    (B) ocular hypertension and open-angle glaucoma
    (C) ocular albinism
    (D) closed-angle glaucoma
    (E) allergic conjunctivitis

CHAPTER 27
Pharmacological Treatment of Respiratory Disorders

Anti-inflammatory Drugs

Corticosteroids
- Fluticasone (FLOVENT, FLONASE)[a]
- Prednisone[b]

Mast cell stabilizers
- Cromolyn sodium[c]

Antileukotriene drugs
- Montelukast (SINGULAIR)
- Zafirlukast (ACCOLATE)
- Zileuton (ZYFLO)

Phosphodiesterase Inhibitor
- Roflumilast (DALIRESP)

Bronchodilators

Selective *beta*$_2$-adrenoceptor agonists
- Albuterol (PROVENTIL, VENTOLIN)
- Arformoterol (BROVANA)
- Formoterol (FORADIL)
- Salmeterol (SEREVENT)[d]

Other bronchodilators
- Ipratropium (ATROVENT)
- Tiotropium (SPIRIVA)
- Umeclidinium (INCRUSE Ellipta)
- Aclidinium (Tudorza Pressair)

- Revefenacin (YUPRELI)
- Theophylline

Monoclonal Antibody Drugs
- Omalizumab (XOLAIR)
- Mepolizumab (NUCALA)
- Resliozumab (CINQAIR)
- Benralizumab (FASENRA)

Antitussives
- Codeine
- Dextromethorphan (DM)
- Hydrocodone

Expectorants
- Guaifenesin (MUCINEX)

Antihistamines
- Diphenhydramine (BENADRYL)
- Fexofenadine (ALLEGRA)[e]

Drugs for Cystic Fibrosis
- Ivacaftor (KALYDECO)[f]
- Dornase alfa (PULMOZYME)
- Aztreonam for inhalation (CAYSTON)[g]

[a] Also as fluticasone furoate (ARNUITY ELLIPTA). Other corticosteroids include budesonide (PULMICORT, RHINOCORT), beclomethasone (QVAR), mometasone (NASONEX), triamcinolone (NASACORT), and ciclesonide (OMNARIS). Combination products with corticosteroids include fluticasone with salmeterol (ADVAIR), fluticasone with azelastine (DYMISTA), and fluticasone with vilanterol (BREO ELLIPTA).
[b] Also prednisolone, and methylprednisolone.
[c] Also lodoxamide (ALOMIDE), and nedocromil (ALOCRIL).
[d] Also levalbuterol (XOPENEX), indacaterol (ARCAPTA), terbutaline, vilanterol, and olodaterol (STRIVERDI RESPIMAT). Combination products include tiotropium with olodaterol (STIOLTO RESPIMAT), glycopyrrolate with indacaterol (UTIBRON NEOHALER), glycopyrrolate with formoterol (BEVESPI AEROSPHERE), and umeclidinium with vilanterol (ANORO ELLIPTA).
[e] Also loratadine (CLARITIN), cetirizine (ZYRTEC), azelastine (ASTELIN) and olopatadine (PAZEO).
[f] Also lumacaftor with ivacaftor (ORKAMBI) tezacaftor with ivacaftor (SYMDECO), and elexacaftor with ivacaftor and tezacaftor (TRIKAFTA).
[g] Also tobramycin inhalation solution (TOBI, BETHKIS, KITABIS PAK) and inhalation powder (TOBI PODHALER).

OVERVIEW

Respiratory Tract Disorders

This chapter is concerned with the pharmacology and clinical use of drugs for common respiratory tract conditions, including asthma, chronic obstructive pulmonary disease (COPD), and the upper respiratory tract symptoms of cough, congestion, and rhinitis (inflammation of the nasal mucosa). The chapter closes with a brief discussion of drugs used for the treatment of cystic fibrosis.

Asthma

Asthma is characterized by airway obstruction caused by inflammation and increased responsiveness to stimuli that cause bronchoconstriction, such as **allergens, cold air, exercise,** and **emotional stress.** The primary symptoms of asthma are difficult breathing, shortness of breath, wheezing, and coughing (Box 27.1).

In susceptible persons, exposure to a stimulus can trigger the release of substances from mast cells, eosinophils, basophils, neutrophils, and macrophages. Some of these substances, such as **histamine, adenosine, bradykinin,** and **major basic protein,** are stored in cell granules. Other substances are formed and immediately released in response to asthmatic stimuli, including those derived from arachidonic acid known as **leukotrienes** and **prostaglandins.** These substances contribute to **inflammation** of the airway, edema and desquamation of the bronchial epithelium, and hypertrophy of smooth muscles in the respiratory tract. The chemical mediators of asthma also increase the responsiveness of smooth muscles and the permeability of bronchioles

CASE PRESENTATION

A 12-year-old boy is brought to his pediatrician after a recent onset of episodes of coughing, wheezing, and shortness of breath. These episodes have occurred two or three times a week while he was playing outdoors, and they gradually subsided after he came indoors and sat down to rest. The family has a history of allergies to molds and pollens, and the boy has been taking an antihistamine for allergic rhinitis. Examination shows an alert, well-developed boy of normal height and weight who is in no distress. His vital signs and breath sounds are normal except for fine wheezes during forced expiration, and there are no signs of infection. Spirometry tests show a forced expiratory volume in 1 second (FEV_1) that is 85% of the predicted value, and the boy's peak expiratory flow (PEF) variability is 20% (normal <20%). These findings are consistent with a diagnosis of mild asthma, which was probably precipitated by exposure to allergens and by exercise. After discussing treatment options with his parents, the boy is started on a daily dose of montelukast, and an albuterol inhaler will be used to control acute episodes. The patient and his parents receive further instructions and training concerning the use of the inhaler, and he is given prescriptions and scheduled for a follow-up evaluation in 3 weeks to determine the need for additional therapy.

CASE DISCUSSION

Asthma typically manifests with wheezing, dyspnea, and coughing and is often associated with a history of respiratory allergies. The history, physical examination findings, and FEV_1 usually provide most of the information needed to diagnose and manage asthma. The patient appears to have mild asthma, which may be intermittent or persistent. Because the severity of his illness is uncertain, the patient is started on a leukotriene receptor antagonist because of its convenience, safety, and demonstrated effectiveness in children. The course of asthma is highly variable. His response to treatment and the future course of his illness will be monitored in order to determine the need for additional tests and treatments.

to allergens, infectious agents, mediators of inflammation, and other irritants. As a result, mucus production increases and leads to mucus plugging of the airways that reduces the ability of the airways to remove noxious substances.

Airway obstruction in asthma results from a combination of bronchial inflammation, bronchoconstriction, and obstruction of the lumen with mucus, inflammatory cells, and epithelial debris. Symptoms of obstruction include dyspnea (difficult breathing), coughing, wheezing, headache, tachycardia, syncope, sweating, pallor, and cyanosis. Patients experience a biphasic reduction in pulmonary function, with an early phase that occurs within 10 to 30 minutes of exposure to an allergen and lasts for 2 to 3 hours, and then a late phase that occurs 2 to 8 hours after exposure. The late phase is believed to be responsible for inducing and maintaining bronchial hyperreactivity in asthmatic patients. Because of the circadian variation in bronchial responsiveness, some patients have up to an eightfold increase in airway hyper-responsiveness at night, and nearly 70% of asthma-related deaths happen at night.

The drugs used to treat asthma include **anti-inflammatory drugs and bronchodilators.** The pathophysiology of asthma and sites of anti-inflammatory drug action are illustrated in Fig. 27.1.

Chronic Obstructive Pulmonary Disease

COPD includes **chronic bronchitis** and **emphysema.** Chronic bronchitis is characterized by a productive cough associated with inflammation of the bronchioles, whereas emphysema is caused by permanent destruction and enlargement of the airspaces distal to the bronchioles. Both conditions result in airway obstruction, dyspnea, decreased blood oxygen concentrations, and elevated blood carbon dioxide concentrations. Patients with these conditions have abnormal pulmonary function test values, such as a decreased forced expiratory volume in 1 second (FEV_1). **Smoking and advanced age** are the primary risk factors for COPD, and smoking cessation can slow disease progression. Although most of the airway obstruction in COPD is irreversible, a portion of the obstruction is caused by smooth muscle spasm and bronchiolar inflammation, and this portion can be reversed by bronchodilator drugs. Patients with COPD often require long-term oxygen therapy, and antibiotics can be used to treat acute exacerbations caused by bacterial infections.

Rhinitis

Rhinitis, or inflammation of the mucous membranes of the nasal passages, is most frequently caused by **allergic reactions** to pollens, mold spores, and dust mites or by a **virus infection** caused by rhinoviruses and other agents of the common cold.

Allergic rhinitis can be seasonal or nonseasonal (perennial), whereas viral rhinitis is an acute, self-limiting condition. Both types of rhinitis are characterized by sneezing, nasal congestion, and rhinorrhea. Nasal pruritus and conjunctivitis are more commonly associated with allergic rhinitis than with viral rhinitis. Malaise, pain, and general discomfort are generally associated with viral rhinitis.

Table 27.1 shows the relative efficacy of various types of respiratory tract drugs, including those used in the treatment of allergic rhinitis and viral rhinitis.

ANTI-INFLAMMATORY DRUGS

Corticosteroids

Corticosteroids (glucocorticoids) are effective in the treatment of a wide variety of inflammatory and other diseases. The discussion here focuses on the use corticosteroids for **asthma, allergic rhinitis,** and **COPD.** The pharmacologic properties and clinical use of these drugs are described more completely in Chapter 33.

The recognition that asthma is primarily an inflammatory disease has increased the role of corticosteroids in asthma therapy. For persons with moderate to severe asthma, steroids have become the cornerstone of therapy, and some patients with mild asthma may derive significant benefit from their use as well. Although corticosteroids are the most efficacious anti-inflammatory drugs available for the treatment of both asthma and allergic rhinitis (see Table 27.1), they have the potential to cause a number of adverse effects if given systemically. The incidence of adverse effects is markedly reduced when these drugs are given by inhalation, so this route of administration is employed whenever possible. Systemic administration is usually reserved for the treatment of severe asthma or for short-term treatment of severe allergic rhinitis.

Among the steroids available as metered-dose inhalers are **beclomethasone, budesonide, fluticasone,** and **triamcinolone.** Beclomethasone and triamcinolone are usually administered three or four times a day, whereas fluticasone

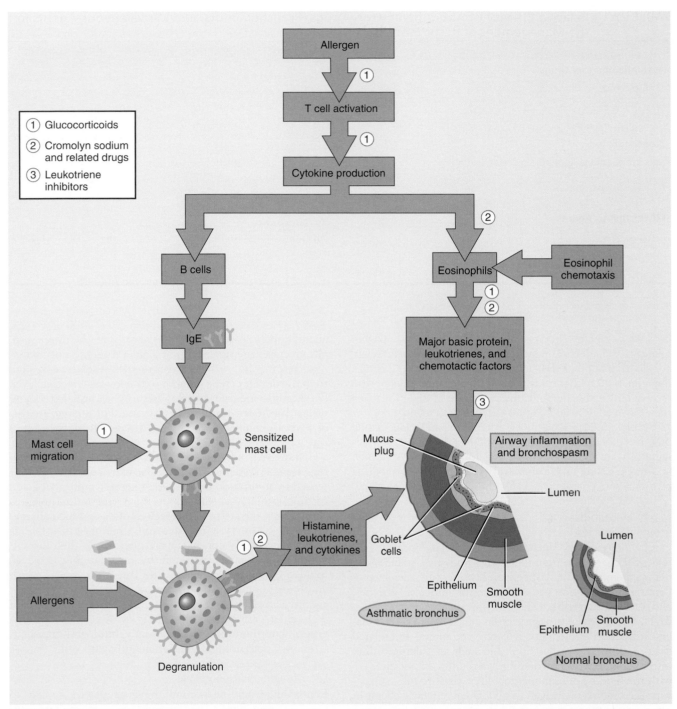

FIG. 27.1 Pathophysiology of asthma and sites of anti-inflammatory drug action. When allergens activate T cells, cytokine production is stimulated. The cytokines, in turn, trigger the recruitment, activation, and release of a variety of cells and mediators. Glucocorticoids (corticosteroids) inhibit numerous steps in this process, including T-cell activation, cytokine production, eosinophil recruitment and activation, and mast cell migration. Glucocorticoids, cromolyn sodium, and other cromolyn-related drugs all inhibit the release of mediators from mast cells and eosinophils. Cromolyn and related drugs also inhibit eosinophil chemotaxis induced by cytokines and other mediators. Leukotriene inhibitors either block leukotriene receptors or inhibit leukotriene synthesis. *IgE*, Immunoglobulin E.

and budesonide need to be administered only twice a day. The proper use of metered-dose inhalers requires considerable skill and the use of a spacer device between the mouth and the inhaler. The spacer decreases the amount of drug that is deposited in the mouth and upper airway and facilitates the delivery of the drug to the bronchioles.

As with other anti-inflammatory drugs, corticosteroids are primarily used on a **long-term basis** to **prevent asthmatic attacks,** rather than to treat acute bronchospasm.

The maximal response to steroids usually requires treatment for up to 8 weeks. Corticosteroids can reduce the number and severity of symptoms and decrease the need for *beta*$_2$-adrenoceptor agonists and other bronchodilators.

Adverse effects associated with inhaled corticosteroids are usually mild. Excessive deposition of the drugs in the mouth and upper airway can lead to **oral candidiasis** (thrush). There has been some concern about the potential for steroids to suppress **growth** in children. This problem is difficult to evaluate

TABLE 27.1   Relative Efficacy of Anti-Inflammatory Drugs, Bronchodilators, and Miscellaneous Agents in the Management of Respiratory Tract Disorders[a]

DRUG	ASTHMA	COPD	ALLERGIC RHINITIS	VIRAL RHINITIS
Anti-inflammatory Drugs				
Corticosteroids	++++	0 to ++	++++	0
Mast cell stabilizers	+++	0 to ++	+++	0
Leukotriene inhibitors	+++	0 to +	Unknown	0
Bronchodilators				
Selective $beta_2$-adrenoceptor agonists	++++	++	0	0
Ipratropium	+	+++	++	++
Theophylline	++ to +++	++ to +++	0	0
Miscellaneous Agents				
Analgesics	0	0	0	+++
Antihistamines	0 to ++	0	++++	+
Decongestants	0 to ++	0 to ++	+++	+++

COPD, Chronic obstructive pulmonary disease (e.g., emphysema).
[a]Ratings range from 0 (not efficacious) to ++++ (highly efficacious).

because asthmatic children may have growth disturbances related to their disease. A meta-analysis of 21 studies, however, concluded that inhaled beclomethasone does not cause growth impairment. Another study showed that 95% of children who received inhaled budesonide for an average of 9 years reached their target adult height despite initial growth retardation.

Several products contain a corticosteroid and a long-acting $beta_2$-receptor agonist (see later), including **fluticasone and salmeterol** (ADVAIR), **budesonide and formoterol** (SYMBICORT), and **mometasone and formoterol** (DULERA). These products provide a convenient method for chronic asthma therapy.

Mast Cell Stabilizers
Cromolyn Sodium

Chemistry and Mechanisms. Cromolyn sodium and related drugs are nonsteroidal compounds that stabilize the plasma membranes of mast cells and eosinophils, thereby preventing degranulation and release of histamine, leukotrienes, and other substances that cause airway inflammation (see Fig. 27.1). Hence, these drugs are often called **mast cell stabilizers.** Inhibition of mediator release by cromolyn and related drugs is thought to result from **blockade of calcium influx** into mast cells. Cromolyn and related drugs do not interfere with the binding of immunoglobulin E (IgE) to mast cells or with the binding of antigen to IgE. Their beneficial effects in asthma and other conditions are largely prophylactic.

Pharmacokinetics. Cromolyn and other mast cell stabilizers are rather insoluble in body fluids, and minimal systemic absorption occurs after oral administration or inhalation of these drugs. In fact, the oral bioavailability of cromolyn is about 1%. When cromolyn is **administered by inhalation,** its major effect is exerted on the respiratory tract and very little is absorbed into the circulation. Most of the drug is swallowed after inhalation, and about 98% is excreted in the feces.

Indications. Cromolyn is administered by inhalation to treat **asthma** or **allergic rhinitis** and is available in an ophthalmic solution to treat **vernal (seasonal) conjunctivitis.** Cromolyn and related compounds are primarily used for the long-term prophylaxis of asthmatic bronchoconstriction and allergic reactions, and they have no role in the treatment of acute bronchospasm. For perennial asthma, the drug is usually given several times a day at regular intervals until symptoms resolve. Improvement can require several weeks, and then the dosage can be reduced to the lowest effective level. For exercise-induced asthma, cromolyn is inhaled 1 hour or less before the anticipated exercise. For allergic rhinitis or vernal conjunctivitis, cromolyn is administered several times a day at regular intervals.

Cromolyn is administered orally before meals and at bedtime to treat **systemic mastocytosis,** a rare condition characterized by infiltration of the liver, spleen, lymph nodes, and gastrointestinal tract with mast cells. A similar dosage schedule has been used to treat **ulcerative colitis** and **food allergy.**

Adverse Effects. Cromolyn and other mast cell stabilizers are **remarkably nontoxic,** partly because of their low solubility and systemic absorption. In some patients, however, inhaled cromolyn can irritate the throat and cause cough and bronchospasm. Administration of a $beta_2$-adrenoceptor agonist can usually prevent or relieve this reaction. Nasal and ocular preparations can cause localized pain and irritation, but these effects are usually mild and transient. Cromolyn does not interact significantly with other drugs.

Lodoxamide and Nedocromil

Lodoxamide and **nedocromil** have properties similar to those of cromolyn and are formulated as ophthalmic solutions to treat ocular allergies, including **vernal keratitis** and **vernal conjunctivitis.** They can cause ocular discomfort but are generally well tolerated.

Leukotriene Inhibitors

Leukotrienes (*leuko* from leukocyte; *trienes* meaning three conjugated double bonds) are a group of arachidonic acid metabolites formed via the **5-lipoxygenase pathway** in mast cells and various types of leukocytes, as shown in Fig. 27.2. **Cysteinyl leukotrienes C4, D4, and E4** activate the **type 1 cysteinyl leukotriene receptor** ($CysLT_1$), and thereby increase recruitment of leukocytes, stimulate mucus secretion, increase vascular permeability, increase collagen, and cause smooth muscle proliferation and contraction. These

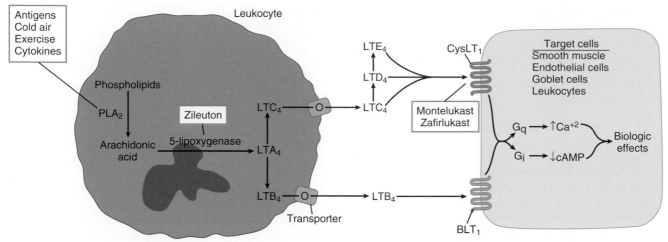

FIG. 27.2 Synthesis and effects of leukotrienes and sites of drug action. Asthmatic stimuli (antigens, cold air, exercise, cytokines, and others) activate phospholipase A_2 (PLA_2), leading to formation of leukotriene A_4 (LTA_4) by 5-lipoxygenase, which is inhibited by zileuton. LTA_4 is converted to leukotriene B_4, which activates B leukotriene receptors, such as BLT_1. LTA_4 is also converted to the cysteinyl leukotrienes C_4, D_4, and E_4, which activate cysteinyl leukotriene receptors, such as $CysLT_1$. These receptors are blocked by montelukast and zafirlukast. Leukotriene receptors are coupled with G_q and G_i, leading to increased intracellular calcium, decreased cAMP, activation of protein kinases, and biologic effects.

effects lead to **airway inflammation** and to **sustained bronchoconstriction**. The effects of leukotrienes are mediated in part by activation of G protein–coupled receptors linked with G_q, which increases intracellular calcium and activates protein kinase C.

Leukotriene Receptor Antagonists

Mechanisms. **Montelukast** and **zafirlukast** have a structure that resembles that of the **cysteinyl leukotrienes,** and they compete with these substances for the $CysLT_1$ receptor. These drugs inhibit both the early and the late phases of bronchoconstriction induced by antigen challenge. However, they do not block the effects of leukotriene B_4, which appear to be important in severe asthma and asthma exacerbations.

Pharmacokinetics. Montelukast and zafirlukast are administered orally and are well absorbed from the gut. **Montelukast** is taken as a single daily dose in the evening and is available in dosage forms for treating adults and pediatric patients as young as 6 months old. **Zafirlukast** is indicated for patients aged 5 years and older and is given twice daily 1 to 2 hours before meals because food retards its absorption. These drugs are highly bound to plasma proteins (>99%) and are extensively metabolized by hepatic cytochrome P450 enzymes.

Effects and Indications. Montelukast and zafirlukast have been shown to improve pulmonary function, control symptoms, reduce the need for short-acting rescue $beta_2$-agonists, decrease asthma exacerbations, and improve overall quality of life of asthmatic patients. Although inhaled corticosteroids are more potent than leukotriene antagonists and are generally preferred for initial therapy, antileukotriene agents can be used in persons who are unable or unwilling to take steroids. Leukotriene receptor antagonists offer the advantages of **convenient oral administration and minimal side effects,** and they often benefit asthmatic patients not adequately controlled by inhaled steroids alone. They are not as effective as long-acting $beta_2$-agonists as add-on therapy to corticosteroids, but they may be safer (see later).

Antileukotriene drugs are effective in persons with **allergic asthma,** including **aspirin-sensitive asthma,** and they may be used to prevent **exercised-induced asthma** when taken at least 2 hours before the precipitating event. The beneficial effects of these drugs are cumulative, and maximal effectiveness may require several weeks to months of therapy. Although they are not indicated for the treatment of acute bronchospasm, they do enhance the bronchodilating effect of $beta_2$-agonists. In general, antileukotriene agents benefit children more than adults with asthma, and younger children more than older children.

Adverse Effects and Interactions. Leukotriene antagonists are relatively free of serious adverse effects, but hypersensitivity reactions and other adverse effects may occur in a small percentage of patients. Rare cases of liver injury have been reported, and a few cases of liver failure have occurred. Rarely, allergic granulomatous vasculitis (Churg-Strauss syndrome), a condition often treated with corticosteroids, has developed in patients being withdrawn from glucocorticoid therapy while a leukotriene antagonist has been substituted. In such cases, corticosteroids should be withdrawn gradually and patients closely monitored.

Zafirlukast inhibits CYP2C9 and CYP3A4 and may interfere with the metabolism of phenytoin and warfarin (metabolized by CYP2C9) and of felodipine, lovastatin, and triazolam (metabolized by CYP3A4). **Montelukast does not inhibit these isozymes** or exhibit significant drug interactions, and its use may be preferred in patients receiving concomitant drug therapy.

Zileuton

Effects and Indications. Leukotriene synthesis increases during an asthmatic attack; this can be prevented by zileuton, which inhibits **5-lipoxygenase** and blocks the formation of all leukotrienes, including LTB_4. Because the $CysLT_1$ receptor antagonists do not block the **leukocyte chemoattractant** and other effects of LTB_4, zileuton might be more effective in severe cases of asthma in which these effects may be particularly important.

Zileuton is indicated for the prophylaxis and treatment of asthma in adults and children 12 years of age and older. The immediate-release formulation should be taken orally four times a day, but a sustained-release preparation is now available for twice-daily administration. Zileuton undergoes some first-pass hepatic inactivation and is almost entirely eliminated as the glucuronide metabolite with a half-life of about 2 hours.

Adverse Effects and Interactions. Mild and transient adverse reactions to zileuton use include a flulike syndrome, headache, drowsiness, and dyspepsia. Zileuton may elevate **hepatic enzyme levels,** so patients taking the drug should be monitored for signs of hepatitis. Patients with transaminase levels greater than three times the upper limit of normal should discontinue zileuton, and it should be used cautiously in patients who consume substantial quantities of alcohol.

Zileuton **inhibits CYP1A2 and CYP3A4,** and it may elevate plasma concentrations of theophylline and warfarin. Doses of these drugs may need to be reduced in individuals taking zileuton.

Phosphodiesterase Type 4 Inhibitors

Phosphodiesterase type 4 (PDE4) is a family of enzymes that hydrolyze **cyclic adenosine monophosphate** (cAMP) and are predominantly found in immune cells. PDE4 inhibitors increase cAMP levels and exert anti-inflammatory actions, and they are being investigated for treatment of a wide range of disorders. **Apremilast** is approved for treatment of psoriatic arthritis (see Chapter 30), while **roflumilast** is used for treatment of COPD.

Roflumilast

Mechanism and Effects. Roflumilast and its active metabolite are selective inhibitors of PDE4 in lung tissue, and it is being employed in the treatment of more severe cases of COPD. A 4-week roflumilast treatment reduced sputum neutrophils and eosinophils by 30% to 40% in COPD patients, while increasing drug FEV_1 by an average of 50 mL across four clinical trials.

Indications. Roflumilast is used to reduce **COPD exacerbations** in patients with chronic bronchitis who have a history of exacerbations. It is **not a bronchodilator** and has no utility in acute episodes.

Adverse Effects and Interactions. The most common side effects of roflumilast are **diarrhea, nausea,** and **weight loss.** The drug causes psychiatric effects in about 5% of patients, particularly anxiety, insomnia, and depression. Roflumilast is metabolized by CYP3A4 and CYP1A2, and strong inducers (e.g., rifampin) and inhibitors (e.g., erythromycin) of CYP enzymes should be used with caution in patients taking roflumilast.

Administration and Kinetics. Roflumilast is administered orally once a day and has **good oral bioavailability.** It is converted to an active N-oxide metabolite by CYP enzymes before undergoing renal excretion. The half-lives of the parent compound and its metabolite are about 17 and 30 hours, respectively.

BRONCHODILATORS

The bronchodilators include selective $beta_2$-adrenoceptor agonists, muscarinic receptor antagonists, and theophylline. All of these drugs relax bronchial smooth muscle and prevent or relieve bronchospasm. The $beta_2$-agonists are the only type of bronchodilator used to terminate acute asthmatic attacks. Muscarinic antagonists are less useful in asthma and are primarily used to treat patients with COPD. Theophylline can be administered on a long-term basis to reduce bronchoconstriction in patients with either asthma or emphysema.

Beta$_2$-Adrenoceptor Agonists

The selective $beta_2$-adrenoceptor agonists are the primary bronchodilators used in the treatment of **asthma.** By activating $beta_2$-receptors, these drugs increase cAMP concentrations in smooth muscle and thereby cause the muscle to relax (Fig. 27.3; see also Fig. 11.3). The selective $beta_2$-agonists relax bronchial smooth muscle without producing as much cardiac stimulation as the nonselective $beta$-receptor agonists (Fig. 27.4). The selectivity of $beta_2$-agonists is limited, however, and higher doses can activate cardiac $beta_1$-receptors and thereby increase heart rate. Furthermore, the human heart contains some $beta_2$-receptors, possibly 10% to 50% of the total cardiac $beta$-receptors, and even highly selective $beta_2$-agonists may increase heart rate and contractility.

Chapter 8 describes the pharmacologic and other properties of various types of adrenoceptor agonists, and Table 27.2 compares the properties of selective $beta_2$-adrenoceptor agonists that are administered by inhalation. All $beta_2$-agonists can cause tachycardia, tremor, and nervousness.

Rapid-acting $beta_2$-agonists (e.g., **albuterol, levalbuterol, fenoterol,** and **terbutaline**) are usually given by the inhalational route to prevent or treat **acute bronchospasm.** Although oral formulations of albuterol and terbutaline are available for children or adults who are unable to use a metered-dose inhaler, the oral formulations have a slower onset of action and cause more systemic side effects.

Levalbuterol, the (R)-enantiomer of racemic albuterol, is claimed to cause less tachycardia, fewer palpitations, and fewer tremors than albuterol, but a study found no significant difference in heart rates or number of emergency department visits between racemic albuterol and levalbuterol.

Salmeterol and formoterol are long-acting $beta_2$-receptor agonists (LABAs) that are given twice daily by inhalation for the long-term treatment of asthma and emphysema. They are particularly useful in preventing **nocturnal asthmatic attacks,** which are sometimes life-threatening. Salmeterol and formoterol inhibit the late phase of **allergen-induced bronchoconstriction,** which usually occurs after the bronchodilating effects of shorter-acting drugs have dissipated. These drugs are not indicated for the treatment of acute bronchospasm, for which a rapid-acting $beta_2$-agonist should be used. Salmeterol and formoterol are available as single ingredients and in combination products that contain fluticasone or budesonide, respectively. **Arformoterol,** the active stereoisomer of formoterol, is administered twice daily by inhalation for treatment of bronchoconstriction in COPD patients with **chronic bronchitis** or **emphysema.**

Indacaterol is an ultralong-acting $beta_2$-receptor agonist that has recently been approved for the treatment of airflow obstruction in patients with COPD. It is the **only once-daily $beta_2$-receptor agonist** bronchodilator available for this purpose. A clinical study found that **indacaterol** may be more effective than twice-daily formoterol in improving FEV_1 in COPD patients.

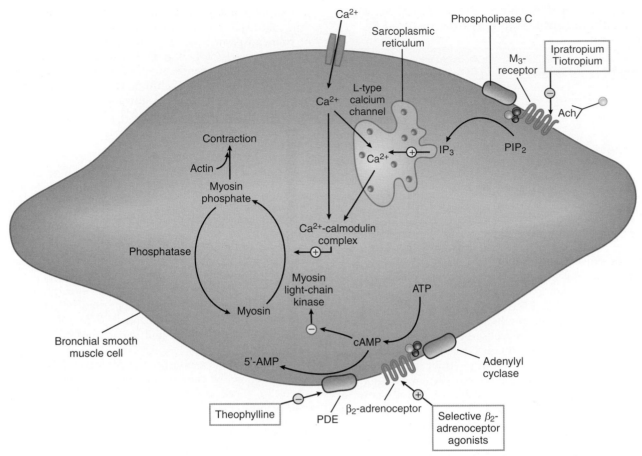

FIG. 27.3 Mechanisms of action of bronchodilators. Selective *beta₂*-adrenoceptor agonists activate *beta₂*-receptors. This increases cAMP concentrations in smooth muscle and causes the muscle to relax. Theophylline inhibits phosphodiesterase *(PDE)* isozymes and blocks the degradation of cAMP to 5′-AMP. Ipratropium and tiotropium block the stimulation of muscarinic receptors by acetylcholine *(ACh)* released from vagus nerves and thereby attenuate reflex bronchoconstriction. The effect of ACh is mediated by IP₃-induced calcium release and leads to smooth muscle contraction. *AMP,* adenosine monophosphate; *ATP,* adenosine triphosphate; *IP3,* inositol triphosphate.

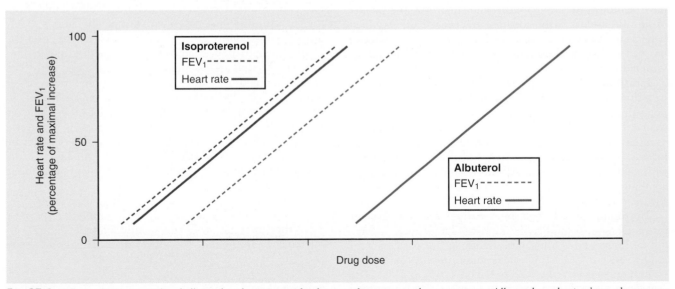

FIG. 27.4 Effects of isoproterenol and albuterol on heart rate and pulmonary function in asthmatic patients. Albuterol, a selective *beta₂*-adrenoceptor agonist, increases the forced expiratory volume in 1 second (*FEV₁*) at doses that produce relatively little cardiac stimulation. Isoproterenol, a nonselective *beta₁*- and *beta₂*-adrenoceptor agonist, has equipotent effects on heart rate and FEV₁.

A **black-box warning** has been added to products containing LABAs, stating that these drugs may increase the **risk of asthma-related death.** However, the two studies on which this warning was based were criticized as not being well controlled, and asthma treatment guidelines still recommend use of LABAs in combination with corticosteroids for persons with moderate to severe asthma not controlled by corticosteroids alone.

TABLE 27.2   Pharmacologic Properties of Selected Beta$_2$-Adrenoceptor Agonists Administered By Inhalation

DRUG	ONSET OF ACTION (MIN)	DURATION OF ACTION (H)	DOSAGE
Albuterol	5	3–8	2 puffs every 4–6 h
Formoterol	5	12	1 inhalation every 12 h
Indacaterol	15	>24	1 inhalation every 24 h
Salmeterol	20	12	2 puffs every 12 h
Terbutaline	5–15	3–6	2 puffs every 4–6 h

Ipratropium and Tiotropium

Ipratropium and tiotropium are **muscarinic receptor antagonists.** Ipratropium is the isopropyl derivative of atropine, whose properties are described in Chapter 7. The addition of the isopropyl group results in a quaternary ammonium compound that is not well absorbed into the circulation. Tiotropium is a synthetic quaternary ammonium compound. Both drugs are administered by oral inhalation for pulmonary disease and produce very few systemic side effects. **Ipratropium** is also available as a **nasal spray for rhinitis**. These drugs produce their bronchodilating effects by blocking the bronchoconstricting effect of vagus (parasympathetic) nerve stimulation (see Fig. 27.3).

In patients with **chronic bronchitis** and **emphysema,** the bronchodilating effect of ipratropium is slower to develop than that of a *beta$_2$*-agonist, but it lasts longer. Investigators found that the effect of ipratropium was sustained after 12 weeks of treatment, whereas the effect of albuterol on FEV$_1$ tended to diminish over a 12-week period. Other studies have demonstrated that ipratropium improves the quality of life in patients with moderate to severe COPD, and it benefits **infants** with **acute bronchitis.** A nasal solution can be used to reduce **rhinorrhea** in patients with **allergic or viral rhinitis.**

Ipratropium is typically less effective than a *beta$_2$*-agonist in asthmatic patients, but combined therapy with ipratropium and a *beta$_2$*-agonist has a greater bronchodilating effect than either drug alone, and this combination is beneficial in some cases of moderate to severe asthma. Ipratropium is useful as a "rescue" therapy, along with other drugs, for children with acute severe asthma. **Albuterol and ipratropium** are combined in a formulation called COMBIVENT indicated for the treatment of COPD.

Tiotropium is the **first once-daily inhaled treatment** for patients with COPD. It improves lung function for a full 24 hours and is a first-line treatment for patients with mild to severe COPD. Clinical studies found that tiotropium increased FEV$_1$ by 0.28 to 0.31 L (28% to 31%) after 1 week of therapy, and this improvement was maintained throughout the 6-month study period. As with ipratropium, the most common adverse effect of tiotropium is dry mouth.

Umeclidinium is another muscarinic receptor antagonist that is given by inhalation, either alone or in combination with **vilanterol,** a *beta$_2$*-agonist, or with **fluticasone,** for once-daily long-term treatment of airway obstruction

in COPD patients. **Aclidinium** is also an antimuscarinic drug approved for the **long-term maintenance treatment of bronchospasm** associated with chronic obstructive pulmonary disease (COPD), including chronic bronchitis and emphysema. Just recently, the long-acting **revefenacin** was approved for treatment of chronic COPD. It also is an **antimuscarinic drug with equal antagonism at the different subtypes of muscarinic family** (M1-M4 receptors).

Theophylline
Chemistry, Mechanisms, and Effects
Like caffeine, **theophylline** is a methylxanthine drug that causes central nervous system (CNS) stimulation, bronchodilation, and diuresis. Compared with caffeine, **theophylline produces less CNS stimulation and more bronchodilation.**

Theophylline has several actions at the cellular level, including inhibition of **PDE** isozymes, blockade of **adenosine receptors,** inhibition of **calcium influx,** and enhancement of **catecholamine secretion.** All of these effects may contribute to the drug's bronchodilating effects, and it has anti-inflammatory and immunosuppressant effects as well. The therapeutic effects of theophylline in pulmonary diseases probably result from multiple actions on several cell types and receptors.

Theophylline is a **nonspecific inhibitor of PDE** isoenzymes in bronchial **smooth muscle** and **inflammatory** cells where it increases cAMP levels and exerts bronchodilating and anti-inflammatory effects (see Fig. 27.3). Its anti-inflammatory effects result from inhibition of cytokine production and T-lymphocyte proliferation, and from reduced numbers of eosinophils, lymphocytes, and monocytes in the airway epithelium. It also reduces the release of **cationic basic protein** and **eosinophil-derived** neurotoxin that damage the epithelial lining of the bronchioles.

Pharmacokinetics
After oral administration, theophylline is well absorbed from the gut with little first-pass inactivation. The drug is widely distributed and crosses the blood-brain barrier to enter the CNS. Theophylline is converted to inactive metabolites by CYP1A2 that are excreted in the urine along with 10% of the parent drug. The half-life of theophylline is about 8 hours in adults who do not smoke, but only 4.5 hours in adults who smoke and in **children from 1 to 9** years of age because they metabolize the drug more rapidly. **Cigarette smoke** contains compounds that **induce CYP1A2 enzyme** synthesis. Hence, children and cigarette smokers usually require larger doses of theophylline per kilogram of body weight than do nonsmoking adults.

Because of theophylline's narrow margin of safety, theophylline serum levels should be monitored, especially when therapy is initiated. Therapeutic serum levels are considered to be in the range of 5 to 15 mg/L. Higher levels are associated with a greater risk of adverse reactions.

Indications
Theophylline is used to treat **COPD, asthma,** and **neonatal apnea.** In patients with **COPD,** theophylline can increase in FEV$_1$ about 20%, with improved minute ventilation and gas exchange. Treatment with theophylline reduces dyspnea, increases diaphragmatic contractility, improves exercise performance, and reduces fatigue. Theophylline

also increases the central respiratory drive and has favorable cardiovascular effects, including a reduction in pulmonary artery pressure, and an increase in ventricular ejection fraction. Theophylline is primarily used to treat COPD patients whose symptoms are not controlled with a *beta*$_2$-agonist and ipratropium or tiotropium.

Although the use of theophylline in the management of **asthma** is declining, the drug may be useful in patients whose symptoms are not adequately controlled by other drugs. **Theophylline** and **caffeine** are both used for the treatment of **recurrent apnea in premature infants.** In this setting, the drugs block **adenosine receptors,** thereby increasing the sensitivity of respiratory centers to carbon dioxide and the contractility of respiratory muscles. Theophylline has also been used to treat **obstructive sleep apnea** and periodic breathing, though it can also reduce sleep quality owing to CNS stimulation.

Adverse Effects

Major adverse effects of theophylline include **gastrointestinal distress, CNS stimulation,** and **cardiac stimulation.** Adverse gastrointestinal effects (e.g., abdominal pain, nausea, and vomiting) may be minimized by taking the drug with food or antacids or with a full glass of water or milk. CNS effects include headache, anxiety, restlessness, insomnia, dizziness, and seizures. A reduction in dosage will often eliminate these problems. Theophylline can adversely affect the cardiovascular system, causing hypotension, bradycardia, premature ventricular contractions, and tachycardia. These events are usually mild and transient, but serious reactions occasionally develop. **Seizures** and **cardiac dysrhythmias** can occur at concentrations over 25 mg/L.

Interactions

Cimetidine and erythromycin inhibit CYP1A2 and **increase theophylline plasma concentrations,** but the interaction is significant only when theophylline concentrations are already in the high therapeutic range. Other drugs that increase theophylline levels include fluoroquinolone antimicrobial drugs, isoniazid, and verapamil. Careful monitoring of patients is important, because it is difficult to predict which patients will require theophylline dosage adjustments when other drugs are given concurrently.

MONOCLONAL ANTIBODIES

As in so many areas of medicine, monoclonal antibody drugs (see Chapter 46) are now available to treat respiratory disorders. **Omalizumab** (Xolair) was the **first monoclonal antibody drug to be approved for moderate to severe chronic asthma** in patients 6 years of age and older with a positive skin test or *in vitro* test to a seasonal allergen, and who are not adequately maintained with inhaled corticosteroids. It also has an indication for chronic idiopathic urticaria in adults and adolescents who suffer despite H$_1$ antihistamine treatment. **Omalizumab** contains **anti-IgE monoclonal antibodies,** which binds the elevated IgE in the blood due to these conditions and prevents IgE from activating mast cells and other immune components.

About a decade or two later, there are now three new monoclonal antibodies specific for the inflammatory cytokine, interleukin-5 (IL-5). **Mepolizumab** was approved as an **add-on (adjunct) drug** for patients over 12 years old with **severe asthma** who have an eosinophilic phenotype. Eosinophilic phenotype refers to a rarer form of asthma that is distinguished by an increase of eosinophils in blood and sputum samples. **Resliozumab** (Cinqair) is also approved as an **adjunct drug for severe asthma.** Both these agents bind to the increased IL-5 in the blood and therefore decrease pro-inflammatory signaling. Finally, the newest monoclonal for asthma, **benralizumab,** bypasses IL-5 itself and instead binds to the interleukin-5 receptor on eosinophils and basophils. After **benralizumab binds to the IL-5 receptor,** natural killer cells can bind to the eosinophil and **cause apoptosis** in a process called antibody-dependent cell-mediated cytotoxicity (ADCC).

As with all subcutaneously administered peptides or protein, the most dire adverse effect is an immunological reaction to the injection. All of the above **monoclonal antibody drugs** come with **strong warnings** to be watchful of **hypersensitivity reactions** (e.g., anaphylaxis, angioedema, bronchospasm, hypotension, urticaria, and/or rash) after administration. Indeed, it is common practice to administer these doses, at least initially, in the clinic to observe the patient for at least 30 minutes to monitor the possible occurrence of hypersensitivity reactions.

MANAGEMENT OF ASTHMA

The management of asthma is based on the severity and frequency of asthmatic episodes, as determined by the number of days and nights with symptoms per week, and by the FEV$_1$ expressed as a percentage of the predicted normal FEV$_1$. Based on these criteria, asthma can be classified as mild **intermittent** or as mild, moderate, or severe **persistent** asthma. A stepwise approach is used to treat asthma, with the doses and frequency of drug administration increased with the level of severity. The pharmacologic therapy for asthma falls into two categories. Some medications are administered daily to suppress airway inflammation and prevent bronchospasm, whereas others are used as rescue therapy to counteract bronchospasm when acute exacerbations occur.

For **mild, intermittent asthma,** no daily medications are required, and acute asthma episodes are treated with a short-acting *beta*$_2$-agonist. For **mild, persistent asthma,** a low dose of an inhaled corticosteroid administered with a nebulizer or a metered-dose inhaler is the preferred therapy for preventing asthma episodes. Alternatives include cromolyn compounds, **anti-leukotriene** drugs, or a sustained-release **theophylline** preparation.

The preferred treatment to prevent acute episodes in persons with **moderate, persistent asthma** is a low-dose or medium-dose inhaled corticosteroid. An LABA can be added if a corticosteroid alone is not adequate. Alternatively, a leukotriene antagonist or theophylline can be added to low to medium doses of an inhaled corticosteroid. Long-term preventive therapy for **severe, persistent asthma** is usually a medium dose of an inhaled corticosteroid plus an LABA.

Mild **acute exacerbations** of asthma are usually managed with one or two treatments of an inhaled *beta*$_2$-agonist (e.g., albuterol or levalbuterol), given 4 to 6 hours apart. Medical attention is required if the patient does not respond to these treatments and may consist of multiple treatments of albuterol alone or in combination with ipratropium, oxygen, and possibly fluid replacement. In addition, short-course "burst" treatments of systemic corticosteroids (e.g., prednisone, prednisolone, or intravenous methylprednisolone) may be initiated for these episodes. Antibiotics should also be prescribed for documented bacterial infections. Severe attacks that do not respond to normal therapy, termed **status asthmaticus,** are more aggressively treated with oxygen, systemic steroids, and back-to-back or continuous *beta*$_2$-agonist treatments.

ANTITUSSIVES

Coughing usually serves a beneficial purpose by expelling irritating substances such as dust, pollen, and accumulated fluids and inflammatory cells from the upper airways. An incessant nonproductive cough, however, can lead to loss of sleep, rib fractures, pneumothorax, rupture of surgical wounds, or even syncope. Antitussive drugs are frequently used to **suppress coughing,** but the first-line therapy consists of controlling the infection, allergy, or other condition responsible for the cough.

The **cough reflex** is initiated by stimulation of sensory receptors on afferent nerve endings located between mucosal cells of the pharynx, larynx, and larger airways. The impulses ascend via the vagus nerve to the dorsal medulla. The efferent limb of the reflex consists of somatic nerves innervating the larynx and thoracoabdominal muscles. Some antitussives act locally to anesthetize the afferent nerves that initiate the cough reflex, whereas others act by inhibiting the cough center in the medulla.

The locally acting antitussives include **menthol and related drugs** that are administered as throat sprays or lozenges. The centrally acting antitussives consist of **opioids,** and these are usually administered orally. Almost all of the opioid agonist drugs will exert an antitussive effect, but opioids that have a higher ratio of antitussive effects to analgesic and euphoric effects are usually used for this purpose. These include **dextromethorphan, codeine, and hydrocodone.**

Dextromethorphan is the D-isomer of a potent opioid agonist. It is an effective antitussive drug but will not cause drowsiness, euphoria, analgesia, or other CNS effects, except at very high doses. For these reasons, dextromethorphan is available in many nonprescription products for cough and other respiratory tract conditions, and it is the most widely used opioid antitussive drug.

Codeine and **hydrocodone** are moderate opioid agonists whose analgesic effects are described in Chapter 23. These drugs exhibit excellent antitussive activity at doses that produce relatively little CNS depression or euphoria. They are available in a number of liquid cough preparations that may also include **guaifenesin, antihistamines,** and **decongestants.**

EXPECTORANTS

An expectorant is a drug that **facilitates the coughing up of mucus** and other material from the lungs. **Guaifenesin** is an oral nonprescription drug that has been used for this purpose for many years. It is purported to reduce the adhesiveness and surface tension of respiratory tract secretions and thereby facilitate their expectoration, but the exact mechanism by which the drug produces this effect is unknown. Through its expectorant effect, guaifenesin can also reduce the frequency of coughing. The drug may be useful in patients with **thick, tenacious respiratory tract secretions;** in patients with **dry, nonproductive coughing;** and in patients with **sinusitis** to increase airway hydration.

MANAGEMENT OF RHINITIS
Allergic Rhinitis

The effective management of allergic rhinitis includes environmental control of allergens, prophylactic use of anti-inflammatory medications, and control of symptoms with antihistamine drugs and decongestants. Most patients with mild symptoms can be adequately treated with an antihistamine drug alone, but patients with moderate to severe rhinitis usually benefit from anti-inflammatory therapy.

Antihistamines are usually employed during peak seasonal exposure to pollens and mold spores. A long-acting, nonsedating drug, such as **cetirizine, loratadine,** or **fexofenadine,** is suitable for most patients (see Chapter 26). Diphenhydramine is highly effective but causes sedation and is best reserved for relief of nocturnal symptoms that do not respond to other antihistamines.

Corticosteroids (glucocorticoids) are the most efficacious anti-inflammatory drugs for allergic rhinitis (see Table 27.1). Formulations of **budesonide, fluticasone, ciclesonide,** and other steroids are available for nasal inhalation for this purpose. These products are convenient and effective, and they cause very few adverse reactions.

If anti-inflammatory drugs and antihistamines do not control nasal congestion, a decongestant drug such as **pseudoephedrine** (see Chapter 8) can also be added to the regimen. Decongestants, however, are often not needed if patients take an anti-inflammatory drug at the onset of seasonal allergies or use an antihistamine drug when symptoms commence.

Ipratropium is used occasionally for the treatment of rhinorrhea associated with rhinitis. A nasal spray formulation is available for this purpose, but it does not relieve nasal itching or congestion.

Ocular inflammation, discomfort, and pruritus can be particularly troublesome aspects of seasonal allergies. **Cromolyn** and **lodoxamide** are available in topical ocular formulations that are effective in preventing symptoms of **allergic conjunctivitis.** Mild ocular symptoms can be treated with topical decongestants and oral or topical antihistamines, such as **azelastine** and **olopatadine.** More severe ocular symptoms may be controlled with a topical nonsteroidal anti-inflammatory drug such as **ketorolac** (see Chapter 30). Topical corticosteroids are not usually used for allergic conjunctivitis because their long-term ocular use is associated with increased intraocular pressure and cataracts.

Viral Rhinitis

Viral rhinitis (the common cold) is a self-limiting condition that is best treated conservatively. Analgesics such as **acetaminophen** or **ibuprofen** (see Chapter 30) can relieve aches and discomfort, while decongestants such as **pseudoephedrine** (see Chapter 8) reduce nasal congestion, and **ipratropium** will control rhinorrhea. Some clinicians advocate short-term use (10 days) of products containing *Echinacea,* which stimulates the immune system and may shorten the duration and severity of viral rhinitis. However, long-term use of *Echinacea* may suppress the immune system.

DRUGS FOR CYSTIC FIBROSIS

Cystic fibrosis (CF) is a genetic disorder that is the **most common inherited disease** in Caucasian populations. It is an autosomal recessive genetic disorder caused by mutations of a chloride ion channel gene, the CF transmembrane conductance regulator (CFTR) gene. There are about 2,000 or more mutations in the CFTR gene associated with CF. The most common mutation in Caucasians leads to the **deletion of a single amino acid, phenylalanine**, at position 508 (F508*del*). The prevalence of **CF is 1 in 2500 newborn infants**, with a heterozygous carrier frequency of 1 in 25. The median age of survival is now 40 years, an improvement over earlier prognoses when CF children did not live to see high school. It is thought that the CF mutation may have had a selective advantage during the advancement of Western civilization as heterozygotes are resistant to typhus and cholera.

The CFTR channel protein normally **transports Cl⁻ ions out of the epithelial cells** on the luminal side, bringing Na⁺ and water with it. Patients with CF and defective CFTR proteins experience excessive mucus build-up in the lungs, pancreas, and other organs. In the lungs, excessive mucus clogs the airways and provides a safe harbor for bacterial growth, leading to infection, lung damage, and progressing to respiratory failure.

Dornase alfa (PULMOZYME) is a **mucolytic agent** that targets and **cleaves the extracellular DNA** from invading neutrophils to decrease mucus viscosity. It is recombinant human deoxyribonuclease I, with a primary amino acid sequence that is identical to the human enzyme. To prevent or treat the inevitable bacterial lung infection, special formulations of antibiotics are available. **Aztreonam** for inhalation and **tobramycin** inhalation solution or inhalation powder are effective therapies for preventing or treating the bacteria that produce lung infections in CF patients.

Two new drugs target the defective CFTR protein itself, called **CFTR modulators**. Because different mutations cause different protein dysfunctions, the CFTR modulators are effective only in people with certain mutations. **Ivacaftor** (KALYDECO) targets mutations such as G551D, R117H, S1251N, and a number of other single amino acid substitutions. In these patients, ivacaftor is a **potentiator of the CFTR protein,** increasing chloride ion transport by **increasing the channel-open probability** (or gating) of the CFTR protein. However, ivacaftor is **not effective in the F508del** mutation, which is the most common CF defect in the United States. To address this issue, **lumacaftor with ivacaftor** (ORKAMBI) was recently approved. **Lumacaftor is a chaperone drug**, bringing the defective CFTR protein to the cell surface. Once there, ivacaftor can potentiate the mutated CFTR protein, which would **not be trafficked to the cell surface** without lumacaftor due to its mutation and misfolding of the protein.

Newer formulations for the treatment of CF include combination drugs such as **tezacaftor with ivacaftor** (SYMDECO), and **elexacaftor with ivacaftor and tezacaftor** (TRIKAFTA). These drug combinations add additional **CFTR modulators** to potentiate their effects on the defective ion channel in CF. Other breakthrough drugs are in the development pipeline which will soon offer the CF patient a chance at a fuller lifespan.

SUMMARY OF IMPORTANT POINTS

- Drugs used in the management of asthma are classified as anti-inflammatory agents or bronchodilators.
- Corticosteroids, the most efficacious anti-inflammatory drugs, are usually given by inhalation on a long-term basis to prevent asthmatic attacks and COPD. Orally or parenterally administered steroids are used for the management of chronic severe asthma or acute exacerbations of asthma.
- Cromolyn sodium and related drugs are used prophylactically in the management of mild to moderate asthma, allergic conjunctivitis, and related disorders. They have few adverse effects.
- Leukotriene inhibitors have anti-inflammatory and bronchodilating activity and offer convenient oral therapy for the prevention of asthmatic attacks. Montelukast and zafirlukast are leukotriene receptor antagonists, and zileuton is a leukotriene synthesis inhibitor.
- Roflumilast is a type 4 phosphodiesterase inhibitor with anti-inflammatory effects that is used in treating exacerbations of chronic bronchitis in patients with COPD.
- Short-acting *beta*₂-adrenoceptor agonists are the most efficacious bronchodilators for the treatment of acute bronchospasm. Examples are albuterol and terbutaline. Long-acting *beta*₂-agonists, salmeterol and formoterol, are used for chronic prevention. Indacaterol is an ultralong-acting *beta*₂-agonist recently approved for once-daily treatment of COPD.
- *Beta*₂-agonists may cause excessive cardiac stimulation and fatalities have resulted from their use.
- Ipratropium and tiotropium are muscarinic receptor antagonists that are primarily used to treat COPD.
- Theophylline has anti-inflammatory and bronchodilating activity and is useful for the treatment of asthma and COPD. The metabolism of theophylline is affected by smoking and by the concurrent administration of drugs that inhibit cytochrome P450. Children and smokers metabolize theophylline more rapidly than nonsmoking adults.
- Theophylline levels should be monitored to ensure efficacy and prevent toxicity. Adverse effects include gastrointestinal, central nervous system, and cardiac toxicity.
- Omalizumab is a monoclonal antibody to IgE that is used by injection for severe allergic asthma, whereas mepolizumab and reslizumab are monoclonal antibodies to interleukin-5 used to treat severe eosinophilic asthma, and benralizumab binds to the IL-5 receptor.
- Antitussives are used to suppress dry, nonproductive coughing. Dextromethorphan is available without a prescription, whereas codeine and hydrocodone are contained in many prescription cough preparations.
- Allergic rhinitis is managed with anti-inflammatory drugs (corticosteroids and cromolyn compounds), antihistamines, and decongestants.
- Pharmacotherapy for treating cystic fibrosis is limited, although there are now a few new agents available that target the defective chloride ion channel protein.

Review Questions

1. Which of the following correctly describes monteleukast?
   (A) blocks receptors for leukotrienes C_4, D_4, and E_4
   (B) inhibits cytochrome P450 enzymes
   (C) is administered twice daily
   (D) inhibits formation of leukotriene A_4
   (E) is excreted unchanged in the urine
2. Which drug used for the treatment of asthma inhibits 5-lipoxygenase?
   (A) theophylline
   (B) zileuton
   (C) zafirlukast
   (D) fluticasone
   (E) roflumilast
3. A woman with allergic conjunctivitis uses a drug that prevents the release of chemical mediators from mast cells. Which mechanism is responsible for this pharmacologic effect?
   (A) activation of *beta*$_2$-adrenoceptors
   (B) decreased cytokine production
   (C) blockade of muscarinic receptors
   (D) inhibition of 5-lipoxygenase
   (E) blockade of calcium influx
4. A 15-year-old girl with severe asthma triggered by seasonal allergies is receiving twice-monthly injections of a monoclonal antibody. Which mediator of asthma is antagonized by this drug?
   (A) immunoglobulin E
   (B) leukotriene C4
   (C) major basic protein
   (D) histamine
   (E) interleukin-2
5. A man being treated for severe asthma experiences an episode of life-threatening tachycardia requiring emergency treatment. Which drug is most likely responsible for this adverse effect?
   (A) budesonide
   (B) ipratropium
   (C) formoterol
   (D) cromolyn
   (E) montelukast

CHAPTER 28 Pharmacological Treatment of Gastrointestinal Disorders

CLASSIFICATION OF GASTROINTESTINAL DRUGS

Drugs for Peptic Ulcer Disease

Histamine H₂ receptor antagonists
- Ranitidine (ZANTAC)
- Famotidine (PEPCID)[a]

Proton pump inhibitors
- Esomeprazole (NEXIUM)
- Omeprazole (PRILOSEC)[b]

Gastric antacids
- Aluminum hydroxide/magnesium hydroxide (MAALOX)
- Calcium carbonate (TUMS)

Cytoprotective drugs
- Sucralfate (CARAFATE)
- Misoprostol (CYTOTEC)

Drugs for inflammatory bowel diseases
- Hydrocortisone (COLOCORT)
- Budesonide (UCERIS)
- (AZULFIDINE)[c]
- Infliximab (REMICADE)[d]

Agents affecting motility
- Metoclopramide (REGLAN)
- Atropine[e]

Drugs for constipation
- Psyllium (METAMUCIL)[f]
- Docusate (COLACE, SURFAK)
- Magnesium oxide (MILK OF MAGNESIA)[g]
- Bisacodyl (DULCOLAX)[h]
- Tegaserod (ZELNORM)[i]
- Lubiprostone (AMITIZA)[j]
- Methylnaltrexone bromide (RELISTOR)[k]

Antidiarrheal agents
- Diphenoxylate (LOMOTIL)
- Loperamide (IMODIUM)[l]
- Rifaximin (XIFAXAN)[m]
- Alosetron (LOTRONEX)

Drugs for nausea and vomiting
- Ondansetron (ZOFRAN)[n]
- Promethazine (PHENERGAN)[o]
- Dimenhydrinate (DRAMAMINE)[p]
- Aprepitant (EMEND)[q]
- Dronabinol (MARINOL)[r]

[a] Also cimetidine (TAGAMET), and nizatidine (AXID).
[b] Also lansoprazole (PREVACID), rabeprazole (ACIPHEX), and pantoprazole (PROTONIX).
[c] Also olsalazine (DIPENTUM), and mesalamine (ASACOL HD).
[d] Also adalimumab (HUMIRA), golimumab (SIMPONI), and vedolizumab (ENTYVIO).
[e] Also hyoscyamine (LEVSIN), dicyclomine (BENTYL), and scopolamine (TRANSDERM SCOP).
[f] Also calcium polycarbophil (FIBERCON), and bismuth subsalicylate (PEPTO-BISMOL).
[g] Also sodium phosphate, lactulose (rectal only), polyethylene glycol (MIRALAX), and lactitol (PIZENSY).
[h] Also senna glycoside (EX-LAX, SENOKOT).
[i] Also prucalopride (MOTEGRITY).
[j] Also linaclotide (LINZESS), and plecanatide (TRULANCE).
[k] Also naldemedine (SYMPROIC), and naloxegol (MOVANTIK).
[l] Also eluxadoline (VIBERZI).
[m] Also rifamycin (AEMCOLO), and crofelemer (FULYZAQ).
[n] Also granisetron, dolasetron (ANZEMET), and palonosetron (ALOXI); odansetron is also available as an oral soluble film (ZUPLENZ).
[o] Also amisulpride (BARHEMSYS), and trimethobenzamide (TIGAN).
[p] Also meclizine (ANTIVERT), and doxylamine with pyridoxine immediate-release (DICLEGIS) and in a new extended-release formulation (BONJESTA).
[q] Also fosaprepitant, rolapitant (VARUBI), and the combination of fosnetupitant with palonosetron (AKYNZEO).
[r] Available also as dronabinol oral solution (SYNDROS); there is a synthetic cannabinoid agonist, nabilone (CESAMET), also marketed for nausea and vomiting.

OVERVIEW

Gastrointestinal (GI) complaints are among the most common reasons that people seek medical care, and a large number of drugs have been developed to treat these conditions. This chapter describes drugs used in the management of peptic ulcer disease, inflammatory bowel diseases, GI motility disorders, and nausea and vomiting.

DRUGS FOR PEPTIC ULCER DISEASE

Peptic ulcer disease is characterized by epigastric pain, loss of appetite, and weight loss caused by inflamed excavations (ulcers) of the mucosa and underlying tissue of the upper GI tract. The ulcers result from damage to the mucous membrane that normally protects the esophagus, stomach, and duodenum from gastric acid and pepsin. This damage is often caused by **Helicobacter pylori** infection, but nonsteroidal anti-inflammatory drugs (NSAIDs) and other factors may cause or contribute to peptic ulcers.

In developed countries, the number of persons who harbor *H. pylori* increases from under 5% at birth to about 20% at the age of 45 years. However, only a small proportion of persons harboring this bacterial organism will develop

BOX 28.1 A CASE OF RECURRENT EPIGASTRIC PAIN

CASE PRESENTATION

A 50-year-old man tells his physician about a burning epigastric pain that has awakened him at night for the past 3 weeks. The pain often begins in the late morning and is relieved by food or antacids but reappears about 3 h after a meal and during sleep. He has been otherwise healthy, and his vital signs and physical examination findings are normal. Blood samples are taken for routine chemistries and blood cell counts. A rapid urease test for *Helicobacter pylori* is positive, and he is scheduled for gastrointestinal endoscopy, which reveals an inflamed ulcer in the wall of the duodenal bulb. A gastric mucosal biopsy confirms the presence of *H. pylori*. The patient denies any drug allergies and is placed on a combination of rabeprazole plus amoxicillin, clarithromycin, and tinidazole for 14 days. His symptoms improve markedly after several days of therapy. After completion of therapy, the result of a rapid urease test for *H. pylori* is negative, and endoscopy confirms ulcer healing.

CASE DISCUSSION

H. pylori infection is responsible for most cases of duodenal ulcers. Epigastric pain is the most common symptom; it is usually relieved by food but often awakens a patient at night. Several tests for *H. pylori* are available, including the rapid urease test. Endoscopy is a valuable tool for determining the type and location of a peptic ulcer and enables biopsy to distinguish simple gastric ulcers from stomach cancer. It can also identify a bleeding ulcer and permit laser probe coagulation to stop bleeding. The treatment of peptic ulcers caused by *H. pylori* has been continuously improved, and current regimens often employ a proton pump inhibitor and two or more antimicrobial agents. Local antibiotic resistance patterns should guide drug selection.

peptic ulcer disease. Those at greatest risk include individuals who smoke, ingest excessive amounts of alcohol or NSAIDs, are elderly, or have GI ischemia. Prolonged use of glucocorticoids also increases the risk of peptic ulcer disease.

H. pylori can be found in the GI tract of almost all patients with **duodenal ulcers** and in about 80% of patients with **gastric** ulcers. *H. pylori*–induced gastritis is believed to precede the development of peptic ulcers in most persons (Box 28.1). The organism attaches to epithelial cells and releases enzymes that damage mucosal cells and cause inflammation and tissue destruction. Eradication of *H. pylori* heals most peptic ulcers and significantly reduces the recurrence rate for gastric and duodenal ulcers.

The agents used to treat peptic ulcer disease include drugs that eliminate *H. pylori*, drugs that reduce gastric acidity, and drugs that exert a cytoprotective effect on the GI mucosa.

Drugs That Reduce Gastric Acidity

Gastric acid promotes the development of peptic ulcers by damaging submucosal tissue and by converting pepsinogen to pepsin, which is a proteolytic enzyme. The physiology of gastric acid secretion and sites of drug action are illustrated in Fig. 28.1. The principal physiologic stimulants of gastric acid secretion are **gastrin, acetylcholine,** and **histamine.** Gastrin is a hormone secreted by G cells in the gastric antrum, whereas acetylcholine is released from vagus nerve terminals. Gastrin and acetylcholine directly **stimulate**

acid secretion by parietal cells, and they also stimulate the release of histamine from paracrine (enterochromaffin-like) cells. Histamine stimulates H_2 receptors located on parietal cells and provokes acid secretion via cyclic adenosine monophosphate (cAMP) stimulation of the proton pump (H^+,K^+-ATPase).

The vagus nerve mediates the cephalic phase of gastric acid secretion evoked by the smell, taste, and thought of food. Gastrin mediates the gastric phase of acid secretion induced by the presence of food in the stomach. Histamine augments the cephalic and gastric phases of acid secretion and mediates basal acid secretion in the fasting state.

The level of gastric acidity can be reduced either by neutralizing gastric acid with antacids or by inhibiting gastric acid secretion with a histamine H_2 receptor antagonist or a proton pump inhibitor (PPI).

Histamine H_2 Receptor Antagonists

The H_2 receptor antagonists (H_2 blockers) include cimetidine, famotidine, ranitidine, and nizatidine.

Chemistry, Mechanisms, and Effects

The structure of H_2 blockers is similar to that of histamine (Fig. 28.2), enabling the drugs to compete with histamine for binding to H_2 receptors on gastric parietal cells (see Fig. 28.1). The H_2 blockers have been shown to be potent inhibitors of both **meal-stimulated secretion** and **basal secretion** of gastric acid. They reduce the volume and concentration of gastric acid, and they produce a proportionate reduction in the production of **pepsin** because gastric acid catalyzes the conversion of inactive pepsinogen to pepsin. The H_2 blockers also reduce the secretion of **intrinsic factor,** but not enough to significantly reduce vitamin B_{12} absorption. They have no effect on gastric emptying time, esophageal sphincter pressure, or pancreatic enzyme secretion.

Pharmacokinetics

The H_2 blockers are well absorbed from the gut and undergo varying degrees of hepatic inactivation before being excreted in the urine. Although the half-life of most H_2 blockers is only 2 to 3 hours, their clinical duration of action is considerably longer (Table 28.1), and these drugs are usually administered once or twice daily.

Indications

The H_2 blockers are used to treat conditions associated with **excessive acid production,** including dyspepsia, peptic ulcer disease, and gastroesophageal reflux disease (GERD). An H_2 blocker is occasionally used in combination with an H_1 blocker for the treatment of **allergic reactions** that do not respond to an H_1 blocker alone.

Dyspepsia, or **heartburn,** is characterized by epigastric discomfort after meals. It is often associated with impaired digestion and excessive stomach acidity. Several low-dose formulations of H_2 receptor antagonists are available without a prescription for the prevention and treatment of dyspepsia. These products are most effective when taken 30 minutes before ingestion of a dyspepsia-provoking meal.

For the treatment of **peptic ulcer disease,** H_2 blockers are administered once or twice daily at doses that raise the gastric pH above 4 for at least 13 hours a day. Most authorities recommend giving a single daily dose at bedtime to ensure

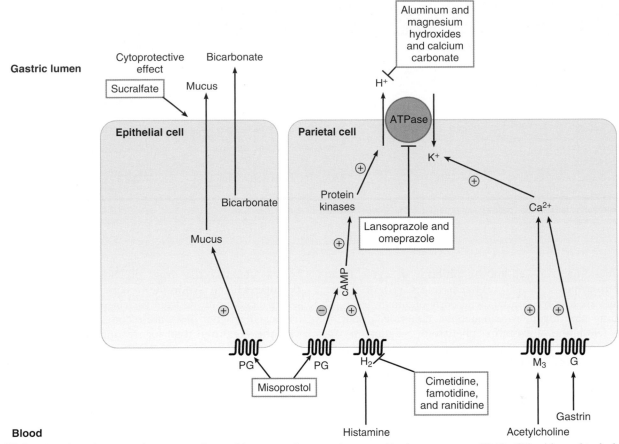

Fig. 28.1 Physiology of gastric acid secretion and sites of drug action. Gastric acid is secreted by the proton pump (H+,K+-ATPase) located in the luminal membrane of parietal cells. H+,K+-ATPase is stimulated by histamine, acetylcholine, and gastrin, and it is irreversibly blocked by the proton pump inhibitors (lansoprazole, omeprazole). The effect of histamine is blocked by H2 receptor antagonists (cimetidine, famotidine, and ranitidine). Prostaglandins (e.g., misoprostol) inhibit gastric acid secretion and stimulate secretion of mucus and bicarbonate by epithelial cells. Sucralfate binds to proteins of the ulcer crater and exerts a cytoprotective effect, whereas antacids (aluminum and magnesium hydroxides and calcium carbonate) neutralize acid in the gastric lumen. *cAMP,* Cyclic adenosine monophosphate; *G,* gastrin receptor; *H2,* histamine H2 receptor; *M3,* muscarinic M3 receptor; *PG,* prostaglandin receptor.

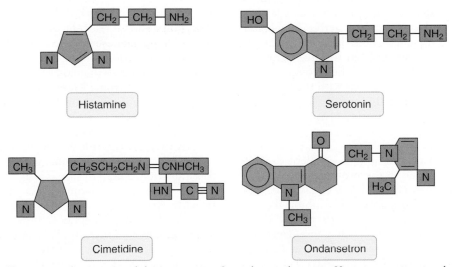

Fig. 28.2 Structures of histamine and serotonin and their antagonists. Cimetidine is a histamine H2 receptor antagonist whose structure is similar to that of histamine. Ondansetron is a serotonin 5-HT3 receptor antagonist whose structure is similar to that of serotonin. The parts of the structures that are similar are unshaded.

that acid secretion is suppressed all night. PPIs are usually preferred for treating peptic ulcer disease because they heal almost 90% of ulcers in 4 weeks (when used alone), whereas H2 blockers require 6 to 8 weeks to achieve this level of efficacy.

Adverse Effects and Interactions

The H2 blockers cause few adverse effects. Cimetidine has weak **antiandrogenic activity** and can cause gynecomastia in elderly men, but this reaction is uncommon with other H2 blockers.

TABLE 28.1   Properties of Drugs for Peptic Ulcer Disease

DRUG CLASS	DURATION OF ACTION	ADVANTAGES	DISADVANTAGES
Antimicrobial agents	Varies	Heal *Helicobacter pylori* infection and peptic ulcer when used with acid secretion inhibitors	Microbial resistance increasing (e.g., clarithromycin resistance)
Cytoprotective drugs (sucralfate)[a]	6–12 h	Few adverse effects; useful when other drugs are not tolerated	Limited utility for *H. pylori*-induced ulcers; can impair absorption of other drugs
Gastric antacids	3–4 h	Few adverse effects; rapid-acting	Primarily for symptomatic relief
Histamine H$_2$ receptor antagonists[a]	12 h	Few adverse effects; well tolerated	Not as effective as PPIs
Proton pump inhibitors (PPIs)[a]	24–48 h	Most efficacious acid inhibitors	More adverse effects and interactions than other drugs

[a]Recurrence rates are high when patients with peptic ulcer disease are not treated for *H. pylori* infection.
PPI, Proton pump inhibitor.

Cimetidine is a well-known **inhibitor of cytochrome P450 isozymes** CYP2C9, CYP2D6, and CYP3A4. These isozymes are involved in the metabolism of numerous drugs, including alprazolam, carbamazepine, cisapride, disopyramide, felodipine, lovastatin, phenytoin, saquinavir, triazolam, and warfarin. The dosage of these drugs may need to be reduced in patients taking cimetidine. Other H$_2$ blockers do not inhibit P450 enzymes significantly and are preferred for patients receiving concomitant drug therapy.

Proton Pump Inhibitors
The PPIs include esomeprazole, lansoprazole, omeprazole, pantoprazole, and rabeprazole.

Chemistry and Pharmacokinetics
The PPIs are acid-labile prodrugs that are administered orally as sustained-release, **enteric-coated** preparations to protect them from stomach acid. After they are absorbed from the gut, the drugs are distributed to the secretory canaliculi in the gastric mucosa and converted to **active metabolites** that bind to the proton pump. These drugs are eventually metabolized to inactive compounds in the liver, primarily by cytochrome P450 (CYP) 2C19, and these compounds are excreted in the urine and feces. Persons with the CYP2C19 **extensive (rapid) and ultrarapid metabolizer phenotypes** may require higher doses of PPIs to cure peptic ulcers.

Mechanisms and Effects
The active metabolites of PPIs form a covalent disulfide link with a cysteinyl residue in the **proton pump (H$^+$,K$^+$-ATPase)** found in the luminal membrane of gastric parietal cells (see Fig. 28.1). The drugs irreversibly inhibit the proton pump and prevent the secretion of gastric acid for an extended period. The drugs can produce a dose-dependent inhibition of up to 95% of gastric acid secretion, and a single dose can inhibit acid secretion for 1 to 2 days. Hence, the PPIs are more efficacious than the H$_2$ blockers for reducing gastric acidity (see Table 28.1).

Indications
PPIs are highly effective in treating **peptic ulcer disease.** They typically heal 80% to 90% of peptic ulcers in 2 weeks or less when used in combination with antibiotics, whereas H$_2$-blocker combinations heal 70% to 80% in 4 weeks.

PPIs are also the drugs of choice for patients with **Zollinger-Ellison syndrome,** a condition characterized by severe ulcers resulting from **gastrin-secreting tumors (gastrinomas).** Higher doses are required for treating patients with this condition than for treating patients with typical peptic ulcer disease.

PPIs are also the most effective drugs for treating GERD and are available without prescription for the treatment of **dyspepsia** and **heartburn.** Finally, PPIs can be used to prevent peptic ulcers and bleeding in persons receiving high-dose or long-term therapy with **NSAIDs** such as diclofenac (see Chapter 30).

Adverse Effects and Interactions
PPIs are usually well-tolerated, and short-term use typically causes few adverse effects. Minor GI and central nervous system (CNS) side effects have occurred in some patients, and skin rash and elevated hepatic enzyme levels have also been reported. Although many patients with GERD have taken PPIs for several years without significant side effects, **hypomagnesemia** (low blood magnesium levels) may occur in persons taking the drug for more than a year. Studies also suggest that long-term use of high dose PPIs may also cause **chronic kidney disease.** High doses of PPIs have also been associated with an **increased risk of osteoporosis,** and there is a small potential for these drugs to cause malabsorption of vitamin B$_{12}$. In addition, PPIs may slightly increase the risk of community-acquired pneumonia and certain **GI infections,** including *Clostridiodes difficile* infection.

PPIs can elevate serum levels of methotrexate, particularly in patients taking higher methotrexate doses. Omeprazole and esomeprazole prevent the activation of **clopidogrel** by inhibiting CYP2C19, leading to lower clopidogrel levels, and these PPIs should not be used with this antiplatelet drug (see Chapter 16). Pantoprazole does not appear to cause this interaction and can be used concurrently with clopidogrel.

Gastric Antacids
Gastric antacids chemically neutralize stomach acid. This raises the GI pH sufficiently to relieve the pain of dyspepsia and acid indigestion and to enable peptic ulcers to heal. The most commonly used antacids are **calcium carbonate** and

a combination of **aluminum and magnesium hydroxides**. These substances are available in chewable tablets and in liquid suspensions. When used alone, aluminum hydroxide can cause constipation, whereas magnesium hydroxide often causes diarrhea. Hence, the combination of aluminum hydroxide and magnesium hydroxide has a relatively neutral effect on GI motility. Calcium carbonate can also cause constipation, and large doses of calcium carbonate can lead to a rebound in acid secretion.

Antacids are available without a prescription and are commonly used to treat **acid indigestion** and dyspepsia. Nonprescription products containing a low dose of a histamine H_2 antagonist and an antacid are also available. Antacids were formerly used to treat peptic ulcers, but they must be taken in large doses at frequent intervals for this purpose, and nocturnal acid secretion is particularly difficult to control with antacids. Hence, they are seldom used alone in treating peptic ulcers today.

Cytoprotective Drugs

Sucralfate and **misoprostol** both protect the GI mucosa, but they do so by different means (see Fig. 28.1).

Sucralfate

Chemistry, Mechanisms, and Effects. Sucralfate is a viscous polymer of sucrose octasulfate and aluminum hydroxide. This sulfated polysaccharide **adheres to ulcer craters** and epithelial cells and inhibits pepsin-catalyzed hydrolysis of mucosal proteins. Sucralfate also **stimulates prostaglandin synthesis** in mucosal cells. These actions form a protective barrier to acid and pepsin and facilitate the healing of ulcers.

Pharmacokinetics. Sucralfate is administered orally as a tablet or suspension. The drug is **not absorbed** significantly from the gut and is primarily excreted in the feces. Patients absorb a small amount of aluminum from the drug, so sucralfate should be used cautiously in patients with renal impairment.

Indications. In the management of **peptic ulcer disease,** sucralfate can be used to treat active ulcers or to suppress the recurrence of ulcers. It is less effective than drugs that inhibit gastric acid secretion and is primarily used in patients who cannot tolerate H_2 blockers or PPIs.

Adverse Effects and Interactions. Although sucralfate causes very **few systemic adverse effects,** constipation and other GI disturbances and laryngospasm have been reported occasionally. The use of sucralfate can **impair the absorption of other drugs** (e.g., digoxin, fluoroquinolones, ketoconazole, and phenytoin). To prevent this problem, sucralfate should be ingested 2 hours before or after these other drugs are taken.

Misoprostol

As discussed in Chapter 26, misoprostol is a **prostaglandin E_1 analog.** The drug exerts a cytoprotective effect by inhibiting gastric acid secretion and promoting the secretion of mucus and bicarbonate. It is primarily indicated for the prevention of **gastric and duodenal ulcers** in patients who are taking NSAIDs on a long-term basis. Misoprostol is expensive and is usually reserved for patients at high risk of NSAID-induced ulcers, including the elderly and those with a history of peptic ulcer disease.

Misoprostol is administered orally four times daily with food for the duration of NSAID therapy. Diarrhea and intestinal cramping are the most common adverse effects, but other GI reactions can also occur.

Misoprostol can stimulate uterine contractions and induce labor in pregnant women, so it is **contraindicated during pregnancy.**

TREATMENT OF *HELICOBACTER PYLORI* INFECTION

Studies show that 80% to 90% of peptic ulcer patients who are only treated with a gastric acid inhibitor have an **ulcer recurrence** within 1 year after discontinuing this therapy. In contrast, less than 10% of patients who receive both a gastric acid inhibitor and antimicrobial agents to eliminate *H. pylori* have a recurrence, and this type of **combination therapy** is now the standard of care. Clinicians should employ regimens that have a 90% cure rate in their locality.

The treatment of *H. pylori* infection has continuously evolved, and the latest guidelines should be consulted for current recommendations. Most regimens now include a PPI plus two or three antimicrobial agents (called triple or quadruple therapy). One recent study found that the combination of **rabeprazole** plus **amoxicillin, clarithromycin,** and **metronidazole** produced a higher cure rate than triple therapy with two of these antibiotics or sequential therapy with rabeprazole plus amoxicillin followed by rabeprazole plus the other two antibiotics. Several other antimicrobial agents have been used to treat *H. pylori* infection, and local resistance patterns have a role in deciding which agents to use. Therapy usually lasts 10 to 14 days and should be continued until the eradication of *H. pylori* is confirmed by a laboratory test. Gastric ulcers often require longer treatment than required for duodenal ulcers.

Histamine H_2 blockers or sucralfate **plus antimicrobial agents** can be used to treat *H. pylori* but often requires 4 or more weeks of treatment and is usually reserved for persons who cannot take a PPI. The properties of antimicrobial agents are discussed in the chapters of Section VII.

DRUGS FOR INFLAMMATORY BOWEL DISEASES

The two most common inflammatory bowel diseases are **ulcerative colitis** and **Crohn disease.** In ulcerative colitis, inflammation of the GI mucosa is limited to the colon and rectum. In Crohn disease, inflammation is transmural and can occur in any part of the GI tract.

Abdominal cramping and diarrhea are the most common complaints of patients with inflammatory bowel disease. Many patients experience acute exacerbations separated by periods of remission, but prolonged illness can occur in persons with severe disease. Ulcerative colitis and Crohn disease are generally treated with **glucocorticoids, mesalamine,** and **infliximab.**

Glucocorticoids

Hydrocortisone and other glucocorticoids (see Chapter 33) have been extensively used for the treatment of both **ulcerative colitis** and **Crohn disease.** In cases of mild ulcerative colitis, they may be effectively administered as rectal enemas. Hydrocortisone rectal suspension (COLOCORT) is indicated as an **adjunct drug in the treatment of ulcerative colitis**, especially distal forms, including ulcerative proctitis, ulcerative proctosigmoiditis, and left-sided ulcerative colitis.

In cases of Crohn disease and more severe ulcerative colitis, hydrocortisone is usually administered orally or parenterally. **Budesonide,** marketed as UCERIS, is a **glucocorticoid** specifically indicated for the treatment of ulcerative colitis. It is formulated under this brand name as an **extended-release tablet or rectal aerosol foam.**

Glucocorticoids are often able to induce the remission of ulcerative colitis or Crohn disease, but they have proved less valuable in maintaining remission, particularly without causing troublesome adverse effects (see Chapter 33).

Aminosalicylates

Sulfasalazine, olsalazine, and their active metabolite **mesalamine** are used to induce and maintain the remission of ulcerative colitis, but they are less effective in maintaining the remission of Crohn disease. **Sulfasalazine** is also used for the treatment of rheumatoid arthritis (see Chapter 30).

Sulfasalazine is a sulfonamide compound that is not well absorbed from the gut. Colonic bacteria convert sulfasalazine to 5-aminosalicylic acid **(mesalamine)** and sulfapyridine. **Olsalazine** is a salicylate compound that is also converted to **mesalamine** by colonic bacteria. **Mesalamine** is believed to exert **anti-inflammatory effects** by inhibiting **prostaglandin synthesis** and possibly by inhibiting the migration of inflammatory cells into the bowel wall. Mesalamine is also a superoxide-free radical scavenger. Besides being the active metabolite of sulfasalazine and olsalazine, **mesalamine is also marketed by itself** and can be administered as a rectal suppository, rectal suspension, or delayed-release oral tablet. It acts primarily in the gut, but about 15% of the drug is absorbed into the circulation.

Monoclonal Antibody Drugs

Immunosuppressive agents may be useful in maintaining remission in patients with Crohn disease and severe ulcerative colitis. **Infliximab, adalimumab,** and **golimumab** are monoclonal antibodies to **tumor necrosis factor alpha (TNFα),** a substance believed to play a role in the pathogenesis of these conditions as well as in rheumatoid arthritis (see Chapter 30). **Vedolizumab** is an **integrin receptor antagonist** indicated for the treatment of ulcerative colitis and Crohn disease. It is a monoclonal antibody to the type of integrin expressed on T-lymphocytes and inhibits their migration across the endothelium and into the inflamed GI parenchymal tissue. By blocking integrin on lymphocytes, **vedolizumab reduces the inflammation of the GI tract.** Monoclonal antibody drugs are discussed as a class in Chapter 46.

Agents Affecting Motility

A number of disorders are characterized by **abnormal GI motility.** These include diarrhea, constipation, GERD, gastroparesis, and irritable bowel syndrome (IBS). GERD is caused by the reflux of gastric acid into the esophagus, leading to **esophagitis.** The disease is often associated with excessive secretion of gastric acid and decreased pressure in the lower esophageal sphincter. Pharmacologic agents used in the treatment of GERD include drugs that reduce gastric acidity (e.g., H_2 receptor antagonists and PPIs) and drugs that increase esophageal sphincter pressure, such as **metoclopramide.** Avoidance of certain foods (e.g.,

chocolate) and bedtime snacks, plus the elevation of the upper body during sleep, is also helpful. Because obesity contributes to GERD, weight reduction can help alleviate symptoms.

Acute gastroparesis is a delay in gastric emptying that is typically seen in patients recovering from surgery, trauma, or abdominal infections. **Chronic gastroparesis** is seen in patients with neuropathies that affect the stomach, such as patients with diabetes mellitus. As with other forms of gastroparesis, **diabetic gastroparesis** can be treated with **prokinetic drugs** such as metoclopramide (see later).

Metoclopramide

Mechanisms and Effects. Metoclopramide is a **prokinetic drug** believed to increase **GI tone and motility** by blocking **dopamine D_2 receptors,** which prevents the relaxation of GI smooth muscle produced by dopamine. Dopamine infusions have been found to reduce gastric muscle tone in human volunteers and cause delayed gastric emptying. In addition to blocking the direct effects of dopamine, metoclopramide increases the release of **acetylcholine** from cholinergic motor neurons in the enteric nervous system by blocking presynaptic dopamine receptors whose activation inhibits acetylcholine release. This increases stimulation of acetylcholine muscarinic receptors and enhances propulsive activity, leading to increased tone and motility in the esophagus and stomach.

Metoclopramide accelerates **gastric emptying** by preventing the relaxation of the gastric body and increasing phasic contractions of the antrum. At the same time, it relaxes the proximal duodenum so that it can accept gastric material as antral contractions arrive at the pyloric sphincter. Metoclopramide also increases the resting pressure of the **lower esophageal sphincter** and thereby **reduces reflux of acid** from the stomach into the esophagus.

Pharmacokinetics and Use. Metoclopramide can be administered orally or parenterally. It is rapidly absorbed from the gut and has an average bioavailability of 85%. The drug is conjugated with sulfate and glucuronate, and these metabolites are excreted in the urine, along with 20% of the parent compound. The terminal half-life is about 4 hours.

Metoclopramide is used to treat **GERD, diabetic gastroparesis,** and **intractable hiccup.** It is sometimes used to facilitate **intubation of the small bowel** during a radiologic examination. In addition, metoclopramide exerts **antiemetic effects** by blocking dopamine D_2 and serotonin 5-hydroxytryptamine ($5-HT_3$) receptors in the chemoreceptor trigger zone (CTZ; see later).

Adverse Effects. The major adverse effects of metoclopramide are **CNS reactions** (e.g., drowsiness, extrapyramidal effects, and seizures). Hyperprolactinemia, diarrhea, and hematologic toxicity have also been reported. Metoclopramide is contraindicated in persons with seizure disorders, mechanical obstruction of the GI tract, GI hemorrhage, or pheochromocytoma.

Antispasmodic Agents

Atropine, hyoscyamine, dicyclomine, and **scopolamine** are used as antispasmodic agents to temporarily relieve **intestinal cramping and pain** due to intestinal hyperactivity and irritability. The pharmacology of these muscarinic acetylcholine receptor antagonists is described in Chapter 7.

DRUGS FOR CONSTIPATION

Constipation is an acute or chronic condition that is characterized by the difficult passage of hard, dry feces. If not treated, it may lead to fecal impaction of the colon and rectum. The treatment of constipation rests on a foundation of increased dietary fiber and fluid intake and regular exercise. Patients should be encouraged to eat fruits, vegetables, and whole-grain foods that add bulk to the diet. If dietary modifications are not sufficient to alleviate constipation, a laxative can be used to increase peristalsis (propulsive movements). Glycerin rectal suppositories may be used to relieve mild acute constipation before resorting to other treatments.

Laxatives

Laxatives are drugs that increase bowel movements and facilitate defecation; they are classified by their mechanism of action as bulk-forming, surfactant, osmotic, and stimulant laxatives. They are used to prevent and treat **constipation,** to **evacuate the bowel** before surgery and diagnostic procedures, and to **remove drugs and poisons** from the intestines.

Bulk-Forming Laxatives

Bulk-forming laxatives are indigestible hydrophilic substances that resemble dietary fiber, such as **psyllium hydrophilic mucilloid** and **calcium polycarbophil.** They absorb and retain water in the intestinal lumen and increase the mass of intestinal material. These actions cause mechanical distention of the intestinal wall and stimulate peristalsis. Bulk-forming laxatives are available in several preparations, including fiber tablets and packets of psyllium granules. They must be taken with a full glass of water to ensure adequate hydration of the preparation and avoid intestinal obstruction. Bulk-forming laxatives are the safest and most physiologic type of laxative, and they rarely cause adverse effects. For this reason, they are the preferred drugs for the management of chronic constipation. Because of their ability to absorb water and irritant substances such as bile salts, these drugs are also used in the **treatment of diarrhea** (see later).

Surfactant Laxatives

The surfactant laxatives include **docusate sodium** and docusate calcium. These laxatives are also called **stool softeners** because they facilitate the incorporation of water into fatty intestinal material and thereby soften the feces. Stool softeners are primarily beneficial when fecal materials are hard or dry and when their passage is irritating and painful (e.g., as occurs with anorectal conditions such as hemorrhoids). They are also useful when patients must avoid straining during defecation (e.g., after having abdominal or other surgery). Surfactants produce few adverse effects.

Osmotic Laxatives

Osmotic laxatives include saline laxatives such as **magnesium oxide** (Milk of Magnesia) and **sodium phosphate,** sugars such as **lactulose,** and **polyethylene glycol (PEG).** These substances retain water in the intestinal lumen and increase intraluminal pressure, stimulating peristalsis. They can be taken orally, and some can be administered as an enema. Magnesium oxide is used to treat or prevent constipation, such as in those receiving opioid analgesics. Sodium phosphate acts rapidly to vigorously stimulate defecation and is used to **evacuate the bowel** in patients scheduled for surgery or diagnostic examination and in those with a drug overdose or poisoning. This agent may cause considerable cramping and discomfort. The newest member of the osmotic laxative family is **lactitol,** which is indicated for the treatment of chronic idiopathic constipation (CIC) in adults.

Excessive use of saline laxatives can lead to **loss of fluids and electrolytes,** and patients with renal impairment may not be able to properly excrete phosphate after sodium phosphate administration. There have been rare episodes of renal impairment and permanent **kidney damage** in persons given sodium phosphate for bowel evacuation. This laxative should be avoided in persons with kidney disease or intestinal disorders, and in those taking drugs affecting renal function. Saline laxatives should be limited to short-term use.

In contrast to saline laxatives, **lactulose** and **PEG** are safe and effective agents for treating **chronic constipation.** Lactulose is a disaccharide composed of fructose and galactose. It is converted to low-molecular-weight acids by colonic bacteria that osmotically attract water and thereby stimulate peristalsis. The acidic metabolites also convert ammonia to ammonium ion that is then excreted. For this reason, lactulose is also used for the treatment of **hepatic encephalopathy** associated with elevated blood ammonia levels. Unlike lactulose, PEG is available without a prescription.

Stimulant (Secretory) Laxatives

The stimulant laxatives include **botanical products** such as **castor oil, senna glycoside** (Ex-Lax, Senokot), and synthetic compounds such as **bisacodyl.** These drugs act directly on the intestinal mucosa to alter fluid secretion and stimulate peristalsis. **Bisacodyl** is available in formulations for oral and rectal administration for **evacuating the bowel** before surgery or examination, as well as for treating constipation. The stimulant laxatives can cause a number of adverse effects, including **abdominal pain and cramping** and electrolyte and fluid depletion. For this reason, the use of these drugs should be limited to the **short-term treatment of constipation** and bowel evacuation. They have been used to treat opioid-induced constipation when a milder laxative is not sufficient.

Opioid Antagonists

As noted above, opioid agonists, such as loperamide, diphenoxylate, and eluxadoline, are effective treatments for diarrhea. It follows that chronic pain patients receiving long-term administration of opioid analgesics would suffer from constipation. To combat this, opioid antagonist drugs that are restricted to the periphery were developed to specifically treat opioid-induced constipation. The classic opioid antagonist naloxone was modified with a methyl group to give **methylnaltrexone bromide,** available as an injection or tablet for opioid-induced constipation. Two other opioid antagonists indicated for opioid-induced constipation are **naldemedine** and **naloxegol.**

ANTIDIARRHEAL AGENTS

Diarrhea is a condition characterized by **increased frequency and liquidity** of bowel movements. It can be acute or chronic, and it can range in severity from mild to life-threatening. Diarrhea has many causes, including microbial and parasitic infections, excessive laxative use, inflammatory bowel diseases, malabsorption syndromes causing steatorrhea (excess fat in the feces), and pancreatic tumors that secrete vasoactive intestinal polypeptide.

Severe diarrhea caused by bacterial infections and other conditions can lead to significant loss of fluids and electrolytes and should be treated promptly. If fever or systemic symptoms are present, patients with diarrhea should be examined for **microbial and parasitic infections.** If cultures are positive, an appropriate antimicrobial or antiparasitic drug should be given. **Chronic diarrhea** is defined as diarrhea lasting for 14 days or longer. This condition requires a more thorough diagnostic workup to determine the underlying cause and enable the selection of appropriate therapy.

Most cases of **mild diarrhea** are self-limiting and subside within 1 or 2 days. It can usually be managed with **dietary restrictions** and **fluid and electrolyte replacement.** Patients should avoid solid food and milk products for 24 hours after onset of illness, and preparations containing glucose and electrolytes for fluid replacement can be taken. If needed, an **antidiarrheal agent** can be given to older children and adults. As bowel movements decrease, a bland diet can be started.

A number of drugs can cause diarrhea, including antibiotics that eradicate the normal intestinal flora. Administration of *Lactobacillus* preparations can help restore the normal bowel flora and reduce diarrhea in these patients.

Opioid Drugs

Opioids are the most efficacious antidiarrheal drugs. They exert a nonspecific effect that can control diarrhea from almost any cause. Opioids act by inducing a sustained segmental contraction of intestinal smooth muscle, which prevents the rhythmic waves of smooth muscle contraction and relaxation that occur with normal peristalsis.

The effects of opioids are mediated by the activation of **opioid receptors** in smooth muscle. All of the opioid receptor agonists are effective antidiarrheal compounds, but those usually employed in treating diarrhea selectively activate intestinal opioid receptors while having relatively little effect on the CNS. **Diphenoxylate** and **loperamide** are the opioid agonists with the greatest ratio of intestinal smooth muscle activity to CNS activity and are widely used for this purpose. Loperamide is available without a prescription and can effectively control mild diarrhea. Excessive use of these drugs can cause constipation. **Eluxadoline** is a new opioid agonist indicated for the treatment of IBS with diarrhea (see later). The pharmacology of opioid drugs is described in Chapter 23.

Antibiotics and Crofelemer

Rifaximin is an antibiotic indicated for the **treatment of travelers' diarrhea** caused by **noninvasive strains of *Escherichia coli* (*E. coli*).** Rifaximin is a semi-synthetic antibacterial derived from **rifamycin.** Like rifamycin and other structural analogs, **rifaximin kills bacteria** by binding to the *beta*-subunit of bacterial DNA-dependent RNA polymerase, which prevents bacterial RNA synthesis (see Chapter 40). Rifaximin demonstrated a significant reduction in the duration of diarrhea and a higher cure rate than placebo.

More recently, the antibiotic **rifamycin** itself was developed in an extended-release formulation for the **treatment of travelers' diarrhea** caused by **noninvasive strains of *E. coli*.** Like rifaximin, rifamycin should not be taken in patients with diarrhea complicated by fever and/or bloody stool or due to pathogens other than noninvasive strains of *E. coli*.

A new antidiarrheal agent, **crofelemer,** is indicated for the symptomatic relief of noninfectious diarrhea in **adult patients with human immunodeficiency virus/acquired immunodeficiency syndrome (HIV/AIDS)** on antiretroviral therapy. Crofelemer is an **inhibitor** of both the cAMP-stimulated cystic fibrosis transmembrane conductance regulator (CFTR) chloride ion channel (see Chapter 27, under CF drugs) and the calcium-activated Cl⁻ channels (CaCC) at the luminal membrane of enterocytes. By blocking Cl⁻ secretion, crofelemer **decreases the excretion of sodium ions and water,** improving stool consistency and reducing diarrhea. Crofelemer is not systemically absorbed following oral administration.

Locally Acting Drugs

Psyllium and **calcium polycarbophil** control diarrhea by acting within the intestines to absorb water and irritant substances such as bile acids. These substances are suitable for the treatment of mild diarrhea as well as for constipation (see earlier).

Bismuth subsalicylate (Pepto-Bismol) appears to produce its antidiarrheal effect by inhibiting intestinal secretions. It is most effective in treating **infectious diarrhea,** which often has a strong secretory component. In patients with travelers' diarrhea and other forms of infectious diarrhea, clinical studies demonstrated that bismuth subsalicylate caused a greater reduction in the number of diarrheal episodes than did a placebo. Bismuth subsalicylate suspension, however, must be given frequently and repeatedly for maximal efficacy (30 mL every 30 minutes for up to eight doses per day). This preparation causes few side effects, but excessively large doses can expose the patient to bismuth or salicylate toxicity.

Agents for Irritable Bowel Syndrome

IBS is a complex **biopsychosocial disorder** characterized by **chronic abdominal pain** relieved by defecation and is associated with altered bowel habits. Some patients complain primarily of **diarrhea,** whereas **constipation** predominates in others. Hence, the disorder is classified as **IBS with diarrhea** or **IBS with constipation.** Many patients also experience nausea, bloating, and flatulence. Mild cases of IBS may respond to stool stabilizers such as **calcium polycarbophil** (Fibercon) that can reduce episodes of diarrhea and constipation. Other drugs are available for more severe cases, but all of these have limitations and potential adverse effects.

Serotonin 5-HT plays a vital role in promoting GI motility, and drugs affecting serotonin are among those used in treating IBS with diarrhea or constipation. Serotonin is produced and released by enterochromaffin cells in the gut, where it activates **5-HT$_3$ and 5-HT$_4$ receptors** on cholinergic neurons and thereby enhances intestinal motility. Activation of 5-HT$_3$ receptors increases the release of acetylcholine from **myenteric neurons,** whereas activation of presynaptic **5-HT$_4$ receptors** increases the release of acetylcholine from **submucosal neurons.** Drugs that activate 5-HT$_4$ receptors increase intestinal motility and have been used in treating constipation, whereas drugs that block 5-HT$_3$ receptors reduce motility and are used in treating diarrhea-predominant IBS. Other drugs affecting serotonin are described in Chapter 26.

Agents for Irritable Bowel Syndrome With Constipation

Tegaserod is a serotonin **5-HT$_4$ receptor agonist** used for treating women with IBS with constipation (IBS-C). It was removed from the open market because of a small but statistically significant increase in **angina, myocardial infarction,** and **stroke** in those taking the drug. It is only available under an emergency treatment, investigational new drug (IND) protocol for patients who cannot be effectively treated with any other agent. To fill this market niche, **prucalopride,** a new **5-HT$_4$ receptor agonist,** was recently approved for the treatment of chronic idiopathic constipation (CIC) in adults. Serotonergic agonists are discussed further in Chapter 26.

Lubiprostone is indicated for treating **IBS-C, chronic idiopathic constipation (CIC),** and some cases of **opioid-induced constipation.** The CIC syndrome is characterized by hard, lumpy stools and appears to result from impaired colonic activity and fecal evacuation. Patients with CIC have minimal abdominal bloating and discomfort compared with patients with IBS-C.

Lubiprostone is poorly absorbed after oral administration and increases intestinal motility by directly activating the **chloride Cl-C$_2$ channel** in the luminal membrane of the intestinal epithelium, resulting in the secretion of a chloride-rich fluid into the intestinal lumen. The increased intestinal fluid stimulates peristalsis and relieves constipation. Clinical studies found that **lubiprostone significantly increased the frequency of spontaneous bowel movements** in persons with CIC. Results in patients with IBS-C were less dramatic, and only 12% of these patients had an "overall response" to the drug, defined as being significantly relieved 2 or more weeks of the month in 2 out of 3 months. The drug caused **nausea** in about 30% of patients, which is reduced by taking it with food, and **diarrhea** occurred in 13% of persons taking the drug.

Linaclotide is another new agent for CIC and IBS-C. It stimulates **guanylate cyclase** on the luminal surface of intestinal epithelium and elevates intracellular cyclic GMP levels, leading to increased secretion of chloride and bicarbonate into the intestines and causing increased intestinal fluid accumulation and motility. Cyclic GMP may also decrease the activity of pain-sensing neurons. **Diarrhea** is the most common side effect of linaclotide. A second guanylate cyclase-C agonist is **plecanatide,** indicated for chronic idiopathic constipation (CIC) and irritable bowel syndrome with constipation (IBS-C).

Agents for Irritable Bowel Syndrome With Diarrhea

Alosetron is a serotonin **5-HT$_3$ receptor antagonist** that is used to treat IBS with diarrhea. Activation of 5-HT$_3$ receptors is coupled with the opening of cation (sodium and potassium) channels in myenteric neurons, leading to neuronal depolarization and release of acetylcholine. This stimulates intestinal motility and contributes to diarrhea and visceral pain in patients with IBS. Alosetron is employed in women whose symptoms have lasted at least 6 months and include diarrhea, abdominal pain, and frequent bowel urgency or incontinence causing disability or restriction of daily activities. In these patients, **alosetron increases colonic transit time** and reduces pain and other symptoms of IBS.

Alosetron may infrequently cause adverse GI effects, including **ischemic colitis,** that rarely require blood transfusions and surgery and that have been fatal in a few cases. Hence, the drug is restricted to treating patients whose condition does not respond to conventional antidiarrheal and antispasmodic medications.

Eluxadoline is a new drug for **diarrhea-predominant IBS** in adults. This opioid drug binds to several subtypes of **opioid receptors,** acting as an agonist at opioid *mu* (**μ**) and *kappa* (**κ**) receptors and an antagonist at opioid *delta* (**δ**) receptors (see Chapter 23). Activation of **μ** receptors leads to decreased intestinal motility and relief of diarrhea, while actions of eluxadoline on other opioid receptors are postulated to reduce the incidence of constipation typically caused by **μ** opioid agonists. In clinical trials, IBS patients had improved stool consistency and reduced pain while taking eluxadoline, which is given orally twice daily with food.

DRUGS FOR NAUSEA AND VOMITING

Emesis, or **vomiting,** is a physiologic response to the presence of irritating and potentially harmful substances in the gut or bloodstream. It sometimes occurs as a result of excessive vestibular stimulation (motion sickness) or psychological stimuli such as fear, dread, or obnoxious sights and odors. Vomiting is frequently preceded by nausea.

Vomiting is initiated by a nucleus of cells located in the medulla that is called the **vomiting** or **emesis center.** This center coordinates a complex series of events involving pharyngeal, GI, and abdominal wall contractions that lead to the expulsion of the gastric contents. These include orally migrating intestinal contractions (reverse peristalsis), gastric contractions, contractions of the diaphragm and abdominal wall, and relaxation of the esophageal sphincter and wall. The reverse intestinal contractions are associated with **nausea,** which is an intensely unpleasant feeling of the imminent need to vomit. Nausea can also occur in the absence of vomiting.

The neural pathways involved in emesis and the sites of antiemetic drug action are shown in Fig. 28.3. The vomiting center can be activated by afferent fibers arising from the gut, **CTZ,** cerebral cortex, or vestibular apparatus. The CTZ is located in the area postrema and responds to blood-borne substances, including cytotoxic cancer chemotherapy drugs. These substances activate the CTZ via stimulation of **serotonin 5-HT3, dopamine D2, or muscarinic M1 receptors.** The vestibular apparatus activates the vomiting center via fibers that project to the cerebellum and release acetylcholine or histamine. Noxious substances in the gut can activate vagal afferent pathways to the solitary tract nucleus, which projects to the vomiting center, as well as pathways to the nerve tracts that stimulate the CTZ. The **D$_2$, 5-HT$_3$,** and **neurokinin 1 (NK1) receptors** also have a major role in these pathways.

Antiemetic drugs act by blocking specific receptors in the emetic pathway described above. Some drugs appear to inhibit several pathways that lead to vomiting center activation. The D_2 and 5-HT$_3$ receptor antagonists inhibit activation of both the CTZ and the solitary tract nucleus. Muscarinic receptor antagonists can block the CTZ, solitary tract, and vestibular pathways involved in emesis. **Dexamethasone,** a glucocorticoid (see Chapter 33), is an effective antiemetic whose mechanism is not well understood. It is particularly effective for preventing delayed nausea and vomiting in persons receiving cancer chemotherapy.

Serotonin 5-HT$_3$ Receptor Antagonists

Whereas alosetron is a serotonin 5-HT$_3$ receptor antagonist for treating diarrhea-predominant IBS (see earlier), **ondansetron** was the first 5-HT$_3$ receptor antagonist developed for the treatment of cancer chemotherapy-induced nausea and vomiting. It significantly reduces the number of episodes of emesis in patients treated with cisplatin, which is one of the most highly emetogenic chemotherapy agents. Other first-generation 5-HT$_3$ antagonists include **granisetron** and **dolasetron.** These drugs have similar pharmacologic properties and clinical efficacies. **Palonosetron** is called a second-generation 5-HT$_3$ antagonist because of its greater affinity for 5-HT$_3$ receptors and its much longer half-life and duration of action.

Mechanisms and Effects

Serotonin contributes to the development of nausea and vomiting at several sites in the emesis pathway. It is released from the enterochromaffin cells of the small intestine, where it activates 5-HT$_3$ receptors on vagal afferent nerves so as to initiate the vomiting reflex (see Fig. 28.3). Serotonin also promotes vomiting by activating 5-HT$_3$ receptors in the solitary tract nucleus and in the CTZ. Ondansetron and other 5-HT$_3$ antagonists are structural analogs of serotonin (see Fig. 28.2) and function as competitive receptor antagonists at these sites to reduce stimulation of the vomiting center.

Pharmacokinetics and Indications

Some of the 5-HT$_3$ receptor antagonists (e.g., ondansetron) can be administered orally or intravenously, whereas others (e.g., palonosetron) are only given intravenously. These drugs are metabolized by cytochrome P450, and the metabolites are primarily eliminated in the urine. The half-lives of granisetron, ondansetron, and dolasetron are 4, 6, and 7 hours, respectively. Palonosetron has a half-life of about 40 hours, which confers a much longer duration of action than other 5-HT$_3$ antagonists.

All of the 5-HT$_3$ antagonists except dolasetron are indicated for the prevention of **cancer chemotherapy-induced emesis** and have been shown to significantly reduce the number of episodes of vomiting in patients treated with highly emetogenic chemotherapy agents. Ondansetron and dolasetron are indicated for the prevention and treatment of **postoperative vomiting,** whereas ondansetron and granisetron are also used to prevent **nausea and vomiting caused by radiation therapy.**

First-generation 5-HT$_3$ antagonists are usually administered just before chemotherapy and continue for 3 to 5 days after the course of chemotherapy is completed. Because of its longer duration of action, a single dose of palonosetron may prevent nausea and vomiting for up to 7 days after chemotherapy. Palonosetron is approved for treating both acute and delayed nausea and vomiting in persons receiving emetogenic chemotherapy.

Other antiemetic drugs exert an additive or synergistic effect with 5-HT$_3$ antagonists. **Dexamethasone** and **neurokinin NK$_1$ antagonists** are often employed in combination with a 5-HT$_3$ antagonist for preventing chemotherapy-induced emesis (see guidelines later).

Studies have also confirmed the usefulness of ondansetron in controlling postoperative nausea and vomiting. In patients who underwent laparoscopic cholecystectomy, for example, ondansetron was found to be more effective than metoclopramide or a placebo in controlling emesis.

Adverse Effects and Interactions

The serotonin 5-HT$_3$ antagonists are generally well tolerated and usually produce few adverse effects. The most common side effects of 5-HT$_3$ antagonists are **headache, constipation,** and **diarrhea.** Less common reactions include hypertension and elevated hepatic enzyme levels. Ondansetron has been associated with a few anaphylactoid reactions consisting of bronchospasm, angioedema, hypotension, and urticaria, but clinically significant drug interactions with 5-HT$_3$ receptor antagonists have not been identified. Higher intravenous doses of **dolasetron** were found to cause **prolongation of the QT interval** of the electrocardiogram and potentially fatal **torsade des pointes** (polymorphic ventricular tachycardia). The Food and Drug Administration has warned that higher doses of dolasetron should be avoided, but lower oral doses may still be used for postoperative emesis because they do not prolong the QT interval significantly.

Neurokinin-1 Receptor Antagonists
Aprepitant and Rolapitant

Substance P is a peptide of the **tachykinin** family that acts as a neurotransmitter in the gut and brain. The neurotransmitter is released from vagal afferent fibers in the solitary tract, where it activates **NK$_1$** receptors and thereby produces emesis (see Fig. 28.3). **Aprepitant** and **rolapitant** are nonpeptide NK$_1$ receptor antagonists that prevent emesis induced by various stimuli. The drugs are most often used in combination with a 5-HT$_3$ antagonist (e.g., ondansetron) and/or dexamethasone to prevent acute and delayed nausea and vomiting during cancer chemotherapy. For this reason, a new combination formulation of the prodrug **fosnetupitant** (see below) **with palonosetron** was marketed.

Aprepitant is administered orally and is metabolized primarily by cytochrome CYP3A4 with a terminal half-life of 9 to 13 hours. Drugs that inhibit CYP3A4 can elevate plasma concentrations of aprepitant. In contrast, rolapitant has an elimination half-life of about 7 days. It is slowly converted to an active metabolite by CYP3A4. **Fosaprepitant** is an aprepitant prodrug intended for intravenous administration.

Although inducers of CYP3A4 can significantly lower plasma levels of rolapitant and should not be given concurrently, inhibitors of this enzyme had no clinically significant effect on rolapitant kinetics. Aprepitant and rolapitant appear to cause few adverse effects during short-term use.

Dopamine D$_2$ Receptor Antagonists

The D$_2$ receptor antagonists include **metoclopramide** (see earlier) and phenothiazine drugs such as **perphenazine** (see Chapter 22) and **promethazine.** As antiemetics, D$_2$ blockers

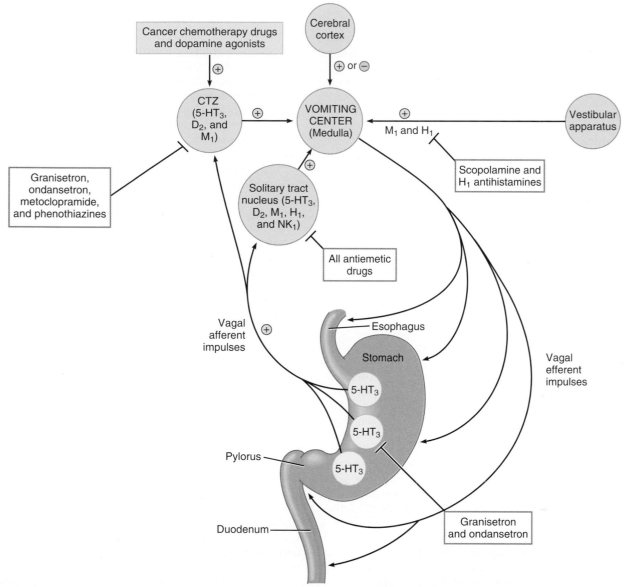

Fig. 28.3 Physiology of emesis and sites of drug action. Emetic stimuli travel from the gastrointestinal tract via the solitary tract nucleus to arrive at the vomiting center in the medulla. Emetic stimuli also reach the vomiting center via afferent fibers from the chemoreceptor trigger zone (CTZ), cerebral cortex, and vestibular apparatus. Granisetron and ondansetron prevent emesis by blocking serotonin 5-HT$_3$ receptors in the gastrointestinal tract, solitary tract nucleus, and CTZ. Metoclopramide and phenothiazines prevent emesis by blocking dopamine D$_2$ receptors in the solitary tract nucleus and CTZ. Aprepitant blocks neurokinin 1 (NK$_1$) receptors in the solitary tract. Scopolamine and the H$_1$ antihistamines prevent emesis by blocking muscarinic M$_1$ receptors, histamine H$_1$ receptors, or both types of receptors in the vestibular tracts that project to the vomiting center and in the solitary tract nucleus and CTZ. Note that cancer chemotherapy drugs and dopamine agonists cause emesis, in part, by stimulating the CTZ.

act primarily on the CTZ to inhibit stimulation of the vomiting center, but they also inhibit afferent impulses from the gut by antagonizing receptors in the solitary tract nucleus. **Promethazine is used in treating emesis in a number of medical conditions,** but it is less effective than other drugs in treating chemotherapy-induced emesis.

Other D$_2$ receptor antagonists indicated for the treatment of nausea and vomiting are **amisulpride**, used alone or with another antiemetic of a different class, and **trimethobenzamide**, indicated for the treatment of postoperative nausea and vomiting and for nausea associated with gastroenteritis.

Other Antiemetics

Dronabinol, an oral formulation of Δ^9-**tetrahydrocannabinol** (the active ingredient of the marijuana plant), is approved

for the treatment of **cancer chemotherapy-induced emesis** when conventional antiemetic drugs have failed. Dronabinol is usually administered several hours before chemotherapy and is then administered every 4 to 6 hours during a 12-hour period after chemotherapy. The drug probably acts on the vomiting center in the medulla. It is less effective than serotonin antagonists and has about the same antiemetic efficacy as perphenazine. Dronabinol is also approved as an **appetite stimulant** for anorexic patients with AIDS. A synthetic cannabinoid called **nabilone** is also available for the treatment of cancer chemotherapy-induced emesis.

Several histamine H$_1$ receptor antagonists (H$_1$ antihistamines) have antiemetic actions and are discussed in Chapter 26. Two of these agents, **dimenhydrinate** and **meclizine,** are used in the management of **motion sickness.** Another of these agents, **promethazine,** besides its D_2 antagonism mentioned above, is more active as an H_1 receptor antagonist and antimuscarinic agent. As mentioned above, **promethazine** is used to prevent and treat **nausea and vomiting** induced by medications, anesthetics, and a wide variety of neurologic, psychogenic, and GI stimuli. Promethazine is usually administered as a rectal suppository or by injection.

After many years off the market due to erroneous lawsuits claiming fetal malformations, a new formulation of **doxylamine with vitamin B6 (pyridoxine)** was approved for the treatment of **morning sickness** in **pregnant women** (see also Chapter 34). It is marketed under the brand name DICLEGIS. This combination antiemetic is also available in a fast-acting and long-lasting formulation called BONJESTA. Doxylamine is a first-generation antihistamine discussed previously (see Chapter 26).

Scopolamine is a muscarinic receptor antagonist similar to **atropine** (see earlier and Chapter 7) and is primarily used to prevent **motion sickness.** It has been used by astronauts in space as well as by persons traveling in cars, planes, or boats. Scopolamine is available as a skin patch that slowly releases the drug over 72 hours.

Cannabinoid Hyperemesis Syndrome

Cannabinoid hyperemesis syndrome (CHS) is a rare condition that occurs in daily long-term users of marijuana or other cannabis products. **CHS** is noted by **severe** and **repeated bouts of vomiting** that can lead to dehydration, electrolyte disturbances, and death. The etiology of CHS is not completely understood; it is a paradoxical effect of **THC (dronabinol)** which is approved for the treatment of nausea and vomiting due to cancer-induced emesis (see above). Interestingly, people with CHS also present to the ER with **severe skin burns as compulsive hot baths** tend to decrease nausea and vomiting due to CHS. The only known cure for CHS is the **cessation of marijuana** or other cannabis product use.

Guidelines for Chemotherapy-Induced Emesis

The Multinational Association for Supportive Care in Cancer recommends a **serotonin antagonist** (e.g., ondansetron) plus **dexamethasone** and/or **aprepitant** for preventing acute emesis caused by highly vomit-inducing (emetogenic) drugs such as **cisplatin, dacarbazine,** and **cyclophosphamide.** Aprepitant and dexamethasone are recommended to be given on days 2 and 3 to prevent delayed emesis. For moderately emetogenic chemotherapy, a serotonin antagonist and dexamethasone are recommended for acute emesis, and dexamethasone alone is recommended for delayed emesis. For minimally emetogenic chemotherapy, a low dose of dexamethasone is recommended.

SUMMARY OF IMPORTANT POINTS

- Drugs used to treat peptic ulcers include inhibitors of gastric acid secretion, cytoprotective agents, and antibiotics for *H. pylori* infection. The histamine H_2 receptor antagonists (famotidine, ranitidine, and others) and the proton pump inhibitors (omeprazole and others) are the primary gastric acid inhibitors. Gastric antacids (aluminum and magnesium hydroxides and calcium carbonate) are used to relieve heartburn and dyspepsia.

- The H_2 receptor antagonists inhibit basal and meal-stimulated acid secretion and can be used to treat GERD and dyspepsia as well as peptic ulcer disease. Cimetidine inhibits cytochrome P450 isozymes and may increase the plasma concentrations of many other drugs, potentially causing adverse effects.

- Omeprazole and related drugs irreversibly inhibit the proton pump (H^+,K^+-ATPase) and acid secretion. They are the most efficacious drugs for treating GERD and peptic ulcers, and they are the drugs of choice for use in patients with gastrin-secreting tumors (gastrinomas) and Zollinger-Ellison syndrome.

- Sucralfate is a cytoprotective drug that binds to the ulcer crater and forms a barrier to acid and pepsin. Misoprostol is a prostaglandin E_1 analog that increases the production of mucus and bicarbonate while reducing the secretion of gastric acid. Misoprostol is used to prevent ulcers caused by long-term therapy with NSAIDs.

- Inflammatory bowel diseases (ulcerative colitis and Crohn disease) are primarily treated with glucocorticoids, mesalamine, infliximab, and other monoclonal antibodies to tumor necrosis factor-α or integrin molecules.

- Metoclopramide inhibits dopamine D_2 receptors and blocks dopamine-induced smooth muscle relaxation while increasing acetylcholine release in the gut. It is used to increase gastrointestinal motility in gastroparesis and to increase lower esophageal pressure in GERD.

- Laxatives are drugs used to facilitate defecation and evacuate the bowels. They include bulk-forming laxatives (psyllium and polycarbophil), surfactant laxatives (docusate sodium), osmotic laxatives (magnesium oxide and sodium phosphate), and stimulant laxatives (bisacodyl and others).

- Bulk-forming laxatives are preferred for the treatment of chronic constipation. Osmotic and stimulant laxatives are used to clear the bowels of patients preparing for intestinal surgery or diagnostic examination and patients being treated for a drug overdose or poisoning.

- Lubiprostone (chloride channel activator), linaclotide (guanylate cyclase activator), and tegaserod (5-HT_4 agonist) are agents for constipation-predominant irritable bowel syndrome (IBS). Alosetron is a serotonin 5-HT_3 antagonist that decreases gastrointestinal motility and relieves diarrhea in IBS, while eluxadoline is an opioid drug for this indication.

- Opioids are the most efficacious antidiarrheal drugs. Loperamide and diphenoxylate have very little central nervous system effects at doses that control diarrhea.

- Serotonin 5-HT_3 receptor antagonists (ondansetron and others) are the most efficacious antiemetics for the management of cancer chemotherapy-induced nausea and vomiting.

- Aprepitant and rolapitant are neurokinin-1 receptor antagonists that prevent chemotherapy-induced emesis. Other antiemetics include metoclopramide and other dopamine D_2 receptor antagonists.

- Promethazine is used for mild nausea and vomiting caused by drugs, infections, and other stimuli. Motion sickness can be prevented by meclizine and dimenhydrinate (histamine H₁ receptor antagonists) or by scopolamine, a muscarinic receptor antagonist.

Review Questions

1. A woman is using a scopolamine skin patch to prevent motion sickness while on a cruise ship. Which is the most common adverse effect of this drug?
   (A) flatulence
   (B) heartburn
   (C) headache
   (D) diarrhea
   (E) dry mouth
2. A woman with irritable bowel syndrome has recurrent episodes of abdominal pain and diarrhea that are not relieved by polycarbophil. Which adverse effect may result from taking alosetron for this condition?
   (A) pulmonary fibrosis
   (B) ischemic colitis
   (C) ischemic heart disease
   (D) gastric ulcer
   (E) muscle rigidity and tremor
3. Which drug combination usually provides the most rapid and effective treatment for a duodenal ulcer caused by *H. pylori* infection?

   (A) sucralfate, amoxicillin, and clarithromycin
   (B) rabeprazole, bismuth subsalicylate, and tetracycline
   (C) famotidine, amoxicillin, and metronidazole
   (D) pantoprazole, amoxicillin, clarithromycin, and metronidazole
   (E) amoxicillin, clarithromycin, tetracycline, and metronidazole
4. A man with chronic heartburn caused by gastric acid reflux is prescribed metoclopramide. Which mechanism is responsible for its pharmacologic effect?
   (A) histamine H2 receptor blockade
   (B) muscarinic receptor blockade
   (C) dopamine D2 receptor blockade
   (D) α-adrenoceptor activation
   (E) chloride ClC-2 channel activation
5. A man is given medication to prevent cisplatin-induced vomiting. Which combination of drugs is recommended for this purpose?
   (A) palonosetron, dexamethasone, and aprepitant
   (B) dexamethasone only
   (C) dexamethasone and aprepitant
   (D) aprepitant only
   (E) palonosetron only

CHAPTER 29

Drugs for Headache Disorders

CLASSIFICATION OF DRUGS FOR HEADACHE DISORDERS

Drugs for Migraine Headaches

Drugs for migraine prevention

Antiepileptic drugs and antidepressants
- Valproic acid (DEPAKENE)
- Fluoxetine (PROZAC) also amitriptyline (ELAVIL)
- Phenelzine (NARDIL)

Nonsteroidal anti-inflammatory drugs
- Naproxen (NAPROSYN, ALEVE)
- Fenoprofen (NALFON)[a]

Beta (β)-adrenoceptor antagonists
- Propranolol (INDERAL)
- Timolol (TIMOLIDE)

Calcium channel blockers
- Verapamil (CALAN)
- Nimodipine (NIMOTOP)

CGRP-targeted monoclonal antibodies
- Galcanezumab (EMGALITY)
- Erenumab (AIMOVIG)[b]

Other agents for preventing migraine
- Gabapentin (NEURONTIN)
- Botulinum toxin A (BOTOX)

Drugs for migraine termination

Serotonin 5-HT receptor agonists
- Dihydroergotamine (DHE, MIGRANAL)[c]
- Sumatriptan (IMITREX)[d]
- Lasmiditan (REYVOW)

CGRP receptor antagonists
- Rimegepant (NURTEC)
- Ubrogepant (UBRELVY)

Other agents for migraine termination
- Isometheptene (MIDRID)
- Tramadol (ULTRAM)
- Butorphanol (STADOL NS)
- Naproxen (NAPROSYN, ALEVE)[e]
- Acetaminophen with codeine (TYLENOL #3)[f]
- Prochlorperazine (COMPAZINE)

Drugs for cluster and tension headaches
- See Table 29.1.

[a] Also flurbiprofen (ANSAID), ketoprofen (ORUDIS), and mefenamic acid (PONSTEL).
[b] Also fremanezumab (AJOVY), and eptinezumab (VYEPTI).
[c] Also ergotamine (ERGOMAR).
[d] Also naratriptan (AMERGE), zolmitriptan (ZOMIG), rizatriptan (MAXALT), frovatriptan (FROVA), almotriptan (AXERT), and eletriptan (RELPAX); sumatriptan is also formulated as a nasal spray (ONZETRA XSAIL) and as a transdermal iontophoresis patch (ZECURITY).
[e] Also flurbiprofen (ANSAID), ketoprofen (ORUDIS), and mefenamic acid (PONSTEL).
[f] Also acetaminophen with caffeine, butalbital, and codeine (FIORICET).

OVERVIEW

An occasional headache for most people is easily remedied by a couple of aspirin or ibuprofen pills and a glass of water. However, for many people, headaches are unremitting, severe, and recurring. The International Headache Society divides headache disorders into two large groups. The first group, primary headache disorders, includes cluster, migraine, and tension headaches. The characteristics and management of these three types of headaches, which together account for about 95% of all headaches, are compared in Table 29.1. The second group, secondary headache disorders, consists of headaches that arise from organic disorders (e.g., hemorrhage, infection, neuropathy, stroke, and tumor). In patients with secondary headaches, management focuses on treating the underlying disorder.

Because migraine is the most serious and common type of headache in patients with a headache disorder, it is the main focus of the discussion. The chapter closes with a brief review of treatment options for cluster and tension headaches.

CHARACTERISTICS AND PATHOGENESIS OF MIGRAINE HEADACHES

In the United States, approximately 24 million people experience migraine headaches (Box 29.1). The pathophysiologic mechanisms of migraines are not completely understood, but migraine headaches appear to result from neurovascular dysfunction caused by an imbalance between excitatory and inhibitory neuronal activity at various levels in the central nervous system (CNS). This imbalance can be triggered by hormones, stress, fatigue, hunger, diet, or drugs.

About 15% of patients who have migraine headache disorder report that they experience an **aura** that precedes each headache attack and lasts for about 15 to 20 minutes. A **visual aura** can take the form of brightly flashing lights or rippling images that spread from the corner of the visual field (teichopsia). A **sensory aura** can take the form of paresthesias that involves the arm and face and tends to *march* sequentially from the fingers to the hand and then to the body. Auras are believed to result from the cerebral vasoconstriction and ischemia that precipitate migraine attacks.

TABLE 29.1 **Classification and Pharmacologic Management of Headache Disorders**

CLASSIFICATION	CHARACTERISTICS	DRUGS FOR PREVENTING HEADACHES	DRUGS FOR ABORTING HEADACHES
Primary Headaches			
Cluster headaches	Severe, unilateral, retro-orbital; clustered over time	Lithium and verapamil	DHE, ergotamine, glucocorticoids, lidocaine, oxygen, and sumatriptan
Migraine headaches	Moderate or severe, often unilateral, usually pulsatile; occur with or without aura	β-adrenoceptor antagonists, anticonvulsants, antidepressants, calcium channel blockers, NSAIDs, and serotonin 5-HT$_2$ receptor antagonists CGRP drugs	DHE, ergotamine, isometheptene, NSAIDs, tramadol, and triptans[a]
Tension headaches	Mild or moderate, bilateral, non-pulsatile; exert bandlike pressure	Amitriptyline	Muscle relaxants and NSAIDs
Secondary Headaches			
	Characteristics vary, depending on the underlying cause[b]	None	None (treat underlying disorder)

DHE, Dihydroergotamine; *NSAIDs,* nonsteroidal anti-inflammatory drugs.
[a]Triptans include naratriptan, rizatriptan, sumatriptan, and zolmitriptan.
[b]Examples of causes are hemorrhage, infection, neuropathy, stroke, and tumor.

BOX 29.1 THE CASE OF THE UNMITIGATING MIGRAINE

CASE PRESENTATION
A 26-year-old woman who has frequent migraine headaches reports to her physician that the drug she has been taking to stop her migraine attacks is not working anymore. The physician looks in her medical record and tells her that he prescribed sumatriptan on her last visit a month ago and that she may be tolerant to its effects. The physician talks to her about trying a drug to prevent migraine attacks as well as a new drug to abort migraines. She agrees to this new strategy and is prescribed valproate for migraine prevention and a new intranasal formulation of dihydroergotamine for aborting a migraine attack.

CASE DISCUSSION
Migraine is an extremely common condition that will affect 12% to 28% of people at some point. It is more common in women than in men, with about 25% of adult women experiencing a migraine headache at least once a year, compared with less than 10% of men. Too-frequent use of an abortive agent for migraine headaches, such as sumatriptan, can lead to loss of effectiveness; another antimigraine agent can be administered and might be effective. In the case presented, an ergot alkaloid, dihydroergotamine (DHE), which is now available in a convenient and rapid-acting nasal inhalation formulation, was prescribed. This class of drugs, however, carries potential risks for serious adverse effects, including ischemic conditions, and the frequency of their use should be limited. Valproate is an antiseizure drug that is commonly used for migraine prophylaxis. It has an onset of action of a couple of weeks, which may be shorter than other agents used to prevent migraine attacks. Propranolol, a β-blocker, is also used to prevent the occurrence of migraine headaches, and its use in controlled clinical studies did not show tolerance in migraine sufferers who used it for at least 6 months. The latest treatments are CGRP antagonists, which are very effective for treating migraine disorders.

A migraine without an aura (previously known as a **common migraine**) is often accompanied by an attack of photophobia, phonophobia, nausea, or vomiting.

Each migraine attack has two phases. The **first phase** is characterized by **cerebral vasoconstriction** and **ischemia.** The release of **serotonin** from CNS neurons and circulating platelets contributes to this first phase. Hence, antiplatelet drugs and serotonin receptor antagonists are efficacious in the prevention of migraine headaches. The **second phase,** which is longer than the first one, is characterized by **cerebral vasodilation** and **pain.** The trigeminal neurovascular system appears to play a central role in the second phase. Neurons in the trigeminal complex release vasoactive peptides, including **substance P** and **calcitonin gene-related peptide** (CGRP). These peptides trigger vasodilation and inflammation of pial and dural vessels, which in turn stimulate nociceptive fibers of the trigeminal nerve and cause pain. Fig. 29.1 depicts these events and the mechanisms of drugs used to terminate migraine headaches.

DRUGS FOR MIGRAINE HEADACHES
The drugs used to manage patients with migraine headaches can be classified **as prophylactic drugs** and **abortive (symptomatic) drugs.** Many prophylactic drugs act by preventing the vasoconstrictive phase of the disorder, whereas abortive drugs reverse the vasodilation phase of migraine or relieve pain and inflammation.

Several drugs for migraine are antagonists or agonists at specific types of **serotonin receptors.** These receptors have been classified into four main types, 5-HT$_1$ through 5-HT$_4$.

The **5-HT$_2$ receptors** are widely distributed in the CNS, smooth muscle, and platelets, where they mediate vasoconstriction and platelet aggregation. Drugs that block 5-HT$_2$ receptors can prevent the vasoconstrictive phase of migraine and are in development as migraine prophylactics.

The **5-HT$_1$ receptors** are the predominant serotonin receptors in the CNS, and many of them function as presynaptic autoreceptors whose activation inhibits the release of serotonin and other neurotransmitters. The 5-HT$_1$ receptors also mediate cerebral vasoconstriction. Drugs that activate these receptors, such as **sumatriptan,** are used to terminate a migraine attack.

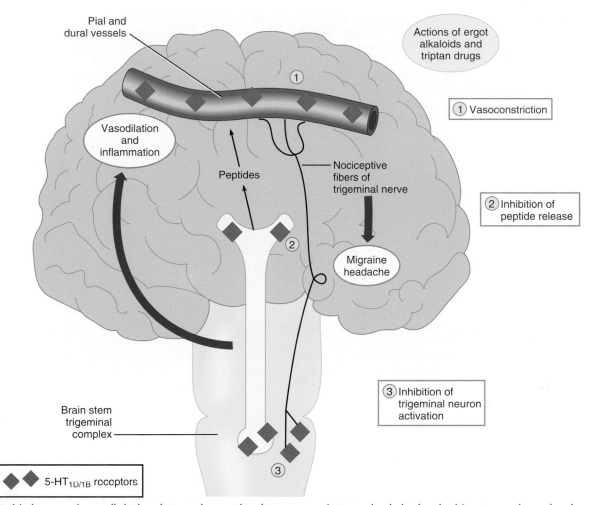

Fig. 29.1 Mechanisms of ergot alkaloids and triptan drugs used in the treatment of migraine headache disorder. Migraine attacks are thought to result from trigeminal neurovascular dysfunction. When neurons in the trigeminal complex release peptides such as substance P and calcitonin gene-related peptide (CGRP), this causes vasodilation and inflammation of pial and dural vessels. These events activate nociceptive trigeminal fibers and cause moderate to severe pain that is characteristic of migraine headaches. Ergot alkaloids and triptan drugs terminate the pain by activating serotonin 5-HT$_{1B/1D}$ receptors at several sites: *(1)* They activate receptors on pial and dural vessels and thereby cause vasoconstriction. *(2)* They activate presynaptic receptors to inhibit the release of peptides and other mediators from trigeminal neurons. *(3)* They activate receptors in the brainstem, which is believed to inhibit the activation of trigeminal neurons responsible for migraine attacks. CGRP antagonists (not shown) are also effective in the treatment of migraine.

The newest targets for migraine prevention and termination are the **CGRP peptide and the CGRP receptor**. Recently approved monoclonal antibody drugs and CGRP receptor antagonists block the activation of the CGRP system in migraine and are highly effective.

DRUGS FOR MIGRAINE PREVENTION

Numerous classes of drugs are used to prevent migraine headaches in persons who experience frequent attacks. These include anticonvulsants, antidepressants, anti-inflammatory drugs, *beta (β)*-adrenoceptor antagonists, calcium channel blockers, and serotonin-receptor antagonists. A trial of several different types of drugs may be useful to determine the most effective drug for a particular patient. Each drug requires several weeks of therapy before its effectiveness can be determined.

Antiepileptic Drugs and Antidepressants

The properties of antiepileptic drugs (AEDs) and antidepressants are described in Chapters 20 and 22, respectively. Studies have shown that these two classes of drugs can

prevent migraine in some patients, but the precise mechanisms underlying their effects are poorly understood.

Valproate (valproic acid, DEPAKENE) is the most widely used AED for migraine prophylaxis. Its onset of efficacy (2 to 3 weeks) is somewhat shorter than that of other prophylactic drugs. Its common adverse effects include sedation, tremor, and weight gain.

Three types of antidepressants can be used to prevent migraine. The first consists of selective serotonin reuptake inhibitors (SSRIs), such as **fluoxetine.** The second consists of tricyclic antidepressants (TCAs). In this second group, tertiary amines such as **amitriptyline** are more potent inhibitors of serotonin reuptake and **may be more effective in preventing migraine** than are secondary amines such as **desipramine.** The third group consists of monoamine oxidase inhibitors (MAOIs), such as **phenelzine.** MAOIs can block serotonin degradation and are occasionally used in persons who fail to respond to other antidepressants.

Patients must take antidepressants for 3 to 4 weeks before the drugs become effective in preventing headaches, as is the case for alleviating the symptoms of depression. The inhibition of serotonin reuptake by the antidepressants leads to **down-regulation** of postsynaptic serotonin receptors and a compensatory increase in the firing rate of serotonin neurons. The relationship between these actions and migraine prophylaxis, however, is not clearly established.

Serotonin reuptake inhibitors sometimes cause anxiety, insomnia, tremor, anorexia, and sexual dysfunction. TCAs can cause drowsiness, tremor, and anticholinergic effects such as dry mouth, blurred vision, and urinary retention. **MAOIs can cause a hypertensive crisis** if they are taken with tyramine-containing foods or with sympathomimetic amine drugs (see Chapter 22).

Nonsteroidal Anti-inflammatory Drugs

Nonsteroidal anti-inflammatory drugs (NSAIDs), including **naproxen and fenoprofen,** can be used for the prevention and treatment of migraine. As discussed in Chapter 30, these drugs act by blocking thromboxane synthesis and platelet aggregation and thereby **reducing the release of serotonin.** NSAIDs can be used continuously or on an intermittent basis to prevent predictable headaches. For example, administration beginning 1 week before menses and continuing through menstruation may prevent migraine headaches associated with the menstrual cycle. Other NSAIDs used for migraine prevention include **flurbiprofen, ketoprofen,** and **mefenamic acid,** but **any NSAID or aspirin may be effective if tolerated by the patient.**

Beta (β)-Adrenoceptor Antagonists

Of the various types of β-adrenoceptor antagonists that are available (see Chapter 9), only the β-blockers that lack intrinsic sympathomimetic activity are effective for the prevention of migraine headaches. One example of effective β-blockers is **timolol.** Another example, **propranolol,** is widely used for migraine prophylaxis but can cause more CNS side effects than timolol.

The mechanism of action of β-blockers in migraine prophylaxis is uncertain. These drugs may attenuate the **second phase** of migraine by **blocking vasodilation** mediated by β_2-adrenoceptors. They may also reduce platelet aggregation and thereby decrease the release of serotonin from platelets.

Calcium Channel Blockers

Although **verapamil, nimodipine,** and other calcium channel blockers are used for migraine prophylaxis, there is evidence that the calcium channel blockers are less effective in preventing migraine attacks than are other classes of drugs.

Calcium channel blockers may be effective in migraines by preventing the **vasoconstrictive phase** of migraine headaches. The properties of these drugs are described in Chapter 11.

CGRP-Targeted Monoclonal Antibodies

Sensory nerve fibers releasing **CGRP** and **CGRP receptors** are found throughout peripheral tissues and centrally in **neurons of the trigeminal nerve that innervate cerebral blood vessels** (the trigeminovascular system). CGRP released from trigeminal neurons is a potent vasodilator and mediates pain transmission when trigeminal sensory nerve fibers are activated. From preclinical and clinical studies, it was found that **CGRP is a potent mediator of migraine headaches.**

Recently, the development and approval of four monoclonal antibody drugs (see Chapter 46) were proven effective in reducing migraine frequency and intensity of migraine episodes. **Galcanezumab** (EMGALITY) was the first monoclonal antibody drug for the preventive treatment of migraine. It is given by subcutaneous injection (SC) on a monthly schedule, with a loading dose of 240 mg initially followed by 120 mg monthly. **Galcanezumab binds CGRP and thereby blocks the binding of CGRP to the CGRP receptor.** Other CGRP monoclonal antibody drugs that target the CGRP peptide are **fremanezumab** (AJOVY), which is longer-lasting and given SC on a quarterly (3 months) schedule, and **eptinezumab** (VYPEPTI) given by an IV infusion on a quarterly basis.

Taking a slightly different approach, the newest monoclonal antibody drug is **erenumab** (AIMOVIG) which **targets the CGRP receptor and not the CGRP peptide.** In this way, the binding of CGRP to its receptor is blocked, and migraine frequency and severity are reduced.

Other Agents for Migraine Prevention

Gabapentin is an agent approved for the treatment of seizure disorders (see Chapter 20) and postherpetic neuralgia. It is moderately effective in preventing the occurrence of migraines with few adverse effects. Although gabapentin is known to enhance *gamma* (γ)-aminobutyric acid (GABA) action in the treatment of seizure disorder, its actions in migraine treatment are unclear.

The cosmetic agent **botulinum toxin A** (BOTOX) was recently approved for the prevention of migraines. Its exact mechanism is unknown; however, BOTOX disrupts the neurotransmission of acetylcholine by preventing vesicle fusion with the membrane of the presynaptic terminal. Drugs made from botulinum toxin are further discussed in Chapter 6 and Chapter 24.

DRUGS FOR MIGRAINE TERMINATION

Numerous drugs can be used to terminate a migraine headache after it has begun. Most of these drugs are serotonin 5-HT$_{1D/1B}$ receptor agonists, and their sites of action are shown in Fig. 29.1.

5-HT Receptor Agonists
Ergot Agents

Ergotamine and **dihydroergotamine (DHE)** are **ergot alkaloids** and are effective in the treatment of migraine headaches and cluster headaches. A number of other ergot alkaloids are available and are used in the treatment of Parkinson disease, hyperprolactinemia, and other disorders. The potent hallucinogen lysergic acid diethylamide (LSD) is also an ergot derivative.

Mechanism of Action. Ergotamine and DHE are isolated from substances produced by *Claviceps purpurea*, a fungus first discovered growing on rye grain. Ergotamine and DHE relieve migraine primarily by activating **serotonin 5-HT$_{1D}$/$_{1B}$ receptors** at several levels in the trigeminal neurovascular system. Agonist activity at 5-HT$_{1D/1B}$ receptors in cerebral blood vessels produces **vasoconstriction,** thereby reversing the vasodilation that contributes to the throbbing migraine headache. Stimulation of presynaptic 5-HT$_{1D/1B}$ receptors on trigeminal nerve endings also inhibits the release of peptides that cause vasodilation, neurogenic inflammation, and pain. Finally, stimulation of 5-HT$_{1D/1B}$ receptors in the brainstem prevents activation of pain fibers in trigeminal nerves involved in migraine headaches.

Pharmacokinetic and Pharmacologic Effects. The ergot alkaloids are most effective when they are given early in a migraine attack. **Ergotamine** is marketed in parenteral, oral, and rectal formulations. When it is given orally, it has a relatively slow onset of action because of its poor oral bioavailability. Although it is available as a rectal suppository for use by patients with nausea and vomiting, it can actually worsen these symptoms by stimulating the vomiting center. Some oral and rectal ergotamine preparations contain caffeine, which appears to increase the absorption of ergotamine and may also exert a mild vasoconstrictive effect that helps relieve migraine.

DHE is available in intranasal and injectable preparations. The intranasal preparation, which was recently approved by the U.S. Food and Drug Administration (FDA), offers patients a convenient method of administering DHE and has a moderately rapid onset of action. The injectable DHE preparation, which is usually more rapid-acting and reliable than the various ergotamine preparations, can be administered subcutaneously, intramuscularly, or intravenously. When administered parenterally, DHE is often given with an antiemetic drug, such as the dopamine receptor antagonist **metoclopramide,** to prevent drug-induced nausea and vomiting.

Adverse Effects. The relatively mild adverse effects of ergot alkaloids include nausea and vomiting, diarrhea, muscle cramps, cold skin, paresthesias, and vertigo.

Ergotamine and DHE can cause peripheral vasoconstriction by stimulating alpha$_1$ (α_1)-adrenoceptors and by directly stimulating vascular smooth muscle. These drugs, therefore, are contraindicated in persons with coronary artery disease or peripheral vascular disease. Excessive doses of ergotamine or DHE can cause severe cerebral vasoconstriction, ischemia, rebound vasodilation, and headache. A rebound headache can last several days, and hospitalization may be required to wean the patient from ergotamine and alleviate the pain. Strict dosage guidelines must be followed to prevent rebound headaches and other forms of toxicity. To prevent cumulative toxicity, daily use of ergotamine should be avoided.

Interactions. Concomitant use of **ergot alkaloids** and **β-adrenoceptor antagonists** can cause severe peripheral ischemia resulting from α-adrenoceptor–mediated vasoconstriction that is unopposed by β_2-adrenoceptor–mediated vasodilation. Hence, this drug combination should be avoided.

Triptan Agents

Sumatriptan was the first of a new group of selective serotonin 5-HT$_{1D/1B}$ agonists to be developed for the treatment of migraines. The class of **triptan drugs** is now quite numerous and includes **naratriptan, rizatriptan,** and **zolmitriptan.** Although these four triptans have amassed the most data on their effectiveness in aborting a migraine attack, newer agents, such as **frovatriptan, almotriptan,** and **eletriptan,** are also available. The newer triptans are similar to sumatriptan, but their improved pharmacokinetic properties may be advantageous in some cases. **Almotriptan** has the distinction of being the first and only triptan agent to be

approved for use in both adults *and* adolescents. It can be used for the acute treatment of migraine headache pain in adolescents ages 12 to 17 years with a history of migraine attacks with or without aura, usually lasting 4 hours or more when untreated.

Mechanism of Action. Sumatriptan and other 5-HT$_{1D/1B}$ agonists are structural analogs of serotonin. Their mechanisms for terminating migraine headaches appear to be similar to those of ergotamine and DHE (see earlier).

Pharmacokinetic and Pharmacologic Effects. A sumatriptan preparation for subcutaneous administration was introduced in 1992, and oral and intranasal preparations were introduced several years later. Peak plasma levels of sumatriptan are achieved most rapidly with subcutaneous administration and least rapidly with oral administration. Relief of migraine usually takes an hour when **sumatriptan** is given subcutaneously using an autoinjector (ALSUMA) but can take up to 2 hours when it is given orally.

Naratriptan, rizatriptan, and **zolmitriptan** are currently limited to oral administration. In comparison with sumatriptan, these newer triptan drugs are more lipophilic, have higher oral bioavailabilities, and achieve higher concentrations in the CNS. The finding that they penetrate the CNS more readily may enable them to inhibit the brainstem mechanisms involved in migraine more effectively than does sumatriptan.

In a clinical trial comparing the effects of sumatriptan treatment with those of DHE treatment in patients with migraine headache disorder, subcutaneously administered sumatriptan was found to relieve 85% of migraine attacks and to be slightly superior to DHE in this regard. Nevertheless, studies show that sumatriptan is not efficacious in 10% to 20% of patients who have migraine headache disorder, and about 40% of patients who initially obtain relief with sumatriptan have a **recurrence** of their headache on the same day. Recurrences are more prevalent in patients who have more severe and longer attacks. If a headache recurs, treatment can be repeated at specified intervals until a maximal daily dose of sumatriptan has been administered. Because sumatriptan and other triptan drugs cost more than ergotamine alkaloids, the need to repeat doses may be a factor in drug selection.

According to some clinical trials, the newer triptans have a 10% to 20% greater efficacy than sumatriptan, and their rates of headache recurrence are lower (30% for newer triptans *versus* 40% for sumatriptan). **Naratriptan** has a **longer half-life** than sumatriptan, and this may explain its lower rate of headache recurrence. Further clinical studies are needed to confirm these differences.

Adverse Effects and Interactions. In clinical trials, the incidence of chest tightness, weakness, somnolence, and dizziness in subjects treated with a triptan agent was nearly 50%, whereas the incidence in subjects treated with a placebo was about 30%. The incidence of adverse effects appears to be similar for all triptan drugs.

The triptans have been reported to cause abnormal tingling or burning sensations (paresthesias) in the skin on various parts of the body. These sensations are benign, but they can be mistaken for a serious adverse effect by the patient.

Triptan drugs can cause **coronary vasospasm** and should not be used in patients with a history of angina pectoris, myocardial infarction, or another coronary artery disease.

As with ergots, triptan agents can increase blood pressure, so they should not be given to patients with uncontrolled hypertension. The triptans should not be used concurrently with MAOIs, nor should they be used within 24 hours of administration of an ergot alkaloid. The use of triptans with SSRI antidepressant agents, such as **duloxetine** or **fluoxetine,** increases the risk of triggering **serotonin syndrome** (see Chapter 22).

Lasmiditan is a first-in-class medication for the acute treatment of migraine with or without aura (a sensory phenomenon or visual disturbance) in adults. **Lasmiditan** is a serotonergic agonist **selective for the 5-HT$_{1F}$ receptor,** whereas the triptans above are selective for 5-HT$_{1D/1B}$ receptors. Clinical trials show that lasmiditan is as effective as sumatriptan in terminating migraine headaches. Importantly, lasmiditan does not exhibit the cardiovascular effects of the triptan agents. The most common **adverse effects** from clinical trials were **dizziness, fatigue**, a burning or prickling sensation in the skin (**paresthesia**), and **sedation.**

CGRP Receptor Antagonists

Ubrogepant was the first **small molecule CGRP receptor antagonist** to be approved and marketed. It is an oral medication indicated for the acute treatment of migraine with or without aura in adults. Ubrogepant should be taken at a dose of 50 or 100 mg and may be repeated in 2 hours if the migraine does not subside. The most common **adverse reactions** from clinical trials (at least 2% and greater than placebo) were **nausea** and **somnolence**. Although clinical trials showed that ubrogepant relieved migraine pain in a greater percentage of treated patients than those in the placebo group, the results were not particularly strong, and there was no comparator group such as sumatriptan. A second CGRP receptor antagonist, **rimegepant**, was very recently approved and is formulated as an **orally disintegrating tablet** for sublingual or oral use. The most common adverse effect of rimegepant was nausea.

Other Drugs for Migraine Termination

An NSAID, such as **naproxen,** can be used either to prevent or to abort a migraine attack. Combination formulations of **acetaminophen, butalbital** (a barbiturate), and **caffeine** are also effective in aborting migraine headaches.

Isometheptene, an agent that acts as a sympathomimetic, can terminate migraine headaches. It is available in a preparation that also contains acetaminophen and a mild sedative drug.

Opioid analgesics can relieve the pain of migraine headaches, but their use should be reserved for patients in whom other agents are contraindicated or ineffective. **Tramadol** has been particularly useful in chronic pain syndromes (see Chapter 23) and is one of the most widely used opioid drugs for the treatment of migraine. Tramadol is an agonist at *mu* (µ) opioid receptors, and it also inhibits norepinephrine and serotonin reuptake in the CNS. The latter action may contribute to the drug's analgesic effect. **Butorphanol** acts as an agonist at *kappa* (κ) opioid receptors and a mixed agonist-antagonist at µ opioid receptors. It is available in a nasal spray formulation for rapid onset of action. **Acetaminophen with codeine** and other NSAID-opioid combinations are also effective in patients resistant to other drug treatments.

In severe cases, the antipsychotic agent **prochlorperazine** is effective in aborting unremitting migraine headaches when given intravenously.

GUIDELINES FOR MANAGING MIGRAINE HEADACHES

Prophylactic Treatment of Migraines

Nonpharmacologic measures can play a significant role in the prevention of migraine attacks. These measures include appropriate patient education; the identification and avoidance of factors that contribute to migraine attacks, including particular foods, beverages, and environmental factors; biofeedback and relaxation therapy; and psychotherapy. Acupuncture and physiotherapy may be beneficial, but their efficacy has not been established in controlled clinical trials.

Many pharmacologic agents are known to **prevent migraine attacks.** The efficacy of these agents varies from patient to patient, however, so finding a drug that works well is largely a matter of trial and error. The characteristics of individual patients should help guide drug selection. For example, β-blockers have negative effects on cardiac output, so they are usually less suitable than other drugs for competitive athletes. The goal of prophylactic drug use is to reduce the frequency of migraine attacks by at least 50%, and the criteria for evaluating the efficacy of particular drugs should be clearly established and understood by the physician and patient. It usually takes 3 to 4 weeks of therapy before the benefit of a given drug is observed, so authorities recommend a trial of 4 to 6 weeks before switching to another drug.

Acute Treatment of Migraines

The ideal drug to terminate migraine headaches would act rapidly, be highly efficacious, and have a low potential to cause serious adverse effects. No available drug meets all of these criteria. The newer serotonin agonists (triptans) appear to be **less toxic** and slightly more effective than the ergot preparations. DHE, however, has the advantage of a longer duration of action than triptan drugs. Intranasal preparations of sumatriptan and DHE offer a more rapid onset of action than do oral preparations, and they are more convenient than parenteral therapy.

The optimal use of abortive treatment requires prudent drug selection and reasonable restrictions on drug use to avoid **toxicity** or **habituation.** The effectiveness of a given drug varies widely from patient to patient, so a judicious trial of several drugs is usually required to determine the most effective drug for a particular patient. Some authorities recommend starting abortive therapy with an NSAID (e.g., naproxen). If the use of an NSAID consistently fails to relieve pain within an hour, then the patient should be encouraged to switch to a different agent, such as a triptan drug or DHE. Although this approach may work well for some patients, others may derive more benefit from the initial use of a triptan or DHE. To evaluate the effects of drug therapy, the patient should be instructed to keep an accurate log of drug dosage and symptom severity, especially during a trial period.

The overuse of abortive drugs can lead to serious toxicity, so patients must be properly instructed about limiting their use of these drugs. According to the guidelines of the National Headache Foundation, patients should limit their use of **ergotamine** to 8 treatment days per month, with an ample interval between treatment days. They should limit their use of **sumatriptan** and other triptan drugs to 6 treatment days per month and 2 treatment days per week, and they should limit their use of opioid drugs to 2 treatment days per week.

CHARACTERISTICS AND TREATMENT OF CLUSTER HEADACHES

Cluster headaches are severe, unilateral, **retro-orbital headaches** that tend to group or cluster over time. Patients often describe a searing or burning pain that arises behind one eye, occurs without warning, and can be excruciating. Pain often lasts from 15 minutes to 3 hours and usually occurs at the same time each day. Unlike patients with migraine headaches who are highly sensitive to movement and external stimuli, those with cluster headaches often pace in an agitated fashion, apply pressure to the orbit, or even strike the face to provide a distraction from the pain. The incidence of cluster headache disorder is low, affecting less than 0.5% of the population.

Drugs to prevent cluster headaches include **verapamil** (see Chapter 11) and **lithium** (see Chapter 22). As with migraine headaches, cluster headaches can be aborted by administering DHE, ergotamine, or sumatriptan. Other agents effective in aborting cluster headaches include inhaled oxygen, intranasal lidocaine, and glucocorticoids. Guidelines for selecting drugs to manage cluster headaches are similar to those outlined previously for migraine headaches.

CHARACTERISTICS AND TREATMENT OF TENSION HEADACHES

Tension headaches are characterized by bilateral, nonpulsatile, **bandlike** pressure that is mild or moderate in intensity. This common type of headache often responds to physiologic approaches that correct cervical or dental alignment or visual refractive error. Nonpharmacologic therapies (e.g., biofeedback, acupuncture, and physiotherapy) are also useful in controlling both episodic and chronic tension headaches. Pharmacologic therapy usually consists of **NSAIDs and muscle relaxants**, but patients with chronic tension headaches may also respond to prophylactic use of **amitriptyline**. This drug is usually tolerated well when therapy is initiated with a low dose at bedtime, and the dosage is gradually increased over a period of several weeks.

SUMMARY OF IMPORTANT POINTS

- Migraine, the most common headache disorder, is believed to result from neurovascular dysfunction at several levels in the CNS. Cerebral vasoconstriction and ischemia are followed by vasodilation; inflammation; and a unilateral, pulsatile headache.
- Drugs for migraine prophylaxis should aim to reduce the frequency of migraine attacks by 50%. These include anticonvulsants (valproate), antidepressants (amitriptyline and fluoxetine), NSAIDs (naproxen), β-adrenoceptor antagonists (propranolol, timolol), and calcium channel blockers (verapamil, nimodipine).
- Prophylactic drugs often must be taken for 3 to 4 weeks before benefits are observed.

- Drugs for aborting migraine headaches include ergot alkaloids (ergotamine and dihydroergotamine) and so-called *triptan* drugs (sumatriptan and others). These drugs act primarily by stimulating serotonin 5-HT$_{1D/1B}$ receptors. This stimulation causes cerebral vasoconstriction, inhibits the release of peptides and other mediators of inflammation and vasodilation from trigeminal neurons, and inhibits activation of the trigeminal nucleus in the brainstem.
- Ergot alkaloids and triptan drugs can cause marked vasoconstriction, so their dosage and frequency of use must be restricted to avoid rebound headaches and adverse effects. Common adverse effects of ergots include nausea, vomiting, and muscle cramps; those of triptans include chest tightness and drowsiness. The use of ergots or triptans is contraindicated in patients with coronary artery disease.
- Other agents for aborting migraine headaches include NSAIDs (e.g., naproxen), opioid analgesics (e.g., tramadol), and a sympathomimetic drug called *isometheptene.*
- The newest agents for the treatment of migraine are monoclonal antibodies that target the CGRP peptide or CGRP receptor for the prevention of migraines and small molecule CGRP receptor antagonists for the termination of migraines.
- Cluster headaches can be prevented with lithium or verapamil. They can be terminated with ergot alkaloids, sumatriptan, inhaled oxygen, intranasal lidocaine, or glucocorticoids.
- Tension headaches often respond to NSAIDs and muscle relaxants. Nonpharmacologic therapies (e.g., biofeedback and physiotherapy) are also useful.

Review Questions

1. Which of the following agents has not shown effectiveness in the prophylactic treatment of migraine headache?
   (A) zolmitriptan
   (B) valproic acid
   (C) verapamil
   (D) naproxen
   (E) amitriptyline
2. Use of sumatriptan is contraindicated in which one of the following groups of patients?
   (A) postpartum women
   (B) patients with uncontrolled hypertension
   (C) patients with moderate to severe unresponsive migraines
   (D) patients with hepatic insufficiency
   (E) patients with renal dysfunction
3. The therapeutic effect of the triptan class of drugs is caused by which mechanism of action?
   (A) antagonism at serotonin 5-HT$_2$ receptors
   (B) stimulation of serotonin 5-HT$_{1D}$ receptors
   (C) antagonism at dopamine receptors
   (D) antagonism at α-adrenoceptors
   (E) direct inhibition of substance P receptors in the vasculature

4. Verapamil is indicated for the treatment of migraine because it has which of the following effects?
   (A) it prevents the release of serotonin
   (B) it is a 5-HT$_{1B/D}$ agonist
   (C) it inhibits the COX-2 enzyme
   (D) it is an antagonist at 5-HT$_2$ receptors
   (E) it blocks calcium channels

5. A 35-year-old woman with a history of migraine reports to her physician that the last time she used her medicine to stop an acute attack, she felt numbness and tingling in her extremities and blanching and cyanosis of her fingers. Which one of the following medications did she take?
   (A) butorphanol
   (B) sumatriptan
   (C) dihydroergotamine
   (D) tramadol
   (E) naproxen

Drugs for Pain, Inflammation, and Arthritic Disorders

CLASSIFICATION OF DRUGS FOR PAIN, INFLAMMATION, AND ARTHRITIC DISORDERS

Nonsteroidal Anti-inflammatory Drugs (NSAIDs)

Nonselective cyclooxygenase inhibitors
- Acetaminophen (Tylenol)[a]
- Aspirin and other salicylates
- Ibuprofen (Motrin, Advil)[b]
- Ketoprofen (Orudis)
- Meloxicam (Mobic)[c]
- Naproxen (Naprosyn, Aleve)[d]

Selective cyclooxygenase-2 inhibitors
- Celecoxib (Celebrex)

Disease-Modifying Antirheumatic Drugs (DMARDs)

Gold salts
- Auranofin (Ridaura)
- Aurothioglucose (Solganal)
- Gold sodium thiomalate (Myochrysine, Aurolate)

Glucocorticoids
- Prednisone (Deltasone)[e]

Other disease-modifying antirheumatic drugs
- Adalimumab (Humira)[f]
- Etanercept (Enbrel)[g]
- Upadacitinib (Rinvoq)[h]
- Hydroxychloroquine (Plaquenil)
- Leflunomide (Arava)
- Methotrexate (Rheumatrex)
- Penicillamine (Cuprimine)
- Sulfasalazine (Azulfidine)

Drugs for Gout

Drugs to prevent gout attacks
- Allopurinol (Zyloprim)
- Febuxostat (Uloric)
- Pegloticase (Krystexxa)
- Rasburicase (Elitek)
- Lesinurad (Zurampic)

Drugs to treat gout attacks
- Colchicine (Colcrys)
- Indomethacin and other NSAIDs

---

[a] Also IV injection formulation of acetaminophen (Ofirmev).
[b] Also IV injection formulation ibuprofen (Caldolor).
[c] Meloxicam also available in a microparticle formulation (Vivlodex).
[d] Also indomethacin in oral and injection formulations (Indocin) and in oral only (Tivorbex), sulindac (Clinoril), ketorolac (Toradol, Acuvail, Sprix), piroxicam (Feldene), nabumetone (Relafen), etodolac (Lodine), diclofenac (Flector, Voltaren Gel, Zipsor, Dyloject), and combination formulations such as ibuprofen with famotidine (Duexis) and naproxen with esomeprazole (Vimovo).
[e] Also available in a prednisone delayed-release formulation (Rayos).
[f] Also infliximab (Remicade), certolizumab (Cimzia), golimumab (Simponi), tocilizumab (Actemra), and sarilumab (Kevzara).
[g] Also abatacept (Orencia), apremilast (Otezla), crisaborole (Eucrisa), and anakinra (Kineret).
[h] Also baricitinib (Olumiant).

OVERVIEW

A variety of medical disorders and injuries are characterized by **pain** and **inflammation.** This chapter describes the pharmacologic properties of **nonsteroidal anti-inflammatory drugs (NSAIDs),** which are widely used to alleviate the symptoms of rheumatoid arthritis (RA), osteoarthritis (OA), and gout, as well as to relieve the pain and fever that accompany many nonarthritic disorders. They are also used by millions on a daily basis for the occasional headache. The chapter also discusses **disease-modifying antirheumatic drugs (DMARDs)** and drugs for the prevention and treatment of gout.

RHEUMATOID ARTHRITIS

RA is an autoimmune disorder of unknown cause. The hallmark symptom of RA is joint inflammation, and most patients with RA experience a chronic, fluctuating course of disease that, despite therapeutic measures, can result in progressive joint destruction, deformity, disability, and premature death.

RA affects 2% to 3% of the US population, making it the most common systemic inflammatory disease (Box 30.1). It is three times more common in women than in men. RA is characterized by **symmetric joint inflammation** that most frequently affects the small joints of the hands, wrists, and feet, but also the joints of the ankles, elbows, hips, knees, and shoulders. Cardiopulmonary, neurologic, and ocular inflammation are also often found in patients with RA, and many patients develop rheumatoid nodules on the extensor surfaces of the elbows, forearms, and hands. In addition, many patients have extra-articular manifestations, such as vasculitis, lymphadenopathy, and splenomegaly.

As shown in Fig. 30.1, RA is triggered by **autoimmune mechanisms** that lead to the destruction of synovial tissue and other connective tissue. Both humoral and cellular immune mechanisms are involved in the pathogenesis of the disease. These mechanisms include the cytokine-mediated activation of T and B lymphocytes and the recruitment and activation of macrophages. The inflammatory

BOX 30.1 THE CASE OF THE ACHING ARTHRITIC

CASE PRESENTATION

A 52-year-old woman reports soreness in her knees and wrists that is not related to physical activity. Her physician notes that both right and left joints are affected and appear reddened and swollen. She has round, painless nodules under the skin and tells her physician that the pain is worse in the morning. The physician orders joint radiographs, a synovial fluid draw, and a blood test for rheumatic factor. All three studies come back positive for rheumatoid arthritis (RA), so the doctor prescribes celecoxib for the pain and inflammation and methotrexate to slow the progression of the disease.

CASE DISCUSSION

RA is a common disease, affecting more than 2 million people in the United States; it is three times more likely to be found in women than in men. RA is an autoimmune disease that causes chronic, symmetric inflammation of the joints. The disease can begin at any age but most often starts after age 40 and before age 60. There are two main classes of medications used in treating RA: the anti-inflammatory agents, such as celecoxib, aspirin, and cortisone, used to reduce pain and inflammation; and the disease-modifying antirheumatic drugs (DMARDs), such as methotrexate, leflunomide, hydroxychloroquine, and others, which promote disease remission and prevent progressive joint destruction. Newer immunomodulating DMARD agents are administered by the intravenous route and include infliximab, anakinra, adalimumab, and others. Methotrexate is the most common DMARD used to treat RA, and the use of the selective COX-2 inhibitor celecoxib is warranted given no stated history of cardiovascular disease in the patient.

leukocytes then release a variety of prostaglandins, cytotoxic compounds, and free radicals that cause joint inflammation and destruction. Patients with RA show elevated levels of immunoglobulin G–rheumatoid factor (IgG-RF) complexes; extracorporeal filtering of these complexes using immunoabsorption apheresis has helped some patients.

In patients with RA, NSAIDs are used to relieve pain and inflammation, and DMARDs are used to suppress the underlying disease process and slow the progression of joint destruction. The sites of action of selected antirheumatic drugs are depicted in Fig. 30.1 and discussed later.

OSTEOARTHRITIS

OA, also called **degenerative joint disease,** is the most common joint disease in the world. It affects about 10% of persons over 60 years of age, and radiographic evidence of OA can be found in most persons over 65. However, the disease is not simply associated with the aging process. Other factors that increase the risk for OA include obesity, osteoporosis, smoking, heredity, repetitive use of joints through work or leisure activities, and joint trauma.

OA primarily affects **weight-bearing joints** and causes deformity, limitation of motion, and progressive disability. The cartilage undergoes thickening, inflammation, splitting, and thinning. Eventually, the cartilaginous layer is completely destroyed, leading to erosion and microfractures in the underlying bone. The major symptoms of OA are pain, stiffness, and muscle weakness around affected joints.

Nonpharmacologic measures for treating OA include joint protection and splinting, physiotherapy, orthotic prostheses to support the feet, and joint replacement surgery. Pharmacologic measures include NSAIDs, local glucocorticoid injections, and experimental chondroprotective drugs (e.g., chondroitin sulfate and glucosamine). Recently, **sodium hyaluronate** (SUPARTZ) was approved for intraarticular injection as a type of joint fluid replacement in the treatment of OA. It is a sterile, viscoelastic solution prepared from chicken combs (the fleshy growths on top of chicken heads). The antidepressant **duloxetine** (see Chapter 22) is also indicated for the management of persistent musculoskeletal pain caused by chronic OA and chronic low back pain.

GOUT

Gout is an arthritic syndrome caused by an inflammatory response to crystals of monosodium urate monohydrate in joints, renal tubules, and other tissues. The deposition of these crystals occurs as a consequence of **hyperuricemia,** which can result from **overproduction** or **underexcretion** of uric acid. Risk factors for gout include **obesity, alcohol** consumption, and **hypertension. Cancer chemotherapy** can also increase plasma uric acid by cell death and lysis, releasing **purines** into the plasma; the purines are subsequently catabolized to uric acid.

Acute gout is treated with an **NSAID** or **colchicine** to relieve joint inflammation. Subsequent attacks of gout can be prevented by long-term therapy with a drug that either increases uric acid excretion or inhibits uric acid formation and thereby reduces the serum level of uric acid, as discussed later.

NONSTEROIDAL ANTI-INFLAMMATORY DRUGS

Mechanism of Action

The NSAIDs make up a large family of weak acidic drugs whose pharmacologic effects result primarily from the **inhibition of** cyclooxygenase (COX), an enzyme that catalyzes the first step in the synthesis of prostaglandins from arachidonic acid and other precursor fatty acids (see Chapter 26). COX is a microsomal enzyme, existing as a dimer (two molecules linked to form a functional unit) in the lumen and membrane of the endoplasmic reticulum. NSAIDs decrease COX activity primarily by competitive inhibition; however, **aspirin** forms a **covalent, irreversible inhibition of COX** (Fig. 30.2). The net effect of NSAID administration is a **decrease in the production of prostaglandins** and other autacoids.

Prostaglandin Effects

Prostaglandins play an important role in the development of **pain, inflammation,** and **fever.** Prostaglandins are released from cells in response to chemical stimuli or physical trauma. They sensitize sensory nerve endings to nociceptive stimuli and thereby amplify the generation of pain impulses. They also promote **tissue** inflammation by stimulating inflammatory cell chemotaxis, causing vasodilation and increasing capillary permeability and edema.

Fever, defined as the elevation of body temperature to a level above 37°C (98.6°F), often results from an alteration of hypothalamic thermoregulatory mechanisms. **Bacterial toxins** and other **pyrogens** stimulate the production of

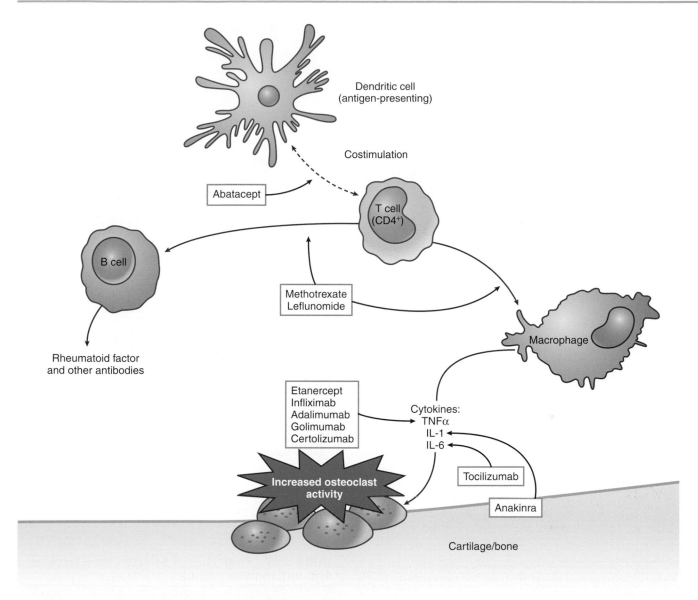

Fig. 30.1 Pathogenesis of rheumatoid arthritis and sites of action of selected antirheumatic drugs. In this simplified view of the immune system, dendritic (antigen-presenting) cells phagocytose antigens and present them to T cells, thereby activating the T cells. Activated T cells stimulate the production of B and T cells. B cells produce plasma cells that form rheumatoid antibodies. Helper T cells activate macrophages and cytotoxic T cells. Together, T cells, macrophages, and cytotoxic T cells produce cytotoxic cytokines (tumor necrosis factor-α [TNFα], interleukin [IL]-1, IL-6, and others) and prostaglandins that cause joint inflammation, synovial proliferation, and bone and cartilage destruction. Abatacept blocks the costimulation of T cells. Methotrexate and leflunomide inhibit the proliferation and activity of T cells and B cells. Etanercept, infliximab, adalimumab, golimumab, and certolizumab inactivate TNFα. Anakinra blocks the action of IL-1, and tocilizumab and sarilumab inactivate IL-6. Not shown are the glucocorticoids that inhibit T-cell activation and IL-2 production by regulation of gene transcription. Glucocorticoids and nonsteroidal anti-inflammatory drugs (NSAIDs) also inhibit the formation of prostaglandins. Immunoglobulin G–rheumatoid factor (IgG-RF) complexes are detected in the blood of patients with rheumatoid arthritis.

cytokines by leukocytes, and these cytokines increase prostaglandin synthesis in the preoptic area of the hypothalamus. The prostaglandins then act to reset the body's thermostat to a new point above 37°C. This in turn activates temperature-raising mechanisms, such as a reduction in heat loss via cutaneous vasodilation, and causes the temperature to rise. All NSAIDs **relieve fever by inhibiting prostaglandin synthesis** in the hypothalamus, but these drugs are not capable of reducing body temperature below normal.

Cyclooxygenase Isozymes
COX is now known to occur in two major isoforms: **COX-1 and COX-2. COX-1 is a constitutive or housekeeping enzyme** found in relatively constant levels in various tissues.

COX-1 participates in the synthesis of prostaglandins that have a cytoprotective effect on the gastrointestinal (GI) tract. It also catalyzes the formation of thromboxane A_2 in platelets, leading to platelet aggregation and hemostasis. In contrast, **COX-2 is an inducible enzyme.** Its levels are normally very low in most tissues but are rapidly upregulated during the inflammatory process by proinflammatory substances (e.g., cytokines, endotoxins, and tumor promoters). Both COX-1 and COX-2 appear to participate in renal homeostasis.

Most of the NSAIDs available today are **nonselective inhibitors of COX-1 and COX-2.** The discovery of COX isozymes led to the development of selective COX-2 inhibitors, the first one being celecoxib. These selective inhibitors

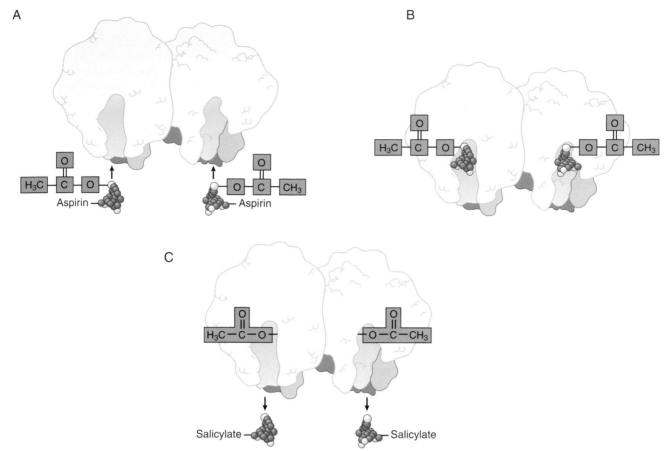

FIG. 30.2 Mechanism of action for aspirin. (A) The cyclooxygenase (COX) enzyme exists as a homodimer with two interlocking identical molecules, each providing an active channel for its substrates. Aspirin is chemically known as *acetylsalicylic acid*. (B) Aspirin molecules enter the active channel of COX and add an acetyl group to an amino acid R-group in the active site of COX. The acetyl group is attached to serine at the 530 position in COX-1 and to serine at the 516 position in COX-2. This produces irreversible or noncompetitive inhibition. (C) The aspirin molecule without the acetyl group is called *salicylic acid* or *salicylate*, which is a competitive inhibitor of COX.

are effective anti-inflammatory drugs, and they produce less GI bleeding and ulcers than do the nonselective COX inhibitors.

A third COX isozyme (COX-3), which was recently discovered, appears to be an alternative splice variant of COX-1. **Acetaminophen** potently inhibits COX-3, and this finding likely explains the reason that acetaminophen has little anti-inflammatory action.

Nonselective Cyclooxygenase Inhibitors

Among the nonselective COX inhibitors are many well-known NSAIDs that are available without a prescription, including **aspirin, ibuprofen, ketoprofen,** and **naproxen.** Acetaminophen is a weak anti-inflammatory agent, but it is also included in this class of drugs because it exerts analgesic and antipyretic effects via inhibition of COX. As shown in Table 30.1, NSAIDs vary greatly in potency and half-life, but most of them are administered two to four times a day with food.

Lower doses of NSAIDs are usually sufficient to treat mild to moderate pain and counteract fever, whereas higher doses are generally needed to relieve inflammation associated with arthritic disorders and injuries. NSAIDs are particularly effective in relieving pain caused by tissue inflammation or bone or joint trauma, and they can be combined with opioid analgesics to obtain a greater analgesic effect and reduce the

TABLE 30.1 Properties of Selected Nonsteroidal Anti-inflammatory Drugs

DRUG	RELATIVE POTENCY	HALF-LIFE (h)	DAILY DOSES
Nonselective COX Inhibitors			
Acetaminophen	1	3	4
Aspirin	1	2[a]	4
Ibuprofen	4	2	2–4
Indomethacin	40	4	1–3
Ketoprofen	20	2	2–4
Ketorolac	100	7	4
Naproxen	4	14	2
Selective COX-2 Inhibitors			
Celecoxib	20	11	2

COX, Cyclooxygenase.
[a]For aspirin, the value shown is the half-life of the active metabolite, salicylic acid.

need for higher doses of opioids. For example, NSAIDs are widely used in the treatment of postoperative pain, either alone or in **combination with an opioid analgesic.**

Although NSAIDs are effective in relieving the pain of chronic disorders, their long-term use is associated with a number of **adverse effects,** including GI bleeding, peptic ulcers, and renal and hepatic dysfunction. **Acetaminophen** produces fewer GI problems than other nonselective COX inhibitors, but it also **lacks significant antiplatelet and anti-inflammatory activity.** Although acetaminophen can be used concurrently with another NSAID for supplemental analgesia, alternative combinations of two NSAIDs should generally be avoided, not only because they increase the risk of GI and other side effects but also because they sometimes have adverse interactions. For example, **aspirin and other salicylates** displace some NSAIDs (e.g., ketorolac) from plasma proteins and thereby increase their serum levels significantly.

The NSAIDs can interact with a large number of other drugs through pharmacokinetic and pharmacodynamic mechanisms. Most **NSAIDs inhibit the renal excretion of** lithium and can increase lithium serum levels and toxicity. NSAIDs can reduce the clearance of methotrexate and aminoglycoside drugs. NSAIDs can also interfere to varying degrees with the antihypertensive effect of diuretics, *beta* (*β*)-adrenoceptor antagonists, angiotensin inhibitors, and other antihypertensive drugs. When given with potassium-sparing diuretics, NSAIDs can cause potassium retention and **lead to hyperkalemia.** Some drug interactions are associated with only a particular NSAID. For example, high doses of salicylates exert a hypoglycemic effect that can alter the effects of antidiabetic drugs. Indomethacin reduces the natriuretic effect of diuretics and can cause nephrotoxicity when given with triamterene.

Low doses of acetaminophen can be safely used for **analgesia and antipyresis during pregnancy.** The use of other NSAIDs during the second half of pregnancy is generally not recommended, however, because of potential adverse effects on the fetus. These effects result from prostaglandin inhibition and include GI bleeding, platelet inhibition, renal dysfunction, and premature closure of the ductus arteriosus.

Aspirin and Other Salicylates

The therapeutic value of salicylates was originally recognized when they were identified as the active ingredients of willow bark and other plant materials used in folk medicine to relieve pain and fever. Aspirin was synthesized in 1899 during a search for a salicylate derivative that would be less irritating to the stomach than salicylic acid. Aspirin soon became widely used around the world as an analgesic, antipyretic, and anti-inflammatory drug.

Salicylic acid derivatives include **aspirin** (acetylsalicylic acid [ASA]) and several nonacetylated drugs, such as salsalate, choline magnesium salicylate, and methyl salicylate (oil of wintergreen).

Pharmacologic Effects and Indications. In adults, the salicylates can be used in the management of pain, fever, and inflammation, as well as in the prophylaxis of myocardial infarction, stroke, and other thromboembolic disorders. In children, the use of salicylates should be avoided because the risk of **Reye syndrome** appears to be increased in virus-infected children treated with these drugs.

The analgesic, antipyretic, and anti-inflammatory effect of aspirin and other salicylates result from **nonspecific** inhibition of COX in peripheral tissues and the CNS. **Aspirin** irreversibly **acetylates platelet COX** and has a longer-lasting effect on thromboxane synthesis than other salicylates.

The antiplatelet effect of aspirin persists for about 14 days, whereas that of most other NSAIDs is much shorter. The effect is long-lived because platelets lack a nucleus and do not make new COX enzymes.

The salicylates are usually administered orally, but formulations are also available for **topical and rectal administration.** The oral dosage of aspirin needed to inhibit platelet aggregation is somewhat lower than the oral dosage needed to obtain analgesic and antipyretic effects, and it is much lower than the oral dosage needed to relieve inflammation caused by arthritic and other inflammatory disorders. Fig. 30.3 shows the relationship between the dosage of aspirin and the pharmacologic and toxic effects of the drug.

Pharmacokinetics. Aspirin is well absorbed from the gut. Although its concurrent administration with antacids may slow its absorption rate, it does not significantly reduce its bioavailability. Aspirin is **rapidly hydrolyzed to salicylic acid** (salicylate) by plasma esterase, and this accounts for its short plasma half-life (about 15 minutes). Most of the pharmacologic effects of aspirin are attributed to its salicylate metabolite, which has a half-life of about 2 hours. Aspirin itself, however, is responsible for irreversible inhibition of platelet COX and platelet aggregation.

Most of the salicylic acid formed from aspirin and other salicylate drugs is **conjugated with glycine** to form salicyluric acid. This substance is then excreted in the urine, along with about 10% of free salicylate and a similar amount of glucuronide conjugates. The rate of excretion of salicylate is affected by urine pH. For this reason, **alkalinization** of the urine by administration of sodium bicarbonate has been used to increase the ionization and elimination of salicylic acid in cases of drug overdose (see Chapter 2).

When a therapeutic dose of aspirin or other salicylate drug is ingested, the rate of metabolism and the rate of excretion of salicylate are proportional to the drug's plasma concentration (first-order elimination). When an excessive dose is taken, the elimination pathways become saturated, giving rise to **zero-order elimination.** For this reason, larger doses can rapidly elevate plasma salicylate concentrations to toxic levels, especially in the elderly, who are at greatest risk of aspirin toxicity.

Adverse Effects. The use of aspirin in children with chickenpox and other viral infections has been associated with Reye syndrome. As mentioned, treatment with salicylates, therefore, should be avoided in children.

Therapeutic doses of aspirin can cause **gastric irritation** and contribute to **GI bleeding** and **peptic ulcers.** Moderately high therapeutic doses can cause tinnitus, which is described as an abnormal auditory sensation or buzzing noise and is considered an early sign of salicylate toxicity.

Excessive doses of aspirin produce the toxic effects shown in Fig. 30.3. **Hyperventilation** is caused by direct and indirect stimulation of the respiratory center in the medulla, and it often leads to increased exhalation of carbon dioxide and respiratory alkalosis. Higher plasma salicylate concentrations can cause **fever, dehydration,** and **severe metabolic acidosis.** If not treated promptly, these events can culminate in shock, coma, organ system failure, and death. Excessive doses of aspirin also cause **hypoprothrombinemia,** which is an impairment of hemostasis and causes bleeding.

Aspirin hypersensitivity is an uncommon but serious condition that can result in severe and potentially fatal

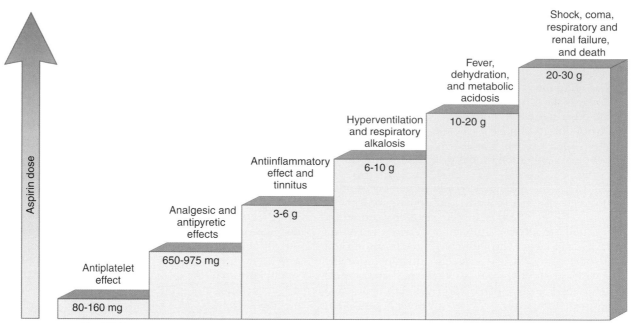

Fig. 30.3 Relationship between the dosage of aspirin and the pharmacologic and toxic effects of the drug.

anaphylactic reactions. Symptoms of aspirin intolerance include vasomotor rhinitis, angioedema, and urticaria (hives). Aspirin sensitivity occurs most frequently in persons with asthma, nasal polyps, or chronic urticaria. Persons who have had a **severe hypersensitivity reaction** to aspirin or another salicylate should not be treated with another type of NSAID because a 5% risk of cross-sensitivity exists between salicylates and other NSAIDs.

Treatment of Salicylate Overdose. The treatment of salicylate poisoning may include the following: (1) induction of vomiting and gastric lavage to remove unabsorbed drug; (2) intravenous administration of sodium bicarbonate to counteract metabolic acidosis, increase the ionization of salicylate in the kidneys, and thereby enhance the rate of excretion of salicylate; and (3) administration of fluids, electrolytes, and other supportive care, as needed.

Acetaminophen

Pharmacologic Effects and Indications. For more than 100 years, acetaminophen (also known as *APAP*, from its chemical name, *N-acetyl-p-aminophenol*) has been available for the treatment of mild pain and fever. Acetaminophen exerts analgesic and antipyretic effects at doses that are well tolerated and produce remarkably few adverse effects during short-term administration. Unlike aspirin use, **acetaminophen use has not been associated with Reye syndrome,** so acetaminophen can be safely given to children with fever caused by viral illnesses.

Acetaminophen has only **weak anti-inflammatory activity,** partly because it is inactivated by peroxides produced in the cells of inflamed tissue. Recent evidence suggests the existence of a third COX isoform, designated COX-3, with roles in mediating pain and fever, and subject to inhibition by acetaminophen. Acetaminophen has little effect on COX-1 or COX-2 and therefore lacks anti-inflammatory activity. Although acetaminophen is not considered a first-line drug for patients with arthritic disorders, it is sometimes used as an analgesic in those with mild arthritis. Because

acetaminophen lacks the ability to inhibit thromboxane synthesis and platelet aggregation, it is not used for the prophylaxis of myocardial infarction, stroke, or other thromboembolic disorders. Owing to the success of **ketorolac** injection for pain (see later), there is now an **injectable form of acetaminophen** (OFIRMEV).

Pharmacokinetics. Acetaminophen is rapidly absorbed from the gut, exhibits minimal binding to plasma proteins, and is widely distributed to peripheral tissues and the CNS.

As shown in Fig. 30.4, acetaminophen is extensively metabolized by several pathways in the liver. Most of the drug is conjugated with sulfate and glucuronide, and these metabolites are excreted in the urine. A small amount of acetaminophen is converted by cytochrome P450 to a **potentially hepatotoxic** quinone intermediate. When a therapeutic dose of acetaminophen is taken, the quinone intermediate is rapidly inactivated by conjugation with glutathione. Toxic doses of acetaminophen, however, deplete hepatic glutathione, cause accumulation of the quinone intermediate, and lead to hepatic necrosis. To prevent liver damage, patients who ingest an overdose and are determined to be at risk for hepatotoxicity can be given acetylcysteine, a sulfhydryl compound that conjugates the quinone intermediate and renders it harmless.

Adverse Effects. Some epidemiologic evidence indicates that long-term use of acetaminophen is associated with an increased **risk of renal dysfunction.** Although therapeutic doses of acetaminophen are remarkably nontoxic, the ingestion of 20 to 30 tablets is sufficient to cause life-threatening hepatotoxicity.

Treatment of Acetaminophen Overdose. Because hepatotoxicity gradually progresses over several days after an acetaminophen overdose, prompt treatment with **acetylcysteine** can prevent or significantly reduce hepatotoxicity.

Ibuprofen, Ketoprofen, and Naproxen

Pharmacologic Effects and Indications. Ibuprofen, **ketoprofen,** and **naproxen** are among the most widely used

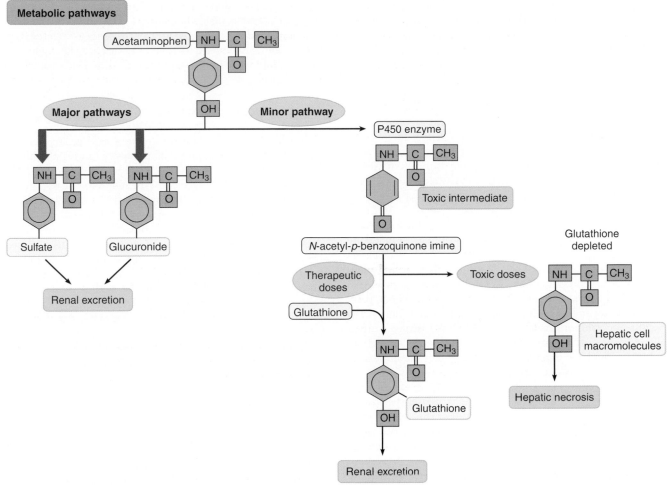

Fig. 30.4   Acetaminophen metabolism and hepatotoxicity. Acetaminophen is primarily metabolized by conjugation with sulfate and glucuronide. A minor pathway involves oxidation of acetaminophen by cytochrome P450 enzymes (CYP1A2, CYP2E1, and CYP3A isozymes) to form a potentially toxic intermediate, *N*-acetyl-*p*-benzoquinone imine. When a therapeutic dose of acetaminophen is taken, this quinone intermediate is conjugated with glutathione and excreted in the urine. When a toxic dose of acetaminophen is taken, glutathione stores are depleted, and the quinone intermediate attacks hepatic cell macromolecules. This process results in hepatic necrosis. Acetylcysteine (Mucomyst) given to treat acetaminophen overdose protects the liver by maintaining or restoring the glutathione levels, or by acting as an alternative substrate for conjugation with and thus detoxification of the reactive metabolite.

NSAIDs for pain and inflammation caused by trauma, infection, autoimmune disorders, neoplasms, joint degeneration, and other causes. By reversibly and **nonselectively** inhibiting COX isozymes, these drugs exert analgesic, antipyretic, and anti-inflammatory effects. Low-dose formulations of the drugs are available without prescription for the treatment of mild pain and inflammation. Formulations with higher doses are used to treat most arthritic disorders and still require a prescription. **Ibuprofen** is combined with the histamine H$_2$-receptor antagonist **famotidine** (see Chapter 28) in a new formulation (Duexis) indicated for RA and OA and shown to decrease the risk of developing GI ulcers. Likewise, a new **naproxen** and **esomeprazole** formulation (Vimovo) is available for the treatment of arthritis. Esomeprazole is a proton pump inhibitor (PPI) that reduces the risk of ulcers, a risk of prolonged NSAID treatment.

Pharmacokinetics.   Ibuprofen, ketoprofen, and naproxen are administered orally, are widely distributed, and are extensively metabolized to inactive metabolites in the liver before undergoing renal excretion. **Naproxen** has a longer half-life (14 hours) than ibuprofen or ketoprofen (2 hours each). For this reason, naproxen is given twice daily, whereas ibuprofen

or ketoprofen is usually administered from two to four times a day. As with **ketorolac** and **acetaminophen,** an injectable form of **ibuprofen** (Caldolor) is available.

Adverse Effects.   Ibuprofen and related drugs produce dose-dependent gastric irritation, nausea, dyspepsia, and bleeding. Long-term administration of high doses has been associated with peptic ulcer disease, but short-term use of low doses causes very few serious adverse effects. Among the serious effects that have been reported are **hepatic toxicity** and **renal toxicity.** In some cases, acute renal failure occurred after short-term use of therapeutic doses by patients who failed to ingest adequate fluids and became dehydrated.

Indomethacin, Sulindac, and Ketorolac

Indomethacin, an indoleacetic acid derivative, is one of the **most potent inhibitors of COX** isozymes. Because of its greater tendency to cause adverse effects, this drug is usually reserved for the management of moderate to severe acute inflammatory conditions. It is also used to treat infants with a **patent ductus arteriosus.** In these infants, indomethacin inhibits the synthesis of prostaglandins and thereby causes closure of the ductus arteriosus.

The incidence of GI and CNS side effects is higher with the use of indomethacin than with the use of many other NSAIDs. Indomethacin therapy is also associated with a risk of serious hematologic toxicity. Hence, therapy should be limited to short-term use whenever possible, and patients should be closely monitored.

Sulindac is actually a **prodrug** converted to an active sulfide metabolite. The parent compound, sulindac sulfoxide, is inactive in COX inhibition assays done *in vitro* as biotransformation in the liver produces the active metabolite. It is noted for having a *renal-sparing* effect such that moderate doses alter renal prostaglandin production less than with other NSAIDs. Besides sulindac use in the treatment of RA, it is also administered to treat adenomas in polyp disease.

Ketorolac has potent analgesic activity and was the first NSAID available for **parenteral use** for either intravenous or intramuscular administration. In studies of mild to moderate postoperative pain, ketorolac produced a level of analgesia comparable to that produced by morphine but caused less nausea, vomiting, and drowsiness. Ketorolac, therefore, has been widely used for the short-term management of moderate pain, such as postoperative pain associated with dental surgery. An ophthalmic solution for **ketorolac** (ACUVAIL) is used to treat allergic conjunctivitis and postoperative ocular inflammation. It is also formulated in a **nasal spray** (SPRIX) for the short-term management of moderate to moderately severe pain.

Ketorolac causes fewer adverse GI and CNS effects than opioid analgesics, but it poses a significant risk of hematologic toxicity and other adverse effects. For this reason, oral, parenteral, or intranasal therapy with ketorolac is limited to 5 or fewer days. In patients with renal or hepatic disease, ketorolac should be used with caution because it is associated with an **increased risk of severe renal or hepatic impairment.** A similar drug, **bromfenac** (DURACT), was withdrawn from the market in 1998 after postmarketing reports of hepatic failure and death.

Piroxicam and Nabumetone

Piroxicam is an effective anti-inflammatory agent with potency equal to aspirin or naproxen for the chronic treatment of RA. The main advantage of piroxicam is its 50-hour plasma half-life. This allows a single daily dose in most patients, although it can take up to 2 weeks for maximal therapeutic effect to be achieved.

One of the few nonacid NSAIDs, **nabumetone** is a ketone prodrug with weak COX inhibitory activity *in vitro*. It is converted to one or more active metabolites *in vivo*, and a potent inhibition of COX activity occurs with these metabolites. It also has the advantage that a half-life of 20 hours allows once-daily administration in most patients.

Etodolac and Meloxicam

Other NSAIDs, including **meloxicam** and **etodolac,** which were marketed in Europe or the United States as safer NSAIDs, were found to be preferential inhibitors of COX-2 after the discovery of this isozyme. They are more selective for COX-2 than typical NSAIDs but not as selective as the remaining COX-2 inhibitor, **celecoxib.**

Diclofenac

Diclofenac is available in a number of preparations, including immediate-release, extended-release, a transdermal patch (FLECTOR), and a new formulation for topical administration (VOLTAREN GEL). The latter formulation contains 1% diclofenac sodium indicated for treating pain associated with OA in joints amenable to topical treatment. Diclofenac is also available in a rapidly soluble oral dose (ZIPSOR), which reaches peak plasma concentrations in 28 minutes.

Selective Cyclooxygenase-2 Inhibitors
Celecoxib, Rofecoxib, and Valdecoxib

The selective COX-2 inhibitors are a new group of drugs that provide potent anti-inflammatory activity without causing significant GI toxicity. **Celecoxib** (CELEBREX), the first selective COX-2 inhibitor to be marketed, was soon followed by the release of rofecoxib (VIOXX) and valdecoxib (BEXTRA). Together, these agents are known as *coxibs*.

In late 2004, the makers of **rofecoxib** voluntarily **withdrew the drug** from the market after data were analyzed from a clinical trial testing rofecoxib's effectiveness in preventing recurrence of colorectal polyps. This study found an increased relative risk of confirmed cardiovascular events (e.g., heart attack and stroke) beginning after 18 months of treatment in the patients taking rofecoxib compared with those taking placebo.

Valdecoxib also showed an **increased risk for cardiovascular events** in patients after heart surgery. Serious skin reactions (e.g., toxic epidermal necrolysis, Stevens-Johnson syndrome, and erythema multiforme) were reported in patients receiving valdecoxib. Some of these reactions resulted in fatalities. For these reasons, the U.S. Food and Drug Administration (FDA) removed valdecoxib from the market in 2005.

With regard to celecoxib, patients in a colon cancer clinical trial who took 400 mg of celecoxib twice daily had a 3.4 times greater risk of cardiovascular events compared with those taking placebo. For patients in the trial who took 200 mg of celecoxib twice daily, the risk was 2.5 times greater. As a result, the FDA strengthened the warnings regarding **cardiovascular risk** of the **only remaining selective COX-2 inhibitor,** celecoxib, and **for all NSAID agents except aspirin.**

Although cardiovascular risk may dampen wider use of coxibs and other NSAID agents, recent studies show that NSAIDs can delay or slow the progress of Alzheimer disease. The neurodegeneration that occurs in this disease is accompanied by inflammatory mechanisms that involve COX and the activation of the complement cascade. In addition, increased expression of COX-2 is seen in some cancer cells, and the angiogenesis essential to tumor growth requires COX-2 activity. Overexpression of COX-2 leads to increased expression of vascular endothelial growth factor, a factor vital to tumor angiogenesis. Regular use of NSAIDs may therefore decrease the risk of developing cancer (particularly colon cancer) and especially so with the use of a COX-2 selective inhibitor.

Pharmacologic Effects and Indications. **Celecoxib** is a potent analgesic, antipyretic, and anti-inflammatory agent. This drug does not inhibit platelet aggregation, because platelets contain only the COX-1 isozyme.

In clinical studies of OA and RA, celecoxib was shown to be as efficacious as naproxen without causing significant side effects. In a study of postoperative pain management, however, celecoxib was reported to provide insufficient analgesia to control pain after general surgery. In laboratory studies, investigators found that celecoxib was more effective than nonselective COX inhibitors in protecting against colon carcinogenesis. This finding suggested a role for prophylactic coxib use in persons with a high risk of colon cancer; however, clinical trials were halted because of cardiovascular events (see earlier).

Pharmacokinetics. Celecoxib is available for oral administration and is usually taken twice daily. The drug is rapidly absorbed from the gut, is metabolized by cytochrome P450 isozyme CYP2C9, and is excreted in the feces and urine. The half-life is about 11 hours.

Adverse Effects and Interactions. Besides the risk of cardiovascular events, celecoxib appears to cause a low incidence of adverse reactions, the most common of which are diarrhea, dyspepsia, and abdominal pain. This drug is associated with a much lower incidence of gastroduodenal ulcers than the nonselective NSAIDs (e.g., ibuprofen and naproxen).

Because celecoxib is metabolized by CYP2C9, drugs such as fluconazole, fluvastatin, and zafirlukast may inhibit its metabolism and increase its serum concentration. Lower doses of celecoxib should be used in patients treated concurrently with these interacting drugs.

DISEASE-MODIFYING ANTIRHEUMATIC DRUGS

DMARDs are agents capable of slowing the progression of joint erosions in patients with RA. Examples of DMARDs are gold salts, glucocorticoids, hydroxychloroquine, methotrexate, a number of newer immunologic agents and monoclonal antibodies, and small molecule inhibitors. These drugs have a delayed onset of action and require several weeks to months before their antirheumatic benefits are observed. Several studies suggest that using a combination of DMARDs is more effective than using a single DMARD in many patients with RA.

DMARDs act by various mechanisms to suppress the proliferation and activity of lymphocytes and polymorphonuclear leukocytes and thereby counteract their ability to cause joint inflammation and destruction. Because joint erosion is usually found within the first 2 years of RA, many rheumatologists prescribe DMARDs at the time of diagnosis. The utility of DMARDs, however, is often limited by their toxicity or by their loss of efficacy over time, and many patients must cease taking them within 5 years of commencing therapy.

Gold Salts

Gold salts were first used to treat RA in the late 1920s, after the finding of Robert Koch in 1890 that elemental gold inhibited the growth of *Mycobacterium tuberculosis* and the mistaken belief that the swollen joints characteristic of RA were caused by these bacteria. They were once used extensively in the management of this disease, but their popularity has declined with the introduction of newer DMARDs, which tend to be more efficacious and less toxic. However, both oral and parenteral gold preparations are still available. The oral compound **auranofin** is poorly absorbed from the gut, however, and may be less efficacious than parenteral preparations, such as **gold sodium thiomalate** (also called *sodium aurothiomalate*). A second preparation of gold for intravenous administration is available as aurothioglucose.

The antirheumatic effects of gold salts are usually not observed until 3 to 6 months after starting therapy. The action of gold salts in RA is not well understood but is suggested to be linked to **antimitochondrial activity and cell apoptosis.**

Gold salts can cause a variety of adverse hematologic, dermatologic, GI, and renal effects. Flushing, hypotension, and tachycardia are sometimes observed. Skin rash and stomatitis are commonly observed and require discontinuation of treatment until they resolve.

Glucocorticoids

For many years, **prednisone** and other **glucocorticoids** have played an important role in the treatment of RA. These drugs induce the formation of **lipocortin,** a protein that **inhibits phospholipase A$_2$** activity. By this mechanism, they inhibit the release of arachidonic acid from cell membranes and the formation of prostaglandins. Glucocorticoids also inhibit the production of numerous cytokines, including **interleukins** and **tumor necrosis factor** (TNF), by the synthesis of proteins that inhibit their action.

Glucocorticoids act more rapidly than other DMARDs, but their long-term use is limited by the development of serious adverse effects. In light of these facts, glucocorticoids have been used in various ways to manage patients with RA or other inflammatory joint diseases. For example, they have been used to induce a remission in the disease at the time that therapy with another (slower-acting) DMARD is started; to provide short courses of therapy during disease flare-ups; and to provide continuous low-dose background therapy in patients being treated with other DMARDs and NSAIDs.

Other Disease-Modifying Antirheumatic Drugs
Methotrexate

Methotrexate is an **antineoplastic** and immunomodulating drug whose properties are discussed in detail in Chapter 45. The drug was first used to treat RA in the 1980s, and it remains the single most effective DMARD available today.

Methotrexate has several mechanisms of action. It **inhibits human folate reductase** and thereby reduces the availability of active forms of folate required for thymidylate and DNA synthesis. It also **inhibits lymphocyte proliferation** and the production of cytokines and rheumatoid factor. In addition, it interferes with polymorphonuclear leukocyte chemotaxis and **reduces the production of cytotoxins** and free radicals that damage the synovial membrane and bone.

Methotrexate is considered the DMARD of choice for most patients with RA. The drug can be given orally or intramuscularly and has a fairly rapid onset of action, with benefits observed as early as 2 to 3 weeks after therapy is started. From 45% to 55% of patients continue therapy for at least 5 to 7 years, and sustained efficacy for up to 15 years has been demonstrated in some patients. The combined use of methotrexate and other DMARDs is often more effective than single-drug therapy.

Treatment with methotrexate is generally well tolerated by patients with RA, but it can cause adverse GI, hematologic, hepatic, and pulmonary reactions. Elevated liver enzyme levels are found in up to 15% of patients treated with methotrexate, but serious hepatotoxicity is rare. The administration of folic acid supplements does not reduce the drug efficacy and may prevent some of these adverse effects. The use of **methotrexate is** contraindicated in pregnancy.

Leflunomide

Leflunomide is a newer immunosuppressive drug that acts as a powerful **inhibitor of leukocyte** and **T-cell proliferation.** The active metabolite of leflunomide inhibits a key enzyme in pyrimidine synthesis, dihydroorotate dehydrogenase, and thereby prevents replication of DNA and synthesis of RNA and protein in immune cells. Leflunomide is converted to its active metabolite, **teriflunomide,** in the intestinal wall and liver. Teriflunomide is further metabolized and excreted in the urine and feces, with an elimination half-life of about 2 weeks. Teriflunomide is also marketed and indicated for the treatment of multiple sclerosis (see Chapter 24).

Leflunomide is marketed as an **alternative to methotrexate** for the first-line management of RA. In a controlled trial, 41% of patients treated with leflunomide showed significant improvement in tender and swollen joints compared with 35% of those treated with methotrexate and 19% given a placebo.

The adverse effects of leflunomide include **diarrhea** and **reversible alopecia** (baldness). The drug can increase serum levels of hepatic enzymes and increase the risk of hepatotoxicity alone and when it is used in combination with methotrexate. The active metabolite of leflunomide inhibits CYP2C9 and may thereby increase the serum level of many drugs, including ibuprofen and some of the other NSAIDs. Leflunomide is **teratogenic,** so its use is **contraindicated in pregnancy.**

Hydroxychloroquine

Hydroxychloroquine, an antimalarial drug related to chloroquine, is extensively used as a DMARD. It reduces the chemotaxis and phagocytosis of polymorphonuclear leukocytes and decreases the production of superoxide radicals by these cells. The drug has a slow onset of action and can require 6 months of therapy before benefits are observed. It does not produce the myelosuppressive, hepatic, and renal toxicities that many other DMARDs produce. Hydroxychloroquine occasionally causes GI disturbances, and patients undergoing hydroxychloroquine treatment must be monitored for adverse ocular effects, including blurred vision, scotomas, and night blindness. Hydroxychloroquine is also famous as a drug touted as an effective treatment for patients infected with the SARS-CoV-2 virus (see Chapter 43).

Immunomodulators

Tumor Necrosis Factor α (TNFα) Blocking Agents. TNFα blocking agents are immunomodulating agents that exert their effects by binding to and **inactivating** TNFα. TNFα is one of the proinflammatory cytokines produced by macrophages and activated T cells. Elevated levels of TNFα are found in the synovial fluid of joints of RA patients and play an important role in both the pathologic inflammation and the joint destruction that are hallmarks of RA. Newer agents have novel mechanisms of action such as preventing interleukin binding and T-cell activation, and are introduced later (see Fig. 30.1).

Etanercept is a protein formed by recombining human **soluble TNFα receptors** with Fc fragments of human immunoglobulin G1 (IgG1). In comparison with the original protein,

the **recombined protein** can antagonize TNFα to a greater extent and has a longer half-life. Experimental studies in several animal models of RA have found etanercept treatment to be effective, as have subsequent clinical trials in patients with this disease. According to a 3-month clinical study, 75% of patients with RA had a significant improvement in the signs and symptoms of their disease. The drug was generally well tolerated, although **injection site reactions** were common. The drug is currently intended for use in patients whose RA is refractory to treatment with methotrexate or other DMARDs. Etanercept can be used alone or in combination with methotrexate in these patients.

Infliximab is a **chimeric human-murine (mouse) monoclonal antibody** (see Chapter 46) that **inactivates** TNFα. It is used in the treatment of **Crohn disease** and **RA.** In one clinical trial, infliximab treatment resulted in an improvement of RA manifestations in 80% of patients whose disease was refractory to other drugs. In another study, infliximab was found to be **more effective when combined with methotrexate** than when used alone. Infliximab is administered intravenously at 4- to 12-week intervals.

Adalimumab is a human **IgG1 monoclonal antibody specific** for human TNFα. It is made by recombinant DNA technology in a mammalian cell expression system and purified to exclude viral particles. For adult patients, adalimumab is administered every other week as a subcutaneous injection. During adalimumab treatment, administration of methotrexate, glucocorticoids, salicylates, NSAIDs, analgesics, or other DMARDs can continue safely. Some patients not taking concomitant methotrexate may see additional benefits by increasing the frequency of adalimumab to 40 mg/week.

Certolizumab is a **pegylated, monoclonal antibody** directed against TNFα. By combining the active molecule with polyethylene glycol (PEG), the resulting product remains in the body longer and provides sustained activity.

Golimumab is a human monoclonal antibody that binds to **both the soluble and transmembrane** forms of human TNFα. This interaction prevents the binding of TNFα to its receptors, thereby inhibiting the biological activity of TNFα. Golimumab, in **combination with methotrexate,** is indicated for the treatment of adult patients with moderately to severely active RA.

All TNFα-blocking agents produced **serious infections and sepsis,** some fatal, during clinical trials. Many of the serious infections were seen in patients on concomitant immunosuppressive therapy that, in addition to their RA, could predispose them to infections. Tuberculosis and invasive opportunistic fungal infections were also noted during treatment with TNF blockers. In September 2011, the FDA mandated a **new block box warning** on the prescribing information for all TNF blockers that warns specifically of the risk of *Legionella* pneumonia (also known as *Legionnaire disease*) and *Listeria* infections.

Lymphomas were also reported in patients **treated with TNFα-blocking agents.** In clinical trials, patients with RA, particularly those with highly active disease, were at increased risk for the development of lymphoma. The role of TNFα blockers in the development of this malignancy is not known.

Small Molecule Inhibitors. Small molecule inhibitors are a new class of pharmaceutical agents that target specific proteins in signaling pathways. Most small molecule inhibitors are employed in the battle against cancer (see Chapter 45). **Upadacitinib is a Janus kinase (JAK) inhibitor** approved for the treatment of adults with moderately to severely active rheumatoid arthritis who cannot take methotrexate or had an inadequate response to it. **Baricitinib is a second JAK inhibitor** indicated for rheumatoid arthritis patients who had inadequate responses to one or more TNFα blockers.

JAK is an intracellular enzyme that initiates the signal transduction pathway from cytokine or growth factor-receptor activation cell membrane to modulate immune cell function. JAK kinase phosphorylates signal transducers and activators of transcription (STAT) proteins which modulate intracellular activity including gene expression. **Upadacitinib** and **baricitinib prevent phosphorylation and activation of STAT** and decrease the immune component of rheumatoid arthritis.

Other Immunomodulating Agents. Anakinra is a recombinant form of the human **interleukin-1 receptor antagonist (IL-1Ra),** differing only by the addition of a single methionine residue at its amino terminus. It blocks the biological activity of IL-1 by competitively inhibiting IL-1 binding to the interleukin-1 type I receptor (IL-1RI). IL-1 production is induced in response to inflammatory stimuli and mediates inflammatory and immunologic responses. IL-1 has a broad range of activities, including cartilage degradation by its induction of the rapid loss of proteoglycans, as well as stimulation of bone resorption. The levels of the naturally occurring IL-1Ra in synovial fluid of patients with RA are not sufficient to compete with the increased production of IL-1. The recommended dose of anakinra is 100 mg/day administered daily by subcutaneous injection. The adverse effects are the same as for the TNF blockers, with serious infections and lymphoma of most concern.

Abatacept is a selective **costimulation modulator** and **inhibits T-cell activation** by binding to cell surface markers (proteins) on leukocytes. Activated T lymphocytes are involved in the cause of RA and are found in the synovial fluid of patients with RA. Abatacept is a recombinant protein made by joining the extracellular domain of human cytotoxic T-lymphocyte–associated antigen 4 (CTLA-4) to the modified Fc portion of human IgG1. It is the CTLA part of the molecule that binds to specific cell surface proteins of T lymphocytes to prevent their activation. Abatacept is the first and only biologic for the treatment of RA available in a self-injectable subcutaneous formulation.

Tocilizumab is a humanized **anti–IL-6 receptor monoclonal antibody** (see Chapter 46). It binds selectively to IL-6 receptors and blocks IL-6 activity. IL-6 is a proinflammatory cytokine produced by a variety of cell types, including T and B cells, lymphocytes, monocytes, and fibroblasts. Tocilizumab is indicated for the treatment of RA and uniquely indicated for the treatment of active systemic **juvenile idiopathic arthritis** in patients 2 years of age and older. **Sarilumab** is a second **anti–IL-6 receptor monoclonal antibody** used for the treatment of adult patients with **moderately to severely active rheumatoid arthritis.**

Apremilast is an **inhibitor of phosphodiesterase type 4** (PDE$_4$), which is the isozyme primarily expressed on immune cells and is specific for breaking down cyclic adenosine monophosphate (cAMP). PDE$_4$ inhibition by apremilast increases cAMP levels, which **decreases expression of TNFα,** and other proinflammatory cytokines. Apremilast is approved for the treatment of psoriatic arthritis. A new topical PDE$_4$ inhibitor, **crisaborole,** is used for mild to moderate **atopic dermatitis** (eczema).

Sulfasalazine and Penicillamine
Sulfasalazine was originally used in the treatment of RA in the 1930s, but only recently was it approved for this indication by the FDA. In the 1920s and 1930s, scientists theorized that RA was an inflammatory disease caused by an infection in the GI tract. Consistent with that hypothesis, **sulfasalazine** was developed and is a **formulation combining an anti-inflammatory drug, 5-amino salicylic acid, with an antibacterial drug, sulfapyridine.** Recent experiments suggest that sulfasalazine is active against RA, but the exact mechanism is not known. Sulfasalazine is also indicated for use in ulcerative colitis (see Chapter 28). Because **sulfasalazine is a sulfa drug,** people who are allergic to sulfa compounds should not take it.

D-**Penicillamine** is a penicillin-derived compound used frequently in the past, but its use today has declined with the increasing use of other DMARDs (e.g., methotrexate). It is not understood exactly how penicillamine provides a benefit in RA, but it is known to reduce the blood levels of inflammatory cytokines. Penicillamine effects can take up to 3 months to manifest; however, if no effect is seen in a year, it should be stopped. Penicillamine is also used as a **copper chelating agent** in the treatment of Wilson disease (see Chapter 5).

DRUGS FOR THE TREATMENT OF GOUT
Drugs for Preventing Gout Attacks
Gout attacks can be prevented by lowering the serum concentration of uric acid. **Probenecid** and **lesinurad** accomplish this goal by increasing the excretion of uric acid, whereas allopurinol and other agents do so by inhibiting the synthesis of uric acid. A third class of agents provides catabolic enzymes to reverse hyperuricemia. Uric acid metabolism and sites of drug action are depicted in Fig. 30.5.

Uricosuric Drugs
A **uricosuric drug,** such as **probenecid,** is used to prevent gout attacks in persons who **underexcrete uric acid,** as indicated by a 24-hour uric acid excretion that is less than 800 mg.

Probenecid is a weak acid that **competitively inhibits the reabsorption of uric acid** by renal tubules and thereby increases the excretion of uric acid. The drug is taken orally and should be swallowed with a full glass of water to ensure adequate fluid intake. Treatment should begin with a low dose, and the dosage should be gradually increased until an adequate uricosuric effect is obtained or the maximal dosage is reached. Probenecid treatment is usually well tolerated.

The use of aspirin and other **salicylates can alter or interfere with the** uricosuric effect of probenecid, so patients should avoid concurrent use of these agents. High doses of salicylates inhibit uric acid reabsorption and exert a uricosuric effect. Low doses of salicylates, however, inhibit uric acid secretion by renal tubules and thereby increase serum concentrations of uric acid.

Lesinurad reduces serum uric acid levels by inhibiting the function of transporter proteins involved in uric acid

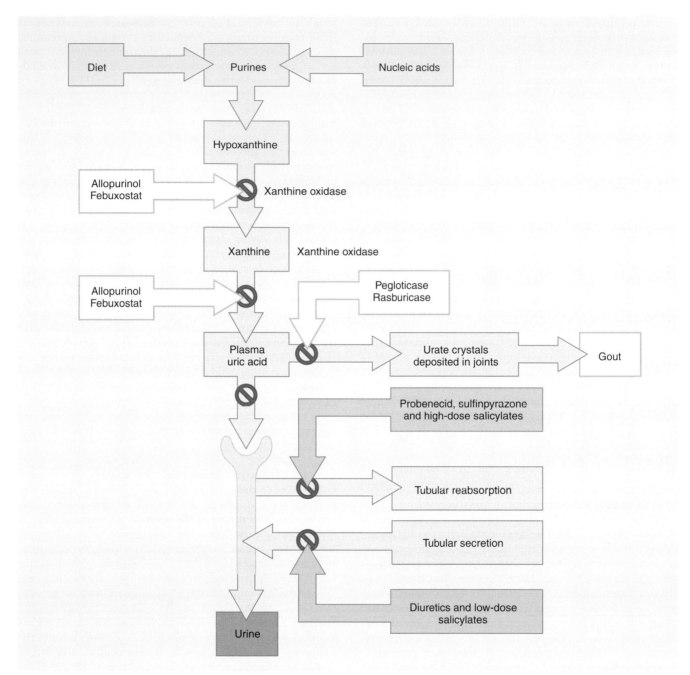

FIG. 30.5 Uric acid metabolism and sites of drug action. Purines obtained from the diet or from catabolism of nucleic acids are converted to hypoxanthine. Under normal conditions, xanthine oxidase converts hypoxanthine to xanthine and then to uric acid. Allopurinol and febuxostat act by inhibiting xanthine oxidase. Pegloticase and rasburicase administration provides a recombinant uricase enzyme that converts uric acid to allantoin, which is then excreted. Probenecid, lesinurad, and high-dose salicylates inhibit the renal tubular reabsorption of uric acid, whereas diuretics and low-dose salicylates inhibit the renal tubular secretion of uric acid.

reabsorption in the kidney. Lesinurad inhibited the function of two apical transporters responsible for uric acid reabsorption, uric acid transporter 1 (URAT1), and organic anion transporter 4 (OAT4). URAT1 is responsible for the majority of the reabsorption of filtered uric acid from the renal tubular lumen.

Xanthine Oxidase Inhibitors

Allopurinol is used to prevent gout attacks in persons who **overproduce uric acid,** as indicated by a 24-hour uric acid excretion greater than 800 mg. It is also sometimes used to

prevent hyperuricemia and gout in persons having cancer chemotherapy and whose **rate of purine catabolism is high** because of the death of neoplastic cells.

Allopurinol and its active metabolite, **oxypurinol** (also called *alloxanthine*), decrease the production of uric acid by **inhibiting xanthine oxidase,** the enzyme that converts hypoxanthine to xanthine and xanthine to uric acid. Allopurinol is a competitive inhibitor of xanthine oxidase. In contrast to uricosuric drugs, allopurinol causes a decrease in uric acid excretion and a corresponding increase in the urinary excretion of hypoxanthine. In addition, allopurinol increases the reutilization of hypoxanthine and xanthine for nucleotide and nucleic acid synthesis via inhibition of hypoxanthine-guanine phosphoribosyltransferase. The resultant increase in nucleotide concentration leads to increased feedback inhibition of de novo purine synthesis. By lowering both serum and urine concentrations of uric acid below its solubility limits, allopurinol prevents or decreases urate deposition, thereby **preventing the occurrence or progression of both gouty arthritis and urate nephropathy.**

Allopurinol is administered orally. Most of the drug is rapidly converted to its active metabolite, oxypurinol, in the liver. Oxypurinol has a half-life of about 20 hours; most of this metabolite is excreted unchanged in the urine.

About 25% of patients are unable to tolerate allopurinol because of its **adverse effects,** which include nausea, vomiting, hepatitis, skin rashes, and other forms of hypersensitivity. Because allopurinol inhibits the catabolism of **azathioprine** and **mercaptopurine,** doses of these drugs may need to be reduced if allopurinol is given concurrently with either of them.

Febuxostat is the first new drug to treat gout in more than 40 years. It is also a **competitive inhibitor of xanthine oxidase** but has the advantage of once-a-day administration and greater efficacy than allopurinol. It is also more **selective for xanthine oxidase** than allopurinol because it is not a purine analog. Adverse effects are minor and rare but include liver enzyme elevations, nausea, arthralgia, and rash.

Catabolic Enzyme Preparations

An intravenous infusion formulation of **pegloticase** was recently approved for patients with **refractory chronic gout.** Pegloticase is **recombinant uricase** and achieves its therapeutic effect by **catalyzing the oxidation of uric acid to allantoin,** thereby lowering serum uric acid. Allantoin is an inert and water-soluble purine metabolite readily eliminated by renal excretion. Pegloticase must be administered in the clinic with supportive measures available nearby, as there is the risk of life-threatening **allergic reactions.**

A similar recombinant uricase enzyme, **rasburicase,** is indicated only for the initial management of plasma uric acid levels in pediatric and adult patients with leukemia, lymphoma, and solid tumor malignancies who are receiving anticancer therapy. As mentioned earlier, cancer chemotherapy results in **tumor lysis** and **cell death** and can cause an abnormal **elevation of plasma uric acid** (tumor lysis syndrome). Its administration by the intravenous route carries the same risks of allergic reactions as pegloticase.

Drugs for Treating Gout Attacks
Indomethacin
In patients with acute gout, a potent anti-inflammatory drug is given for the rapid relief of pain. Although indomethacin (see earlier) is widely used for this purpose, other NSAIDs are often effective when used in an adequate dosage. If these drugs do not provide relief or cannot be tolerated by the patient, colchicine can be given orally or parenterally.

Colchicine
Colchicine was traditionally used to treat acute gout, but it is less frequently used today because of its unpleasant side effects, which include nausea, vomiting, diarrhea, and

abdominal cramps. The drug is believed to act by **disrupting microtubules** and inhibiting the motility of inflammatory leukocytes and thereby blocking their ability to cause urate crystal-induced joint inflammation. Colchicine is rapidly absorbed after oral administration. It is partly metabolized in the liver, and the drug and its metabolites are excreted by the biliary and fecal routes. If colchicine treatment causes the adverse effects noted previously, treatment should be stopped to avoid more serious toxicity.

SUMMARY OF IMPORTANT POINTS

- NSAIDs act primarily by inhibiting COX and the synthesis of prostaglandins. The drugs exhibit varying degrees of analgesic, anti-inflammatory, and antipyretic activity. Most of them also inhibit platelet aggregation. Long-term use of NSAIDs can lead to renal or hepatic toxicity.
- Nonselective COX inhibitors include acetaminophen, aspirin, ibuprofen, indomethacin, ketoprofen, ketorolac, and naproxen. Except for acetaminophen, the agents in this group can cause gastric irritation and bleeding, and their long-term use can lead to peptic ulcers.
- Acetaminophen is an effective analgesic and antipyretic agent, but it lacks significant anti-inflammatory and antiplatelet activity. A minor metabolite of acetaminophen is a potentially hepatotoxic quinone. This quinone metabolite is normally inactivated by conjugation with glutathione, but toxic doses of acetaminophen can deplete glutathione and cause fatal liver failure.
- Acetylcysteine, a sulfhydryl compound that conjugates and inactivates the quinone metabolite of acetaminophen, is used as an antidote for acetaminophen hepatotoxicity.
- Low doses of aspirin have potent antiplatelet effects because they acetylate and irreversibly inhibit platelet COX. Low doses of aspirin also produce analgesic and antipyretic effects, but higher doses are needed to counteract inflammation.
- High therapeutic doses of aspirin can cause tinnitus. Toxic doses cause hyperventilation and respiratory alkalosis, followed by metabolic acidosis. In cases of severe aspirin toxicity, sodium bicarbonate can be given to counteract acidosis and increase urinary excretion of salicylic acid.
- Ibuprofen, ketoprofen, and naproxen are potent NSAIDs that are widely used as analgesic, antipyretic, and anti-inflammatory agents. Ketorolac is a potent analgesic that can be given orally or parenterally. To avoid hematologic toxicity, ketorolac use should be limited to a few days.
- Indomethacin is a potent COX inhibitor that can be used to treat moderate to severe acute inflammatory conditions. It is also used to cause closure of the ductus arteriosus in infants.
- Celecoxib, the first and only selective COX-2 inhibitor now available, is a potent analgesic, antipyretic, and anti-inflammatory drug. The incidence of GI bleeding and peptic ulcers with this agent is lower than that of nonselective COX inhibitors. Increased risk of

cardiovascular events for celecoxib and all nonaspirin NSAIDs is now a concern with chronic administration.

- DMARDs are agents capable of slowing the progression of joint erosions in patients with RA. These drugs have a slow onset of action and can cause considerable toxicity. DMARDs act by inhibiting the proliferation and activity of lymphocytes and polymorphonuclear leukocytes.
- Methotrexate, the most widely used and effective DMARD, can be combined with other drugs in this class for enhanced activity. It is generally well tolerated and can be used effectively for many years.
- Etanercept, infliximab, and adalimumab are DMARDs that bind to and inactivate TNF. Abatacept decreases T-cell activation. Anakinra blocks the biological activity of IL-1 by competitively inhibiting IL-1 binding to IL-1RI. These drugs are administered intermittently by injection and appear to benefit many patients with RA, but all carry the risk of increased infections.
- Other DMARDs include gold salts, glucocorticoids, leflunomide, hydroxychloroquine, sulfasalazine, and penicillamine.
- Gout is caused by hyperuricemia and the deposition of urate crystals in joints. Uricosuric drugs (e.g., probenecid and lesinurad) increase uric acid excretion, whereas allopurinol inhibits uric acid formation. These drugs are used to prevent gout attacks.
- Acute gout is treated with an NSAID (e.g., indomethacin) or colchicine. Colchicine inhibits the motility of leukocytes and thereby prevents their migration into joints and their ability to cause urate crystal-induced joint inflammation.

Review Questions

1. Aspirin is often used in low doses to prevent platelet aggregation by inhibiting the synthesis of which substance?
   (A) leukotriene
   (B) prostacyclin (PGI2)
   (C) thromboxane A2
   (D) arachidonic acid
   (E) phospholipase A

2. Acetaminophen is a potent analgesic and antipyretic NSAID but differs from other agents in that it has no anti-inflammatory action. Which of the following reasons explains this unique aspect of acetaminophen?
   (A) the distribution of acetaminophen does not reach peripheral sites of inflammation
   (B) acetaminophen is not an inhibitor of the COX enzyme
   (C) anti-inflammatory doses of acetaminophen are too high and toxic
   (D) it is selective for a newly discovered isozyme of COX
   (E) acetaminophen undergoes significant first-pass metabolism

3. Which of the following agents augments the physiologic concentration of IL-1Ra proteins in the treatment of RA?
   (A) adalimumab
   (B) leflunomide
   (C) etanercept
   (D) infliximab
   (E) anakinra

4. With respect to antigout therapy, inhibition of tubulin polymerization into microtubules is important given the role of which process in which aspect of the disease?
   (A) leukotriene synthesis
   (B) uric acid production
   (C) kidney reabsorption of uric acid
   (D) leukocyte migration
   (E) plasma binding of uric acid

5. A 45-year-old obese man with a history of alcohol abuse and hypertension develops joint swelling and pain. His urate excretion rate is 950 mg/day. Which of the following agents is the best treatment for his condition?
   (A) probenecid
   (B) allopurinol
   (C) piroxicam
   (D) lesinurad
   (E) colchicine

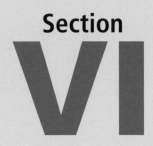

Section

VI

ENDOCRINE PHARMACOLOGY

CHAPTER 31

Hypothalamic and Pituitary Hormone Drugs

OVERVIEW

The hypothalamus and pituitary gland constitute an important neuroendocrine system that regulates growth, reproduction, metabolic rates, and other critical body functions. The pituitary gland (hypophysis) is divided into two major lobes: the **adenohypophysis** (anterior lobe) and the **neurohypophysis** (posterior lobe). Various hormones are secreted by each of these lobes and by the hypothalamus. These hormones and their antagonists have both diagnostic and therapeutic uses.

The two lobes of the pituitary are distinguished not only by which hormones they secrete but also by their neuronal connections. The posterior lobe is interconnected with adjacent brain tissue, hence the name, neurohypophysis. This provides it with information and substances that input information about the body and the environment. The anterior lobe is more or less dependent on the bloodstream for its input and connections to the state of the body and the outside world.

Neuropeptides and Dopamine Released From the Hypothalamus

The secretion of hormones from the anterior lobe of the pituitary is controlled by several hormone-releasing and hormone-inhibiting factors produced in the hypothalamus. They include the following: (1) **corticotropin-releasing factor (CRF)**; (2) **growth hormone–releasing hormone** (GHRH); (3) **somatostatin** (growth hormone–inhibiting hormone); (4) **gonadotropin-releasing hormone** (GnRH); (5) thyrotropin-releasing hormone (TRH); and (6) **dopamine (prolactin-inhibiting hormone [PIH])**. Evidence also suggests the presence of one or more prolactin-releasing factors. The various hypothalamic neuropeptides and dopamine are **released by neurons** projecting from the **arcuate** and other hypothalamic nuclei. The neuropeptides and dopamine are transported to the anterior pituitary via the **hypophysioportal circulation.**

Hormones Released From the Anterior Lobe of the Pituitary

In response to the neuropeptides and dopamine released from the hypothalamus, and other factors yet to be identified, the adenohypophysis secretes six protein hormones. They are: (1) **corticotropin** (i.e., adrenocorticotropic hormone [ACTH]), (2) **somatotropin** (growth hormone); (3) **follicle-stimulating hormone** (FSH); (4) **luteinizing hormone** (LH); (5) **thyrotropin** (thyroid-stimulating hormone [TSH]); and (6) **prolactin.** The actions of these anterior pituitary hormones are summarized in Fig. 31.1.

The hormones released from the anterior pituitary are transported to their target organs via the bloodstream. In their target organs, the hormones stimulate growth, development, and/or the secretion of other hormones. For example, ACTH released from the anterior lobe of the pituitary stimulates the production of corticosteroids in the adrenal cortex. These target organ hormones, like corticosteroids from the adrenal cortex, stimulate their own effects in target tissues. Most importantly, target organ hormones **exert negative feedback inhibition** to the production and release of their own regulatory hormones produced in the hypothalamic and anterior lobe. Continuing the example, **corticosteroids** released from the adrenal cortex into the bloodstream provide **negative feedback by inhibiting CRF** production in the hypothalamus and **ACTH production** in the anterior lobe of the pituitary.

Hormones Released From the Posterior Lobe of the Pituitary

The neurohypophysis secretes oxytocin and vasopressin. These posterior pituitary hormones are synthesized in the

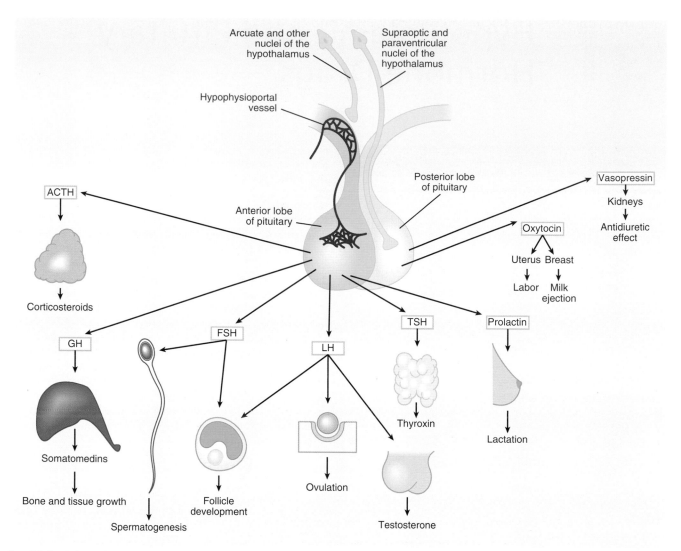

FIG. 31.1 Relationships among hypothalamic hormones, pituitary hormones, and target organs. Numerous hormone-releasing and hormone-inhibiting factors formed in the arcuate and other hypothalamic nuclei are transported to the anterior pituitary by hypophysioportal vessels. In response to hypothalamic hormones, the anterior pituitary secretes the following: corticotropin, which evokes corticosteroid secretion by the adrenal cortex; growth hormone (*GH*), which elicits production of insulin-like growth factors by the liver; follicle-stimulating hormone (*FSH*), which stimulates spermatogenesis and facilitates ovarian follicle development; luteinizing hormone (*LH*), which elicits testosterone secretion by the testes, facilitates ovarian follicle development, and induces ovulation; thyroid-stimulating hormone (*TSH*), which stimulates thyroxin secretion by the thyroid gland; and prolactin, which induces breast tissue growth and lactation. The posterior pituitary hormones, which are formed in the supraoptic and paraventricular nuclei, are transported by nerve axons to the posterior lobe, where they are released by physiologic stimuli. Oxytocin induces milk ejection by the breast and stimulates uterine contractions during labor. Vasopressin increases water and sodium reabsorption by the kidneys.

cell bodies of neurons in the supraoptic and paraventricular nuclei of the hypothalamus. The hormones are transported down the nerve axons to their endings in the posterior pituitary, where they are released in response to depolarization of the nerve terminals.

Clinical Uses of Hypothalamic and Pituitary Hormones

Drugs that mimic or block hypothalamic and pituitary hormones are used for several purposes. Hypothalamic hormone-releasing factors are helpful in assessing the functional capacity of the anterior pituitary to secrete particular pituitary hormones. Anterior pituitary hormones are used to evaluate the function of their target organs, to stimulate hypofunctional target organs, and to provide replacement therapy in hormone-deficiency states. Some agents are

used to reduce hormone production when it is excessive. Posterior pituitary hormones are used to activate specific physiologic functions.

Most of the hypothalamic and pituitary hormones are protein hormones that are extensively degraded in the gut after oral administration. These hormones are administered parenterally, and several are available as a nasal spray. See Table 31.1 for agents and uses.

ANTERIOR PITUITARY HORMONES
Corticotropin and Related Drugs

Corticotropin or ACTH is a 39–amino-acid peptide released from the anterior pituitary in response to CRF stimulation. Corticotropin stimulates the adrenal cortex to produce cortisol, aldosterone, and adrenal androgens by

TABLE 31.1 Select Hypothalamic and Pituitary Drugs and Their Uses

ANTERIOR PITUITARY HORMONES AND RELATED DRUGS		
Corticotropin and Its Releasing Hormone		
Corticotropin	H.P. Acthar Gel	Infantile spasms, MS, and rheumatic, collagen, dermatologic, allergic states, ophthalmic, and respiratory disorders
Cosyntropin	Cortrosyn	Diagnostic test for adrenal insufficiency
Corticorelin ovine triflutate	Acthrel	Diagnostic test for Cushing syndrome
Growth Hormone and Related Drugs		
Somatropin	Humatrope, Nutropin	Pediatric patients who lack adequate endogenous GH secretion, chronic renal insufficiency, Turner syndrome
Somapacitan	Sogroya	Replacement of endogenous growth hormone in adults with growth hormone deficiency
Mecasermin	Increlex	Growth failure in children with severe IGF-1 deficiency unresponsive to growth hormone administration
Octreotide	Sandostatin	Patients with acromegaly
Lanreotide acetate	Somatuline Depot	Patients with acromegaly
Pegvisomant	Somavert	Acromegaly in patients who are resistant to somatostatin analogs
Gonadotropins and Related Drugs		
Menotropins	Menopur	Infertility and hypogonadism in men and women
Leuprolide	Lupron	prostate and breast cancer, endometriosis, uterine fibroids, precocious puberty
Ganirelix	Antagon	Advanced prostate cancer
Agents Inhibiting Prolactin Secretion		
Cabergoline		Hyperprolactinemia
Posterior Pituitary Hormones and Related Drugs		
Desmopressin	DDAVP	Diabetes insipidus, children with nocturnal enuresis, hemorrhagic conditions
Conivaptan	Vaprisol	Euvolemic and hypervolemic hyponatremia
Tolvaptan	Samsca	Euvolemic and hypervolemic hyponatremia
Oxytocin	Pitocin	induce contractions during labor, prevent postpartum hemorrhage, and to stimulate milk let-down in nursing mothers

increasing the activity of the enzyme that converts cholesterol to pregnenolone (cholesterol side-chain cleavage enzyme), which is the rate-limiting enzyme in corticosteroid production.

Corticotropin Preparations

Two corticotropin preparations are available for clinical use: **porcine corticotropin** and a synthetic form of human corticotropin called **cosyntropin.** Cosyntropin contains the first 24 amino acids of human corticotropin necessary for biologic activity and is preferred for clinical use because it produces fewer allergic reactions than porcine corticotropin.

Porcine **corticotropin** is available as a gel formulation for depot intramuscular (IM) injection. It is used for the treatment of infantile spasms, for exacerbations of multiple sclerosis in adults, and may also be used for rheumatic, collagen, dermatologic, allergic states, ophthalmic, and respiratory disorders. The depot injection of corticotropin stimulates the adrenal cortex to secrete cortisol, corticosterone, aldosterone, and some androgenic substances. The exact mechanism of corticotropin in the treatment of infantile spasms is unknown; it may help in other disorders by the **increased corticosteroid release** and the effects of this hormone (see Chapter 33).

Cosyntropin is used in two diagnostic tests. First, it is used to distinguish congenital adrenal hyperplasia from ovarian hyperandrogenism. Second, and more commonly, it is used to diagnose **adrenal insufficiency** in a test that measures plasma cortisol levels before and after a cosyntropin injection. Cosyntropin increases cortisol levels in healthy individuals but fails to increase cortisol levels in persons with adrenal insufficiency. Then, to distinguish primary adrenal insufficiency from secondary adrenal insufficiency, endogenous plasma corticotropin concentrations are measured. In patients with primary adrenal insufficiency, corticotropin concentrations are high because of the lack of negative feedback inhibition of the hypothalamus and pituitary gland by the adrenal corticosteroids. In patients with secondary adrenal insufficiency, corticotropin concentrations are low because of inadequate production of corticotropin by the pituitary gland.

Corticotropin-Releasing Hormone

Corticorelin ovine triflutate is a recombinant form of ovine corticotropin-releasing hormone. Intravenous administration of this preparation stimulates secretion of corticotropin and cortisol in normal subjects. Corticorelin is used in the diagnostic test to determine the cause of excessive levels of cortisol in persons with **Cushing syndrome.**

Growth Hormone and Related Drugs

Growth hormone **(somatotropin),** a large peptide that contains 191 amino acids, is produced by the anterior pituitary and has both direct and indirect actions on target organs. Growth hormone acts directly to stimulate lipolysis and antagonize insulin to elevate blood glucose levels. Most of the effects of growth hormone are mediated by **insulin-like growth factor-1** (IGF-1), a protein produced in the liver and cartilage structurally similar to insulin. IGF-1 stimulates skeletal growth, amino acid transport, protein synthesis, nucleic acid synthesis, and cell proliferation.

The secretion of growth hormone is stimulated by growth hormone–releasing hormone (GHRH) and is inhibited by somatostatin. Several preparations of growth hormone, GHRH, and somatostatin are available for use in the diagnosis and treatment of growth disorders associated with excessive or inadequate secretion of growth hormone.

Growth Hormone Preparations

Growth hormone preparations obtained from animal sources are not active in humans. In the past, growth hormone obtained from human cadavers was used to treat patients with growth hormone deficiency and short stature, but some of the patients subsequently developed Creutzfeldt–Jakob disease. This fatal disease is characterized by spongiform encephalopathy, as are other such afflictions such as bovine spongiform encephalopathy (BSE) and *kuru kuru,* the local term from the New Guinea cannibals they gave to a characteristic brain disease seen in some tribal members after eating raw human brains. These bizarre disorders are due to unconventional neurotoxic agents called *prions.* Prions are nasty, misfolded pieces of proteins that have gone rogue and gained the ability to self-replicate and transmit like a virus. Basically, the misfolded prion protein goes into cells and interacts with the same protein as the prion, but not misfolded. Then, the prion protein forms a misfolded template, and the normal protein becomes misfolded. Transmission and infection of the misfolded prions occurs exponentially as additional normal proteins turn into misfolded proteins and prions. The degree of encephalopathy produced by an infection with prions was dramatically seen in English cattle whose affliction and behavior suggested the name of "mad-cow disease." After linking the onset of Creutzfeldt–Jakob disease to administration of growth hormone obtained from human cadavers, this practice was stopped and synthetic hormones were developed.

A biosynthetic form of human growth hormone known as recombinant **somatropin** is now used to treat children with various forms of **growth hormone deficiency,** including idiopathic growth hormone deficiency, Turner syndrome, chronic renal failure, Prader-Willi syndrome, and others. **Somatropin** preparations have been clearly shown to **improve height velocity** and **final height** in these conditions. Children who received craniospinal irradiation for treatment of a childhood malignancy are less responsive to growth hormone replacement than children with idiopathic growth hormone deficiency, and they have a tendency to enter puberty at an earlier age. These children may respond to supraphysiologic doses of growth hormone preparations

and suppression of early puberty using a GnRH analog (see later). Somatropin is usually administered subcutaneously once daily to children with growth hormone deficiency and is usually well tolerated. Growth hormone deficiency is often accompanied by other pituitary hormone deficiencies that should be treated with appropriate hormones.

Somapacitan is a recently approved growth hormone (somatotropin) analog that differs from the natural sequence of somatotropin by one amino acid and the attachment of albumin. **Somapacitan improves** upon the daily injection of previous growth hormone analogs because it is **injected weekly.** It has a **long elimination half-life of 2–3 days** with steady-state concentrations in the blood after two injections.

Mecasermin is a recombinant form of **human IGF-1.** It is produced by *Escherichia coli* bacteria that have been transfected with the human gene for IGF-1. Mecasermin is indicated for the treatment of **growth failure in children** with severe IGF-1 deficiency unresponsive to growth hormone administration, including those with a growth hormone receptor mutation and those who have developed neutralizing antibodies to growth hormone. The main adverse effect is **hypoglycemia,** which is controlled by eating a meal or snack before or soon after the time of the injection.

Growth Hormone–Inhibiting Hormone Preparations

Somatostatin (growth hormone–inhibiting hormone) is a 14-amino acid peptide that inhibits the secretion of growth hormone as well as certain hormones of the pancreas, pituitary, and gastrointestinal tract. Somatostatin's multiple actions and short half-life of a few minutes led to the development of **octreotide,** a somatostatin analog of eight amino acids that is 45 times more potent in inhibiting growth hormone secretion but only twice as potent in inhibiting insulin secretion. In addition, it has a much longer half-life of about 80 minutes.

Octreotide is used to treat patients with **acromegaly,** which is an uncommon condition caused by excessive growth hormone secretion most often due to a pituitary adenoma. Acromegaly is characterized by acral enlargement (pertaining to peripheral body parts) with soft tissue overgrowth of the hands and feet. Other features include coarsening of facial features, thickening and oiliness of the skin, and increased sweating. Acromegaly is often accompanied by other metabolic and endocrine abnormalities (Box 31.1). Octreotide is also used to treat tumors secreting insulin, glucagon, gastrin, thyrotropin, and vasoactive intestinal peptide, and **carcinoid tumors** secreting serotonin and kallikrein. Octreotide is administered subcutaneously every 8 hours, and its adverse effects include nausea, vomiting, abdominal cramps, steatorrhea (excessive fat in the feces), and gallstones.

Lanreotide acetate is a prolonged-release formulation of a cyclic octapeptide analog of somatostatin. It is administered by deep subcutaneous injection every 4 weeks and has similar uses and effectiveness as octreotide.

In patients with acromegaly, the use of **cabergoline** (see later) and other dopamine agonists can reduce circulating levels of growth hormone, IGF-1, and prolactin. These drugs are particularly useful in the treatment of persons with elevated growth hormone and prolactin secretion.

BOX 31.1 A CASE OF FACIAL ENLARGEMENT, SWEATING, AND TIGHT SHOES

CASE PRESENTATION

A 42-year old man complained to his health care provider of the gradual onset of headaches, arthralgia of the hands and feet, and changes in his facial appearance over the previous several years. His hands had become enlarged with thickened fingers, and unexplained palmar sweating had developed and intensified. His brow ridge and jaw had thickened and protruded over time, and he had noticed wider gaps between his teeth and a swollen tongue. His shoe size and glove size had also increased, and he was no longer able to wear his wedding ring. His examination revealed an elevated blood pressure (148/92 mm Hg), and his chest x-ray showed cardiac enlargement. Laboratory studies found an elevated serum growth hormone level of 1.65 (normal 0.01–0.97 ng/mL) and an elevated IGF-1 of 490 (normal 62–184 ng/mL). A subsequent MRI of the pituitary revealed an 8 mm × 9 mm pituitary microadenoma, and the patient was started on octreotide injections to reduce pituitary growth hormone secretion and normalize IGF-1 levels. He was also prescribed lisinopril to control hypertension. The patient was also referred to a neurosurgeon for further treatment. Following successful transsphenoidal surgery to remove the pituitary microadenoma, his growth hormone level decreased to a normal level of 0.55 ng/mL on day 2, and his 6-week IGF-1 level was normal at 165 ng/mL. His headaches, arthralgia, and abnormal physical features gradually resolved over several months, and his blood pressure returned to normal without medication. His growth hormone and IGF-1 levels will be monitored periodically, and a repeat MRI of the pituitary gland will be performed after 3 months. Additional treatments with octreotide will not be needed unless the tumor returns in the future.

CASE DISCUSSION

Acromegaly (enlargement of the extremities) is an uncommon condition (40–70 cases per million in the United States) that is almost always due to a benign growth hormone-secreting pituitary adenoma. If the onset occurs before puberty, it leads to gigantism, and body heights of over 7 feet are often achieved. After puberty, the condition results in the characteristic enlargement of the extremities and other physical features observed in this patient. It can also lead to hypertension, heart failure, kidney failure, visual field defects, diabetes, and premature death. Surgical removal of the pituitary tumor is the definitive treatment and often is curative, with growth hormone levels usually falling immediately after surgery, while normalization of IGF-1 levels may take several weeks. Patients are sometimes given a somatostatin analog such as octreotide, a dopamine agonist such as cabergoline, or pegvisomant to reduce excessive growth hormone secretion before surgery. These treatments can also be used on a long-term basis to control growth hormone levels in patients who are not able to undergo surgery.

Growth Hormone Receptor Antagonist

Pegvisomant is a pegylated analog of growth hormone that acts as a growth hormone receptor antagonist in target organs and normalizes serum IGF-1 concentrations in 97% of persons with acromegaly. However, growth hormone secretion is not reduced by the drug, and growth levels may increase. Pegylation (addition of polyethylene glycol to the drug) is responsible for its long serum half-life, which is about 6 days. Pegvisomant improves signs and symptoms of growth hormone excess in persons with **acromegaly** and is used primarily to treat patients who are wholly or partially resistant to somatostatin analogs such as octreotide. In one study, pegvisomant reduced serum IGF-1 levels and finger ring size in a dose-dependent manner while improving symptoms of tissue swelling, arthralgia, headache, perspiration, and fatigue. The drug appears to have a good safety profile, but it may elevate serum levels of liver enzymes, which should be monitored.

Gonadotropins and Related Drugs

The pituitary secretes two gonadotropins, FSH and LH, in response to pulsatile stimulation by GnRH, a decapeptide produced by neurons in the preoptic area of the hypothalamus. The frequency and amplitude of the GnRH pulses determine which gonadotropin is secreted at that time. In females, FSH stimulates ovarian follicle maturation and estrogen production, whereas LH assists FSH in follicle development, induces ovulation, and stimulates the corpus luteum to produce progesterone and androgens. In males, FSH stimulates spermatogenesis, whereas LH stimulates Leydig cells in the testes to produce testosterone.

Gonadotropin Preparations

A large number of gonadotropin preparations are available for the treatment of infertility and hypogonadism in men and women. These include **menotropins** (human menopausal gonadotropins), which contain both **FSH** and **LH** and are obtained from the urine of menopausal women.

Other preparations have either FSH or LH activity. **Preparations of FSH** include recombinant forms of human FSH called **follitropin alfa** and **follitropin beta,** whereas **urofollitropin** is highly purified FSH obtained from the urine of postmenopausal women. **Preparations of LH** include **chorionic gonadotropin** (human chorionic gonadotropin [hCG]), which is isolated from the urine of pregnant women and is essentially identical to **LH** in structure and function. **Choriogonadotropin alfa** is a recombinant form of hCG, and **lutropin alfa** is a recombinant form of human LH that has similar uses as the hCG preparations.

In women with **infertility,** FSH and LH are used sequentially for the induction of ovulation before natural insemination and for the induction of multiple follicles for patients participating in an **assisted reproductive technology** and *in vitro* fertilization program. A preparation containing FSH, such as menotropins or follitropin, is administered each day, typically for 9 to 12 days, to stimulate maturation of the ovarian follicle. On the day after the last dose is given, a single dose of an LH preparation such as chorionic gonadotropin is administered to induce ovulation followed by insemination or oocyte retrieval for *in vitro* fertilization procedures.

In men with infertility due to inadequate gonadotropin secretion, menotropins can be administered to stimulate **spermatogenesis.** Chorionic gonadotropin, having LH activity, was formerly used in prepubertal boys with hypogonadism and cryptorchidism (undescended testes) to stimulate testosterone production and descent of the testes, but this treatment is inferior to surgical methods and has potential adverse effects on germ cells.

Gonadotropin-Releasing Hormone Agonists

The GnRH agonists, known as **goserelin, histrelin, leuprolide, nafarelin,** and **triptorelin,** are synthetic GnRH analogs that have longer half-lives than the natural decapeptide hormone. These drugs activate pituitary G protein-coupled receptors for gonadotropin-releasing hormone and thereby influence the secretion of FSH and LH. The way in which they are administered determines their effects on gonadotropin secretion. **Pulsatile administration** of these drugs mimics the natural secretion of GnRH and is used therapeutically to stimulate the release of FSH and LH from the anterior pituitary. In contrast, **continuous administration** of GnRH agonists leads to **down-regulation** of GnRH receptors and decreases the secretion of FSH and LH, leading to decreased testosterone and estrogen secretion.

The various uses of GnRH agonists include the treatment of advanced prostate and breast cancer, endometriosis, and uterine fibroids. They are also used in the treatment of **central precocious puberty** in boys or girls to retard premature development of secondary sex characteristics and ensure adequate final height. In addition, a GnRH agonist is used to suppress the premature estrogen-induced LH surge that would otherwise occur during the use of gonadotropins in the treatment of infertility.

Nafarelin is administered as a nasal spray to manage **endometriosis** in women and central **precocious puberty** (CPP) in children. **Histrelin** is available as a subcutaneous implant that lasts for 12 months for the treatment of children with CPP. **Leuprolide** and **goserelin** are available as pellets that slowly release the drug after subcutaneous implantation and are used to treat advanced **prostate cancer, breast cancer,** and **endometriosis.** Because these drugs cause a transient increase in testosterone levels when treatment of prostate cancer is begun, they should be given in combination with a testosterone antagonist (e.g., **flutamide** or **bicalutamide**) until testosterone levels fall (see Chapter 34). These drugs can cause a number of adverse effects because of decreased sex steroid levels including hot flashes.

Gonadotropin-Releasing Hormone Antagonists

Ganirelix, cetrorelix, and **degarelix** are synthetic peptides that act as **competitive antagonists at GnRH receptors** in the pituitary gland. They dose-dependently inhibit the secretion of FSH and LH. In women undergoing ovarian stimulation as an infertility treatment, ganirelix and cetrorelix are used to inhibit premature LH surges in the same manner as the GnRH agonists. **Degarelix** is indicated for the treatment of **advanced prostate cancer** in men. By blocking pituitary GnRH receptors, degarelix inhibits the secretion of gonadotropins and subsequent release of testosterone. All of the agents are absolutely **contraindicated during pregnancy.** As with other injectable peptides and proteins, the major adverse effects of these agents are **hypersensitivity** and **allergic reactions,** including anaphylaxis.

Prolactin and Related Drugs

Prolactin contains 198 amino acids and acts on the mammary gland to stimulate tissue growth and promote lactation (milk production) in the presence of adequate levels of estrogens, progestins, and other hormones. Prolactin does not have any current clinical use.

The secretion of prolactin is inhibited by dopamine (the prolactin-inhibiting hormone) and is stimulated by hypothalamic prolactin-releasing factors. Excessive prolactin secretion causes **hyperprolactinemia** and often leads to galactorrhea (excessive milk production), hypogonadism, and infertility. In some cases, hyperprolactinemia results from prolactin-secreting pituitary adenomas.

Both the idiopathic and secondary forms of hyperprolactinemia can be treated with a dopamine agonist such as **cabergoline** or **bromocriptine.** These drugs mimic the action of dopamine and reduce prolactin secretion. In patients with prolactin-secreting adenomas, treatment produces a significant reduction in tumor size.

Bromocriptine and cabergoline are both **ergot alkaloid derivatives.** The pharmacologic properties of bromocriptine, a drug that is also used to treat Parkinson disease, are described in Chapter 24. In comparison with bromocriptine, cabergoline appears to be more effective and better tolerated in patients with hyperprolactinemia. Cabergoline selectively activates **dopamine D2 receptors** in the pituitary gland and suppresses the secretion of prolactin. It is also useful in persons with a mixed growth hormone and prolactin-secreting pituitary adenoma. The drug has an elimination half-life of about 65 hours and a long duration of action. The most common adverse effects of cabergoline are nausea, headache, and dizziness.

POSTERIOR PITUITARY HORMONES

Oxytocin and vasopressin are nine–amino-acid peptides released from the posterior pituitary in response to specific physiologic stimuli (see Fig. 31.1).

Oxytocin and Related Drugs

Oxytocin is a hormone that increases the strength of uterine contractions and causes milk ejection (milk let-down) by contracting myoepithelial cells that line the ducts of the breast. The hormone is released via a reflex that is triggered by dilation of the uterine cervix, uterine contractions, or breast suckling. During late pregnancy, the uterus becomes highly sensitive to the actions of oxytocin owing to an increased number of oxytocin receptors. The sensitivity of the uterus is enhanced by estrogen and is inhibited by progesterone.

Synthetic **oxytocin (PITOCIN)** has several uses in obstetrics (see Chapter 34). The drug is given to induce contractions during **labor,** to prevent **postpartum uterine hemorrhage,** and to stimulate **milk let-down** in nursing mothers.

Vasopressin and Related Drugs

Vasopressin (arginine vasopressin [AVP]) is secreted by the posterior pituitary in response to a decrease in extracellular fluid volume or an increase in plasma osmotic pressure. The hormone interacts with two types of vasopressin receptors to exert its **antidiuretic** and **vasoconstrictive effects.** Vasopressin causes vasoconstriction in several vascular beds by stimulating **V1 receptors** in vascular smooth muscle.

The renal actions of vasopressin are mediated by **V2 receptors** via the production of cyclic adenosine monophosphate. Activation of V_2 receptors increases water reabsorption by the kidney by causing the insertion of water channels (aquaporins) in the luminal membranes of renal tubule cells in the collecting ducts. This action expands extracellular fluid volume and concentrates the urine. For this reason, vasopressin is also called **antidiuretic hormone.**

A deficiency of pituitary vasopressin secretion leads to **diabetes insipidus,** a condition characterized by excessive water excretion (polyuria) and increased water intake (polydipsia). Diabetes insipidus is usually treated with **desmopressin,** a long-acting synthetic analog of vasopressin. This agent has potent antidiuretic activity but causes less vasoconstriction than natural vasopressin. Desmopressin solutions are available for injection and as a nasal spray that is used to prevent nocturnal urine production and enuresis in patients with diabetes insipidus. Desmopressin overdose can result in dilutional hyponatremia.

Desmopressin is also used in treating children with **nocturnal enuresis.** This condition is often caused by a nocturnal diuresis volume that exceeds the functional bladder capacity. Not all children with nocturnal enuresis respond to desmopressin therapy, but it has been helpful in many cases.

Intravenous desmopressin is used in treating a variety of **hemorrhagic conditions,** including **von Willebrand disease,** mild **hemophilia A,** and other congenital or drug-induced platelet function defects. It can also be used to **control bleeding** caused by esophageal varices or colonic diverticula. Because of its vasoconstrictive effect, desmopressin should be used cautiously in persons with coronary artery disease.

Conivaptan is a **dual AVP antagonist** with nanomolar affinity for human V_1 and V_2 receptors *in vitro*. It is indicated for the treatment of euvolemic and hypervolemic **hyponatremia** in hospitalized patients. It is available for intravenous administration only. **Tolvaptan** is a similar agent but is a **selective antagonist at V2 receptors** and is available in an oral formulation. It is indicated for the treatment of clinically significant hypervolemic and euvolemic hyponatremia, including patients with heart failure, cirrhosis, and syndrome of inappropriate antidiuretic hormone (SIADH). By blocking V_2 receptors, both agents increase free water clearance (aquaresis), decrease urine osmolality, and increase serum sodium concentrations.

SUMMARY OF IMPORTANT POINTS

- Cosyntropin is a synthetic corticotropin analog used to diagnose adrenal insufficiency, whereas corticorelin ovine triflutate is a corticotropin-releasing hormone used as a diagnostic test in persons with Cushing's syndrome.
- Recombinant somatropin is a growth hormone preparation used to treat growth hormone deficiency in children with a low growth rate. Other growth hormone analogs are also now available.
- Octreotide is a synthetic growth hormone–inhibiting hormone (somatostatin) analog used in the treatment of acromegaly, carcinoid syndrome, pituitary adenomas that secrete thyrotropin, and tumors that secrete vasoactive intestinal polypeptide.
- Pegvisomant is a growth hormone analog and growth hormone receptor antagonist used to treat acromegaly.
- Menotropins, chorionic gonadotropin, follitropin, lutropin, and others are natural or recombinant human gonadotropin preparations used to induce ovulation in women and spermatogenesis in men.

- Goserelin, leuprolide, and others are synthetic GnRH preparations administered continuously to suppress gonadotropin secretion in children with precocious puberty and in adults with prostate cancer, breast cancer, endometriosis, and uterine fibroids.
- Nafarelin is a GnRH preparation administered as a nasal spray to treat precocious puberty in children and endometriosis in women.
- Ganirelix, cetrorelix, and degarelix are competitive GnRH receptor antagonists used to treat prostate cancer and suppress a premature LH surge during ovulation induction.
- Dopamine agonists—cabergoline and bromocriptine—are used to suppress prolactin secretion in women with hyperprolactinemia. This condition is often associated with galactorrhea, hypogonadism, and infertility. Cabergoline may also reduce excessive growth hormone secretion in some persons with acromegaly and hyperprolactinemia.
- Oxytocin, which stimulates uterine contractions at term, is used to induce or augment labor, to prevent postpartum uterine hemorrhage, and to stimulate milk let-down in nursing women.
- Desmopressin is a synthetic vasopressin analog that retains the antidiuretic activity of the natural hormone but has a less vasoconstrictive effect. It is administered parenterally and intranasally to treat diabetes insipidus resulting from deficient vasopressin secretion. Desmopressin is also used to control gastrointestinal bleeding by causing vasoconstriction and to treat hemophilia A and von Willebrand disease.
- Conivaptan and tolvaptan are arginine vasopressin receptor antagonists used to treat hypervolemic and euvolemic hyponatremia.

Review Questions

1. Which drug is used to reduce the secretion of gonadotropins and gonadal steroids in children with precocious puberty?
   (A) cabergoline
   (B) menotropins
   (C) leuprolide
   (D) gonadorelin
   (E) octreotide

2. Which drug for treating acromegaly acts by blocking receptors for growth hormone?
   (A) pegvisomant
   (B) somatropin
   (C) octreotide
   (D) leuprolide
   (E) cabergoline

3. By which mechanism does cabergoline relieve symptoms of hyperprolactinemia in persons with a prolactin-secreting pituitary adenoma?
   (A) blocks prolactin receptors
   (B) blocks receptors for prolactin-releasing hormone
   (C) exerts a cytotoxic effect on pituitary adenoma cells
   (D) activates receptors for prolactin-inhibiting hormone
   (E) stimulates the breakdown of prolactin

4. Octreotide is correctly described by which of the following statements?
   (A) It is identical to naturally occurring somatostatin.
   (B) It is used to treat growth hormone deficiency.
   (C) It is administered orally.
   (D) It is a more potent inhibitor of growth hormone secretion than is somatostatin.
   (E) It contains more than 100 amino acids.

5. Which sequence of gonadotropin preparations is used to induce ovulation?
   (A) choriogonadotropin alfa then lutropin alfa
   (B) follitropin alfa then lutropin alfa
   (C) choriogonadotropin alfa then follitropin beta
   (D) chorionic gonadotropin (hCG) then lutropin alfa
   (E) follitropin alfa then follitropin beta

Drugs for the Treatment of Thyroid Disorders

OVERVIEW

Thyroid hormones are necessary for normal growth and development and timely sexual maturation. They affect every organ system and have a crucial role in metabolic processes, including those involved in the synthesis and degradation of essentially all other hormones. Thyroid hormones also augment sympathetic nervous system function, primarily by increasing the number of adrenoceptors in target tissues.

Thyroid Hormone Secretion

The thyroid gland synthesizes and secretes the hormones **triiodothyronine (T_3)** and **tetraiodothyronine (T_4, thyroxine).** The secretion of thyroid hormones is initiated by a hypothalamic hormone called thyrotropin-releasing hormone (TRH) and is increased by cold exposure and regulated other physiologic factors. TRH increases secretion of an anterior pituitary hormone called **thyrotropin (thyroid-stimulating hormone, [TSH]).** TSH is the prime regulator of **iodide uptake** and thyroid hormone formation by the thyroid gland. It fulfills this role by **inducing the expression of three genes** for proteins involved in iodide uptake and hormone production: (1) the **sodium/iodide symporter** that transports iodide into the thyroid gland, (2) **thyroglobulin,** and (3) **thyroperoxidase.** The secretion of TRH and TSH is regulated, in turn, by feedback inhibition from T_4 and T_3 (Fig. 32.1).

Thyroid hormones are synthesized in a process that involves the uptake and *organification* (below) of iodide and the subsequent coupling of iodotyrosine residues of thyroglobulin. These steps are depicted in Fig. 32.2.

After iodide is actively transported into thyroid follicle cells, it diffuses across the cells to the apical membrane, where it is **oxidized to iodine** and then attached to tyrosine residues of thyroglobulin. This process is called **iodide organification.** The iodinated tyrosine residues, monoiodotyrosine and diiodotyrosine, are then coupled to form T_3 and T_4. Iodide organification and the coupling reactions are catalyzed by thyroperoxidase, an enzyme **inhibited by iodides and thioamide drugs** (see later).

Thyroglobulin is stored as colloid in the follicular lumen. During the release of thyroid hormones, thyroglobulin reenters the follicular cell by endocytosis and undergoes proteolysis. The release of T_4 and T_3 is stimulated by TSH via the formation of cyclic adenosine monophosphate (cAMP) in thyroid follicular cells.

T_4 accounts for about 80% of the hormones secreted by the thyroid, and T_3 accounts for the remainder. These hormones are transported to target organs by thyroid-binding globulin, thyroid-binding prealbumin, and albumin. In peripheral tissues, some of the T_4 is converted to T_3 and reverse T_3 (rT_3) by 5′-deiodinase and 5-deiodinase, respectively. T_3 is about five times more active than T_4, whereas rT_3 is completely inactive. For this reason, the deiodinase enzymes have an important role in controlling the level of thyroid activity. The rate of conversion of T_4 to T_3 is also affected by a variety of other hormones, nutrients, and disease states. T_3 and rT_3 are eventually metabolized by deiodinase and sulfotransferase reactions to diiodothyronine sulfate.

When T_3 enters the target cell, it binds to thyroid hormone receptors (TR) that **activate gene transcription,** leading to increased synthesis of proteins necessary for growth, development, and calorigenesis (heat production). In this complex process, binding of T_3 to its receptor (TR) causes disruption of the native TR receptor homodimer (containing two identical receptors), forming a **heterodimer** consisting of TR bound to a retinoid X receptor (RXR). The TR-RXR heterodimer enters the nucleus and acts as a **transcription factor,** leading to the activation of multigene transcription.

THYROID DISORDERS

Normal thyroid function, or euthyroidism, is maintained via feedback inhibition of TSH secretion so as to keep the plasma concentration of free (circulating or unbound) T_4 within a narrow range. Abnormally low or high T_4 and T_3 levels result in clinical manifestations of **hypothyroidism** or **hyperthyroidism,** respectively.

Hypothyroidism is characterized by low T_4 levels and leads to impaired growth and development, decreased physiologic and metabolic activity, and decreased heat

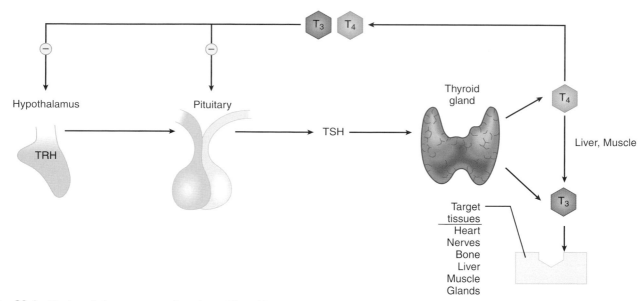

Fig. 32.1 The hypothalamic-pituitary-thyroid axis. Thyroid hormone synthesis is initiated by the release of thyroid-releasing hormone (*TRH*) from the hypothalamus, which stimulates the pituitary to release thyroid-stimulating hormone (*TSH*). TSH acts on the thyroid gland to increase iodide uptake and the synthesis of thyroid hormones triiodothyronine (T$_3$) and tetraiodothyronine (T$_4$, thyroxine). T$_4$ is converted to T$_3$ in liver and muscle and other tissues. T$_3$ activates thyroid receptors in target tissues. Both T$_4$ and T$_3$ exert feedback inhibition of TRH and TSH secretion.

production (calorigenesis). In contrast, hyperthyroidism is characterized by high T$_4$ levels, leading to hyperactivity of organ systems (particularly the nervous and cardiovascular systems) and an increased metabolic rate and calorigenesis.

Thyroid disorders are relatively common. In many cases, patients seek medical attention because they notice a diffuse or nodular thyroid gland enlargement (**goiter**) or experience other manifestations of abnormal thyroid function. Thyroid disorders are diagnosed primarily on the basis of their clinical manifestations and plasma T$_4$ and TSH levels. In most cases, TSH levels are abnormally high in persons with hypothyroidism and low in persons with hyperthyroidism.

Hypothyroidism

In infants and children, **hypothyroidism** causes irreversible **mental retardation** and impairs growth and development. In adults, hypothyroidism is associated with impairment of physical and mental activity and with slowing of cardiovascular, gastrointestinal, and neuromuscular functions. Hypothyroid patients may note lethargy, cold intolerance, weight gain, and constipation. The skin may become coarse, dry, and cold. Eventually, hypothyroidism causes **myxedema,** which is described as a dry, waxy swelling of the skin with nonpitting edema. **Myxedema coma** is characterized by hypothermia, hypoglycemia, weakness, stupor, and shock, and is the end stage of long-standing, untreated hypothyroidism.

Many patients with mild hypothyroidism have a T$_4$ level within the normal range. As the disease progresses, however, the T$_4$ level usually falls below normal.

The most common cause of hypothyroidism in adults is **autoimmune thyroiditis (Hashimoto disease).** Other causes include thyroid surgery or **radioactive iodine** (RAI) treatment for hyperthyroidism, dietary iodine deficiency, and thyroid hypoplasia or enzymatic defects. Pituitary or hypothalamic dysfunction can cause **secondary hypothyroidism.**

Several types of drugs can induce thyroid disorders. **Lithium** inhibits the release of thyroid hormones by the thyroid gland (see Fig. 32.1) and can cause hypothyroidism by this mechanism. **Amiodarone** is an iodine-containing antiarrhythmic drug that can cause either hypothyroidism or hyperthyroidism through a variety of mechanisms that alter several thyroid functions. Most commonly, amiodarone causes hypothyroidism by inhibiting conversion of peripheral T$_4$ to T$_3$.

The treatment for all forms of hypothyroidism is **replacement therapy** with a thyroid hormone preparation.

Hyperthyroidism

Manifestations of hyperthyroidism, or **thyrotoxicosis,** can include nervousness, emotional lability, weight loss despite an increased appetite, heat intolerance, palpitations, proximal muscle weakness, increased frequency of bowel movements, and irregular menses.

Most cases of hyperthyroidism are associated with **overproduction of thyroid hormones** by the thyroid gland, as indicated by the finding of increased RAI uptake. Excessive thyroid hormone production can result from excessive TSH, as occurs in patients with TSH-secreting pituitary adenomas, or it can result from gland stimulation by thyroid antibodies, as occurs in patients with **Graves disease.**

Graves disease is the most common cause of hyperthyroidism and results from the formation of **antibodies directed against the TSH receptor** on the surface of thyroid cells. These antibodies stimulate the receptor in the same manner as TSH, resulting in overproduction of thyroid hormones. Graves disease is characterized by hyperthyroidism, thyroid enlargement, and exophthalmos (abnormal protrusion of the eyeball). **Exophthalmos** results from stimulation of orbital muscles by thyroid antibodies causing retraction of the upper lid.

Excessive thyroid hormone production also occurs in persons with thyroid nodules that are independent of pituitary

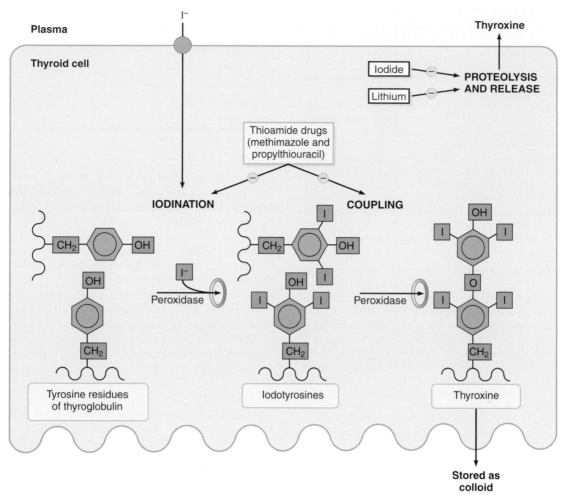

FIG. 32.2 Thyroid hormone synthesis and sites of drug action. Iodide is accumulated by thyroid follicular cells by the sodium/iodide symporter. Thyroperoxidase catalyzes the iodination of tyrosine residues of thyroglobulin and the coupling of iodotyrosines to form triiodothyronine (T_3) and tetraiodothyronine (T_4, thyroxine). Thyroglobulin is stored as colloid in thyroid follicles and undergoes proteolysis to release T_4 and T_3 when stimulated by thyroid-stimulating hormone *(TSH)* or thyrotropin. Thioamide drugs inhibit the synthesis of thyroid hormones by inhibiting iodination and coupling of tyrosine residues. Elevated iodide concentrations and lithium inhibit the release of thyroid hormones.

gland control. Inflammatory thyroid disease **(subacute thyroiditis)** can cause a transient form of hyperthyroidism caused by the release of preformed thyroid hormone from thyroid follicles.

Three treatment modalities are used in hyperthyroidism: **antithyroid agents, surgery,** and **RAI treatment.** The goals of therapy are to eliminate excessive thyroid hormone production and to control the symptoms of hyperthyroidism. The choice of treatment depends on the type and severity of hyperthyroidism and on the individual characteristics of the patient. Antithyroid agents are primarily used for the short-term treatment of hyperthyroidism, either to induce remission of Graves disease or to control the symptoms of hyperthyroidism before thyroid surgery or RAI treatment. Surgery or RAI treatment can permanently cure hyperthyroidism, but both of these treatments often result in chronic hypothyroidism, necessitating lifelong thyroid hormone replacement therapy.

THYROID HORMONE PREPARATIONS

Synthetic thyroid hormone preparations include levothyroxine (T_4), liothyronine (T_3), and a mixture of both hormones in a 4:1 ratio of T_4 to T_3 called liotrix. **Levothyroxine**

is widely considered the drug of choice for thyroid hormone replacement therapy because of its stability, standardized purity and potency, predictable effects, and long half-life (Box 32.1). Clinical studies indicate that **liotrix** is not superior to T_4 alone with respect to various measures of clinical efficacy, and it is more expensive than T_4. **Thyroid desiccated** is a preparation of thyroid glands from pigs that contains both T_4 and T_3, but it is not recommended by most endocrinologists because of concerns about its stability, purity, and potency, and difficulty of laboratory monitoring.

The pharmacologic and pharmacokinetic properties of levothyroxine and liothyronine are shown in Table 32.1.

Levothyroxine
Pharmacokinetics
The oral bioavailability of levothyroxine is typically about 70% to 80%. Different brands and generic formulations of levothyroxine may **vary in their bioavailability,** and formulations should not be substituted for one another without monitoring T_4 and TSH levels. Certain foods, including coffee, soy, and dietary fiber, can reduce absorption of levothyroxine, and it is recommended that levothyroxine be taken **on an empty stomach,** either 1 hour before or 4 hours after

CASE PRESENTATION

A 42-year-old woman reports to her health care provider that she has gained 10 pounds over the last 6 months and has a low energy level despite getting plenty of sleep. She has also had more trouble than usual with constipation and dry skin, and she has wanted to keep her home warmer than do other members of her family. On physical examination, her temperature is 97.3° F, her skin is dry, and she is found to have an enlarged thyroid gland (goiter). Laboratory tests are ordered and show that her thyroid-stimulating hormone (TSH) level is 20 mU/L (normal is 0.4–5.5 mU/L), her free tetraiodothyronine (T$_4$, thyroxine) level is 0.6 ng/dL (normal is 0.8–2.7 ng/dL), and her thyroperoxidase antibody level is 150. She is started on a low dose of levothyroxine and instructed to have a TSH level obtained in 6 weeks.

CASE DISCUSSION

The patient's enlarged thyroid and thyroid autoantibodies are consistent with chronic autoimmune thyroiditis (Hashimoto thyroiditis). Her symptoms and laboratory values are indicative of mild hypothyroidism. Her treatment goals are to relieve her symptoms and normalize her TSH level. The serum TSH concentration is the primary test used to evaluate replacement therapy in persons with hypothyroidism. This test is very sensitive to minute changes in free T$_4$ levels. A twofold change in the free T$_4$ level can cause a 100-fold change in the TSH level. In patients who have had their dose or brand of levothyroxine changed, the TSH level should be measured after 2 to 3 months. When the optimum replacement dose has been attained, clinical and laboratory monitoring should be performed every 6 to 12 months or whenever there is a change in the patient's status.

meals, or at bedtime, to achieve consistent blood levels. Because the half-life of levothyroxine is about 7 days, once-daily administration of the drug produces a stable hormone pool with little fluctuation in plasma hormone levels. It takes 6 to 8 weeks after starting or changing a dose to achieve steady-state blood levels. Because about 35% of T$_4$ is converted to T$_3$ in peripheral tissues, levothyroxine administration produces physiologic levels of both T$_4$ and T$_3$.

Indications

Levothyroxine is the **drug of choice** for thyroid hormone replacement in patients with hypothyroidism for reasons cited earlier. Levothyroxine tablets are available in a wide range of doses to accommodate individualized therapy based on clinical and laboratory data. Therapy is often begun with a lower dose, particularly in elderly patients and those with long-standing or more severe hypothyroidism. The dose is then increased at monthly intervals until a full replacement dose is achieved. A gradual increase in the dose prevents excessive stress on the cardiovascular and other organ systems and thereby causes fewer adverse reactions. Younger persons with minimal disease can usually be started at full replacement doses. Children typically require higher doses per kilogram of body weight than do adults.

The maintenance dose of levothyroxine is determined on the basis of the patient's clinical response, TSH levels, and T$_4$ levels. The **TSH level** is the most sensitive test for determining thyroid replacement dosage, and an elevated

TABLE 32.1 Pharmacologic and Pharmacokinetic Properties of Levothyroxine (T$_4$) and Liothyronine (T$_3$)

PROPERTY	LEVOTHYROXINE	LIOTHYRONINE
Relative potency	1	4
Oral bioavailability	80% (variable)	95%
Elimination half-life	7 days	1 day
Daily doses	1	1–3

TSH level indicates that the levothyroxine dose is not sufficient. The expected range of T$_4$ levels in patients receiving thyroid replacement therapy is higher than that in healthy individuals, because a higher level of T$_4$ is required in patients to maintain adequate T$_3$ levels in the absence of endogenous T$_3$ production by the thyroid gland.

Levothyroxine is also the drug of choice for suppressive therapy in patients with **thyroid nodules, diffuse goiters,** or **thyroid cancer.** In these conditions, levothyroxine acts to suppress TSH production and reduce stimulation of abnormal thyroid tissue. Suppressive therapy thereby reduces goiter size and thyroid gland volume.

Myxedema coma is a medical emergency that requires **intravenous administration** of a loading dose of levothyroxine or liothyronine followed by smaller maintenance doses.

Adverse Effects

Thyroid hormone preparations rarely cause adverse reactions if dosage is appropriate and carefully monitored during the initial treatment of hypothyroidism and periodically thereafter. Excessive doses produce symptoms of **hyperthyroidism.**

Interactions

Aluminum hydroxide, calcium supplements, cholestyramine, ferrous sulfate, and sucralfate are among the drugs that **interfere with the absorption of levothyroxine.** These drugs should be administered 2 hours before or after levothyroxine is administered. Estrogens, androgens, and glucocorticoids can alter thyroid-binding globulin and total T$_4$ and T$_3$ levels, but free T$_4$ and TSH levels usually remain normal in patients taking these steroid hormones. For this reason, the dosage of levothyroxine usually does not need to be adjusted in persons who are taking steroid hormones.

Liothyronine

As shown in Table 32.1, liothyronine (the synthetic name for T$_3$) is more potent than levothyroxine (T$_4$) and has a **higher oral bioavailability.** However, it is seldom used in the treatment of hypothyroidism because it has several disadvantages. Liothyronine has a much **shorter half-life** than levothyroxine, and multiple daily doses may be needed to obtain a smooth response during hormone replacement therapy. Liothyronine does not increase plasma T$_4$ levels, so it is more difficult to monitor the response to treatment. Finally, liothyronine also causes more **adverse cardiac effects** and is more expensive than levothyroxine.

ANTITHYROID AGENTS

Antithyroid agents used in the treatment of hyperthyroidism include thioamide drugs, *beta* (β)-adrenoceptor antagonists, iodide salts, and RAI.

The thioamide drugs inhibit the synthesis of thyroid hormones, whereas sufficient doses of iodide salts inhibit the release of these hormones. The β-blockers are used to control the cardiovascular symptoms of hyperthyroidism until definitive treatment becomes effective. β-blockers, propylthiouracil (PTU), corticosteroids, amiodarone, and some iodinated contrast agents (ipodate) also inhibit the peripheral conversion of T_4 to T_3.

Thioamide Drugs

The thioamide drugs are **methimazole** and **PTU.**

Mechanisms

As discussed earlier in this chapter, the synthesis of thyroid hormones requires oxidation of trapped iodide, formation of iodotyrosines, and the coupling of iodotyrosines to form T_3 and T_4. Methimazole and PTU **inhibit thyroperoxidase-catalyzed** steps in this process (see Fig. 32.1). In addition, PTU (but not methimazole) **inhibits the conversion** of T_4 to T_3 in peripheral tissues. The contribution of this action to the therapeutic efficacy of PTU is uncertain, however, because PTU and methimazole appear to be therapeutically equivalent.

Pharmacokinetics

The thioamide drugs are well absorbed from the gut after oral administration. They are actively concentrated in the thyroid gland, which may account for their relatively long duration of action despite having relatively short half-lives. The thioamide drugs are extensively metabolized before undergoing renal excretion.

Indications

In patients with **Graves disease,** a thioamide drug can be used in an attempt to induce remission or as a means to control symptoms before surgery or RAI treatment. The **effects of thioamide drugs are delayed** because it takes about 4 to 8 weeks of therapy before the glandular hormone stores are depleted and circulating hormone levels start to return to the normal range. At this time, doses can be gradually tapered at monthly intervals to achieve the desired steady-state thyroid hormone level. If the objective is long-term remission of Graves disease, patients usually remain on the drug for 12 to 24 months. About 45% of patients will eventually achieve a permanent remission. The mechanisms responsible for remission are uncertain but may involve a reduction in the thyroid-stimulating activity of thyroid antibodies or an alteration of the immunologic defect that stimulated antibody production. Persons with persistent thyroid-stimulating antibodies have a higher incidence of relapse than do persons without persistent antibodies.

Adverse Effects

Pruritic **maculopapular rash,** arthralgia, and fever occur in up to 5% of persons treated with a thioamide drug. Less frequently, a lupus erythematosus–like syndrome, hepatitis, or gastrointestinal distress is reported. Many patients experience benign and **transient leukopenia,** with a white blood cell count of less than 4,000/μL. This condition is distinct from the more severe **agranulocytosis** that sometimes occurs and is characterized by a granulocyte count of less than 250/μL. Severe agranulocytosis usually develops during the first 3 months of therapy and can be managed by advising patients to stop treatment and immediately contact their physician if they experience fever, malaise, sore throat, or other flulike symptoms. Both methimazole and PTU may cause liver injury and **fatal liver failure,** but an analysis of adverse drug reactions by the US Food and Drug Administration (FDA) indicates that PTU is associated with a higher incidence of **liver failure** than methimazole, and it recommends that PTU be reserved for patients who are allergic or intolerant of methimazole. When therapy with PTU is initiated, patients should be monitored for liver toxicity for the first 6 months. Because methimazole and PTU exhibit cross-sensitivity (allergic hypersensitivity) in about 50% of patients, persons switched to the other drug should be carefully monitored.

Specific Drugs

Although **methimazole** and **PTU** appear to be clinically equivalent, they have minor differences. The plasma half-lives of methimazole and PTU are about 7 and 2 hours, respectively. Either drug, however, can be administered once or twice a day. Unlike methimazole, PTU inhibits the peripheral conversion of T_4 to T_3. Nevertheless, the clinical effects of the drugs are primarily related to inhibition of hormone synthesis and depletion of glandular stores.

About 70% of PTU is bound to plasma proteins. Methimazole is not bound to plasma proteins, and it readily crosses the placenta and appears in breast milk. According to a recent analysis by the FDA, methimazole is about 3 times more likely to cause **birth defects** than PTU. Hence, PTU appears to be the drug of choice just before and during the first trimester of pregnancy.

Beta-Adrenoceptor Antagonists

Thyroid hormones and the sympathetic nervous system act synergistically on cardiovascular function. This explains why increased levels of thyroid hormones cause **tachycardia, palpitations,** and arrhythmias. *Beta*-adrenoceptor antagonists such as propranolol are used to reduce cardiovascular stimulation associated with hyperthyroidism. They act immediately and are particularly useful during severe acute **thyrotoxicosis (thyroid storm).** *Beta*-blockers are also used to control symptoms of hyperthyroidism in patients awaiting surgery or for the effects of RAI treatment to ensue.

Other Antithyroid Agents

Iodide Salts

Iodide salts are contained in **potassium iodide tablets** and solutions, such as saturated solution of **potassium iodide** and **Lugol solution** (elemental iodine and potassium iodide). Potassium iodide is used on a short-term basis to treat patients with acute thyrotoxicosis, to prepare patients for thyroid surgery, and to inhibit the release of thyroid hormones after RAI treatment.

When administered in sufficient doses, iodide salts act immediately to inhibit the release of thyroid hormones from the thyroid gland. Plasma hormone levels then gradually decline as the circulating hormones are degraded.

Patients with hyperthyroidism usually obtain symptomatic improvement within 2 to 7 days after starting iodide therapy. This effect is **limited to several weeks,** however, because the thyroid gland eventually escapes from the inhibitory effects of iodide salts. A thioamide drug can be used concurrently with iodide salts to further inhibit thyroid function and to provide a longer-lasting antithyroid effect.

In patients scheduled for **thyroid surgery,** a potassium iodide solution is usually administered preoperatively for 7 to 14 days to reduce the size and vascularity of the thyroid gland. As an adjunct to RAI treatment, potassium iodide is given 3 to 7 days after the administration of RAI.

The **adverse effects** of iodide salts are usually mild and can include skin rashes and other hypersensitivity reactions, salivary gland swelling, metallic taste, sore gums, and gastrointestinal discomfort.

Radioactive Iodine

RAI is usually administered as a colorless and tasteless solution of sodium iodide I-131 (^{131}I). The isotope is rapidly absorbed from the gut and concentrated by the thyroid gland. In the gland, it emits β-**particles** that **destroy thyroid tissue**. The particles have a tissue penetration of 2 mm, and the isotope has a half-life of 8 days. As thyroid tissue is destroyed, the circulating thyroid hormone levels gradually return to normal over several weeks.

Beta-adrenoceptor antagonists are used to control symptoms of hyperthyroidism while the patient is awaiting the response to RAI treatment. Methimazole or PTU can be used if *Beta*-blockers alone are not adequate to control these symptoms. Pretreatment with thioamide drugs before RAI treatment, however, appears to reduce the cure rate and cause a higher incidence of posttreatment recurrence or persistence of hyperthyroidism. For this reason, thioamide drugs should be withdrawn several days before RAI treatment and reinstituted several days after it.

Iodide salts are used after RAI treatment to inhibit radioactive thyroid hormone release. They should not be used before RAI treatment, however, because nonradioactive iodide would compete with iodine-131 (^{131}I) for uptake by the thyroid gland.

Treatment with RAI is absolutely contraindicated in pregnant women because it destroys fetal thyroid tissue.

Thyrotropin

A preparation of recombinant human thyrotropin, **thyrotropin alfa** (THYROGEN), is used to increase thyroid gland **uptake of RAI** in the diagnosis and treatment of thyroid conditions. It is used to facilitate RAI ablation of thyroid tissue remnants after thyroidectomy for **thyroid cancer,** and it is used in the follow-up evaluation of thyroid function in thyroid cancer patients.

DRUGS FOR THYROID TREATMENT AFTER NUCLEAR REACTOR ACCIDENT OR NUCLEAR BOMB EXPLOSION

As previously noted, RAI-131 is used clinically to destroy thyroids tissue in Graves disease. However, exposure to the radioactive nuclear fission product ^{131}I **after a nuclear bomb** or **nuclear reactor meltdown** affects people with or without Graves disease. As previously discussed, the thyroid concentrates circulating iodine, and incorporation of the hot ^{131}I isotope destroys thyroid tissue. Iodide salts can also be used to competitively block RAI uptake by the thyroid gland in the event of a nuclear reactor accident or other accidental exposure to toxic levels of RAI. **Potassium iodide** preparations are available without prescription for this purpose (THYROSAFE, THYROSHIELD). In emergency situations, potassium iodide preparations can be made at home by adding the KI salt into water until saturated.

SUMMARY OF IMPORTANT POINTS

- The thyroid gland synthesizes and secretes T_3 and T_4. The steps in thyroid hormone synthesis consist of iodide uptake by the thyroid gland, incorporation of iodide into thyroglobulin, and coupling of mono- and diiodotyrosine to form T_3 and T_4. The secretion of T_3 and T_4 is modulated by TSH and by TRH.
- In target cells, cytoplasmic T_4 is converted to T_3, which enters the cell nucleus and activates T_3 receptors, leading to gene transcription for synthesis of enzymes that increase the metabolic rate and accelerate a wide range of cellular activities required for growth and development, hormone secretion, and maintenance of normal metabolism.
- Levothyroxine (synthetic T_4) is the drug of choice for all forms of hypothyroidism. It has a long half-life (7 days) and can be administered orally once a day.
- Liothyronine (synthetic T_3) is more potent than levothyroxine and has a higher oral bioavailability. It has a shorter half-life and may need to be given several times a day, and it may cause excessive cardiac stimulation.
- Methimazole and PTU are thioamide drugs that inhibit peroxidase-catalyzed steps in the synthesis of thyroid hormone. PTU also inhibits the peripheral conversion of T_4 to T_3. The onset of action of these drugs is delayed because of the time required to deplete glandular stores of thyroid hormone.
- In patients with Graves disease, methimazole or PTU is used in an attempt to induce remission or as a means to control symptoms before surgery or RAI treatment.
- A β-adrenoceptor antagonist, usually propranolol, is used to control the cardiovascular symptoms of hyperthyroidism in patients who are suffering from acute thyrotoxicosis or who are awaiting surgery or a response to RAI treatment.
- The iodide salts in potassium iodide solutions act rapidly to inhibit the release of thyroid hormones from the thyroid gland. They produce symptomatic improvement in 2 to 7 days as circulating levels of thyroid hormones decline.
- Potassium iodide solutions are used to control symptoms of acute thyrotoxicosis, to reduce the vascularity and size of the thyroid gland before surgery, to inhibit thyroid hormone release following RAI treatment, and to competitively inhibit uptake of RAI after a nuclear reactor accident.
- RAI (^{131}I) is concentrated by the thyroid gland and emits β-particles that destroy thyroid tissue. It is used

in the treatment of Graves disease and other forms of hyperthyroidism. RAI treatment is absolutely contraindicated in pregnant women.

Review Questions

1. A man is given a drug to reduce thyroid gland size and vascularity before surgical thyroidectomy. Which mechanism is responsible for its use in this setting?
   (A) inhibition of the sodium/iodide symporter
   (B) inhibition of thyroperoxidase
   (C) inhibition of TSH secretion
   (D) inhibition of thyroid hormone release
   (E) destruction of thyroid tissue
2. A woman with weight loss, nervousness, heat intolerance, and exophthalmos is prescribed methimazole to induce a remission in her disease. Which adverse effect is most often associated with this medication?
   (A) hypotension and bradycardia
   (B) thromboembolism
   (C) pruritic rash
   (D) liver failure
   (E) agranulocytosis
3. After total thyroidectomy, a woman is placed on levothyroxine to maintain normal thyroid levels. Which attribute is correctly associated with this drug?
   (A) partly converted to T_3 in the body
   (B) administered several times a day
   (C) the most potent thyroid hormone
   (D) half-life of 1 day
   (E) oral bioavailability of 95%
4. After exposure to radioactive fallout containing ^{131}I, which agent could be administered to prevent destruction of thyroid tissue?
   (A) liothyronine
   (B) methimazole
   (C) propranolol
   (D) potassium iodide
   (E) levothyroxine
5. Treatment of hyperthyroidism by propylthiouracil (PTU) shows clinical effects due to:
   (A) blocking β-adrenergic receptors
   (B) inhibiting enzymes forming T_3 and T_4
   (C) destroying thyroid tissue
   (D) inhibiting release of T_3 and T_4
   (E) acting on thyroid hormone receptors

Adrenal Steroids and Related Drugs

CLASSIFICATION OF ADRENAL STEROIDS AND RELATED DRUGS

Adrenal Steroid Drugs

Mineralocorticoids
- Fludrocortisone (FLORINEF)

Glucocorticoids
- Cortisone and Hydrocortisone
- Dexamethasone[a]
- Deflazacort (EMFLAZA).
- Prednisone (PREDNISONE INTENSOL)[b]
- Desoximetasone (TOPICORT)[c]

Adrenal androgens
- Dehydroepiandrosterone (DHEA)

Adrenal Steroid Inhibitors

Corticosteroid synthesis inhibitors
- Metyrapone (METOPIRONE)
- Osilodrostat (ISTURISA)
- Ketoconazole (NIZORAL)
- Fluconazole (DIFLUCAN)

Corticosteroid receptor antagonists
- Mifepristone (MIFEPREX)[d]
- Spironolactone (ALDACTONE)

[a] Also betamethasone (DIPROLENE), beclomethasone (BECONASE), mometasone (NASONEX), budesonide (RHINOCORT), and triamcinolone (ARISTOCORT).
[b] Also prednisolone (PRELONE), methylprednisolone (MEDROL), loteprednol (LOTEMAX), and difluprednate (DUREZOL).
[c] Also desonide (TRIDESILON), fluticasone (FLONASE), fluocinonide (FLUONEX), ciclesonide (OMNARIS, ALVESCO), and clobetasol (CLOBEVATE).
[d] Mifepristone was given an additional brand name when approved for treatment of hyperglycemia in patients with Cushing syndrome (KORLYM).

OVERVIEW

The adrenal glands are situated on top of the kidneys (as obvious from their name) and are essential for life. The adrenal glands are composed of two major parts: the adrenal cortex and the adrenal medulla, also called *chromaffin tissue*, owing to its brightly staining characteristics. The adrenal medulla produces epinephrine (adrenaline) as its main hormone and is an integral part of the sympathetic nervous system (see Chapter 8). This chapter describes the drugs that serve as replacements or alter the effects of steroid hormones produced by the adrenal cortex.

SYNTHESIS AND SECRETION OF ADRENAL STEROIDS

The adrenal cortex occupies about 90% of the adrenal gland, consists of three layers, and produces three types of steroid hormones, or **adrenocorticosteroids.** These hormones are classified as **mineralocorticoids, glucocorticoids,** and **adrenal androgens.** The mineralocorticoids are primarily produced in the outer layer (zona glomerulosa), whereas the glucocorticoids and adrenal androgens are produced in the middle layer (zona fasciculata) and inner layer (zona reticularis), respectively.

The major pathways for mineralocorticoid, glucocorticoid, and androgen biosynthesis are shown in Fig. 33.1. Also shown is the site of action of drugs that inhibit **adrenocorticoid** synthesis. In humans, **aldosterone** is the major mineralocorticoid, **cortisol** is the major glucocorticoid, and **dehydroepiandrosterone (DHEA)** is the major adrenal androgen.

The regulation of corticosteroid secretion is depicted in Fig. 33.2. The secretion of cortisol and adrenal androgens is primarily controlled by **corticotropin (i.e., adrenocorticotropic hormone [ACTH])** secreted by the pituitary gland, whereas the secretion of aldosterone is chiefly regulated by the **renin-angiotensin system.** Various types of physical and mental stress are powerful activators of corticotropin-releasing hormone secretion, leading to increased corticotropin and cortisol production. Cortisol exerts several effects that increase the body's **resistance to stress.**

As shown in Fig. 33.2, cortisol and other glucocorticoids act as **feedback inhibitors** of both corticotropin-releasing hormone and corticotropin. This is why exogenously administered glucocorticoids can suppress the hypothalamic-pituitary-adrenal axis and inhibit endogenous cortisol production, leading to **adrenal insufficiency** when the exogenous glucocorticoid is withdrawn.

PHYSIOLOGIC EFFECTS OF ADRENAL STEROIDS

The adrenal steroids act on target tissues by binding to specific cytoplasmic steroid receptors, which are then translocated to the cell nucleus, a common mechanism for all steroid hormones (see Fig. 3.4 in Chapter 3). In the nucleus, the activated receptors stimulate the transcription of specific genes and thereby increase the translation of specific proteins. These actions lead to the various **metabolic** and **anti-inflammatory effects** of glucocorticoids, which are described later. In the renal tubules, activation of the mineralocorticoid receptor stimulates the synthesis of sodium channels and sodium-potassium adenosine triphosphatase, which are needed for **sodium reabsorption.** This mechanism is responsible for the salt-retaining effects of mineralocorticoids.

The **glucocorticoid receptor** has a high affinity for cortisol but a much lower affinity for aldosterone, whereas the **mineralocorticoid receptor** has a high affinity for both aldosterone and cortisol. This enables cortisol to exert both glucocorticoid and mineralocorticoid actions.

Glucocorticoids induce enzymes involved in **gluconeogenesis** (the formation of glucose from amino acids) and have an **antiinsulin effect.** For this reason, glucocorticoid insufficiency can lead to **hypoglycemia** during stress. Glucocorticoids also activate enzymes involved in **protein**

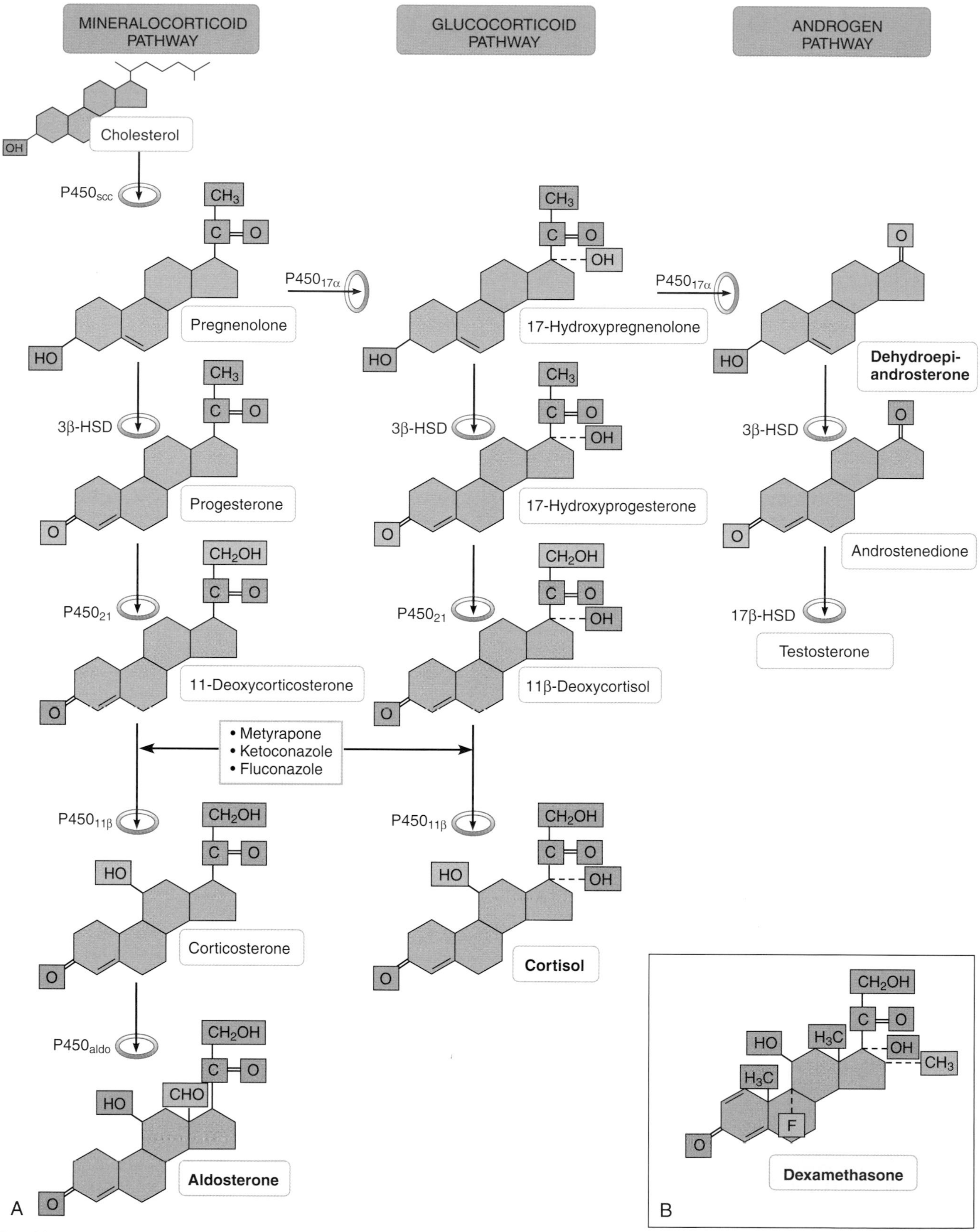

FIG. 33.1 (A) Biosynthetic pathways for adrenal steroids. Major pathways for Mineralocorticoid, glucocorticoid, and androgen biosynthesis are shown. Important enzymes include 3β-hydroxysteroid dehydrogenase (3β-HSD), steroid 21-hydroxylase (P450$_{21}$), steroid 11β-hydroxylase (P450$_{11β}$), aldosterone synthase (P450$_{aldo}$), steroid 17α-hydroxylase (P450$_{17α}$), and 17β-hydroxysteroid dehydrogenase (17β-HSD). The structural changes produced by each reaction are unshaded. Metyrapone, ketoconazole and fluconazole inhibit P450$_{11β}$. The most common defect causing congenital adrenal hyperplasia is P450$_{21}$ deficiency. (B) (*inset*) The structure of dexamethasone is shown in the inset in the lower right corner. In synthetic steroids, glucocorticoid potency is enhanced by the introduction of a double bond at the 1,2 position or the introduction of a hydroxyl or methyl group at the 16 position. Both glucocorticoid and mineralocorticoid activities are increased by a fluorine substitution at the 9 position.

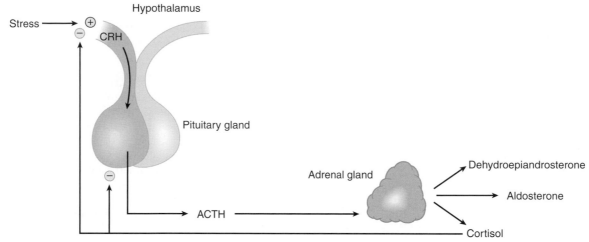

Fig. 33.2   Regulation of the secretion of cortisol by the adrenal cortex. Stress and other stimuli increase the release of corticotropin-releasing factor *(CRF)* from hypothalamic paraventricular nuclei, and CRF is carried by hypophysioportal vessels to the anterior pituitary, where it stimulates the release of corticotropin *(ACTH)*. Corticotropin acts on the adrenal cortex to increase the release of adrenal steroids, although the release of aldosterone is primarily regulated by the renin-angiotensin system. Cortisol exerts feedback inhibition on the hypothalamus and pituitary to inhibit the release of CRF and corticotropin. *CRH,* Corticotropin-releasing hormone.

TABLE 33.1   Pharmacologic Properties of Selected Corticosteroids

DRUG[a]	ROUTE OF ADMINISTRATION	DURATION OF ACTION (HOURS)	MINERALOCORTICOID (SALT-RETAINING) POTENCY	GLUCOCORTICOID (ANTI-INFLAMMATORY) POTENCY
Short-acting drugs				
Hydrocortisone (cortisol)	Oral, parenteral, or topical	8–12	1	1
Cortisone	Oral, parenteral, or topical	8–12	0.8	0.8
Fludrocortisone	Oral	8–12	200	10
Intermediate-acting drugs				
Methylprednisolone	Oral, parenteral, or topical	12–36	0.5	5
Prednisone	Oral	12–36	0.7	3.5
Triamcinolone	Oral, parenteral, or topical	12–36	0	5
Long-acting drugs				
Betamethasone	Oral, parenteral, or topical	24–72	0	30
Dexamethasone	Oral, parenteral, or topical	24–72	0	30

[a]Fludrocortisone is classified as a mineralocorticoid; the other drugs are classified as glucocorticoids.

catabolism, thereby increasing the supply of amino acids needed for gluconeogenesis. Glucocorticoids **stimulate lipolysis** and inhibit the uptake of glucose by adipose tissue. By this mechanism, excessive glucocorticoid levels can lead to **abnormal fat distribution** and **muscle wasting** (see later).

CORTICOSTEROID DRUGS

A large number of semisynthetic **glucocorticoid** drugs are available; they are most frequently employed to attain the anti-inflammatory effects produced by supraphysiologic doses of these drugs. Less commonly, corticosteroids are used as replacement therapy in the treatment of **adrenal insufficiency** and in the treatment of **adrenogenital syndromes** that produce excessive quantities of adrenal androgens and insufficient quantities of other corticosteroids. **Mineralocorticoids** are primarily used as replacement therapy in persons with adrenal insufficiency. The properties of selected corticosteroids are listed in Table 33.1.

Mineralocorticoids

Aldosterone, the major mineralocorticoid in humans, is not suitable for clinical use owing to the potential for electrolyte disturbances. **Fludrocortisone** is a mineralocorticoid that is used as replacement therapy in patients with **primary adrenal insufficiency (Addison disease).** The drug's salt-retaining potency is about 20 times greater than its anti-inflammatory potency.

Glucocorticoids

A large number of glucocorticoid preparations are available for oral, parenteral, inhalational, or topical administration for the treatment of a wide range of inflammatory, allergic, autoimmune, and other disorders. Whenever possible, **topical** or **inhalational** administration is preferred because it is usually well tolerated and avoids most systemic adverse effects. Topical administration is widely used in the treatment of **allergic or inflammatory conditions** affecting the skin, mucous membranes, or eyes (see later). For example, topical ocular glucocorticoids are used to treat acute uveitis (inflammation of the iris, ciliary body, or choroid). Glucocorticoids are given by inhalation to treat allergic rhinitis, aspiration pneumonia, asthma, and other respiratory conditions (see Chapter 27).

Classification

The glucocorticoids are usually classified according to their **potency and duration of action** (see Table 33.1). When given systemically, the duration of action of glucocorticoids is primarily determined by their potency at the **glucocorticoid receptor,** rather than by their elimination half-life. This is because the highly potent drugs evoke a longer-lasting **stimulation of gene transcription** than do less-potent glucocorticoids. The potency of specific topical corticosteroids is discussed under the treatment of dermatologic conditions (see later).

Low-Potency, Short-Acting Glucocorticoids

Cortisol, the major glucocorticoid in humans, is called **hydrocortisone** when used as a pharmaceutical. **Cortisone** is rapidly metabolized to hydrocortisone by the liver after oral administration. Hydrocortisone has a duration of action of 8 to 12 hours, with equal glucocorticoid and mineralocorticoid effects. Hydrocortisone and cortisone are the preferred glucocorticoids when **replacement therapy** is needed for patients with **adrenal insufficiency.** These drugs are also used as anti-inflammatory agents, but more potent glucocorticoids are often preferred for treating most inflammatory, allergic, and autoimmune disorders.

Medium-Potency, Intermediate-Acting Glucocorticoids

Prednisone, prednisolone, methylprednisolone, and **triamcinolone** are the glucocorticoids used most often for systemic treatment. In the body, **prednisone** is rapidly **converted to prednisolone,** a substance that is itself available

as a drug. The intermediate-acting glucocorticoids have a duration of action of 12 to 36 hours and are often used to treat cancer, inflammation, allergy, and autoimmune disorders.

High-Potency, Long-Acting Glucocorticoids

Betamethasone and **dexamethasone** are stereoisomers that differ only in the configuration of a methyl group. **Betamethasone** is available for systemic use, and it is also used in the topical treatment of a number of skin disorders, including psoriasis, seborrheic or atopic dermatitis, and neurodermatitis. **Dexamethasone** is used in diagnostic **dexamethasone suppression tests** and in the treatment of a variety of neoplastic, infectious, and other inflammatory conditions that require the use of a potent and long-acting drug. **Budesonide** is a long-acting glucocorticoid administered by inhalation. Budesonide is also approved for the **treatment of ulcerative colitis** (see Chapter 28).

Deflazacort is a **corticosteroid prodrug,** whose **active metabolite,** 21-desDFZ, acts through the glucocorticoid receptor to exert anti-inflammatory and immunosuppressive effects. It is approved for the **treatment of Duchenne muscular dystrophy (DMD)** in patients 5 years of age and older.

Anti-inflammatory Effects

The anti-inflammatory effects of glucocorticoids are primarily attributable to their multiple actions on several types of leukocytes (see Fig. 33.3). First, glucocorticoids suppress the activation of T lymphocytes by interleukins and nuclear factor κB (NF-κB), a **transcription factor for proinflammatory cytokine genes.**

Second, they suppress the production of cytokines by activated helper T cells. Cytokines play a major role in inflammation by recruiting and activating eosinophils and by stimulating antibody production by B cells. Glucocorticoids inhibit the production of proinflammatory cytokines by

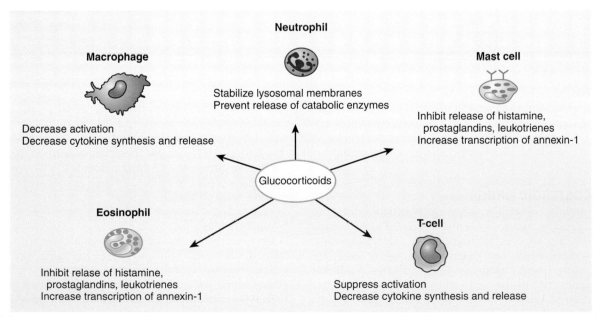

Fig. 33.3 Anti-inflammatory actions of glucocorticoids. Glucocorticoids act by suppressing T-cell activation, decreasing cytokine production and release, and preventing mast cells and eosinophils from releasing various chemical mediators of inflammation, including histamine, prostaglandins, leukotrienes, and other substances that cause tissue damage, vasodilation, and edema. They also have a number of actions on neutrophils and macrophages that reduce the chemical mediators of inflammation. Glucocorticoids have additional anti-inflammatory effects described in the text.

increasing the transcription of a gene for a protein that blocks NF-κB, as noted earlier.

Third, glucocorticoids decrease the release of various chemical mediators of inflammation, including histamine, prostaglandins, leukotrienes, and other substances from mast cells, eosinophils, and inflamed tissue. They decrease the synthesis of prostaglandins and leukotrienes by increasing the **transcription of annexin-1** (previously named *lipocortin-1*), which **inhibits phospholipase A,** the first step in the eicosanoid pathway (see Chapter 26).

Fourth, glucocorticoids **stabilize lysosomal membranes** of neutrophils and prevent the release of catabolic enzymes (e.g., acid phosphatase) from these organelles; this limits cytotoxic effects of inflammation.

Fifth, glucocorticoids cause vasoconstriction and decrease capillary permeability by **increased synthesis of annexin-1** leading to **decreased prostacyclin** by the mechanism outlined previously. They also decrease the synthesis of proinflammatory cytokines and other substances released from eosinophils in blood vessels as noted previously, and both actions **reduce the vasodilation and plasma extravasation** that are the signs of inflammation.

Finally, glucocorticoids decrease activation of macrophages and decrease the synthesis and release of cytokines from these cells.

Glucocorticoids also have multiple effects on **circulating leukocytes.** Pharmacologic doses of glucocorticoids suppress lymphoid tissue and reduce the number of circulating lymphocytes. They also reduce the concentration of circulating eosinophils, basophils, and monocytes, while at the same time increasing the concentration of erythrocytes, platelets, and polymorphonuclear leukocytes.

Indications

Glucocorticoids are used for the diagnosis and treatment of adrenal diseases and for the treatment of a diverse group of nonadrenal disorders.

Inflammation, Allergy, and Autoimmune Disorders

The glucocorticoids are frequently used to **suppress inflammation and immune dysfunction** associated with diseases affecting almost every organ in the body. Glucocorticoids counteract inflammation evoked by physical trauma, extreme temperatures, noxious chemicals, radiation damage, and microbial pathogens. They also suppress inflammation caused by allergic and autoimmune reactions and other disease states. Examples of diseases treated with corticosteroids include systemic **lupus erythematosus, autoimmune thrombocytopenia purpura, polyarteritis nodosa, multiple sclerosis, ulcerative colitis,** and **polymyositis.**

Several glucocorticoids, including **beclomethasone** and **mometasone,** are available for nasal insufflation or oral inhalation to treat **allergic rhinitis** or **asthma,** respectively. Inhaled glucocorticoids are often first-line therapy for these disorders, and their administration and use are described in Chapter 27. **Ciclesonide** is a newer agent also indicated for hay fever or allergic rhinitis.

For corneal inflammation and keratitis, many glucocorticoids are available in eyedrops, including a new combination of **loteprednol** and the antibiotic **tobramycin** (ZYLET). **Difluprednate** is a new eyedrop formulation indicated for the inflammation and pain associated with ocular surgery.

There are also combinations for the treatment of superficial bacterial infections of the external auditory canal (swimmer's ear) containing **hydrocortisone** and **neomycin** (CORTISPORIN).

Cancer

Because of their lymphotoxic effects, glucocorticoids are used in the treatment of **lymphocytic leukemias** and **lymphomas** (see Chapter 45). **Dexamethasone** is a long-acting glucocorticoid used in combination with other drugs to prevent emesis during cancer chemotherapy.

Respiratory Distress Syndrome

Betamethasone is used to prevent respiratory distress syndrome in premature infants. It acts by promoting fetal lung maturation in the same manner as endogenous cortisol does. Betamethasone is used because it is not highly protein bound and will readily enter the placental circulation.

Adrenal Insufficiency

In primary adrenal insufficiency **(Addison disease),** all regions of the adrenal cortex are destroyed. This gives rise to deficiencies in cortisol and aldosterone and to a reduction in androgen secretion. **Secondary adrenal insufficiency** has several causes, but it most commonly results when steroid drugs are used for a prolonged time, thereby suppressing the hypothalamic-pituitary-adrenal axis. Secondary disease is characterized by low levels of cortisol and androgens but normal levels of aldosterone.

Acute adrenal insufficiency (adrenal crisis, addisonian crisis) is a medical emergency that must be treated promptly with intravenously administered hydrocortisone for up to 48 hours. Once the patient's condition is stabilized, long-term oral hydrocortisone treatment can be instituted.

In the treatment of **chronic adrenal insufficiency,** hydrocortisone is administered orally in a manner that mimics the circadian secretion of cortisol by the normal adrenal gland, with two-thirds of the daily dose given in the morning and one-third given in the evening. If hyperkalemia is still present after the oral hydrocortisone dose is stabilized, the addition of a mineralocorticoid to the treatment regimen is usually required. A single daily dose of **fludrocortisone,** given in the morning, is often used for this purpose.

Congenital Adrenal Hyperplasia

Congenital adrenal hyperplasia (CAH) refers to a group of disorders caused by specific enzyme deficiencies that **impair the synthesis of cortisol and aldosterone.** Impaired synthesis leads to a compensatory increase in corticotropin secretion by the pituitary and results in adrenal hyperplasia. Because of the enzyme deficiencies, the steroid biosynthetic pathway **shifts** to the production of adrenal androgens, thereby resulting in virilization (masculinization) and pseudohermaphroditism in girls, and precocious development of secondary sex characteristics, including the genitals (macrogenitosomia), in boys. The most common defect is **21-hydroxylase deficiency,** which accounts for 90% of cases of CAH. The second most common defect is **11β-hydroxylase deficiency,** which accounts for 9% of cases. CAH is treated by giving **hydrocortisone** to suppress the secretion of corticotropin. **Fludrocortisone** can be given to provide additional mineralocorticoid activity for salt-losing patients with CAH.

Cushing Syndrome

Adrenocortical hyperfunction (Cushing syndrome), which is caused by excessive levels of circulating corticotropin, is treated with surgery, irradiation, and adrenal steroid inhibitors (Box 33.1). Cushing syndrome most often results from a **pituitary adenoma** that produces excessive quantities of corticotropin, leading to adrenal hyperplasia and excessive cortisol production. Other causes of Cushing syndrome include adrenal adenomas, adrenal carcinomas, and ectopic corticotropin (ACTH)-secreting tumors.

The diagnosis of Cushing syndrome is often based on the free cortisol level in urine samples and on the results of testing with dexamethasone. In the **low-dose dexamethasone suppression test,** a single dose of dexamethasone is given orally at 11:00 PM, and cortisol levels in plasma are measured at 8:00 AM the following morning. In healthy individuals, dexamethasone will suppress corticotropin secretion by the pituitary and cause plasma cortisol levels to be under 5 mcg/dL. In persons with Cushing syndrome, dexamethasone will not suppress corticotropin secretion, so the cortisol level will usually exceed 10 mcg/dL. The **high-dose dexamethasone suppression test** can be used to differentiate adrenal hyperplasia from other causes of hyperadrenocorticism.

Cushing syndrome is usually treated by surgical excision of the pituitary adenoma or the hyperplastic adrenal glands. Patients must receive hydrocortisone parenterally in large doses during the surgical procedure. The dose is then gradually tapered to normal replacement levels.

BOX 33.1 THE CASE OF THE MOON-FACED MAN

CASE PRESENTATION

A 49-year-old man with a history of cigarette smoking notices recent weight gain of about 15 pounds in the last few months. He is puzzled by this as he watches his diet and gets moderate exercise in his job as a construction foreman. His wife says that his face looks "puffy" and he has stretch marks on his stomach. On questioning by his physician, he admits to having felt tired lately, and physical examination reveals a small fatty hump on his back. The physician orders a low-dose dexamethasone suppression test, which results in no change of the man's elevated levels of cortisol; a similar finding is found after a high-dose dexamethasone test. Given the history of smoking, imaging studies including chest radiographs and computed tomography (CT) scans are done and reveal small cell (oat cell) carcinoma of the lungs. He is prescribed metyrapone to treat Cushing syndrome and is told he has less than a year to live.

CASE DISCUSSION

Pituitary adenomas, which are benign tumors of the pituitary gland, are the cause of most cases of noniatrogenic Cushing syndrome. This form of Cushing syndrome, known as *Cushing disease,* affects women five times more frequently than men. Corticotropin (ACTH) can also be produced outside ("ectopic") the pituitary from benign or malignant tumors. In many cases, more frequently in men than in women, small oat cell lung tumors are the cause. More rarely, an abnormality of the adrenal glands, most often an adrenal tumor, causes Cushing syndrome. In the case of the moon-faced man, both suppression tests came back with no change in the elevated cortisol levels, suggesting that a pituitary adenoma was not the cause. Many cancer cells secrete excess levels of adrenal cortical hormones, including cortisol and adrenal androgens. Given the patient's history of smoking, it is likely his Cushing syndrome was related to an ectopic ACTH-producing tumor. Metyrapone inhibits the synthesis of glucocorticoids by inhibiting the 11β-hydroxylase enzyme that catalyzes the final step in the glucocorticoid pathway. Metyrapone is occasionally used to treat Cushing syndrome in patients whose condition is refractory to other treatments and who are not candidates for surgery, as in this case. An alternative is aminoglutethimide, which inhibits the conversion of cholesterol to pregnenolone, an early and rate-limiting step in adrenal steroid biosynthesis.

Dermatologic Conditions

Corticosteroids are often used to treat a wide range of dermatologic conditions, including **atopic (contact)** and **seborrheic dermatitis, pruritus** (itching) from various causes, psoriasis, sunburn, and a number of other conditions. Topical corticosteroids are grouped according to their relative anti-inflammatory potency (high, medium, and low). Low-potency drugs are preferred for treating areas with thinner skin (e.g., the face, eyes) and intertriginous areas where skin is folded or overlapped. Low- to medium-potency steroids can be used on the ears, trunk, arms, legs, and scalp. Medium- to very-high-potency drugs may be needed to treat disorders in areas of thicker skin (e.g., the palms and soles).

The type of lesion influences the choice of vehicle for drug administration. Ointments are preferred to treat disorders involving dry, cracked, scaly, or hardened skin. Lotions and creams are best for treating moist, weeping lesions or conditions with intense inflammation. Lotions and gels are usually more convenient for applying steroids to hairy areas.

Low-potency topical steroids include hydrocortisone, which is available without prescription for treating minor allergic reactions (e.g., insect bites). Other low-potency topical steroids include desonide and dexamethasone. **Medium-potency topical steroids** include triamcinolone and fluticasone. Desoximetasone and fluocinonide are **high-potency steroids,** whereas betamethasone dipropionate and clobetasol are **very-high-potency steroids.**

Other Disorders

Glucocorticoids are used to treat **hypercalcemia,** and they are the drugs of choice for managing **sarcoidosis** (a systemic granulomatous disorder). Glucocorticoids are also used as immunosuppressant drugs to prevent **organ graft rejection** (see Chapter 45).

Systemic Administration and Pharmacokinetics

Glucocorticoids are highly lipid soluble and are well absorbed from the gut after oral administration. In the circulation the glucocorticoids are highly bound to corticosteroid-binding globulin and albumin. Glucocorticoids are oxidized by cytochrome P450 enzymes and conjugated with sulfate or glucuronide in the liver before undergoing renal excretion.

Glucocorticoids are administered orally to treat **allergic reactions, autoimmune disorders, neoplastic diseases,** and many other conditions. For acute disorders, glucocorticoids are often more effective when they are initially given in large doses that are gradually tapered over several days until treatment is discontinued. For severe autoimmune and inflammatory disorders (e.g., systemic lupus erythematous and polymyositis with dermatomyositis), large doses of prednisone must be given daily for several months until a remission is achieved, and then the dose is slowly tapered and continued for 1 to 2 years or longer. In some conditions, it may be possible to convert the patient to **alternate-day therapy,** in which all or most of the dose is given on alternate days. This dosage schedule appears to reduce the severity of adverse effects and produces less suppression of the hypothalamic-pituitary-adrenal axis by allowing more time for recovery between doses.

Glucocorticoids are administered parenterally to treat **acute adrenal crises, acute allergic reactions,** and **similar emergencies.** In some cases, the drugs are given intravenously. In other cases, they are given intramuscularly, either as a rapidly absorbed solution or as a slowly absorbed drug suspension (depot preparation). Depot preparations are useful in providing a sustained level of the drug for several weeks, as is sometimes necessary in the treatment of a severe allergic reaction.

Adverse Effects

Administration of supraphysiologic doses of glucocorticoids for more than 2 weeks produces a series of tissue and metabolic changes that result in a form of **Cushing syndrome.** The face becomes rounded and puffy ("moon face") as fat is redistributed to the face and trunk from the extremities. Fat accumulation in the supraclavicular and dorsocervical areas contributes to the development of a buffalo hump. Increased hair growth (hirsutism), weight gain, and muscle wasting and weakness are often observed. Dermatologic changes can include acne (steroid acne), bruising, and thinning of the skin.

Other metabolic and physiologic changes caused by glucocorticoid administration include **hyperglycemia, glucose intolerance,** and **hypertension.** Some changes, such as sodium retention, potassium loss, and hypertension, are more common when cortisone or hydrocortisone is used because these drugs have greater mineralocorticoid activity than do other glucocorticoids.

Glucocorticoids increase bone catabolism and antagonize the effect of vitamin D on calcium absorption, thereby contributing to the development of **osteoporosis** (see Chapter 36). Glucocorticoids also have several effects on the central nervous system. They alter the mood in some persons and can cause **euphoria** or **psychosis.** Large doses of glucocorticoids stimulate gastric acid and pepsin production and may thereby exacerbate peptic ulcers. Glucocorticoids can also reduce the secretion of thyroid-stimulating hormone and follicle-stimulating hormone by the pituitary gland.

Long-term use of glucocorticoids can cause posterior subcapsular **cataracts** and **glaucoma,** and it can mask the symptoms and signs of mycotic and other infections. In children, long-term use can cause growth retardation.

For these reasons, glucocorticoids should be avoided or used with caution in patients with psychoses, peptic ulcers, heart diseases, hypertension, diabetes, osteoporosis, and certain infections.

ADRENAL ANDROGENS

DHEA is the major androgen secreted by the adrenal cortex. Smaller quantities of **androstenedione** and **testosterone** are also secreted by the adrenal gland.

DHEA is an extremely weak androgen, but it is partly converted to testosterone in the body. In humans, studies show that the production of DHEA by the adrenal gland **declines in a linear fashion** after the age of 20 years. In animals, studies indicate that DHEA protects against the development of diabetes mellitus, immune disorders, and cancer. DHEA also appears to prevent weight gain and prolong life in some species. For these reasons, the use of DHEA supplements has been adopted uncritically by the alternative medicine–health store culture. Although some evidence suggests beneficial effects of DHEA in the elderly and other people, much remains to be learned about the clinical utility of this steroid (see below).

Because DHEA is a weak androgen, it should **not be used by men with prostate cancer.**

CORTICOSTEROID SYNTHESIS INHIBITORS

Fig. 33.1 also shows the sites of action of three inhibitors of corticosteroid synthesis: **metyrapone, ketoconazole,** and **fluconazole.**

Metyrapone

Metyrapone inhibits the synthesis of glucocorticoids by **inhibiting the 11β-hydroxylase** enzyme that catalyzes the final step in the glucocorticoid pathway. As a result of this action, the steroid biosynthetic pathway is shifted to the production of adrenal androgens. Metyrapone is occasionally used to treat **Cushing syndrome** in patients whose condition is refractory to other treatments and who are not candidates for surgery. Metyrapone is also sometimes used in tests of adrenal function and for preparing patients for surgery.

Osilodrostat is a cortisol synthesis inhibitor indicated for the treatment of adult patients with Cushing disease for whom pituitary surgery is not an option or has not been curative. **Osilodrostat, like metyrapone** inhibits the synthesis of glucocorticoids by **inhibiting the 11β-hydroxylase** enzyme that catalyzes the final step in the glucocorticoid pathway.

Ketoconazole and Fluconazole

Ketoconazole and **fluconazole** are antifungal drugs (see Chapter 42) that inhibit several cytochrome P450 enzymes involved in steroid biosynthesis, **including 11β-hydroxylase.** When used in the treatment of **Cushing syndrome,** the drugs can lower the amount of cortisol to the normal range for some patients. They also inhibit androgen synthesis, however, and may cause **gynecomastia** in male patients.

CORTICOSTEROID RECEPTOR ANTAGONISTS

Spironolactone

Spironolactone is a synthetic steroid that competes with aldosterone for the mineralocorticoid (aldosterone) receptor in the renal tubules. It is used as a **potassium-sparing diuretic** (see Chapter 13) and as an agent for the treatment of hyperaldosteronism. Spironolactone is the drug of choice for **primary hyperaldosteronism** caused by bilateral adrenal hyperplasia, whereas surgery is the treatment of choice for hyperaldosteronism caused by an aldosterone-producing adenoma. **Secondary hyperaldosteronism**

associated with heart failure, Bartter syndrome, and other conditions may also be improved by the administration of spironolactone.

Mifepristone

Mifepristone is an antagonist at both progesterone and glucocorticoid receptors (see Chapter 34). It has been studied for the treatment of **Cushing syndrome** and is effective in reversing some effects of **hyperadrenocorticism,** including high blood sugar. **Mifepristone** (as KORLYM) was recently approved for the treatment of hyperglycemia in patients with Cushing syndrome.

DHEA USE IN OLDER MEN

DHEA has the status of a dietary supplement in the United States and is freely available over-the-counter in health-food stores or other overpriced venues. **DHEA** is touted as the "fountain of youth" by the supplement industry and widely used as an **antiaging medicine.** The plasma levels of DHEA do decrease with age in men, reaching a low of only 10% to 20% the amount present in a young adult male. Studies show a **positive relationship between DHEA levels and muscle mass, muscle strength, mobility, and a lower risk for falls.** Decreased levels of DHEA were correlated to erectile dysfunction in men.

Administration of DHEA supplements was shown to **increase muscle mass and strength,** as well as endurance and other physical performance parameters in elderly men. Sexual function was also improved. As **DHEA precedes testosterone in the biosynthetic pathway** (see Fig. 33.1), it can be considered a **prodrug,** and it is likely that many of the health benefits are **due to additional testosterone,** as well as DHEA itself. The side effects of DHEA include mild acne, seborrhea, and facial hair growth, much like testosterone. Although the popularity of DHEA self-administration is likely to continue as long as it is freely available, there are no long-term studies on its chronic use and the resulting risks of cardiovascular disease and malignancies.

SUMMARY OF IMPORTANT POINTS

- The adrenal gland secretes mineralocorticoids (primarily aldosterone), glucocorticoids (primarily cortisol), and adrenal androgens (primarily dehydroepiandrosterone [DHEA]).
- Mineralocorticoids have salt-retaining activity. They include fludrocortisone, a short-acting drug used to supplement hydrocortisone (cortisol) treatment in patients with adrenal insufficiency.
- Glucocorticoids increase gluconeogenesis, protein and lipid catabolism, and the body's resistance to stress. They reduce inflammation by inhibiting the migration of leukocytes and the production and release of cytokines, prostaglandins, leukotrienes, and other mediators of inflammation. They also stabilize lysosomal membranes and cause vasoconstriction.
- Glucocorticoids are chiefly used as anti-inflammatory and immunosuppressive drugs in the treatment of a wide range of allergic, inflammatory, and autoimmune disorders. They are also used as replacement therapy in the treatment of primary adrenal insufficiency (Addison disease) and CAH.
- Glucocorticoids include short-acting drugs (cortisone and hydrocortisone), intermediate-acting drugs (methylprednisolone, prednisone, and triamcinolone), and long-acting drugs (betamethasone and dexamethasone).
- In comparison with cortisol, most synthetic glucocorticoids have increased glucocorticoid potency and decreased mineralocorticoid potency.
- Glucocorticoids are generally administered topically to treat skin, mucous membrane, and ocular disorders and by inhalation to treat allergic rhinitis and asthma.
- Topical steroids for treating dermatologic conditions include desonide (low potency), triamcinolone and fluticasone (medium potency), desoximetasone (high potency), and clobetasol (very high potency).
- In patients with acute allergic reactions, glucocorticoids are initially given in large doses. The doses are rapidly tapered and eventually discontinued. In patients with severe autoimmune and inflammatory diseases, large doses of prednisone or other glucocorticoids may be required for several months. Alternate-day therapy is preferred for their long-term administration.
- Adverse effects of glucocorticoids include fat accumulation in the face and trunk, muscle wasting, skin changes, glucose intolerance, potassium depletion, osteoporosis, hypertension, and cataracts.
- Aminoglutethimide, metyrapone, and ketoconazole inhibit various steps in corticosteroid biosynthesis and are occasionally used to diagnose and treat adrenal hyperplasia.

Review Questions

1. After receiving a low dose of dexamethasone, a patient is found to have a plasma cortisol level of 20 mcg/dL the next morning. Which disorder is most likely in this patient?
   (A) congenital adrenal hyperplasia
   (B) chronic adrenal insufficiency
   (C) 11β-hydroxylase deficiency
   (D) Cushing syndrome
   (E) pituitary insufficiency
2. A boy experiences a moderately severe reaction to a wasp sting. Which method of corticosteroid administration is appropriate for this patient?
   (A) continuous high-dose therapy for several weeks
   (B) continuous low-dose therapy for several weeks
   (C) gradually increasing doses over several days
   (D) gradually decreasing doses over several days
   (E) intermittent every-other-day therapy until symptoms resolve

3. A patient with Addison disease continues to have hyperkalemia despite receiving adequate replacement doses of hydrocortisone (cortisol). Which drug should be added to the treatment regimen to reduce serum potassium levels?
   (A) dexamethasone
   (B) fludrocortisone
   (C) triamcinolone
   (D) prednisone
   (E) aldosterone

4. The long-term administration of large doses of prednisone will cause the least reduction in the secretion of which hormone?
   (A) cortisol
   (B) corticotropin
   (C) corticotropin-releasing hormone
   (D) aldosterone

5. A woman has developed a moderately severe contact dermatitis reaction to a cosmetic preparation on her face and eyes. Which topical corticosteroid would be most suitable for treating this condition?
   (A) desonide
   (B) prednisone
   (C) clobetasol
   (D) fluocinonide
   (E) desoximetasone

Fertility and Reproduction Drugs

CLASSIFICATION OF DRUGS AFFECTING FERTILITY AND REPRODUCTION

Estrogens

- Estradiol (ALORA, CLIMARA)[a]
- Conjugated equine estrogens (MENEST, PREMARIN)

Progestins

- Medroxyprogesterone (PROVERA, DEPO-PROVERA)
- Hydroxyprogesterone caproate (MAKENA)[b]
- Norethindrone (AYGESTIN, CAMILA, ERRIN)[c]

Long-Acting Reversible Contraceptives (LARCs)

- Etonongestrel/ethinyl estradiol vaginal ring (NUVARING)[d]
- Norelgestromin/ethinyl estradiol transdermal system (XULANE)
- Etonogestrel implant (NEXPLANON)
- Copper intrauterine device (PARAGARD T 380A)
- Levonorgestrel intrauterine device (MIRENA)

Emergency Contraceptives

- Ulipristal acetate (ELLA)
- Levonorgestrel (PLAN B)

Selective Estrogen Receptor Modulators (SERMs)

- Clomiphene (CLOMID)[e]
- Ospemifene (OSPHENA)[f]

Selective Estrogen Receptor Degrader (SERD)

- Fulvestrant (FASLODEX)

Antiprogestins

- Mifepristone (MIFEPREX)

Aromatase Inhibitors

- Anastrozole (ARIMIDEX)
- Letrozole (FEMARA)

Androgens

- Testosterone (AndroGel, Androderm, Delatestryl, Striant)[g]
- Testosterone cypionate (Depo-Testosterone)
- Methyltestosterone (Testred)
- Danazol (Danocrine)

Antiandrogens

- Flutamide[h]
- Finasteride (PROPECIA, PROSCAR)[i]

Agents for Treating Dysmenorrhea and Female Sexual Dysfunction

- Mefenamic acid (PONSTEL)[j]
- Elagolix (ORILISSA)[k]
- Bremelanotide (VYLEESI)
- Flibanserin (ADDYI)

Drugs Used in Obstetrics

- Methyldopa (ALDOMET)[l]
- Terbutaline (BRETHINE)
- Dinoprostone (CERVIDIL)[m]
- Oxytocin (PITOCIN)
- Doxylamine with vitamin B_6 (DICLEGIS)[n]
- Brexanolone (ZULRESSO)

---

[a] Also ethinyl estradiol, estradiol cypionate, estradiol valerate, and mestranol.
[b] Also megestrol (MEGACE) and progesterone (PROMETRIUM).
[c] Also desogestrel, drospirenone, levonorgestrel, norelgestromin, norethynodrel, and norgestimate.
[d] Also seqesterone/ethinyl estradiol vaginal ring (Annovera).
[e] Also raloxifene (Evista), tamoxifen (Soltamox), and toremifene (Fareston).
[f] Also a formulation of conjugated estrogens with baxedoxifine (Duavee).
[g] Also oxandrolone (Oxandrin) and fluoxymesterone (Androxy).
[h] Also bicalutamide (Casodex), enzalutamide (Xtandi), apalutamide (Erleada), darolutamide (Nubeqa), and nilutamide (Nilandron).
[i] Also dutasteride (Avodart).
[j] Also diclofenac, ibuprofen, ketoprofen, meclofenamate, and naproxen.
[k] Also in a combination formulation of elagolix, estradiol, and norethindrone (Oriahnn).
[l] Also labetalol, nifedipine, hydralazine, and magnesium sulfate.
[m] Also misoprostol (Cytotec).
[n] Also in higher dosage, the extended-release form Bonjesta.

OVERVIEW

Human reproduction involves a cascade of hormonal secretions, beginning with the secretion of gonadotropin-releasing hormone (GnRH) from the hypothalamus. As described in Chapter 31, GnRH stimulates the pituitary to release two gonadotropins: follicle-stimulating hormone (FSH) and luteinizing hormone (LH). These gonadotropins then stimulate the production of **steroid hormones** and **gametes** (germ cells) by the ovary in females and by the testis in the males.

The three categories of steroids secreted by the gonads are (1) **estrogens,** which include **estradiol, estrone,** and **estriol;** (2) **progestins,** which include **progesterone;** and (3) **androgens,** which include **testosterone.** Estrogens, progesterone, and testosterone are produced in both males and females, but the relative amounts and patterns of secretion differ markedly between the sexes. Females primarily secrete estrogens and progesterone, whereas males primarily produce testosterone.

Biosynthesis of Gonadal Steroids

As shown in Fig. 34.1, **pregnenolone** is the precursor to progesterone. It is also the precursor to dehydroepiandrosterone and androstenedione (two androgens secreted by the adrenal gland and discussed in Chapter 33) and to testosterone (the major androgen in males). The adrenal and gonadal androgens are converted to estrogens by **aromatase,** an enzyme that forms the aromatic A-ring necessary for the selective high-affinity binding of estradiol, estrone, and estriol to **estrogen receptors (ERs).**

In females, **ovarian thecal cells** secrete small quantities of testosterone. In males, approximately 95% of testosterone is produced by **Leydig cells** in the testes, and the remainder is derived from the **adrenal cortex.** Testosterone is synthesized in the testes by the same pathways as in the ovaries. Testosterone is subsequently converted to **dihydrotestosterone** (DHT) by **5α-reductase** in the prostate, hair follicles, and skin. In the plasma, testosterone is primarily bound to sex steroid–binding globulin. In the liver, it is converted to androstenedione and other metabolites, including sulfate and glucuronide conjugates of testosterone. Approximately 90% of these metabolites are excreted in the urine.

Although both testosterone and DHT activate **androgen receptors,** DHT has greater receptor affinity and forms a more stable receptor-ligand complex than testosterone. If DHT formation is inhibited, this significantly reduces androgenic stimulation of the prostate gland and hair follicles. The androgen receptor located in target cells interacts with **response elements in target genes** and thereby stimulates gene transcription and protein synthesis in the same manner as other gonadal steroids (see ERs later).

Hormonal Actions of Estrogens and Progesterone

In females, estrogens and progesterone have multiple actions and interactions that are necessary for reproductive activity. Estrogens are formed in the **granulosa cells** of the ovary, whereas progesterone is primarily produced by the **corpus luteum** in response to LH secretion. Estrogens promote the development and growth of the fallopian tubes, uterus, and vagina, as well as secondary sex characteristics such as breast development, skeletal growth, and axillary and pubic hair patterns.

The pattern of hormonal changes occurring during the **menstrual cycle** is depicted in Fig. 34.2. During the **follicular phase** of the cycle, ovarian follicles are recruited and a dominant estrogen-secreting follicle develops. Estrogen levels gradually increase, whereas progesterone levels remain very low. A surge of LH is released at midcycle in response to **positive estrogen feedback** to the pituitary gland, and this **LH surge** triggers ovulation. During the **luteal phase** of the cycle, the follicle becomes the *corpus luteum* ("yellow body") that secretes both estrogen and progesterone in response to LH. Together, these hormones prepare the uterus for implantation of a fertilized egg as the endometrium becomes more vascular and secretory. If pregnancy does not occur, the corpus luteum ceases to produce estrogen and progesterone, resulting in endometrial sloughing and menstruation. If pregnancy occurs, the placenta produces human chorionic gonadotropin, which maintains the production of progesterone by the corpus luteum. After approximately 3 months, the placenta becomes the predominant source of progesterone. This hormone serves to maintain pregnancy and prevents endometrial sloughing and miscarriage.

Estrogens have a number of other actions important in reproduction and other bodily functions. They sensitize the myometrium to oxytocin at parturition, and this facilitates labor. They stimulate protein synthesis in the brain and may thereby affect mood and emotions. Estrogens influence the distribution of body fat and thereby contribute to the development of feminine body contours. They enhance blood coagulation by increasing the synthesis of clotting factors, and they prevent osteoporosis by inhibiting bone resorption. Estrogens are responsible for epiphyseal closure in both males and females, which halts linear bone growth.

Estrogens and progestins have different effects on serum lipoprotein levels. Estrogens decrease the levels of **low-density lipoprotein (LDL) cholesterol** and **lipoprotein (a)** while increasing the levels of **high-density lipoprotein (HDL) cholesterol.** In contrast, progestins produce a dose-related increase in LDL levels and a decrease in HDL levels.

Progesterone and other progestins increase basal body temperature by 0.5°C to 0.8°C (1.0°F to 1.5°F) at ovulation and throughout the luteal phase, which enables timing of ovulation. They also affect the emotional state and have mild mineralocorticoid (salt-retaining) properties. Some of the synthetic progestins have other effects attributed to their androgenic activity (see later).

Hormonal Actions of Testosterone

LH stimulates testosterone synthesis in **Leydig cells,** whereas FSH promotes spermatogenesis by **Sertoli cells** in the seminiferous tubules. These cells provide an environment rich in testosterone, which is necessary for germ cell development. Sertoli cells also produce a protein called **inhibin,** which acts in concert with DHT as a feedback regulator of FSH secretion by the pituitary.

Testosterone is responsible for the development of primary and secondary **sex characteristics** in males during **puberty.** It promotes sexual function by stimulating growth of the penis, scrotum, seminal vesicles, and prostate gland, and it causes growth of the larynx, thickening of the vocal cords, and growth of facial, axillary, and pubic hair. Testosterone and other androgens also increase lean body mass and skeletal growth and eventually accelerate epiphyseal closure. In addition, testosterone contributes to the development of acne in both sexes by increasing sebaceous gland activity and sebum production. **Androgens** also increase the production of **erythropoietin** in the kidneys and **decrease levels of HDL cholesterol.**

ESTROGENS AND PROGESTIN DRUGS

An estrogen or progestin preparation can be used alone for the treatment of various disorders, or the two preparations can be used in combination for **hormone replacement therapy** (HRT) in postmenopausal women or for **contraception** in women of childbearing age.

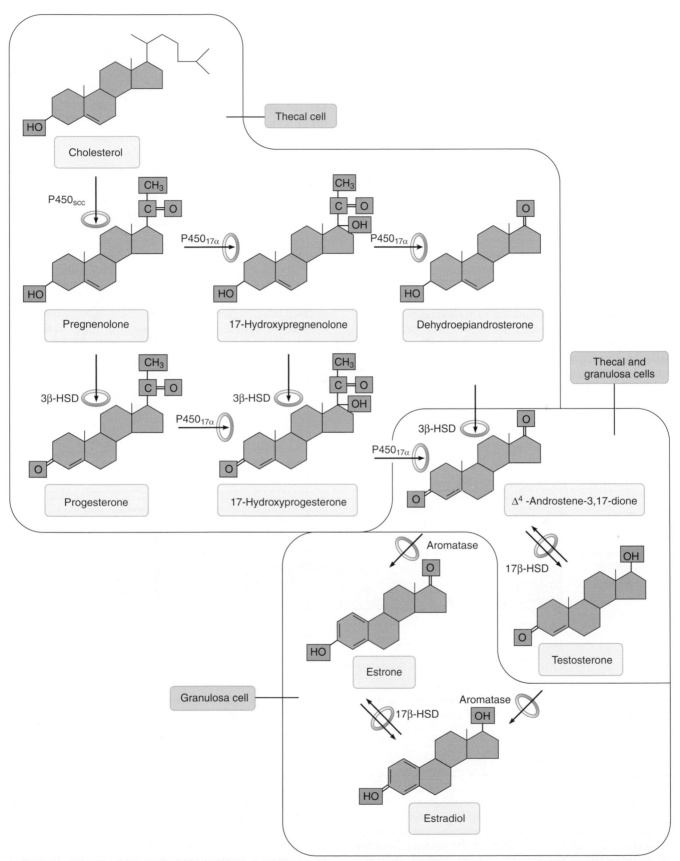

Fig. 34.1 Biosynthesis of sex steroids. In the ovary, pregnenolone is converted to androstenedione and testosterone in thecal cells. These steroids are then converted to estrone and estradiol in granulosa cells. Enzymes involved in these steps include the cholesterol side-chain cleavage enzyme *(P450scc)*, steroid 17α-hydroxylase *(P450$_{17\alpha}$)*, 3β-hydroxysteroid dehydrogenase *(3β-HSD)*, 17β-hydroxysteroid dehydrogenase *(17β-HSD)*, and aromatase. Estrone and estradiol are partly converted to estriol by other enzymes. After ovulation, the major product of thecal cells is progesterone, owing to the development of a relative deficiency of 17α-hydroxylase activity.

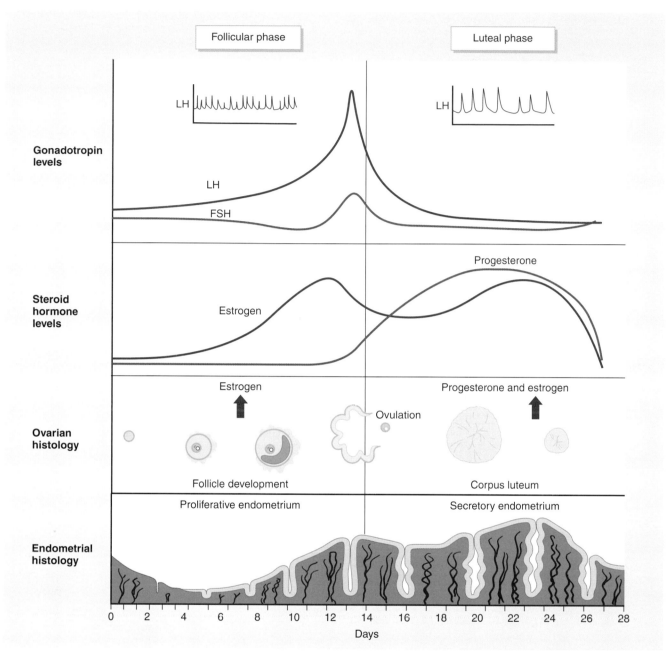

FIG. 34.2 Hormone secretion during the human menstrual cycle. Luteinizing hormone *(LH)* and follicle-stimulating hormone *(FSH)* are released in a pulsatile manner from the pituitary gland in response to the pulsatile secretion of gonadotropin-releasing hormone (GnRH) from the hypothalamus. FSH stimulates ovarian follicle development and the secretion of estrogen during the follicular phase of the cycle. After ovulation, the corpus luteum produces both estrogen and progesterone during the luteal phase. Estrogen decreases FSH and LH secretion during most of the cycle (feedback inhibition) while provoking the midcycle LH and FSH surge that triggers ovulation. Progesterone decreases the frequency of hypothalamic GnRH pulses and the frequency of pulsatile LH and FSH secretion *(inset in top panel)*. During the luteal phase, progesterone increases the amount of LH released (pulse amplitude). Estrogen stimulates the proliferation of the endometrium during the follicular phase, whereas progesterone causes the endometrium to become more vascular and secretory during the luteal phase.

Estrogens

Mechanism of Action

Estradiol and other estrogens bind to ERs found inside and on the surface of target cells of the reproductive system and elsewhere. The ERs are members of the **nuclear hormone receptor family,** which includes adrenal steroid, androgen, progesterone, and thyroid hormone receptors. There are two molecular forms of the cytosolic ER, which combine to form homodimers and heterodimers upon activation by estrogen. The ER dimers translocate to the nucleus, bind to estrogen response elements of DNA, and interact with coactivators and corepressors of **gene transcription,** leading to expression of proteins mediating estrogen's hormonal effects.

Preparations and Disposition

A variety of substances have estrogenic activity, including steroidal estrogens produced by vertebrate animals as well as nonsteroidal estrogens obtained from plants (phytoestrogens). Estrogens contained in pharmaceutical preparations include **estradiol, estradiol esters,** and **sulfate esters of**

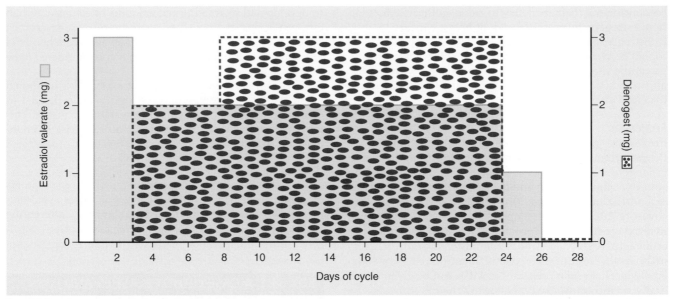

FIG. 34.3 The estrogen and progestin content of a multiphasic oral contraceptive (NATAZIA). In this preparation, the amount of estrogen (estradiol valerate) is sequentially stepped down during the administration cycle, while the amount of progestin (dienogest) is stepped up.

estrone, and **equilin** obtained from the **urine of pregnant mares** and known as **conjugated or esterified equine estrogens.** In addition, semisynthetic derivatives of estradiol are available and described later.

Estradiol, or more precisely **17β-estradiol,** is the **predominant estrogen in humans** and many other animals. It is an 18-carbon steroid with a phenolic (fully unsaturated) A-ring (see Fig. 34.1). Estradiol preparations are available for oral, parenteral, topical, and transdermal administration. Orally administered estradiol preparations such as ESTRACE contain micronized estradiol particles that improve oral bioavailability. Vaginal estradiol tablets and a topical emulsion are also available, as well as a vaginal ring that slowly releases estradiol.

Several long-acting formulations of estradiol are available for intramuscular or transdermal administration. **Estradiol cypionate** and **estradiol valerate** are esters of estradiol that are slowly absorbed after **intramuscular injection.** They are hydrolyzed to estradiol in the liver and blood and provide effective plasma concentrations of estradiol for **several weeks.** Estradiol valerate is also contained in a variable dose oral contraceptive (NATAZIA), in which the estrogen dose is stepped up and the progestin dose is stepped down during each menstrual cycle (Fig. 34.3). **Transdermal estradiol systems** slowly release estradiol for absorption through the skin. These preparations are formulated for twice-weekly or weekly application.

Ethinyl estradiol and **mestranol** are **semisynthetic** derivatives of estradiol modified by the addition of an ethinyl group, which reduces first-pass metabolism, increases the **half-life to approximately 20 hours,** and results in greater oral potency compared with native estradiol. These agents are primarily used in estrogen-progestin **oral contraceptives.**

Conjugated equine estrogens are hydrolyzed to **estrone** and **equilin** before absorption from the gut. They undergo relatively little first-pass metabolism and can be converted in the liver to sulfate and glucuronide conjugates excreted in the urine. In addition, estrone is partly **converted to the more active estradiol.** After their absorption, estrogens are

highly bound to sex steroid–binding globulin in the plasma and are widely distributed to tissues and concentrated in fat. Estrogens undergo enterohepatic cycling, in which conjugated metabolites are excreted in the bile and converted to free estrogens by intestinal bacteria. The free estrogens are then reabsorbed into the circulation. As with estrone and equilin, estradiol is metabolized to sulfate and glucuronide conjugates in the liver, which are primarily excreted in the urine with small amounts excreted in the feces.

Indications

Estrogen preparations are used in the treatment of **primary hypogonadism,** including cases caused by surgical oophorectomy, menopause, and other causes. Micronized estradiol, transdermal estradiol, and conjugated equine estrogens are primarily used for **HRT** (see later) in postmenopausal women. New low-dose and ultralow-dose preparations are available for this purpose, containing 0.3 mg conjugated estrogens or 0.5 mg estradiol, respectively. **Combination estrogen-progestin preparations** contain either ethinyl estradiol or mestranol. These estrogen-progestin combinations are used for **oral contraception** (birth control pills) and for the treatment of **acne vulgaris** and **dysmenorrhea** (see later). For example, the combination of **estradiol valerate and dienogest** (a synthetic progestin) effectively **controls heavy or prolonged menstrual bleeding** (dysmenorrhea).

Adverse Effects

Estrogens occasionally cause **breast tenderness, headache, edema, nausea, vomiting, anorexia,** and **changes in libido.** These effects are less likely to occur in women using the lower-dose preparations now recommended for **HRT.**

The more serious adverse effects of estrogens include **hypertension, thromboembolic disorders,** and **gallbladder disease.** The hypertensive effect of estrogens has been partly attributed to increased angiotensinogen synthesis and formation of angiotensin II, whereas thromboembolic complications result from increased hepatic synthesis of clotting factors. Estrogens increase cholesterol excretion in the bile, accounting for their tendency to cause gallstones. In addition, **estrogens increase the risk of breast cancer**.

Estrogens are contraindicated during pregnancy and should be avoided in women with uterine fibroids. Estrogens should be used with great caution in women with hepatic diseases, endometriosis, thromboembolic diseases, or hypercalcemia.

Progestins

Progestins refers to progesterone and its derivatives. **Progesterone** is the primary natural progestin in mammals. Progesterone undergoes extensive first-pass metabolism after oral administration and has a short plasma half-life. To extend the oral bioavailability and half-life, esters of progesterone have been developed. These include **megestrol, hydroxyprogesterone caproate,** and **medroxyprogesterone acetate (MPA).** Megestrol is administered orally, whereas hydroxyprogesterone caproate is administered as a long-acting intramuscular preparation. **MPA can be given either orally or intramuscularly.** Following their absorption, the progesterone esters are bound to albumin in the circulation. The esters are converted to several hydroxylated metabolites and to pregnanediol glucuronide in the liver, and these metabolites are excreted in the urine.

Progesterone esters are used to suppress ovarian function in the treatment of **dysmenorrhea, endometriosis,** and **uterine bleeding.** In this setting, the progesterone derivatives produce feedback inhibition of gonadotropin secretion by the pituitary gland. In **HRT** (see later), the progesterone esters are used in combination with estrogens to decrease the incidence of estrogen-induced irregular bleeding and to prevent uterine hyperplasia and endometrial cancer. **Hydroxyprogesterone caproate once-weekly injections** are approved by the US Food and Drug Administration (FDA) to reduce the risk of **preterm delivery** in women with a history of at least one spontaneous preterm birth. Studies found that women treated with the drug had significantly fewer preterm deliveries (see section "Drugs used in Obstetrics," later).

Synthetic Progestins

Synthetic progestins are primarily used as **oral contraceptives** (see later), but they are also used to treat **dysmenorrhea, endometriosis,** and **uterine bleeding** in the same manner as the progesterone esters.

Most of the synthetic progestins are derivatives of 19-nortestosterone (testosterone without a methyl group on carbon-19) and stimulate varying degrees of estrogenic, antiestrogenic, and androgenic activity. **Norgestrel initiates more androgenic** activity than other progestins, whereas desogestrel and norgestimate have less androgenic and more progestational activity. **Drospirenone** is a spironolactone derivative with significant **antiandrogenic** effects. The synthetic progestins also contain molecular entities that increase their oral bioavailability and duration of action. Their half-lives range from 7 to 24 hours, whereas the half-life of progesterone is only approximately 5 minutes.

Hormone Replacement Therapy

Menopause refers to the cessation of menstruation that occurs in most women between the ages of 45 and 55. Before menopause, the supply of eggs in a woman's ovaries declines and ovulation becomes irregular. The ovarian follicles fail to develop and secrete normal amounts of estrogen. When estrogen levels are no longer sufficient to suppress FSH secretion by the pituitary gland, FSH levels rise. When FSH levels are greater than 40 IU/L, a woman is considered to be in menopause.

Although estrogens can be used alone for HRT in women who have had a hysterectomy, estrogen should be used in combination with a progestin for women with a uterus. This is because giving **estrogen alone increases the risk of endometrial cancer** in these women.

Therapeutic Effects

Studies consistently show that estrogens relieve **symptoms of menopause** in up to 90% of women. These symptoms include **hot flashes (flushes)** that consist of alternating chills and sweating accompanied by nausea, dizziness, headache, tachycardia, and palpitations (Box 34.1). Episodes of

---

BOX 34.1 A CASE OF HOT FLASHES AND LOSS OF SLEEP

CASE PRESENTATION

A 50-year-old woman tells her health care provider about episodes of hot flashes that occur mostly at night accompanied by sweating and interrupted sleep. She has also noticed vaginal dryness and feeling slightly depressed. Her periods have been increasingly infrequent over the past year. She suspects that she is entering menopause and asks about hormone replacement therapy (HRT). The woman has been healthy throughout her adult life and adheres to a good diet and a regular exercise program. Her mother developed osteoporosis after menopause, and the patient is concerned about maintaining healthy bones. She does not have a family history of premature cardiovascular disease or of reproductive tract cancer. Her physical examination findings and laboratory test results are normal, and she is scheduled for a bone density determination. She is started on a low dose of oral estrogen and a vaginal estrogen cream along with cyclic medroxyprogesterone. Her bone density will be monitored and appropriate therapy provided. She is encouraged to maintain a high level of calcium intake and to increase her vitamin D supplementation. This case is continued in Chapter 36.

CASE DISCUSSION

Menopause is defined as the absence of menstruation for 12 consecutive months and is caused by cessation of estrogen production by the ovaries. Common symptoms of menopause include hot flashes, mood swings, sleeplessness, vaginal dryness, and urinary incontinence. Many women experience irregular periods and other symptoms of menopause for several months preceding menopause. Tachycardia, depression, and other symptoms of estrogen withdrawal may also occur. Low doses of estrogens control most menopausal symptoms, and vaginal estrogen preparations effectively relieve vaginal atrophy. Clinical trials have produced conflicting data with respect to HRT and the risk of cardiovascular disease. In some cases, the findings of trials involving older women with heart disease have been erroneously extrapolated to healthy younger women. Recent analysis of these trials suggests that hormonal replacement in younger menopausal women 50–59 years of age may protect against cardiovascular disease as well as osteoporosis and reduces the risk of colorectal cancer. For most healthy menopausal women, short-term HRT is a relatively safe and effective method of controlling menopausal symptoms.

these symptoms often occur several times a day, and night sweats are particularly common. These symptoms occur in association with **surges in GnRH and gonadotropins** that result from the lack of estrogen feedback inhibition. The gonadotropin surges alter hypothalamic thermoregulatory centers, leading to the symptoms described earlier.

Estrogens also **relieve other menopausal symptoms,** including urogenital, vulvar, and vaginal atrophy, and they **protect against osteoporosis.** Estrogens may improve mood and reduce cognitive difficulties, possibly secondary to improved sleep.

Although some epidemiologic studies suggest that HRT reduces the risk of cardiovascular disease, recent clinical trials of estrogen replacement in postmenopausal women have reached the opposite conclusion. The **Nurses' Health Study** was an observational study of a cohort of women that obtained information about the relationship between cardiovascular disease and lifestyle, lipid levels, and HRT. This study concluded that HRT decreased the risk of coronary artery disease. This study has the same limitations as all cohort observational studies, and it has been postulated that the women who sought HRT were also more likely to adopt a healthy lifestyle that reduced their risk of heart disease.

The **Postmenopausal Estrogen/Progestin Interventions** study was a randomized, prospective trial of HRT in 875 women aged 45 to 64. It demonstrated beneficial effects of HRT on risk factors for heart disease by showing that **HRT reduced cholesterol and fibrinogen levels.** The relatively short duration of the trial (3 years) was not sufficient to determine long-term effects of HRT on morbidity and mortality, but it does provide useful information about short-term estrogen therapy.

The **Heart and Estrogen-Progestin Replacement Study** investigated the effects of HRT in **older postmenopausal women** with **existing heart disease.** This study found a lack of benefit of HRT on fatal or nonfatal myocardial infarction. In fact, the study found that women were at an increased risk of myocardial infarction during the first year of HRT, although the risk of myocardial infarction decreased in subsequent years. After an additional 3 years of study, no significant differences were noted in cardiovascular outcomes between women on HRT and those not receiving HRT. This trial has been criticized because women in the study were already receiving cardioprotective medications and were allowed to begin or change statin therapy during the study. In addition, the average age of women in the study was 67, which is much older than the age when women enter menopause.

The **Women's Health Initiative** included a randomized trial of more than 16,000 women who received **conjugated equine estrogen** plus **MPA** or a placebo. After 5 years, the study was halted because the data showed that women receiving HRT had increased risk of **coronary artery disease, stroke,** and **pulmonary embolism.** However, HRT reduced the risk of **colorectal cancer** and **hip fractures.** Another arm of this study looked at the effect of estrogen by itself in women without a uterus. This study was stopped when it was reported that estrogen increased the risk of stroke but did not affect the incidence of coronary artery disease in these women. The Women's Health Initiative study has been criticized for the **older age** of the participants.

More recently, a trial conducted by the Women's Health Initiative in younger and generally healthier **50- to 59-year-old** women found that both estrogen alone and estrogen and progestin in combination provided **cardioprotective effects** with a reduction in coronary events and total mortality. This study added to the growing evidence that HRT is safe and effective in younger menopausal women, particularly when used with the lowest doses and for the shortest duration required to relieve menopausal symptoms.

In summary, **low-dose estrogen preparations** are still a very useful treatment for relieving menopausal symptoms in younger menopausal women. Estrogens also protect against **osteoporosis** and certain cancers and may reduce the risk of cardiovascular disease in younger women. The role of estrogens in older women remains uncertain. Older women with existing heart disease should not be placed on estrogen therapy. Other medications are available to prevent osteoporosis in menopausal women and should be used when HRT is discontinued.

In addition to this, other medications are available and effective to **decrease postmenopausal vasomotor symptoms (VMSs) in women** when estrogen therapy is contraindicated. **Low-dose paroxetine,** a serotonin-selective reuptake inhibitor (SSRI) antidepressant, was recently approved for the treatment of VMS ("hot flashes" and night sweats) in postmenopausal women. It was given the brand name of BRISDELLE for this indication (see Chapter 22). Other medications already on the market and used "off label" for the treatment of VMSs include **clonidine,** a centrally acting $alpha2$ (α_2)-adrenergic agonist used for treatment of hypertension and other conditions (see Chapter 8). In addition, **gabapentin,** a gamma-aminobutyric acid (GABA) analog used as an antiepileptic drug (AED), is often prescribed for the treatment of postmenopausal VMSs (see Chapter 20).

Treatment Considerations

Most women with an **intact uterus** should begin **HRT with a combination of a progestin and a low-dose estrogen.** Doses should be titrated to provide symptom relief without causing side effects such as headache, nausea, weight gain, breast tenderness, or vaginal bleeding. The dose of estrogen can then be gradually reduced to the lowest level required and for the shortest duration of time to prevent hot flashes and other symptoms. HRT should not be used in women with a history of **endometrial cancer** or in **breast cancer survivors.**

Estrogens can be administered using a wide variety of dosage forms and routes of administration, enabling women to try alternative preparations and determine which one is most effective and tolerable for them. Oral tablets are convenient and relatively inexpensive, whereas transdermal skin patches require less frequent administration. Women with mainly **vulvovaginal symptoms may prefer a vaginal cream, tablet, or ring.** Other options include intramuscular injections and subcutaneously implanted pellets.

HRT can be given as **cyclic** or **continuous hormonal therapy.** In cyclic therapy, estrogen is given for 25 days, a progestin (e.g., medroxyprogesterone) is given for the last 10 to 13 days of estrogen treatment, and then no therapy is given for 5 to 6 days. In continuous therapy, estrogen is given every day, and a progestin is added for the first 10 to 13 days of each month. The addition of a progestin suppresses endometrial growth and diminishes the risk of endometrial hyperplasia or endometrial cancer.

CONTRACEPTIVES

Contraceptives are drugs, devices, or devices that release drugs that are used to prevent conception, the fertilization of an egg by the sperm and resulting pregnancy. Some contraceptives act locally in the female reproductive tract. These include agents that kill sperm on the way to the egg, called **spermicides.** Most spermicides contain **nonoxynol-9,** a detergent that disrupts the cell membrane of the sperm. Spermicides **increase the contraceptive efficacy** of condoms and other barrier methods. They are moderately effective and well tolerated, although they can cause local irritation in some women. **Spermicides are available without prescription** in the form of a gel, foam, film, or sponge. There are devices that prevent sperm from reaching the uterus and fertilizing the ovum, called **barrier methods.** Barrier methods include condoms (for both men and women) and diaphragms and cervical caps in women. **Intrauterine devices** (IUDs) are available that prevent implantation of the blastocyst; some of them **release progestin drugs.** Other contraceptives are administered orally or by injection. **Oral contraceptives** (birth control pills) contain female sex hormones that prevent ovulation. Most of the oral contraceptives contain both an estrogen and a progestin, whereas a few contain only a progestin. Progestin-only contraceptives are also available for administration as **intramuscular injections** or **subdermal implants** or released from **IUDs.** This last group of agents is called **long-acting reversible contraceptives (LARCs).** Drugs that are available to prevent pregnancy after unprotected sex are called **emergency contraceptives.** Table 34.1 lists the estrogen and progestin components of various hormonal contraceptive preparations.

TABLE 34.1 Estrogen and Progestin Components of Selected Hormonal Contraceptive Preparations

PREPARATION TYPE AND TRADE NAMES	ESTROGEN	PROGESTIN
Monophasic Oral Contraceptives		
Brevicon, Loestrin, Norinyl, Ovcon-35, and others	Ethinyl estradiol	Norethindrone
Kelnor	Ethinyl estradiol	Ethynodiol diacetate
Desogen, Ortho-Cept, and others	Ethinyl estradiol	Desogestrel[a]
Yasmin, *and others*	Ethinyl estradiol	Drospirenone
Lo/Ovral-28, *and others*	Ethinyl estradiol	Norgestrel
Nordette, Seasonale, Seasonique, Lybrel	Ethinyl estradiol	Levonorgestrel
Norinyl 1 + 35, *and others*	Mestranol	Norethindrone
Multiphasic Oral Contraceptives		
Mircette and others (biphasic)	Ethinyl estradiol	Desogestrel[a]
Ortho-Novum 7/7/7, Tri-Norinyl, and others (triphasic)	Ethinyl estradiol	Norethindrone
Tri-Levlen, Triphasil, and others (triphasic)	Ethinyl estradiol	Levonorgestrel
Ortho Tri-Cyclen, Tri-Sprintec (triphasic)	Ethinyl estradiol	Norgestimate
Natazia (quadriphasic) and others.	Estradiol valerate	Dienogest
Progestin-Only Oral Contraceptives		
Micronor, Nor-QD		Norethindrone
Contraceptive Implant		
Nexplanon		Etonogestrel[a]
Intrauterine Contraceptive		
Mirena		Levonorgestrel
Injectable Contraceptives		
Depo-Provera		Medroxyprogesterone acetate
Transdermal Contraceptive		
Xulane	Ethinyl estradiol	Norelgestromin
Vaginal Ring Contraceptive		
NuvaRing	Ethinyl estradiol	Etonogestrel[a]
Emergency (Postcoital) Contraceptive		
Plan B, Plan B One-Step, Next Choice		Levonorgestrel
Ella		Ulipristal

[a]Etonogestrel is the active metabolite of desogestrel.

Estrogen-Progestin Contraceptives

Classification

The combination estrogen-progestin oral contraceptives include monophasic and multiphasic preparations. **Monophasic contraceptives** contain the same amount of progestin throughout the administration cycle, whereas **multiphasic contraceptives** increase the amount after 7 and 14 days of the cycle. The amount of progestin is increased in multiphasic preparations to mimic the natural ratio of estrogen to progestin during the menstrual cycle. The estrogen content is constant in all monophasic and in most multiphasic contraceptives. NATAZIA is a newer contraceptive that sequentially steps down the estradiol valerate dose while the progestin dose is stepped up (see Fig. 34.3). The dose of estrogen may be consistent within each pack, but different amounts of estrogen are available.

Mechanisms and Pharmacologic Effects

The estrogen-progestin contraceptives act primarily by feedback inhibition of GnRH secretion from the hypothalamus, leading to decreased gonadotropin secretion and **inhibition of ovulation.** The **estrogen** component is believed to **reduce FSH secretion** and the selection and maturation of the dominant follicle, whereas the **progestin** component **inhibits the midcycle LH** surge required for ovulation. Neither the estrogen nor the progestin dose used in oral contraceptives is sufficient to prevent ovulation by itself, but used together they act synergistically to suppress ovulation. Other effects that contribute to contraception include delayed maturation of the endometrium, which prevents implantation of the blastocyst, and the development of viscous cervical mucus, which retards sperm motility. Tubal motility is also a factor. The actions on the **endometrium and cervical mucus** are believed to be the mechanisms of progestin preparations used for **emergency (postcoital) contraception.**

Administration

Estrogen-progestin **oral contraceptives** usually contain 21 active ingredient tablets that are administered once a day, beginning on day 5 of the menstrual cycle. Many preparations also include seven inert pills taken for the remainder of the cycle as a method of reinforcing daily pill administration. The tablets are packaged in a calendar format to facilitate proper use. **Extended-cycle** (menstrual suppression) preparations are now available for continuous daily administration for 84 days followed by 7 days of inactive tablets (SEASONALE, SEASONIQUE). These preparations contain ethinyl estradiol and levonorgestrel and allow for withdrawal bleeding only four times a year, whereas other oral estrogen-progestin contraceptives result in 13 withdrawal bleeding episodes a year. The extended-cycle preparation is as effective as 28-day cycle products. Whether the longer exposure to hormones could increase the risk of adverse effects (e.g., thromboembolism) is uncertain.

Preparations containing **drospirenone** and **ethinyl estradiol** are available for either a 21-day or 24-day hormone regimen. Recent studies found that the 24-day regimen is associated with slightly lower rates of contraceptive failure.

Estrogen-progestin preparations are also used to treat **acne vulgaris** and produce a significant improvement in facial acne lesions. They are also useful in managing **dysmenorrhea,** a condition characterized by episodic pain that is believed to result from a local increase in uterine prostaglandins (PGs). The release of PGs is a reaction to the ischemia caused by vasoconstriction of small arteries in the uterine wall at the time of menstruation. For this condition, oral contraceptives are started a number of days before the onset of menstruation. Nonsteroidal antiinflammatory drugs (NSAIDs, e.g., ibuprofen and naproxen) can be used instead, especially by women desiring to maintain the ovulatory cycle.

Another estrogen-progestin contraceptive is formulated as a **transdermal skin patch** (ORTHO EVRA). This preparation uses a 4-week administration cycle; a new patch is applied on the same day each week for 3 weeks, and week 4 is patch-free to allow for withdrawal bleeding. Its association with **venous thromboembolism (VTE)** is described later.

Adverse Effects

Box 34.2 lists the common adverse effects resulting from estrogen or progestin excess or deficiency. Less frequent effects of oral contraceptives include **hypertension, thromboembolic complications,** and **gallstones.**

Oral contraceptives have been associated with an increased risk of **stroke, myocardial infarction, deep vein thrombosis,** and other thromboembolic complications. The increased risk of thromboembolism in healthy women using preparations containing a low dose of estrogen (<50 μg of ethinyl estradiol) is extremely small, although approximately threefold higher than in women not taking an oral contraceptive. **Smokers older than 35 years** of age have a greater risk of thromboembolic complications from oral

---

BOX 34.2 COMMON ADVERSE EFFECTS OF ORAL CONTRACEPTIVES

EFFECTS OF ESTROGEN EXCESS
- Breast enlargement
- Dizziness
- Dysmenorrhea
- Edema
- Headache
- Irritability
- Nausea and vomiting
- Weight gain (cyclic)

EFFECTS OF PROGESTIN EXCESS
- Acne
- Depression
- Fatigue
- Hirsutism
- Libido change
- Oily skin
- Weight gain (noncyclic)

EFFECTS OF ESTROGEN DEFICIENCY
- Atrophic vaginitis
- Continuous bleeding
- Early or midcycle bleeding
- Hypomenorrhea
- Vasomotor symptoms

EFFECTS OF PROGESTIN DEFICIENCY
- Dysmenorrhea
- Hypermenorrhea
- Late-cycle bleeding

contraceptives and should use other forms of contraception. Healthy nonsmokers who are 35 to 44 years old may continue to use oral contraceptives, according to the American College of Obstetricians and Gynecologists. The **contraceptive skin patch** containing norelgestromin/ethinyl estradiol (Xulane) produced greater systemic exposure to these steroids and caused a greater incidence of **VTE,** and possibly other thromboembolic disorders, compared with oral administration of these steroids. Xulane was less effective in women weighing greater than 198 pounds. However, it should be kept in mind that the **risk of VTE** is sixfold greater for **pregnant women** than for nonpregnant women.

Contraceptives containing estrogen should be used with caution in women with **gallbladder disease.** They are contraindicated in women with thromboembolic disease or a history of myocardial infarction or coronary artery disease. They are also contraindicated in women with active liver disease, breast cancer, or carcinoma of the reproductive tract. On the positive side, oral contraceptives have been found to **reduce the incidence of endometrial and ovarian cancer,** and the lifetime incidence of **breast cancer does not appear to be increased.** Oral contraceptives have also been associated with a very low risk of hepatic adenoma.

The progestin component of oral contraceptives can cause adverse effects that can be attributed to excessive androgenic activity. The androgenic side effects of progestins include **acne, hirsutism, increased libido,** and **oily skin. Norgestrel** is one of the most androgenic progestins, whereas **desogestrel** is one of the least androgenic. **Norethindrone** appears to have an intermediate androgenic potency. **Drospirenone** is a newer progestin derived from spironolactone (see Chapter 13). Drospirenone is an **aldosterone antagonist** with a weak **antiandrogenic effect.** It lowers blood pressure by reducing salt and water retention, and a contraceptive containing this progestin has improved tolerability with respect to weight gain, mood changes, and acne in comparison with contraceptives containing other progestins.

Interactions

Carbamazepine, phenytoin, and other drugs that **increase the hepatic metabolism of oral contraceptives** may reduce the plasma levels of contraceptive steroids and lead to contraceptive failure. **Antibiotics,** including penicillins and tetracyclines, can eradicate intestinal flora involved in the enterohepatic cycling of contraceptive steroids and **thereby diminish their effectiveness** (see Fig. 34.3). Estrogens can inhibit the metabolism and potentiate the effects of cyclosporine, antidepressants, and glucocorticoids. Estrogens increase the synthesis of vitamin K–dependent clotting factors and may thereby antagonize the effect of warfarin. Estrogens also appear to increase the hepatotoxicity of dantrolene.

Progestin-Only Contraceptives

The progestin-only contraceptives include **norethindrone** products administered orally (sometimes called *minipills*), subdermal implants and IUDs that slowly release **progestin,** and long-acting intramuscular or subcutaneous injections of **MPA** (Depo-Provera).

MPA is also used far "off label" as a **chemical castration agent** in men convicted of pedophilia, serial rape, and other sex crimes. In some states, courts can mandate such pharmacologic treatment of these sex offenders or offer treatment of MPA to offenders in exchange for a shorter prison sentence.

The systemic progestin-only contraceptives may prevent pregnancy through several mechanisms. They act on the hypothalamus to decrease the frequency of the GnRH pulse generator and thereby blunt the midcycle LH surge that produces ovulation. Progestin-only pills thicken and decrease the amount of cervical mucus, making it more difficult for sperm to penetrate. Progestins also create a thin, atrophic endometrium that is **hostile to implantation of the blastocyst.** IUDs are believed to prevent pregnancy by producing localized effects on the endometrium.

The **progestin-only contraceptives** are particularly suited for women who smoke, **older women,** and women in whom an **estrogen is contraindicated.** However, the estimated failure rates are slightly higher with perfect use of progestin-only contraceptives than with perfect use of estrogen-progestin products (rates of 0.5% and 0.1%, respectively). However, the Nexplanon subdermal **etonogestrel implant** is the **most effective form of birth control** now available (see later). Progestin-only contraceptives are associated with **frequent spotting and amenorrhea** and with an increased risk of ectopic pregnancy. An irregular or unpredictable menstrual cycle is one of the most common reasons that women stop using these preparations. Unlike the estrogen-progestin preparations, the progestin-only preparations must be taken daily without interruption to prevent pregnancy.

Long-Acting Reversible Contraceptives

A number of drug-eluting contraceptive devices are available to provide greater efficacy by offering lower pregnancy rates and fewer contraceptive failures. Patient compliance is higher with LARCs, thus proving them to be more effective forms of contraception than a daily birth control pill. These LARCs provide from 1 week (estradiol transdermal patch) to 10 years (copper IUD) of highly effective contraception that rivals that of many permanent sterilization procedures.

With many LARC methods, the **incidence of ectopic pregnancy is often increased** if pregnancy does occur. In addition, each device or contraceptive system has its own unique profile in regard to mechanism of action, common side effects, and bleeding profile that may limit their use in certain populations of women.

The **etonongestrel/ethinyl estradiol vaginal ring** (Nuvaring) is a pliable rubber-like ring that is inserted into the vagina for 3 weeks. The ring is removed for 1 week during which a woman will usually have a menstrual period. Side effects of Nuvaring are similar to other combination estrogen/progestin birth control formulations. A second vaginal ring was marketed containing **seqesterone/ethinyl estradiol** (Annovera). Both vaginal rings are similar in that they are removed 1 week per month for menustration. However, the Annovera ring is good for 1 year instead of 1 month, is a little bigger and thicker, and can be stored unopened at room temperature. Both products have the same effectiveness as oral contraceptives, with approximately 9% of women getting pregnant while using vaginal rings.

The **norelgestromin/ethinyl estradiol transdermal system** (Xulane) is a combination estrogen/progestin hormone contraceptive device in the form of a patch applied to the skin. A new patch is applied to the skin of the upper arm, buttock, or abdomen each week for 3 weeks. No patch is applied during week 4 to allow for menstruation to occur. The transdermal patch may be less effective in the prevention of pregnancy in women weighing more than 198 pounds. The transdermal patch has **higher area under the curve (AUC) values, higher steady state concentrations, and lower peak concentrations** than oral contraceptives.

Etonogestrel Implant (NEXPLANON) is a flexible, 4-cm plastic rod containing 68 mg of etonogestrel and 15 mg of barium sulfate. The barium sulfate is added to the implant to make it radiopaque for easier removal after the 3-year lifespan of the implant is over. The etonogestrel implant emits a steady dose of progestin, which works to prevent pregnancy by interfering with ovulation, by thickening cervical mucus, and by altering the endometrial lining that prevents implantation of the blastocyst.

The **copper IUD** (PARAGARD T 380A) was one of the first LARCs to be developed. It works to prevent pregnancy by mechanisms that take place both before and after fertilization occur. Alterations in the viability and transport of both the sperm and the ovum prevent pregnancy before fertilization. The copper released from this IUD is also known to cause damage or destruction to the ovum after fertilization but before implantation.

Similar in structure to the copper IUD, the **levonorgestrel IUD** (MIRENA, SKYLA, LILETTA) is a T-shaped device inserted into the uterus and emits progestin causing prevention of pregnancy. These IUDs provide contraceptive effects from 3 to 5 years after placement and may continue to work effectively for up to 7 years, depending on the device. Patient satisfaction is often increased with this method of contraception due to the desirable effect of less frequent menses or amenorrhea. Both IUDs are the most effective forms of contraception (other than sterilization), with fewer than 1 out of 100 women using them getting pregnant.

Emergency Contraceptives

Drugs that are available to prevent pregnancy after unprotected sex are called **emergency contraceptives.** Preparations containing **levonorgestrel** are also available **with or without prescription** for use as an **emergency (postcoital) contraceptive** in women who have not been taking another contraceptive. These preparations consist of a either a single 1.5-mg dose of the progestin **levonorgestrel** (PLAN B, ONE-STEP), or two 0.75-mg doses (PLAN B, NEXT CHOICE), with the first dose taken within 72 hours of intercourse and a second dose taken 12 hours later. Use of an emergency contraceptive usually causes **nausea and vomiting** that can be reduced by administration of an antiemetic agent (e.g., promethazine). It can also cause **headache, dizziness, leg cramps,** and **abdominal cramps.** A urine pregnancy test can be used to verify the prevention of pregnancy.

A second emergency contraceptive is available as **ulipristal acetate** (ELLA). **Uliprsital** is a **progestin agonist/antagonist** approved for emergency contraception after unprotected sex or a known contraceptive failure. Currently, it is available by prescription only.

SELECTIVE ESTROGEN RECEPTOR MODULATORS

Most drugs act as an agonist at a receptor and activate the receptor and its signaling pathway, or as an antagonist and block agonist access to the receptor, stopping the signaling pathway. However, this simple binary classification of drug-receptor action does not hold for all drugs. A number of drugs acting at ERs exhibit either agonist or antagonist action, **depending on the tissue that expresses the ERs**. After ligands bind to the ERs, the signaling pathway is regulated by protein cofactors, either **coactivators to give an estrogenic response (agonist) or corepressors to yield an antiestrogenic (antagonist) response**. The ratio of coactivators and corepressors differs in ER tissues, and the predominant cofactor determines the agonist or antagonist response. For example, **tamoxifen** is used for breast cancer prophylaxis where it **antagonizes estrogen effects in breast tissue** while at the same time exerting estrogen agonist effects on the endometrial lining of the uterus and can cause **endometrial hyperplasia** (see Chapter 45).

SERMs that are currently approved for pharmacotherapy include clomiphene, raloxifene, ospemifene, baxedoxifine, tamoxifen, and toremifene.

Clomiphene
Pharmacokinetics
Clomiphene is well absorbed after oral administration. It undergoes hepatic biotransformation and biliary excretion, and it is mostly eliminated in the feces. Its long elimination half-life of approximately 5 days is caused by extensive plasma protein binding, enterohepatic cycling, and accumulation in fatty tissues.

Mechanisms and Indications
Clomiphene is a weak estrogen agonist and a moderate estrogen antagonist. It is used to treat anovulatory infertility, including infertility associated with polycystic ovary disease (PCOS). Clomiphene blocks ERs in the hypothalamus and pituitary and prevents estrogen's feedback inhibition of gonadotropin secretion (Fig. 34.4). This increases FSH and LH secretion, which induces ovarian follicle development and ovulation.

Suitable patients for clomiphene therapy often have an anovulatory disorder dating back to puberty but have a functional hypothalamic-pituitary-ovarian axis. Clomiphene is less successful in women who have reduced estrogen levels, and it is unlikely to benefit women with FSH levels at or greater than 40 IU/L or women with absent or resistant ovarian follicles.

Clomiphene treatment is usually begun on or about the fifth day of the cycle after the start of uterine bleeding and continues for 5 days. Ovulation is expected 5 to 10 days after the last dose of clomiphene and can be detected by monitoring basal body temperature, urinary LH secretion, plasma progesterone levels, or endometrial histology. However, **only approximately 15% of women achieve pregnancy with clomiphene therapy**. Aromatase inhibitors have recently been used to treat infertility and appear to have a **better pregnancy rate** (see later).

Adverse Effects
Approximately 5% to 7% of women treated with clomiphene have multiple births (twins in the vast majority of cases). The risk of multiple births is reduced if women are started on a lower dose of clomiphene. The dose can then be increased each cycle until ovulation occurs.

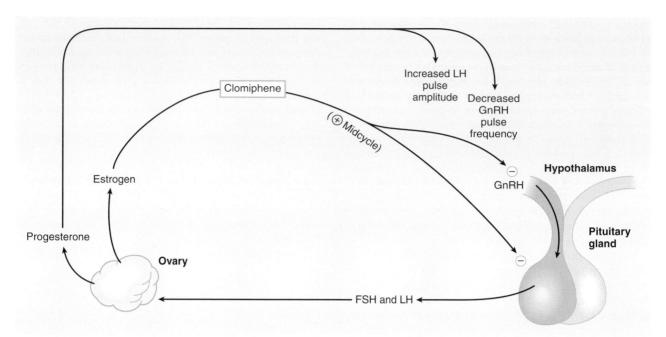

Fig. 34.4 The hypothalamic-pituitary-ovarian axis. Follicle-stimulating hormone (FSH) and luteinizing hormone (LH) are released from the pituitary gland in response to gonadotropin-releasing hormone (GnRH) produced by hypothalamic neurons. During the follicular phase of the menstrual cycle, FSH stimulates the development of an ovarian follicle and the secretion of estrogen. Estrogen increases the synthesis of LH but inhibits its release until midcycle, when a surge in LH is accompanied by a smaller surge in FSH secretion, leading to ovulation. During the luteal phase, progesterone produced by the corpus luteum feeds back to the hypothalamus to decrease the frequency of GnRH pulses while acting on the pituitary to increase the amplitude of LH secretion. Together, these actions produce less-frequent LH pulses of greater amplitude. Clomiphene inhibits estrogen feedback and thereby increases gonadotropin secretion in anovulatory women.

Raloxifene

Raloxifene is a SERM indicated for the prevention of **osteoporosis** (see Chapter 36) and for **reducing the risk of breast cancer** in postmenopausal women. Raloxifene acts in a manner similar to that of tamoxifen by producing **estrogen-like effects on bone** and **lipid metabolism** while **antagonizing the effects of estrogen on breast tissue**. However, unlike tamoxifen, raloxifene also acts as an **estrogen antagonist in uterine** tissue. Raloxifene increases the risk of **stroke, pulmonary emboli,** and **deep vein thrombosis.**

Ospemifene

Ospemifene is indicated for the treatment of **moderate to severe dyspareunia** (pain during intercourse), a symptom of **vulvar and vaginal atrophy** due to **menopause**. It is a new type of more potent estrogen agonist/antagonist (SERM) with tissue selective effects. Like all SERMs, its biologic actions are mediated through binding to ERs. This binding results in activation of estrogenic pathways in some tissues (agonism) and blockade of estrogenic pathways in others (antagonism).

Bazedoxifene

Bazedoxifene is the newest SERM in the same chemical class as ospemifene. It is not available as a single agent but only in combination formulation of **conjugated estrogens with baxedoxifine** (DUAVEE). It is approved for the treatment of **moderate to severe VMSs** associated with menopause and for the **prevention of osteoporosis.**

Selective Estrogen Receptor Degrader

Fulvestrant is a first-in-class **ER antagonist** that acts as a selective estrogen receptor degrader (SERD). Unlike SERMs which may have agonist or antagonist effects at ERs depending on the tissue, **fulvestrant is a pure ER antagonist** in all tissues tested. It binds to the ER monomer, preventing dimerization of the receptor, and causes internalization and degradation of the ER by proteasomes within the tumor cell. **Fulvestrant is indicated for ER-positive, metastatic breast cancer** and is given by intramuscular injection every 2 weeks for three times then monthly thereafter (see Chapter 45). Given the success of **fulvestrant** in treating women with **tamoxifen-resistant breast cancer**, there is vigorous development of additional SERDs that will be orally available.

ANTIPROGESTINS

Mifepristone is a synthetic steroid compound that acts as a progesterone receptor antagonist when progesterone is present. In the absence of progesterone, it acts as a partial agonist. It is also a competitive antagonist at the glucocorticoid receptor (see Chapter 33). Mifepristone is approved for **medical termination of pregnancy** through 70 days of gestation, when given in a regimen with the PG **misoprostol** (see Chapter 26). **Mifepristone causes breakdown of the decidua** (the endometrium of the pregnant uterus), leading to detachment of the blastocyst from the endometrium.

    Mifepristone is administered as a single oral dose of 200 mg followed by **misoprostol** given in an 800 mg buccal dose 24 to 48 hours after mifepristone **to stimulate uterine contractions and expel the products of conception.** Mifepristone has good oral bioavailability. Following absorption, the drug is highly bound to plasma proteins, which contributes to its long half-life of approximately 22 hours. Mifepristone is metabolized in the liver, is excreted in the bile, undergoes enterohepatic cycling, and is eventually excreted in the feces.

The major adverse effects of mifepristone include anorexia, nausea, vomiting, abdominal pain, fatigue, and heavy uterine bleeding. When **mifepristone and misoprostol** are taken as directed, **termination of pregnancy occurs without complications** in more than 97% of women.

AROMATASE INHIBITORS

Breast cancer is often hormonally responsive—including breast cancer classified as estrogen and/or progesterone receptor positive. This type of breast cancer has responded to a variety of efforts to decrease estrogen levels (e.g., removal of the ovaries, an oophorectomy) or to inhibit estrogen effects, such as with SERMs. These interventions lead to decreased tumor mass, delayed progression, and improved survival in many patients.

In postmenopausal women, estrogens are derived from adrenal androgens, primarily testosterone and androstenedione, which are **converted to estrogens in peripheral tissues and in cancer tissue** by the **enzyme aromatase** (see Fig. 34.1). **Anastrozole** and **letrozole** are nonsteroidal **aromatase inhibitors** that **reduce circulating levels of estrogen** and are indicated as first-line treatments for locally advanced or **metastatic breast cancer** in postmenopausal women (see Chapter 45).

Recently, **letrozole** has been used to treat infertility in anovulatory women, either alone or in combination with gonadotropins. Letrozole appears to result in better pregnancy rates than clomiphene.

ANDROGENS
Testosterone and Methyltestosterone

When given orally, testosterone undergoes extensive first-pass metabolism, and it must be given by other routes to achieve effective blood levels. **Methyltestosterone** can be given orally, but it is seldom used because long-term use can cause hepatic damage and liver failure.

Gels and skin patches are available for transdermal administration of testosterone, and long-acting esters of testosterone (e.g., **testosterone cypionate**) provide effective plasma levels for several weeks after intramuscular injection. A **buccal system** (STRIANT) has been developed that adheres to the gum or inner cheek and provides a sustained release of testosterone for absorption through the buccal mucosa throughout the day. All of these preparations can be used to treat **hypogonadism** caused by primary testicular failure or occurring secondary to pituitary insufficiency. In patients with **hypopituitarism, testosterone should be given in combination with growth hormone** to obtain a maximal effect on skeletal growth. In these patients, the androgen is added to the treatment regimen at the time of puberty, and the dosage is gradually increased. Testosterone therapy may also **benefit older men** with testosterone deficiency by preventing osteoporosis and improving overall quality of life.

Testosterone is occasionally used in **gynecologic disorders.** It is sometimes combined with estrogens for **HRT** in postmenopausal women who experience endometrial bleeding when only an estrogen is used.

Anabolic Steroids

Testosterone and its derivatives **increase muscle mass and strength** when used in a weight-training program. Anabolic steroids are synthetic derivatives of testosterone that have more anabolic than androgenic activity. The ratio of anabolic activity to androgenic activity for testosterone is 1:1, whereas the ratio for some synthetic androgens is as high as 3:1. Examples of anabolic steroids include **oxandrolone** and **fluoxymesterone.**

Oxandrolone is approved as an adjunct drug to **increase weight gain after weight loss** of surgery, chronic infections, or severe trauma. It is also indicated to **reverse the catabolism** after chronic administration of corticosteroids and for the **relief of bone pain** that may occur with osteoporosis.

Fluoxymesterone is a synthetic androgen and indicated for replacement therapy in conditions associated with a deficiency or absence of endogenous testosterone. It is approved for treatment of **primary hypogonadism** (congenital or acquired); **testicular failure** due to cryptorchidism, bilateral torsion, orchitis, vanishing testis syndrome, or orchidectomy; **hypogonadotropic hypogonadism** (congenital or acquired); **idiopathic gonadotropin or luteinizing hormone–releasing hormone (LHRH) deficiency**; or **delayed puberty.**

Anabolic steroids have been used by athletes to **increase body mass, strength,** and **physical performance.** This type of use has been banned by sports organizations such as the International Olympic Committee. The large doses of anabolic steroids often used for this purpose can lead to a number of adverse effects, including **tendon rupture,** hepatic dysfunction or failure, cholestatic jaundice, increased aggressiveness, psychotic symptoms, acne, decreased testicular size and function, and impotence. In adolescents, androgenic drugs can cause **closing of epiphyses** and premature cessation of growth. In women, excessive use of androgens can cause masculinization, hirsutism, deepening of the voice, and menstrual irregularities. The issue of **anabolic steroid abuse** is further discussed in Chapter 25.

Danazol

Danazol is a synthetic steroid with weak androgenic activity. It is used in the treatment of several gynecologic disorders because of its ability to cause **feedback inhibition of pituitary gonadotropin secretion and decreased secretion of estrogen.** Danazol was used in treating **endometriosis,** a condition characterized by the presence of endometrial tissue outside the endometrial cavity, although it has been largely replaced for this purpose by the GnRH agonists (see Chapter 31). Danazol causes **atrophy of ectopic endometrial tissue** and relieves disease symptoms.

Danazol has also been used to treat **fibrocystic breast disease** due to its ability to decrease estrogen production and the growth of abnormal breast tissue. In women with **heavy menstrual bleeding,** danazol treatment leads to endometrial atrophy and reduced menstrual blood loss. In addition, danazol is also used to treat **hereditary angioedema,** a disorder caused by deficiency of an inhibitor of the first component of complement (a cascade of plasma proteins involved in immunity to pathogens) that causes **swelling of the face, airways, arms, and legs.** Danazol prevents attacks of this disorder in both males and females by increasing levels of **first-component esterase inhibitor** by an unknown mechanism.

Common adverse effects of danazol include mild hirsutism, oily skin, acne, and menstrual irregularities. The drug can also cause hypercholesterolemia, hepatotoxicity, and thromboembolic events, including stroke. Danazol is **teratogenic** and should not be given to pregnant women.

ANTIANDROGENS

Several types of androgen antagonists have been developed and used in the **treatment of prostate disorders, male pattern baldness,** and other conditions. These drugs act through a variety of mechanisms, including inhibition of LH secretion, testosterone synthesis, **DHT synthesis,** and antagonism of androgen receptors.

Gonadotropin-Releasing Hormone Analogs

When a GnRH analog is administered in a continuous rather than a pulsatile fashion, it reduces LH secretion by the pituitary and thereby reduces testosterone production by the testes.

The GnRH analogs include **leuprolide,** an agent discussed in Chapter 31. Leuprolide has been successfully used in the treatment of inoperable **prostate cancer** (see Chapter 45). Because leuprolide increases the production of LH and testosterone when it is first administered, the drug is sometimes given in combination with an androgen receptor antagonist (e.g., **flutamide**).

Androgen Receptor Antagonists

Flutamide, bicalutamide, enzalutamide, and **nilutamide** are nonsteroidal agents that compete with testosterone for the androgen receptor. These drugs are used in combination with a synthetic GnRH analog to treat inoperable **prostate cancer** (see Chapter 45). For example, bicalutamide is used with a GnRH analog for treatment of stage D2 metastatic **carcinoma of the prostate.** In one study, enzalutamide produced a 12-month progression-free survival of 65% versus 14% in those receiving a placebo. After 22 months of treatment, 28% of men receiving enzalutamide had died versus 35% of the placebo group. The adverse effects of these drugs include **nausea, gynecomastia, impotence, hot flashes,** and **hepatitis.**

5α-Reductase Inhibitors

Finasteride and **dutasteride** are synthetic testosterone derivatives that block 5α-reductase and decrease the synthesis of DHT in the prostate gland, skin, and other target tissues. The drugs are administered orally, undergo hepatic metabolism, and are eliminated in the feces. Finasteride has a half-life of approximately 8 hours, and it reduces DHT synthesis for approximately 24 hours.

Finasteride and dutasteride are used to treat symptomatic **benign prostatic hyperplasia (BPH).** The drugs reduce prostate volume and can retard the progression of BPH. In men with BPH, they improve urinary flow and decrease the risk of urinary retention. The reductase inhibitors are used in combination with an α-adrenoceptor antagonist, such as tamsulosin (see Chapter 9). Finasteride is also used off-label for the treatment of **male pattern baldness.**

The **adverse effects** of finasteride and dutasteride include **erectile dysfunction, decreased libido,** and **gynecomastia,** but these effects are not common and tend to decrease over time.

AGENTS FOR TREATING DYSMENORRHEA AND FEMALE SEXUAL DYSFUNCTION

Treatment of Dysmenorrhea

Pain associated with **menstruation** is called **dysmenorrhea.** Primary dysmenorrhea, known as "menstrual cramps," is due to local **PGs synthesized and released from the lining of the uterus,** which can produce painful uterine contractions. **Secondary dysmenorrhea is pain caused by disorders** of the reproductive system such as **endometriosis, adenomyosis,** or **fibroids.**

Because **NSAIDs inhibit the production of PG** (Chapter 30), they are the first drug of choice for primary dysmenorrhea. Although most NSAIDs would be effective, **mefenamic acid, diclofenac, ibuprofen, ketoprofen, meclofenamate,** and **naproxen** are the NSAIDs specifically approved by the FDA for treatment of dysmenorrhea.

Elagolix (ORILISSA) is the **only GnRH receptor antagonist** (see Chapter 31) indicated for the management of **moderate to severe pain associated with endometriosis.** The major adverse effect is dose- and duration-dependent decreases in bone mineral density that may not be completely reversible. **Elagolix** is also found in **combination** with **estradiol and norethindrone** (ORIAHNN) approved for the management of **heavy menstrual bleeding associated with uterine leiomyomas** (a.k.a. fibroids) in premenopausal women.

Treatment of Female Sexual Dysfunction

Female sexual dysfunction is a catch-all term that includes persistent problems with lack of sexual response, low desire for sexual activity, difficulty in achieving orgasm, or pain during sexual intercourse. The most common of female sexual dysfunction is low sexual desire characterized by lack of sexual interest and unwillingness to participate in sexual activity.

Bremelanotide

Bremelanotide (VYLEESI) is a **first-in-class melanocortin receptor agonist** to treat acquired, generalized **hypoactive sexual desire disorder (HSDD)** in premenopausal women. HSDD is characterized by low sexual desire that causes distress or interpersonal difficulty and is not caused by adverse effects of a medication or drug substance, a coexisting medical or psychiatric condition, or problems in the relationship with their sexual partner. **Melanocortins include** peptides cleaved from proopiomelanocortin (POMC) such as **ACTH (corticotropin)** and **melanocyte-stimulating hormone (MSH).** POMC-containing neurons are found in the hypothalamus and project to many areas of the brain and spinal cord. POMC is also expressed and processed in pituitary corticotrophs. **Melanocortin receptors are typical GPCRs** that come in five types, MCR1 to MCR5; all melanocortin receptors signal by increasing intracellular cAMP.

Although the exact mechanism of the **increased libido** produced by **bremelanotide** is not clear, clinical trials show a **significant improvement in sexual desire scores.** Patients are instructed to inject **bremelanotide** in the abdomen or thigh at least 45 minutes before anticipated sexual activity. **Bremelanotide cannot be used more than once in 24 hours** or more than eight doses per month. The most common adverse effects are nausea and vomiting, flushing reaction, injection site pain and swelling, and headaches.

Flibanserin

Flibanserin (ADDYI) has the exact same indication as **bremelanotide,** and like that drug, the FDA label adds that **flibanserin is not indicated** for the treatment of HSDD **in postmenopausal women or in men** and is **not indicated to enhance sexual performance.** Flibanserin has **black-box warnings** for **severe syncope when taken with alcohol,** for use in individuals with hepatic dysfunction, and for certain drug-drug interactions that inhibit flibanserin metabolism. In vitro, **flibanserin** demonstrates high affinity as an **agonist at 5-HT$_{1A}$ receptors** and an **antagonist at 5-HT$_{2A}$ receptors.** The exact mechanism that produces increased sexual desire in women treated with flibanserin is not known.

DRUG THERAPY FOR HIRSUTISM AND GENDER TRANSITION

Treatment of Hirsutism

The increased growth of hair in **women that follows a male distribution is called hirsutism.** Hirsutism affects approximately 10% of reproductive-age women and is caused by excess androgenic steroids. It is benign in most women, although severe cases cause **virilization** marked by **deepening voice, male pattern baldness, increased muscles, and clitoromegaly.** Elevated androgens can be caused by disorders such as PCOS, adrenal hyperplasia, and Cushing syndrome.

Treatment of hirsutism is aimed at reducing androgen production. Initial treatment consists of oral **combination contraceptive pills which reduces gonadotropin release** and production of ovarian androgens. Continuous administration of **GnRH agonists such as goserelin and leuprolide** leads to downregulation of GnRH receptors and decreased release of FSH and LH which also leads to decreased testosterone and estrogen secretion. In patients who fail to adequately respond to this treatment, **flutamide or other androgen receptor antagonists** can be used.

Female to Male Transition

The main medication used in female to male gender transition is administration of a long-lasting androgen injection, such as **testosterone enanthate or cypionate,** or **androgen gels.** Blood testing should be used to reach the target testosterone levels of the normal male range. If breakthrough bleeding occurs, a long-lasting injection of **depot medroxyprogesterone** (150 mg every 3 months) can be used until bleeding ceases.

Male to Female Transition

The primary medication in **male to female transitioning patients is some form of estrogen.** Oral estradiol, transdermal estradiol, or long-acting estradiol injections can be used. Patients should be aware of the **increased risk of thrombosis and breast cancer,** although controlled clinical studies have not yet been done in this patient population. **Antiandrogens and GnRH agents can be coadministered;** this allows the estradiol dose to be lowered.

DRUGS USED IN OBSTETRICS

Treatment of Pregnancy-Induced Hypertension and Preeclampsia

Pregnancy-induced hypertension or **preeclampsia** most often occurs after 20 weeks of gestation and presents as a new onset hypertension with proteinuria. Preeclampsia involves placental factors that alter vascular integrity and endothelial function in the mother; peripheral edema, renal and hepatic dysfunction, and in severe cases, seizures can result. Although several drugs exist to treat pregnancy-induced hypertension and preeclampsia, the only way to stop it entirely is delivery of the child.

There are numerous antihypertensive drugs available for use in nonpregnant patients (Chapter 10). However, many of these drugs (e.g., ACE inhibitors, ARBs) cannot be used in pregnant patients due to strong evidence of adverse fetal effects. **Methyldopa,** a centrally acting *alpha*-adrenoceptor agonist is often used because it appears safe during pregnancy. Methyldopa is metabolized to **methylnorepinephrine, which is selective for the alpha$_2$-adrenoceptors** on neurons that control sympathetic outflow from the brainstem medulla. Other drugs include the **alpha$_1$-selective and *beta* nonselective antagonist labetalol** (see Chapter 8) and the **calcium channel blocker nifedipine.**

If the preceding agents are not effective, the **direct-acting vasodilator hydralazine** (Chapter 10) can be given intravenously or intramuscularly with repeated doses after 20 minutes if needed. In addition to drugs to lower blood pressure, women with more severe cases as noted by **central nervous system (CNS) disturbance** (headache, visual disturbances, or altered mental status) are administered with **magnesium sulfate. Magnesium sulfate** has documented efficacy in **preventing seizures** and is safe to mother and baby. This treatment should also be considered for postpartum patients with CNS manifestations as up to 20% of women experience onset of eclampsia more than 2 days after delivery.

Prevention of Preterm Labor

More than 10% of pregnancies result in preterm birth, defined as delivery before 37 weeks of gestation. Preterm birth is associated with significant complications such as neonatal respiratory distress syndrome, pulmonary hypertension, and intracranial hemorrhage.

Hydroxyprogesterone caproate once-weekly injections are approved by the FDA to **reduce** the risk of **preterm delivery** in women with a history of at least one spontaneous preterm birth. Administration of progesterone inhibits the release of proinflammatory cytokines and delays cervical ripening. Vaginal administration of progesterone also significantly delays preterm birth.

Drugs that **inhibit uterine contractions** are called **tocolytics. Terbutaline,** a *beta$_2$*-adrenoceptor agonist (see Chapter 8) is used "off label" to relax the smooth muscle of the uterus and delay preterm birth. However, it is effective only during the first 48 hours of treatment and its use is associated with significant adverse effects in the mother, including tachycardia, hypotension, and pulmonary edema. **Calcium channel blockers** (e.g., **nifedipine**) and **magnesium sulfate** reduce uterine contractions by **inhibition of calcium ion influx** in uterine muscle cells. **NSAIDs** such as **indomethacin block the production of PGs** and are used to inhibit uterine contractions based on the role of PGs in stimulating contractions.

Despite a number of clinical trials, an effective tocolytic agent that is devoid of adverse maternal and fetal effects is not available.

Initiation of Labor

The induction of labor is indicated when the risk to the mother or fetus of continued pregnancy is greater than the risks of delivery and pharmacologic induction. Labor is also induced for nonmedical reasons, such as the patient residing at a great distance from the hospital or a history of rapid birth. This is called **elective induction and should not occur before 39 weeks of pregnancy,** although other medical issues may warrant earlier induction.

Dinoprostone

PGs are among the natural triggers to start labor and begin the process of cervical ripening and cervical dilation. Because PGs also stimulate uterine contractions, they are useful in the treatment of postpartum hemorrhage.

Dinoprostone (Cervidil) is the same entity as natural **prostaglandin E$_2$ (PGE$_2$;** see Chapter 26) and is formulated as s a thin, flat slab with rounded corners encased in a pouch attached to a long tape for easy retrieval. Each slab contains 10 mg of **dinoprostone in a slow-releasing hydrogel,** releasing approximately 0.3 mg/h. PGE$_2$ stimulates the production of PGF$_2$*alpha* which in turn sensitizes the myometrium to endogenous or exogenously administered oxytocin. At concentrations used for labor induction, **dinoprostone by itself does not affect uterine contraction** to any appreciable degree. This consideration lends credence to the clinical practice of treating cervical ripening and uterine contraction, usually with oxytocin (see next) as two separate events.

Because of cost issues, **misoprostol (Cytotec) is often used "off label" for cervical ripening.** Misoprostol is a synthetic PGE$_1$ analog and approved for use in prevention of NSAID-induced gastric ulcers (see Chapter 26). Misoprostol is also approved as an **abortifacient** when **used together with mifepristone** (see earlier in this chapter).

Oxytocin

Oxytocin (Pitocin) is a hormone secreted from the posterior lobe of the pituitary that stimulates uterine contractions during labor and induces milk ejection from the breast (see Chapter 31). The drug is given intravenously to **induce or enhance uterine contractions** during labor, and it is injected intramuscularly to **prevent postpartum uterine hemorrhage** by causing the uterine muscle to contract. In addition, a nasal spray preparation of oxytocin is available to **stimulate milk let-down in nursing mothers.** The spray is inhaled 2 to 3 minutes before breast-feeding. Adverse reactions to oxytocin are uncommon. They include cardiac arrhythmias, CNS stimulation, excessive uterine contraction, and hyponatremia. Use of synthetic oxytocin is contraindicated in instances of fetal distress, abnormal fetal presentation, prematurity, or cephalopelvic disproportion.

Drugs for Morning Sickness and Hyperemesis Gravidarum

Affecting more than half of pregnant women, **nausea and vomiting ("morning sickness")** usually begins by the fourth week and abates by the 16th week of pregnancy. The etiology of pregnancy-induced nausea and vomiting is unknown; some studies suggest that it may be caused by the increase in human chorionic gonadotrophin (hCG). In less than 1% of women, the condition progresses to **hyperemesis gravidarum,** which is noted by prolonged and severe nausea and vomiting, dehydration, and weight loss.

Doxylamine With Vitamin B$_6$

Doxylamine is a first-generation H$_1$ antihistamine, and vitamin B$_6$ is also known as pyridoxine. Diclegis is a fixed-dose combination drug product of 10 mg of doxylamine and 10 mg of pyridoxine indicated for the treatment of nausea and vomiting of pregnancy in women who do not respond to conservative management. Although **antihistamine drugs such as doxylamine** do have some antinausea and antiemetic effects (see Chapter 26), the addition of pyridoxine appears to be a holdover from the FDA approval of the first medication (Bendectin) that contained the same two ingredients. Bendectin was subsequently removed from the market due to increased pressure and costs from litigation claiming fetal defects with use; this litigation was subsequently shown to be based on "junk science." Very recently, the manufacturers of Diclegis formulated a **higher-dose combination** (20 mg each of doxylamine and pyridoxine) claimed to be faster-acting and longer-lasting and gave it the new brand name of Bonjesta.

Because these drugs are expensive, many obstetricians will recommend using over-the-counter substitution for these agents with the sleeping aid Unisom (doxylamine) and vitamin B$_6$ (pyridoxine) supplements.

Cannabinoid Hyperemesis Syndrome

The increased use of cannabinoids during pregnancy has led to the rise of **cannabinoid hyperemesis syndrome (CHS)** among pregnant patients. CHS was first described approximately 10 years ago and is characterized by **chronic cannabis use, cyclic episodes of nausea and vomiting,** and the learned behavior of **hot bathing** (see Chapter 28). The only known cure for CHS is cessation of marijuana or other cannabis product use. In severe cases, the pregnant patient with CHS will need to be hospitalized and given parenteral nutrition.

Treatment of Postpartum Depression

Postpartum depression (PPD) affects approximately 10% of women after birth of their child. PPD is diagnosed when women meet the Diagnostic and Statistical Manual of Mental Disorders (DSM)-5 criteria for a major depressive episode with onset of symptoms in within 4 weeks of delivery.

Brexanolone was the **first drug specifically approved for the treatment of PPD** and has a mechanism of action unlike any other antidepressant on the market. **Brexanolone** is a **positive allosteric modulator of GABA$_A$ receptors** in a manner similar to that of barbiturates and benzodiazepines but binds to multiple types of different subunit containing GABA$_A$ receptors at a different binding site. The mainstay of PPD treatment is the same as other types of depression that respond to pharmacotherapy (e.g., an SSRI antidepressant such as fluoxetine [Prozac]).

The main advantage of **brexanolone,** like **esketamine** (see Chapter 22), is that **antidepressant effects take place immediately;** SSRIs and other antidepressants typically take 2 to 4 weeks to be effective. The main disadvantage (besides astronomic cost) is the method of administration.

Brexanolone is given by a 60-hour continuous intravenous (IV) infusion (2.5 days) in which the patient must be admitted to the hospital and under supervision. Antidepressant effects were shown to last at least 30 days. Most common adverse effects of **brexanolone** were excessive **sedation and sudden loss of consciousness**.

SUMMARY OF IMPORTANT POINTS

- Estradiol preparations include skin patches for transdermal administration, micronized estradiol for oral administration, and estradiol cypionate and estradiol valerate for intramuscular or oral administration.
- Conjugated equine estrogens are sulfate esters of estrone and equilin. They are used for HRT in postmenopausal women and to treat other forms of hypogonadism.
- In menopausal women, estrogens relieve VMSs and protect against osteoporosis. Clinical trials suggest estrogens may prevent cardiovascular disease in healthy, younger menopausal women but may increase cardiovascular disease in older women.
- Ethinyl derivatives of estradiol (ethinyl estradiol and mestranol) have higher oral bioavailability and longer half-lives than estradiol. They are used primarily in oral contraceptives.
- Progesterone derivatives (e.g., MPA) are primarily used in combination with estrogens in HRT to reduce endometrial hyperplasia and the risk of endometrial cancer. They are also used to suppress ovarian function in the treatment of dysmenorrhea, endometriosis, and uterine bleeding, as well as for contraception.
- Synthetic progestins, including norethindrone, are primarily used in contraceptives, including combination estrogen-progestin contraceptives and progestin-only contraceptives.
- Norgestrel is the most androgenic progestin, desogestrel is one of the least androgenic, and drospirenone has antiandrogenic and antimineralocorticoid activity.
- Hormonal contraceptives act primarily by inhibiting gonadotropin secretion and ovulation. They also affect mucus viscosity, sperm transport, and endometrial histology.
- Contraceptives have been associated with an increased risk of hypertension, thromboembolic disorders, and gallstones. The risk of thromboembolism is substantially reduced with preparations containing low doses of estrogen.
- Some of the progestin-only contraceptives are administered as long-acting implants or injections, and others are given as oral tablets for both preventive and emergency contraception. Adverse effects include frequent spotting and amenorrhea.
- Tamoxifen, an antiestrogen primarily used to treat breast cancer, is given in combination with surgery and other chemotherapy.
- Anastrozole and letrozole, aromatase inhibitors that decrease estrogen synthesis, are used to treat breast cancer in postmenopausal women.
- Clomiphene is an antiestrogen used to treat anovulatory infertility. By reducing estrogen feedback inhibition of gonadotropin secretion, clomiphene increases gonadotropin secretion and stimulates ovulation.
- Raloxifene is a selective ER modulator that acts as an estrogen antagonist in breast and uterine tissue. The drug produces estrogen-like effects on bone metabolism and reduces the risk of osteoporosis.
- Mifepristone is an antiprogestin used for medical termination of intrauterine pregnancy.
- Testosterone preparations are primarily used to treat hypogonadism.
- Flutamide and other androgen receptor antagonists are used to treat prostate cancer, often in combination with a GnRH agonist (e.g., leuprolide).
- Finasteride and dutasteride are 5α-reductase inhibitors that block the formation of DHT. They are used to treat BPH and male pattern baldness and to prevent prostate cancer.
- Drugs used in obstetrics include dinoprostone and oxytocin for cervical ripening and labor induction, doxylamine and pyridoxine for morning sickness, and brexanolone for PPD.

Review Questions

1. Raloxifene is indicated for the treatment of which disorder?
   - (A) thromboembolism
   - (B) osteoporosis
   - (C) menopausal symptoms
   - (D) endometriosis
   - (E) contraception
2. A progestin is included in regimens for HRT to prevent which of the following adverse effects?
   - (A) breast cancer
   - (B) endometrial cancer
   - (C) myocardial infarction
   - (D) stroke
   - (E) elevated cholesterol levels
3. A man is taking nilutamide for prostate cancer. Which adverse effect is most likely to occur in persons taking this drug?
   - (A) breast tenderness
   - (B) alopecia
   - (C) glaucoma
   - (D) deep vein thrombosis
   - (E) hot flashes
4. A woman is taking norethindrone daily for contraception. Which adverse effect is associated with this agent?
   - (A) venous thromboembolism
   - (B) irregular menstrual cycles
   - (C) hot flashes
   - (D) breast enlargement
   - (E) hypertension
5. Which hormone receptors are blocked by drospirenone?
   - (A) aldosterone and androgen receptors
   - (B) estrogen and progestin receptors
   - (C) only progestin receptors
   - (D) only gonadotropin receptors
   - (E) only glucocorticoid receptors

CHAPTER 35

Drugs for the Treatment of Diabetes

CLASSIFICATION OF ANTIDIABETIC AGENTS

Insulin Preparations
- See Table 35.1

Antidiabetic Agents

α-glucosidase inhibitors
- Acarbose (PRECOSE)
- Miglitol (GLYSET)

Amylin analog
- Pramlintide (SYMLIN)

Biguanides
- Metformin (GLUCOPHAGE)

Dipeptidyl peptidase-4 inhibitors
- Sitagliptin (JANUVIA)[a]
- Linagliptin (TRADJENTA)

Glucagon-like peptide-1 receptor agonists
- Semaglutide (OZEMPIC)
- Dulaglutide (TRULICITY)[b]

Meglitinides
- Repaglinide (PRANDIN)
- Nateglinide (STARLIX)

Sodium-glucose cotransporter 2 inhibitors
- Canagliflozin (INVOCANA)
- Dapagliflozin (FARXIGA)[c]

Sulfonylureas
- Glipizide (GLUCOTROL)
- Glyburide (DIABETA)[d]

Thiazolidinediones
- Pioglitazone (ACTOS)
- Rosiglitazone (AVANDIA)

Dopamine agonist
- Bromocriptine (CYCLOSET)

[a] Also saxagliptin (ONGLYZA), and alogliptin (NESINA). The combination products of linagliptin with metformin (JENTADUETO), and sitagliptin with metformin (JANUMET and JANUMET XR), as well as sitagliptin with the statin drug simvastatin (JUVISYNC) are also available.
[b] Also exenatide (BYETTA), albiglutide (TANZEUM), liraglutide (VICTOZA), and lixisenatide (ADLYXIN); exenatide extended-release for injection is marketed as BYDUREON, and first newly formulation in this class for oral administration (tablet) is semaglutide (RYBELSUS).
[c] Also empagliflozin (JARDIANCE), and the combination products canagliflozin with metformin (INVOKAMET), empagliflozin with metformin (SYNJARDY), and dapagliflozin with metformin (XIGDUO XR); ertigliflozin (STEGLATRO) is a new sodium glucose co-transporter 2 (SGLT2) inhibitor, in combination with metformin as SEGLUROMET and in combination with sitagliptin as STEGLUJAN.
[d] Also glimepiride (AMARYL), and the combo formulation of glyburide with metformin (GLUCOVANCE).

OVERVIEW

Pancreatic Hormones

The hormones secreted by the endocrine pancreas are produced in clusters of cells called **islets of Langerhans.** These islets contain three major types of hormone-secreting cells.

The α cells produce **glucagon,** the β cells produce **insulin** and **amylin,** and the δ cells secrete **somatostatin.** Insulin promotes the uptake, usage, and storage of glucose and thereby lowers the plasma glucose concentration, whereas glucagon increases the hepatic glucose output and blood glucose concentration. **Diabetes mellitus** (hereafter, diabetes) results from inadequate insulin secretion or insulin activity that is not sufficient to maintain normal blood glucose concentrations.

Insulin

As shown in Box 35.1, **proinsulin** is converted to **insulin** and **C peptide.** Insulin consists of two peptide chains (the A chain and the B chain), which are linked by two disulfide (-S-S-) bridges. Although both insulin and C peptide are released in response to rising glucose concentrations, the physiologic role of C peptide remains unknown.

Secretion

Insulin secretion has meal-stimulated and basal components. Insulin release is activated by the **rise in blood glucose** concentration that follows the digestion and absorption of carbohydrates (Fig. 35.1A and B). Insulin is released at the rate of 1 unit (U) per 10 g of dietary carbohydrate, and its level usually peaks within 1 hour of eating. **Insulin promotes the uptake and storage of glucose** and other ingested nutrients, and the postprandial (postmeal) plasma concentrations of both insulin and glucose return to preprandial (premeal) levels within 2 hours. Basal secretion, which usually ranges from 0.5 to 1 U of insulin per hour, serves to retard hepatic glucose output during the postabsorptive state.

Physiologic Effects

Insulin is sometimes referred to as the "**storage hormone**" because it promotes the formation of glycogen, triglycerides, and protein while inhibiting their breakdown.

Insulin has several important actions on the **liver,** the organ that normally serves as the major source of blood glucose to supply the brain in the fasting state. The liver provides blood glucose through the processes of gluconeogenesis (the formation of glucose from amino acids) and glycogenolysis (the breakdown of glycogen). Insulin stimulates enzymes involved in glycogen synthesis while inhibiting glycogenolytic and gluconeogenic enzymes, thereby reducing glucose output by the liver.

Insulin promotes the uptake of glucose by **skeletal muscle** and **adipose tissue** by activating a glucose transporter in these tissues called GLUT4. Skeletal muscle and adipose tissue are dependent on insulin for glucose uptake, whereas the brain can use blood glucose in the absence of insulin. By promoting glucose uptake, insulin facilitates the metabolism of glucose to provide energy for skeletal muscle contraction and stimulates glycogen synthesis. In adipose tissue, insulin increases the conversion of glucose to fatty acids for storage

TABLE 35.1 Onset of Action, Peak Effect, and Duration of Action of Insulin Preparations After Subcutaneous Administration or Inhalation

TYPE OF INSULIN	ONSET	PEAK	DURATION
Rapid-acting insulin			
Insulin aspart (NovoLog)	10–20 min	40–50 min	3–5 h
Insulin lispro (Humalog)	15–30 min	30–90 min	3–5 h
Insulin glulisine (Apidra)	20–30 min	30–90 min	1–2.5 h
Short-acting insulin			
Regular insulin (Humulin R)	30–60 min	2–5 h	5–8 h
Intermediate-acting insulin			
Isophane (NPH) insulin	1–2 h	4–12 h	18–24 h
Long-acting insulin			
Insulin glargine (Lantus)	1–1.5 h	None	20–24 h
Insulin detemir (Levemir)	1–2 h	6–8 h	Up to 24 h
Insulin degludec (Tresiba)	1–2 h	None	>24 h
Inhaled insulin			
Human insulin powder (Afrezza)	5–10 min	1 h	5–10 h

NPH, Neutral protamine Hagedorn.

as triglyceride. It also promotes the uptake and esterification of fatty acids and inhibits lipolysis (the conversion of triglyceride to fatty acids). In skeletal muscle, insulin inhibits protein catabolism and amino acid output.

Mechanisms of Action

Insulin binds to **insulin receptors** located in the plasma membrane of target cells, which are primarily cells of the liver, skeletal muscle, and adipose tissue. The intracellular domain of the insulin receptor has **tyrosine kinase** (phosphate transferring) activity, and activation of these receptors leads to tyrosine **phosphorylation of insulin receptor substrate proteins** (ISP). In turn, the phosphorylated ISP regulate the **expression and activity of key enzymes** of carbohydrate, lipid, and protein metabolism as well as enzymes involved in cardiovascular and other physiologic functions. For example, activated insulin substrate proteins increase the synthesis of ribosomal proteins and promote the translation of messenger RNA encoding metabolic enzymes. In addition, ISP phosphorylation increases the **insertion of GLUT4 glucose transporter** molecules into cell membranes of muscle and adipose tissue, enabling **increased glucose uptake** into these cells.

Glucagon

Glucagon is produced by α cells of the pancreas in response to **decreased blood glucose** concentrations. It activates glycogenolysis and gluconeogenesis and increases hepatic glucose production. Patients with diabetes continue to produce glucagon, and the imbalance between glucagon and insulin is one factor that contributes to the metabolic derangements of this disease. Glucagon is available in a formulation for **subcutaneous injection** used to counteract hypoglycemic reactions in patients with diabetes.

DIABETES
Classification

Diabetes is characterized by elevated basal and postprandial blood glucose concentrations. It affects about 25 million people in the United States and about 350 million worldwide. The two major forms of diabetes are type 1 and type 2, with the latter accounting for about 85% of cases of diabetes.

Type 1 diabetes usually has its onset before 30 years of age, with a median onset of 12 years of age. It is believed to be an autoimmune disease triggered by a viral infection or other environmental factors. The resulting destruction of pancreatic β cells leads to severe insulin deficiency and excessive production of ketones, causing **ketonemia and ketoacidosis.** Persons with type 1 diabetes require exogenous insulin for survival.

Type 2 diabetes (Box 35.2) is a heterogeneous disease that usually has its onset after the patient reaches 30 years of age and is often associated with a significant degree of **insulin resistance** and **obesity.** Insulin resistance can be caused by the presence of insulin antibodies or by defects in insulin receptors and signal transduction mechanisms in target organs. Patients with type 2 diabetes are less susceptible to developing ketonemia and ketoacidosis than type 1 patients. Most patients with type 2 diabetes have normal or elevated concentrations of insulin and do not require exogenous insulin for survival. Type 2 diabetes is usually treated with oral antidiabetic medications in combination with dietary modifications and exercise, but some patients benefit from insulin treatment. A large number of genetic mutations have been identified that influence the development of type 2 diabetes.

Additional forms of diabetes include **gestational diabetes,** which has its onset during pregnancy, and **secondary diabetes,** which occurs in association with other endocrine disorders or with exposure to drugs or chemical agents toxic to the pancreas.

Pathophysiology

The early manifestations of diabetes are metabolic abnormalities resulting from lack of insulin, whereas the long-term complications of diabetes result in part from nonenzymatic glycosylation of proteins, primarily in the cardiovascular system, leading to endothelial and cardiac dysfunction, atherosclerosis, and other problems. The percentage of **glycosylated hemoglobin** (hemoglobin A_{1c}) is used as a clinical marker of long-term control of glycemia in individuals with diabetes.

The **acute metabolic abnormalities** that occur in untreated diabetes result from decreased glucose uptake by muscle and adipose tissue, increased hepatic output of glucose, increased catabolism of proteins in muscle tissue, and increased lipolysis and release of fatty acids from adipose tissue. A reduction in glucose use combined with an increase in hepatic glucose production leads to hyperglycemia. Hyperglycemia can then cause glycosuria (glucose in the urine), osmotic diuresis, polyuria (excessive urine formation), and polydipsia (excessive water intake). These derangements lead to dehydration and the loss of calories and weight. For these reasons, diabetes has been described as "starvation in the midst of plenty."

In patients with type 1 diabetes, the absence of insulin accelerates lipolysis, and this leads to increased production of ketones (acetoacetic acid, acetone, and β-hydroxybutyric acid) in the liver. When the body is no longer able to metabolize these ketones, the keto acids are excreted in the urine. These derangements can eventually lead to ketoacidosis, acetone breath, abnormal respiration, electrolyte depletion,

BOX 35.1 STRUCTURES OF PROINSULIN AND INSULIN MOLECULES

Preproinsulin is synthesized in the rough endoplasmic reticulum of pancreatic β cells, and proinsulin is formed by enzymatic cleavage of this precursor molecule. Proinsulin is then transported to the Golgi apparatus and converted to insulin and C peptide (connecting peptide) by the removal of four amino acids (dipeptide linkage). Insulin and C peptide are packaged in storage granules until released in equimolar amounts in response to rising glucose concentrations.

Insulin consists of a 21-amino-acid A chain and a 30-amino-acid B chain linked by two disulfide bridges.

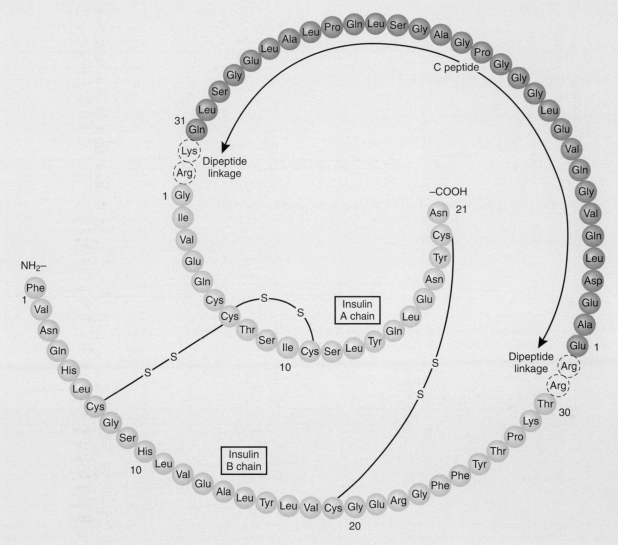

Differences in the amino acid composition of insulins are shown in the following table.

Type of Insulin	CHAIN POSITION				
	A-21	B-3	B-28	B-29	B-30
Human insulin	Asparagine	Asparagine	Proline	Lysine	Threonine
Insulin aspart	Asparagine	Asparagine	Aspartate	Lysine	Threonine
Insulin lispro	Asparagine	Asparagine	Lysine	Proline	Threonine
Insulin glulisine	Asparagine	Lysine	Proline	Glutamate	Threonine
Insulin glargine	Glycine	Asparagine	Proline	Lysine	Threonine[a]
Insulin detemir	Asparagine	Asparagine	Proline	Lysine[b]	None
Insulin degludec	Asparagine	Asparagine	Proline	Lysine[c]	None

[a]Two additional arginine residues are attached to threonine at B-30.
[b]A 14-carbon fatty acid chain is attached to this amino acid, and threonine is omitted at B-30.
[c]Glutamic acid and a 16-carbon fatty acid are attached to this amino acid, and threonine is omitted at B-30.

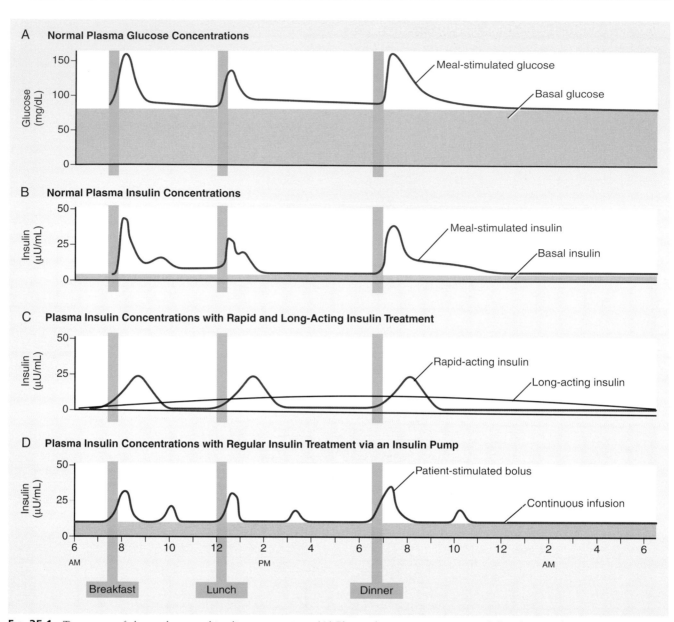

FIG. 35.1 Time course of plasma glucose and insulin concentrations. (A) Plasma glucose concentrations result from hepatic glucose output in the fasting state and the digestion and absorption of carbohydrates after meals. (B) Plasma insulin levels result from a basal level of insulin secretion throughout the day and glucose-stimulated secretion after meals. (C) Insulin levels resulting from daily injections of long-acting insulin to provide the basal insulin requirement and premeal injections of rapid-acting insulin to control postprandial glycemia in individuals with type 1 diabetes. (D) Insulin levels obtained with an insulin pump. The pump delivers a constant infusion of regular insulin to fulfill the basal insulin requirement, and the patient activates small bolus injections of insulin before meals, before snacks, and at bedtime.

vomiting, coma, and death. Insulin deficiency also leads to increased catabolism of proteins and increased loss of nitrogen in the urine.

The **long-term complications** of diabetes include microvascular complications, such as **nephropathy** and **retinopathy;** macrovascular complications, such as **cerebrovascular disease, coronary artery disease,** and **peripheral vascular disease;** and neuropathic complications, such as **sensory, motor,** and **autonomic neuropathic disorders.**

Although all of the complications of diabetes contribute significantly to morbidity, the most prevalent cause of death is coronary artery disease. Patients with diabetes often develop **hypertension** and **dyslipidemia,** characterized by a decrease in the high-density lipoprotein (HDL) cholesterol level and an increase in the triglyceride level. Furthermore,

diabetes appears to be a risk factor for coronary artery disease independent of other risk factors such as smoking, hypertension, and dyslipidemia. For these reasons, patients with diabetes should exercise regularly, adhere closely to dietary guidelines, and comply with pharmacologic interventions to control hypertension and dyslipidemia and to achieve near-normal blood glucose concentrations.

INSULIN PREPARATIONS

Insulin preparations are used to treat all patients with type 1 diabetes and about one-third of patients with type 2 diabetes. Insulin is also used to treat pregnant women with gestational diabetes.

For many years, insulin was obtained from pork and beef pancreas. More recently, **human insulin** has been

BOX 35.2 A CASE OF POSTPRANDIAL HYPERGLYCEMIA

CASE PRESENTATION

A 52-year-old man with an 8-year history of type 2 diabetes is concerned that his diabetes is not well controlled. He has started a regular exercise program and has lost 12 lb. His A_{1c} level is now 8.0%, down from 8.4% at the previous determination. He is already taking maximal doses of metformin and glipizide and has been taking insulin glargine every evening for the past 3 months. His self-monitored blood glucose (SMBG) values show that his fasting blood glucose (FBG) values are fairly good, but his postprandial glucose (PPG) values are often high after breakfast and lunch, ranging from 158 to 230 mg/dL (normal values are less than 140). His evening PPG values are usually acceptable. Based on these findings, his health care provider suggests that he reduce carbohydrate intake at breakfast and lunch or add a rapid-acting insulin preparation before these meals. After considering his diet and activity level, the man decides to use insulin aspart before breakfast and lunch and to adjust the dose based on PPG values.

CASE DISCUSSION

SMBG is one of the most effective tools available to assist patients in achieving optimal glycemic control and target A_{1c} levels. However, studies show that a large percentage of people with diabetes fail to follow recommended guidelines for SMBG. Obstacles to the effective use of SMBG include patient denial and unwillingness to adopt changes indicated by SMBG data, lack of patient confidence in their ability to use SMBG data, and the cost, inconvenience, and physical discomfort of SMBG. It is no surprise that patient education is the largest factor determining the successful use of SMBG. Blood glucose monitors enable patients to obtain a record of glucose levels on which to base dietary and treatment decisions. Premeal and postmeal glucose values can be used to guide the selection and adjustment of insulin therapy. Rapid-acting insulins such as insulin aspart and insulin lispro can help patients control PPG levels, whereas long-acting insulins such as insulin glargine and insulin detemir can improve FBG values and overall glycemic control.

produced by expression of the human insulin gene in *Escherichia coli* or yeast using recombinant DNA technology. Human insulin is less likely than pork or beef insulin to elicit insulin antibodies leading to insulin resistance, and it is less likely to cause allergic reactions or lipodystrophy at injection sites. The latest innovation in insulin therapy has been the development of **human insulin analogs** that overcome some of the limitations of native human insulin as a therapeutic agent. These analogs have improved pharmacokinetic properties and provide more physiologic insulin levels than native insulin preparations. The insulin analogs are discussed later.

The concentration of insulin preparations is expressed as the number of units of insulin per milliliter of solution or suspension. The *United States Pharmacopeia* (USP) defines 1 unit (U) as the amount of insulin needed to decrease the blood glucose concentration by a defined amount in a fasting rabbit. The insulin preparations used by most people with diabetes contain 100 U/mL. Regular insulin is also available in a concentrated preparation containing 500 U/mL for use by persons with insulin resistance who require more than 100 U as a single injection.

Administration and Absorption

Insulin is usually **injected subcutaneously** or administered by **continuous subcutaneous infusion** with an insulin pump. Insulin preparations for inhalation are also available. Insulin absorption is most rapid from an abdominal injection site and is progressively slower from sites on the arm, thigh, and buttock. Because repeated injections at the same site can contribute to tissue reactions (lipodystrophy) that affect the rate of insulin absorption, patients should be taught to rotate injection sites within a particular anatomic area. Newer, silicone-covered needles are painless and have reduced patient aversion to insulin injections.

Based on their onset and duration of action, insulin preparations are classified as short-acting, rapid-acting, intermediate-acting, and long-acting (see Table 35.1).

Rapid-Acting Insulin

Three rapid-acting preparations are now available to control postprandial glycemia. **Insulin lispro, insulin aspart,** and **insulin glulisine** are human insulin analogs with amino acid substitutions in the B chain, as shown in Box 35.1. These modifications reduce the aggregation of insulin molecules and enable more rapid absorption after subcutaneous injection compared with regular insulin. An ideal insulin for premeal administration would have an onset of action in 10 to 20 minutes, would peak at 1 hour, and would have a duration of action of less than 3 hours. Hence, the rapid-acting insulin analogs are well suited for this purpose. Because the hypoglycemic effect of these insulins begins 10 to 20 minutes after subcutaneous injection, patients can easily coordinate insulin injections and mealtimes. These insulins are often used as part of a regimen that includes a long-acting insulin to provide basal insulin requirements.

Short-Acting Insulin

Regular insulin (insulin injection USP) has a slower onset and a longer duration of action than the rapid-acting insulin analogs after subcutaneous administration. It can also be given intravenously to treat diabetic ketoacidosis. Regular insulin consists of insulin hexamers crystallized around a zinc molecule. After subcutaneous injection, the hexamers dissociate into dimers and monomers that are absorbed into the circulation. Because of the time required for this process, the onset of action of regular insulin occurs 30 to 60 minutes after an injection, and the duration of action is 5 to 8 hours. For this reason, regular insulin is not ideally suited to control **postprandial glycemia.** It is often absorbed too slowly to prevent postprandial hyperglycemia, causing hypoglycemia later, thereby necessitating a snack and contributing to weight gain. Hence, a rapid-acting insulin preparation is usually more effective for premeal use and may contribute to a greater reduction in A_{1c} levels than regular insulin.

Intermediate-Acting Insulin

Neutral protamine Hagedorn (NPH) insulin is the **only intermediate-acting insulin** still available for human use, though a veterinary formulation of pork insulin zinc suspension recently became available to treat diabetic dogs. NPH insulin consists of particles of insulin combined with zinc and protamine that slowly dissolve after subcutaneous injection, enabling sustained absorption and blood levels. NPH is more prone to erratic absorption and intrapatient variability than the long-acting insulin analogs, and it must be gently rolled or inverted before each use to ensure uniform dosage. However, it offers a lower-cost alternative to insulin analogs to meet basal insulin requirements, especially in people with type 2 diabetes.

Long-Acting Insulin

Long-acting insulin preparations provide basal levels of insulin and facilitate control of glycemia throughout the day. These preparations are formulated to slowly release insulin for absorption into the circulation after a subcutaneous injection. In comparison with NPH insulin, the long-acting insulins provide a slower and more prolonged absorption and duration of action with less of a peak effect. However, some clinical trials found that the efficacy and incidence of hypoglycemia with long-acting insulins was no better than obtained with NPH insulin. Diabetic patients are usually started on a lower dose of a long-acting insulin, and the dose is gradually titrated upward to achieve the targeted fasting blood glucose levels. The long-acting insulins typically supply about one-third of the total daily insulin requirement, with the remainder filled by a rapid-acting insulin administered at mealtimes.

Insulin glargine contains amino acid substitutions in the A and B chains that enable it to be slowly released and absorbed after subcutaneous injection. It is formulated as a solution at a pH of 4, but it is less soluble at body pH and forms microprecipitates after subcutaneous injection. These precipitates slowly release insulin glargine for absorption over a 24-hour period, providing a relatively constant hypoglycemic effect over this time period. Hence, it does not exhibit a peak effect (see Table 35.1). Insulin glargine is administered subcutaneously once or twice daily. It is often used in combination with rapid-acting insulin given at mealtimes and is suitable for both type 1 and type 2 diabetes.

Insulin detemir is a solution of recombinant human insulin that has been chemically modified by deletion of threonine at B-30 and the attachment of a 14-carbon fatty acid chain to the amino acid at B-29 (see Box 35.1). After subcutaneous injection, insulin detemir reversibly binds to albumin in extracellular fluid and plasma, from which it is slowly released for absorption. It provides a consistent duration of action of about 24 hours with little intrapatient variability. Insulin detemir is administered once or twice daily to meet basal insulin requirements.

Insulin degludec is an ultra-long-acting recombinant insulin preparation that has similar structural modifications as insulin detemir. Its duration of action is over 24 hours, and it is injected subcutaneously once a day to meet basal insulin requirements.

Inhaled Insulin

A product containing **powdered human insulin** (Afrezza) is available for administration using an inhaler. It is used at mealtimes to **control postprandial glycemia** in type 1 diabetics and should be used in combination with a long-acting insulin preparation to meet basal insulin requirements. When a patient inhales through the device, the **insulin powder is aerosolized and delivered to the lungs.** The amount of insulin delivered may vary somewhat according to inhalation technique. Patients are instructed to exhale fully, then insert the device in the mouth and inhale deeply,

holding their breath as long as comfortable after inhaling before removing the inhaler. The product is available in cartridges containing 4, 8, or 12 units of **recombinant regular human insulin.**

OTHER ANTIDIABETIC AGENTS

A growing number of noninsulin agents are now available to treat diabetes. Most of these drugs are only employed in treating type 2 diabetes, but an amylin analog can be used for both type 1 and type 2 diabetes. The noninsulin antidiabetic drugs include the **insulin secretagogues,** the **insulin-sensitizing agents,** drugs that **decrease intestinal glucose absorption** (α-glucosidase inhibitors) or that **increase urinary glucose excretion** (*gliflozins*), and an **amylin analog called pramlintide.** Insulin secretagogues can cause hypoglycemia if carbohydrate intake is not sufficient to balance the increased insulin secretion produced by these agents, whereas other noninsulin antidiabetic agents are not typically associated with hypoglycemia. The pharmacologic properties of these drugs are depicted in Tables 35.2 and 35.3 and Fig. 35.2.

Insulin Secretagogues
Sulfonylurea Drugs

Of the currently used drugs, the sulfonylurea drugs were the earliest oral antidiabetic agents to be developed. The original sulfonylureas, such as tolbutamide, are no longer used because of their lower potency and their greater tendency to cause side effects. The second-generation drugs, which are at least 100 times more potent than first-generation drugs, include **glimepiride, glipizide,** and **glyburide.**

Pharmacokinetics. The sulfonylurea drugs are administered orally and undergo varying degrees of hepatic metabolism followed by renal and biliary elimination of the metabolites.

Mechanisms and Pharmacologic Effects. Sulfonylurea drugs act primarily by increasing the secretion of insulin and secondarily by decreasing the secretion of glucagon.

Sulfonylureas increase the release of insulin from pancreatic β cells by inhibiting **adenosine triphosphate (ATP)–sensitive potassium channels** in the plasma membrane. The potassium channel contains a pore-forming subunit through which potassium moves out of the cell and a subunit that functions as the sulfonylurea receptor. When a sulfonylurea drug binds to this receptor, it closes the potassium channel. This prevents potassium efflux and leads to β cell depolarization, an influx of calcium, and activation of the secretory machinery that releases insulin. Sulfonylureas increase the pulsatile secretion of insulin by increasing the amount of insulin secreted during each pulse, but they have no effect on basal secretion.

Sulfonylurea drugs **decrease glucagon secretion** as a result of increasing insulin and pancreatic somatostatin secretion, both of which inhibit the release of glucagon from pancreatic α cells. This action tends to normalize the ratio of insulin to glucagon in individuals with diabetes. Sulfonylurea drugs may also increase insulin sensitivity in patients with type 2 diabetes.

In contrast to some of the antihyperglycemic drugs, sulfonylureas do not have beneficial effects on lipoprotein levels, and their use has been associated with **weight gain.**

Indications. A sulfonylurea drug can be used alone to treat type 2 diabetes that is not controlled with dietary

TABLE 35.2   Properties of Antidiabetic Drugs

DRUG	HYPOGLYCEMIA AND WEIGHT GAIN	OTHER ADVERSE EFFECTS	ADVANTAGES
Acarbose and miglitol	No	Frequent bloating and flatulence; decreased iron absorption	Lack of systemic adverse effects
Metformin	No	Frequent diarrhea; rare lactic acidosis	Modest weight loss and cardiovascular benefits
Repaglinide and nateglinide	Yes, but less than sulfonylureas		Good for variable meal schedules
Glipizide and other sulfonylureas	Yes	Skin rash, hematologic reactions	Inexpensive add-on drug
Pioglitazone and rosiglitazone	No	Edema, heart failure, osteoporosis	Uncertain
Sitagliptin and other dipeptidyl peptidase-4 inhibitors	No	Pancreatitis, joint and muscle pain	Oral administration, well tolerated, few adverse effects
Exenatide and other glucagon-like peptide-1 agonists	No	Nausea is common, pancreatitis, must be injected	Weight loss
Canagliflozin and other sodium-glucose cotransporter 2 inhibitors	No	Genital and urinary tract infections, diuresis, increased risk of acute renal failure	Weight loss, blood pressure reduction
Pramlintide	No	Transient nausea	

TABLE 35.3   Metabolic Effects of Antidiabetic Drugs

DRUG	GLYCEMIC EFFECTS			LIPID EFFECTS			
	FPG	PPG	A_{1C} (%↓)	LDL	HDL	TG	BODY WEIGHT
Acarbose and miglitol	→ or ↓	↓	0.3–1.0	→	→	↓	→ or ↓
Metformin	↓	↓	1.5–2.0	↓	↑	↓	→ or ↓
Repaglinide and nateglinide	→	↓	1	→	→	→	↑
Glimepiride and other sulfonylureas	↓	↓	1.5–2.0	→	→	→ or ↓	↑
Pioglitazone	↓	↓	0.8–1.8	→ or ↑	↑	↓	→ or ↑
Sitagliptin and other DDP-4 inhibitors	↓	↓	0.7	→	→	→	→
Exenatide and other glucagon-like peptide-1 agonists	↓	↓	1–1.1	→	↓	↓	↓
Canagliflozin and other sodium-glucose cotransporter 2 inhibitors	↓	↓	0.7	→	→	→	↓

A_{1c}, Glycosylated hemoglobin; *FPG,* fasting plasma glucose concentration; *HDL,* high-density–lipoprotein cholesterol level; *LDL,* low-density–lipoprotein cholesterol level; *PPG,* postprandial glucose concentration; *TG,* triglyceride level; →, unchanged; ↓, decreased; ↑, increased.

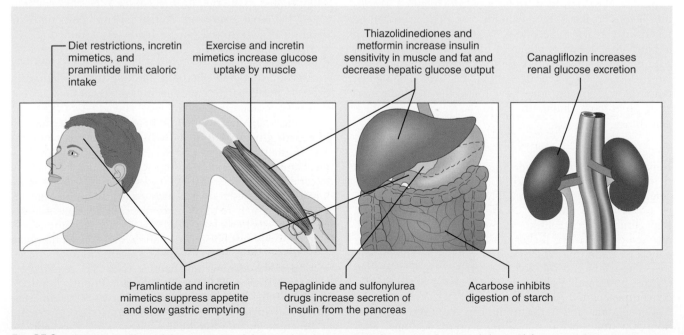

Fig. 35.2 Therapeutic effects of diet, exercise, and drugs used in the treatment of patients with type 2 diabetes. If these treatment measures are not adequate, insulin can be used to control glycemia.

restrictions, exercise, and weight reduction. A sulfonylurea can also be given in combination with **metformin,** and this combination may provide better control of blood glucose concentrations while causing fewer adverse reactions.

Adverse Effects. Hypoglycemia, the most common adverse effect of sulfonylurea drugs, can result from skipped or delayed meals, inadequate ingestion of carbohydrates, excessive doses, or renal or hepatic disease. Other adverse effects include skin rashes (which occur in up to 3% of patients), nausea, vomiting, and cholestasis. Less commonly, sulfonylureas cause hematologic reactions such as leukopenia, thrombocytopenia, and hemolytic anemia.

Interactions. Health care providers should be aware that sulfonylureas can interact with many other drugs. Although the clinical significance of many of these interactions is usually minimal, dosage adjustments may be required. Thiazide diuretics, corticosteroids, estrogens, thyroid hormones, phenytoin, and other drugs decrease the effectiveness of sulfonylureas and may necessitate a dosage increase.

Angiotensin-converting enzyme (ACE) inhibitors, sulfonamides, salicylates, and other nonsteroidal anti-inflammatory drugs, gemfibrozil, and **alcohol** are among the agents that can **increase the hypoglycemic effect** of sulfonylureas. Excessive ingestion of alcohol by patients treated with sulfonylureas or insulin can cause significant hypoglycemia. A disulfiram-like reaction can also result when alcohol is taken with sulfonylureas. Individuals with diabetes should be counseled to use alcohol moderately and to limit consumption to about 2 oz (60 mL) of distilled beverage per day.

Specific Drugs

The second-generation sulfonylurea drugs consist of **glimepiride, glipizide,** and **glyburide.** Glyburide is called *glibenclamide* in some countries.

Sulfonylurea therapy usually begins with a low dose given once a day. The dose is then increased every 1 to 2 weeks until adequate glycemic control is achieved, side effects occur, or the maximal dose is reached. The absorption of glipizide is slowed by food, and it should be ingested 30 minutes before breakfast, but glyburide and glimepiride can be taken with breakfast. Second-generation sulfonylureas have a duration of action of about 24 hours, and many patients require only a single **daily dose to control glycemia,** but if larger doses are required, they should be divided and given twice daily. Clinical studies have found that second-generation drugs have similar efficacy in the treatment of type 2 diabetes.

Meglitinide Drugs

Repaglinide and **nateglinide** are meglitinide compounds that are rapidly absorbed and promptly produce a hypoglycemic effect of short duration. These drugs are intended to be taken **before meals** to control postprandial glycemia. Repaglinide and nateglinide increase the amount of insulin released by pancreatic β cells during and immediately after a meal by inhibiting **ATP-sensitive potassium channels** in the same manner as sulfonylurea compounds. These drugs control postprandial glycemia and decrease blood glucose concentrations and A_{1c} levels.

Repaglinide and nateglinide can be taken anytime from 30 minutes before a meal right up to mealtime. They achieve peak effectiveness in about 1 hour, which coincides with the time when postprandial glucose concentrations are rising toward their peak. Repaglinide and nateglinide are completely metabolized and inactivated by the liver in about 3 to 4 hours. For this reason, their duration of action is relatively short, and insulin concentrations return to basal levels before the next meal.

Repaglinide and nateglinide are indicated to treat type 2 diabetes in conjunction with diet and exercise, and they can be used in combination with metformin when either agent alone does not adequately control postprandial glycemia. They are particularly useful for patients whose meal schedules vary from day to day, a factor that increases their risk of hypoglycemic reactions to sulfonylureas. They should not be used with other oral antidiabetic drugs or with insulin.

The primary adverse effect of meglitinide drugs is **hypoglycemia.** Hypoglycemic reactions are not often serious, but they have caused 1.4% of patients to discontinue their use of repaglinide. This is about half the rate of discontinuation attributed to hypoglycemic reactions in patients taking sulfonylureas. Mild hypoglycemia can be treated with oral glucose, and severe hypoglycemia with intravenous D50W (50% dextrose in water) followed by a more dilute dextrose solution infusion.

Insulin Sensitizing Agents

The insulin-sensitizing agents include metformin, thiazolidinedione compounds such as pioglitazone, and the glucagon-like peptide-1 (GLP-1) receptor agonists (incretin mimetic).

Metformin

Chemistry and Pharmacokinetics. Metformin is the only **biguanide** type of oral antidiabetic medication currently available in the United States. Another biguanide, **phenformin,** was removed from the market in the 1970s because of an unacceptable risk of it causing fatal lactic acidosis (see later).

The immediate-release formulation of metformin is administered orally two to three times a day and is eliminated by **renal excretion** of the parent compound. Its duration of action is about 18 hours. A sustained-release metformin preparation is given as a single daily dose with the evening meal.

Mechanisms and Pharmacologic Effects. Metformin exerts its antihyperglycemic effects primarily in the liver, but it also has actions in skeletal muscle and adipose tissue. The most important effect of metformin appears to be a **reduction of hepatic glucose output** due to inhibition of **gluconeogenesis** (formation of new glucose) in the liver. The primary mechanism responsible for this effect is uncertain. One effect of metformin is that it reduces the expression of genes for gluconeogenesis enzymes such as glucose-6-phosphatase, which may partly result in metformin's activation of 5′adenosine monophosphate (AMP)-activated protein kinase. The drug also inhibits mitochondrial glycerol-3-phosphate dehydrogenase, an enzyme enabling regeneration of reduced nicotinamide adenine dinucleotide (NADH) required for electron transport and energy production in mitochondria.

In peripheral tissues, metformin **increases insulin sensitivity** by increasing insulin binding to its receptors, and it enhances **glucose uptake** in skeletal muscle and adipose tissue by inducing phosphorylation of a **GLUT4 enhancing**

factor. (GLUT4 is the insulin-sensitive membrane transporter that transfers glucose into cells of these tissues.) Metformin also inhibits glucose absorption from the intestines. Unlike the insulin secretagogues, metformin does not stimulate insulin secretion or cause hypoglycemia or weight gain.

Indications. **Metformin is a first-line drug** for the treatment of type 2 diabetes. It is particularly appropriate for obese patients with insulin resistance and for patients with hyperlipidemia. Metformin often controls hyperglycemia in patients who do not adequately respond to another antidiabetic drug, and it typically has a favorable effect on **plasma lipid levels** and may enable the **loss of weight** (see Table 35.3). Metformin can be used alone or in combination with a sulfonylurea, meglitinide, α-glucosidase inhibitor, or incretin mimetic for patients whose diabetes is not controlled with a single drug. For this purpose, metformin is available in combination products containing metformin and another agent.

Adverse Effects. The most common adverse effects of metformin are gastrointestinal disturbances. **Diarrhea** occurs in up to 30% of patients and causes about 4% of them to stop taking metformin, but this effect usually subsides over time. Unlike phenformin, metformin does interfere with glucose oxidation, and it causes **lactic acidosis** rarely (in only 3 cases per 100,000 patient-years of use). Patients with **renal or hepatic disease,** alcoholism, or a predisposition to metabolic acidosis should not be treated with metformin, however, because they are at increased risk of this serious adverse effect.

Interactions. Metformin has few drug interactions, though cimetidine can inhibit the drug's metabolism and elevate its plasma concentrations.

Thiazolidinediones
Chemistry and Pharmacokinetics
Pioglitazone and **rosiglitazone** are members of the thiazolidinedione (glitazone) class of insulin-sensitizing antihyperglycemic agents. In contrast to metformin, these drugs have a greater effect on **skeletal muscle** and **adipose tissue** and a lesser effect on the liver. These drugs are taken orally once or twice daily with or without food and are well absorbed from the gut and almost entirely metabolized by the liver. Two metabolites of pioglitazone have pharmacologic activity, but metabolites of rosiglitazone are inactive.

Mechanisms and Pharmacologic Effects
The thiazolidinedione drugs are agonists at the **peroxisome proliferator-activated receptor-γ (PPAR-γ)** in adipose tissue, skeletal muscle, and the liver. The various PPARs were discovered because of their role in causing the proliferation of peroxisomes, which are organelles involved in the metabolism of amino acids, fatty acids, phospholipids, and carbohydrates. Activation of PPAR-γ increases transcription of insulin-responsive genes that control glucose metabolism, leading to **increased insulin sensitivity** and decreased insulin resistance in patients with type 2 diabetes. Thiazolidinediones (glitazones) increase the insulin sensitivity of **skeletal muscle** and **adipose** by about 60%. Specifically, the drugs increase the number of **GLUT4 glucose transporters** in cell membranes of muscle and adipose tissue, which increases the

uptake and usage of glucose in these tissues. Pioglitazone and rosiglitazone also suppress hepatic glucose output. The glitazones can decrease plasma glucose concentrations by 40 to 80 mg/dL and decrease insulin requirements by 5% to 30%. However, their maximal effectiveness usually does not occur until **4 to 6 weeks** after initiation of treatment or an increase in dosage.

The glitazone drugs also activate the PPAR-α receptor and alter serum lipids in a manner similar to gemfibrozil and other fibrate drugs (see Chapter 15), though **rosiglitazone** and **pioglitazone** have somewhat different effects on **serum lipids.** Pioglitazone has a more favorable effect on serum lipids, as it increases HDL cholesterol more than does rosiglitazone while it increases low-density–lipoprotein (LDL) cholesterol less than rosiglitazone. Pioglitazone also reduces serum triglycerides more than does rosiglitazone.

Adverse Effects
Pioglitazone and rosiglitazone can cause **edema,** increase plasma volume, and increase the risk of developing heart failure in individuals with diabetes. Hence, they should not be used in persons with heart failure or a high risk of developing heart failure. An earlier meta-analysis of short-term studies of rosiglitazone suggested it increased cardiovascular mortality, but a more recent long-term, prospective, randomized controlled trial found that rosiglitazone does not increase cardiovascular risk more than metformin or sulfonylurea drugs such as glimepiride.

The glitazones tend to **increase body weight** rather than reduce it as metformin does. In addition, a French study suggested that pioglitazone may be associated with a slightly increased risk of **bladder cancer.** Finally, studies show that glitazones may **decrease bone mineral density** and increase the risk of osteoporosis and fractures in older women, possibly because PPAR-γ activation diverts bone stem cells from the osteogenic to the adipocytic cell lineage.

Indications
Given the potential adverse effects and limitations of glitazones, the role of these drugs in treating type 2 diabetes is uncertain. They are not first-line agents for most patients, but the glitazones might be employed as an adjunct to diet and lifestyle changes for patients who cannot control their diabetes with other oral drugs and who are unable or unwilling to use injectable agents.

G Glucagon-Like Peptide-1 Agonists
This class of antidiabetic drugs is also called **incretin mimetics. Incretins** are **intestinal peptide hormones** released in response to glucose and lipids derived from nutrients. Levels of these hormones are low in the fasting state but increase rapidly after ingestion of food. The incretins include glucose-dependent insulinotropic polypeptide and **GLP-1.** These effects of these peptides include **stimulation of glucose-dependent insulin secretion** and **inhibition of glucagon secretion** by the pancreas, increased **glucose uptake** by muscle and adipose tissue, **slowed gastric emptying,** and **decreased appetite and food intake.** Because these effects are beneficial to individuals with diabetes, two kinds of drugs have been developed that mimic the effects of endogenous incretins, namely GLP-1–like peptides and drugs that inhibit the breakdown of GLP-1.

GLP-1 stimulates insulin secretion in part by binding to a pancreatic G-protein-coupled receptor (GLP-1 receptor) that is coupled with the $G_{\alpha s}$ subunit, resulting in increased production of cyclic AMP. Cyclic AMP then stimulates protein kinase A, which phosphorylates pancreatic β-cell proteins leading to the closure of ATP-dependent potassium channels (see earlier) and insulin secretion. Other mechanisms also contribute to the stimulation of insulin secretion and other effects of GLP-1.

GLP-1 itself is not suited for therapeutic use because it is **rapidly degraded by dipeptidyl peptidase-4 (DPP-4)** and has a half-life of only 2 minutes. **Exenatide** is a GLP-1 receptor agonist derived from Gila monster lizard's saliva that resists degradation by DPP-4 and has a half-life of 12 to 14 hours. Exenatide is administered **subcutaneously twice daily** within 60 minutes of the morning and evening meals, whereas the longer-acting **liraglutide** and **lixisenatide** are injected **once a day. Sustained-release preparations** of exenatide, albiglutide, dulaglutide, and **semaglutide** are available for **once-weekly injection.** These drugs are primarily used to treat type 2 diabetics that do not respond adequately to oral agents. Clinical trials found that using a GLP-1 mimetic in combination with a sulfonylurea drug or metformin improved A_{1c} values and decreased body weight. The drugs can also be used in patients taking insulin, but the insulin dose should be reduced 20% when starting a GLP-1 mimetic and then titrated upward as needed.

Very recently, **semaglutide** (Rybelsus) was formulated as the **first oral GLP-1 receptor agonist** product approved for the treatment of type 2 diabetes. The FDA label includes instructions to convert from once-weekly semaglutide to the oral formulation of daily semaglutide tablets. Because the absorption of semaglutide is influenced by food and beverages, patients should take oral semaglutide with only 4 oz. of plain water, first thing in the morning at least 30 minutes before breakfast or coffee. Dosages start at 3 mg/day for a month, then escalate to 7 mg/day thereafter. Reported **adverse effects** from clinical trials were **nausea, abdominal pain, diarrhea, decreased appetite, vomiting, and constipation.**

Exenatide and other GLP-1 agonists may cause mild to moderate **nausea** and slightly increase the risk of **pancreatitis,** particularly in persons with hypertriglyceridemia or gallstones. Patients taking these drugs should be instructed to report severe abdominal pain that might be a symptom of pancreatitis. However, it should be kept in mind that untreated type 2 diabetics already have an increased risk of pancreatitis. **Liraglutide** also caused dose-dependent and treatment-duration–dependent thyroid C-cell tumors in laboratory rodents. There is no evidence that this occurs in humans, but patients with a personal or family history of medullary thyroid cancer should avoid these drugs until additional data is available.

Dipeptidyl Peptidase-4 Inhibitors

Sitagliptin, alogliptin, linagliptin, and saxagliptin (*gliptins*) are DPP-4 inhibitors intended for once-daily oral administration. These drugs cause over 80% inhibition of DPP-4, resulting in a twofold increase in plasma GLP-1 levels. Clinical trials found that gliptins increase plasma insulin levels and reduce postprandial glucose levels in type 2 diabetics, resulting in a dose-dependent reduction of A_{1c}

levels. In one study, 45% of patients taking the highest dose achieved A_{1c} levels below 7%. The gliptins are used to improve glycemic control in individuals with type 2 diabetes as monotherapy or in combination with metformin or another antidiabetic agent. However, they do not facilitate bodyweight loss as much as the GLP-1 agonists.

Sitagliptin and related drugs are generally **well tolerated** and do not cause hypoglycemia or gastrointestinal side effects, and they can be used in patients with renal insufficiency. Hence, they are usually well suited for older or frail patients. However, there is recent evidence that the **DDP-4 inhibitors** can cause **joint and skeletal muscle pain,** which is occasionally severe and disabling. Fortunately, patients recover from this condition when the medication is stopped.

Drugs Affecting Glucose Absorption or Excretion

α-Glucosidase Inhibitors

Mechanisms and Pharmacologic Effects. The digestion of dietary starch and disaccharides (e.g., sucrose) is dependent on the action of **α-glucosidase,** an enzyme located in the brush border of the intestinal tract. This enzyme converts oligosaccharides and disaccharides to glucose and other monosaccharides. **Acarbose** and **miglitol** competitively inhibit this enzyme and delay the digestion of starch and disaccharides. This action **decreases the rate of glucose absorption** and lowers postprandial blood glucose concentrations, thereby reducing postprandial hyperglycemia. Studies have shown that acarbose and miglitol reduce A_{1c} levels, although the reduction is usually less than that obtained with other oral antidiabetic drugs (see Table 35.3).

Indications and Pharmacokinetics. Acarbose and **miglitol** are **usually used in combination** with another oral antidiabetic agent in the treatment of type 2 diabetes. **Acarbose** and **miglitol** should be administered **with the first bite of a meal.** Acarbose is not absorbed systemically, and it is eliminated in the feces, whereas miglitol is partly absorbed from the gut. Both drugs, however, act locally to inhibit α-glucosidase in the gastrointestinal tract.

Adverse Effects and Interactions. The most common side effects of acarbose and miglitol are increased **flatulence** and **abdominal bloating.** These reactions probably result from the delivery of greater amounts of carbohydrate to the lower intestinal tract, where they exert an osmotic attraction for water and are metabolized by bacteria. These drugs do not inhibit lactase or cause lactose intolerance.

Acarbose can increase the oral bioavailability of metformin and cause a decrease in iron absorption. Miglitol can decrease the absorption of ranitidine and propranolol.

If concurrent administration of insulin or a sulfonylurea drug results in hypoglycemia in patients taking acarbose, this reaction **should be treated with glucose (dextrose) rather than sucrose** because sucrose requires α-glucosidase activity for digestion.

Sodium-Glucose Cotransporter 2 Inhibitors

Sodium-glucose cotransporter 2 (SGLT2) inhibitors are also known as **renal glucose reabsorption inhibitors.** The kidney has an important role in glucose homeostasis. Blood glucose is filtered at the renal glomerulus and reabsorbed into the bloodstream from the proximal tubule of the nephron by the action of the **SGLT2.** This transport protein is responsible for 90% of renal glucose reabsorption, which is increased in diabetics as a result of increased plasma and urinary glucose levels and increased expression and activity of SGLT2.

The SGLT2 inhibitors, known as *gliflozins*, are the newest type of oral agent for type 2 diabetes. The gliflozins include **canagliflozin, dapagliflozin,** and **empagliflozin.** By inhibiting SGLT2, the gliflozins decrease renal glucose reabsorption, increase urinary glucose excretion, and lower blood glucose levels. However, the typical reduction in A_{1c} levels produced by these drugs (0.7%) is less than achieved with many other oral agents. The efficacy of gliflozins is dependent on renal glomerular filtration, and these drugs should not be used in patients with glomerular filtration rates below 50 mL/min.

In their favor, these agents cause a loss of body weight averaging about 5 lb, and they tend to lower blood pressure. A recent study found that empagliflozin significantly reduces the progression to renal disease in type 2 diabetics with a high risk of cardiovascular events. This long-term renal benefit is in contrast to the acute risk of renal injury associated with gliflozins, as described in the next paragraph.

The **adverse effects** of canagliflozin and other gliflozins include an increased incidence of **urinary tract infections** and **genital yeast infections** because they increase urinary glucose levels and thereby facilitate microbial growth. They may also cause **volume depletion** resulting from osmotic diuresis. Canagliflozin and dapagliflozin have been associated with cases of **acute renal injury,** which is more likely to occur in patients who are dehydrated, have heart failure or low blood pressure, or are taking other drugs affecting the kidneys such as diuretics and ACE inhibitors. The acute renal injury was manifested as **azotemia** (elevated serum creatinine and uric acid) and was usually reversible. In addition, gliflozins may rarely lead to diabetic **ketoacidosis.** Gliflozins also increase the risk of **osteoporosis** and **bone fractures,** most likely because they increase urinary calcium excretion.

Amylin Analog

Amylin is a pancreatic hormone that is co-secreted with insulin by pancreatic β cells in response to elevated blood glucose levels. Amylin reduces the rate of rising blood glucose after a meal by several mechanisms. It **slows gastric emptying,** thereby retarding digestion and absorption of nutrients, and it **suppresses glucagon secretion** and glucose output by the liver. Amylin also **reduces appetite** by an effect on the appetite centers in the brain. Because secretion of both insulin and amylin is impaired in individuals with diabetes, administration of amylin may improve glycemic control and lead to weight loss in these persons.

Pramlintide acetate is a synthetic analog of human amylin for use in patients with **type 1** or **type 2 diabetes** who are being treated with insulin. It exerts an antihyperglycemic effect in these patients by slowing the rate at which food is delivered from the stomach to the intestines, and it reduces the rate of rising plasma glucose for about 3 hours after a meal. However, the overall absorption of ingested carbohydrates is not changed. Pramlintide also reduces caloric intake and may lead to weight loss.

Pramlintide is given **subcutaneously** at mealtimes and is indicated for individuals with type 1 or type 2 diabetes who use mealtime insulin and have failed to achieve optimal glucose control. Coadministration of insulin and pramlintide increases the risk of hypoglycemia. Patients should begin treatment with low doses of pramlintide that are gradually increased over time, and mealtime insulin doses should be initially lowered 50% and gradually retitrated. Pramlintide may cause **nausea, anorexia,** and **headache,** though these often subside over time. It should be discontinued if recurrent hypoglycemic episodes or significant nausea occurs.

DOPAMINE AGONIST

Bromocriptine is a dopamine D2 receptor agonist that has been used for many years in the treatment of hyperprolactinemia and Parkinson disease. Research suggests that deficient dopamine neurotransmission in the hypothalamus is associated with disturbances in the hypothalamic **circadian rhythm** that can lead to the development of insulin resistance, obesity, and diabetes. Early morning administration of bromocriptine was subsequently found to reset disturbed circadian rhythms and to reduce hepatic glucose output and serum triglycerides and free fatty acids, whose elevation was associated with insulin resistance and diabetes. Clinical trials found that a **quick-release formulation of bromocriptine** (CYCLOSET) taken early in the morning reduced **insulin resistance** and decreased A_{1c} levels by 0.6% to 1.2% in individuals with type 2 diabetes, and the drug has been approved as an adjunct to diet and exercise to improve glycemic control in this population. Bromocriptine should be taken within 2 hours after waking in the morning and should be taken with food to reduce nausea. Doses of bromocriptine used for this purpose are much lower than those used for Parkinson disease, and patients are started on one tablet per day and titrated upward by one additional tablet per week until the optimum dose has been achieved. The drug has been well tolerated except for **nausea.**

MANAGEMENT OF DIABETES
Type 1 Diabetes
All patients with type 1 diabetes require insulin therapy to achieve a high degree of glycemic control. Clinical trials have found that achieving and maintaining near-normal blood glucose concentrations in patients with type 1 diabetes reduces the incidence of nephropathy, neuropathy, and retinopathy and may lower the risk of cardiovascular disease.

Objectives of Insulin Therapy
The specific objectives of insulin therapy are to maintain the **fasting plasma glucose concentration** below 140 mg/dL (normal is less than 100 mg/dL); to maintain the **2-hour postprandial glucose concentration** below 175 mg/dL (normal is less than 140 mg/dL); and to maintain the **A1c concentration** below 6.5% or 7% (the recommendation varies among diabetes and endocrinology groups). The A_{1c} concentration, which is normally 4% to 6%, provides a cumulative indication of overall glycemic control and is believed to indicate the extent to which glycosylation of tissue proteins contributes to microvascular and other complications of diabetes.

Insulin Requirements and Administration Schedules
In patients with type 1 diabetes, multiple daily injections of insulin are required to obtain acceptable control of glycemia without causing hypoglycemia. The total amount of insulin

required by most of these patients is 0.5 to 1 U/kg per day. This amount, however, usually decreases during the *honeymoon phase* of diabetes (during the first several months after the initial episode of illness).

The preferred regimens for most patients with type 1 diabetes consist of a daily injection of a **long-acting insulin analog** to meet the basal insulin requirement and multiple injections of **rapid-acting insulin** at mealtimes to control postprandial glycemia (see Fig. 35.1). A subcutaneous **insulin pump** is an option for patients who are sufficiently motivated to properly use and maintain the device. Some studies show that insulin pump therapy improves glycemic control and reduces rates of hypoglycemia compared with multiple daily injections. However, there have also been reports of pump failures and hypoglycemic episodes when these devices fail or are not used properly. **Inhaled insulin** offers a needle-free alternative that may be used in place of rapid-acting insulin at mealtimes. Inhaled insulin could be advantageous to patients who have injection site reactions, needle aversion, or difficulty using injectable insulin. **Pramlintide,** an amylin analog, may be useful in patients who have failed to achieve optimal glucose control with insulin therapy alone.

Diabetic Ketoacidosis

Diabetic ketoacidosis is a common and life-threatening complication of type 1 diabetes, with a mortality as high as 6% to 10%. It is the most common cause of death in children with type 1 diabetes. Diabetic ketoacidosis can also occur in individuals with type 2 diabetes, particularly those who are hospitalized for other medical or surgical conditions. Therapy must be individualized based on the clinical and laboratory status of the patient. **Intravenous fluids** are given to restore fluid volume that has been depleted by osmotic diuresis and vomiting. A **continuous intravenous infusion of insulin** is given to decrease the plasma glucose concentration at a rate of 50 to 100 mg/dL per hour. Intravenous administration of **potassium chloride** is usually required to counteract hypokalemia that results from the correction of dehydration and acidosis. **Dextrose** (glucose) should be added to the intravenous infusion when glucose levels fall to 250 mg/dL because hyperglycemia is usually corrected more rapidly than is acidosis. Insulin should be continued until acidosis is resolved and the plasma bicarbonate level is above 15 mEq/L.

Type 2 Diabetes

Treatment of type 2 diabetes rests on a foundation of a nutritious diet and appropriate exercise. Dietary recommendations should attempt to limit calories and saturated fat. **Overweight patients should be encouraged to exercise and lose weight** to improve glycemic control, reduce insulin resistance, and lower plasma lipid levels. If nonpharmacologic measures are inadequate, as indicated by fasting blood glucose concentrations **exceeding 140 mg/dL** or **A1c concentrations exceeding 7%,** the next step is usually to add an oral antidiabetic medication.

Metformin, oral incretin mimetics, sulfonylureas, and meglitinide drugs are considered first-line drugs for type 2 diabetes, but **metformin is preferred for most patients.** In obese patients with type 2 diabetes who have insulin resistance or hyperlipidemia, metformin is a logical choice to begin drug therapy unless contraindicated because it lowers elevated lipid levels and does not cause weight gain. Metformin does not cause hypoglycemia and can be combined with another oral drug when metformin alone does not adequately control blood glucose levels. An incretin mimetic such as sitagliptin or liraglutide could be used for patients who do not tolerate metformin.

Insulin can be used to treat type 2 diabetes when other drugs are not effective or not tolerated. The insulin regimens used to treat type 2 diabetes are usually less complicated than those used to treat type 1 diabetes. Patients with type 2 diabetes are less susceptible to ketoacidosis, and most of them have significant endogenous insulin production. Hence, the insulin requirement is often less than 20 U/day. Insulin therapy is usually started with a single daily dose of a long-acting insulin analog. Giving a single dose at bedtime may be sufficient for patients who experience only early-morning hyperglycemia. Some patients also benefit from using a rapid-acting insulin analog before meals to control postprandial glycemia (see Box 35.2). Inhaled insulin at mealtimes is another option for individuals with type 2 diabetes.

SUMMARY OF IMPORTANT POINTS

- All patients with type 1 diabetes require insulin. Most patients with type 2 diabetes can be managed with diet, exercise, and oral antidiabetic drugs. Oral antidiabetic drugs have no role in the treatment of type 1 diabetes.
- Insulin increases glucose uptake by muscle and fat, decreases hepatic glucose output, and controls postprandial glycemia.
- Type 1 diabetes is typically treated with a long-acting insulin to meet basal insulin requirements and a rapid-acting insulin at mealtimes to control postprandial glycemia. Alternatively, an insulin pump can be used to provide basal and mealtime injections of insulin.
- Insulin lispro, insulin aspart, and insulin glulisine are rapid-acting insulin preparations. Insulin glargine and insulin detemir are used as long-acting insulins.
- Other antidiabetic drugs include hypoglycemic agents (sulfonylureas and meglitinides) and antihyperglycemic agents (α-glucosidase inhibitors, metformin, thiazolidinediones, incretin mimetics, and an amylin analog).
- Sulfonylurea (glipizide, glyburide, and glimepiride) and meglitinide drugs (repaglinide and nateglinide) increase insulin release from pancreatic β cells. Hypoglycemia is the main side effect of these drugs, and they tend to cause weight gain.
- Acarbose and miglitol inhibit α-glucosidase and slow digestion and absorption of glucose but may cause bloating and flatulence.
- Metformin, pioglitazone, and rosiglitazone decrease hepatic glucose output and increase insulin sensitivity in muscle and fat.
- Metformin, sulfonylureas, meglitinides, and DPP-4 inhibitors are first-line drugs for the treatment of type 2 diabetes. Metformin can be used alone or in

combination with most other antidiabetic agents and is often the first drug used to treat type 2 diabetics.

- Incretin mimetics (exenatide, sitagliptin, and others) slow gastric emptying, decrease appetite, increase insulin secretion, and reduce glucagon secretion. They also increase glucose uptake by muscle and adipose tissue in type 2 diabetes. Pramlintide is an amylin analog that slows gastric emptying and the rate of rising plasma glucose and is used in individuals with type 1 or 2 diabetes who take insulin.
- Canagliflozin and other renal glucose reabsorption inhibitors block the sodium-glucose cotransporter-2 in the proximal tubule and increase glucose and water excretion.
- Bromocriptine is a dopamine agonist that can reset the disturbed hypothalamic circadian rhythm that is associated with the development of insulin resistance and diabetes.

Review Questions

1. A patient takes nateglinide before each meal. Which mechanism is responsible for the therapeutic effect of this drug?
   (A) closing of potassium channels
   (B) slowed gastric emptying
   (C) inhibition of α-glucosidase
   (D) inhibition of DPP-4
   (E) insertion of glucose transporters in cell membranes

2. A patient with type 1 diabetes injects pramlintide at mealtimes. Which adverse effect may result from this drug?
   (A) increased appetite
   (B) nausea and anorexia
   (C) flatulence and bloating
   (D) weight gain
   (E) increased risk of heart failure

3. A diabetic patient takes pioglitazone. Which effect is produced by this drug?
   (A) increased insulin secretion
   (B) lowered high-density lipoprotein cholesterol levels
   (C) increased serum triglyceride levels
   (D) insertion of glucose transporters in cell membranes
   (E) weight loss

4. Which of the following phrases correctly describes insulin glargine?
   (A) it is injected at mealtimes
   (B) proline and lysine are transposed in the B chain
   (C) aspartate is substituted for proline in the B chain
   (D) it is slowly absorbed over 24 hours
   (E) it is administered by inhalation

5. A type 2 diabetic patient is prescribed metformin. Which adverse effect often occurs when taking this drug?
   (A) heart failure
   (B) weight gain
   (C) diarrhea
   (D) lactic acidosis
   (E) hypoglycemia

Drugs Affecting Calcium and Bone Formation

OVERVIEW

The strength and structure of bone result from the deposition of calcium phosphate salts called *hydroxyapatite* (Ca$_5$[PO$_4$]$_3$OH) on bone matrix proteins, a process called *mineralization*. Normal bone is constantly undergoing **remodeling** by sequential demineralization and mineralization. During remodeling, bone calcium is in dynamic equilibrium with ionized calcium in extracellular fluid. Hence bone mineralization increases as the extracellular calcium concentration increases, and demineralization increases as it decreases. The proper extracellular calcium concentration is also required for normal function of nerves and muscles, gland secretion, blood coagulation, enzyme activities, and other physiologic functions.

Calcium and Bone Metabolism

Control of the extracellular calcium concentration depends on hormonal regulation of the absorption and excretion of calcium, as well as on the exchange of ionized calcium with bone. As shown in Fig. 36.1, the hormones involved in this regulation include **vitamin D, parathyroid hormone (PTH)**, and **calcitonin.**

Vitamin D stimulates calcium absorption by increasing the synthesis of a calcium-binding protein that mediates the gastrointestinal absorption of calcium. Vitamin D also stimulates bone resorption and the closely coupled process of bone formation through its actions on osteoclasts and osteoblasts, respectively.

PTH has four actions that increase the extracellular calcium concentration. First, it stimulates resorption of calcium by renal tubules. Second, it decreases resorption of phosphate by renal tubules. This decreases the extracellular phosphate concentration, which in turn tends to increase the extracellular calcium concentration. Third, PTH stimulates the hydroxylation of vitamin D in the kidneys (Fig. 36.2). Fourth, PTH increases bone resorption by stimulating osteoclast activity, which enables bone calcium to enter the extracellular pool.

Calcitonin is released by parafollicular cells of the thyroid gland in response to **increased plasma calcium levels,** and it acts to inhibit bone resorption and decrease plasma calcium levels. The physiologic significance of calcitonin is unclear because normal calcium balance is maintained in the absence of calcitonin in persons who undergo thyroidectomy.

Bone remodeling (Fig. 36.3) consists of a sequence of events involving the dynamic interaction of **osteoclasts** (bone-resorbing cells) and **osteoblasts** (bone-forming cells). The recruitment and activation of osteoclasts is mediated by compounds released from osteoblasts and peripheral leukocytes called **bone cell cytokines.** The cytokines include **interleukins, tumor necrosis factor, colony-stimulating factors,** and other factors such as ligand for receptor activator of nuclear factor κB (**RANKL,** described later) that alter gene expression. After the osteoclasts are activated, they adhere to the bone surface and release hydrogen ions and proteases to break down the bone. The destroyed bone releases growth factors that increase osteoblast production and decrease osteoclast activity. The osteoblasts then lay down new bone in the cavity created by osteoclasts. The entire remodeling process takes approximately 100 days on average. Trabecular bone (internal, spongy, cancellous bone) undergoes more remodeling than cortical (hard compact outer layer) bone (25% versus 3% annually).

The balance between **bone resorption** and **bone formation** is usually maintained until the third or fourth decade of life, when a slow, age-related imbalance begins and favors resorption over formation. Hormonal and nutritional deficiencies can contribute to this imbalance.

Bone Disorders

Osteoporosis, the most common bone disorder, is characterized by a gradual reduction in bone mass that weakens

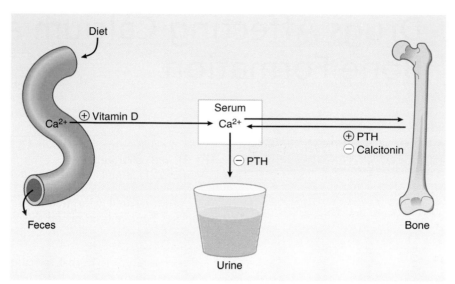

FIG. 36.1 Calcium and bone metabolism. Vitamin D facilitates calcium absorption from the gut. Parathyroid hormone *(PTH)* decreases calcium excretion in the urine but increases phosphorus excretion (not shown). Endogenously secreted PTH increases bone resorption (and also bone formation), whereas calcitonin decreases bone resorption.

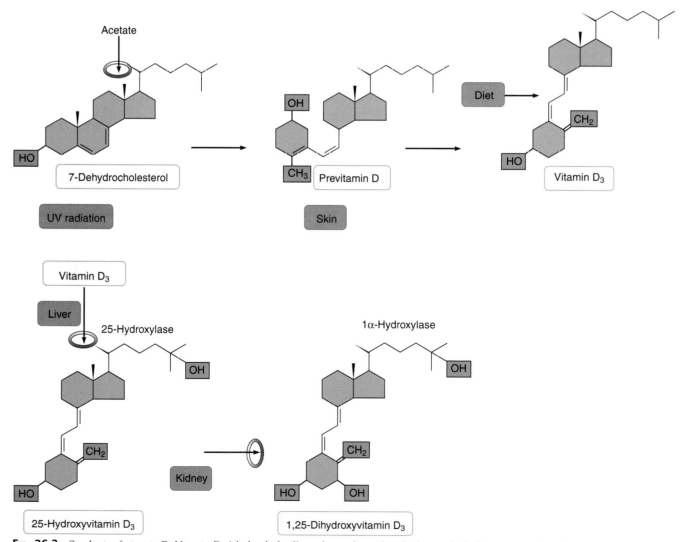

FIG. 36.2 Synthesis of vitamin D. Vitamin D_3 (cholecalciferol) can be synthesized in the human body from acetate through a pathway that requires ultraviolet radiation. Diet and vitamin supplements also provide vitamin D_3, which is activated by specific hydroxylation steps in the liver and kidneys to form 1,25-dihydroxyvitamin D_3 (calcitriol).

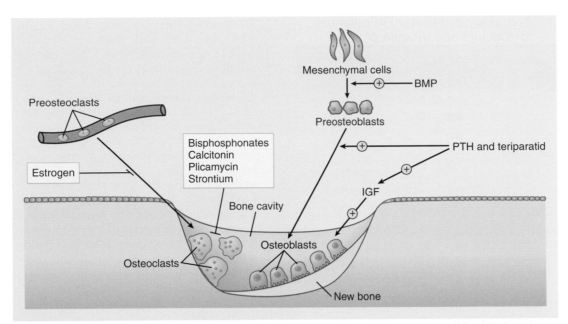

FIG. 36.3 Effects of drugs and hormones on bone remodeling. Bone remodeling consists of two phases: bone resorption followed by bone formation. In the first phase, growth factors such as RANKL (ligand for receptor activator of nuclear factor κB) induce circulating preosteoclasts to differentiate to osteoclasts and attach to bone. Osteoclasts erode the mineral and matrix of bone surfaces, creating small cavities. In phase two, bone morphogenetic protein *(BMP)* and other factors induce mesenchymal cells to differentiate into preosteoblasts. Under the influence of parathyroid hormone *(PTH)*, preosteoblasts become osteoblasts and are further stimulated by insulin-like growth factor *(IGF)* to fill the cavities with new bone matrix that is subsequently mineralized. Short-term intermittent administration of teriparatide mimics the effect of PTH on bone formation and increases bone mass, but continuous long-term administration of these hormones increases bone resorption.

bones and leads to the occurrence of fractures with minimal trauma, such as falls. **Vertebral fractures** are the most frequent type of fracture in patients with **postmenopausal osteoporosis,** a disorder partly caused by decreased estrogen secretion in this population; **hip, humerus,** and **pelvis fractures** are also major causes of immobility, morbidity, and mortality in older persons. In the United States, the annual cost of osteoporotic hip fractures is approximately $11 billion, and the cost is projected to rise to $240 billion by the year 2040 if more effective methods of prevention and treatment are not developed and implemented (Box 36.1).

Paget disease of bone, or osteitis deformans, is the second most common bone disorder. Characterized by excessive bone turnover, this disease is characterized by localized bone deformities, pain, and fractures. Its cause remains uncertain, although genetic mutations may have a role and certain virus infections have been implicated.

Osteomalacia is characterized by abnormal mineralization of new bone matrix. The condition has numerous causes, the most common of which include vitamin D deficiency, abnormal vitamin D metabolism, phosphate deficiency, and osteoblast dysfunction. In children, osteomalacia usually results from vitamin D deficiency and is called **rickets.** This disorder is uncommon nowadays because of vitamin D–supplemented foods and sun exposure. In adults, factors such as aging, malabsorption, chronic renal impairment, and use of phenytoin or other **anticonvulsant drugs** can interfere with vitamin D absorption, metabolism, or target organ response and result in osteomalacia.

Calcium and Vitamin D
An adequate intake of calcium and vitamin D is essential for optimal bone formation in children and to prevent

BOX 36.1 A CASE OF LOW BONE DENSITY

CASE PRESENTATION
A healthy 50-year-old woman has returned to her physician to assess hormone replacement therapy. She recently entered menopause and for the past 3 months has been taking a low dose of oral estrogen and a vaginal estrogen cream along with cyclic medroxyprogesterone to relieve menopausal symptoms. The treatment has reduced hot flashes and sleep disruption, but she still has an occasional episode. Because her mother had osteoporosis and fractured her hip, she asks about preventive therapy. She has been taking an adequate amount of calcium and has increased her intake of vitamin D. Her physician arranges for a bone mineral density (BMD) test, which reveals that her BMD T-score is −2 (normal is greater than −1). Based on her T-score and family history of osteoporosis, her physician suggests that she begin therapy with alendronate. She will be scheduled for a follow-up BMD test in 6 months.

CASE DISCUSSION
BMD typically increases until approximately age 35 and then levels off until menopause. After menopause, BMD usually undergoes a sharp decline, and the risk of fractures increases with age. BMD is often determined using dual energy x-ray absorptiometry. The T-score compares a woman's BMD in grams per square centimeter with that of healthy young adults. The T-score is calculated as the patient's BMD minus the average young adult BMD, divided by 1 standard deviation of young adult BMDs. A normal T-score is greater than −1, whereas scores of −1 to −2.5 indicate low bone mass (osteopenia) and a risk of developing osteoporosis. Scores less than −2.5 indicate osteoporosis. Treatment guidelines recommend that women with risk factors receive preventive therapy if their T-score is less than −1.5. The risk factors include a previous fragility fracture, a family history of fracture, cigarette smoking, and low body weight (<127 pounds). Hence the woman meets the criteria for preventive treatment, and a bisphosphonate drug is usually selected for this purpose. If this treatment does not improve her BMD, calcitonin therapy might be considered.

TABLE 36.1 Recommended Dietary Allowances for Calcium and Vitamin D[a]

AGE GROUP	DAILY ELEMENTAL CALCIUM (MG)	DAILY VITAMIN D$_3$ OR EQUIVALENT (IU)
Infants		
0–6 months	400	400
7–12 months	600	400
Children, Adolescents		
1–3 years	700	600
4–8 years	1000	600
9–18 years	1300	600
Men		
19–70 years	1000	600
>70 years	1200	800
Women		
25–50 years	1000	600
>50 years	1200	600
>70 years	1200	800
Pregnant and nursing	1000–1300	600

[a]Food and Nutrition Board, Institute of Medicine of the National Academies.

osteoporosis in adults. All persons should be encouraged by health professionals to meet the recommendations of the National Academy of Medicine, or similar agencies in other countries, for daily calcium and vitamin D intake (Table 36.1). These recommendations can be met by ingesting **calcium-rich foods, which are primarily dairy products,** and by taking oral calcium and vitamin D supplements if dietary intake is inadequate. Studies have shown that adequate calcium and vitamin D intake prevents loss of bone mass and osteoporosis. For example, nursing-home residents who were given 800 International Units (IU) of vitamin D$_3$ and 1200 mg of calcium were found to have an **increased bone density and a decreased incidence of hip and nonvertebral fractures** in comparison with those who were given placebos. In another study, administration of vitamin D$_3$ was found to **decrease the incidence of vertebral and nonvertebral fractures** in women with previous fractures.

Calcium

In the United States, it is estimated that two-thirds of women age 18 and older have an inadequate calcium intake, which predisposes them to postmenopausal osteoporosis. Most people get 300 mg of calcium daily in their diet from nondairy sources, and adding two servings of dairy products typically brings the total calcium intake to 900 mg. Supplementing with just 300 mg of calcium or adding another high-calcium dairy product would provide approximately 1200 mg and thereby fulfill the daily requirement for all adults and children except adolescents (see Table 36.1).

Pharmacokinetics. Calcium absorption from the gut is incomplete. Even with ingesting adequate amounts of vitamin D, only approximately 30% of calcium is absorbed from milk and other dairy products, and calcium absorption from supplements is often less than 30%. The absorption of **calcium carbonate** requires stomach acid, whereas the absorption of **calcium citrate** does not. Because elderly persons can have decreased stomach acid secretion, they may benefit more from using calcium citrate, as do persons taking proton pump inhibitors such as omeprazole that inhibit gastric acid secretion.

Indications. In addition to their role in the prevention and treatment of **osteoporosis,** calcium and vitamin D are also the primary treatment for **hypocalcemia.** For this purpose, calcium can be given orally or intravenously.

Adverse Effects and Interactions. The most common adverse effect of calcium supplements is constipation. This is best managed by ingesting adequate amounts of fruits and vegetables. Calcium can decrease the absorption of ciprofloxacin, fluoride, phenytoin, levothyroxine, and tetracycline, so calcium supplements should be taken at least 2 hours before or after taking these drugs. Clinical trials have found that use of calcium supplements appears to modestly increase the risk of **myocardial infarction.** Hence persons should estimate their dietary intake and take only the amount of supplemental calcium required to meet their recommended daily allowance (RDA).

Vitamin D

Chemistry and Pharmacokinetics. Vitamin D is a fat-soluble substance similar to cholesterol. The form of the vitamin obtained from the diet and can be synthesized in skin exposed to ultraviolet radiation is called **vitamin D3,** or **cholecalciferol.** It is a relatively inactive precursor of **1,25-dihydroxyvitamin D3,** which is called **calcitriol,** and is the most active form of the vitamin in the human body. The formation of calcitriol involves hydroxylation of vitamin D$_3$ at the 25 position in the liver to form **calcifediol** (25-hydroxycholecalciferol), which is then hydroxylated at the 1 position in the kidneys to form calcitriol (see Fig. 36.2). PTH stimulates the renal hydroxylation of vitamin D, as shown in Fig. 36.2.

Indications. Vitamin D preparations are used for the following purposes: (1) to ensure adequate vitamin D intake to prevent rickets and to develop and maintain sufficient bone mass and strength to prevent osteoporosis; (2) to treat **vitamin D–dependent rickets, familial hypophosphatemia** (vitamin D–resistant rickets), **hypocalcemia from hypoparathyroidism,** and postoperative and idiopathic **tetany;** and (3) to prevent vitamin D deficiency in persons with **chronic renal failure.** Patients with chronic renal failure must be treated with **calcitriol** because they lack the 1α-hydroxylase enzyme required to synthesize the active form of vitamin D (see Fig. 36.2). In addition, an ointment preparation of calcitriol (VECTICAL) is indicated for treatment of **plaque psoriasis** (raised silvery flaking of the skin) because it reduces the rate of excessive skin cell replication present in this condition.

Doxercalciferol and **paricalcitol** are analogs of calcitriol for oral or parenteral treatment of secondary hyperparathyroidism (HPT) due to chronic renal disease. Their advantage over calcitriol itself is that they reduce PTH levels with less risk of causing hypercalcemia. A third agent, **calcifediol,** is an analog of vitamin D$_3$ in an extended-release formulation also approved for treatment of secondary HPT in adults with stage 3 or 4 chronic kidney disease (CKD).

Many vitamin D preparations are available to enable adequate intake for infants, children, and adults. Most of these preparations contain vitamin D$_3$ **(cholecalciferol),** vitamin D$_2$ **(ergocalciferol),** or **calcitriol.** Multivitamin preparations contain at least 400 IU of vitamin D, and milk and milk substitutes as well as foods prepared from milk (e.g., yogurt, ice cream) are supplemented with vitamin D. Until recently, it was possible for adults to obtain the RDA for vitamin D (formerly 400 IU) from their diet, but the National Academy of Medicine and similar organizations in other countries have increased the RDA for vitamin D to 600 IU for people up to age 70 and to 800 IU for those older than 70 (see Table 36.1). Most individuals will need to supplement their diet with a vitamin D preparation to obtain the RDA, and many authorities argue that healthy adults should receive even higher amounts of 800 to 2000 IU/day to maintain optimal bone mass and other health benefits. For example, adequate vitamin D intake appears to reduce the risk of **cardiovascular disease, cancer,** and **autoimmune disorders** such as multiple sclerosis (MS) and type 1 diabetes. Vitamin D has been found to interact with cell receptors associated with cancer and autoimmune diseases so as to alter gene expression, and a study showed that adequate vitamin D intake may slow progression of MS.

Adverse Effects and Interactions. Doses of vitamin D in excess of 5000 IU/day can cause **hypercalcemia** and **hypercalciuria.** The absorption of vitamin D is inhibited by cholestyramine, and administration of these preparations should be separated by at least 2 hours. Phenytoin and barbiturates can induce enzymes that metabolize vitamin D and lead to vitamin D deficiency. Patients taking these drugs often require vitamin D supplementation and may benefit from determination of serum vitamin D levels.

PHARMACOLOGIC AGENTS

Most of the drugs used in treating bone disorders **inhibit bone resorption by osteoclasts.** These agents include the bisphosphonate drugs, calcitonin, estrogen and raloxifene, and denosumab. In contrast, **teriparatide stimulates bone formation by osteoblasts.** Strontium has a dual mechanism of action, inhibiting bone resorption while increasing bone formation.

Bisphosphonates

A number of bisphosphonate compounds are available to treat several disorders of calcium metabolism and bone. These compounds are classified according to their ability to inhibit bone resorption. The original bisphosphonate, etidronate, is the least potent inhibitor of bone resorption. It is not used extensively because long-term administration causes osteomalacia. Second-generation bisphosphonates, **alendronate, pamidronate,** and **risedronate,** are approximately 100-fold more potent than etidronate, and third-generation drugs, such as **ibandronate** and **zoledronic acid,** are almost 1000-fold more potent than etidronate.

Chemistry and Pharmacokinetics

Bisphosphonate drugs are pyrophosphate analogs in which the phosphorus-oxygen-phosphorus structure (P–O–P) is replaced with a phosphorus-carbon-phosphorus (P–C–P) moiety resistant to enzymatic hydrolysis. Pamidronate and zoledronic acid are given intravenously, but other bisphosphonates are administered orally, and ibandronate can be given orally or intravenously. After oral administration, less than 5% of a bisphosphonate is absorbed when taken on an empty stomach, and absorption is further reduced by food, certain drugs, and liquids other than water. Patients should take bisphosphonates with a full glass of water 30 minutes before ingesting anything else in the morning.

Once absorbed, approximately half of the drug is **deposited in bone** where bisphosphonates adsorb to hydroxyapatite and become a permanent part of the bone structure, and the remainder is excreted in the urine. Bisphosphonates are slowly released from bone during bone remodeling, and the terminal half-life appears to be greater than 10 years.

Mechanisms and Pharmacologic Effects

Bisphosphonates appear to **inhibit bone resorption** through several mechanisms, and it has been difficult to establish which actions are most important. It seems clear that bisphosphonates reduce **osteoclast metabolic activity** and survival, and evidence suggests that inhibition of the **mevalonate pathway** is at least partly responsible for this effect. This pathway, which leads to cholesterol synthesis, is involved in subcellular protein trafficking that maintains the cytoskeletal shape required for contact between osteoclasts and the bone surface. **Statin drugs** used in treating hypercholesterolemia also inhibit the mevalonate pathway and appear to inhibit bone resorption, although to less extent than bisphosphonates.

Indications

Bisphosphonate compounds are used in the treatment of **osteoporosis, Paget disease of bone, hypercalcemia,** and **osteolytic bone lesions of metastatic cancer,** as described later in Specific Drugs. As a side benefit of bisphosphonate therapy, clinical trials have found that bisphosphonates are associated with a reduced risk of developing **breast cancer** as well as reduced breast cancer mortality in postmenopausal women. This effect remained significant regardless of a woman's body mass index, or use of aspirin, statins, vitamin D, or postmenopausal hormones.

Adverse Effects

The bisphosphonate compounds produce varying degrees of **gastrointestinal distress.** Orally administered bisphosphonates can cause **esophageal erosion,** but this can be prevented by remaining upright after taking these drugs. Pamidronate is not given orally because it causes more gastric irritation than other bisphosphonates. Alendronate and risedronate seldom cause gastric distress except when high doses are used to treat Paget disease. Occasionally, alendronate causes mild nausea, dyspepsia, constipation, or diarrhea. Clinical trials have shown that long-term use of bisphosphonates (usually more than 5 years) increases the risk of **atypical femur fractures** called subtrochanteric and diaphyseal fractures, which occur just below the hip joint or in the long part of the bone, respectively. Both are uncommon and account for less than 1% of all femur fractures. Most patients who develop these fractures experience a **dull, aching pain in the thigh or groin** for weeks or months before a fracture occurs. Prescribers should discontinue bisphosphonate therapy if a patient reports this symptom until the cause is determined. Finally, bisphosphonates may increase the risk of **osteonecrosis of the jaw,** especially in persons with poor oral health or following oral surgery, and in those taking higher doses.

Interactions

The bisphosphonates have few interactions with other drugs. Calcium supplements and antacids decrease the absorption of bisphosphonates and should be taken at least 2 hours before or after a bisphosphonate compound, which is also prudent for other medications taken concurrently.

Specific Drugs

Alendronate was the first bisphosphonate to be developed for the treatment of osteoporosis. It is effective in all forms of this disorder, including glucocorticoid-induced osteoporosis, and serves to prevent bone loss and produce a sustained increase in bone mass. A study of women with low bone mass and preexisting vertebral fractures found that alendronate reduced new vertebral fractures by 47% over a 3-year period. Alendronate is available in oral formulations for once-daily or once-weekly administration.

Ibandronate and risedronate are both indicated for the **prevention and treatment of osteoporosis in postmenopausal women. Risedronate** is also approved for osteoporosis in men and for treatment of glucocorticoid-induced osteoporosis. Ibandronate is formulated for once-monthly oral administration, whereas risedronate formulations are available for daily, weekly, or monthly oral administration.

Alendronate, pamidronate, and **risedronate** are also approved for the treatment of **Paget disease of bone.** Before treatment, imaging and laboratory studies usually show evidence of increased bone turnover (remodeling), bone hypertrophy, and abnormal bone structure. By inhibiting abnormal osteoclast activity in patients with this disease, the bisphosphonates help to normalize biochemical indices of bone remodeling and restore normal bone structure. Patients who are symptomatic or who require orthopedic surgery are candidates for bisphosphonate therapy. Treatment should be initiated as early as possible to halt disease progression. Bisphosphonate compounds may require 6 months to be effective. If a relapse occurs, another course of treatment can be given after a 6-month interval.

In patients with **bone cancer,** bisphosphonates are useful in the management of **osteolytic bone disease** and resulting **hypercalcemia.** Intravenous administration of **pamidronate** or **zoledronic acid** is the most effective treatment for hypercalcemia associated with cancer. Bisphosphonate treatment inhibits bone resorption, reduces the tumor burden in bone, decreases bone pain, and reduces the risk of fractures in patients whose cancer has metastasized to bone. For example, pamidronate reduces skeletal complications in women with stage IV breast cancer with bone metastases. In men, pamidronate inhibits the adhesion of prostate carcinoma cells to bone, and **zoledronic acid** prevents bone loss and increases bone mineral density (BMD) in patients with prostate cancer.

Parathyroid Hormone and Related Drugs

Parathyroid Hormone

PTH itself is available on the market as the full 84-amino-acid protein manufactured by genetic engineering in vat-grown bacteria (NATPARA). PTH is indicated for the treatment of hypoparathyroidism as an adjunct to calcium and vitamin D to reverse hypocalcemia.

Teriparatide

Teriparatide is a **recombinant form of human PTH** that consists of the 34 biologically active amino acids of the hormone. In contrast to drugs that inhibit bone resorption, teriparatide is an anabolic agent that **increases bone formation** and has the potential to reverse bone loss (see Fig. 36.3).

The skeletal effects of teriparatide depend on the frequency and duration of administration. **Daily subcutaneous administration** of teriparatide for **up to 2 years** stimulates bone formation on trabecular and cortical bone surfaces by preferentially **stimulating osteoblastic activity** more than osteoclastic activity. Teriparatide increases markers of bone formation, skeletal mass, and bone strength. In contrast, **long-term exposure** to excessive amounts of PTH as occurs in HPT can **stimulate bone resorption** more than bone formation and have a detrimental effect on the skeleton. Hence the duration of teriparatide treatment must be limited.

Clinical trials of teriparatide in postmenopausal women and hypogonadal men with osteoporosis found that the drug increased vertebral and femoral neck BMD while reducing the risk of vertebral and nonvertebral fractures. Teriparatide is indicated for the treatment of **postmenopausal women with osteoporosis who are at high risk for bone fracture.** These include women with a history of osteoporotic fracture, women who have multiple risk factors for fracture, and women who are intolerant of other therapy. Teriparatide is also used to increase bone mass in **hypogonadal men** with a high risk of fracture, such as those receiving gonadotropin-releasing hormone therapy for prostate cancer. Cessation of teriparatide therapy may be followed by a rapid loss of bone, and teriparatide should be followed by a bisphosphonate or other antiresorptive agent. Teriparatide is contraindicated in persons with an increased risk of osteosarcoma, including those with **Paget disease** or elevated serum alkaline phosphatase activity, because the drug itself appears to increase the risk of this malignancy.

Abaloparatide is a human PTH analog that shares only about half of the natural sequence of human PTH. Like teriparatide, **abaloparatide binds to and activates PTH receptors** to produce its effects on bone and kidney. It carries the same black box **warning of osteosarcoma** and is indicated for the **treatment of postmenopausal women with osteoporosis** at high risk for fracture.

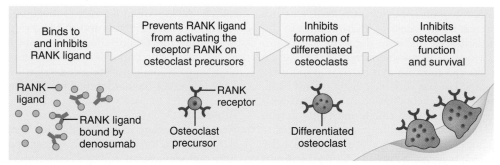

FIG. 36.4 Inhibition of osteoclast activity by denosumab. Denosumab is an immunoglobulin G2 monoclonal antibody that binds and inactivates a membrane protein called RANK ligand (ligand for receptor activator of nuclear factor κB, or RANKL), which is a member of the tumor necrosis factor superfamily. Unless inactivated by denosumab, RANKL activates the RANK receptor, leading to gene expression required for cell fusion and the formation of mature osteoclasts. By inactivating RANKL, denosumab prevents osteoclast-mediated bone resorption.

Cinacalcet and Etelcalcetide

Cinacalcet is a first-in-class new drug entity that brings a novel mechanism of action for the treatment of hypercalcemia. It works by an agonist action at the **calcium-sensing receptor** in the parathyroid gland, **increasing the activation of these calcium-sensing receptors** to extracellular calcium. This leads to **decreased secretion of PTH and lowering of serum calcium** levels. The clinical aspects of cinacalcet use are discussed later. **Etelcalcetide** is the second calcium-sensing receptor agonist recently approved. It is indicated for **secondary hyperparathyroidism (HPT) in adult patients with chronic kidney disease (CKD)** on hemodialysis.

RANKL Antibody
Denosumab

Denosumab is a unique approach to the treatment of osteoporosis through the **inactivation of gene transcription** required for osteoclast viability and function (Fig. 36.4).

Mechanism of Action. Denosumab is a human **monoclonal antibody** produced in genetically engineered mammalian cells (see Chapter 46) that binds and inactivates a **transmembrane protein called RANKL.** RANKL augments the formation, function, and survival of osteoclasts and their participation in bone resorption. Inactivation of RANKL prevents activation of RANK, the receptor activator of nuclear factor *kappa*-B (NF-κB). **NF-κB** is a **transcription factor** and is **rapid-acting gene transcription modifier** that functions as a "first responder" to factors that alter gene expression such as RANK.

Inactivation of the RANKL pathway by denosumab **inhibits gene expression** required for osteoclast formation and activity, as shown by its ability to reduce a serum marker of bone resorption called *type-1 telopeptide* by 85%. Denosumab decreases bone resorption in both cortical and trabecular bone.

Clinical Use and Effects. Denosumab is given by **subcutaneous injection every 6 months** for the **treatment of osteoporosis.** This regimen gradually increases bone mass and strength and reduces the risk of bone fractures. In clinical studies, the drug increased BMD 8.8% at the lumber spine, 6.4% at the hip, and 5.2% at the femoral neck after 3 years treatment, and these effects were consistently observed regardless of differences in patient age, race, weight, and baseline BMD.

In a 3-year placebo-controlled trial of women with osteoporosis and a baseline T-score of −2.5 to −4.0, denosumab reduced new vertebral fractures at 2 years from 5% in the placebo group to 1.4% in the denosumab group, for a relative risk reduction of 71%. The drug also **significantly reduced hip and other nonvertebral fractures.**

XGEVA is a formulation of **denosumab** that is indicated for the **prevention of skeletal-related events,** such as pathologic fractures and spinal cord compression, in patients with **bone metastases from breast cancer, prostate cancer, and other solid tumors.** Clinical trials showed that the drug was equivalent to zoledronic acid for this indication. A second monoclonal antibody drug for the treatment of osteoporosis is **romosozumab. Romosozumab inhibits the action of sclerostin,** a regulatory factor in bone metabolism, increasing bone formation.

Adverse Effects. The most common **adverse effect** of denosumab is muscle and joint pain. The drug also appears to increase the risk of **infections,** particularly skin and soft tissue infections, possibly owing to the role of RANKL in immune cell function. **Hypocalcemia** may be worsened by denosumab treatment, possibly because more serum calcium is being used for bone formation than is being released by bone resorption. Patients should have normal **calcium and vitamin D levels** before beginning denosumab therapy and receive supplements of these nutrients during treatment. Similarly to bisphosphonates, denosumab may increase the risk of osteonecrosis of the jaw following teeth extraction or oral surgical procedures.

Other Agents
Calcitonin

Chemistry and Pharmacokinetics. Human calcitonin is a 32-amino-acid peptide hormone secreted by the parafollicular cells of the thyroid gland. **Salmon calcitonin** is at least 40 times more potent than human calcitonin and is available as a synthetic peptide for subcutaneous injection (MIACALCIN) and as a recombinant DNA-produced hormone for nasal inhalation (FORTICAL). The higher potency of salmon calcitonin appears to result from its greater structural flexibility that increases its affinity for the calcitonin receptor. The drug is not reliably absorbed after oral administration.

Mechanisms and Effects. Calcitonin binds to G protein–coupled receptors on osteoclasts and increases **cyclic adenosine monophosphate** (cAMP) and **inositol triphosphate** (IP_3) levels via activation of G_s and G_q, respectively. When given on a short-term basis, calcitonin inhibits osteoclast activity, decreases bone resorption, lowers serum calcium concentrations, and reduces bone pain. However, its long-term effects on bone mass are uncertain.

Indications. Because of its ability to inhibit osteoclast activity and decrease bone turnover, calcitonin is used to treat **osteoporosis, Paget disease of bone,** and **hypercalcemia.**

In patients with osteoporosis, calcitonin treatment has been shown to **increase bone mass** at multiple sites in the body during treatment of up to 2 years duration. Calcitonin treatment is usually reserved for women who cannot tolerate other treatments. Studies indicate that calcitonin increases the BMD in the spine but has variable effects on the BMD in the hips. Patients with osteoporosis can be treated with either **subcutaneous** or **intranasal calcitonin.** In those who have had fractures, treatment in the immediate postfracture period appears to be particularly useful because of the drug's ability to reduce bone pain. Patients taking calcitonin should have **adequate calcium and vitamin D intake** to support bone formation during calcitonin therapy.

In patients with **Paget disease,** calcitonin is administered subcutaneously every 1 to 3 days. The nasal spray is not used for this indication. Calcitonin treatment inhibits osteoclast activity and reduces markers of abnormal bone turnover, such as serum alkaline phosphatase activity and urine hydroxyproline levels. Alleviation of bone pain usually occurs 2 to 8 weeks after calcitonin therapy has begun.

Hypercalcemia can be treated with subcutaneous or intramuscular injections of calcitonin that are administered every 12 hours until a satisfactory response occurs, which usually takes 5 days or less.

Estrogen and Raloxifene

Estrogen **reduces bone resorption** by inhibiting the production of **bone cell cytokines** that stimulate osteoclast formation and activation. These cytokines include interleukin-1, tumor necrosis factor, and granulocyte-macrophage colony-stimulating factor produced by peripheral blood monocytes, and interleukin-6 and osteoclast-stimulating factors secreted by osteoblasts.

Estrogen is often used to relieve menopausal symptoms such as hot flashes, but the lower doses of estrogen used for this purpose may not provide sufficient protection against bone loss, and **higher doses of estrogen** appear to increase the risk of breast cancer and thromboembolic disorders.

Raloxifene is a selective **estrogen receptor modulator** that mimics the effects of estrogen on bone. It increases BMD in postmenopausal women and decreases **vertebral fractures** in women with osteoporosis. At the same time, raloxifene has **antiestrogen effects** in breast and uterine tissues and can cause or intensify **hot flashes** and other symptoms of estrogen withdrawal in menopausal women. As with estrogens, raloxifene increases the risk of stroke, pulmonary emboli, and deep vein thrombosis, and the main advantage of raloxifene is that it reduces the risk of invasive **breast cancer** in postmenopausal women. Estrogen preparations and raloxifene are discussed in greater detail in Chapter 34.

Sodium Fluoride

Sodium fluoride is used to prevent tooth decay and dental caries, a condition in which localized destruction of calcified tissue on the tooth surface is followed by enzymatic lysis of organic material and the development of cavities. After oral administration, fluoride is stored in bone and teeth, where it replaces the hydroxyl group in calcium phosphate salts (hydroxyapatite) to form **fluorapatite.** Fluorapatite deposited on the tooth surface is more resistant to erosion than hydroxyapatite. Fluoride has been added to the drinking water supply in many localities as a method of caries prevention, and it can be applied directly to the tooth surface as a gel or rinse. Liquid and chewable sodium fluoride formulations are available to provide fluoride to infants and children.

Fluoride has potential application in the treatment of osteoporosis, but clinical studies of current formulations have failed to demonstrate a reduction in fractures, and it can cause excessive hardening of bone (osteosclerosis).

Strontium

Strontium ranelate is another anabolic agent currently available in Europe for the treatment of osteoporosis (PROTELOS). After oral administration, strontium is laid down on the surface of newly formed bone, where it decreases osteoclastic activity and reduces **bone resorption.** At the same time, strontium induces the differentiation of preosteoblasts to osteoblasts and increases markers of **bone formation.** Overall, strontium **increases bone mass and strength.** Clinical trials found that strontium ranelate reduced the risk of new vertebral fractures by approximately 25% and nonvertebral fractures by 15%. Strontium typically causes only minor gastrointestinal side effects such as nausea and diarrhea, but recent evidence suggests that it can increase the risk of venous and pulmonary thromboembolism and myocardial infarction. Due to its effectiveness and popularity in other parts of the world, strontium ranelate may soon be approved for use in the United States.

MANAGEMENT OF CALCIUM AND BONE DISORDERS

Osteoporosis

The prevention of osteoporosis rests on a foundation of **lifelong calcium** and **vitamin D** intake in an amount sufficient to maximize bone formation during development and to sustain bone mass during adulthood. Weight-bearing exercise reduces bone loss and helps improve strength and balance. Endogenous estrogen in women and testosterone in men also reduce bone resorption. After menopause, the absence of estrogen accelerates bone loss in women. Although all postmenopausal women are at risk for developing osteoporosis, BMD measurements can be used to identify those who are at greatest risk and guide pharmacologic therapy.

In most postmenopausal women, osteoporosis can be prevented by ensuring an adequate intake of calcium and vitamin D, exercising, and taking antiresorptive agents when required to maintain BMD. Bisphosphonates are often used for this purpose because they can be taken orally, have proven efficacy, and exhibit a low incidence of adverse effects. Calcitonin is a good option for women who have taken a bisphosphonate for an extended period of time and need alternative therapy and for women who cannot tolerate a bisphosphonate. Teriparatide and denosumab can be effective in women with very low or rapidly decreasing BMD measurements, women who have had fractures, and women who are at an increased risk for developing osteoporosis because they require chronic corticosteroid therapy or because they had natural or surgical menopause at an early age.

Paget Disease of Bone

The goals of treating patients with Paget disease are to control bone pain and to prevent progressive bone deformity and other manifestations of the disease. **Calcitonin** or a bisphosphonate drug such as **zoledronic acid** is usually used for this purpose, and the combination of calcitonin and a bisphosphonate may be useful in more severe cases.

Hypercalcemia

The treatment of hypercalcemia depends on the cause and severity of the condition. The major causes of hypercalcemia are HPT and cancer.

Saline diuresis is usually the preferred method of managing acute hypercalcemia that is severe enough to cause symptoms. A saline infusion is used for this purpose; it serves to increase renal calcium excretion and to counteract the dehydration that often accompanies hypercalcemia. A **loop diuretic** (e.g., **furosemide**) can be added to increase calcium excretion, but evidence for its effectiveness for this purpose is lacking.

Bisphosphonates are useful in the treatment of hypercalcemia associated with cancer, sometimes in combination with calcitonin. As a last resort, intravenous phosphate infusions can be used to control hypercalcemia, but these infusions place the patient at considerable risk for acute hypocalcemia, hypotension, renal failure, and tissue calcification.

Cinacablcet is used for the treatment of **hyperparathyroidism** in adult patients with CKD who are on dialysis and for treatment of **hypercalcemia** in patients with **parathyroid cancer.** The drug appears to be safe and effective for these conditions.

SUMMARY OF IMPORTANT POINTS

- The extracellular calcium concentration is regulated by vitamin D, PTH, and calcitonin. Vitamin D increases calcium absorption from the gut; PTH increases calcium reabsorption from renal tubules and increases bone resorption; and calcitonin decreases bone resorption.
- A lifelong intake of adequate amounts of calcium and vitamin D is essential for optimal bone formation and maintenance and for the prevention of osteoporosis.
- Vitamin D is converted to its most active form, calcitriol, by hydroxylation in the liver and kidneys. This active form must be supplied to patients with renal impairment. Dietary vitamin D is essential to prevent rickets in children.
- Osteoporosis, the most common bone disorder, is characterized by a gradual loss of bone mass that leads to skeletal weakness and fractures.
- Osteoporosis can be treated with a bisphosphonate drug, calcitonin, teriparatide, estrogen, raloxifene, denosumab, or strontium ranelate. Most drugs reduce bone resorption, teriparatide stimulates bone formation, and strontium appears to do both.
- Bisphosphonates are also used to treat Paget disease of bone, hypercalcemia, and osteolytic bone lesions associated with cancer.
- Calcitonin reduces osteoclast activity and is used to treat Paget disease of bone and hypercalcemia.

- Denosumab is a monoclonal antibody to a protein ligand called *RANKL*, the inactivation of which prevents gene transcription required for osteoclast formation, survival, and function.

Review Questions

1. A 52-year-old postmenopausal woman is placed on a drug that decreases osteoclast activation but may cause hot flashes. Which drug was most likely given to this patient?
   - (A) alendronate
   - (B) denosumab
   - (C) calcitonin
   - (D) raloxifene
   - (E) teriparatide
2. A woman with osteolytic bone cancer is treated with a drug that reduces the serum calcium level. Which drug is indicated for this purpose?
   - (A) calcitonin
   - (B) ibandronate
   - (C) calcitriol
   - (D) zoledronic acid
   - (E) cinacalcet
3. A woman with a BMD T-score of −3 is given daily subcutaneous injections to increase bone formation. Which effect is most likely produced by this treatment?
   - (A) increased absorption of dietary calcium
   - (B) increased serum levels of vitamin D
   - (C) decreased activation of osteoclasts
   - (D) increased activation of osteoblasts
   - (E) adsorption of the drug to bone
4. A man with bone pain and deformities is placed on a drug that increases cAMP levels in osteoclasts. Which beneficial effect may result from this treatment?
   - (A) increased serum alkaline phosphatase activity
   - (B) decreased urine hydroxyproline levels
   - (C) increased bone turnover
   - (D) increased serum calcium levels
   - (E) increased osteoblast activity
5. A woman with osteoporosis is prescribed a drug that adsorbs to hydroxyapatite and remains in bone for years. Which drug is she most likely taking?
   - (A) risedronate
   - (B) teriparatide
   - (C) calcitonin
   - (D) denosumab
   - (E) vitamin D$_3$

Principles of Antimicrobial Chemotherapy

OVERVIEW

Chemotherapy is defined as the use of drugs to eradicate pathogenic organisms or neoplastic cells in the treatment of infectious diseases or cancer. Chemotherapy is based on the principle of **selective toxicity.** According to this principle, a chemotherapeutic drug inhibits a vital function of invading organisms or neoplastic cells that differs qualitatively or quantitatively from the functions of host cells. The chemotherapeutic drugs include antimicrobial drugs (introduced in this chapter and discussed further in Chapters 38 to 43), antiparasitic drugs (discussed in Chapter 44), and antineoplastic and immunopharmacology drugs (discussed in Chapters 45 and 46).

Antibiotics and Chemotherapy

The **antimicrobial drugs** can be subclassified as **antibacterial, antifungal, and antiviral agents.** These agents include natural compounds, called *antibiotics*, as well as synthetic compounds. An **antibiotic** is a substance produced by a microbe that can inhibit the growth or viability of another microbe. The earliest use of antibiotics was probably in the treatment of skin infections with **moldy bean curd** by ancient Chinese, Egyptians, and other cultures. The development of modern antibiotics can be traced to the work of Louis Pasteur and his pupil, Paul Vuillemin, who observed the antagonism of one bacterium against another (**antibiosis**) and predicted that substances derived from microbes would someday be used to treat infectious diseases.

Several decades later, **Alexander Fleming** observed that the growth of his staphylococcal cultures was inhibited by a *Penicillium* contaminant. Fleming postulated that the fungus produced a substance, which he called **penicillin,** and that this substance inhibited the growth of staphylococci. His observations eventually led to the isolation and use of penicillin for treating bacterial infections. The discovery of penicillin stimulated the discovery and development of many other antibiotics and revolutionized the treatment of infectious diseases.

Synthetic drugs have also provided major advances in the treatment of infectious diseases and cancer. During the Renaissance, **Paracelsus** used **mercury compounds** for the treatment of syphilis. In the late 19th and early 20th centuries, **Paul Ehrlich** pioneered the search for selectively toxic compounds. After many failed attempts, he discovered **arsphenamine** (SALVARSAN), an arsenical compound for the treatment of syphilis. Ehrlich, who became known as the father of chemotherapy, also studied bacterial stains as potential antimicrobial agents. He reasoned that a stain's selective affinity for bacteria could be coupled with an inhibitory action to halt microbial metabolism and destroy invading organisms. This concept led to the discovery of **sulfonamides,** drugs that were originally derived from a bacterial stain called PRONTOSIL. The sulfonamides were the first effective drugs for the treatment of systemic bacterial infections, and their development accelerated the search for other antimicrobial agents.

CLASSIFICATION OF ANTIMICROBIAL DRUGS

Antimicrobial drugs are usually classified on the basis of their site and mechanism of action and are subclassified on the basis of their chemical structure. The antimicrobial drugs include **cell wall synthesis inhibitors, protein synthesis inhibitors, metabolic and nucleic acid inhibitors,** and **cell membrane inhibitors.** The sites of action of these drugs are depicted in (Fig. 37.1), and their mechanisms of action, pharmacologic properties, and clinical uses are described in subsequent chapters.

ANTIMICROBIAL ACTIVITY

The antimicrobial activity of a drug can be characterized in terms of its bactericidal or bacteriostatic effect, its spectrum of activity against important groups of pathogens, and its concentration- and time-dependent effects on sensitive organisms.

Bactericidal or Bacteriostatic Effect

A **bactericidal drug** kills sensitive organisms so that the number of viable organisms falls rapidly after exposure to the drug (Fig. 37.2). In contrast, a **bacteriostatic drug** inhibits the growth of bacteria but does not kill them. For this reason, the number of bacteria remains relatively constant in the presence of a bacteriostatic drug, and immunologic mechanisms are required to eliminate organisms during treatment of an infection with this type of drug. (The same principle applies to a drug that kills or inhibits the growth of fungi and is referred to as a **fungicidal drug** or a **fungistatic drug,** respectively.)

A bactericidal drug is usually preferable to a bacteriostatic drug for the treatment of most bacterial infections. This is because bactericidal drugs typically produce a more rapid microbiologic response and more clinical improvement and are less likely to elicit microbial resistance. Bactericidal drugs have actions that induce lethal changes in microbial metabolism or block activities that are essential for microbial viability. For example, drugs that inhibit the synthesis of the bacterial cell wall (e.g., **penicillins**) prevent the formation of a structure required for the survival of bacteria. In contrast, bacteriostatic drugs usually inhibit a metabolic reaction needed for bacterial growth but is not necessary for survival. For example, **sulfonamides** block the synthesis of folic acid, which is a cofactor for enzymes that synthesize DNA components and amino acids.

Drugs that reversibly inhibit bacterial protein synthesis (e.g., **tetracyclines**) are also bacteriostatic, whereas drugs

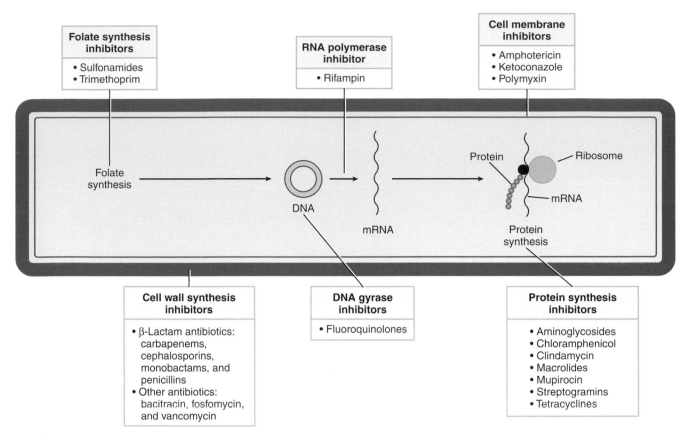

Fig. 37.1 Sites of action of antimicrobial drugs. Antimicrobial drugs include cell wall synthesis inhibitors, protein synthesis inhibitors, metabolic and nucleic acid inhibitors (e.g., inhibitors of folate synthesis, DNA gyrase, and RNA polymerase), and cell membrane inhibitors.

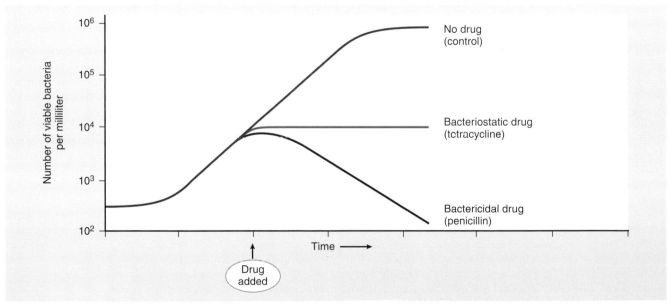

Fig. 37.2 *In vitro* effects of bactericidal and bacteriostatic drugs. In the absence of an antimicrobial drug, bacteria exhibit logarithmic growth in a broth culture. The addition of a bacteriostatic drug (tetracycline) inhibits further growth but does not reduce the number of bacteria. The addition of a bactericidal drug (penicillin) reduces the number of viable bacteria.

that irreversibly inhibit protein synthesis (e.g., **streptomycin**) are usually bactericidal.

Some antibiotics, such as erythromycin, can be either bactericidal or bacteriostatic, depending on their concentration and the bacterial species against which they are used.

Antimicrobial Spectrum

The spectrum of antimicrobial activity of a drug is the primary determinant of its clinical use. Antimicrobial agents that are active against a single species or a limited group of pathogens (e.g., gram-positive bacteria) are called

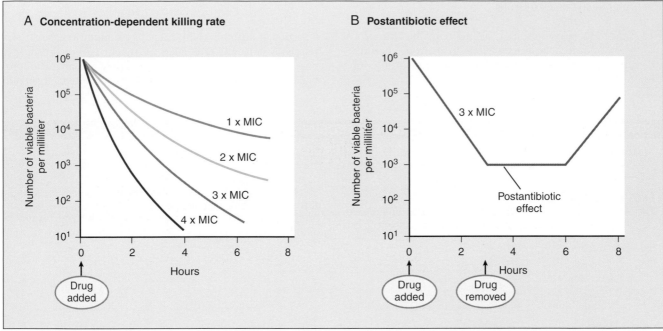

Fig. 37.3 Concentration- and time-dependent effects of antimicrobial drugs. (A) When an aminoglycoside (e.g., tobramycin) is added to a culture of a gram-negative bacterium (e.g., *Escherichia coli*), it will exhibit a concentration-dependent killing rate. In this example, 10^6 bacteria were incubated with different concentrations of tobramycin, ranging from one to four times the minimal inhibitory concentration *(MIC)*. (B) When tobramycin is removed from the culture, bacterial growth continues to be inhibited for several hours.

narrow-spectrum drugs, whereas agents that are active against a wide range of pathogens are called **broad-spectrum drugs.** Agents that have an intermediate range of activity are sometimes called **extended-spectrum drugs.** Narrow-spectrum drugs are usually preferred because they target a specific pathogen without disturbing the normal flora of the gut or respiratory tract. Broad-spectrum drugs are sometimes preferred for the initial treatment of an infection when the causative pathogen is not yet identified.

Concentration- and Time-Dependent Effects
Antimicrobial drugs exhibit various concentration- and time-dependent effects that influence their clinical efficacy, dosage, and frequency of administration. Examples of these effects are the **minimal inhibitory concentration** (MIC), the **concentration-dependent killing rate** (CDKR), and the **postantibiotic effect** (PAE).

The MIC is the lowest concentration of a drug that inhibits bacterial growth. Based on the MIC, a particular strain of bacteria can be classified as susceptible or resistant to a particular drug (see later).

An example of a CDKR is shown in Fig. 37.3A. Some **aminoglycosides** (e.g., tobramycin) and some **fluoroquinolones** (e.g., ciprofloxacin) exhibit a CDKR against a large group of gram-negative bacteria, including *Pseudomonas aeruginosa* and members of the family Enterobacteriaceae. In contrast, **penicillins** and **other *beta* (β)-lactam antibiotics** usually do not exhibit a CDKR.

After an antibacterial drug is removed from a bacterial culture, evidence of a persistent effect on bacterial growth may exist. This effect (Fig. 37.3B) is the PAE. Most bactericidal antibiotics exhibit a PAE against susceptible pathogens. For example, penicillins and macrolide antibiotics

show a PAE against gram-positive cocci, and aminoglycosides show a PAE against gram-negative bacilli. Because aminoglycosides exhibit both a CDKR and a PAE, treatment regimens have been developed in which the entire daily dose of an aminoglycoside is given at one time. Theoretically, the high rate of bacterial killing produced by these regimens would more rapidly eliminate bacteria, and the PAE would prevent any remaining bacteria from replicating for several hours after the drug has been eliminated from the body.

MICROBIAL SENSITIVITY AND RESISTANCE
Laboratory Tests for Microbial Sensitivity
Microbial sensitivity to drugs can be determined by various means, including the **broth dilution test,** the **disk diffusion method (Kirby-Bauer test),** and the **E-test method.** These laboratory procedures are described in Box 37.1.

Either the broth dilution test or the E-test method can be used to determine the **MIC** of a drug, which is the lowest drug concentration that prevents growth of bacteria. The E-test method offers reliability, convenience, and easy interpretation, and it is more commonly used than the broth-dilution test.

On the basis of the MIC, the organism is classified as having **susceptibility, intermediate sensitivity,** or **resistance** to the drug tested. These categories are based on the **relationship between the MIC and the peak serum concentration** of the drug after administration of typical doses. In general, the peak serum concentration of a drug should be 4 to 10 times greater than the MIC for a pathogen to be susceptible to a drug (see later). Pathogens with intermediate sensitivity may respond to treatment with maximal doses of an antimicrobial agent.

Microbial Resistance to Drugs
Origin of Resistance

Resistance to antimicrobial agents can be innate or acquired. Acquired drug resistance arises from **spontaneous mutation** or from the **transfer of plasmids** that confer drug resistance.

Mutation and Selection

Microbes can spontaneously mutate to a form resistant to a particular antimicrobial drug. These mutations occur at a relatively constant rate, such as in 1 in 10^{12} organisms per unit of time. If the organisms are exposed to an antimicrobial drug during this time period, the sensitive organisms

---

BOX 37.1 LABORATORY DETERMINATION OF MICROBIAL SENSITIVITY TO ANTIBIOTICS

Microbial sensitivity to drugs can be determined by various means, including the broth dilution test, the disk diffusion method, and the E-test method.

BROTH DILUTION TEST

Tubes that contain a nutrient broth are inoculated with equal numbers of bacteria and serially diluted concentrations of an antibiotic. After incubation, the minimal inhibitory concentration (MIC) is identified as the lowest antibiotic concentration that prevents visible growth of bacteria. On the basis of the MIC, the organism is classified as having susceptibility, intermediate sensitivity, or resistance to the drug tested. In the following example, the MIC is 1 µg/mL, and the organism is susceptible to the drug.

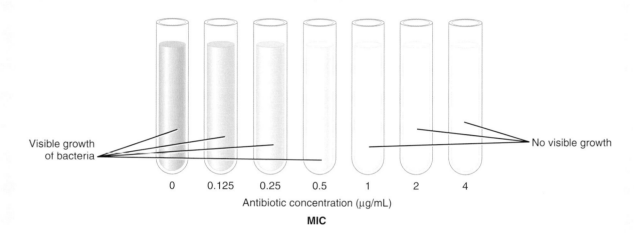

DISK DIFFUSION METHOD (KIRBY-BAUER TEST)

Each disk used in the disk diffusion method is impregnated with a different antibiotic. The disks are placed on agar plates seeded with the test organism. During the incubation period, the antibiotic diffuses from the disk and inhibits bacterial growth. After incubation, the zone inhibited by each antibiotic is measured. The zone diameter for each antibiotic is compared with standard values for that particular antibiotic. The organism is thereby determined to be susceptible, intermediate, or resistant to the various antibiotics tested.

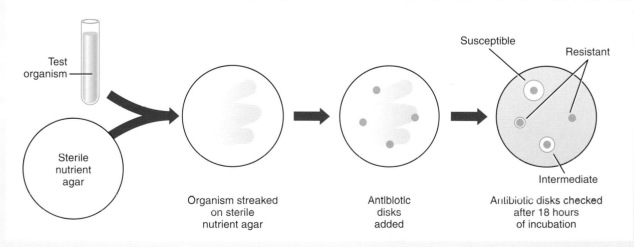

E-TEST METHOD

The E-test strip is a proprietary device that uses a diffusion method to determine the MIC of an organism. The device is a plastic strip that is impregnated with a gradient of antibiotic concentrations. After the strip is placed on an agar culture of the organism, the culture is incubated. During incubation, a tear-shaped zone of inhibition is formed. The point of intersection between the zone of inhibition and the scale displayed on the strip is the MIC. In the following example, the MIC is 0.125 µg/mL.

BOX 37.1 LABORATORY DETERMINATION OF MICROBIAL SENSITIVITY TO ANTIBIOTICS—CONT'D

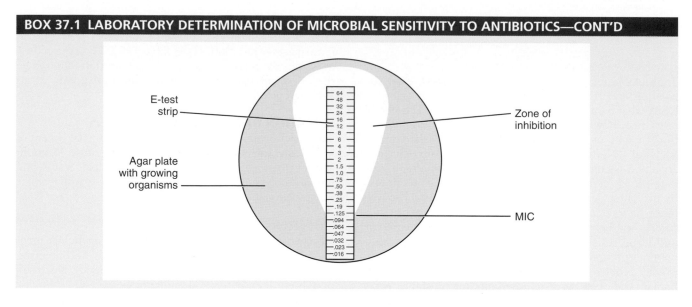

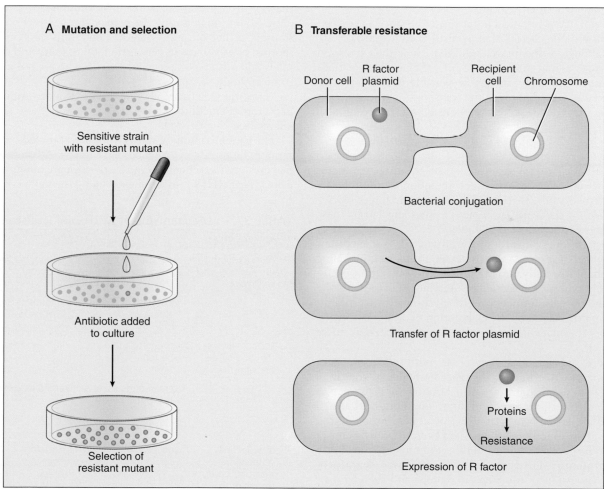

FIG. 37.4 Acquired resistance to antimicrobial drugs can arise by mutation and selection or by transferable resistance. (A) Exposure of an organism to an antibiotic can result in the selection of a resistant mutant. (B) The most common mechanism of transferable resistance is bacterial conjugation and exchange of plasmids containing resistance factors (R factors).

may be eradicated, enabling the resistant mutant to multiply and become the dominant strain (Fig. 37.4A).

The probability that mutation and selection of a resistant mutant will occur is increased during the exposure of an organism to suboptimal concentrations of an antibiotic, and it is also increased during prolonged exposure to an antibiotic. Laboratory tests should be used to guide the selection of an antimicrobial drug, and the dosage and duration of therapy should be adequate for the type of infection being treated. Whenever possible, the bacteriologic response to drug therapy should be verified by culturing samples of appropriate body fluids.

Transferable Resistance

Transferable resistance usually results from bacterial conjugation and the transfer of **plasmids** (extrachromosomal DNA) that confer drug resistance (Fig. 37.4B). Transferable resistance, however, can also be mediated by transformation (uptake of naked DNA) or transduction (transfer of bacterial DNA by a bacteriophage). Bacterial conjugation enables a bacterium to donate a plasmid containing genes that encode proteins responsible for resistance to an antibiotic. These genes are called **resistance factors.** The resistance factors can be transferred both within a particular species and between different species, so they often confer **multidrug resistance.** The various species need not all be present during the period in which the antibiotic is administered. Studies have shown that resident microflora of the human body can serve as reservoirs for resistance genes, allowing the transfer of these genes to organisms that later invade and colonize the host.

Several genes responsible for drug resistance have been cloned, and the factors that control their expression are being studied. In the future, drugs that block the expression of these genes may find use as adjunct therapy for infectious diseases. For example, it may be possible to develop antisense nucleotides that block the transcription or translation of genes that encode proteins responsible for drug resistance.

Mechanisms of Resistance

The three primary mechanisms of microbial resistance to an antibiotic are (1) inactivation of the drug by microbial enzymes, (2) decreased accumulation of the drug by the microbe, and (3) reduced affinity of the target macromolecule for the drug. Examples of drugs affected by these mechanisms are provided in Table 37.1.

Inactivation of the drug by enzymes is an important mechanism of resistance to β-lactam antibiotics, including the penicillins. This form of resistance results from bacterial elaboration of β-lactamase enzymes that destroy the β-lactam ring. Resistance to aminoglycosides (e.g., gentamicin) is partly caused by the elaboration of drug-inactivating enzymes that acetylate, adenylate, or phosphorylate these antibiotics.

Decreased accumulation of an antibiotic can result from **increased efflux** or **decreased uptake** of the drug. Both of these mechanisms contribute to the resistance of microbes to tetracyclines and fluoroquinolones. Increased drug efflux is often mediated by membrane proteins that transport antimicrobial drugs out of bacterial cells. Some of these transport proteins are similar to human **permeability glycoprotein** (P-glycoprotein), which transports antineoplastic drugs out of human cancer cells and thereby confers resistance to the drugs (see Chapter 45). Compounds that inhibit these transport proteins are being investigated as potential agents to reduce drug resistance. Decreased uptake of antimicrobial drugs can result from altered bacterial **porins.** Porins are membrane proteins containing channels through which drugs and other compounds enter bacteria. Resistance to penicillins by gram-negative bacilli is partly caused by altered porin channels that do not permit penicillin entry.

Reduced affinity of target molecules for antimicrobial drugs is a common mechanism of microbial resistance to most classes of antibiotics (see Table 37.1). This type of drug resistance often results from bacterial mutation followed by the selection of resistant mutants during exposure to an antimicrobial drug.

SELECTION OF ANTIMICROBIAL DRUGS

The selection of an antimicrobial agent for the treatment of a particular infection is largely based on the cause, location, and severity of an infection; the age, physiologic status, and immune competency of the patient; and the pharmacologic properties of antimicrobial drugs.

Host Factors

Host factors that influence the choice of a drug include pregnancy, drug allergies, age and immune status, and the presence of renal impairment, hepatic insufficiency, abscesses, or indwelling catheters and similar devices.

Most antimicrobial drugs cross the placenta and can thereby affect the fetus. For example, administering tetracyclines to a woman during **pregnancy** can cause permanent staining of her offspring's teeth. Penicillins and cephalosporins, however, cause very little fetal toxicity and can be safely administered to pregnant women who are not allergic to these drugs.

Many individuals are allergic to one or more antimicrobial drugs. Penicillins are the most common cause of drug allergy (see Chapter 38).

The patient's **immune status** is an important factor determining the success of antimicrobial therapy. **Advanced age, diabetes, cancer chemotherapy,** and **human immunodeficiency virus (HIV) infection** are among the more common

TABLE 37.1   Mechanisms of Microbial Resistance

MECHANISM	EXAMPLES
Inactivation of the drug by microbial enzymes	Inactivation of aminoglycosides by acetylase, adenylate synthetase, and phosphorylase enzymes
	Inactivation of penicillins and other β-lactam antibiotics by β-lactamase enzymes
Decreased accumulation of the drug by the microbe	Decreased uptake of β-lactam antibiotics owing to altered porins in gram-negative bacteria
	Decreased uptake and increased efflux of fluoroquinolones
	Decreased uptake and increased efflux of tetracyclines
Reduced affinity of the target macromolecule for the drug	Reduced affinity of DNA gyrase for fluoroquinolones
	Reduced affinity of folate synthesis enzymes for sulfonamides and trimethoprim
	Reduced affinity of ribosomes for aminoglycosides, chloramphenicol, clindamycin, macrolides, or tetracyclines
	Reduced affinity of RNA polymerase for rifampin
	Reduced affinity of transpeptidase and other penicillin-binding proteins for penicillins and other β-lactam antibiotics

causes of impaired immunity. Immunocompromised individuals should be treated with larger doses of bactericidal drugs and may require a longer duration of therapy than immunocompetent individuals.

Antibiotic access to an **abscess** (collection of pus in a tissue) is poor, and the concentration of an antibiotic in an abscess is usually lower than in the surrounding tissue. Moreover, immune function is often impaired in an abscess. For these reasons, it is often necessary to surgically drain an abscess before the infection can be cured.

Foreign bodies, such as **indwelling catheters,** provide sites where microbes can become covered with a glycocalyx coating (biofilm) that protects them from antibiotics and immunologic destruction.

Many antibiotics are excreted unchanged by the kidneys, and lower doses must be used if the patient has significant **renal impairment.** Less commonly, **hepatic insufficiency** may require dosage adjustment for antimicrobial drugs that are extensively metabolized in the liver. For example, neonates cannot metabolize chloramphenicol, so their dosage of this drug per kilogram of body weight must be lower than the dosage given to older children or adults.

Antimicrobial Activity

Antimicrobial agents can be selected on the basis of **laboratory tests** described earlier or based on knowledge of the most common organisms causing various types of infections and the preferred drugs for these organisms (empiric selection). **Empiric therapy** may be used to treat serious infections until test results are available or to treat minor upper respiratory and urinary tract infections because of the predictability of causative organisms and their sensitivity to drugs. In these situations, the cost of microbial culture and drug sensitivity tests is usually not justified.

Most infections are caused by a single microbial pathogen and are treated with a single drug. This is because monotherapy is less expensive, has less effect on normal host flora, and causes few adverse effects than combination therapy. A few situations in which combination therapy is preferable are described later. The preferred drugs for treatment of infections caused by specific bacteria are listed in Table 37.2.

Pharmacokinetic Properties

The pharmacokinetic properties that influence antibiotic selection include oral bioavailability, peak serum concentration, distribution to particular sites of infection, routes of elimination, and elimination half-life. An ideal antimicrobial drug for ambulatory patients would have good oral bioavailability and a long plasma half-life so that it would need to be taken only once a day. Azithromycin is an example of an antibiotic that meets these criteria.

As described previously, the peak serum concentration of an antimicrobial drug should be several times greater than the MIC of the pathogenic organism for the drug to eliminate the organism. This is partly because the tissue concentrations of a drug are sometimes lower than the plasma concentration. The relationship between the plasma concentration of a typical antimicrobial drug and the drug's MIC for several organisms is shown in Fig. 37.5. The urine concentration of an antimicrobial drug can be 10 to 50 times the peak serum concentration. For this reason, infections of the urinary tract can be easier to treat than are infections at other sites.

Sites of infection that are not readily penetrated by many antimicrobial drugs include the **central nervous system, bone, prostate gland,** and **ocular tissues.** The treatment of meningitis requires that drugs achieve adequate concentrations in the cerebrospinal fluid. Some antibiotics (e.g., penicillin G) penetrate the blood-cerebrospinal fluid barrier when the meninges are inflamed, but the aminoglycosides do not. For this reason, aminoglycosides can be given **intrathecally** for the treatment of meningitis. Because antimicrobial drug concentrations are low in bone, patients with osteomyelitis must usually be treated with antibiotics for several weeks to produce a cure. The prostate gland restricts the entry of some antimicrobial drugs because the drugs have difficulty crossing the prostatic epithelium and because prostatic fluid has a low pH. These characteristics favor the entry and accumulation of weak bases (e.g., trimethoprim) and tend to exclude the entry of weak acids (e.g., penicillin).

The route of elimination affects both the selection and the use of antimicrobial drugs. Drugs that are eliminated by renal excretion (e.g., fluoroquinolones) are more effective for urinary tract infections than drugs that are largely metabolized or undergo biliary excretion (e.g., erythromycin). Antibiotics that are eliminated by the kidneys (e.g., the aminoglycosides) can accumulate in patients whose renal function is compromised, however, and their dosage must be reduced in these patients.

Adverse Effect Profile

Any antimicrobial drug can cause mild to severe adverse effects, but the incidence of these effects varies greatly among different classes of drugs, and it is important to consider the probable risk-to-benefit ratio when selecting drugs for treatment. The β-lactam (e.g., penicillins and cephalosporins) and macrolide (e.g., erythromycin) antibiotics cause a relatively low incidence of organ system toxicity and are often used to treat minor infections, including infections in pregnant women. In contrast, the aminoglycosides (e.g., gentamicin) cause a relatively high incidence of adverse effects and are reserved for the treatment of more serious or life-threatening infections. Fluoroquinolones and tetracyclines are intermediate in their adverse effect profile.

COMBINATION DRUG THERAPY

Drug combinations are used to treat certain types of infections. These include infections that are known or suspected to be caused by more than one pathogen (mixed infections), such as intraabdominal infections caused by both aerobic and anaerobic organisms derived from the intestinal tract. In some cases, life-threatening infections, such as hospital-acquired **(nosocomial)** pneumonia, are treated with a combination of antibiotics until the causative organism can be identified.

When antimicrobial drugs are given in combination, they can exhibit antagonistic, additive, synergistic, or indifferent effects against a particular microbe (Fig. 37.6). The relationship between two drugs and their combined effect is as follows: **antagonistic** if the combined effect is less than the effect of either drug alone; **additive** if the combined effect is equal to the sum of the independent effects; **synergistic** if

TABLE 37.2   Antimicrobial Drugs Most Often Used for the Treatment of Infections Caused by Selected Bacteria[a]

BACTERIA	ANTIMICROBIAL DRUGS
Gram-Positive Cocci	
Enterococcus species	Penicillin G or ampicillin plus gentamicin; vancomycin plus gentamicin; quinupristin + dalfopristin, linezolid, daptomycin, tigecycline
Staphylococcus aureus	Penicillin G (if sensitive), nafcillin, oxacillin, vancomycin, trimethoprim-sulfamethoxazole, linezolid, daptomycin, tigecycline
Streptococcus pyogenes	Penicillin G or V, a cephalosporin, a macrolide, clindamycin
Viridans group streptococci	Penicillin G ± gentamicin; a cephalosporin, vancomycin
Streptococcus pneumoniae	Penicillin G (if sensitive), a cephalosporin 2 or 3, amoxicillin + clavulanate, antipneumococcal fluoroquinolone, azithromycin, telithromycin
Gram-Positive Bacilli	
Bacillus anthracis (anthrax)	Ciprofloxacin or doxycycline, + clindamycin or rifampin
Clostridiodes difficile (diarrhea, pseudomembranous colitis)	Metronidazole, oral vancomycin
Clostridiodes perfringens, Clostridiodes tetani	Penicillin G ± clindamycin, doxycycline
Corynebacterium diphtheriae	Erythromycin or clindamycin
Listeria monocytogenes	Ampicillin (± aminoglycoside), trimethoprim-sulfamethoxazole
Nocardia asteroides and other species	Trimethoprim-sulfamethoxazole, minocycline, imipenem, amikacin, linezolid
Gram-Negative Cocci	
Moraxella catarrhalis	Amoxicillin + clavulanate, a cephalosporin 2 or 3, a macrolide, a fluoroquinolone
Neisseria gonorrheae	Ceftriaxone, cefixime, cefpodoxime
Neisseria meningitides	Penicillin G, ceftriaxone or other cephalosporin 2 or 3, chloramphenicol
Gram-Negative Bacilli	
Bacteroides species (anaerobes)	Metronidazole, cefoxitin, carbapenem, penicillin + β-lactamase inhibitor
Bordetella pertussis (whooping cough)	A macrolide (azithromycin), trimethoprim-sulfamethoxazole
Helicobacter pylori (peptic ulcer disease)	Clarithromycin, amoxicillin, metronidazole, bismuth compounds, tinidazole, proton pump inhibitors
Haemophilus influenzae	Upper respiratory infections: amoxicillin + clavulanate, oral cephalosporin 2 or 3, azithromycin; serious infections: cefotaxime or ceftriaxone
Pseudomonas aeruginosa	Tobramycin, ceftazidime, a carbapenem, aztreonam, piperacillin + tazobactam or quinolone
Most Enterobacteriaceae (*Escherichia coli; Klebsiella, Proteus, Serratia, Enterobacter, Citrobacter, Providencia* species, and others)	Parenteral cephalosporin 2 or 3, an aminoglycoside, piperacillin + tazobactam, a carbapenem, aztreonam, a fluoroquinolone, trimethoprim + sulfamethoxazole (urinary tract infections)
Salmonella and *Shigella* species	A fluoroquinolone; ceftriaxone *(Salmonella)*, azithromycin *(Shigella)*
Campylobacter jejuni	Azithromycin or erythromycin, quinolone
Yersinia pestis (plague); *Francisella tularensis* (tularemia)	Gentamicin, doxycycline
Actinomycetes	
Chlamydiae, *Ehrlichia,* rickettsiae	Doxycycline (all); azithromycin (chlamydiae)
Spirochetes	
Borrelia burgdorferi (Lyme disease)	Doxycycline, amoxicillin, parenteral cephalosporin 2 or 3
Borrelia recurrentis (relapsing fever)	Doxycycline, penicillin G
Treponema pallidum (syphilis, yaws)	Benzathine penicillin G, doxycycline

[a]Recommended drug(s) listed first, followed by alternates in no particular order. 2 or 3 refers to second or third generation cephalosporin.

the combined effect is greater than the sum of the independent effects; and **indifferent** if the combined effect is similar to the greatest effect produced by either drug alone. Some bacteriostatic drugs (e.g., chloramphenicol or tetracycline) are antagonistic to bactericidal drugs. Bactericidal drugs are usually more effective against rapidly dividing bacteria, and their effect may be reduced if bacterial growth is slowed by a bacteriostatic drug.

If two bactericidal drugs that target different microbial functions are given in combination, they can exert **additive or synergistic effects** against susceptible bacteria (Box 37.2). For example, penicillins, which are cell

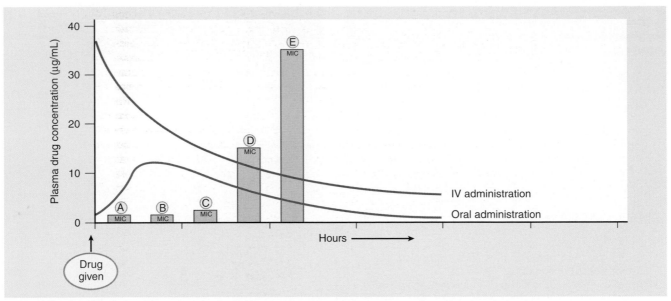

FIG. 37.5   Relationship between the plasma concentration of a typical antimicrobial drug and the drug's minimal inhibitory concentration (MIC) for five bacterial organisms. The *curves* represent typical plasma concentrations over time after intravenous (*IV*) or oral administration of the drug. Each bar represents the MIC of a particular organism: *Streptococcus pneumoniae*, *Staphylococcus aureus*, and *Escherichia coli* (shown as A, B, and C, respectively, in this example) are susceptible to the drug; *Enterobacter cloacae* (shown as D) is intermediate in sensitivity; and *Pseudomonas aeruginosa* (shown as E) is resistant.

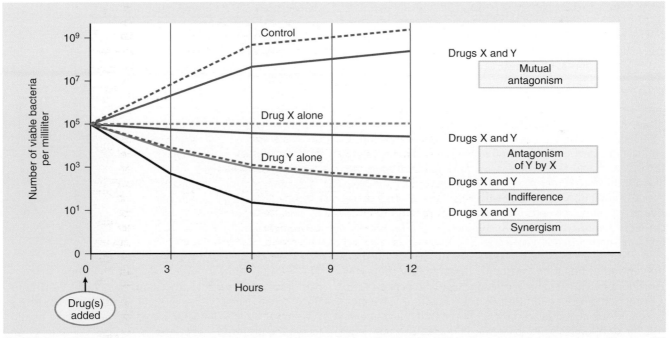

FIG. 37.6   Comparison of several possible interactions of two antimicrobial drugs combined *in vitro*. *Curves* show the results when cultures containing 10^5 bacteria per milliliter are incubated with no drug (control), with drug *X* alone, with drug *Y* alone, and with a combination of drugs *X* and *Y*. In this example, drug *X* is bacteriostatic, whereas drug *Y* is bactericidal. In an antagonistic interaction, the combined effect is less than the effect of either drug alone. In an indifferent interaction, the combined effect is similar to the greatest effect produced by either drug alone. In a synergistic interaction, the combined effect is greater than the sum of the independent effects.

wall synthesis inhibitors, can have additive or synergistic effects with aminoglycosides, which inhibit protein synthesis, against gram-negative bacilli such as *P. aeruginosa*, and against gram-positive enterococci and staphylococci. Likewise, **sulfamethoxazole** and **trimethoprim** inhibit sequential steps in bacterial folate synthesis and have

synergistic activity against organisms that may be resistant to either drug alone.

Combination therapy may also serve to reduce the emergence of resistant organisms, such as in the treatment of tuberculosis (see Chapter 41). This is because about 1 in 10^6 *Mycobacterium tuberculosis* organisms will mutate to a

BOX 37.2 *IN VITRO* ACTIVITY OF ANTIMICROBIAL DRUG COMBINATIONS

SYNERGISTIC COMBINATIONS
- Aminoglycoside plus ampicillin or penicillin G against enterococci
- Aminoglycoside plus broad-spectrum penicillin against gram-negative bacilli
- Aminoglycoside plus cephalosporin against gram-negative bacilli
- Amphotericin B plus flucytosine against *Cryptococcus neoformans*
- Vancomycin plus aminoglycoside against staphylococci
- Reverse transcriptase inhibitor plus protease inhibitor against human immunodeficiency virus

ANTAGONISTIC COMBINATIONS
- Aminoglycoside plus chloramphenicol against members of the family Enterobacteriaceae
- Broad-spectrum penicillin plus chloramphenicol against *Streptococcus pneumoniae*
- Broad-spectrum penicillin plus imipenem against gram-negative bacilli

BOX 37.3 EXAMPLES OF ANTIMICROBIAL PROPHYLAXIS

- Prevention of Infection during Surgical and Invasive Procedures

Infection	Pathogens	Preferred Drugs
Endocarditis in persons with valvular heart disease undergoing oral, dental or upper respiratory procedures		Amoxicillin or clindamycin
Surgical wound infections	*Staphylococcus aureus*, enteric gram-negative rods	Cefazolin
Surgical abdominal infections	Enteric gram-negative bacilli and anaerobes	Cefoxitin, cefotetan, ertapenem, or cefazolin + metronidazole

- Prevention of Disease Transmission in Persons at Increased Risk

Infection	Preferred Drugs
Genital or perinatal herpes simplex	Acyclovir
HIV infection in newborns	Highly active antiretroviral therapy (HAART)[a]
Influenza, type A and B	Oseltamivir or zanamivir
Malaria	Chloroquine, or atovaquone + proguanil, doxycycline, or mefloquine
Meningococcal disease	Rifampin, ciprofloxacin, or ceftriaxone
Tuberculosis	Isoniazid or rifampin; isoniazid + rifapentine

[a]See Chapter 43.

resistant form during treatment with any single drug. The rate of mutation to a form resistant to two drugs is the product of the individual drug resistance rates, or about 1 in 10^{12} organisms. Because fewer than 10^{12} organisms are usually present in a patient with tuberculosis, it is unlikely that a resistant mutant will emerge during combination therapy. In the case of tuberculosis, combination therapy can delay emergence of resistance even though the drugs may not exhibit a synergistic effect against the microbe.

PROPHYLACTIC THERAPY

The prevention of infections requires the sterilization of diagnostic and surgical instruments, the use of disinfectants to reduce environmental pathogens in hospitals and clinics, and the disinfection of skin and mucous membranes before invasive procedures. In some cases, antimicrobial drugs are also administered prophylactically either to reduce the incidence of infections associated with surgical and other invasive procedures or to prevent disease transmission to close contacts of infected persons. Recommendations for prophylaxis are summarized in Box 37.3.

Prevention of Infection Caused by Invasive Procedures

Antibiotics are used to prevent **endocarditis** in persons with a history of valvular heart disease, such as mitral valve prolapse and rheumatic heart disease. These individuals are at risk for developing acute bacterial endocarditis caused by viridans streptococci and other streptococci that can be acquired during dental, oral, or upper respiratory tract procedures and surgery. Amoxicillin is currently considered the drug of choice, but endocarditis can be prevented by using an alternative drug (e.g., clindamycin, cephalexin, azithromycin, or clarithromycin).

Antibiotics are routinely used to prevent **wound and tissue infections** that can be acquired during a wide range of surgical procedures. The choice of antibiotic depends on the most likely sources of bacterial pathogens during a particular procedure. The skin is the most common source of pathogens, especially staphylococci, during most types of surgery.

The gastrointestinal tract is also an important source of pathogens when surgical procedures involve the gastrointestinal system. Surgery to repair contaminated wounds (e.g., gunshot or knife wounds) presents the most severe requirements for prophylaxis because of the greater number and variety of bacteria often associated with this type of trauma.

Prevention of Disease Transmission

Antimicrobial drugs are occasionally used to prevent the transmission of a highly contagious disease, such as **meningococcal infection,** from an infected person or insect vector to an exposed individual. Drugs are also used to prevent **malaria** in persons who are traveling to regions of the world where malaria is endemic and to prevent **influenza type A** in populations at increased risk for these diseases. Prophylactic drugs are discussed more thoroughly in subsequent chapters.

SUMMARY OF IMPORTANT POINTS

- Antibiotics are substances produced by one microbe that inhibit the growth or viability of pathogenic organisms. These include cell wall synthesis inhibitors, protein synthesis inhibitors, metabolic and nucleic acid inhibitors, and cell membrane inhibitors.
- Antimicrobial drugs can be characterized as bactericidal (able to kill microbes) or bacteriostatic (able to slow the growth of microbes). They can also be characterized as narrow-spectrum, broad-spectrum, or extended-spectrum based on their range of antimicrobial activity.
- Laboratory tests used to determine microbial sensitivity to drugs include the broth dilution test, the disk diffusion method (Kirby-Bauer test), and the E-test method. The broth dilution test and E-test method are used to determine the MIC, which is the lowest drug concentration that inhibits microbial growth *in vitro*.
- Acquired microbial resistance arises by mutation and selection or by transfer of genes encoding resistance factors. The most common mechanism of transferable resistance is bacterial conjugation followed by the exchange of plasmids containing resistance genes.
- The mechanisms responsible for microbial resistance to a drug include inactivation of the drug by microbial enzymes, decreased uptake or increased efflux of the drug by the microbe, and reduced affinity of the target macromolecule for the drug.
- The selection of an antimicrobial drug for treating a particular infection requires consideration of host factors (pregnancy, drug allergies, age and immune status, and the presence of concomitant diseases) and drug characteristics (antimicrobial activity, pharmacokinetic properties, adverse effect profile, cost, and convenience).
- Combinations of antimicrobial agents can be used for the treatment of infections caused by more than one organism, the empiric treatment of serious infections, and the prevention of antibiotic resistance. A combination of two synergistic drugs is sometimes employed to treat an infection caused by a single microbe.
- Antibiotic prophylaxis is used to prevent infections during surgical and other invasive procedures and to prevent the transmission of infectious diseases to persons at risk.

Review Questions

For each numbered description, select the corresponding term from the lettered choices.

1. A cell membrane constituent that transports chemotherapeutic drugs out of a target cell.
   - (A) plasmid
   - (B) porin
   - (C) resistance factor
   - (D) β-lactamase
   - (E) P-glycoprotein
2. The continued suppression of bacterial growth after an antibiotic has been eliminated from the body.
   - (A) bacteriostatic
   - (B) postantibiotic effect
   - (C) time-dependent killing
   - (D) concentration-dependent killing
   - (E) synergistic effect
3. The combined antibacterial effect of two drugs is greater than the sum of their individual effects.
   - (A) mutual antagonism
   - (B) indifference
   - (C) synergism
   - (D) additive
   - (E) competition
4. The most frequent mechanism of transferable drug resistance.
   - (A) transduction
   - (B) transformation
   - (C) transmission
   - (D) plasmid exchange
   - (E) mutation and selection
5. An antibiotic diffusion method for determining the MIC of an antibiotic.
   - (A) E-test strip method
   - (B) broth dilution method
   - (C) disk diffusion method
   - (D) growth rate method
   - (E) turbidity method

Antibiotics That Inhibit Bacterial Cell Wall Synthesis

CLASSIFICATION OF CELL WALL SYNTHESIS INHIBITORS

Narrow-Spectrum Penicillins

- Penicillin G
- Penicillin V

Penicillinase-Resistant Penicillins

- Dicloxacillin
- Nafcillin
- Oxacillin

Extended-Spectrum Penicillins

- Amoxicillin
- Ampicillin
- Piperacillin

Beta (β)-Lactamase Inhibitors

- Clavulanate with amoxicillin (AUGMENTIN)
- Tazobactam with piperacillin (ZOSYN)[a]

First-Generation Cephalosporins

- Clavulanate with amoxicillin (AUGMENTIN)
- Clavulanate with amoxicillin (AUGMENTIN)

Second-Generation Cephalosporins

- Clavulanate with amoxicillin (AUGMENTIN)
- Clavulanate with amoxicillin (AUGMENTIN)
- Clavulanate with amoxicillin (AUGMENTIN)

Third-Generation Cephalosporins

- Ceftriaxone[b]
- Cefdinir
- Cefpodoxime

Fourth-Generation Cephalosporins

- Cefepime (MAXIPIME)

Advanced-Generation Cephalosporins

- Ceftaroline (TEFLARO)
- Cefiderocol (FETROJA)

Monobactam

- Aztreonam (AZACTAM)

Carbapenems

- Meropenem (MERREM)
- Ertapenem (INVANZ)
- Imipenem (with cilastatin as PRIMAXIN)[c]

Other Bacterial Cell Wall Synthesis Inhibitors

- Bacitracin
- Fosfomycin (MONUROL)
- Vancomycin (VANCOCIN)
- Telavancin (VIBATIV)

[a] Also sulbactam with ampicillin (UNASYN).
[b] Also cefotaxime (CLAFORAN), cefixime (SUPRAX), ceftazidime (FORTAZ), and ceftazidime with avibactam (AVYCAZ).
[c] Other combination drugs include meropenem and vabomactam (VABOMERE), and imipenem with cilastatin and relebactam (RECARBIO).

OVERVIEW

Several classes of antibiotics inhibit the synthesis of the bacterial cell wall, including the penicillins and cephalosporins. The penicillins were the first antibiotics to be discovered, and their development inaugurated the modern era of antimicrobial chemotherapy in the 1940s. Despite the growing problem of microbial resistance to these drugs, the cell wall inhibitors have remained one of the most widely used groups of antibiotics for more than 70 years. This chapter describes the structure and function of the bacterial cell envelope and the pharmacologic properties and clinical use of the bacterial cell wall inhibitors.

Cell Envelope

The cell envelope of both gram-positive and gram-negative bacteria consists of a **cytoplasmic membrane** surrounded by a **cell wall** (Fig. 38.1). Gram-negative bacteria also have an **outer membrane** not found in other types of bacteria. The cell wall is much thicker in gram-positive bacteria than in gram-negative bacteria.

Cytoplasmic and Outer Membranes

The cytoplasmic membrane is a trilaminar membrane. It contains several **transport proteins** that facilitate the uptake of substances used by bacteria, and it contains the enzymes that synthesize the bacterial cell wall. These enzymes are inhibited by penicillins and other beta (β)-lactam antibiotics and are collectively known as **penicillin-binding proteins (PBPs)**.

The outer membrane of gram-negative bacteria is also a trilaminar membrane. It contains species-specific forms of a complex **lipopolysaccharide** and various types of protein channels called **porins.** One portion of lipopolysaccharide (the lipid A portion) is the **endotoxin** responsible for gram-negative sepsis. This endotoxin activates immunologic mechanisms that lead to fever, platelet aggregation, increased vascular permeability, and other adverse effects

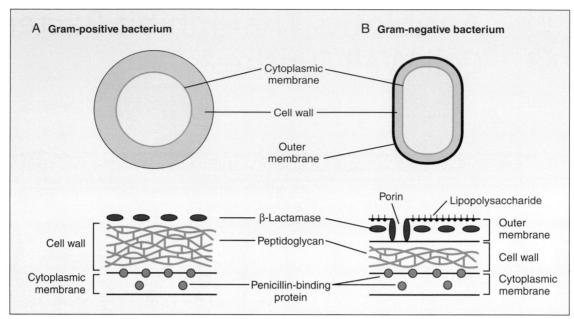

FIG. 38.1 Comparison of the cell envelopes of gram-positive and gram-negative bacteria. (A) The gram-positive bacterium has a thick cell wall but does not have an outer membrane. β-lactamases are located in the outer portion of the cell wall. Penicillin-binding proteins are found in the cytoplasmic membrane. (B) The gram-negative bacterium has a thin cell wall. It also has an outer membrane that contains lipopolysaccharide and protein channels called *porins*.

on tissues. Porins allow ions and other small molecules to pass through the outer membrane, including various antibiotics. Alterations in porin structure can lead to bacterial resistance to antibiotics, such as may occur with resistance to carbapenem antibiotics, such as imipenem.

The inner bacterial cytoplasmic membrane is the target of two peptide antibiotics, **daptomycin** and **polymyxin.** These drugs act directly on the cell membranes to increase membrane permeability and thereby cause the cytoplasmic contents to leak out of the cell. The properties and uses of these antibiotics are discussed in Chapter 40.

Cell Wall

The cell wall consists primarily of **peptidoglycan,** a polymer constructed from repeating disaccharide units of **N-acetylglucosamine** (GlcNAc) and **N-acetylmuramic acid** (MurNAc). Each disaccharide is attached to others through glycosidic bonds. Each molecule of MurNAc has a peptide containing two molecules of D-alanine and a pentaglycine side chain (Fig. 38.2). The strands of peptidoglycan in the cell wall are cross-linked by a transpeptidase reaction in which the glycine pentapeptide of one strand is attached to the penultimate D-alanine molecule of another strand. During this reaction, the terminal D-alanine is removed.

The cell wall maintains the shape of the bacterium and protects it from **osmotic lysis** if it is placed in a hypotonic solution. Without a cell wall, the bacterium is unprotected and inhibition of cell wall synthesis by antibiotics is often bactericidal. Because a cell wall is not found in higher organisms, inhibition of cell wall synthesis has no effect on host cells. The cell wall is synthesized during bacterial replication, and drugs that inhibit cell wall synthesis are more active against **rapidly dividing bacteria** than they are against bacteria in the resting or stationary phase. For the same reason, the effectiveness of cell wall inhibitors is

sometimes reduced by concurrent administration of bacteriostatic antibiotics that slow the growth of bacteria.

Sites of Drug Action
β-Lactam Drugs
The β-lactam antibiotics inhibit bacterial enzymes known as the **PBPs.** These enzymes are anchored in the cytoplasmic membrane and extend into the periplasmic space. The PBPs are responsible for the assembly, maintenance, and regulation of the peptidoglycan portion of the bacterial cell wall. Some of the PBPs have **transpeptidase** activity, whereas others have carboxypeptidase and transglycosylase activity.

The β-lactam antibiotics form a covalent bond with PBPs and inhibit the catalytic activity of these enzymes. Inhibition of some PBPs prevents **elongation** or **cross-linking of peptidoglycan** (see Fig. 38.2), while inhibition of other PBPs leads to the bacterium's **autolysis** or to its change to a **spheroplast** or a **filamentous form.**

Each bacterial species has a unique set of PBPs to which particular β-lactam antibiotics bind with different affinities. This partly accounts for the variation in the sensitivity of different organisms to different antibiotics.

Other Drugs
Bacitracin and **fosfomycin** inhibit cell wall peptidoglycan synthesis by blocking specific steps in the formation of the disaccharide precursor, MurNAc-GlcNAc. As shown in Fig. 38.2, bacitracin inhibits the dephosphorylation of bactoprenol pyrophosphate (C_{55}-isoprenyl pyrophosphate), which is the carrier of the building-blocks of the peptidoglycan.

Fosfomycin inhibits **enolpyruvyl transferase,** the enzyme that catalyzes the condensation of uridine diphosphate–GlcNAc (UDP-GlcNAc), with phosphoenolpyruvate to synthesize UDP-MurNAc. **Vancomycin** binds tightly to the **d-alanyl-d-alanine** portion of the peptidoglycan precursor and prevents bonding of the penultimate D-alanine to the

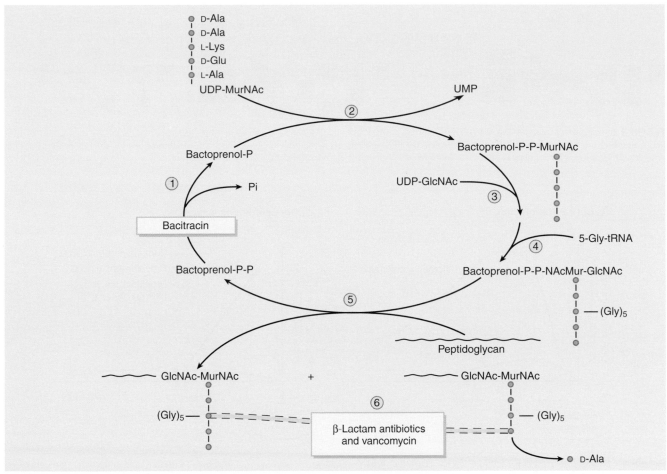

FIG. 38.2 Sites of action of bacterial cell wall synthesis inhibitors. The bacterial cell wall consists primarily of peptidoglycan, a polymer constructed from repeating disaccharide units of N-acetylglucosamine (*GlcNAc*) and N-acetylmuramic acid (*MurNAc*). Numbers indicate the steps involved in the synthesis of the cell wall of *Staphylococcus aureus*. In step 1, bactoprenol pyrophosphate (*bactoprenol-P-P*; also known as C_{55}-isoprenyl pyrophosphate) is dephosphorylated to regenerate the carrier molecule, bactoprenol phosphate (*bactoprenol-P*). In step 2, uridine diphosphate-MurNAc (*UDP-MurNAc*) is added. In steps 3 and 4, UDP-GlcNAc and a glycine pentapeptide (*5-Gly tRNA*) are added. In step 5, the disaccharide peptide is transferred to the peptidoglycan growth point. In step 6, the cross-linking of peptidoglycan strands is catalyzed by transpeptidase, a type of penicillin-binding protein. In this reaction a glycine of one strand forms a peptide bond with the penultimate D-alanine of an adjacent strand, and the terminal D-alanine is released. Bacitracin blocks step 1, and β-lactam antibiotics and vancomycin block step 6 by different mechanisms. Fosfomycin (not shown) inhibits enolpyruvyl transferase, the enzyme that catalyzes the condensation of UDP-GlcNAc with phosphoenolpyruvate to synthesize UDP-MurNAc.

pentaglycine peptide during cross-linking of peptidoglycan strands.

β-LACTAM ANTIBIOTICS

The β-lactam antibiotics include penicillins, cephalosporins, carbapenems, and a monobactam antibiotic called aztreonam.

Penicillins

Penicillin was the first antibiotic to be isolated and used to treat systemic bacterial infections. Alexander Fleming discovered penicillin when he recognized that a *Penicillium* fungus contaminating his bacterial cultures produced a substance that inhibited bacterial growth. Fleming investigated the antimicrobial activity of crude extracts of penicillin but was unable to isolate the antibiotic in sufficient purity and quantity for clinical use. Later, Chain and Florey extracted enough penicillin from fungal cultures to establish its clinical effectiveness, and advances in microbial fermentation technology enabled the production of sufficient quantities of penicillin for widespread use during and after WWII.

Penicillins can be grouped according to their antimicrobial activity. **Narrow-spectrum penicillins** (penicillin G and penicillin V) are active against many gram-positive cocci. **Penicillinase-resistant penicillins** (nafcillin, oxacillin) are active against some strains of penicillinase-producing staphylococci, while **extended-spectrum penicillins** (ampicillin, piperacillin) are active against some gram-negative bacilli and anaerobic bacteria, as well as gram-positive organisms.

Chemistry and Pharmacokinetics

The penicillin antibiotics consist of a β-lactam ring fused to a thiazolidine ring with a unique side chain (R group) for each antibiotic, as shown in Fig. 38.3. The penicillin family includes natural penicillins (e.g., penicillin G) isolated from strains of *Penicillium notatum* and other species, as well as semisynthetic derivatives of natural penicillins (e.g., amoxicillin).

Some of the penicillins, such as amoxicillin and penicillin V, are stable in gastric acid and can be given orally, whereas others are acid-labile and must be given parenterally, such as piperacillin. The penicillins are widely distributed to organs

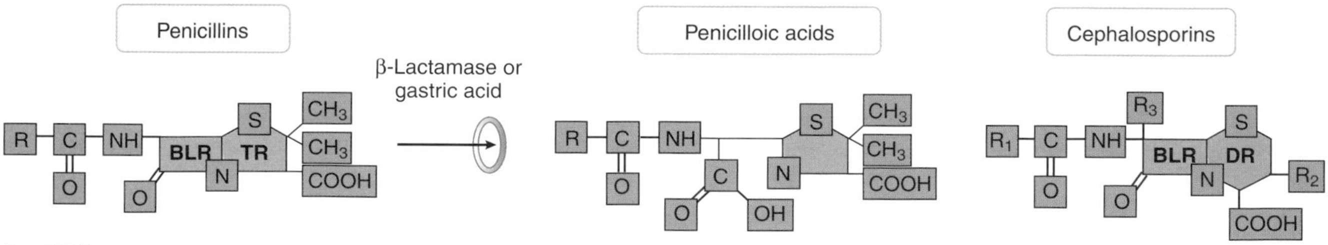

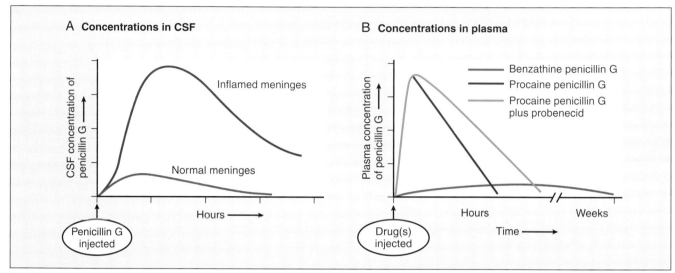

FIG. 38.3 Structures of β-lactam drugs. Penicillins contain a β-lactam ring *(BLR)* and a thiazolidine ring *(TR)*, whereas cephalosporins contain a BLR and a dihydrothiazine ring *(DR)*. β-lactamases hydrolyze the BLR and convert penicillins to penicilloic acids, which may react with body proteins to form antigens. β-lactamases convert cephalosporins to inactive cephalosporanic acids (not shown).

FIG. 38.4 Pharmacokinetics of penicillin G preparations. (A) When penicillin G is administered to patients with normal meninges, the concentration in cerebrospinal fluid *(CSF)* remains low, but when it is administered to patients with meningitis, the CSF concentration is much higher because meningeal inflammation increases meningeal permeability to penicillin G. (B) Administration of benzathine penicillin G produces low plasma concentrations of the drug for several weeks. Administration of procaine penicillin G produces higher plasma concentrations for about 24 hours. Probenecid inhibits the renal excretion of penicillin G, prolongs its half-life, and increases its plasma concentrations.

and tissues except the central nervous system. Because penicillins penetrate the cerebrospinal fluid when the meninges are inflamed (Fig. 38.4), they can be administered intravenously for the treatment of meningitis. Most penicillins are eliminated by active renal tubular secretion and have short half-lives of about 0.5 to 1.3 hours (Table 38.1), though a few penicillins (e.g., ampicillin and nafcillin) are excreted primarily in the bile. The renal tubular secretion of penicillins is inhibited by **probenecid,** a drug that competes with penicillins for the organic acid transporter located in the proximal tubule. Probenecid has been used to slow the excretion and prolong the half-life of penicillin G (see Fig. 38.4).

Penicillin G is available in two long-acting forms for intramuscular administration, **procaine penicillin G** and **benzathine penicillin G.** Penicillin G is slowly released from these two preparations for absorption into the circulation after an intramuscular injection. Benzathine penicillin G provides very low plasma concentrations of the drug for a few weeks. Procaine penicillin G produces higher plasma concentrations of penicillin for about 24 hours (see Fig. 38.4B). A few preparations contain both of these formulations.

Spectrum and Indications

Table 38.2 outlines the spectrum and major clinical uses of penicillins.

The **narrow-spectrum penicillins,** penicillins G and V, are used to treat infections caused by sensitive strains of streptococci (including pneumococci), meningococci, and spirochetes (e.g., *Treponema pallidum*). For example, penicillin G is used to treat group A **streptococcal infections** and to treat **syphilis.** Penicillin G is also active against *Clostridium perfringens*, the cause of **gas gangrene,** and other pathogens. Most staphylococci and gonococci, and some strains of pneumococci, are now resistant to penicillin G.

The **penicillinase-resistant penicillins** (e.g., dicloxacillin and nafcillin) were developed to treat penicillin-resistant strains of **staphylococci** that express penicillinase (a type of β-lactamase). These penicillins are not active against most other species of penicillinase-producing bacteria. Nafcillin is usually preferred when parenteral administration is required, whereas dicloxacillin can be given orally for less severe infections.

The penicillinase-resistant drugs are used to treat serious staphylococcal infections, such as acute endocarditis and osteomyelitis, as well as skin and soft tissue infections. Staphylococci that are resistant to these penicillins are designated **methicillin-resistant *Staphylococcus aureus* (MRSA),** though methicillin itself is seldom used today because of its tendency to cause interstitial nephritis. Bacteria resistant to methicillin are also cross-resistant to

TABLE 38.1   Pharmacokinetic Properties of Selected Bacterial Cell Wall Synthesis Inhibitors

DRUG	ROUTE OF ADMINISTRATION	ELIMINATION HALF-LIFE (H)	PRIMARY ROUTE OF ELIMINATION
β-lactam Antibiotics			
Narrow-Spectrum Penicillins			
Penicillin G	Oral or parenteral	0.5	Renal (TS)
Penicillin V	Oral	1.0	Renal (TS)
Penicillinase-Resistant Penicillins			
Dicloxacillin	Oral	0.6	Renal (TS)
Nafcillin	Oral or parenteral	0.5	Biliary
Extended-Spectrum Penicillins			
Amoxicillin	Oral	1.0	Renal (TS)
Ampicillin	Oral or parenteral	1.0	Renal (TS) and biliary
Piperacillin	Parenteral	1.2–1.3	Renal (TS)
First-Generation Cephalosporins			
Cefazolin	Parenteral	2.0	Renal (TS)
Cephalexin	Oral	0.5	Renal (TS)
Second-Generation Cephalosporins			
Cefotetan	Parenteral	4.0	Renal (TS)
Cefoxitin	Parenteral	0.8	Renal (TS)
Cefprozil	Oral	1.3	Renal (TS)
Cefuroxime	Oral or parenteral	1.7	Renal (TS)
Third-, Fourth-, and Advanced-Generation Cephalosporins			
Cefdinir	Oral	1.7	Renal (TS)
Cefotaxime	Parenteral	1.6[a]	Renal (TS)
Ceftaroline	Parenteral (IV)	2.6	Renal (GF)
Ceftazidime	Parenteral	1.8	Renal (GF)
Ceftriaxone	Parenteral	8.0	Biliary
Cefepime	Parenteral	2.0	Metabolized
Monobactam			
Aztreonam	Parenteral	1.7	Metabolized
Carbapenems	Parenteral	1.0–1.2	Renal (TS)
Other Bacterial Cell Wall Synthesis Inhibitors			
Bacitracin	Topical	NA	NA
Fosfomycin	Oral	6.0	Renal (GF)
Vancomycin	Oral or parenteral	6.0	Renal (GF)

GF, Glomerular filtration; *IV,* intravenous; *NA,* not applicable; *TS,* tubular secretion.
[a]For cefotaxime, the value shown is the half-life of the metabolite.

nafcillin and all other penicillinase-resistant penicillins. Most strains of MRSA are also resistant to cephalosporins.

The **extended-spectrum penicillins** include amoxicillin and ampicillin. **Amoxicillin** can be used alone to treat respiratory tract infections caused by sensitive bacteria, including **otitis media, sinusitis, bronchitis,** and **community-acquired pneumonia,** but some strains of pneumococci (*Streptococcus pneumoniae*) have developed intermediate resistance to amoxicillin, and larger doses are required to treat infections caused by these organisms. Amoxicillin is also used alone for prophylaxis of bacterial endocarditis in persons with heart valve defects.

Many strains of *Haemophilus influenzae* and *Moraxella catarrhalis* produce **penicillinase** (β-lactamase), and

infections caused by these organisms should be treated with amoxicillin in combination with, **clavulanate,** a β-lactamase inhibitor. Formulations of amoxicillin-clavulanate are available to treat **respiratory tract infections** (pneumonia, sinusitis) caused by these organisms, including a liquid suspension for treating children with **otitis media** (Box 38.1). Amoxicillin-clavulanate is also indicated for treating **bite wound infections** because it is active against the common pathogens causing these infections, including ***Pasteurella multocida*** and *S. aureus,* and it is used to treat impetigo due to gram-positive cocci.

Ampicillin is active against ***Listeria monocytogenes*** and is used to treat meningitis and other infections caused by

CASE PRESENTATION

A previously healthy 18-month-old infant is brought to her pediatrician with cough, nasal congestion, and irritability. Examination reveals a temperature of 39°C (102°F) and redness and bulging of the tympanic membrane under pneumatic otoscopy, suggesting acute otitis media (AOM). Because of the possibility of an infection caused by pneumococci with intermediate penicillin resistance, she is placed on amoxicillin at a dose of 90 mg/kg/day in three divided doses for 10 days. Her mother is instructed to contact the pediatrician if the infant does not respond to treatment.

CASE DISCUSSION

Otitis media is a common infection of infants and children. Distinguishing AOM from otitis media with effusion is important because antibiotics are seldom indicated for the latter condition. An important diagnostic criterion is the position of the tympanic membrane, which is usually bulging in AOM and in a neutral or retracted position in otitis media with effusion.

Antibiotic treatment of AOM is recommended for children less than 2 years of age in order to decrease inflammation in the middle ear and eustachian tube, particularly during the first episode. Amoxicillin is a good choice because of its superior penetration in the middle ear. *Streptococcus pneumoniae* with intermediate penicillin resistance necessitates an amoxicillin dose of 90 mg/kg/day. In recurrent AOM with β-lactamase–producing *Haemophilus influenzae* or *Moraxella catarrhalis,* amoxicillin should be combined with clavulanic acid, or an oral cephalosporin or azithromycin may be used. In children over 2 years of age with AOM, antibiotic administration should be postponed a few days to counteract overuse of antibiotics and increased bacterial resistance. In such cases, children are given topical otic and systemic analgesics for a few days until either the infection resolves or antibiotic treatment is instituted.

this organism (listeriosis). It is also used in combination with **sulbactam** (a β-lactamase inhibitor) to treat infections caused by penicillinase-producing strains of bacteria, including bite wounds and diabetic foot ulcers. Ampicillin can be combined with an **aminoglycoside** (e.g., gentamicin) for the treatment of enterococcal infections, such as enterococcal endocarditis. Other uses for ampicillin and amoxicillin are listed in Table 38.2.

Piperacillin is active against many gram-positive and gram-negative aerobic and anaerobic bacteria, including some strains of *Pseudomonas aeruginosa*. Piperacillin combined with a β-lactamase inhibitor, **tazobactam,** is effective for the treatment of patients with intraabdominal, skin and soft tissue, lower respiratory tract, complicated urinary tract, and gynecologic infections, as well as febrile neutropenia. In some cases, piperacillin is given in combination with an aminoglycoside antibiotic.

Bacterial Resistance

As shown in Table 38.3, bacteria exert resistance to β-lactam antibiotics through three general mechanisms. Resistance can result from **decreased affinity of PBPs** for β-lactam drugs. Gram-positive bacteria are innately resistant to aztreonam because their PBPs do not bind to this

drug. Resistance of other bacteria to penicillins can be acquired when the structure of PBPs is altered in a manner that reduces the affinity of PBPs for the drugs. This mechanism has been responsible for the emergence of pneumococci resistant to penicillin G and of staphylococci resistant to methicillin.

Resistance to penicillins and other β-lactam drugs can result from changes in the structure of **porins** in their outer membrane that become **impermeable** to these antibiotics. This is an important mechanism of acquired resistance of *P. aeruginosa* to imipenem.

The production of β-**lactamases** is the major cause of bacterial resistance to penicillins and other β-lactam antibiotics. These enzymes cleave the β-lactam ring and thereby inactivate the drugs (see Fig. 38.3). β-lactamases are expressed by both chromosomal and plasmid genes. Some β-lactamases are constitutive, whereas others can be induced by β-lactam antibiotics. In gram-positive bacteria, β-lactamases are secreted as exoenzymes and act extracellularly. β-lactamases remain in the periplasmic space in gram-negative bacteria, where they attack the antibiotic before it can bind to PBPs.

The β-lactamases are classified in two ways. The **functional classification** of Bush-Jacoby-Medeiros contains four groups of β-lactamases (groups 1 through 4). The **molecular classification** based on amino acid sequences includes classes A through D, with A and C found most frequently in bacteria. Functional **group 1 β-lactamases** (molecular class C) are enzymes that hydrolyze cephalosporins (cephalosporinases). **Group 2 β-lactamases** (molecular classes A and D) include enzymes that hydrolyze penicillins, cephalosporins, and carbapenems. These enzymes are expressed by β-lactamase genes such as *TEM* (obtained from a patient named Temoneira) and *SHV* (sulfhydryl variable). **Class A enzymes** are the only β-lactamases that are inhibited by **clavulanic acid, sulbactam,** or **tazobactam.**

Group 3 β-lactamases (molecular class B) are zinc metalloenzymes that destroy most penicillins, cephalosporins, and carbapenems (but not aztreonam). **Group 4 β-lactamases** are other penicillinases not inhibited by clavulanate.

The staphylococci were the first major group of bacterial pathogens to acquire β-lactamases that rendered them resistant to penicillin. Later, gonococci and other gram-negative bacteria acquired β-lactamases. Resistance of *H. influenzae* to amoxicillin and other penicillins is primarily caused by these enzymes as well. Many strains of Enterobacteriaceae, including *Escherichia coli* and *Klebsiella pneumoniae*, have acquired plasmid-mediated *TEM* and *SHV* β-lactamases. In addition, **extended-spectrum β-lactamases** (ESBL) have emerged and spread globally. ESBLs are expressed by mutated *TEM* and *SHV* genes and can hydrolyze a wider range of substrates, including third-generation cephalosporins.

β-Lactamase Inhibitors

Clavulanate, sulbactam, and **tazobactam** are β-lactam drugs that **inhibit class-A β-lactamases,** but do not inhibit class-B, -C, and -D enzymes. These drugs have no antimicrobial activity by themselves. They serve as surrogate β-**lactamase** substrates when given with a penicillin antibiotic to protect the penicillin from destruction, and they are sometimes called *suicide inhibitors*. The penicillin–β-lactamase inhibitor combinations include orally administered **amoxicillin**

TABLE 38.2 Major Clinical Uses of Selected Bacterial Cell Wall Synthesis Inhibitors

DRUG	INFECTIONS	MAJOR PATHOGENS
Penicillins		
Penicillin G	Syphilis Endocarditis Meningitis Pneumonia Various	*Treponema pallidum* Viridans streptococci, enterococci Meningococci Pneumococci Streptococci
Penicillin V	Pharyngitis	*Streptococcus pyogenes*
Nafcillin, oxacillin	Osteomyelitis, endocarditis, pneumonia, skin and soft tissue infections	*Staphylococcus aureus*
Amoxicillin ± clavulanate	Otitis, upper respiratory tract infections, pneumonia, skin and soft tissue infections, urinary tract infections	Pneumococci, streptococci, staphylococci, *Haemophilus influenzae, Moraxella catarrhalis, Escherichia coli, Pasteurella multocida*
Ampicillin ± sulbactam	Meningitis Decubitus and diabetic foot ulcers Endocarditis Lyme disease	*Listeria monocytogenes* Gram-positive and anaerobic organisms Streptococci, enterococci *Borrelia burgdorferi*
Piperacillin ± tazobactam	Intraabdominal infections, skin and soft tissue infections, pneumonia, and other infections	Aerobic and anaerobic organisms, including *Pseudomonas aeruginosa*
Cephalosporins		
Cephalexin	Skin and soft tissue infections	Streptococci, staphylococci
Cefazolin	Perioperative prophylaxis	Staphylococci, *E. coli*
Cefotetan	Intraabdominal, gynecologic, biliary tract infections	Aerobic and anaerobic bacilli
Cefdinir, cefprozil, cefuroxime axetil	Respiratory tract, skin and soft tissue infections	Pneumococci, *H. influenzae, M. catarrhalis*
Ceftriaxone	Gonorrhea, urinary tract infections, otitis, meningitis, pneumonia, Lyme disease	Gonococci, pneumococci, meningococci, *B. burgdorferi, H. influenzae,* other gram-negative bacilli
Ceftazidime	Urinary tract infections, pneumonia, others	*P. aeruginosa* and other gram-negative bacteria
Ceftazidime with avibactam	Complicated intraabdominal and urinary tract infections including pyelonephritis	*E. coli, P. aeruginosa,* and species of *Citrobacter, Enterobacter, Klebsiella, Proteus,* and other bacteria
Cefepime	Intraabdominal infections, urinary tract infections, pneumonia, skin and soft tissue infections	Drug-resistant gram-negative bacilli, including *Citrobacter* and *Enterobacter* species
Ceftaroline	Community-acquired pneumonia, skin and soft tissue infections	Methicillin-resistant *S. aureus,* drug-resistant pneumococci
Carbapenems	Intraabdominal infections, pneumonia, meningitis, febrile neutropenia, sepsis	Aerobic, anaerobic, and drug-resistant gram-negative bacilli
Monobactam (aztreonam)	Urinary tract, gynecologic, intraabdominal, skin, lung, and other infections	Aerobic, gram-negative bacilli including *P. aeruginosa*
Vancomycin	Bone and joint infections, skin and soft tissue infections, pneumonia, septicemia, endocarditis, and others	Methicillin-resistant staphylococci, enterococci, and others
Bacitracin	Skin and eye infections	Staphylococci, streptococci
Fosfomycin	Lower urinary tract infections	*E. coli, Enterococcus fecalis,* others

plus clavulanate (AUGMENTIN), parenterally administered **ampicillin plus sulbactam** (UNASYN), and injectable **piperacillin plus tazobactam** (ZOSYN). The major uses of these preparations are listed in Table 38.2.

Avibactam is a new β-lactamase inhibitor with a unique **non-β-lactam structure.** It is active against several types of β-lactamases, including the AmpC (ampicillin C) β-lactamases and other extended spectrum β-lactamases expressed by cephalosporin-resistant gram-negative bacteria. Avibactam is available in **combination with ceftazidime**

for treating complicated infections caused by these organisms (see later). It is the first β-lactamase inhibitor to be used in combination with a cephalosporin.

Adverse Effects

Penicillins are a common cause of **drug-induced hypersensitivity reactions.** However, it has been determined that true penicillin allergy occurs in only 7% to 23% of patients who give a history of penicillin allergy. Hypersensitivity reactions occur when penicillin is degraded to penicilloic

TABLE 38.3 Bacterial Resistance to β-Lactam Antibiotics

MECHANISM	EXAMPLES
Inactivation of the drug by β-lactamase enzymes	Resistance of gonococci and staphylococci to penicillin G Resistance of gram-negative bacteria to carbapenems, extended-spectrum penicillins, cefoxitin, and other cephalosporins Resistance of *Haemophilus influenzae* to amoxicillin and other penicillins
Reduced affinity of PBPs for the drug	Resistance of enterococci to cephalosporins Resistance of gram-positive bacteria to aztreonam Resistance of meningococci, pneumococci, and streptococci to penicillin G Resistance of staphylococci to methicillin
Decreased entry of the drug into bacteria through outer membrane porins	Resistance of gram-negative bacteria to various β-lactam antibiotics Resistance of *Pseudomonas aeruginosa* to imipenem

PBP, Penicillin-binding protein.

acid and other compounds that combine with body proteins to form antigens that elicit antibody formation.

An immediate hypersensitivity reaction, which is a type of reaction mediated by immunoglobulin E, can lead to **urticaria** (hives) or anaphylactic shock. Other types of hypersensitivity reactions can lead to serum sickness, interstitial nephritis, hepatitis, and various skin rashes. Hepatitis is more common with antistaphylococcal and extended-spectrum penicillins and is usually reversible when use of the drug is discontinued. Ampicillin is likely to cause a maculopapular skin rash in patients with certain viral infections, such as mononucleosis. This reaction is mediated by sensitized lymphocytes, and its frequency in ampicillin-treated patients with mononucleosis is over 90%.

Penicillin allergy can be confirmed by the use of commercial preparations of penicillin antigens. These preparations contain the major or minor antigenic determinants of penicillin that are formed in the body during penicillin degradation. These preparations are injected intradermally and cause erythema at the injection site in allergic persons. The preparations should be administered by personnel prepared to provide treatment for anaphylactic shock in the event that the patient develops a severe hypersensitivity reaction after the injection.

Except for drug hypersensitivity reactions, the penicillins are **remarkably nontoxic** to the human body and produce very few other adverse effects. High concentrations of penicillins can be irritating to the central nervous system and elicit seizures in patients who have received very large doses of these drugs. As with other antibiotics, penicillins can disturb the normal flora of the gut and produce diarrhea and superinfections with penicillin-resistant organisms, such as staphylococci and *Clostridioides difficile*.

Cephalosporins

The cephalosporins are one of the largest and most widely used groups of antibiotics. Based on differences in their antimicrobial spectrum, they have been divided into four generations. Table 38.2 lists examples of each. The first-generation cephalosporins are primarily active against gram-positive cocci and a limited number of gram-negative bacilli. Subsequent generations of cephalosporins have increased activity against gram-negative bacilli and less activity against some species of gram-positive cocci.

Chemistry

The cephalosporins are semisynthetic drugs, most of which are derived from cephalosporin C, a substance obtained from a species of *Cephalosporium* discovered near a sewage outlet off the coast of Sardinia. Cephalosporins consist of a β-lactam ring fused to dihydrothiazine ring, plus two or three side chains (R groups) attached to the dihydrothiazine moiety (see Fig. 38.3), enabling greater structural diversity and the development of antibiotics that are more resistant to β-lactamases and have a wider range of antimicrobial activity.

Pharmacokinetics

Several of the cephalosporins are given orally, whereas others are given by intravenous or intramuscular injection. **Cefuroxime** is available for both oral and parenteral administration. The orally administered cephalosporins are well absorbed from the gut, and their bioavailability is not significantly affected by food. Most cephalosporins are excreted primarily by renal tubular secretion, which is inhibited by probenecid. Ceftriaxone is excreted primarily in the bile and has a longer half-life than other cephalosporins. Compared with penicillins, the cephalosporins are more stable in the body and are less likely to form antigens that evoke hypersensitivity reactions.

Clinical Use

The pharmacokinetics and clinical uses of cephalosporins are shown in Tables 38.1 and 38.2. The **first-generation cephalosporins** have good activity against streptococci and methicillin-sensitive staphylococci. They are also active against a few gram-negative enteric bacilli, including *E. coli* and *K. pneumoniae.* The orally administered drugs (e.g., **cephalexin**) are primarily used to treat skin and soft tissue infections caused by gram-positive cocci, such as impetigo, and to treat uncomplicated urinary tract infections. However, many strains of *E. coli* are now resistant to cephalexin, and it is used less often for this purpose today. Parenterally administered **cefazolin** is used to treat more serious infections caused by these organisms and is widely employed for **prophylaxis of surgical infections** caused by staphylococci and aerobic gram-negative enteric bacilli.

In comparison with first-generation cephalosporins, the **second-generation cephalosporins** have similar activity against gram-positive cocci while demonstrating increased activity against gram-negative bacilli. For example, the second-generation drugs are active against many strains of *H. influenzae* and have been used to treat respiratory tract and other infections caused by this organism. Oral second-generation drugs, including **cefprozil** and **cefuroxime axetil,** are used to treat otitis media, particularly when it is caused by *H. influenzae* strains resistant to amoxicillin and other drugs. **Cefuroxime sodium,** a parenteral preparation, has been used as empiric therapy for patients with community-acquired pneumonia. **Cefotetan** is active against both aerobic and anaerobic gram-negative bacilli, including *Bacteroides fragilis*, and it is used to treat intraabdominal, gynecologic, and biliary tract infections caused by these organisms. **Cefoxitin** has activity similar to that of cefotetan and is used for surgical prophylaxis of infections caused by gram-negative bacteria.

In comparison with second-generation cephalosporins, the **third-generation cephalosporins** have greater activity against a wider range of gram-negative organisms, including enteric gram-negative bacilli (Enterobacteriaceae), *H. influenzae*, and *M. catarrhalis*. In addition, **ceftazidime** is active against some strains of *P. aeruginosa*. Several third-generation drugs, including **cefpodoxime, cefotaxime,** and **ceftriaxone,** are active against gonococci and have been used as a single-dose treatment for gonorrhea. Other clinical indications for third-generation drugs include otitis media, pneumonia, meningitis, intraabdominal or urinary tract infections, and advanced Lyme disease.

Ceftazidime with avibactam (AVYCAZ) is the first cephalosporin/β-lactamase inhibitor combination to be developed. Avibactam is resistant to some Class-C β-lactamases, such as AmpC cephalosporinases, as well as some extended spectrum β-lactamases (*TEM, SHV,* and others). The drug combination is active against a large number of gram-negative bacteria (see Table 38.2) and is indicated for treating complicated **intraabdominal and urinary tract infections.** It is usually given parenterally for 7 to 14 days to treat these infections.

Cefepime has been called a **fourth-generation cephalosporin** because it is active against many gram-negative bacilli that are often resistant to other cephalosporins, including *Citrobacter freundii* and *Enterobacter cloacae*. This is attributed to its more rapid penetration of bacteria, its ability to target multiple PBPs, and its lower affinity for several β-lactamases. Cefepime is resistant to plasmid-encoded β-lactamase and relatively resistant to inducible chromosomally encoded β-lactamase. It has been used in treating a variety of systemic infections, including intraabdominal and urinary tract infections and pneumonia. However, a recent analysis of clinical trials found that cefepime is associated with **higher all-cause mortality** than are other β-lactam antibiotics, possibly because of drug-induced encephalopathy; thus, its use should be carefully monitored.

Ceftaroline (TEFLARO) is a new **advanced-generation cephalosporin** whose unique antimicrobial activity does not allow it to be assigned to one of the traditional cephalosporin classes. It is effective against **MRSA** and **drug-resistant pneumococci,** as well as common gram-negative pathogens. It is administered intravenously and is approved for the treatment of skin and **soft tissue infections** and **community acquired pneumonia.** The drug's activity against MRSA is a result of its high-affinity binding to PBP-2a, which results in more efficient inhibition of this enzyme compared with other β-lactam antibiotics.

Cefiderocol is a very recently approved cephalosporin bactericidal antibiotic for the treatment of gram-negative microorganisms as the causative agent in complicated urinary tract infections (cUTI), including pyelonephritis, and hospital-acquired bacterial pneumonia and ventilator-associated bacterial pneumonia. Cefiderocol is the first antibiotic to kill gram-negative bacteria with one or more primary mechanisms of resistance to β-lactams (porin

channel alterations, β-lactamase inactivation, and efflux pump upregulation). Like ceftaroline, cefiderocol can also be classified as an advanced-generation cephalosporin.

Bacterial Resistance

Bacteria acquire resistance to cephalosporins through the same three mechanisms by which they acquire resistance to penicillins (see Table 38.3). The cephalosporins are more resistant to β-lactamases than are the penicillins, and resistance to gram-negative β-lactamases increases with successive generations of cephalosporins. Many cephalosporins, however, are susceptible to the **extended-spectrum β-lactamases,** and some cephalosporins induce certain β-lactamase enzymes. Worldwide resistance to cephalosporins is increasing, as evidenced by the alarming development of gonococcal resistance to cephalosporins. There is a growing need for additional inhibitors of extended-spectrum β-lactamase enzymes that could be administered with cephalosporins.

Adverse Effects

The cephalosporins cause little toxicity to the host and have an excellent safety record. Although cephalosporins can elicit hypersensitivity reactions, the incidence is lower than with penicillins. Cephalosporins exhibit some **cross-sensitivity** with penicillins, and about 5% of persons allergic to penicillin will also be allergic to cephalosporins. Persons who have had a mild hypersensitivity reaction to penicillin usually do not cross-react to a cephalosporin. However, a person who has had a severe hypersensitivity reaction to penicillin (e.g., a documented anaphylactic reaction) has a greater risk of cross-reacting and should usually not be given a cephalosporin.

Monobactam

Aztreonam is a monocyclic β-lactam (monobactam) antibiotic. It is active against many aerobic **gram-negative bacilli,** including strains of *Enterobacter, Citrobacter, Klebsiella,* and *Proteus* species, as well as *P. aeruginosa*. Aztreonam is used to treat serious infections caused by susceptible organisms and is particularly useful for infections caused by multidrug-resistant strains of these organisms. The drug is administered intravenously and is extensively metabolized before undergoing renal excretion. Aztreonam can cause hypersensitivity reactions and thrombophlebitis. It only rarely shows cross-sensitivity with penicillins and cephalosporins, however, and can usually be used in persons allergic to other β-lactam antibiotics.

Carbapenems

Carbapenems are penicillin-like antibiotics in which the sulfur atom of the thiazolidine ring is replaced with a carbon atom. These agents are bactericidal to a wide range of gram-positive and gram-negative bacteria, including many aerobic and anaerobic gram-negative bacilli, and they are resistant to many β-lactamases. However, the bacterial expression of **extended-spectrum β-lactamases** that inactivate penicillins, cephalosporins, and carbapenems is a growing problem that has resulted in increasing resistance to carbapenems.

Imipenem has high affinity for PBP-2, whereas **meropenem** binds to both PBP-2 and PBP-3. The greater affinity of meropenem for PBP-3 may account for its superior activity against *P. aeruginosa* and other gram-negative organisms. **Ertapenem** has good *in vitro* activity against some extended-spectrum β-lactamase–producing organisms, while **doripenem** has been called an ultrabroad-spectrum antibiotic that is particularly active against *P. aeruginosa.*

Carbapenems are used to treat a wide range of systemic infections, including endocarditis, pneumonia, and infections of the urinary tract, pelvis, skin and soft tissue, and intraabdominal. They are particularly useful for infections caused by multidrug-resistant organisms and for mixed infections caused by aerobic and anaerobic enteric bacilli.

Carbapenems are administered intravenously. Imipenem is rapidly inactivated by renal dehydropeptidase and is available in a formulation containing a dehydropeptidase inhibitor called **cilastatin.** Other combination drugs with carbapenems are available and include **meropenem** and **vabobactam** (VABOMERE), and **imipenem** with **cilastatin** and **relebactam** (RECARBIO). The addition of **relebactam**, a β-**lactamase inhibitor**, gives RECARBIO effective antibacterial action against **resistant gram-negative microorganisms**. It is indicated for treatment of hospital-acquired bacterial pneumonia and ventilator associated bacterial pneumonia (HABP/VABP), complicated urinary tract infections, including pyelonephritis (cUTI), and complicated intraabdominal infections (cIAI) in patients who have limited or no alternative treatment options.

The **carbapenems** are eliminated by **renal tubular secretion**, which can be inhibited by **probenecid.** Dosage adjustments are required when these drugs are given to persons with renal impairment. The carbapenems exhibit cross-sensitivity with penicillins and other β-lactam antibiotics and should not be administered to patients who are allergic to these drugs. Though generally well tolerated, they can cause seizures in patients with epilepsy. Less commonly, carbapenems may cause anemia, leukopenia, thrombocytopenia, and altered bleeding time.

OTHER BACTERIAL CELL WALL SYNTHESIS INHIBITORS

Vancomycin and Telavancin

Vancomycin is a glycopeptide antibiotic that is active, while telavancin is a semisynthetic derivative to vancomycin. These agents are active against many **gram-positive cocci** and gram-positive bacilli, including some strains of **MRSA.** Vancomycin is usually the first choice for treating skin and soft tissue infections and other MRSA infections. Other drugs for MRSA are listed in Table 39.4. Vancomycin is also used to treat streptococcal and enterococcal infections caused by penicillin-resistant organisms, including endocarditis and necrotizing fasciitis. However, some strains of staphylococci and enterococci have acquired resistance to vancomycin through mutations that alter the amino acid sequence of the cell wall pentapeptide containing D-alanine. **Telavancin** is also approved for the treatment of skin and soft tissue infections caused by methicillin-sensitive *S. aureus* and MRSA, and infections due to vancomycin-sensitive *Enterococcus fecalis*. The drug appears to be equivalent to vancomycin in most respects.

Vancomycin is also active against *Bacillus, Clostridium,* and *Corynebacterium* species. Although it has been used to treat diarrhea and **pseudomembranous colitis** caused by *C. difficile,* metronidazole is usually preferred for this infection.

Vancomycin is poorly absorbed from the gut and must be administered parenterally to treat systemic infections, though it is given orally to treat gastrointestinal *C. difficile* infections. Vancomycin is distributed to most body fluids and tissues, and it is excreted in the urine by the process of glomerular filtration. The half-life of vancomycin is normally about 6 hours (see Table 38.1), but the half-life is markedly prolonged in patients with renal failure.

Improvements in the manufacturing of vancomycin preparations have reduced the incidence of **nephrotoxicity** and **ototoxicity** associated with their use. Vancomycin, however, should be used cautiously with other nephrotoxic drugs, including aminoglycosides and amphotericin B. The ototoxic effects of vancomycin can include both **vestibular dysfunction** (ataxia, vertigo, nystagmus, and nausea) and **cochlear dysfunction** (tinnitus and hearing loss). Ototoxicity is usually caused by excessive serum concentrations and is reversible when these concentrations are reduced.

If vancomycin is infused at an excessive rate, it can cause hypotension and an **erythematous rash** on the face and upper body known as **red neck syndrome.**

Bacitracin

Bacitracin is an antibiotic derived from a *Bacillus subtilis* strain isolated from a girl named Tracy. The drug inhibits cell wall peptidoglycan synthesis by blocking the regeneration of C55-isoprenyl phosphate (bactroprenol phosphate), the lipid carrier molecule (see Fig. 38.2). Bacitracin is active against **gram-positive cocci,** including staphylococci and streptococci, and it is primarily used for the topical treatment of minor skin and ocular infections. It is often combined with polymyxin or neomycin in ointments and creams. Bacitracin is very **nephrotoxic** and is not used systemically.

Fosfomycin

Fosfomycin is a unique antibiotic that blocks one of the first steps in cell wall peptidoglycan synthesis, the formation of UDP-MurNAc. Fosfomycin is structurally similar to phosphoenolpyruvate. By irreversibly inhibiting the enzyme enolpyruvyl transferase, fosfomycin blocks the addition of phosphoenolpyruvate to UDP-GlcNAc, thereby preventing the synthesis of UDP-MurNAc.

Fosfomycin is active against enterococci and many gram-negative enteric bacilli, including *E. coli, Citrobacter* species, *Klebsiella* species, *Proteus* species, and *Serratia marcescens*. The drug is specifically approved for the treatment of **uncomplicated urinary tract infections** caused by *E. coli* or *E. fecalis*. For this purpose, fosfomycin can be administered orally as a single large dose. The drug is excreted unchanged in the urine and feces and has a half-life of about 6 hours. Fosfomycin sometimes causes diarrhea but is otherwise well tolerated and is associated with few adverse effects.

SUMMARY OF IMPORTANT POINTS

- β-lactam antibiotics, vancomycin, bacitracin, and fosfomycin are drugs that inhibit bacterial cell wall synthesis.
- The β-lactam antibiotics inhibit the transpeptidase reaction that cross-links the peptidoglycan component of the cell wall. These antibiotics include penicillins, cephalosporins, aztreonam, and carbapenems.

- β-lactamase inhibitors (avibactam, clavulanate, sulbactam, or tazobactam) are administered in combination with a β-lactam antibiotic to prevent degradation of the antibiotic by bacteria.
- Narrow-spectrum penicillins (e.g., penicillin G) are primarily active against gram-positive cocci and spirochetes; penicillinase-resistant penicillins (e.g., dicloxacillin and nafcillin) are used to treat staphylococcal infections; and extended-spectrum penicillins (e.g., amoxicillin) are active against various gram-negative bacilli.
- Acid-stable penicillins (e.g., penicillin V, amoxicillin, and dicloxacillin) can be given orally, whereas acid-labile drugs (piperacillin) must be given parenterally.
- Most penicillins are eliminated primarily by renal tubular secretion, a process that is inhibited by probenecid. Two long-acting forms of penicillin G (procaine and benzathine penicillin G) are available for intramuscular administration.
- Penicillins can elicit any of the four types of hypersensitivity reactions, including anaphylactic shock and other immediate hypersensitivity reactions mediated by immunoglobulin E.
- Cephalosporins are semisynthetic antibiotics that are subdivided into four generations on the basis of their antimicrobial spectrum. The activity against gram-negative organisms increases from the first to the fourth generation.
- Some cephalosporins (e.g., cefazolin) are eliminated by renal tubular secretion, whereas others (e.g., ceftriaxone) are eliminated in the bile. Ceftriaxone has a much longer half-life than other cephalosporins, enabling it to be used as single-dose treatment for certain infections, including gonorrhea.
- Carbapenems (e.g., imipenem and meropenem) are active against a broad spectrum of bacteria, including many strains of gram-negative bacteria resistant to other antibiotics. Aztreonam is a monobactam antibiotic that is active against aerobic gram-negative bacilli. It does not show cross-sensitivity with other β-lactam drugs.
- Vancomycin is a glycopeptide antibiotic that is active against gram-positive organisms, including methicillin-resistant staphylococci, enterococci, and *Clostridiodes difficile*.
- Bacitracin is used topically for infections caused by gram-positive cocci. Fosfomycin is administered as a single-dose treatment for uncomplicated urinary tract infections caused by *E. coli* or enterococci.

Review Questions

1. Aztreonam is used for the treatment of infections caused by which organism?
   - (A) *Staphylococcus aureus*
   - (B) *Enterococcus faecium*
   - (C) *Streptococcus pneumoniae*
   - (D) *Pseudomonas aeruginosa*
   - (E) *Bacillus anthracis*
2. Which drug inhibits extended-spectrum β-lactamases including some cephalosporinases?
   - (A) avibactam
   - (B) clavulanate
   - (C) sulbactam
   - (D) tazobactam
   - (E) monobactam
3. Higher doses of vancomycin used to treat methicillin-resistant staphylococci may cause which adverse effect?
   - (A) hepatitis
   - (B) alopecia
   - (C) hallucinations
   - (D) hypertension
   - (E) impaired hearing
4. Fosfomycin is given as a large single dose to treat which infection?
   - (A) gonorrhea
   - (B) syphilis
   - (C) urinary tract infection
   - (D) impetigo
   - (E) traveler's diarrhea
5. Cilastatin is used to inhibit the metabolism of which antibiotic by dehydropeptidase?
   - (A) ceftazidime
   - (B) imipenem
   - (C) piperacillin
   - (D) vancomycin
   - (E) bacitracin

Antibiotics That Inhibit Bacterial Protein Synthesis

OVERVIEW

After the discovery of penicillin, scientists searched for antibiotics that could inhibit penicillin-resistant bacteria. Several new classes of antibiotics were eventually isolated from the *Streptomyces* species, including the aminoglycosides, tetracyclines, and macrolides, and these antibiotics were found to inhibit bacterial protein synthesis. Streptomycin was one of the first antibiotics discovered in this process and was the first effective treatment for tuberculosis.

Bacterial Protein Synthesis

Several classes of antibiotics selectively block one or more steps in bacterial protein synthesis. These drugs have little effect on the protein synthesis of mammals and other animals because of differences in the structure and function of ribosomes in bacteria (prokaryotes) and animals (eukaryotes).

Each ribosome has two subunits. The **ribosome in prokaryotes** is composed of a 30S subunit and a 50S subunit

(with S denoting the Svedberg unit of flotation, which forms the basis for the separation and isolation of ribosomal subunits from cells). In contrast, the **ribosome in eukaryotes** is composed of a 40S and a 60S subunit, and the proteins that initiate and carry out translation of messenger RNA (mRNA) in eukaryotic systems are more complex and function differently than the proteins of bacterial systems.

The basic steps in bacterial protein synthesis are illustrated in Fig. 39.1. These steps include the binding of aminoacyl transfer RNA (tRNA) to the ribosome, the formation of a peptide bond, and translocation. Aminoacyl tRNA binds to the 30S ribosomal subunit, whereas peptide bond formation and translocation involve components of the 50S ribosomal subunit.

SITES OF DRUG ACTION

As shown in Fig. 39.1, each type of antibiotic discussed in this chapter acts at a specific site on the ribosome to inhibit one or more steps in protein synthesis. Tetracyclines and aminoglycosides act at the **30S ribosomal subunit.** Macrolides, chloramphenicol, dalfopristin, and clindamycin act at the **50S ribosomal subunit.**

Tetracyclines competitively block binding of tRNA to the 30S subunit and thereby prevent the addition of new amino acids to the growing peptide chain. The reversibility of this effect accounts for the bacteriostatic action of tetracyclines.

Aminoglycosides also bind to the 30S subunit, where they interfere with the initiation of protein synthesis and cause misreading of the genetic code so that the wrong amino acid is inserted into the protein structure. These irreversible actions account for the bactericidal effects of these antibiotics.

Macrolides, chloramphenicol, and **dalfopristin** block peptidyl transferase, the enzyme that catalyzes the formation of a peptide bond between the latest amino acid and the nascent peptide. **Macrolides** and **clindamycin** prevent translocation of the nascent peptide from the acceptor or aminoacyl site (A site) to the peptidyl site (P site) on the ribosome, which in turn prevents binding of the next aminoacyl tRNA to the ribosome.

DRUGS THAT AFFECT THE 30S RIBOSOMAL SUBUNIT

Aminoglycosides

The aminoglycosides include amikacin, gentamicin, tobramycin, neomycin, paromomycin, streptomycin, and plazomicin. Aminoglycosides exhibit concentration-dependent killing and have a long postantibiotic effect (see Chapter 37). Hence aminoglycosides are sometimes administered as a large single daily dose rather than the standard regimen of smaller doses three times a day (see later). The properties and major clinical uses of these drugs are compared in Tables 39.1 and 39.2.

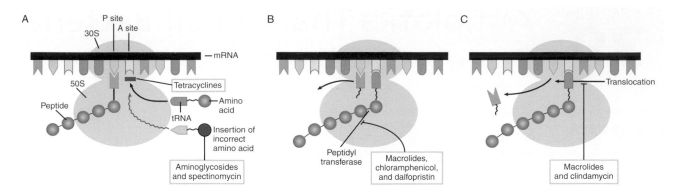

FIG. 39.1 Bacterial protein synthesis and sites of drug action. The bacterial ribosome is composed of a 30S subunit and a 50S subunit. The steps in protein synthesis and translation of messenger RNA (*mRNA*) include the binding of aminoacyl transfer RNA (*tRNA*) to the ribosome, the formation of a peptide bond, and translocation. (A) Under normal circumstances, the nascent peptide is attached to the ribosome at the peptidyl site (*P site*), and the next aminoacyl tRNA binds to the acceptor or aminoacyl site (*A site*). Tetracyclines block aminoacyl tRNA from binding to the *A site*. Aminoglycosides cause misreading of the genetic code, which leads to binding of the wrong aminoacyl tRNA and insertion of the wrong amino acid into the nascent peptide. (B) Macrolides, chloramphenicol, and dalfopristin block peptidyl transferase, the enzyme that catalyzes the formation of a peptide bond between the nascent peptide and the amino acid attached to the *A site*. (C) Macrolides and clindamycin block the translocation step in which the nascent peptide is transferred from the *A site* to the *P site* after the formation of a new peptide bond.

TABLE 39.1 Pharmacokinetic Properties of Bacterial Protein Synthesis Inhibitors[a]

DRUG	ROUTE OF ADMINISTRATION	ORAL BIOAVAILABILITY	ELIMINATION HALF-LIFE (HOURS)	PRIMARY ROUTE OF ELIMINATION
Aminoglycoside antibiotics				
Amikacin	IV	NA	2.5	Renal excretion
Gentamicin	IV or topical	NA	1.5	Renal excretion
Neomycin	Topical	NA	NA	NA
Streptomycin	IM	NA	2	Renal excretion
Tobramycin	IV or topical	NA	2.5	Renal excretion
Tetracycline and related antibiotics				
Doxycycline	Oral or IV	90%	20	Fecal and renal excretion
Minocycline	Oral or IV	95%	20	Biliary and renal excretion
Tetracycline	Oral	70%	10	Renal excretion
Tigecycline	IV	NA	40	Biliary, fecal, and renal excretion
Macrolide and ketolide antibiotics				
Azithromycin	Oral or IV	37%	12	Biliary excretion
Clarithromycin	Oral	62%	5	Biliary and renal excretion
Erythromycin	Oral or topical	35% ± 25%	2	Biliary excretion
Other antibiotics				
Chloramphenicol	IV	NA	3	Hepatic metabolism; renal excretion
Clindamycin	Oral, IV, or topical	95%	2.5	Hepatic metabolism; renal, biliary, and fecal excretion
Linezolid	Oral or IV	100%	6	Hepatic metabolism; renal excretion
Mupirocin	Topical	NA	NA	NA
Quinupristin-dalfopristin	IV	NA	0.8 and 0.4[b]	Hepatic metabolism; biliary excretion

IM, Intramuscular; *IV,* intravenous; *NA,* not applicable.
[a]Values shown are the mean of values reported in the literature.
[b]The half-lives for quinupristin and dalfopristin are 0.8 and 0.4 hour, respectively. The drugs are given in combination.

Chemistry and Pharmacokinetics

Aminoglycoside antibiotics consist of amino sugars linked through glycosidic bonds. The amino groups become protonated and **ionized in body fluids.** For this reason, the aminoglycosides are poorly absorbed from the gut and must be administered parenterally for the treatment of systemic infections. Occasionally, they are administered orally to treat gastrointestinal infections such as neonatal necrotizing enterocolitis. They are also administered topically to treat infections of the skin, mucous membranes, and ocular tissues.

TABLE 39.2   Major Clinical Uses of Selected Bacterial Protein Synthesis Inhibitors

DRUG	INFECTIONS
Streptomycin	Plague, tularemia, drug-resistant tuberculosis
Gentamicin, tobramycin, and amikacin	Infective endocarditis; infections with aerobic gram-negative bacilli, including *Pseudomonas aeruginosa*
Tetracycline antibiotics	Lyme disease, Rocky Mountain spotted fever, ehrlichiosis, granuloma inguinale, brucellosis, cholera, relapsing fever, peptic ulcer disease from *Helicobacter pylori,* chlamydial urethritis, acne, MRSA, gonorrhea (doxycycline in combination with ceftriaxone)
Tigecycline	Skin and soft tissue infections with MRSA; intraabdominal infections with various organisms; community-acquired pneumonia
Erythromycin	Respiratory tract infections with streptococci, pneumococci, *Legionella pneumophila, Mycoplasma pneumoniae,* or *Chlamydia pneumoniae*
Azithromycin, clarithromycin	Respiratory tract infections with organisms sensitive to erythromycin plus *Haemophilus influenzae, Moraxella catarrhalis, Mycobacterium avium-intracellulare.* Gonorrhea in combination with ceftriaxone.
Clarithromycin	Peptic ulcer disease from *H. pylori*
Chloramphenicol	Meningitis, brain abscess
Clindamycin	Streptococcal, staphylococcal, and anaerobic infections
Quinupristin-dalfopristin	Skin and soft tissue infections with *Staphylococcus aureus* or *Streptococcus pyogenes;* infections with *Enterococcus faecium*
Linezolid	Infections with vancomycin-resistant *E. faecium,* streptococci, and methicillin-resistant staphylococci
Mupirocin	Impetigo from streptococci, staphylococci; eradication of nasal colonization of MRSA

MRSA, Methicillin-resistant Staphylococcus aureus.

Because of their ionized structure, aminoglycosides do not penetrate tissue cells and their volumes of distribution are similar to extracellular fluid volume. Aminoglycosides also have poor penetration of the meninges, even when the meninges are inflamed. They are **excreted unchanged** by renal glomerular filtration, with little tubular reabsorption. The renal clearance of aminoglycosides is approximately equal to the creatinine clearance because creatinine is also filtered at the glomerulus but is not secreted or reabsorbed significantly by the tubules. Because the clearance of aminoglycosides is proportional to the glomerular filtration rate, the dosage of aminoglycosides must be reduced in patients with **renal impairment.** In most cases, this is accomplished by increasing the interval between doses.

The plasma concentrations of aminoglycosides are routinely measured to ensure adequate dosage and to minimize toxicity. The peak concentration is found approximately 30 minutes after completing an intravenous infusion of an aminoglycoside, whereas the trough concentration is found immediately before administration of the next dose. Optimal **peak and trough concentrations** have been established and can be used to guide dosage adjustments for individuals receiving the standard regimen of three daily doses given at 8-hour intervals. For example, therapeutic concentrations of gentamicin and tobramycin are usually between 4 and 8 mg/L. A peak concentration greater than 12 mg/L or a trough concentration greater than 2 mg/L indicates the need to reduce the dosage of these antibiotics. Therapeutic concentrations of amikacin are between 16 and 32 mg/L, and the toxic peak and trough concentrations are greater than 35 mg/L and 10 mg/L, respectively.

Spectrum and Indications

The aminoglycosides are active against a wide range of **aerobic gram-negative bacilli.** Streptomycin is the least active against most gram-negative bacilli and is primarily used to treat tuberculosis and infections caused by *Yersinia pestis* (plague) and *Francisella tularensis* (tularemia).

Tobramycin is the most active aminoglycoside against many strains of **Pseudomonas aeruginosa,** whereas gentamicin is more active against *Escherichia coli, Klebsiella* species, and other species of **Enterobacteriaceae.** Gentamicin is also used in combination with a penicillin to treat serious **enterococcal, staphylococcal, or viridans group streptococcal infections** such as **endocarditis.** Amikacin is more resistant to bacterial enzymes that inactivate aminoglycosides, and it is active against some strains resistant to gentamicin and tobramycin.

The newest aminoglycoside is **plazomicin,** used for the treatment of patients 18 years of age or older with complicated urinary tract infections (cUTIs), including pyelonephritis. **Plazomicin is not degraded by most aminoglycoside-modifying enzymes (AMEs)** known to affect gentamicin, amikacin, and tobramycin, such as acetyltransferase, phosphotransferases, and nucleotidyltransferases. **Plazomicin,** like other aminoglycosides, is **inactive against resistance** bacterial isolates that **overproduce 16S ribosomal RNA (rRNA) methyltransferases.** Plazomicin also has reduced activity against *Enterobacteriaceae* that **upregulate drug efflux pumps.**

Bacterial Resistance

Resistance to aminoglycosides is primarily caused by **inactivation of the drugs by bacterial enzymes** that combine the drugs with acetate, phosphate, or adenylate. Resistance to aminoglycosides can also be caused by **decreased binding** of the drugs to the 30S ribosomal subunit or to **decreased uptake** of the drugs by porins in bacterial membranes (Table 39.3). Both plasmid and chromosomal genes are involved in resistance to aminoglycosides. A diagram shows the eight different mechanisms of resistance to ribosome-targeting antibiotics (Fig. 39.2).

Adverse Effects

The most serious adverse effects of aminoglycosides are **nephrotoxicity** and **ototoxicity.** The risk of toxicity is related to the dosage and duration of treatment and varies with the specific drug. Irreversible toxicity can occur, even after use of the drug is discontinued, but serious toxicity is less likely if the offending drug is discontinued at the earliest sign of dysfunction.

Aminoglycosides are one of the most common causes of **drug-induced renal failure.** When the drugs accumulate in proximal tubule cells, they can cause **acute tubular necrosis.** Aminoglycosides also cause **glomerular toxicity.** These effects impair renal function and lead to an increase in plasma concentrations of the aminoglycosides. The elevated drug concentrations can further impair renal function and contribute to ototoxicity. Hence it is important to monitor renal function and plasma aminoglycoside concentrations and to adjust the aminoglycoside dosage accordingly. Increasing the interval between doses to 24 hours or longer in persons with impaired renal function decreases the likelihood of toxicity.

Ototoxicity is associated with the accumulation of aminoglycosides in the **labyrinth** and **hair cells of the cochlea** and has been attributed to activation of caspase-dependent apoptosis (programmed cell death) in hair cells. Patients can experience both **vestibular and cochlear toxicity.** Manifestations of vestibular toxicity include dizziness, impaired vision, nystagmus, vertigo, nausea, vomiting, and problems with postural balance and walking. Cochlear toxicity is characterized by tinnitus and hearing impairment and can lead to irreversible deafness. Often, a delay occurs between drug administration and the onset of symptoms, and many hospitalized patients are ambulatory before signs of toxicity appear.

The aminoglycosides vary in their tendency to cause cochlear or vestibular toxicity. Amikacin produces more cochlear toxicity (deafness), whereas gentamicin and streptomycin cause more vestibular toxicity. Tobramycin appears to cause similar degrees of cochlear and vestibular toxicity.

Neomycin is the most nephrotoxic aminoglycoside, and its use is limited to topical treatment of **superficial infections.** Neomycin is available in ointments and creams in combination with bacitracin and polymyxin. These **triple-antibiotic** preparations have been shown to prevent infections after minor skin trauma. Bacitracin provides gram-positive coverage, polymyxin provides gram-negative coverage, and neomycin is active against both gram-positive and gram-negative organisms. Neomycin can elicit hypersensitivity reactions, especially with long-term administration, and products containing only bacitracin and polymyxin are also available.

TABLE 39.3 Bacterial Resistance to Protein Synthesis Inhibitors

MECHANISM	EXAMPLES
Inactivation of the drug by bacterial enzymes	Inactivation of aminoglycosides by acetylase, adenylase, and phosphorylase enzymes
	Inactivation of chloramphenicol by acetyltransferase
Decreased binding of the drug	Decreased binding of aminoglycosides to the 30S ribosomal subunit
	Decreased binding of macrolides and clindamycin to the 50S ribosomal subunit
Decreased accumulation of the drug by bacteria	Active removal of macrolides from bacteria via membrane proteins
	Decreased uptake of aminoglycosides via porins in bacterial membranes
	Decreased uptake of tetracyclines via porins in bacterial membranes

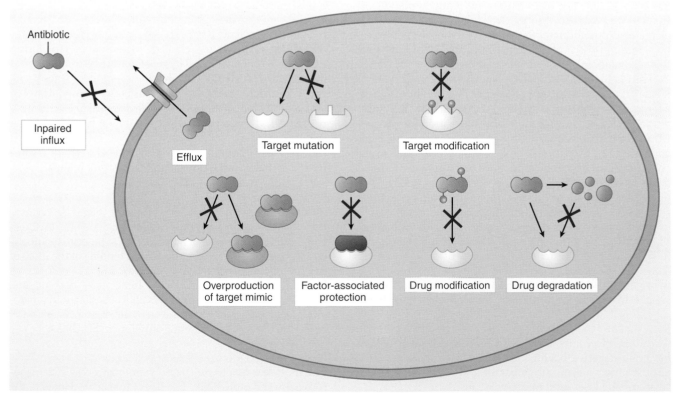

Fig. 39.2 Mechanisms of resistance to ribosome-targeting antibiotics. Note the eight different mechanisms identified in ribosome-targeting antibiotics.

TABLE 39.4 Agents for Methicillin-Resistant *Staphylococcus aureus* Infections

DRUG	INFECTION	CLINICAL RESPONSE[A]	ADVERSE EFFECTS
Oral agents			
Clindamycin	Community-acquired SSTIs	Excellent if strains are susceptible	Diarrhea
Trimethoprim-sulfamethoxazole ± rifampin	Community-acquired SSTIs	Most strains are susceptible	Nausea, vomiting, rash, photosensitivity, thrombocytopenia
Doxycycline, minocycline	Community-acquired SSTIs	83% in one study	Nausea, vomiting, photosensitivity
Rifampin	Community-acquired SSTIs	Must combine with another antibiotic	Drug interactions, discoloration of body fluids, abnormal liver function
Parenteral agents			
Vancomycin	SSTIs	67%–87%	Flushing and hypotension
Linezolid[b]	SSTIs	89%	Thrombocytopenia, anemia, neutropenia
Linezolid	Nosocomial pneumonia	80%	Same as previous entry
Linezolid	Bacteremia	56%	Same as previous entry
Tigecycline	SSTIs	84% responded	Nausea, vomiting, photosensitivity
Daptomycin	SSTIs	75%–83%	Muscle toxicity
Daptomycin	Bacteremia and endocarditis	44%	Muscle toxicity
Quinupristin-dalfopristin	SSTIs	Uncertain	Arthralgia, myalgia, gastrointestinal effects
Telavancin (VIBATIV)	SSTIs	82%–89%	Gastrointestinal effects

SSTIs, Skin and soft tissue infections.
[a]Reported as cure rate, response rate, success rate, or survival rate.
[b]Can also be given orally.

Tetracyclines
Chemistry and Pharmacokinetics
The tetracycline antibiotics are semisynthetic derivatives of anthracycline compounds produced by various *Streptomyces* species. This class of antibiotics includes **doxycycline, tetracycline minocycline,** and **tetracycline,** a newer derivative of minocycline called **tigecycline,** and the recently approved **omadacycline, and eravacycline.** The properties and clinical uses of these drugs are outlined in Tables 39.1 and 39.2.

The oral bioavailability of the tetracyclines varies from 70% for tetracycline to greater than 90% for doxycycline and minocycline. Tetracycline antibiotics bind divalent and trivalent cations, including calcium, aluminum, and iron. For this reason, their **oral bioavailability is reduced if they are taken with foods or drugs containing these ions.** Dairy products reduce the oral bioavailability of tetracycline but have little effect on the bioavailability of doxycycline and minocycline. However, none of the tetracyclines should be taken with antacids or iron supplements.

The tetracycline drugs undergo minimal biotransformation and are excreted primarily in the urine and feces. Unlike other tetracyclines, **doxycycline is not dependent on renal elimination, and doses do not need to be adjusted in persons** with renal insufficiency.

Spectrum and Indications
The **tetracyclines** are **broad-spectrum, bacteriostatic drugs** that inhibit the growth of many gram-positive and gram-negative organisms, rickettsiae, spirochetes, mycoplasmas, chlamydiae, and protozoa. The unique antibacterial activity of tigecycline is described later.

Tetracyclines are the drugs of choice for **Rocky Mountain spotted fever** and other infections caused by *Rickettsia* species. They are also used for the treatment of two spirochetal infections, **Lyme disease** and relapsing fever, which are caused by *Borrelia burgdorferi* and *Borrelia recurrentis,* respectively. Tetracyclines are alternatives to macrolides to treat infections caused by *Mycoplasma pneumoniae.* For most **genital infections** caused by *Chlamydia trachomatis,* a 7-day course of oral doxycycline is effective. For pelvic inflammatory disease caused by chlamydiae, intravenous doxycycline may be necessary. Doxycycline (and azithromycin) can be used in combination with ceftriaxone for the treatment of **gonorrhea.**

Tetracyclines are used in the management of **acne vulgaris** and may be the most effective drugs for the treatment of moderately severe acne. In this condition, antibiotics suppress the growth of *Propionibacterium acnes,* an organism found on the skin that can infect sebaceous glands. This organism converts sebum triglycerides to fatty acids, which then cause skin irritation and contribute to sebaceous gland inflammation and the formation of comedones. **Minocycline** is sometimes used for the treatment of **acne** because of its **excellent penetration of the skin.** Doxycycline and minocycline have also been used to treat skin and soft tissue infections caused by methicillin-resistant *Staphylococcus aureus* (MRSA) (Table 39.4).

Tetracyclines are also used in the treatment of **brucellosis, ehrlichiosis,** and **granuloma inguinale.** Although oral rehydration therapy is the most important treatment modality for persons with severe diarrhea caused by *Vibrio cholerae,* a tetracycline can be used to shorten the course of **cholera** and reduce the risk of disease transmission to other persons. A tetracycline is included in some regimens to treat **peptic ulcers** caused by *Helicobacter pylori.*

Tigecycline is a glycylglycine derivative of minocycline that has increased affinity for the 30S ribosomal subunit and lower minimum inhibitory concentrations against many gram-positive and gram-negative organisms compared with older tetracyclines. It also has decreased susceptibility to resistance mechanisms affecting other tetracyclines. Tigecycline is used for the treatment of **complicated skin and soft tissue infections** caused by methicillin-sensitive *S. aureus* (MSSA) and MRSA, *E. coli*, *Enterococcus fecalis*, various streptococci, and *Bacteroides fragilis*. It is also approved for treating community-acquired pneumonia and complicated **intra-abdominal infections** caused by various gram-positive and gram-negative organisms. Unlike other tetracyclines that are often given orally, tigecycline is given only **intravenously** every 12 hours. Dose-related nausea and vomiting are the most common adverse effects. However, the US Food and Drug Administration (FDA) issued a black box warning because of an **increased mortality** in persons taking the drug **compared with other treatments,** and the drug should be used only when other treatments are not suitable.

The two newest tetracycline class antibiotics are **omadacycline** and **eravacycline. Omadacycline** was active **in vitro** against gram-positive bacteria that carried ribosomal protection genes and efflux genes and in *Enterobacericeae* that carried the resistant-producing efflux gene. In addition, omadacycline was active against some *S. aureus*, *S. pneumoniae*, and *H. influenzae* strains carrying macrolide resistance genes, or ciprofloxacin resistance genes, and beta(β)-lactamase–positive *H. influenza*.

Eravacycline contains structural substitutions that are not present in any naturally occurring or semisynthetic tetracyclines. These substitutions give pattern **eravacycline** activity against gram-positive and gram-negative strains expressing tetracycline-specific resistance mechanism(s) including efflux pumps and ribosomal protection. **Eravacycline** is also active against *Enterobacteriaceae* in the presence of **increased β-lactamases,** including **extended spectrum β-lactamases.**

Bacterial Resistance

Although tetracyclines inhibit the growth of a wide range of bacteria, they are no longer used to treat infections caused by many common pathogens because strains of these organisms have become resistant. Resistance to tetracyclines is caused by the transmission of plasmids containing resistance factors by bacterial conjugation. The **resistance factors** include genes that express **modified bacterial porins** that do not permit uptake of the tetracyclines. Resistance can also result from **increased drug efflux, decreased ribosomal binding,** and **enzymatic inactivation.** The practice of including tetracyclines in **animal feeds** to promote weight gain has contributed to the development and transmission of tetracycline resistance around the world. This practice continues to promote microbial resistance to other antimicrobial agents.

Adverse Effects

Tetracyclines can cause many adverse effects, including several that are potentially life-threatening. However, these effects can be avoided in most cases by avoiding their use in susceptible patients.

Tetracyclines are concentrated in growing teeth and bone. Their use by pregnant women or children younger than 8 years of age can cause **discoloration of the teeth**

and hypoplasia of the enamel. In affected children, yellow-brown or gray mottling of a significant portion of the enamel of the front teeth can be seen.

Tetracyclines can cause **nephrotoxicity** and **hepatotoxicity** in the form of fatty degeneration. Both of these reactions are rare, but pregnant women are at increased risk of hepatotoxicity, and this is another reason for not administering tetracyclines to this population. Use of tetracyclines potentiates the nephrotoxicity of aminoglycosides and other nephrotoxic drugs and should be avoided in patients undergoing treatment with these other drugs. Tetracyclines are slowly degraded in pharmaceutical preparations to products that are more nephrotoxic than the parent drug. For this reason, tetracycline preparations must be **used or discarded** by their expiration date.

Tetracyclines can produce **photosensitivity** in persons exposed to the sun during treatment. This reaction results from the absorption of ultraviolet radiation by the tetracycline after its accumulation in the skin. The activated drug then emits energy at a lower frequency that damages skin tissue, leads to erythema, and either exacerbates sunburn or causes a reaction similar to sunburn. Doxycycline is more frequently associated with photosensitivity than tetracycline and minocycline.

DRUGS THAT AFFECT THE 50S RIBOSOMAL SUBUNIT

Macrolide Antibiotics

The macrolides include **azithromycin, clarithromycin,** and **erythromycin.** The properties and major clinical uses of these drugs are compared in Tables 39.1 and 39.2.

Chemistry and Pharmacokinetics

Each macrolide antibiotic is composed of a large lactone ring with two attached sugars. Erythromycin, the first-discovered macrolide, is produced by *Saccharopolyspora erythraea* (formerly *Streptomyces erythreus*). Azithromycin and clarithromycin are semisynthetic derivatives of erythromycin that have improved pharmacokinetic properties and antibacterial activity.

Macrolides are usually administered orally, but azithromycin is available in intravenous formulations for treating serious infections such as Legionnaire disease. Erythromycin can also be administered topically to treat acne. When given orally, the bioavailability of erythromycin is low and variable. Azithromycin and clarithromycin have a greater oral bioavailability and achieve higher tissue concentrations than erythromycin (see Table 39.1). Erythromycin also has a shorter half-life than other macrolides, necessitating two to four doses a day, whereas clarithromycin is administered twice daily and azithromycin is given once a day. The macrolides undergo variable degrees of hepatic metabolism and are excreted in the bile and urine.

Spectrum and Indications

The macrolides are active against many gram-positive and gram-negative bacteria that cause upper **respiratory tract infections** and **community-acquired pneumonia,** including group A streptococci, pneumococci, chlamydiae, *M. pneumoniae*, and *Legionella pneumophila*. Azithromycin is also active against pathogens responsible for sinusitis, otitis media, and bronchitis. Macrolides have little activity against gram-negative bacteria such as *Klebsiella pneumoniae* that typically cause pneumonia in neonates, elderly persons, and chronic alcoholics.

As shown in Table 39.2, some macrolides are active against **chlamydiae** and are effective in treating pneumonia and genitourinary tract infections caused by *Chlamydia pneumoniae* and *C. trachomatis*, respectively. In fact, azithromycin is an effective single-dose treatment for uncomplicated **chlamydial urethritis** and is used in combination with ceftriaxone to treat **gonorrhea.** Either azithromycin or clarithromycin can be used to treat *Mycobacterium avium-intracellulare* infections, such as those occurring in patients with acquired immunodeficiency syndrome. Clarithromycin is the most active macrolide against *H. pylori*, an organism frequently associated with **peptic ulcer disease.** As discussed in Chapter 28, clarithromycin is used in combination with other antibiotics and a gastric acid inhibitor to treat this condition.

Bacterial Resistance

Resistance to macrolide antibiotics has gradually increased over several decades. Acquired resistance to macrolides can result from decreased binding to the 50S ribosomal subunit, enzymatic inactivation, and increased **bacterial efflux.** Most strains of staphylococci are now resistant, and pneumococci are increasingly resistant to macrolides. Approximately 30% of pneumococcal isolates from around the world are resistant to macrolides. Many **pneumococcal strains** express the **macrolide efflux (*mef*A) transporter.** Pneumococcal and other bacterial resistance is also caused by antibiotic induction of the ***erm* gene,** which expresses an enzyme that methylates the bacterial ribosome and **reduces antibiotic binding.** This gene confers resistance to macrolides, clindamycin, and quinupristin.

Adverse Effects

The most common adverse effects of macrolides are stomatitis (inflammation of mouth), heartburn, nausea, anorexia, abdominal discomfort, and diarrhea. Erythromycin activates **receptors for motilin,** a gastric hormone that **activates peristalsis,** leading to anorexia, nausea, and vomiting. Azithromycin and clarithromycin have less affinity for motilin receptors and cause less gastrointestinal distress than erythromycin. The macrolides seldom cause serious adverse reactions.

Drug Interactions

Erythromycin and clarithromycin inhibit **cytochrome P450 3A4** (CYP3A4) and can elevate the plasma concentration of a large number of drugs metabolized by this isozyme. For example, concurrent administration of erythromycin or clarithromycin with carbamazepine can lead to life-threatening **carbamazepine toxicity,** and this combination should be avoided. Erythromycin and clarithromycin also inhibit the metabolism of lovastatin and simvastatin, and concurrent use with these statin drugs can lead to elevated statin levels and rhabdomyolysis. In contrast, azithromycin has little effect on P450 drug metabolism and may be the preferred macrolide antibiotic for persons taking other drugs metabolized by CYP3A4.

Clindamycin

Clindamycin is a chlorinated aminosugar antibiotic structurally unrelated to other antibiotics. It is active against

---

BOX 39.1 A CASE OF ABSCESS AND DRAINAGE

CASE PRESENTATION

A 26-year-old man requests evaluation of a painful lesion on his abdominal wall, which developed after he sustained an injury while playing basketball. There is a 4-day history of drainage from this abscess, which has increased in size and become more painful. His temperature is 38.5°C, and his pulse is 115 beats/min. On examination, the lesion is tender and erythematous with a fluctuant area at the center. Purulent material is obtained by aspiration, and a culture yields methicillin-resistant *Staphylococcus aureus* (MRSA) that is susceptible to clindamycin. The D-zone test result is negative. Incision and drainage are performed on the lesion, and he is placed on oral clindamycin, 300 mg three times daily. The infection responds to a 7-day course of clindamycin therapy.

CASE DISCUSSION

The number of community-acquired MRSA infections has increased dramatically in the past 5 years. MRSA is currently the most common pathogen isolated from skin and soft tissue infections in emergency departments. These infections may be managed by incision and drainage if systemic signs such as fever and tachycardia are absent. The optimal antibiotic therapy for these infections has not been established, but clindamycin, trimethoprim-sulfamethoxazole, and other oral agents are usually effective (see Table 39.4). Clindamycin susceptibility test results may be misleading because of the occurrence of inducible clindamycin resistance expressed by the *erm* gene (see text). The D-zone test can be used to detect this form of resistance. This test result is positive if a D-shaped or blunted area of inhibition surrounds the clindamycin disk on a culture of the clinical isolate. In the present case, the D-zone test result was negative, and the patient was effectively treated with clindamycin.

---

gram-positive cocci and **anaerobic organisms** such as *B. fragilis* and *Clostridiodes perfringens* (the cause of gas gangrene). It has gained importance as a treatment for infections caused by **methicillin-resistant staphylococci** and penicillin-resistant streptococci, including necrotizing fasciitis (Box 39.1).

Clindamycin can be administered orally, parenterally, or topically. It is generally well tolerated, but it is associated with a higher rate of occurrence of gastrointestinal superinfections caused by *Clostridioides difficile* than other antibiotics, which can lead to **severe diarrhea** and life-threatening **pseudomembranous colitis.** The pseudomembrane present in this condition can be observed with proctoscopic examination and consists of mucus, desquamated epithelial cells, and inflammatory cells. Persons who develop diarrhea during clindamycin therapy should discontinue use of the drug and be closely monitored for superinfection and colitis.

Chloramphenicol

Chloramphenicol is a unique nitrobenzene antibiotic that is lipophilic and well absorbed from the gut. It also crosses the blood-brain barrier and achieves high concentrations in the central nervous system, even in the absence of inflamed meninges. This property contributes to the drug's effectiveness in the treatment of meningitis, although it is infrequently used for this purpose nowadays.

Chloramphenicol is partly metabolized by glucuronate conjugation, and the unchanged drug and metabolites are excreted in the urine. Neonates have a reduced capacity to metabolize chloramphenicol due to low levels of glucuronyl transferase, and doses per kilogram body weight must be reduced in neonates to avoid the **gray baby syndrome** characterized by cyanosis, weakness, respiratory depression, and shock.

Other adverse effects of chloramphenicol include two distinct forms of anemia. One form is a **reversible, dose-dependent anemia** caused by blockade of iron incorporation into heme. The other form of anemia is a rare but potentially fatal **aplastic anemia** affecting 1 in 20,000 to 40,000 individuals exposed to the drug. Because safer antibiotics are currently available, little justification exists for the use of chloramphenicol for most infections.

Chloramphenicol is a broad-spectrum antibiotic that is active against pathogens causing **meningitis,** including pneumococci, meningococci, and *H. influenzae*. It has also been used to treat *Salmonella* and *Bacteroides* infections. Chloramphenicol should be used to treat only meningitis and other infections caused by organisms resistant to other drugs, and it is seldom used nowadays.

Quinupristin-Dalfopristin

Quinupristin and dalfopristin are **streptogramin** antibiotics that synergistically inhibit bacterial protein synthesis when administered in a 30:70 ratio. Quinupristin and dalfopristin bind sites on the bacterial 50S ribosomal subunit and inhibit **peptidyl transferase** and peptide bond formation in the same manner as the macrolides.

Quinupristin and dalfopristin are bactericidal against susceptible strains of staphylococci and streptococci but are bacteriostatic against *Enterococcus faecium*. Given in combination, the drugs are active against many gram-positive bacteria, including **multidrug-resistant staphylococci, penicillin-resistant pneumococci,** and **vancomycin-resistant E. faecium** but not *E. fecalis*. The combination has been used to treat bacteremia, pneumonia, and skin and soft tissue infections caused by these organisms. For example, it has been successfully used in cases of bacteremia, peritonitis, endocarditis, and aortic graft infections caused by vancomycin-resistant organisms.

Following intravenous administration, quinupristin and dalfopristin are partly converted to active metabolites, and these are distributed to most tissues except the central nervous system. The drugs and metabolites are primarily excreted in the bile. Quinupristin-dalfopristin can cause inflammation of veins at the infusion site, arthralgia, myalgia, diarrhea, and nausea. The drugs inhibit the metabolism of other drugs by CYP3A4.

Lefamulin is the first antibiotic approved in more than 20 years with a **new mechanism of action at the bacterial ribosome.** Lefamulin inhibits bacterial protein synthesis through molecular interactions (hydrogen bonds, hydrophobic interactions, and Van der Waals forces) with the A- and P-sites of the peptidyl transferase center (PTC) in domain V of the 23S rRNA of the 50S subunit. Lefamulin binding **prevents correct positioning of tRNA and shuts down strand elongation.** Lefamulin is bactericidal in vitro and in clinical infections against *S. pneumoniae, H. influenzae,* and *M. pneumoniae* (including macrolide-resistant strains); it is bacteriostatic against *S. aureus* and *S. pyogenes* at clinically relevant concentrations. **Lefamulin** is indicated for the treatment of adults with **community-acquired bacterial pneumonia** (CABP) caused by susceptible microorganisms.

OTHER PROTEIN SYNTHESIS INHIBITORS

Linezolid

Linezolid is a synthetic **oxazolidinedione** compound that prevents formation of the bacterial protein synthesis **initiation complex.** This is accomplished by inhibiting binding of N-formylmethionyl-tRNA to the 70S ribosome. Because of its unique mechanism, cross-resistance with other classes of antibiotics has not been observed.

Linezolid is active against aerobic gram-positive bacteria. It is bacteriostatic against enterococci and staphylococci and bactericidal against most strains of streptococci. Linezolid is indicated for the treatment of infections caused by **vancomycin-resistant E. faecium; pneumonia** caused by MSSA and **MRSA;** and **skin and soft tissue infections** caused by methicillin-sensitive or methicillin-resistant staphylococci, *Streptococcus pyogenes,* or *Streptococcus agalactiae*. The drug is administered intravenously for serious infections, such as necrotizing fasciitis and pneumonia, and can be given orally for mild to moderate skin and soft tissue infections. Its oral bioavailability is approximately 100%, and it is widely distributed. Approximately 70% of linezolid is metabolized, and the remainder is excreted unchanged in the urine.

Linezolid may cause reversible **thrombocytopenia,** and less commonly anemia and neutropenia, in patients with renal insufficiency or during prolonged therapy. It is a weak inhibitor of monoamine oxidase and may cause **serotonin toxicity** (serotonin syndrome) when combined with a selective serotonin reuptake inhibitor such as fluoxetine. This drug combination should be avoided whenever possible.

Mupirocin

Mupirocin is an antibiotic obtained from *Pseudomonas fluorescens*. The drug has structural resemblance to the amino acid isoleucine. It competes with isoleucine for binding to isoleucyl tRNA synthetase and prevents formation of **isoleucyl** tRNA and bacterial protein synthesis. Because of its unique mechanism of action, it does not exhibit cross-resistance with other antimicrobial drugs.

Mupirocin is active against gram-positive cocci, including most strains of methicillin-resistant staphylococci. It also inhibits most β-hemolytic streptococci, including *S. pyogenes*. Mupirocin is the first effective topical therapy for **impetigo,** a skin disease caused by streptococci and staphylococci. In cases of impetigo, it is applied as a cream to affected areas for 5 days. Mupirocin is also used to eradicate **nasal colonization of methicillin-resistant staphylococci** in infected patients and in health care workers, but the ability of this treatment to prevent future infections is variable. The drug is rapidly inactivated in the body and is not used systemically.

SUMMARY OF IMPORTANT POINTS

- Inhibitors of bacterial protein synthesis act by selectively binding to components of the 30S or 50S ribosomal subunits. Aminoglycosides and tetracyclines inhibit 30S ribosomal function. Macrolides, clindamycin, chloramphenicol, and dalfopristin inhibit 50S ribosomal function.

- Aminoglycosides are poorly absorbed from the gut and do not penetrate the central nervous system. They are excreted unchanged in the urine. Aminoglycosides are active against many aerobic gram-negative bacilli, including *P. aeruginosa.* These drugs often cause renal and otic toxicity.
- Tetracyclines are broad-spectrum, bacteriostatic drugs used to treat infections caused by rickettsiae, chlamydiae, mycoplasmas, and methicillin-resistant *S. aureus.* They are concentrated in growing teeth and bone and can cause permanent staining of teeth if administered during pregnancy or in children younger than the age of 8 years.
- Most tetracyclines are excreted primarily in the urine, but doxycycline is excreted by other routes and can be used without dosage adjustment in patients with renal failure.
- Macrolides, which are active against most pathogens causing respiratory tract infections, are used to treat otitis media and pneumonia caused by pneumococci, chlamydiae, *M. pneumoniae,* and *L. pneumophila.* Azithromycin is particularly effective against *H. influenzae,* whereas clarithromycin is active against *H. pylori* and can be used in the treatment of peptic ulcer disease.
- Clindamycin, which is active against gram-positive cocci, is useful in treating infections caused by gram-positive cocci and anaerobes resistant to penicillin and other drugs. It causes a higher rate of occurrence of pseudomembranous colitis than do other antibiotics.
- Chloramphenicol is used to treat only meningitis and other serious infections when other antibiotics cannot be used. It rarely causes aplastic anemia.
- Quinupristin-dalfopristin and linezolid are active against gram-positive cocci, including methicillin and vancomycin-resistant staphylococci and vancomycin-resistant enterococci.
- Mupirocin is active against streptococci and staphylococci. It is administered topically to treat impetigo and to eradicate nasal carriers of methicillin-resistant staphylococci.

Review Questions

1. A man with a skin infection due to methicillin-resistant *S. aureus* is treated with linezolid. Which adverse effect is associated with this antibiotic?
   (A) myalgia and arthralgia
   (B) nystagmus and vertigo
   (C) thrombocytopenia
   (D) discoloration of body fluids
   (E) flushing and hypotension
2. An infant with enterocolitis due to *E. coli* is treated with oral gentamicin. Which step in bacterial protein synthesis is inhibited by this antibiotic?
   (A) initiation
   (B) peptide bond formation
   (C) isoleucine transfer RNA synthesis
   (D) peptide translocation
   (E) transfer RNA binding to 30S subunit
3. A man being treated for chlamydial urethritis presents with severe erythema over his upper body after sun exposure. Which antibiotic is most likely responsible for this adverse effect?
   (A) azithromycin
   (B) clindamycin
   (C) doxycycline
   (D) erythromycin
   (E) mupirocin
4. Which antibiotic is highly ionized in body fluids and must be given parenterally for systemic infections?
   (A) doxycycline
   (B) azithromycin
   (C) clindamycin
   (D) tobramycin
   (E) linezolid
5. Which antibiotic is active against some strains of vancomycin-resistant *E. faecium*?
   (A) azithromycin
   (B) doxycycline
   (C) chloramphenicol
   (D) clindamycin
   (E) quinupristin-dalfopristin

CHAPTER 40

Other Antimicrobial Agents Such as Quinolones and Antifolate Drugs

OVERVIEW

This chapter discusses several classes of antibacterial drugs used in treating a wide range of infections. Some of these drugs inhibit bacterial folate formation, whereas others impair bacterial DNA topology, disrupt the bacterial cell membrane, or affect bacterial RNA synthesis.

ANTIFOLATE DRUGS

Antifolate drugs treat bacterial infections, protozoal infections (see Chapter 44), and cancer (see Chapter 45). All of these drugs inhibit the synthesis of folate in target cells. This chapter describes the sulfonamides and trimethoprim used in treating bacterial infections.

Mechanisms of Action

The sulfonamides and trimethoprim inhibit sequential steps in the synthesis of bacterial folate (Fig. 40.1). **Sulfonamides** are structural analogs of *para*-aminobenzoic acid (PABA) and competitively inhibit the enzyme that combines PABA with pteridine to form dihydropteroate. Dihydropteroate is then converted to dihydrofolate by the addition of glutamate. **Trimethoprim** inhibits **dihydrofolate reductase** and the formation of **tetrahydrofolate.**

Mammals must obtain folic acid from their diet because they cannot synthesize dihydrofolate, accounting for the lack of effect of sulfonamides on mammalian cells. Once absorbed, dihydrofolate is converted to tetrahydrofolate, and the active folate derivatives (methyl, formyl, and methylenetetrahydrofolate) that donate single-carbon atoms during the synthesis of purine bases and other components of DNA (see Chapter 17). Although folate reductase is found in both microbial and mammalian cells, the affinity of trimethoprim for the bacterial enzyme is about 100,000 times greater than its affinity for the mammalian enzyme.

Sulfonamides

In the 1930s, **sulfanilamide** was found to be the active metabolite of PRONTOSIL, a dye developed in the search for bacterial stains with antimicrobial properties. This discovery led to the synthesis and development of a large number of sulfonamide compounds to treat bacterial infections. Only a few of these are still used today.

Chemistry and Pharmacokinetics

The sulfonamides are a group of benzene sulfonic acid amide derivatives. Most sulfonamides are adequately absorbed from the gut and are widely distributed to tissues and fluids throughout the body, including the cerebrospinal fluid. The half-lives of sulfonamides vary greatly (Table 40.1), but the most widely used compounds for treating human infections, such as **sulfacetamide** and **sulfamethoxazole,** have half-lives ranging from 6 to 10 hours.

Sulfonamides are converted to inactive compounds by *N*-acetylation, and the parent drug and its metabolites are excreted in the urine. The acetylated metabolites are less soluble than the parent compound in urine, and they can precipitate in the renal tubules, causing **crystalluria.** Therefore, it is important for patients treated with a sulfonamide to consume adequate quantities of water.

Spectrum, Indications, and Bacterial Resistance

The sulfonamides were once active against a wide range of organisms, including streptococci, gonococci, meningococci, many gram-negative bacilli, and chlamydiae. Over the years, significant resistance to sulfonamides developed in many species, and the antimicrobial spectrum of these drugs gradually declined. Today, sulfonamides are primarily used to prevent or treat urinary tract infections, partly because of their high urinary concentration (Table 40.2).

Sulfamethoxazole is administered with trimethoprim (see the section on trimethoprim-sulfamethoxazole [TMP-SMX]).

Sulfadiazine is available in the form of **silver sulfadiazine** (SILVADENE) ointment to prevent or treat **burn infections** and other superficial skin infections. The silver ions in this preparation have antibacterial activity and contribute to its efficacy in this setting.

Sulfacetamide is administered topically to treat blepharitis and conjunctivitis, **common ocular infections**

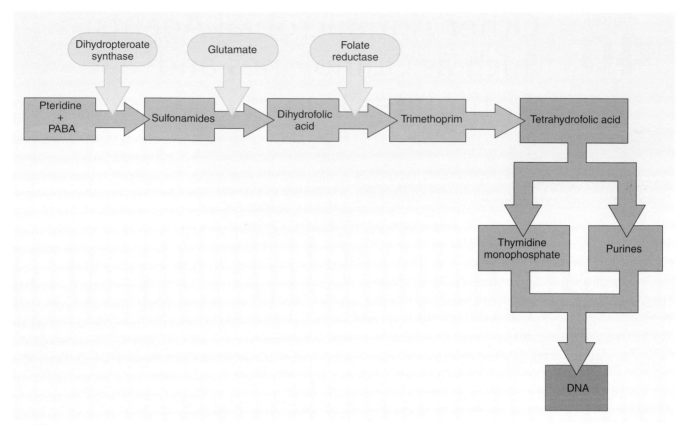

FIG. 40.1 Mechanisms of action of antifolate drugs. Sulfonamides inhibit the action of dihydropteroate synthase and thereby block the synthesis of dihydrofolate. Trimethoprim inhibits the action of dihydrofolate reductase and thereby blocks the formation of tetrahydrofolate. *PABA*, P-aminobenzoic acid.

TABLE 40.1   Pharmacokinetic Properties of Selected Antifolate Drugs, Fluoroquinolones, and Other Agents[a]

DRUG	ROUTE OF ADMINISTRATION	ORAL BIOAVAILABILITY (%)	ELIMINATION HALF-LIFE (HOURS)	ROUTES OF ELIMINATION
Antifolate drugs				
Sulfacetamide	Topical ocular	NA	10	Metabolism; renal excretion
Trimethoprim	Oral	Approximately 100	10	Metabolism; renal excretion
Trimethoprim-sulfamethoxazole	Oral or IV	Approximately 100	10	Metabolism; renal excretion
Fluoroquinolones				
Ciprofloxacin	Oral, IV, or topical ocular	75	4	Metabolism; renal excretion
Levofloxacin	Oral or IV	99	8	Metabolism; renal excretion
Norfloxacin	Oral	35	3.5	Metabolism; renal excretion
Moxifloxacin	Oral or IV	90	12	Metabolism; renal excretion
Gatifloxacin	Topical ocular	NA	NA	Metabolism; renal excretion
Gemifloxacin	Oral	71	7	Metabolism, renal excretion
Other antibacterial drugs				
Nitrofurantoin	Oral	87	0.5	Metabolism; renal excretion
Polymyxin B	IV or topical	NA	5	NA
Daptomycin	IV	NA	9	Renal excretion

[a]Values shown are the mean of values reported in the literature.
IV, Intravenous; *NA,* not applicable.

TABLE 40.2   Major Clinical Uses of Selected Fluoroquinolones, Antifolate Drugs, and Other Antibacterial Drugs

DRUG	MAJOR CLINICAL USES
Fluoroquinolones	
Ciprofloxacin	Bacterial diarrhea; intraabdominal infections; infections of the urinary tract, prostate, bone and joints, skin, and eye; anthrax exposure
Levofloxacin	Bronchitis and community-acquired pneumonia; infections of the urinary tract, prostate, skin, and eye
Gatifloxacin	Bacterial conjunctivitis
Gemifloxacin, moxifloxacin	Community-acquired pneumonia, sinusitis, bronchitis, tuberculosis
Norfloxacin	Urinary tract infections
Antifolate drugs	
Trimethoprim-sulfamethoxazole	Urinary tract and prostatic infections; pulmonary infections caused by *Pneumocystis jiroveci (carinii)* and *Nocardia* species
Silver sulfadiazine	Burn infections, other skin infections
Sulfacetamide	Ocular infections
Other antibacterial drugs	
Nitrofurantoin	Lower urinary tract (bladder) infections
Polymyxin B	Superficial infections of skin and mucous membranes
Daptomycin	Infections caused by methicillin- or vancomycin-resistant staphylococci or vancomycin-sensitive enterococci
Rifaximin	Travelers diarrhea, hepatic encephalopathy, irritable bowel syndrome

worldwide. It is also effective in treating **trachoma,** a highly contagious ocular infection caused by *Chlamydia trachomatis* prevalent in Asia and the Middle East.

Adverse Effects

In some patients, sulfonamides cause skin rashes, which are hypersensitivity reactions that can progress from a mild reaction to a serious or life-threatening form, such as erythema multiforme **(Stevens-Johnson syndrome).** Other adverse effects of sulfonamides include crystalluria (discussed previously), gastrointestinal reactions, headaches, hepatitis, and hematopoietic toxicity. In persons with **glucose-6-phosphate dehydrogenase deficiency,** sulfonamides can cause **hemolytic anemia.**

Trimethoprim

Trimethoprim is a synthetic amino-pyrimidine drug. It is well absorbed from the gut and is widely distributed to tissues. After extensive hepatic metabolism, the remaining parent compound and metabolites are excreted in the urine.

Trimethoprim is a weak base concentrated in acidic prostate tissues and vaginal fluids via **ion trapping** (see Chapter 2). This makes trimethoprim particularly useful in the treatment of **bacterial prostatitis** and **vaginitis.**

Trimethoprim is active against many aerobic gram-negative bacilli and a few gram-positive organisms. It is usually administered in **combination with sulfamethoxazole** to prevent or treat urinary tract infections (see section on TMP-SMX), but it is occasionally used alone for these purposes. The adverse effects of trimethoprim include nausea, vomiting, and epigastric distress; rashes and other hypersensitivity reactions; hepatitis; and thrombocytopenia, leukopenia, and other **hematologic disorders,** including megaloblastic anemia.

Trimethoprim-Sulfamethoxazole

Pharmacokinetics

Sulfamethoxazole and trimethoprim have synergistic activity against susceptible organisms and are available in fixed-dose combinations to treat bacterial infections. Sulfamethoxazole has been combined with trimethoprim because it has a similar half-life (10 hours). *In vitro* tests show that maximal synergistic activity occurs when the concentration of sulfamethoxazole is 20 times greater than the concentration of trimethoprim. To obtain plasma drug concentrations in a ratio of 20:1, the drugs are administered in a ratio of five parts of sulfamethoxazole to one part of trimethoprim. The 5:1 dose ratio produces a 20:1 plasma concentration ratio because trimethoprim has a greater distribution volume than sulfamethoxazole.

Spectrum and Indications

TMP-SMX exhibits bactericidal activity against some organisms that are not susceptible to either drug given alone. TMP-SMX is active against members of the family *Enterobacteriaceae*, including strains of *Escherichia coli*, *Klebsiella pneumoniae*, *Proteus* species, and *Enterobacter* species. TMP-SMX is often used to prevent or treat **urinary tract** and **prostate infections** caused by these organisms (Box 40.1). Because of increased bacterial resistance to TMP-SMX, it is not recommended for the empiric treatment of urinary tract infections in locations where greater than 20% of *E. coli* isolates are resistant to TMP-SMX. In these locations, nitrofurantoin or fosfomycin can treat these infections. TMP-SMX is not active against *Pseudomonas aeruginosa*, which can cause urinary tract infections in hospitalized and nursing home patients.

TMP-SMX is also the drug of choice for treating pulmonary infections caused by **Pneumocystis jiroveci (carinii)** and **Nocardia asteroides,** which most often occur in immunocompromised patients. TMP-SMX is active against *Burkholderia cepacia* and some strains of *Haemophilus influenzae* and *Moraxella catarrhalis*.

TMP-SMX is active against some strains of *Salmonella* and *Shigella*, but other strains are resistant. Currently, a fluoroquinolone (see the section on fluoroquinolones) is usually preferred to treat most infections caused by these organisms.

BOX 40.1 A CASE OF URINARY FREQUENCY AND URGENCY

CASE PRESENTATION

An otherwise healthy 27-year-old woman presented to the outpatient clinic complaining of a 2-day history of worsening suprapubic pain, urinary urgency and frequency, and a burning pain with urination. She reported no fever, chills, back pain, or vaginal irritation or discharge. Urinalysis revealed bacteriuria, pyuria, and hematuria. Her physical examination was otherwise normal. The woman had a previous history of acute bacterial cystitis, but the most recent episode was more than 2 years ago. She was instructed to increase fluid intake and was prescribed a 3-day course of trimethoprim-sulfamethoxazole because the prevalence of bacterial resistance to this agent in the community was less than 20%. A heating pad was suggested for acute pain relief. She completed the treatment as prescribed, and her symptoms resolved by the end of the treatment period.

CASE DISCUSSION

Acute bacterial cystitis (inflammation of the bladder) is a common infection in women, leading to more than 7 million physician visits in the United States each year. The vast majority of these infections are caused by *Escherichia coli.* Most infections are designated as uncomplicated because they occur in women with a structurally and functionally normal urinary tract. Women are much more likely to develop this infection than men, probably because the urethral opening is near the anus and vagina, the primary sources of bacteria causing this infection. These infections usually respond to a short course of treatment with trimethoprim-sulfamethoxazole, nitrofurantoin, a fluoroquinolone, or other agent. Trimethoprim-sulfamethoxazole is often used when the prevalence of bacterial resistance to this agent is low. Fluoroquinolones are not considered first-line agents because of a greater risk of adverse effects.

Adverse Effects

The adverse effects of TMP-SMX are similar to those of the individual drugs. TMP-SMX can cause **megaloblastic anemia** in persons with a low dietary intake of folic acid, but this adverse effect is uncommon.

FLUOROQUINOLONES

Fluoroquinolones are synthetic drugs that inhibit bacterial DNA gyrase (topoisomerase) and have been used to treat a wide range of infections due to their potent bactericidal activity and attractive pharmacokinetic properties. At the same time, these drugs can cause **serious adverse effects.** Some agents, such as ciprofloxacin, are primarily active against gram-negative bacteria, whereas newer broad-spectrum drugs, such as **levofloxacin,** are active against both gram-positive and gram-negative organisms.

In all organisms, DNA topology (referring to a shape preserved under deformation) is regulated by a family of enzymes, the **DNA topoisomerases.** Every organism requires at least one type I and one type II topoisomerase enzyme to manage DNA supercoiling during DNA transcription and replication. Fluoroquinolones inhibit two types of **bacterial type IIA** topoisomerase, of which one is called **DNA gyrase,** and the other is designated **type IV topoisomerase.** These topoisomerase enzymes are essential for maintaining DNA in a stable and biologically active form. DNA gyrase introduces **negative supercoils** (superhelical twists) into closed circular bacterial DNA. These negative supercoils eliminate the **positive supercoils** that occur ahead of the DNA replication fork during DNA replication. DNA replication cannot proceed without DNA gyrase activity. As shown in Fig. 40.2, DNA gyrase produces supercoiling by breaking doubled-stranded DNA, moving a section of double-stranded DNA through the break, and resealing the broken strands of DNA. DNA gyrase is a tetramer composed of two A and two B subunits. Fluoroquinolones

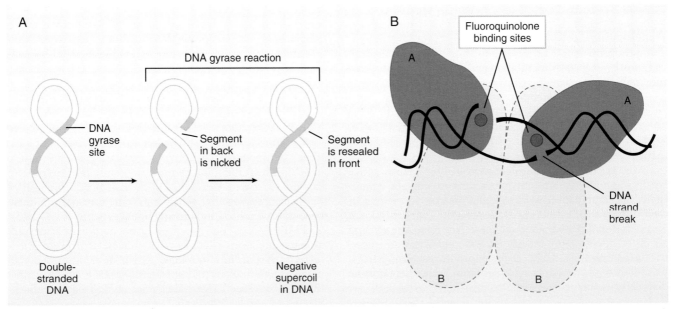

Fɪɢ. 40.2 Effect of fluoroquinolones on DNA gyrase. (A) In the absence of fluoroquinolones, DNA gyrase catalyzes the formation of negative supercoils in the double-stranded DNA of bacteria. After both strands of one segment are nicked, the broken strands are passed across the other strands of DNA and then are resealed. This reaction requires energy in the form of adenosine triphosphate (ATP). (B) DNA gyrase is a tetramer composed of two A subunits and two B subunits. Fluoroquinolones inhibit DNA gyrase by binding to the catalytic sites on the A subunits. ATP binds to the B subunits.

selectively bind to the **A subunits,** which contain the catalytic site of the breaking and resealing reactions.

Type IV topoisomerase is responsible for separating the DNA of daughter chromosomes once DNA replication is completed. This process is called **decatenation.** In general, DNA gyrase is the primary target of fluoroquinolones in gram-negative bacteria, whereas topoisomerase IV is the primary target in gram-positive organisms.

Pharmacokinetics

The pharmacokinetic properties of fluoroquinolones are shown in Table 40.1. Fluoroquinolones are usually given orally, and ciprofloxacin, levofloxacin, and moxifloxacin can also be administered intravenously. Ciprofloxacin has a half-life of 4 hours and is usually administered every 12 hours. Levofloxacin, gemifloxacin, and moxifloxacin have half-lives of 7 to 12 hours and are given once every 24 hours to treat most infections.

Fluoroquinolones are well absorbed from the gut, but, like the tetracyclines, the fluoroquinolones chelate (bind) **divalent and trivalent cations,** including calcium, iron, magnesium, and zinc, forming nonabsorbed compounds. Orally administered fluoroquinolones should be taken 2 hours before or after ingesting foods and drugs containing these metallic cations.

Fluoroquinolones are widely distributed to tissues, and their concentrations in the lungs, kidneys, liver, gallbladder, prostate, and female reproductive tissues are often two to five times greater than their plasma concentrations. Fluoroquinolones undergo varying degrees of hepatic biotransformation, and they are excreted unchanged in the urine, along with their metabolites.

Spectrum and Indications

Fluoroquinolones have **bactericidal activity** against a wide range of gram-positive and gram-negative bacteria and acid-fast bacilli. The drugs exhibit **concentration-dependent-killing,** and the maximum bactericidal effect occurs when the ratio of the peak serum drug level to the organism's minimal inhibitory concentration is at least 10 to 1. Fluoroquinolones have a long **postantibiotic effect,** with some organisms failing to resume growth for 2 to 6 hours after drug levels are no longer detectable. Because of their favorable properties, fluoroquinolones can be given orally to treat some infections that formerly required parenteral therapy with other drugs (see Table 40.2).

Ciprofloxacin and other fluoroquinolones have excellent activity against gram-negative bacteria and are used to treat infections caused by enteric gram-negative bacilli, gonococci, chlamydia, and *P. aeruginosa,* including **urinary tract infections, prostatitis,** and **pelvic inflammatory disease.** Although fluoroquinolones are often used to treat urinary tract infections, the Infectious Diseases Society of America (IDSA) recommends that TMP-SMX, **nitrofurantoin,** and **fosfomycin** (see later and Chapter 38) should be used to treat **acute uncomplicated cystitis** (urinary bladder infection). The IDSA found that fluoroquinolones are prescribed too frequently and often for too long a duration for this infection, leading to excessive adverse effects and contributing to microbial resistance. **Fluoroquinolones** should be reserved for treating serious urinary tract infections and those not responding to other drugs.

Fluoroquinolones are also used to treat **bacterial diarrhea** caused by *Campylobacter, Salmonella,* and *Shigella* species, as well as *Yersinia enterocolitica,* and they are effective in treating **travelers diarrhea** (see rifaximin later). Fluoroquinolones

are also used, sometimes in combination with other drugs, to treat intraabdominal infections, bone and joint infections, skin infections, and febrile neutropenia. In addition, ciprofloxacin can be used to treat **anthrax** and postexposure prevention of inhalational anthrax during a bioterrorism event. Anthrax is caused by *Bacillus anthracis,* a gram-positive rod that can be transmitted via the intestines, lungs, or skin, causing infections at the site of entry into the body.

Several broad-spectrum fluoroquinolones (**levofloxacin, moxifloxacin,** and **gemifloxacin**) have good activity against **pneumococci** while retaining activity against gram-negative organisms. These agents are used to treat mild to moderate **community-acquired pneumonia** caused by pneumococci, *Chlamydia pneumoniae, K. pneumoniae, Mycoplasma pneumoniae,* and *Legionella pneumophila,* as well as sinusitis and bronchitis caused by pneumococci, *H. influenzae,* or *M. catarrhalis.* Fluoroquinolones are also active against mycobacteria and are used to treat *Mycobacterium avium-intracellulare* infections and **drug-resistant tuberculosis** (see Chapter 41). These agents achieve high concentrations in neutrophils, contributing to their effectiveness in mycobacterial infections.

The newest fluoroquinolone antibiotic is **delafloxacin.** The antibacterial activity of delafloxacin arises from the **inhibition** of both **bacterial topoisomerase IV and DNA gyrase** (topoisomerase II) enzymes. These enzymes are required for bacterial DNA replication, transcription, repair, and recombination. Delafloxacin has some activity in bacteria that are resistant to other fluoroquinolones. Delafloxacin shows a **concentration-dependent bactericidal activity against gram-positive and gram-negative bacteria** *in vitro.*

Several fluoroquinolones (ciprofloxacin, gatifloxacin, levofloxacin, moxifloxacin, and ofloxacin) are available in formulations for topical ocular administration treat bacterial **conjunctivitis.** These drugs are the most commonly prescribed treatment for bacterial **corneal ulcers.**

Bacterial Resistance

Resistance to fluoroquinolone drugs has increased among both gram-positive and gram-negative pathogens. This resistance develops through two primary mechanisms: **alterations in the target enzymes** (topoisomerases) and alterations in drug access to the target enzymes. Alterations in bacterial DNA gyrase occur most commonly in gram-negative bacteria, whereas alterations in type IV topoisomerase are more prevalent in gram-positive organisms. Resistance by DNA gyrase mutations is usually caused by decreased affinity of the A subunit of DNA gyrase for the drugs, but B subunit mutations can also lead to resistance. Topoisomerase IV mutations also lead to reduced fluoroquinolone binding affinity.

Resistance to fluoroquinolones can also occur through expression of membrane transport proteins or **efflux pumps** that actively transport a number of antibacterial agents out of bacterial cells and thereby confer **multidrug resistance.** In addition, some gram-negative bacteria have decreased levels of **porins** in their outer membrane, resulting in decreased fluoroquinolone uptake by these bacteria.

ADVERSE EFFECTS AND INTERACTIONS

Fluoroquinolones can cause a number of serious adverse effects, including **tendonitis** and **tendon rupture.** These drugs have a high affinity for cartilage and tendons, where they exert direct toxic effects on the tendon matrix and cause tendon cell death by activating apoptosis pathways (programmed cell death). The risk of tendinitis and tendon rupture is increased in persons over 60 years of age, in those taking corticosteroids, and in those with kidney, heart, or lung transplants. Fluoroquinolones can also cause a potentially serious **peripheral neuropathy** that may begin within a few days of starting systemic therapy and last for months or even be permanent. Typical symptoms of neuropathy include numbness, tingling, weakness, and shooting pain in the limbs, hands, and feet. Because of potential adverse effects, fluoroquinolones should not be prescribed to children, adolescents, nursing mothers, and pregnant women.

Other adverse effects of fluoroquinolones include **alterations in blood glucose** (both hypoglycemia and hyperglycemia), seizures, **phototoxicity** (dermatitis after sun exposure), and **prolongation of the QT interval** (the time between the start of the **Q** wave and the end of the **T** wave of the electrocardiogram) leading to ventricular tachycardia (see Chapter 14). These effects are more likely to occur in persons with other risk factors for these conditions, such as those with diabetes.

Ciprofloxacin inhibits the metabolism of **caffeine** and theophylline by cytochrome P450 1A2. Persons taking these drugs should reduce their caffeine intake to avoid excessive central nervous system stimulation, and theophylline doses may need to be reduced. Even in the absence of caffeine, fluoroquinolones can cause restlessness, anxiety, light-headedness, confusion, and insomnia. Because of the plethora of adverse effects caused by these drugs, fluoroquinolones should only be used when alternative treatments are not available or effective.

OTHER ANTIBACTERIAL DRUGS
Nitrofurantoin
Nitrofurantoin is a synthetic nitrofuran derivative administered orally that is rapidly excreted in the urine. For this reason, its clinical use is limited to the treatment of **lower urinary tract infections** leading to cystitis (inflammation of the bladder). Ingesting nitrofurantoin with food enhances its absorption and reduces the risk of gastrointestinal irritation.

Nitrofurantoin is bactericidal against gram-positive and gram-negative bacteria that commonly cause acute lower urinary tract infections, including *E. coli, Enterococcus fecalis, K. pneumoniae,* and *Staphylococcus saprophyticus.* It is recommended that nitrofurantoin be used to treat acute cystitis when resistance to TMP-SMX exceeds 20% in the local community. In this setting, the drug is taken for 5 days. Nitrofurantoin is not active against *Proteus* species, *Serratia* species, or *P. aeruginosa,* but acquired microbial resistance to nitrofurantoin has not been a significant clinical problem.

Nitrofurantoin is usually well tolerated, but it can cause gastrointestinal irritation, nausea, vomiting, and diarrhea. A **macrocrystalline formulation** of the drug is employed to avoid these adverse effects. The large drug crystals in this formulation dissolve slowly in the gut, producing less gastrointestinal distress than other formulations. Less common adverse effects of nitrofurantoin include pulmonary fibrosis, hepatitis, and hematologic toxicity.

Daptomycin
Daptomycin is a **cyclic lipopeptide** antibiotic that exerts a rapid bactericidal effect against most **gram-positive organisms,** including many drug-resistant strains. Its antibacterial effect results from insertion of the lipophilic daptomycin tail into the **bacterial cell membrane,** causing membrane depolarization and potassium efflux and leading to the arrest of nucleic acid and protein synthesis and cell death.

Daptomycin is active against strains of **methicillin-resistant *Staphylococcus aureus*** (MRSA), **vancomycin intermediate** and **resistant *S. aureus,*** and some strains of **vancomycin-resistant enterococci.** Daptomycin has been approved for the treatment of MRSA skin and skin-structure infections that are a complication of surgery, diabetic foot ulcers, and burns. It has also been approved for MRSA bacteremia and for right-sided infective endocarditis (but not left-sided) caused by susceptible organisms. Daptomycin binds to lung surfactant and should not be used for treating pneumonia. Other agents used to treat infections caused by drug-resistant, gram-positive organisms include vancomycin, quinupristin-dalfopristin, linezolid, and tigecycline, as described in Chapter 39.

Daptomycin is generally well tolerated but may cause **muscle toxicity.** The risk of this adverse effect is diminished by giving the drug once a day intravenously to minimize trough drug levels.

Polymyxin B
Polymyxin B is a polypeptide antibiotic that interacts with the phospholipid component of bacterial **cell membranes** to disrupt cell membrane integrity and permit cytoplasmic components to leak out of the cell. The antibiotic is active against most **gram-negative bacilli,** including *Pseudomonas aeruginosa,* but it is not active against *Proteus* species. Polymyxin B is formulated in creams and ointments with other agents active against gram-positive species, such as bacitracin, neomycin, and trimethoprim. These preparations are used for the topical treatment of minor **skin and ocular infections.**

Polymyxin B can cause considerable **nephrotoxicity** and **neurotoxicity** when given parenterally. Although the drug has been used to treat systemic infections caused by gram-negative organisms, safer drugs are usually employed.

Rifaximin
Rifaximin is a nonabsorbed orally administered antibiotic derived from rifampin. It is used to treat **travelers diarrhea** in patients 12 years of age or older, to reduce recurrences of **hepatic encephalopathy,** and to relieve symptoms of **irritable bowel disease (IBS).** Patients with IBS often have disturbed intestinal microflora, which may be improved by rifaximin treatment. In a 10-week trial of the drug in IBS, rifaximin reduced abdominal pain and discomfort and improved stool consistency compared with a placebo.

Travelers diarrhea is usually a self-limited illness lasting several days acquired by drinking water or eating foods contaminated with various intestinal bacteria. The most common causes are enterotoxigenic or enteroaggregative **strains of *E. coli.*** Clinical trials indicate that rifaximin is about as effective as ciprofloxacin for travelers diarrhea caused by *E. coli,* but it is not effective in patients with fever or blood in the stool or in persons infected with *Campylobacter jejuni.* For mild to moderate travelers diarrhea, nonprescription loperamide or bismuth subsalicylate usually relieves symptoms in less than 24 hours. Hence, rifaximin and other antibacterial agents should be reserved for treating prolonged or severe travelers diarrhea.

For patients at risk of **hepatic encephalopathy** because of hepatic cirrhosis or other liver disease, rifaximin is believed to decrease colonic bacteria that convert foodstuffs to ammonia and other waste products. Ammonia is normally absorbed into the circulation and metabolized by the liver, but it may accumulate in persons with liver disease and impair brain function, causing confusion, lethargy, disturbed sleep, and other signs of neuropsychological impairment (encephalopathy). Lactulose is also used for this purpose, as described in Chapter 28.

In clinical trials, the side effects of rifaximin were similar in nature and frequency to those observed in persons taking a placebo.

Fidaxomicin

Fidaxomicin (Dificid) is used to treat diarrhea caused by *Clostridiodes difficile* infection. The drug is an orally effective macrolide antibiotic that inhibits **RNA polymerases** and RNA synthesis in susceptible bacteria. Some experts suggest using metronidazole for mild to moderate C. *difficile* infections, vancomycin for severe infections, and fidaxomicin to prevent recurrences after treatment.

SUMMARY OF IMPORTANT POINTS

- Sulfonamides and trimethoprim inhibit sequential steps in bacterial folic acid synthesis. Sulfonamides inhibit dihydropteroate synthase and the synthesis of dihydrofolate, whereas trimethoprim inhibits folate reductase and the formation of tetrahydrofolate.
- The combination of sulfamethoxazole and trimethoprim (TMP-SMX) is primarily used to treat urinary tract infections, upper respiratory tract infections, and infections caused by *P. carinii* or *N. asteroides*.
- Fluoroquinolones inhibit DNA topoisomerase and have bactericidal activity against a wide range of pathogens. Many fluoroquinolones, including ciprofloxacin, are used to treat a variety of infections, including urinary tract and gastrointestinal tract infections, bone and joint infections, skin infections, and anthrax exposure.
- Broad-spectrum fluoroquinolones (e.g., moxifloxacin) are also used to treat community-acquired pneumonia caused by pneumococci, *Chlamydia pneumoniae*, *Klebsiella pneumoniae*, *Mycoplasma pneumoniae*, and *Legionella pneumophila*.
- Fluoroquinolones can cause tendonitis, tendon rupture, and peripheral neuropathy and should not be prescribed for children, adolescents, and nursing or pregnant women.
- Nitrofurantoin is a urinary tract antiseptic that is effective in treating uncomplicated urinary tract infections.

- Polymyxin B is primarily used in combination with other drugs to treat superficial ocular and skin infections.
- Daptomycin, a unique lipopeptide antibiotic, is used to treat infections caused by methicillin and vancomycin-resistant staphylococci and vancomycin-sensitive and resistant enterococci.
- Rifaximin is a nonabsorbed rifampin derivative used to treat travelers diarrhea, prevent hepatic encephalopathy, and relieve symptoms of irritable bowel syndrome.

Review Questions

1. A woman being treated for an infection complains of heel pain and is found to have an inflamed Achilles tendon. Which agent most likely caused this adverse effect?
   (A) trimethoprim
   (B) daptomycin
   (C) sulfacetamide
   (D) ciprofloxacin
   (E) polymyxin B
2. Which antimicrobial drugs disrupt the bacterial cell membrane?
   (A) trimethoprim and sulfamethoxazole
   (B) polymyxin B and daptomycin
   (C) rifaximin and fidaxomicin
   (D) ciprofloxacin and moxifloxacin
   (E) nitrofurantoin and fosfomycin
3. Which condition predisposes a person to drug-induced hemolytic anemia?
   (A) immunodeficiency
   (B) folate deficiency
   (C) glucose-6-phosphate dehydrogenase deficiency
   (D) iron deficiency
   (E) thiamine deficiency
4. A woman with travelers diarrhea was treated with an agent that is not absorbed from the gut. Which agent was most likely used for this condition?
   (A) ciprofloxacin
   (B) rifaximin
   (C) trimethoprim-sulfamethoxazole
   (D) daptomycin
   (E) nitrofurantoin
5. Mutations to the alpha subunit of DNA gyrase may cause bacterial resistance to which drug?
   (A) trimethoprim
   (B) gatifloxacin
   (C) sulfamethoxazole
   (D) daptomycin
   (E) nitrofurantoin

CHAPTER 41

Antimycobacterial Drugs for Treating Tuberculosis and Other Diseases

CLASSIFICATION OF ANTIMYCOBACTERIAL DRUGS

Drugs for Tuberculosis

- Isoniazid[a]
- Pyrazinamide
- Rifampin (RIFADIN)
- Ethambutol (MYAMBUTOL)

Drugs for Mycobacterium Avium-Intracellulare Infections

- Azithromycin (ZITHROMAX)
- Clarithromycin (BIAXIN)[b]
- Ciprofloxacin (CIPRO)
- Rifabutin (MYCOBUTIN)

Drugs for Leprosy

- Dapsone
- Rifampin (RIFADIN)
- Clofazimine (LAMPRENE)
- Thalidomide (THALOMID)

[a] Also amikacin, streptomycin, capreomycin, ciprofloxacin, ethionamide, kanamycin, rifapentine (PRIFTIN), bedaquiline (SIRTURO), and pretomanid (PRETOMANID TABLET).
[b] Also amikacin.

OVERVIEW

This chapter focuses on drugs used to treat **tuberculosis (TB)**, *Mycobacterium avium-intracellulare* infections, and **leprosy (Hansen disease).** TB claims a life every 10 seconds, and global mortality rates are increasing despite the use of chemotherapy. Apathy, poverty, and drug resistance are all contributing to our inability to fight this chronic disease, especially in developing countries where it is most prevalent. The global TB–human immunodeficiency virus (HIV) coepidemic poses an additional challenge to public health and health care professionals. Effective treatment of TB now requires the use of increasingly complex drug regimens for at least 6 months and often much longer. TB drug research has increased in recent years, and new agents are being tested, but a breakthrough has yet to occur. There is an urgent need for drugs that are active against dormant and sequestered organisms to shorten the course of treatment.

MYCOBACTERIAL INFECTIONS

Mycobacteria are acid-fast bacilli that cause a variety of diseases, including TB, leprosy, and localized or disseminated *M. avium-intracellulare* infections (Box 41.1).

TB is caused by *Mycobacterium tuberculosis*, which initially infects the lungs after transmission via aerosol droplets

expelled from an infected person by sneezing and coughing. After infecting pulmonary alveoli, the organism invades macrophages that aggregate with connective tissue to form granulomas and caseous lesions that protect the organism from the immune system and chemotherapy drugs. These often **dormant, sequestered organisms** contribute to the chronic nature of the infection and its long, difficult treatment.

Atypical mycobacteria, including *Mycobacterium kansasii* and members of the *M. avium-intracellulare* complex, can cause infections resembling TB. About one-third of the world's population has a latent (asymptomatic) *M. tuberculosis* infection, and about 10% of these will eventually develop active TB, contributing to the 9 million new cases and nearly 2 million deaths that occur annually. In Western countries, the incidence of TB declined after the advent of effective drug therapy and improved public health measures, but the emergence of highly drug-resistant organisms has posed new challenges to clinicians.

M. avium-intracellulare infections are seen most frequently in immunocompromised patients (e.g., those with acquired immunodeficiency syndrome [AIDS]) and often take the form of **pulmonary disease, lymphadenitis,** or **bacteremia.** In immunocompetent persons with chronic bronchitis or emphysema, exposure to *M. avium-intracellulare* can also result in pulmonary infections.

Leprosy, or Hansen disease, results from infection of the **skin and peripheral nervous system** with *Mycobacterium leprae.* This organism grows slowly, and the disease exhibits a progressive course over several decades. Leprosy is not highly contagious, and transmission of infection requires prolonged close contact with an infected individual. The disease occurs in two primary forms, **lepromatous leprosy** and **tuberculoid leprosy,** each of which has a characteristic pathophysiology and clinical presentation. If leprosy is not treated, it ultimately causes severe **deformities and disabilities.** Treatment of leprosy can require **years of therapy** with antimycobacterial agents, although the introduction of newer drugs has enabled the use of shorter courses of therapy for many patients. Largely due to the World Health Organization's global strategy to treat and prevent leprosy, the worldwide **prevalence of leprosy has declined** from tens of millions of cases in the 1960s to several hundred thousand cases today.

Drug Regimens

The goals of TB chemotherapy are to kill tubercle bacilli rapidly, eliminate dormant and sequestered bacilli, and prevent disease relapse and transmission. Current treatment recommendations for TB and other mycobacterial

BOX 41.1 A CASE OF COUGH, NIGHT SWEATS, AND LETHARGY

CASE PRESENTATION

A 42-year-old man is seen at a public health clinic. He reports a productive cough, chills, fever, night sweats, loss of appetite, and feeling tired for the past month. He has a history of knife wounds and was jailed for 3 months after a barroom fight 2 years ago. His chest radiograph shows patchy infiltrates in both upper lobes, and a sputum sample is found to contain acid-fast bacilli. He is given a Mantoux tuberculin skin test, which has a positive result with a 15-mm induration 72 h later. After completing laboratory work that will include a complete blood count, liver function tests, and chemistry profile, he will begin standard four-drug therapy for tuberculosis (TB) because the incidence of multiple-drug–resistant TB in his community is low. Liver function tests and a red-green color discrimination test will be conducted every 2 to 4 weeks throughout his treatment. The patient will be isolated until his sputum is negative for tubercle bacilli, and a public health nurse will visit him regularly to provide care and verify adherence to the treatment regimen.

CASE DISCUSSION

Tubercle bacilli are transmitted on microdroplets expelled by coughing from persons with active infections. Person-to-person transmission requires close contact with an active case and usually leads to a latent infection. Active infections typically occur months or years later when latent TB emerges as a result of decreased immune function, poor nutrition, physical stress, or other insults. The man in the present case has classic signs and symptoms of TB. The definitive diagnosis is based on finding acid-fast bacilli in sputum and a positive tuberculin test result. Effective therapy will sterilize respiratory secretions in a few weeks or less, but eradication of dormant organisms from infected tissues requires lengthy exposure to antitubercular drugs. The prolonged therapy for this disease often leads to drug toxicity and emergence of drug-resistant organisms. There is an urgent need for new drugs that rapidly kill dormant and sequestered organisms.

infections are listed in Table 41.1. Treatment should be guided by **drug susceptibility testing** of the patient's infecting organism at the start of therapy, when treatment fails to sterilize the patient's sputum, and when a relapse of TB occurs after previous treatment. **Isolation of patients** with TB in single-person rooms is essential until sputum cultures are negative, and extended isolation may be required to prevent the spread of drug-resistant strains. **Multidrug therapy** for at least 6 months is required to cure TB. Because of the long duration of treatment and difficulties with patient adherence, **directly observed therapy (DOT),** in which a health care provider observes each drug administration, is the recommended treatment protocol.

Because of the long duration of therapy required to treat TB, attempts have been made to simplify drug regimens and improve adherence to prescribed treatments. **Intermittent administration of drugs** has been found to enable better supervision of drug administration at less cost and with no reduction in efficacy. However, intermittent therapy does increase the risk of acute, dose-related adverse reactions. Clinical studies have found that TB treatments may be given three times a week throughout the full course of therapy, and just twice a week during the continuation phase without loss of effectiveness. The only exception is

for patients with advanced HIV coinfection, who should receive daily TB therapy.

Since the 1980s, the prevalence of **multidrug-resistant TB** (MDR-TB) and **extensively drug-resistant TB** (XDR-TB) has been increasing at an alarming rate. MDR-TB is defined as resistance to at least isoniazid and rifampin, and XDR-TB is defined as MDR-TB plus resistance to fluoroquinolones and at least one of the **second-line injectable drugs** (amikacin, capreomycin, or kanamycin). The treatment of drug-resistant TB necessitates administration of second-line drugs that are less effective and more toxic than first-line drugs. In some cases of resistant TB, it may take up to 2 years of therapy to eradicate the pathogen, and many cases of drug-resistant TB are fatal.

DRUGS FOR MYCOBACTERIAL INFECTIONS

Drugs for Tuberculosis

The drugs initially used to treat most patients with TB are referred to as **first-line** drugs and consist of **isoniazid, ethambutol,** and **pyrazinamide** (which are synthetic drugs), and **rifampin** which is an antibiotic. These drugs are described later, and their properties are shown in Table 41.2.

Second-line drugs are reserved to treat patients infected with organisms that are resistant to first-line drugs and patients with HIV coinfection. They include rifabutin and rifapentine, several fluoroquinolone drugs (see Chapter 40), capreomycin, ethionamide, amikacin, kanamycin, and others. Most of the second-line drugs are not discussed further in this chapter.

Isoniazid

The introduction of isoniazid (**isonicotinic acid hydrazide [INH]**) in the 1950s revolutionized the treatment of TB, and it has remained the mainstay of most drug regimens for 60 years.

Pharmacokinetics. Isoniazid is usually given orally, though a parenteral formulation is available. It is well absorbed from the gut and widely distributed to tissues where it reaches intracellular concentrations sufficiently high to be effective against organisms in caseous granulomas.

Isoniazid is extensively metabolized, and the parent compound and its metabolites are excreted in the urine. The primary metabolite, **acetylisoniazid,** is formed by conjugation of acetate with isoniazid in a reaction catalyzed by **acetyltransferase,** an enzyme whose activity is genetically determined. **Slow acetylation** is an autosomal recessive trait, and persons with the slow phenotype are homozygous for the slow allele. Persons with the fast phenotype are either heterozygous or homozygous dominant. Because of the different rates of acetylation of isoniazid, persons with the fast phenotype have lower plasma isoniazid concentrations than persons with the slow phenotype (Fig. 41.1), though fast acetylators can eradicate M. *tuberculosis.* Persons with the slow phenotype have higher drug levels and are more likely to experience certain adverse drug reactions (see later).

The prevalence of phenotypes varies from population to population. The slow phenotype predominates in some Middle Eastern populations, whereas the fast phenotype predominates in Japanese populations. In the United States, about half the population exhibits each phenotype.

A small amount of acetylisoniazid is converted to isonicotinic acid and **acetylhydrazine.** Investigators believe

TABLE 41.1   Regimens for Treating Mycobacterial Infections

SITUATION	PREFERRED THERAPY	ALTERNATIVE THERAPY
Prevention of tuberculosis in neonates and children <5 years of age exposed to tuberculosis	Isoniazid 10 mg/kg/day for 3 months	
Latent tuberculosis (formerly called *prophylaxis*)	Isoniazid for 9 months (adults: 5 mg/kg/day; children: 10 mg/kg/day)	Rifampin for 4 months (for isoniazid resistant strains)
Active tuberculosis[a]		
Isoniazid resistance <4%	Isoniazid, rifampin, pyrazinamide, and ethambutol for 2 months, followed by 4 months of isoniazid and rifampin	Rifabutin preferred for HIV-infected patients; rifapentine may be used in place of rifampin
Isoniazid resistance >4%	Rifampin, pyrazinamide, ethambutol ± a fluoroquinolone for 6 months	Rifabutin or rifapentine in place of rifampin
Rifampin resistance	Isoniazid, ethambutol, and a fluoroquinolone for 12–18 months, with pyrazinamide for 2 months	
Isoniazid and rifampin resistance	A fluoroquinolone, pyrazinamide, ethambutol, and amikacin for 18–24 months	Other second-line drugs
Multidrug resistance	4–5 drugs to which the organism is susceptible for 18–24 months; may include bedaquiline	Second-line drugs, such as capreomycin, amikacin, and kanamycin
Mycobacterium avium-intracellulare prophylaxis	Azithromycin weekly or clarithromycin twice daily	Rifabutin
M. avium-intracellulare treatment	Clarithromycin or azithromycin plus ethambutol and/or rifabutin	Preferred therapy plus ciprofloxacin and/or amikacin
Leprosy		
Tuberculoid	Dapsone + rifampin	
Lepromatous	Dapsone + rifampin + clofazimine	

HIV, Human immunodeficiency virus.
[a]Preferred regimens are listed, but alternatives are available.

TABLE 41.2   Pharmacokinetic Properties of Antimycobacterial Drugs[a]

DRUG	ROUTE OF ADMINISTRATION	ORAL BIOAVAILABILITY	ELIMINATION HALF-LIFE	ROUTES OF ELIMINATION
Azithromycin	Oral	37%	12 h	Biliary excretion
Bedaquiline	Oral	Increased by food	5–6 months	Metabolism
Ciprofloxacin	Oral or IV	75%	4 h	Metabolism; renal excretion
Clarithromycin	Oral	62%	5 h	Biliary and renal excretion
Clofazimine	Oral	55%	70 days	Biliary and fecal excretion
Dapsone	Oral	Approximately 100%	28 h[b]	Metabolism; renal excretion
Ethambutol	Oral	Approximately 100%	3.5 h	Metabolism; renal and fecal excretion
Isoniazid	Oral or IM	Approximately 100%	2.5 h[b]	Metabolism; renal excretion
Pyrazinamide	Oral	Approximately 100%	9.5 h	Metabolism; renal excretion
Rifabutin	Oral	16%	45 h	Metabolism; renal and biliary excretion
Rifampin	Oral or IV	Approximately 100%	2.75 h	Metabolism; renal and biliary excretion
Rifapentine	Oral	70%	13 h	Metabolism (active metabolite); renal and biliary excretion
Streptomycin	IM	NA	2 h	Renal excretion
Thalidomide	Oral	Approximately 90%	6 h	Metabolism; renal excretion

[a]Values shown are the mean of values reported in the literature.
[b]The half-lives of dapsone and isoniazid exhibit genetic variation.
IM, Intramuscular; *IV,* intravenous; *NA,* not applicable.

that acetylhydrazine is responsible for the **hepatic toxicity** of the drug.

Mechanism of Action and Resistance. Isoniazid acts by inhibiting the synthesis of **mycolic acid,** a cell wall component responsible for the **acid-fast staining property** of mycobacteria. The mechanism of action of isoniazid and other anti-TB drugs is shown in Fig. 41.2. Isoniazid is activated by mycobacterial **catalase-peroxidase** encoded

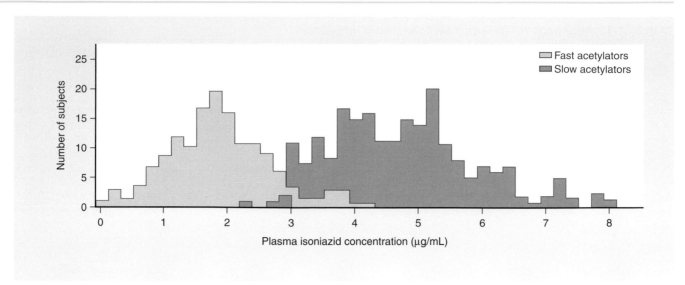

FIG. 41.1 Bimodal distribution of plasma isoniazid concentrations. Plasma concentrations of isoniazid were measured 2 h after the administration of a single 300-mg dose of isoniazid to each member of a general population of human subjects. Subjects with the fast acetylation phenotype showed lower plasma drug concentrations than did subjects with the slow acetylation phenotype.

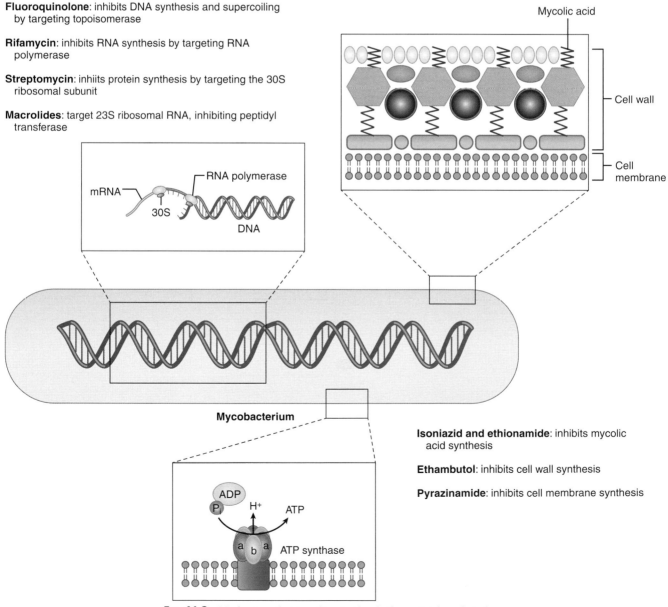

Fluoroquinolone: inhibits DNA synthesis and supercoiling by targeting topoisomerase

Rifamycin: inhibits RNA synthesis by targeting RNA polymerase

Streptomycin: inhiits protein synthesis by targeting the 30S ribosomal subunit

Macrolides: target 23S ribosomal RNA, inhibiting peptidyl transferase

Isoniazid and ethionamide: inhibits mycolic acid synthesis

Ethambutol: inhibits cell wall synthesis

Pyrazinamide: inhibits cell membrane synthesis

FIG. 41.2 Mechanism of action of Isoniazid and other anti-tuberculosis drugs.

by the **katG gene** and forms a complex with reduced nicotinamide adenine dinucleotide (NADH) that inhibits a reductase enzyme involved in the synthesis of mycolic acid. Mycobacterial **resistance to isoniazid** is increasingly prevalent and is often due to mutations to the katG gene.

Spectrum and Indications. Isoniazid is bactericidal against sensitive strains of M. *tuberculosis* and some strains of M. *kansasii*. It has little activity against M. *avium-intracellulare* and is not active against M. *leprae* and other bacteria.

Isoniazid is part of the standard four-drug regimen for TB for persons without resistance to isoniazid (see Table 41.2). These drugs are believed to kill different populations of TB bacilli, which include rapidly growing organisms and dormant (stationary phase) bacteria. Isoniazid, together with rifampin and pyrazinamide, eradicates rapidly growing organisms during the first 2 months of therapy. During the next 4 months of treatment, isoniazid and rifampin act against dormant bacteria that slowly revert to actively growing forms.

Isoniazid is also given to treat **latent TB** (formerly called *prophylaxis*) in persons with a positive reaction to the tuberculin skin test who meet one of the following criteria: HIV positive; recently infected (conversion from a negative to a positive tuberculin skin test result in the past 2 years); chest x-ray study showing nonprogressive tuberculous disease; or predisposing conditions including illicit injected drug use, diabetes mellitus, immunosuppression, or certain diseases. The preferred duration of treatment for latent TB is 9 months, but 6 months may be sufficient in some cases. Rifampin can be used to treat latent TB if isoniazid is contraindicated or if the mycobacterial strain is known to be resistant to isoniazid (see Table 41.2).

Isoniazid is given to prevent TB in neonates and children who have had close contact with persons in whom active TB was recently diagnosed.

Adverse Effects. Isoniazid is fairly well tolerated by most patients, but it causes elevation of serum transaminase levels and potentially life-threatening **hepatitis** in some individuals. The risk of developing hepatitis during isoniazid therapy is low in persons under 35 years of age, is moderate in persons aged 35 to 50 years, and is highest in persons over 50 years of age. Isoniazid treatment of latent TB, however, appears to have a positive risk-benefit ratio in patients over 35 years of age if they are monitored appropriately for hepatotoxicity. Patients who have TB and are being treated with isoniazid should have their serum transaminase levels monitored periodically and should be told to inform their health care provider if they develop symptoms of hepatitis.

Isoniazid can also cause **peripheral neuritis** resulting from drug-induced **pyridoxine (vitamin B6) deficiency** due to direct inactivation of pyridoxine by the drug. Symptoms of this neuritis include paresthesia and numbness of the fingers and toes. This adverse effect is more likely to occur in individuals with the **slow acetylator phenotype** because they have higher plasma concentrations of isoniazid. It can be prevented or treated by administering pyridoxine supplements to patients who are taking isoniazid.

In rare circumstances, isoniazid causes toxic encephalopathy or seizures. Hematologic abnormalities, such as granulocytosis, anemia, or thrombocytopenia, can occur.

Ethambutol

Ethambutol is a butanol (butyl alcohol) derivative that has bacteriostatic activity against mycobacterial organisms. As shown in Table 41.2, it is used in combination with other drugs to treat TB or M. *avium-intracellulare* infections. Ethambutol inhibits the enzyme **arabinosyl transferase** and the synthesis of arabinogalactan required for mycobacterial **cell wall formation,** leading to increased permeability of the cell wall. Mutations to the gene for arabinosyl transferase may confer resistance to ethambutol.

Ethambutol is administered orally, undergoes hepatic biotransformation, and is excreted in the urine and feces. The drug is generally well tolerated, but it can produce dose-dependent **optic neuritis** and **impaired red-green color discrimination.** It can also cause hyperuricemia, gout, hepatitis, and thrombocytopenia.

Pyrazinamide

Pyrazinamide is an important drug in TB therapy because of its more **rapid bactericidal action** and sterilizing effect compared with other agents. Including pyrazinamide in initial treatment regimens made it possible to reduce the treatment duration to 6 months, whereas other therapies required 9 to 12 months. Pyrazinamide is usually **given in combination** with isoniazid, rifampin, and ethambutol (see Table 41.2).

Pyrazinamide is a nicotinamide derivative converted in mycobacteria to an active metabolite, **pyrazinoic acid,** by the enzyme pyrazinamidase. Mutations to this enzyme may confer bacterial resistance to the drug. Pyrazinoic acid inhibits the growth of M. *tuberculosis* by inhibiting fatty acid synthesis required for cell membrane function. It may also inhibit ribosomal translation of messenger RNA, a mechanism proposed to explain its ability to kill dormant, nongrowing organisms.

Pyrazinamide is given orally, is widely distributed to tissues, and is largely converted to pyrazinoic acid in the liver. A small amount of the drug is excreted unchanged in the urine, along with its metabolite. Adverse reactions to pyrazinamide include arthralgia, hyperuricemia and **gout,** hematologic toxicity, fever, **hepatitis,** and an increase in the serum iron concentration.

Rifampin

Chemistry and Pharmacokinetics. Rifampin (also known as **rifampicin**) is a derivative of the antibiotic called **rifamycin** that has improved pharmacokinetic properties compared with the natural antibiotic. Rifampin is rapidly absorbed after oral administration and is converted in the liver to an active metabolite, desacetyl-rifampin. The drug and its metabolite are widely distributed to tissues and fluids, including lung tissue, saliva, and peritoneal and pleural fluids. Rifampin undergoes significant enterohepatic cycling. It is primarily excreted in the feces via biliary elimination, but up to 30% is excreted in the urine.

Mechanisms, Spectrum, and Indications. Rifampin is a **broad-spectrum antibiotic** that has significant activity against many gram-positive, gram-negative, and acid-fast bacilli, including M. *tuberculosis*, M. *avium-intracellulare*, M. *kansasii*, and M. *leprae*. The drug acts by binding to the β subunit of **DNA-dependent RNA polymerase.** This prevents the enzyme from binding to DNA and inhibits DNA transcription and RNA synthesis. Rifampin does not bind to the RNA polymerase of eukaryotic cells.

Rifampin is usually combined with isoniazid, ethambutol, and pyrazinamide to treat **TB,** and it can be combined with a sulfone (e.g., dapsone) or with clofazimine to treat leprosy (see later). Rifampin penetrates inflamed meninges and reaches levels in the cerebrospinal fluid that are 10% to 20% of levels in the serum. Hence, it can be used in the treatment of tubercular meningitis.

Rifampin is also given prophylactically to prevent several types of diseases. It is used as an alternative to isoniazid for latent TB when resistance to isoniazid is known or suspected. Rifampin is also given to individuals who have been exposed to *Haemophilus influenzae* type b and are at risk of transmitting infection to unvaccinated children 4 years of age or younger. Rifampin has been used to prevent meningococcal disease in individuals who have had close contact with a *Neisseria meningitidis*–infected person or an asymptomatic meningococcal carrier, though ciprofloxacin or ceftriaxone are often preferred. Rifampin is also used to eliminate staphylococcal carriage and to treat staphylococcal infections in combination with vancomycin and gentamicin, such as staphylococcal endocarditis. Rifampin is occasionally used to treat *Legionella pneumophila* infections in combination with a macrolide or a fluoroquinolone drug.

Bacterial Resistance. The major drawback of rifampin is the tendency for microbes to acquire resistance during exposure to the drug. Resistance is usually caused by the decreased affinity of RNA polymerase for rifampin. Because of the potential for the emergence of resistance during treatment, rifampin is **never used alone** to treat active infections.

Adverse Effects and Interactions. The adverse effects of rifampin are usually mild, but the drug can impair liver function, elevate serum bilirubin and transaminase levels, and cause **hepatitis.** Liver function should be tested during treatment, and rifampin should be discontinued if signs or symptoms of hepatic dysfunction become evident. Alcohol consumption appears to increase the risk of hepatitis and should be avoided in persons being treated for TB.

A **hypersensitivity reaction,** manifesting as a flulike illness with chills, fever, fatigue, and headache, develops in as many as 50% of persons taking rifampin. This reaction is more common in those who take large doses once or twice a week. High-dose intermittent therapy can also cause renal disease, leukopenia, and thrombocytopenia. Rifampin should be discontinued if purpura develops in persons taking the drug. Rifampin can also cause a reddish-orange to brown **discoloration of saliva, tears, and urine,** and it may cause permanent staining of soft contact lenses.

Rifampin **induces cytochrome P450 isozymes** CYP1A2, CYP2C9, and CYP3A4 and can thereby accelerate the metabolism of other drugs and reduce their serum concentrations and therapeutic effectiveness. The affected drugs include macrolide antibiotics, benzodiazepines, calcium channel blockers, digoxin, estrogens, sulfonylureas, theophylline, and warfarin.

Rifapentine and Rifabutin

Rifapentine is a longer acting rifamycin derivative whose microbiologic activity is similar to that of rifampin. It is indicated for the treatment of pulmonary TB caused by *M. tuberculosis,* typically in a two-phase regimen in which twice-weekly rifapentine is combined with isoniazid, ethambutol, and pyrazinamide for 2 months followed by once-weekly rifapentine and isoniazid for an additional 4 months.

Rifabutin is a semisynthetic antibiotic derived from rifamycin. As with rifampin, it inhibits DNA-dependent RNA polymerase in susceptible bacteria. The drug is active against *M. avium-intracellulare* and most strains of *M. tuberculosis.* It is used for the treatment of **TB** in persons infected with **HIV** and for the prevention of **M. avium-intracellulare** infections (see later). Rifabutin is now preferred over rifampin for treating TB in HIV-infected persons because protease inhibitors can continue to be used to treat HIV infection in persons taking rifabutin but not in persons taking rifampin.

Rifabutin is administered orally once a day with food to reduce gastrointestinal irritation. The drug is highly lipophilic, is widely distributed to tissues, and reaches substantial intracellular concentrations. As with rifampin, rifabutin induces cytochrome P450 enzymes and may reduce serum concentrations of drugs metabolized by these enzymes.

Other Drugs

Amikacin, kanamycin, and **streptomycin** are aminoglycoside antibiotics used to treat TB in cases in which resistance to other drugs is known or suspected. Amikacin is more active than streptomycin against some strains of *M. tuberculosis.* These drugs must be administered parenterally and are not as convenient as other drugs in the treatment of TB.

New Drugs for Tuberculosis

The treatment of TB is desperately in need of new agents active against resistant TB strains and against the dormant and sequestered organisms that contribute to the chronic nature of this infection. **Bedaquiline** is the first unique drug for TB to be developed in more than 40 years and acts by blocking the **proton pump for ATP synthase** in *M. tuberculosis.* It is approved for treating **MDR-TB** in adults and children when another effective treatment regimen cannot be provided. It is administered once daily for 2 weeks and then 3 times per week for an additional 22 weeks, and it should only be used in combination with at least 3 other drugs to which the patient's isolate is susceptible. Patients taking bedaquiline must have an electrocardiogram before treatment is begun and at regular intervals thereafter because the drug can cause prolongation of the QT interval leading to **arrhythmias and sudden death** as a result of blocking the delayed repolarizing potassium channel (*IKr*) in the heart. Patients should also be monitored for adverse liver reactions, and it may cause nausea, headache, and other side effects. The drug interacts with cytochrome P450 enzymes, and dosage adjustments may be needed if other drugs affecting or metabolized by P450 enzymes are given concurrently. For example, rifampin and related antibiotics significantly reduce plasma levels of bedaquiline due to induction of CYP 3A4.

Pretomanid (PRETOMANID TABLET) is the 2nd new molecular entity developed for TB. **Pretomanid destroys actively replicating M. tuberculosis by blocking cell wall production,** as it inhibits mycolic acid biosynthesis. Pretomanid is only **approved for pulmonary extensively drug-resistant (XDR) or treatment-intolerant or nonresponsive multidrug-resistant (MDR) TB** and only when used as part of a combination regimen with **bedaquiline** (see above) **and linezolid,** a protein synthesis inhibitor (see Chapter 39).

DRUGS FOR M. AVIUM-INTRACELLULARE INFECTIONS

Drugs that are active against M. *avium-intracellulare* (*Mycobacterium avium* complex [MAC]) include

ethambutol, rifampin, and **rifabutin; azithromycin** and **clarithromycin** (described in Chapter 39); **ciprofloxacin** (described in Chapter 40); streptomycin and amikacin (described in Chapter 39); and clofazimine. Azithromycin, clarithromycin, or rifabutin is often used alone to prevent MAC infection in HIV-infected and other immunocompromised patients. Various drug combinations are used to treat MAC infections. A current recommendation to treat pulmonary and other MAC infections consists of azithromycin, ethambutol, and rifabutin or rifampin, with rifampin preferred for immunocompetent patients and rifabutin for immunocompromised patients. Effective treatments often require 16 to 24 weeks of drug therapy. Clofazimine, streptomycin, or amikacin is an alternative drug for treating MAC infections in **immunocompromised patients** when other drugs are ineffective or not tolerated.

DRUGS FOR LEPROSY

The treatment of leprosy requires the administration of antimycobacterial drugs for **long periods of time,** ranging from several months to a person's lifetime. The World Health Organization now recommends multidrug therapy for most persons with leprosy. **Multidrug therapy** has been shown to hasten the eradication of bacteria, reduce the duration of active disease, and prevent worsening of disabilities in persons with leprosy. In addition, multidrug therapy appears to reduce overall costs, increase patient compliance, and increase the motivation and availability of leprosy workers.

Sulfones

The sulfones have served as the foundation of drug therapy for leprosy for several decades. These compounds are related to the sulfonamides and have a similar mechanism of action. They **inhibit the synthesis of folic acid** by M. *leprae,* and they exhibit a bacteriostatic action against this organism.

Dapsone, or **diaminodiphenylsulfone,** is the sulfone that is most commonly used in the treatment of leprosy. It is given orally in combination with other drugs (see Table 41.2), is metabolized by acetylation, and is excreted in the urine. Adverse reactions are usually minimal, but dapsone can cause gastrointestinal disturbances, peripheral neuropathy, optic neuritis and blurred vision, proteinuria and nephrotic syndrome, lupus erythematosus–like syndrome, and hematologic toxicity. Individuals who have **glucose-6-phosphate dehydrogenase deficiency** may exhibit **hemolytic anemia** resulting from the oxidation of erythrocyte membranes by dapsone.

Rifampin

Rifampin is the drug with the greatest bactericidal activity against M. *leprae*. For the treatment of leprosy, rifampin is usually combined with dapsone or with dapsone plus clofazimine. It is never used alone because of the probability that organisms will become resistant to it during treatment.

Clofazimine

Clofazimine is a phenazine dye that has antimycobacterial and anti-inflammatory effects. The drug is bactericidal against M. *tuberculosis*, is bacteriostatic against M. *leprae*, and is active against M. *avium-intracellulare*. Clofazimine has little activity against other bacteria. In addition to its antimicrobial effects, the drug enhances the phagocytic activity of neutrophils and macrophages. Clofazimine is

used in combination with dapsone and rifampin to treat lepromatous leprosy.

The anti-inflammatory and immunologic effects of clofazimine may contribute to the drug's efficacy in the prevention and treatment of **erythema nodosum leprosum,** a type II hypersensitivity reaction that may occur during the treatment of patients with lepromatous leprosy. This reaction is characterized by tender erythematous skin nodules with inflammation of subcutaneous fat and acute vasculitis. Clofazimine is usually combined with corticosteroids to treat leprosy that is complicated by erythema nodosum leprosum.

Clofazimine is slowly and incompletely absorbed from the gut, with a bioavailability of about 55%. The highly lipophilic drug is widely distributed to tissues and macrophages, has a long half-life (about 70 days), and remains in the body for years. It slowly undergoes biliary and fecal excretion.

Adverse effects of clofazimine include gastrointestinal distress (anorexia, nausea, vomiting, abdominal pain, and diarrhea), photosensitivity, and discoloration of body secretions and the skin. Because clofazimine can elevate hepatic enzyme levels and cause hepatitis, use of the drug is avoided in persons with hepatic disease.

Thalidomide

Thalidomide was once banned because it caused **phocomelia** (congenital abnormalities of the limbs) in the offspring of women who took it during pregnancy. Subsequent investigations have shown that the drug has immunomodulating actions (see Chapter 45) that are beneficial in the management of several conditions. Thalidomide currently has orphan drug status in the United States and can be used adjunctively to treat TB, leprosy, or erythema nodosum leprosum. The drug can be effective in alleviating the manifestations of erythema nodosum leprosum, possibly because of its ability to stimulate human T cells (particularly the CD8+ cell subset of T cells).

SUMMARY OF IMPORTANT POINTS

- Tuberculosis (TB) and leprosy are chronic mycobacterial infections that often require treatment with multiple drugs for months or years. Combination drug therapy accelerates the eradication of bacteria and reduces the emergence of microbial drug resistance during therapy.
- Most patients with TB are initially treated with a combination of isoniazid, rifampin, ethambutol, and pyrazinamide. Second-line drugs are used to treat TB caused by organisms resistant to first-line drugs.
- Most patients with leprosy are treated with a combination of dapsone and rifampin or a combination of dapsone, rifampin, and clofazimine.
- Isoniazid (isonicotinic acid hydrazide [INH]) is activated by catalase-peroxidase encoded by the *katG* gene and inhibits mycolic acid synthesis. The rate of acetylation of the drug exhibits genetic polymorphism, with some persons showing fast acetylation and some showing slow acetylation.
- Isoniazid can cause age-dependent hepatitis and drug-induced peripheral neuritis due to inactivation of pyridoxine.

- Rifampin is a semisynthetic antibiotic with broad-spectrum activity. It is used in the treatment of TB and leprosy, in the prevention of meningococcal and *H. influenzae* type b infections, and in the treatment of staphylococcal and *L. pneumophila* infections. Adverse effects of rifampin include hepatitis and discoloration of body fluids.
- Pyrazinamide is a bactericidal drug that shortens the duration of therapy for TB.
- Rifabutin, a semisynthetic antibiotic, is used for the prevention and treatment of *M. avium-intracellulare* diseases in individuals who are infected with human immunodeficiency virus or are immunosuppressed. For treatment, rifabutin is usually given in combination with azithromycin or clarithromycin and ethambutol.
- Bedaquiline is a new drug for multidrug-resistant tuberculosis that blocks the proton pump for ATP synthase. The drug may cause adverse cardiac effects and liver toxicity.
- Dapsone is a sulfone drug that forms the foundation of therapy for leprosy. It is used in combination with rifampin and clofazimine.
- Clofazimine is a synthetic dye that has antimycobacterial and anti-inflammatory activity. As with rifampin, it can discolor body fluids.

Review Questions

1. Which drug is recommended for treatment of most persons with latent TB?
   (A) rifampin
   (B) isoniazid
   (C) streptomycin
   (D) ethambutol
   (E) pyrazinamide

2. Which drug inhibits RNA polymerase in *Mycobacteria*?
   (A) rifampin
   (B) ethambutol
   (C) isoniazid
   (D) amikacin
   (E) pyrazinamide

3. A woman being treated for a mycobacterial infection develops optic neuritis. Which agent most likely caused this reaction?
   (A) isoniazid
   (B) rifampin
   (C) pyrazinamide
   (D) ethambutol
   (E) streptomycin

4. Mutations to the *katG* gene may confer resistance to which agent?
   (A) isoniazid
   (B) pyrazinamide
   (C) amikacin
   (D) rifampin
   (E) ethambutol

5. Persons with a high acetyltransferase activity will have comparatively lower plasma levels of which drug?
   (A) pyrazinamide
   (B) rifabutin
   (C) amikacin
   (D) ethambutol
   (E) dapsone

CHAPTER 42

Drugs for the Treatment of Fungal Infections

CLASSIFICATION OF ANTIFUNGAL DRUGS

Polyene Antibiotics

- Amphotericin B (ABELCET, AMBISOME, AMPHOTEC)[a]

Azole Derivatives

- Clotrimazole (GYNE-LOTRIMIN, MYCELEX)
- Fluconazole (DIFLUCAN)
- Itraconazole (SPORANOX)
- Ketoconazole (NIZORAL)
- Efinaconazole (JUBLIA)[b]

Oxaborole Derivatives

- Tavaborole (KERYDIN)

Allylamine Drugs

- Terbinafine (LAMISIL)[c]

Echinocandin Drugs

- Caspofungin (CANCIDAS)[d]

Other Antifungal Drugs

- Ciclopirox (LOPROX, PENLAC)
- Flucytosine (ANCOBON)
- Griseofulvin (GRIS-PEG)
- Tolnaftate (TINACTIN)

[a] Also natamycin (NATACYN) and nystatin (MYKACET); the combination of nystatin and triamcinolone is also available.
[b] Also butoconazole (GYNAZOLE-1), econazole (SPECTAZOLE), oxiconazole (OXISTAT), sulconazole (EXELDERM), terconazole, voriconazole (VFEND), posaconazole (NOXAFIL), secnidazole (SOLOSEC), benznidazole, and isavuconazonium (CRESEMBA).
[c] Also naftifine (NAFTIN), and butenafine (MENTAX).
[d] Also micafungin (MYCAMINE), and anidulafungin (ERAXIS).

OVERVIEW

Fungal Infections

A fungal infection can be described in terms of the causative organism, site of infection, clinical findings, treatment, and prognosis. Pathogenic fungi include yeasts (exist as single cells), molds (multicellular filamentous forms or hyphae), and dimorphic organisms that exist in both yeast and mold forms. Fungal infections (mycoses) include superficial (mucocutaneous), subcutaneous, and systemic infections.

The most common fungal infections are the superficial mucocutaneous mycoses. **Superficial mycoses** include infections of the skin, hair, and nails caused by dermatophyte fungi, most commonly *Epidermophyton*, *Microsporum*, and *Trichophyton* species that feed on keratin in the outer layer of these tissues. Dermatophyte skin and hair infections typically present as a pruritic (itchy) rash and erythema. Examples include **tinea pedis** ("athlete's foot"),

tinea capitis ("ringworm of the scalp"; Box 42.1), **tinea corporis** ("ringworm of the body"), and **tinea cruris** ("jock itch"). **Ringworm** is a colloquial term for an annular (ring-shaped) lesion with a scaling rash and a clear center. Nail dermatophyte infections are known as **tinea unguium** or **onychomycosis.**

Mucocutaneous mycoses are usually caused by **yeasts,** most often *Candida albicans* and other *Candida* species. Affected patients may have oral candidiasis ("thrush"), vaginal candidiasis, or *Candida* infections of the axilla, groin, and gluteal folds (including so-called "diaper rash" in infants). Less common yeasts causing mucocutaneous infections include *Malassezia furfur* (formerly called *Pityrosporum orbiculare*), which causes **tinea versicolor,** a skin infection characterized by hypopigmented and hyperpigmented macules, typically in the shoulder girdle area. *M. furfur* can also cause a form of **seborrheic dermatitis,** characterized by scaling and erythema on the ears, eyebrows, nose, and chest.

The **subcutaneous mycoses** involve the dermis, subcutaneous connective tissue, and muscle. These infections are usually caused by puncture wounds contaminated with soil fungi and include **chromomycosis, pseudallescheriasis,** and **sporotrichosis.**

Systemic mycoses are fungal infections of the internal organs and tissues and include **urinary tract infections, pneumonia, meningitis, esophageal infections,** and **septicemia** (blood infection). Some systemic infections also involve the skin, muscle, joints, and other tissues. These diseases can be chronic and indolent, or invasive and life-threatening. The systemic mycoses are most commonly caused by members of the genera *Aspergillus*, *Blastomyces*, *Candida*, *Coccidioides*, *Cryptococcus*, and *Histoplasma*. Some infections (e.g., **blastomycosis, coccidioidomycosis,** and **histoplasmosis**) endemic to certain geographic regions are found in both immunocompetent and immunocompromised individuals. Other infections (e.g., **aspergillosis, candidiasis, cryptococcosis,** and **mucormycosis**) are more likely to occur in immunocompromised or debilitated patients, such as those receiving immunosuppressive drugs, those with indwelling catheters or prostheses, or those with human immunodeficiency virus (HIV) infection, diabetes, or chronic renal, hepatic, or cardiac diseases. These conditions either suppress cellular immunity or facilitate colonization and infection by fungi. For example, there has been an increased incidence of invasive infections caused by *Aspergillus*, *Scedosporium*, and *Fusarium* species in recipients of hematopoietic stem cell transplants in recent decades.

CLINICAL USES AND MECHANISMS OF ANTIFUNGAL DRUGS

Fungi are eukaryotic organisms whose growth is not inhibited by antibacterial or antiviral drugs. However, drugs that are selectively toxic to fungi have been developed and are available

Polyene antibiotics selectively bind to ergosterol in fungal membranes. This action increases fungal plasma membrane permeability and allows the cytoplasmic contents to leak from the cell. The polyene drugs also bind to a lesser degree to cholesterol in mammalian cells, and this may account for their ability to damage renal cell membranes and cause toxicity.

The mechanism of action of **ciclopirox** is not well understood and appears to involve inhibition of cellular enzymes, DNA repair, and possibly cell division.

The **allylamine drugs** and the **azole derivatives** block distinct steps in ergosterol biosynthesis, but these groups of drugs have little effect on cholesterol biosynthesis in humans. Allylamine drugs, such as terbinafine, inhibit **squalene epoxidase,** which converts squalene to squalene-2,3-oxide, the immediate precursor of lanosterol. The azoles, such as fluconazole, inhibit **14α-demethylase,** a fungal cytochrome P450 enzyme that converts lanosterol to ergosterol.

The **echinocandin drugs** (e.g., caspofungin) represent a new class of antifungal agents that inhibit the synthesis of a **fungal cell wall** component, β-(1,3)-D-glucan. The fungal cell wall surrounds the plasma membrane and normally protects the cell from osmotic and mechanical stress.

Flucytosine, a pyrimidine antimetabolite, affects fungal nucleic acid metabolism. Flucytosine is converted to **5-fluorouracil (5-FU)** in fungal cells by cytosine deaminase, an enzyme not found in mammalian cells. 5-FU is then incorporated into fungal RNA, and this inhibits fungal protein synthesis.

Griseofulvin acts by binding to fungal microtubules, thereby inhibiting microtubule function and mitosis. The mechanism of action of **tolnaftate** is uncertain, but it appears to inhibit squalene epoxidase in a manner similar to allylamine drugs such as terbinafine.

ANTIFUNGAL DRUGS
Polyene Antibiotics
The polyene antibiotics are produced by various soil organisms of the family *Streptomycetaceae* and include amphotericin B, natamycin, and nystatin. Each of these compounds consists of a macrolide (large lactone) ring containing conjugated (side-by-side) double bonds (polyene), with acidic and basic side groups. These drugs are amphoteric because the acidic and basic groups are capable of either donating or accepting a proton (hydrogen ion, H^+), respectively.

Amphotericin B has greater antifungal activity than amphotericin A, which is not used clinically. Amphotericin B is the only polyene drug used to treat systemic and subcutaneous mycoses. The other polyene drugs are limited to topical application for the treatment of superficial and mucocutaneous mycoses.

Amphotericin B
Pharmacokinetics. The pharmacokinetic properties of amphotericin B are listed in Table 42.2. Amphotericin B is available as a deoxycholate complex and as three **lipid formulations** for parenteral administration. As with other polyene antibiotics, it is not absorbed from the gastrointestinal tract.

The dosage of amphotericin B depends on the site and severity of the infection and on the immune status of the

to treat fungal infections in humans and animals. Most of the antifungal drugs inhibit the biosynthesis or function of either the **fungal cell membrane** or the **fungal cell wall.**

As shown in Table 42.1, drugs used in the treatment of systemic and subcutaneous mycoses include a polyene antibiotic (amphotericin B), a number of azole derivatives, three echinocandin drugs (e.g., caspofungin), and flucytosine. The other drugs listed are used in the treatment of superficial mycoses. Amphotericin B tends to be used for treating severe mycoses, whereas the azoles are used for less severe infections. Newer antifungal agents (e.g., voriconazole and caspofungin) can be used to treat invasive *Candida* and *Aspergillus* infections. Flucytosine is usually administered in combination with amphotericin B for the treatment of systemic *Cryptococcus* or *Candida* infections.

Many antifungal drugs act by impairing **plasma membrane function** in fungal cells. The selective toxicity of these drugs is a result of the difference in the sterols found in fungal and mammalian cell membranes. Fungal cell membranes contain **ergosterol,** whereas mammalian cell membranes contain **cholesterol.** Some antifungal drugs bind to ergosterol and thereby increase plasma membrane permeability, whereas other drugs inhibit the synthesis of ergosterol (Fig. 42.1; see Table 42.1).

TABLE 42.1   Clinical Uses and Mechanisms of Antifungal Drugs

	MAJOR CLINICAL INDICATIONS			
DRUG	**SYSTEMIC AND SUBCUTANEOUS INFECTIONS**	**DERMATOPHYTE INFECTIONS**	**MUCOCUTANEOUS INFECTIONS**	**MECHANISM OF ACTION**
Polyene Antibiotics				
Amphotericin B	Infections due to most pathogenic fungi, including *Candida, Cryptococcus, Histoplasma,* and *Aspergillus* species	Not used	Not used	Binds ergosterol in fungal cell membrane; increases membrane permeability
Natamycin	Not used	Not used	*Candida* and *Fusarium* infections	Same as amphotericin B
Nystatin	Not used	Not used	*Candida* infections	Same as amphotericin B
Azole Derivatives				
Clotrimazole	Not used	Infections due to *Epidermophyton, Microsporum,* and *Trichophyton* species	*Candida* infections	Inhibits ergosterol synthesis
Econazole	Not used	Same as clotrimazole	Infections due to *Candida* species and *Malassezia furfur* (tinea versicolor)	Same as clotrimazole
Fluconazole	*Candida* species and *Cryptococcus neoformans*	Not used	*Candida* species	Same as clotrimazole
Itraconazole	*Blastomyces, Histoplasma, Sporothrix* infections	Same as clotrimazole	Not used	Same as clotrimazole
Ketoconazole	Not used	Not used	Seborrheic dermatitis	Same as clotrimazole
Posaconazole	Invasive aspergillosis (salvage therapy), mucormycosis, and *Candida* infections	Not used	Not used	Same as clotrimazole
Voriconazole	Invasive aspergillosis and *Candida* infections	Not used	Not used	Same as clotrimazole
Allylamine Drugs				
Naftifine and terbinafine	Not used	Same as clotrimazole	Not used	Inhibits synthesis of precursor to ergosterol
Other Antifungal Drugs				
Anidulafungin, caspofungin, and micafungin	*Candida* infections and aspergillosis (salvage therapy)	Not used	*Candida* infections	Inhibits fungal cell wall synthesis
Ciclopirox	Not used	Same as clotrimazole	Tinea versicolor (*Malassezia* species)	Inhibits multiple enzymes
Flucytosine	With amphotericin B for cryptococcal meningitis	Not used	Not used	Inhibits nucleic acid synthesis
Griseofulvin	Not used	Tinea capitis and other dermatophyte infections	Not used	Inhibits microtubule function and mitosis
Tolnaftate	Not used	Same as clotrimazole	Not used	Inhibits ergosterol synthesis

patient. Higher doses of amphotericin B are used to treat infections caused by more resistant fungi, especially the *Aspergillus* species, and lower doses are generally used to treat esophageal and urinary tract infections. Concentrations of the drug in cerebrospinal fluid are only 2% to 3% of those in plasma, because amphotericin B does not penetrate the blood-brain barrier very well. Nevertheless, the drug is usually administered intravenously to treat fungal meningitis because of the problems associated with intrathecal administration of the drug. Amphotericin B is extensively metabolized in the liver, and the metabolites are slowly excreted

in the urine. The drug exhibits a biphasic half-life, with an initial half-life of about 24 hours and a terminal half-life of about 15 days.

Spectrum and Indications. Amphotericin B is active against a wide variety of fungi (Table 42.3), and it has been the standard for comparison of other drugs in the treatment of serious fungal infections. It is also active against certain pathogenic protozoa and is used in the treatment of leishmaniasis and amebic encephalitis (see Chapter 44).

Fungal Resistance. Although polyene antibiotics have been used to treat fungal infections for nearly 50 years,

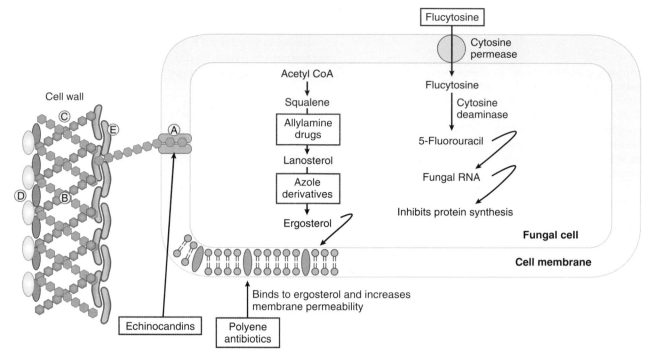

Fig. 42.1 Mechanisms of action of antifungal drugs. The synthesis of ergosterol is inhibited by allylamine drugs and by azole derivatives. Amphotericin B and other polyene antibiotics bind to ergosterol in fungal cell membranes and increase membrane permeability. Ciclopirox may increase membrane permeability by another mechanism (not shown). Flucytosine is accumulated by fungal cells and converted to 5-fluorouracil (5-FU). When 5-FU is incorporated into fungal RNA, protein synthesis is inhibited. Griseofulvin interferes with microtubule function and blocks mitosis (not shown). Caspofungin prevents fungal cell wall synthesis by inhibiting β-1,3 glucan synthase (A) and the synthesis of β-1,3 glucan (B). Other components of the fungal cell wall include β-1,6 glucan (C), mannoproteins (D), and chitin (E).

TABLE 42.2 Pharmacokinetic Properties of Antifungal Drugs[a]

DRUG	ROUTE OF ADMINISTRATION	ORAL BIOAVAILABILITY	ELIMINATION HALF-LIFE	ROUTES OF ELIMINATION
Polyene Antibiotics				
Amphotericin B	Topical, IV, intrathecal, or intraventricular	NA	24 h or 15 days[b]	Metabolism; renal excretion
Natamycin	Topical ocular	NA	NA	NA
Nystatin	Oral or topical	None	NA	NA
Azole Derivatives				
Clotrimazole	Topical	NA	NA	NA
Econazole	Topical	NA	NA	NA
Fluconazole	Oral or IV	95%	35 h	Renal excretion
Itraconazole	Oral	55%	60 h	Biliary, fecal, and renal excretion
Ketoconazole	Oral or topical	Highly variable	8 h	Biliary and fecal excretion
Posaconazole	Oral or IV	Highly variable	28 h	Fecal excretion
Voriconazole	Oral or IV	96%	Dose dependent	Metabolism, renal excretion
Allylamine Drugs				
Naftifine	Topical	NA	2.5 days	Renal and fecal excretion
Terbinafine	Oral or topical	40%	12.5 days	Metabolism; renal excretion
Other Antifungal Drugs				
Caspofungin	IV	NA	11 h	Metabolism
Ciclopirox	Topical	NA	NA	NA
Flucytosine	Oral	82%	3.5 h	Renal excretion
Griseofulvin	Oral	Variable	16 h	Metabolism; renal excretion
Tolnaftate	Topical	NA	NA	NA

[a]Values shown are the mean of values reported in the literature.
[b]For amphotericin B, the values represent the initial and terminal half-life, respectively.
IV, Intravenous; *NA,* not applicable.

relatively few cases of clinical resistance to these drugs have been reported. Fungi that do become resistant to polyenes often have a reduced content of ergosterol in their cell membranes.

Adverse Effects. Amphotericin B has been called "ampho-terrible" because it is one of the most toxic antibiotics in use today. It causes some degree of renal toxicity in about 80% of patients who receive it. Renal toxicity reduces the glomerular filtration rate and contributes to the development of hypokalemia and hypomagnesemia. It also leads to accumulation of creatinine and urea in the blood (azotemia). Electrolytes (especially sodium, potassium, and magnesium) should be monitored weekly during treatment and replacements administered as needed. The toxicity is usually reversible on drug discontinuation.

Lipid formulations of amphotericin B cause less renal toxicity and should be used in persons with renal impairment and those who are intolerant of the traditional deoxycholate formulation. Many clinicians prefer these formulations for treating most systemic fungal infections. These preparations include amphotericin B cholesteryl sulfate (AMPHOTEC), amphotericin B phospholipid complex (ABELCET), and amphotericin B liposomal complex (AMBISOME). The lipid formulations have unique pharmacokinetic characteristics that reduce renal drug concentrations and toxicity. After intravenous administration, the lipid formulations are sequestered by cells of the reticuloendothelial system in the liver and spleen, which slowly release amphotericin B into the circulation over several days, resulting in lower but more sustained plasma levels of the drug.

In addition to causing nephrotoxicity, amphotericin B can cause acute liver failure, cardiac arrhythmias, and hematopoietic disorders such as anemia, leukopenia, and thrombocytopenia. The drug frequently causes less severe but unpleasant infusion-related effects, including **chills, fever, headache, nausea,** and **vomiting.** The severity of these minor adverse effects can be lessened by pretreatment with corticosteroids, antipyretic drugs (e.g., acetaminophen), and antihistamine drugs.

Nystatin and Natamycin

Nystatin, which is active against *Candida* species, is available in various topical formulations, including the following: creams, ointments, and powders for mucocutaneous candidiasis; orally administered tablets and suspensions for intestinal candidiasis; and vaginal tablets for vaginal candidiasis.

Natamycin is active against *Aspergillus, Candida, Fusarium,* and *Penicillium* species and is available as an ophthalmic suspension for the treatment of fungal blepharitis, conjunctivitis, or keratitis.

Azole Derivatives

The azole antifungal agents are synthetic drugs used in the treatment of various mycoses (see Table 42.1). These drugs possess a five-member ring containing two or three nitrogen atoms, which constitute the diazole (imidazole) and triazole compounds, respectively. The **diazole compounds** include butoconazole, clotrimazole, econazole, ketoconazole, oxiconazole, and sulconazole. The **triazole congeners** include efinaconazole, fluconazole, itraconazole, posaconazole, terconazole, and voriconazole.

A closely related analog to the azole derivatives is the new drug **tavaborole,** an oxaborole derivative. Tavaborole is available as an ointment indicated for the topical treatment of onychomycosis of the toenails.

Pharmacokinetics and Drug Interactions
The pharmacokinetic properties of azole antifungal drugs are compared in Table 42.2. Some azoles are applied topically to treat superficial fungal infections, whereas others are given orally to treat the more stubborn superficial mycoses (e.g., onychomycosis). Several of the azole drugs are given orally to treat onychomycosis and systemic and subcutaneous mycoses. Fluconazole, posaconazole, and voriconazole are administered intravenously to treat serious infections.

Most azole drugs are well absorbed from the gut, with the exception of posaconazole. The absorption of ketoconazole, itraconazole, and posaconazole requires the presence of gastric acid, so other drugs that reduce gastric acid should not be administered concurrently. Azoles are widely distributed to tissues and body fluids, but only fluconazole achieves significant concentrations in the cerebrospinal fluid (about 50% of concentrations in the plasma). For this reason, only fluconazole is used in the prophylaxis and treatment of **fungal meningitis.**

The azole derivatives undergo considerable hepatic biotransformation, and the parent compound and metabolites are excreted in the urine and feces.

Many azoles **inhibit human CYP3A4** and their concurrent use with other drugs may cause **drug interactions** when they are given systemically. Drugs whose metabolism is inhibited by azoles include 3-hydroxy-3-methylglutaryl-coenzyme A (HMG-CoA) reductase inhibitors (statins), some benzodiazepines, quinidine, and warfarin. The dosage of these drugs may need to be reduced during concurrent treatment with an azole such as itraconazole. Fluconazole has less affinity for mammalian P_{450} enzymes and causes fewer drug interactions than other azoles.

Spectrum and Indications
Azole drugs can be either fungistatic or fungicidal, depending on the particular organism and the drug concentration. The drugs are active against a wide range of fungi (see Table 42.3) and serve as alternatives to amphotericin B for the treatment of systemic and subcutaneous mycoses. However, recent guidelines recommend testing for drug sensitivity in cases of severe infections, such as with *Candida* blood infections (candidemia). Azoles are also active against most **dermatophytes** that cause tinea infections, including *Epidermophyton floccosum, Microsporum canis, Microsporum gypseum, Trichophyton mentagrophytes, Trichophyton rubrum,* and *Trichophyton tonsurans.* Azoles also inhibit the growth of **yeasts,** including *Candida* and *Malassezia* species. The specific uses of particular azole drugs are discussed later (see the discussion of specific drugs).

Adverse Effects
Azole derivatives are usually well tolerated, but systemic administration can cause **skin rash, elevated hepatic enzyme levels,** hepatic injury, hematopoietic toxicity, or gastrointestinal distress (nausea, vomiting, and diarrhea). A recent US Food and Drug Administration (FDA) warning showed an **increased risk of birth defects** associated with

TABLE 42.3   Pathogens and Management of Selected Systemic and Subcutaneous Mycoses

MYCOSIS	PATHOGENS	TREATMENTS
Aspergillosis	*Aspergillus fumigatus*	Voriconazole, posaconazole, an echinocandin,[a] amphotericin B
Blastomycosis	*Blastomyces dermatitidis*	Itraconazole or amphotericin B; fluconazole for central nervous system disease
Candidiasis, systemic	*Candida albicans, Candida glabrata, Candida parapsilosis, Candida tropicalis, Candida krusei*	An echinocandin,[a] voriconazole, fluconazole, amphotericin B ± flucytosine
Candidiasis, mucocutaneous	*Candida* species	Topical azole (clotrimazole and others), nystatin, oral fluconazole
Coccidioidomycosis[b]	*Coccidioides immitis*	Itraconazole or fluconazole; amphotericin B (severe disease); fluconazole for meningitis
Cryptococcosis	*Cryptococcus neoformans*	Amphotericin B + flucytosine followed by fluconazole for meningitis; fluconazole or amphotericin B for nonmeningeal infections
Fusariosis	*Fusarium* species	Amphotericin B; voriconazole, posaconazole
Histoplasmosis	*Histoplasma capsulatum*	Itraconazole for moderate disease; amphotericin B for severe disease and meningitis ± prednisone or methylprednisolone
Mucormycosis	*Absidia, Rhizopus,* and *Rhizomucor* species	Amphotericin B, posaconazole
Pseudallescheriasis	*Pseudallescheria boydii (Scedosporium apiospermum)*	Voriconazole or itraconazole with surgery
Sporotrichosis	*Sporothrix schenckii*	Superficial: itraconazole or saturated potassium iodide solution; systemic: amphotericin B

[a]Anidulafungin, caspofungin, or micafungin
[b]No treatment needed for uncomplicated pulmonary infection in normal host ("valley fever").

chronic use of fluconazole in high doses (400 to 800 mg/day) during the first trimester of pregnancy. On this basis, the FDA has changed the pregnancy category for fluconazole indications (other than vaginal candidiasis) from category C to category D. Single-dose or short-term use of fluconazole for vaginal candidiasis remains category C.

Specific Drugs

Itraconazole is used to treat blastomycosis and histoplasmosis, but it has poor cerebrospinal fluid penetration and is not used in treating fungal meningitis. Itraconazole is also administered orally to treat **onychomycosis** (fungal infection of the nails). It is available as a capsule and as a liquid formulation in which the drug is packaged in a cyclodextrin (oligosaccharide) ring. Food and cola beverages enhance the absorption of the capsule formulation but not the liquid. Itraconazole has **many drug interactions** due to inhibition of cytochrome P_{450} 3A4 (see earlier).

Fluconazole achieves excellent penetration of the cerebrospinal fluid and is used for prevention of **cryptococcal meningitis** in patients with acquired immunodeficiency syndrome (AIDS), and as follow-up therapy in patients successfully treated with amphotericin B to prevent relapse. Higher doses of fluconazole are recommended for **coccidioidal meningitis.** Fluconazole is also used to treat mucocutaneous (oropharyngeal and esophageal) and disseminated **candidiasis,** such as endocardial candidiasis. Because the drug is excreted in the urine, it is effective for urinary tract infections caused by *Candida* species. A single dose of fluconazole can eradicate acute **vaginal candidiasis.** Fluconazole has **fewer drug interactions** than itraconazole and ketoconazole.

Voriconazole, posaconazole, and **isavuconazonium** have been called **second-generation triazoles** because of their enhanced activity against *Aspergillus* and *Candida*

species. Voriconazole has demonstrated good efficacy in **esophageal and invasive candidiasis.** It is 60 to 100 times more potent than fluconazole against *Candida* species, and it is active against non-*Candida albicans* species that are inherently resistant to fluconazole, such as *Candida krusei.* Voriconazole is also useful in treating **invasive aspergillosis** and has greater fungicidal activity against *Aspergillus fumigatus* than amphotericin B. In addition, voriconazole has been used to treat infections caused by *Cryptococcus, Fusarium, Coccidioides,* and *Pseudallescheria* species.

Although voriconazole is administered intravenously to treat serious fungal infections, patients can be switched to oral voriconazole as they improve because the oral bioavailability of the drug is approximately 96%.

Voriconazole is usually well tolerated. The most common adverse effects are **visual disturbances,** such as altered perception of light, abnormally colored vision (chromatopsia), and photophobia. These events are usually mild and transitory. Elevated serum levels of hepatic enzymes, primarily alanine aminotransferase and aspartate aminotransferase, occurred in 12% to 20% of patients treated with voriconazole and are the dose-limiting adverse effect of this drug. These elevations are usually transitory and reversible, but a few cases of **hepatic failure** and death have been reported. Hence, hepatic enzymes should be routinely monitored during voriconazole therapy.

Posaconazole and **isavuconazonium** are other options for intravenous and oral therapy of systemic infections refractory to other agents, including species of *Aspergillus* and *Fusarium,* and zygomycetes such as *Rhizopus* and *Mucor* species (mucormycosis). Their adverse effects appear to be similar to those of other systemic azole agents.

Ketoconazole is available in oral and topical formulations, but its use has declined with the development of newer agents with greater efficacy and fewer drug interactions. The topical formulation is still used for treating **seborrheic dermatitis.**

Clotrimazole is available in topical formulations for treatment of the mucocutaneous infections, such as **Candida infections** of the mouth, throat, vagina, and vulva; **M. furfur** infection of the skin (tinea versicolor); and **dermatophyte infections** (e.g., tinea pedis and tinea cruris). Likewise, **econazole** and **butoconazole** are available in topical formulations for the treatment of *Candida* and/or dermatophyte infections. **Efinaconazole** (JUBLIA) is the first triazole agent for **topical treatment of onychomycosis** of the toenails. It is applied as a 10% solution with a brush. Although not very effective and extremely expensive, this agent is probably the best topical treatment now available for this infection, and it is a reasonable option for adult patients with mild to moderate infections who cannot take systemic medications. Efinaconazole cured 17% of toenail infections (vs. 3% of those on placebo) and is about two to three times more effective than the next best topical agent, ciclopirox (see later).

Allylamine Drugs

Naftifine and **terbinafine** are allylamines that inhibit ergosterol synthesis (see Fig. 42.1). Although they are primarily used to treat superficial dermatophyte infections, they are also fungistatic against *Candida* species.

Both drugs are available in topical formulations, and terbinafine is also available for oral administration. Terbinafine is often administered orally once a day to treat **onychomycosis.** Fingernail infections usually require 6 weeks of therapy, whereas toenail infections can require 12 weeks of treatment.

Naftifine and terbinafine are well tolerated and rarely cause serious adverse effects.

Echinocandin Drugs

The echinocandin drugs are a class of **semisynthetic antibiotics** that inhibit **fungal cell wall synthesis.** The fungal cell wall is a rigid structure located just outside the plasma membrane. It is composed of chitin and various glucans and glycoproteins and serves to protect fungal cells from osmotic and mechanical stress. The echinocandin drugs inhibit the formation of the cell wall by noncompetitive inhibition of the β-1,3 glucan synthase enzyme complex and formation of β-1,3 glucan (see Fig. 42.1). This action leads to fungal cell lysis and death. Because mammalian cells do not have cell walls, inhibition of glucan synthesis has no direct effect on human cells.

Caspofungin is a semisynthetic derivative of pneumocandin, a fermentation product of a fungus called *Glarea lozoyensis.* Caspofungin has excellent activity against *Candida* species and good activity against *Aspergillus* species, but it is not effective against *Cryptococcus* species. It is active against *Candida albicans, C. glabrata, C. tropicalis,* and *C. krusei,* including strains resistant to azole compounds. Caspofungin is very effective in treating esophageal, oropharyngeal, and invasive candidiasis (74% to 96% response rate). It was moderately effective in treating invasive aspergillosis in one study (45% response rate), but most of these patients had previously failed treatment with amphotericin B or azole drugs.

Caspofungin produces **few adverse effects.** The most common problems have been headache, fever, phlebitis at the site of drug administration, and abnormal liver function tests. Compared with amphotericin B, caspofungin has been very well tolerated. Because of its **poor oral bioavailability,** it must be administered intravenously. Caspofungin has a long half-life and is administered once daily. It appears to provide effective levels in the cerebrospinal fluid in patients with fungal meningitis.

Micafungin and **anidulafungin** are newer echinocandin drugs recommended for prophylaxis and treatment of systemic candidal infections and invasive aspergillosis. They appear to be equivalent to caspofungin in most respects.

Other Antifungal Drugs

Flucytosine

Flucytosine is an orally administered fluorinated pyrimidine analog used in combination with amphotericin B to treat severe fungal infections. The drug is accumulated by fungal cells and is converted to its active metabolite, 5-FU, by cytosine deaminase. The metabolite is incorporated into fungal RNA, and this interferes with fungal protein synthesis (see Fig. 42.1). Unlike fungal cells, human cells lack cytosine deaminase and are unable to activate the drug.

Fungal resistance to flucytosine can result from mutations in genes encoding cytosine deaminase, cytosine permease, or enzymes that incorporate 5-FU into fungal RNA. Because **drug resistance develops rapidly** when flucytosine is given alone, the drug is always given with amphotericin B. This combination produces a synergistic effect against *Candida* and *Cryptococcus* species and is effective in the treatment of pneumonia, meningitis, endocarditis, or septicemia caused by these organisms.

The adverse effects of flucytosine are usually mild. In some patients, however, hematologic toxicity and cardiopulmonary arrest have occurred.

Griseofulvin

Griseofulvin is a fungistatic antibiotic derived from *Penicillium griseofulvum.* It is active against numerous dermatophytes, including *Epidermophyton floccosum, Microsporum audouinii, M. canis, M. gypseum, Trichophyton rubrum, T. tonsurans,* and *T. verrucosum,* but it is not active against Candida or other fungi. Griseofulvin is sometimes used for treatment of **tinea capitis,** which is often caused by *T. tonsurans* (see Box 42.1).

Griseofulvin is a lipophilic drug that is not very soluble in water, and its absorption is increased when it is taken with a high-fat meal. To enhance its dissolution in the gut, microsized (microcrystalline) forms of the drug are used, and the ultramicrosized formulation of griseofulvin is almost completely absorbed. The drug is deposited in keratin precursor cells of the skin, hair, and nails, where it **disrupts microtubule function** and inhibits the mitosis of susceptible dermatophytes. The infected cells are gradually exfoliated and replaced by noninfected tissue. After being metabolized in the liver, griseofulvin is excreted in the urine as inactive metabolites. Some infections respond to griseofulvin therapy in 2 to 8 weeks, but persistent nail infections may require 3 to 6 months of treatment.

Griseofulvin is usually well tolerated, but it can cause dizziness, headache, insomnia, and, rarely, gastrointestinal bleeding, hepatitis, skin rash, or leukopenia. Griseofulvin **induces CYP3A4** and can reduce plasma concentrations of warfarin, oral contraceptives, and barbiturates that are taken concurrently.

Ciclopirox

Ciclopirox is a unique pyridone compound that is active against **dermatophytes,** C. albicans, and M. furfur. It is applied topically twice a day to treat skin infections caused by these organisms, including **tinea versicolor** due to M. furfur. A nail lacquer solution (PENLAC) is available for topical treatment of mild **onychomycosis,** though it is less effective than systemic agents for this infection.

Tolnaftate

Tolnaftate is a nonprescription thiocarbamate drug used to treat **tinea versicolor and mild dermatophyte infections** of the skin. The drug is usually applied twice daily to the affected areas for 2 to 6 weeks as a powder or cream. As with most other topical antifungal drugs, tolnaftate is not reliable for treating infections of the scalp or nail beds.

SUMMARY OF IMPORTANT POINTS

- Polyene antibiotics (amphotericin B, nystatin) increase the permeability of the fungal cell membrane. Azole derivatives and allylamine drugs inhibit synthesis of plasma membrane ergosterol, and caspofungin inhibits cell wall glucan synthesis.
- Flucytosine is converted to 5-FU by fungal cells and is then incorporated into fungal RNA, where it inhibits protein synthesis. Flucytosine is used in combination with amphotericin B for cryptococcal meningitis and candidiasis.
- Amphotericin B is used to treat severe systemic and subcutaneous mycoses, but it often causes chills, fever, nephrotoxicity, and other adverse effects. Lipid formulations have less toxicity and similar efficacy compared with nonlipid formulations.
- Several azole derivatives are used to treat systemic mycoses. Itraconazole can be used to treat blastomycosis, coccidioidomycosis, histoplasmosis, and sporotrichosis. Fluconazole is used to treat candidiasis and cryptococcosis.
- Voriconazole and caspofungin are used to treat invasive candidiasis and aspergillosis. Caspofungin inhibits the synthesis of a fungal cell wall component, β-(1,3)-D-glucan.
- Superficial Candida infections can be treated with nystatin, azole derivatives, or ciclopirox.
- Dermatophyte infections or the skin can be treated by topical or oral administration of an azole derivative

or terbinafine; by oral administration of griseofulvin; or by topical administration of ciclopirox, naftifine, or tolnaftate.
- Itraconazole and terbinafine are given orally to treat onychomycosis, whereas efinaconazole is a topical agent for this infection.
- Griseofulvin interferes with microtubule function and blocks mitosis. It is given orally in treating tinea capitis and other dermatophyte infections.

Review Questions

1. A woman is placed on fluconazole to treat renal candidiasis. Which pharmacologic property is associated with this drug?
   (A) poor oral bioavailability
   (B) low cerebrospinal fluid concentrations
   (C) primarily excreted in the urine
   (D) short elimination half-life
   (E) must be given parenterally
2. Which drug exerts a fungicidal effect by inhibiting synthesis of the fungal cell wall?
   (A) micafungin
   (B) posaconazole
   (C) flucytosine
   (D) nystatin
   (E) terbinafine
3. Which drug is most likely to cause drug interactions due to inhibition of human cytochrome P450 enzymes?
   (A) amphotericin B
   (B) fluconazole
   (C) caspofungin
   (D) naftifine
   (E) itraconazole
4. A child with tinea capitis is treated with griseofulvin. Which adverse effect most often results from taking this drug?
   (A) sedation
   (B) constipation
   (C) nausea and vomiting
   (D) blurred vision
   (E) headache and dizziness
5. Which infection is correctly treated with caspofungin?
   (A) pulmonary blastomycosis
   (B) invasive aspergillosis
   (C) systemic histoplasmosis
   (D) cryptococcal meningitis
   (E) mucormycosis

CHAPTER 43

Drugs for the Treatment of Viral Infections

CLASSIFICATION OF ANTIVIRAL DRUGS

DRUGS FOR HERPESVIRUS INFECTIONS

Nucleoside Analogs

- Acyclovir (ZOVIRAX)[a]
- Ganciclovir (CYTOVENE)

Other Drugs

- Foscarnet (Foscavir)

Drugs for Human Immunodeficiency Virus (HIV) Infection

Nucleoside and nucleotide reverse transcriptase inhibitors

- Abacavir (Ziagen)[b]
- Emtricitabine (Emtriva)
- Lamivudine (Epivir)
- Tenofovir (Viread)

Non-nucleoside reverse transcriptase inhibitors

- Efavirenz (Sustiva)
- Rilpivirine (Edurant)[c]

HIV protease inhibitor

- Darunavir (Prezista)[d]

Fusion and entry inhibitors

- Enfuvirtide (Fuzeon)
- Maraviroc (Selzentry)
- Fostemsavir (Rukobia)
- Ibalizumab (Trogarzo)

Integrase strand transfer inhibitors

- Raltegravir (Isentress)
- Dolutegravir (Tivicay)[e]

Combination drugs for HIV

- Emtricitabine with Tenofovir (Truvada)
- Emtricitabine with Tenofovir and Rilpivirine (Odefsey)
- Elvitegravir with Cobicistat, Emtricitabine, and Tenofovir (Genvoya)[f]

Drugs for Influenza

- Oseltamivir (Tamiflu)
- Zanamivir (Relenza)[g]

Drugs for Hepatitis B Infection

- Entecavir (Baraclude)
- Adefovir (Hepsera)[h]

Drugs for Hepatitis C and Other Viral Infections

- Ribavirin (Virazole)
- Sofosbuvir (Solvaldi)
- Peginterferon alfa (Pegasys, Pegintron)
- Palivizumab (Synagis)

Combination drugs for hepatitis C infection

- Sofosbuvir with Velpatasvir (Epclusa)
- Ledipasvir with Sofosbuvir (Harvoni)[i]

Drug for Smallpox Virus Infection

- Tecovirimat (Tpoxx)

Treatment of SARS-CoV-2 Infection

- Hydroxychloroquine (Plaquenil)
- Remdesivir (Veklury)
- Dexamethasone

---

[a] Also cidofovir, famciclovir (FAMVIR), penciclovir (DENAVIR), trifluridine (VIROPTIC), valacyclovir (VALTREX), and valganciclovir (VALCYTE); acyclovir is also formulated in a buccal tablet (SITAVIG)

[b] Also didanosine (VIDEX), stavudine (ZERIT), and zidovudine (RETROVIR).

[c] Also etravirine (Intelence), nevirapine (Viramune) and doravirine (Pifeltro).

[d] Also atazanavir, fosamprenavir, lopinavir, ritonavir, saquinavir, and tipranavir.

[e] Also elvitegravir (VITEKTA).

[f] Also emtricitabine with tenofovir (DESCOVY), atazanavir with cobicistat (EVOTAZ), darunavir with cobicistat (PREZCOBIX), abacavir with dolutegravir and lamivudine (TRIUMEQ), doravirine with lamivudine and tenofovir (DELSTRIGO), and bictegravir with emtricitabine and tenofovir (BIKTARVY).

[g] Also amantadine (SYMMETREL), rimantadine (FLUMADINE), peramivir (RAPIVAB), and baloxavir (XOFLUZA).

[h] Also telbivudine (TYZEKA), lamivudine (3TC, EPIVIR), and tenofovir (VIREAD).

[i] Also daclatasvir (DAKLINZA) and simeprevir (OLYSIO), both to be taken along with sofosbuvir with or without ribavirin; combination products include elbasvir with grazoprevir (ZEPATIER), glecaprevir and pibrentasvir (MAVYRET), ombitasvir with paritaprevir and ritonavir (TECHNIVIE), sofosbuvir with velpatasvir and voxilaprevir (VOSEVI), and dasabuvir with ombitasvir, paritaprevir, and ritonavir (VIEKIRA XR).

OVERVIEW

Viruses are **obligate intracellular parasites** that use the host cell's metabolic pathways for reproduction. Viruses are considered one of the first forms of life on Earth if you can call viruses "alive" at all. Some might argue that they are not "alive" as they are just self-replicating bits of RNA or DNA encased in a protein shell. Despite the obstacles to discovering drugs that prevent viral replication without harming host cells, effective antiviral compounds have been developed for a limited number of viral infections, including herpesvirus infections, human immunodeficiency virus (HIV) infection, influenza, and hepatitis. The majority of antiviral drugs interfere with the **synthesis of viral nucleic acids**. Other agents prevent the attachment or entry of a

491

virus, inhibit the incorporation of viral nucleic acid into the host cell genome, or prevent the release and spread of a virus.

DRUGS FOR HERPESVIRUS INFECTIONS

All of the drugs used to treat herpesvirus infection act by inhibiting **viral DNA polymerase** and DNA replication. With the exception of **foscarnet,** these drugs are analogs of endogenous nucleoside precursors to DNA.

After the virus enters a host cell, the viral DNA is uncoated and enters the cell nucleus, where it is transcribed to messenger RNA by the host cell's RNA polymerase. The RNA is then translated into virus-specific proteins, including **viral DNA polymerase** and structural proteins. Finally, new viral DNA is synthesized and assembled with viral proteins to form virions that are released from the host cell to invade other cells.

The most common herpesviruses causing human infections are **herpes simplex virus (HSV), varicella-zoster virus (VZV),** and **cytomegalovirus (CMV).** HSV most often causes **herpes genitalis** (genital herpes infection), **herpes labialis** (infection of the lips and mouth), and **herpetic keratoconjunctivitis** (infection of the cornea and conjunctiva). Less commonly, HSV causes **herpetic encephalitis,** a potentially fatal disease.

VZV is the cause of **chickenpox (varicella)** and **shingles (herpes zoster).** Chickenpox occurs primarily in young children. Shingles, which occurs more frequently in persons over 60 years old, results from activation of latent VZV in dorsal root ganglia. In patients with shingles, pain and skin lesions occur in areas where the virus travels peripherally along sensory nerves to the corresponding cutaneous or mucosal surfaces. The skin lesions eventually heal but can leave residual scars. Postherpetic neuralgia is a common and disabling complication of shingles. A vaccine that has been available since 1995 has reduced the incidence of chickenpox by about 95% in the United States. A similar but more potent vaccine to prevent shingles in adults has reduced the incidence of this infection by about 50%, and of postherpetic neuralgia about 60%, in those who are inoculated (see Chapter 46 for more information on vaccines).

CMV infections in immunocompetent individuals are usually asymptomatic. Symptomatic **CMV diseases,** such as **retinitis, esophagitis,** and **colitis,** are seen most often in immunocompromised patients, such as those with HIV infection.

Nucleoside Analogs

Several nucleoside analogs, such as acyclovir, are available to treat herpesvirus infections. Most of these drugs are given orally or intravenously, while a few are administered topically to treat mucocutaneous infections.

Chemistry and Mechanisms

The nucleoside drugs must be activated by viral and host cell kinases before they can inhibit viral DNA polymerase. The drugs are first converted to monophosphate derivatives by a **viral thymidine kinase,** thereby enabling the drugs to inhibit viral DNA polymerase in infected cells while having little effect on normal host cells (Fig. 43.1). **Host cell kinases** then convert the monophosphate derivatives to **active triphosphate metabolites** that competitively inhibit

viral DNA polymerase. Some nucleoside analogs (e.g., acyclovir) are incorporated into nascent viral DNA and cause DNA chain termination because they lack the 3'-hydroxyl group required for attachment of the next nucleoside (see Fig. 43.1). Other analogs (e.g., ganciclovir and penciclovir) inhibit viral DNA polymerase but do not cause DNA chain termination by this mechanism.

PHARMACOKINETICS AND INDICATIONS

The properties and clinical uses of individual drugs for herpesvirus infections are compared in Tables 43.1 and 43.2.

Viral Resistance

The incidence of resistance to the nucleoside analogs varies with the drug and viral pathogen. Resistance of HSV and VZV to acyclovir is not common, and resistant strains are usually less infective than are sensitive strains. Furthermore, most acyclovir-resistant HSV and VZV strains are not resistant to other nucleoside analogs or to foscarnet. Most acyclovir-resistant strains have been recovered from immunocompromised patients. Loss of **thymidine kinase activity** is the major cause of innate and acquired resistance to acyclovir.

Resistance of CMV to ganciclovir is a more serious clinical problem than is HSV resistance. Most ganciclovir-resistant CMV strains are sensitive to cidofovir and foscarnet. Loss of a virus-specific protein kinase is the major cause of resistance to **ganciclovir.**

Acyclovir, Famciclovir, and Valacyclovir

Acyclovir, famciclovir, and **valacyclovir** are nucleoside analogs that are effective in the treatment of various HSV and VZV infections (see Table 43.2). These drugs are not sufficiently active against CMV to be effective in treating CMV infections, but valacyclovir can be used for **prophylaxis of CMV infections,** such as in bone marrow and organ transplant recipients and in persons with HIV infection. All three drugs are available for oral use. In addition, acyclovir is available for intravenous and topical use.

The **intravenous form of acyclovir** is the most effective treatment for serious herpesvirus infections, including herpetic encephalitis and severe HSV and VZV infections in immunocompromised patients.

The **topical form of acyclovir** can be used to treat herpes genitalis and mild mucocutaneous infections in immunocompromised patients. In cases of herpes genitalis, however, the topical form is less effective than the oral form of acyclovir.

Acyclovir has relatively low oral bioavailability (22%), whereas **valacyclovir** is a prodrug that is rapidly converted to acyclovir by intestinal and hepatic enzymes and is more completely absorbed than acyclovir. Because of its greater bioavailability (55%), valacyclovir requires less frequent administration than acyclovir. **Famciclovir** has greater bioavailability (80%) and is rapidly hydrolyzed to **penciclovir** after its absorption.

In the treatment of herpes genitalis, acyclovir, famciclovir, and valacyclovir reduce pain, shorten the time to healing, and decrease the amount of viral shedding. These drugs do not eliminate the virus, and recurrent episodes of infection are common. Shorter courses of therapy are usually sufficient for these episodes because recurrent infections

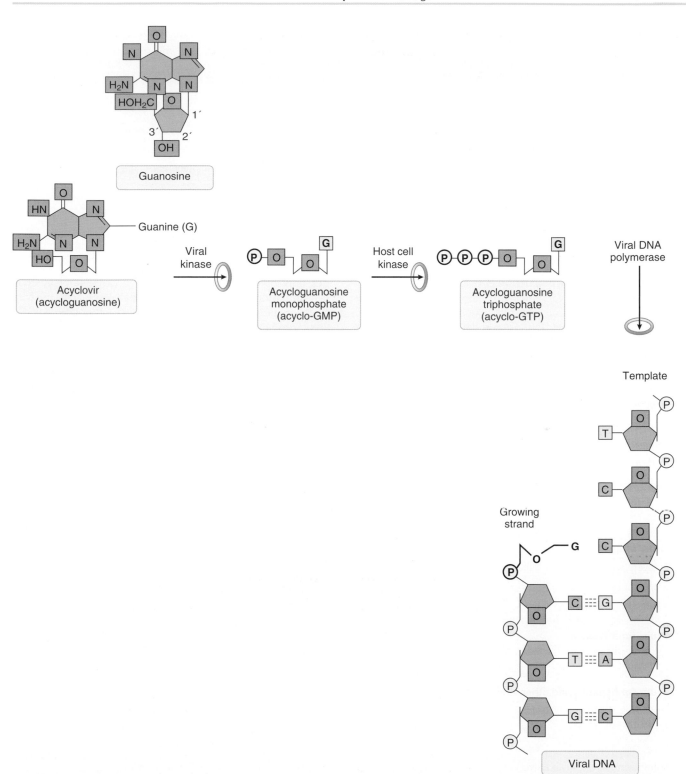

FIG. 43.1 Mechanisms of action of nucleoside analogs used in the treatment of viral infections. Acyclovir and other nucleoside analogs are converted to active nucleoside triphosphates by viral and host cell kinases. These active nucleoside triphosphates compete with the corresponding endogenous nucleoside triphosphates and competitively inhibit viral DNA polymerase. Acyclovir and the nucleoside reverse transcriptase inhibitors (NRTIs) are incorporated into viral DNA and cause chain termination because they lack the 3′-hydroxyl group required to attach the next nucleoside. Ganciclovir and penciclovir do not cause chain termination.

are usually milder. Severe herpes genitalis may require **intravenous acyclovir** therapy.

When acyclovir, famciclovir, and valacyclovir are used for the treatment of **shingles,** they shorten the duration of acute illness, acute pain, and postherpetic pain (neuralgia).

Famciclovir and valacyclovir produce similar rates of healing and appear to be more effective than acyclovir in this infection. They also enable less-frequent administration and provide higher serum drug levels because of their greater oral bioavailability. Acyclovir is available in an oral suspension

TABLE 43.1 **Pharmacokinetic Properties of Selected Antiviral Drugs**

DRUG	ROUTES OF ADMINISTRATION	ORAL BIOAVAILABILITY (%)	ELIMINATION HALF-LIFE (HOURS)	ROUTES OF ELIMINATION
Drugs for herpesvirus infections				
Acyclovir	Oral, IV, or topical	22	3	Renal excretion
Cidofovir	IV	NA	2.5	Renal excretion
Famciclovir	Oral	80	2	Metabolism; renal and fecal excretion
Ganciclovir	IV	NA	4	Renal excretion
Penciclovir	Topical	NA	NA	NA
Trifluridine	Topical ocular	NA	NA	NA
Valacyclovir	Oral	55	3	Renal excretion
Foscarnet	IV	NA	5	Renal excretion
Drugs for HIV infection				
NRTIs				
Abacavir	Oral	83	1.5	Metabolism
Emtricitabine	Oral	93	10	Renal excretion
Lamivudine	Oral	85	6	Renal excretion
Tenofovir disoproxil fumarate	Oral	25 (active metabolite)	17	Renal excretion
Zidovudine	Oral or IV	65	1	Metabolism; renal excretion
NNRTIs				
Efavirenz	Oral	50	65	Metabolism; fecal excretion
Rilpivirine	Oral	Unknown	38	Metabolism; fecal excretion
Protease inhibitors				
Atazanavir	Oral	Dose dependent	7	Metabolism
Darunavir	Oral	37 (alone) 82 (with ritonavir)	15	Metabolism; fecal excretion
Ritonavir	Oral	80	4	Metabolism; fecal excretion
Other drugs				
Enfuvirtide	Subcutaneous	NA	3	Metabolism
Maraviroc	Oral	25	16	Metabolism
Raltegravir	Oral	Unknown	9	Fecal and renal excretion of glucuronide metabolite
Drugs for influenza				
Oseltamivir	Oral	75	8	Metabolism; renal excretion
Zanamivir	Inhalation	NA	U	Metabolism; renal excretion
Drugs for hepatitis and other viral infections				
Daclatasvir	Oral	67	12	Excretion
Ledipasvir	Oral	Well absorbed	47	Biliary-fecal excretion
Simeprevir	Oral	60	41	Metabolism
Sofosbuvir	Oral	92	0.4	Renal excretion
Interferon alfa	Subcutaneous	NA	7	Metabolism
Peginterferon alfa	Subcutaneous	NA	40	Metabolism
Ribavirin	Oral, inhalational, or IV	55	9.5	Renal excretion

HIV, Human immunodeficiency virus; *IV,* intravenous; *NA,* not applicable; *NNRTI,* non-nucleoside reverse transcriptase inhibitor; *NRTIs,* nucleoside reverse transcriptase inhibitor; *U,* unknown.

for the treatment of children with **chickenpox**, though it should be noted that the incidence of this infection has decreased dramatically since the advent of the vaccine.

Acyclovir, famciclovir, and valacyclovir are well-tolerated and do not have significant interactions with other drugs. Gastrointestinal disturbances, headache, and rash

TABLE 43.2   Use of Drugs for Treating Herpesvirus Infections

DRUG	HERPES GENITALIS	HERPES LABIALIS	HERPETIC KERATOCON-JUNCTIVITIS	HERPETIC ENCEPHALITIS	CHICKENPOX	SHINGLES	CYTOMEGALO-VIRUS DIS-EASES
Acyclovir	Yes	Yes	No	Yes	Yes	Yes	No[a]
Cidofovir	No	No	No	No	No	No	Yes[b]
Famciclovir	Yes	Yes	No	No	No	Yes	No
Foscarnet	Yes[b]	No	No	No	No	Yes[b]	Yes[b]
Ganciclovir	No	No	Yes	No	No	No	Yes
Penciclovir	No	Yes	No	No	No	No	No
Trifluridine	No	No	Yes	No	No	No	No
Valacyclovir	Yes	Yes	No	No	No	Yes	No[a]
Valganciclovir	No	No	No	No	No	No	Yes

[a]Can be used for prophylaxis but not for treatment.
[b]For treating patients with intolerance of or resistance to other drugs.

are the most common side effects. Intravenous administration of acyclovir can produce phlebitis and reversible renal dysfunction.

Penciclovir

Penciclovir, the **active metabolite of famciclovir,** is available as a topical cream for the treatment of **herpes labialis** (cold sores). In patients with frequent episodes of herpes labialis, penciclovir was found to decrease the time to healing and the duration of pain and viral shedding by about a day compared to placebo.

Ganciclovir, Valganciclovir, and Cidofovir

Ganciclovir is an intravenously administered nucleoside analog that is used to prevent and treat **CMV** diseases, including retinitis, esophagitis, and colitis. Ganciclovir is about 100 times more active against CMV than is acyclovir. Ganciclovir is also active against **herpes simplex** and is available as an **ophthalmic gel** to treat acute epithelial **keratitis** (infection of the corneal epithelium) caused by HSV-1 and HSV-2. Other treatments for this ocular infection include **trifluridine.**

Ganciclovir produces a higher incidence of **adverse effects** than do acyclovir and famciclovir. The most common serious adverse effects are **leukopenia** and **thrombocytopenia.** Severe myelosuppression is more likely if the drug is given concurrently with zidovudine (ZDV). Other adverse effects of ganciclovir include retinal detachment, liver and renal dysfunction, rash, fever, and gastrointestinal disturbances.

Valganciclovir is an orally administered **prodrug** that is rapidly metabolized to ganciclovir in the gut wall and liver, with a bioavailability of 60%. It is used for the prevention and treatment of less severe CMV infections, including those occurring in renal and heart transplant patients.

Cidofovir is a nucleoside analog that is reserved for treating infections that are resistant to ganciclovir because it can cause **nephrotoxicity,** neutropenia, metabolic acidosis, and other serious adverse effects. About 25% of patients discontinue cidofovir because of adverse reactions. The drug is contraindicated in patients who are taking other nephrotoxic drugs, such as aminoglycosides or amphotericin B.

Trifluridine

Trifluridine is administered topically to treat ocular herpesvirus infections, primarily **herpetic epithelial keratitis** and **keratoconjunctivitis.** Herpetic keratitis typically presents as a dendritic (branching) lesion in the cornea. The drug is generally well tolerated but can cause superficial ocular irritation and hyperemia.

Foscarnet

Foscarnet is a pyrophosphate derivative that blocks the pyrophosphate-binding sites on viral **DNA polymerase** and prevents the attachment of nucleotide precursors to DNA. Unlike the nucleoside analogs used to treat herpesvirus infections, foscarnet does not require activation by viral or host cell kinases.

Foscarnet is active against CMV, VZV, and HSV. It must be administered **intravenously** and is used to treat CMV retinitis in patients with AIDS and to treat acyclovir-resistant HSV infections and shingles. Foscarnet can be combined with ganciclovir to treat infections that are resistant to either drug alone because of their synergistic effect on viral DNA polymerase.

Adverse reactions to foscarnet include renal impairment and acute **renal failure,** hematologic deficiencies, cardiac arrhythmias and heart failure, seizures, and pancreatitis. Renal toxicity can be minimized by administering intravenous fluids to induce diuresis before and during foscarnet treatment.

DRUGS FOR HUMAN IMMUNODEFICIENCY VIRUS INFECTION

Remarkable advances have been made in the treatment of HIV infection and AIDS, and there has been a veritable explosion of new drugs for HIV infection in recent years. This chapter will focus on drugs that are currently recommended for the initial treatment of HIV infections. The combined use of two or more drugs from different classes has been shown to markedly reduce viral loads and improve survival in HIV-positive individuals. This type of multidrug treatment has been called **highly active antiretroviral therapy (HAART).** At first, HAART regimens were complicated and required multiple doses of several drugs every day, but the development of longer-acting combination drug products has enabled effective treatment with only a single or a few doses per day. The guidelines for treating HIV infection continue to evolve as new drug regimens are developed and tested. The current recommendations for previously untreated (therapy-naïve) adult HIV patients are listed in Table 43.3.

Sites of Drug Action

HIV is an RNA **retrovirus.** Its replication and sites of drug action are depicted in Fig. 43.2. Viral replication begins when **glycoprotein 120** on the surface of HIV type 1 (HIV-1) binds to the cell differentiation 4 (CD4) antigen on the

---

TABLE 43.3   Regimens for Initial Treatment of Human Immunodeficiency Virus Infection in Adults and Adolescents (for Patients Without Previous Human Immunodeficiency Virus Therapy)ᵃ

Integrase strand transfer inhibitor–based regimens

- Raltegravir plus tenofovir/emtricitabineᵇ
- Dolutegravir/abacavir/lamivudineᵇ (only for HLA-B 5701 negative patients)
- Dolutegravir plus tenofovir/emtricitabineᵇ
- Elvitegravir/cobicistat/tenofovir/emtricitabineᵇ (only for patients with creatinine clearance ≥30 mL/min)
- Elvitegravir/cobicistat/tenofovir/emtricitabineᵇ (only for patients with creatinine clearance ≥70 mL/min)

Protease inhibitor–based regimen

- Darunavir/ritonavir + tenofovir/emtricitabineᵇ

Regimen for pregnant women

- Lopinavir/ritonavir + zidovudine + emtricitabineᶜ

ᵃGuidelines for the use of antiretroviral agents in HIV-1-infected adults and adolescents, updated January 20, 2022, Department of Health and Human Services (see http://aidsinfo.nih.gov).
ᵇLamivudine can substitute for emtricitabine or vice versa.

---

surface of HIV-specific helper lymphocytes (CD4 cells). The binding of glycoprotein 120 to CD4 causes a conformational change in glycoprotein 120, enabling it to interact with the **chemokine co-receptor** (CCR5 or CXCR4) on the lymphocyte surface. These events expose a virus fusion protein, **glycoprotein 41,** which undergoes a conformational change so it can insert a hydrophobic tail into the host cell membrane and bind host cell integrins, leading to fusion of the viral and host cell membranes and transfer of the viral genome into the cytoplasm.

Once HIV enters the CD4 cell, viral RNA serves as a template to produce a complementary double-stranded DNA in a reaction catalyzed by viral **reverse transcriptase** (RT) (RNA-dependent DNA polymerase). The viral DNA then enters the host cell nucleus and is incorporated into the host genome in a reaction catalyzed by **HIV integrase.** Eventually, the viral DNA is transcribed and translated to produce large, nonfunctional polypeptides called **polyproteins.** These polyproteins, along with a copy of the viral RNA, are packaged into immature virions at the cell surface. An enzyme called **HIV protease** cleaves the polyproteins into smaller, functional proteins in a process called **viral maturation** as the virions are released into the plasma.

The drugs now available for the treatment of HIV infection include those that inhibit fusion and entry, RT, integrase strand transfer, and HIV protease.

Nucleoside Reverse Transcriptase Inhibitors
Mechanism of Action

There are two types of RT inhibitors, nucleoside RT inhibitors (NRTIs) and non-nucleoside RT inhibitors (NNRTIs).

The NRTIs are converted to triphosphate metabolites (nucleotides) by host cell kinases. These drug nucleotides compete with endogenous nucleotides for incorporation into viral DNA. Once incorporated into nascent DNA, the NRTIs cause DNA chain termination in the same manner

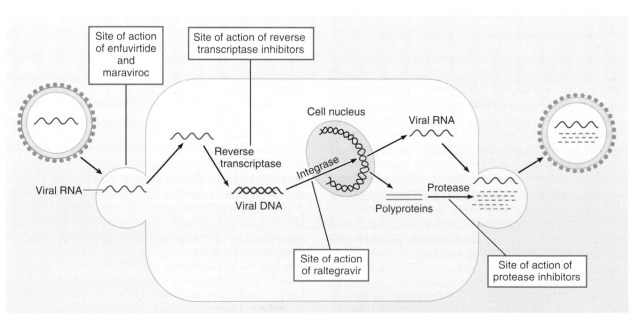

Fɪɢ. 43.2   Sites of action of drugs for human immunodeficiency virus (HIV) infection. Enfuvirtide inhibits the fusion of HIV with host CD4 cell membranes. After the virus penetrates the host cell and becomes uncoated, the viral RNA is transcribed by reverse transcriptase to form viral DNA. Viral DNA is incorporated into the host genome in the cell nucleus by HIV integrase. The viral DNA is then transcribed to RNA. Viral RNA is incorporated into new virions and is translated to synthesize polyproteins. The polyproteins are cleaved into viral proteins by HIV protease as the new virions are released from the cell.

as described earlier for acyclovir (see Fig. 43.1). The NRTIs, particularly ZDV, inhibit host cell DNA polymerase to varying degrees, which may account for some of their toxic effects (e.g., anemia).

Tenofovir disoproxil fumarate (TDF) is a **nucleotide prodrug** that has a slightly different mode of action from NRTIs. TDF is hydrolyzed in the body to form tenofovir, and then tenofovir is converted to tenofovir diphosphate by host (CD4) cell kinases. **Tenofovir diphosphate** competes with deoxyadenosine 5′-triphosphate and is incorporated into viral DNA by RT, causing DNA chain termination.

Chemistry and Pharmacokinetics

The **NRTIs** are synthetic derivatives of naturally occurring **nucleosides**. All of the NRTIs can be given orally, and ZDV can also be given intravenously. The NRTIs cross the blood-brain barrier and are distributed to the cerebrospinal fluid. Most of the NRTIs are eliminated by renal excretion, and renal impairment will prolong their plasma elimination half-life and may necessitate a reduction in dosage.

Clinical Use

The **NRTIs** were the **first class of drugs to be developed for HIV infection** and are included in most HIV treatment regimens. Because the NRTIs are antimetabolites of different purine and pyrimidine bases of DNA, they are more effective when given in combination than when used alone. They are typically combined with either an **integrase strand transfer inhibitor** (INSTI) or a **protease inhibitor** (PI), as shown in Table 43.3. In addition to inhibiting the replication of human and animal retroviruses, some of the NRTIs have demonstrated activity against hepatitis B virus (HBV) and Epstein-Barr virus.

Viral Resistance. Resistance to NRTIs can develop during therapy and is more likely to occur in persons receiving single-drug therapy for 6 months or longer. Studies of ZDV indicate that HIV-1 acquires resistance to the drug in a stepwise manner involving four or five specific mutations in the gene that encodes the RT enzyme. Because the virus undergoes frequent mutations, the only way to prevent resistance is to prevent HIV replication by using combination drug therapy.

Adverse Effects and Interactions. As shown in Table 43.4, the NRTIs differ in their major toxicities and in their interactions with other drugs. ZDV produces bone marrow suppression and can cause anemia and neutropenia. Didanosine and stavudine can cause pancreatitis, and didanosine can also cause peripheral neuropathy. Abacavir (ABC) is more likely to cause a hypersensitivity reaction, whereas tenofovir produces renal impairment in some patients.

Specific Drugs

ZDV was the first NRTI to be developed, and it is available in products containing ZDV with lamivudine, emtricitabine, and other agents. Early studies found that ZDV treatment significantly reduced **in utero transmission of HIV** from infected pregnant women to their offspring when administered from the 14th to the 34th weeks of gestation, and the drug is often used to treat pregnant women with HIV infection (see Table 43.3).

TABLE 43.4 Most Important Adverse Effects and Interactions of Drugs for Human Immunodeficiency Virus Infection

DRUG	ADVERSE EFFECTS AND INTERACTIONS
NRTIs	
All NRTIs	Lactic acidosis, hepatic steatosis, and lipodystrophy (all higher with stavudine)
Abacavir	Hypersensitivity reactions
Didanosine	Pancreatitis, peripheral neuropathy, gastrointestinal intolerance
Emtricitabine	Headache, nausea, diarrhea, fatigue, depression, insomnia
Stavudine	Pancreatitis, peripheral neuropathy
Tenofovir	Headache, gastrointestinal intolerance, renal impairment
Zidovudine	Headache, gastrointestinal intolerance, bone marrow suppression
NNRTIs	
All NNRTIs	Rash, drug interactions
Efavirenz	Neuropsychiatric reactions, teratogenic effects
Etravirine	• Diarrhea, peripheral neuropathy, redistribution of body fat
Nevirapine	Hepatotoxicity, rash including Stevens-Johnson syndrome; increases metabolism of protease inhibitors, contraceptive steroids, and other drugs
Rilpivirine	• Insomnia and sleep disturbances, headache, dizziness, redistribution of body fat
Protease inhibitors	
All protease inhibitors	Lipodystrophy (fat accumulation), hyperlipidemia, insulin resistance and diabetes, liver dysfunction and hepatitis; inhibit metabolism of other drugs including protease inhibitors, antiarrhythmic agents, opioids, and tricyclic antidepressants
Atazanavir	PR interval prolongation
Fosamprenavir	Gastrointestinal intolerance, rash
Lopinavir, ritonavir	Gastrointestinal intolerance
Other drugs	
Enfuvirtide	Injection site reactions, hypersensitivity reactions
Maraviroc	Upper respiratory symptoms, possible hepatotoxicity
Raltegravir	Headache, diarrhea, nausea, vomiting

NNRTI, Nonnucleoside reverse transcriptase inhibitor; *NRTI,* nucleoside reverse transcriptase inhibitor.

Newer NRTIs are now recommended for the initial treatment of HIV infection, including ABC, **TDF,** and **emtricitabine**, as shown in Table 43.3. Several combination drug products containing these NRTIs are available to simplify treatment regimens. **Lamivudine** causes relatively few adverse effects and is also recommended for the initial treatment of HIV infection. **Stavudine** and **didanosine** are used in cases in which a first-line drug is not tolerated or when viral resistance occurs. ZDV and stavudine are not used together because they appear to be antagonistic.

Didanosine is used in combination with lamivudine or emtricitabine.

Nonnucleoside Reverse Transcriptase Inhibitors

The NNRTIs include **efavirenz, rilpivirine etravirine, nevirapine**, and **doravirine**. These drugs do not require metabolic activation and directly inhibit RT.

Pharmacokinetics

The NNRTIs have good oral bioavailability (see Table 43.1). They are highly lipophilic, and the concentrations that they reach in the central nervous system are adequate for antiviral activity. The drugs are extensively metabolized before undergoing fecal and renal excretion.

Activity, Indications, and Viral Resistance

In vitro studies show that NNRTIs act synergistically with NRTIs and other agents against HIV. The NNRTIs are not typically employed in the initial treatment of HIV infections and are used in **alternative regimens** for patients who cannot tolerate or do not respond to the primary drugs listed in Table 43.3. As with other drugs, the NNRTIs are never used alone to treat HIV infection because viral resistance develops rapidly, unless they are combined with other drugs.

Adverse Effects and Interactions

NNRTIs are moderately well tolerated. **Rash** is the most common side effect of these drugs. In patients with a mild rash, the drugs can usually be continued or restarted. Patients should be monitored, however, because the rash can progress to Stevens-Johnson syndrome. Efavirenz is teratogenic in primates and should be avoided in pregnant women and women who may become pregnant. Efavirenz can also cause neuropsychiatric reactions. Nevirapine induces CYP3A4 and CYP2B6 and accelerates the metabolism of certain drugs (see Table 43.4). In addition to skin rash, it can also cause hepatotoxicity and should not be used in patients with hepatic impairment. Drug interactions and other common adverse effects of NNRTIs are listed in Table 43.4.

Protease Inhibitors

HIV protease cleaves the **gag-pol** (group-specific antigen-polymerase) polyprotein to provide functional viral proteins and is essential for the **maturation** of the virus. PIs bind the active site of the enzyme and inhibit proteolytic activity, resulting in the production of immature, noninfectious viral particles.

Saquinavir, the first HIV PI, was approved in 1995, ushering in a new era in the treatment of HIV infection and AIDS. Other PIs were subsequently developed, including **lopinavir** and **ritonavir.** More recently, PIs that are better tolerated and have improved pharmacokinetic properties were introduced, including **atazanavir, darunavir,** and **fosamprenavir.** Darunavir is currently preferred for the initial treatment of most HIV patients (see Table 43.3).

Because ritonavir inhibits the metabolism of other PIs, it is combined with other PIs to increase their plasma levels and duration, and this is known as **boosted therapy.** Combination drug products containing ritonavir and another PI are available and have become the standard mode of PI administration in HIV therapy (see Table 43.3).

Ritonavir is also used to increase serum levels of paritaprevir in the treatment of hepatitis C infection (see later).

Tables 43.1 and 43.4 compare information on the properties, effects, and interactions of selected PIs. Fig. 43.2 shows the site of action of these drugs.

Pharmacokinetics

PIs are given orally and are extensively metabolized by cytochrome P450 enzymes before undergoing fecal excretion.

Activity, Indications, and Viral Resistance

PIs are synergistic with NRTIs and are often combined in treatment regimens. Administration of a PI and two NRTIs significantly reduces viral load, increases CD4 cells, and slows the clinical progression of disease and the emergence of drug resistance. Resistance to PIs is associated with the accumulation of mutations resulting in amino acid substitutions in the viral protease structure. Varying degrees of cross-resistance occur between different PIs, but cross-resistance between PIs and RT inhibitors is rare. The preferred PI and NRTI combinations are listed in Table 43.3.

Adverse Effects and Interactions

All PIs can cause lipid accumulation in tissues **(lipodystrophy)** and hyperlipidemia, insulin resistance and diabetes, elevated liver function test results, and drug interactions. Ritonavir appears to produce the highest incidence of adverse effects, whereas **darunavir** appears to be better tolerated than most other PIs and has a lower propensity to cause diarrhea, lipodystrophy, and hyperlipidemia.

PIs interact with a number of other drugs (see Table 43.4) via inhibition of cytochrome P450 enzymes. They have the greatest effect on drugs metabolized by the CYP3A4 isozyme and can increase the plasma concentration of these drugs and other PIs. The NNRTI nevirapine increases the metabolism and decreases the therapeutic effect of PIs.

Fusion and Entry Inhibitors

Enfuvirtide, maraviroc, fostemsavir, and **ibalizumab** are antiviral agents that **inhibit the fusion and entry of HIV.** They are active against HIV strains that are resistant to RT and PIs, and they are approved for the treatment of HIV infection caused by drug-resistant strains. In this setting, these drugs have been shown to decrease viral loads, increase CD4 cells, and improve symptoms.

Maraviroc is an **antagonist** of **chemokine co-receptor 5 (CCR5).** Maraviroc binds to CCR5 and prevents interaction with HIV-1 glycoprotein 120 (see earlier), which is necessary for CCR5-tropic HIV-1 to enter cells. The drug does not bind CXCR4 and is active only against CCR5-tropic HIV strains. It has been shown to have a **synergistic effect with enfuvirtide.**

Enfuvirtide (T-20) is a large peptide that **binds to HIV glycoprotein 41** and thereby blocks the fusion process. When used in combination with other drugs, **enfuvirtide reduces viral loads and increases CD4 cell counts.** The drug is most often used when resistance or intolerance to other drugs occurs. Because of its peptide structure, enfuvirtide is not given orally and must be injected subcutaneously twice daily. It may cause injection site reactions but is otherwise well-tolerated and is approved for use in both adults and children.

Fostemsavir is a prodrug without antiviral activity that is hydrolyzed to the active agent, **temsavir**. Temsavir is an HIV-1 attachment inhibitor that works by binding to the gp120 subunit within the HIV-1 envelope glycoprotein gp160 and selectively inhibits the interaction between the virus and cellular CD4 receptors.

Ibalizumab is a monoclonal antibody drug (see Chapter 46) classified as a **CD4-directed post-attachment HIV-1 inhibitor**. Ibalizumab, in combination with other antiretrovirals, is indicated for the treatment of HIV type 1 (HIV-1) infection in **heavily treatment-experienced adults with multidrug-resistant HIV-1 infection failing their current antiretroviral regimen.**

Integrase Strand Transfer Inhibitor

Integrase incorporates the viral DNA formed by RT into the DNA of CD4 cells through a multistep process. First, integrase removes the last nucleotide from both 3′ ends of the viral DNA strand to enable the formation of a preintegration complex of viral DNA, integrase, and other viral and host cell proteins. This complex is able to pass from the cell cytoplasm into the nucleus, where integrase randomly incorporates viral DNA into the host chromosome by DNA strand transfer.

Raltegravir was the first **integrase strand inhibitor** developed for treating HIV infections, while **dolutegravir** and **elvitegravir** are newer agents in this class. All of these drugs are included in the preferred regimens for the initial treatment of HIV infection (Table 43.3). These agents prevent DNA strand transfer by **binding divalent cations** in the catalytic core of integrase that are required for interaction of the enzyme with host cell DNA. When used in combination with other antiretroviral agents, the INSTIs decrease viral loads and increase CD4 cells. The drugs are given orally and produce few serious adverse effects, though they may cause headache, diarrhea, and nausea. They are not substrates for cytochrome P450 enzymes and do not appear to inhibit or induce these enzymes.

Treatment Considerations

It is now recommended that antiretroviral therapy be initiated in HIV-positive patients as soon as possible before immunodeficiency becomes evident, with the goal of **reducing plasma viral concentrations** as much as possible and for as long as possible. The patient's **viral load** (expressed in terms of the number of **HIV RNA copies per milliliter**) should be determined at the outset of therapy and 2 to 8 weeks after therapy is begun, and then every 3 to 4 months thereafter. The response to drug therapy is highly variable, and viral suppression can take months in patients with high viral loads. The **CD4 count** (expressed in terms of the number of T cells per microliter [μL]) can be used to assess a patient's immune status.

The currently **preferred drug regimens** for treating HIV infection in adults and adolescents are listed in Table 43.3 and consist of either an INSTI **or a PI, each combined with two NRTIs.** Alternative regimens are available from public health agencies for patients who do not respond to the preferred regimens. The main reasons for changing drug therapy after treatment has begun are **treatment failure and drug toxicity.** Treatment failure is indicated by increased viral loads and decreased CD4 cells. If the patient fails to respond to a drug regimen, the new regimen should include at least two new drugs. **Drug resistance testing** can provide useful information concerning the selection of alternative therapy. If drug toxicity occurs, alternative drugs can be chosen that have fewer adverse effects experienced by the patient.

To increase patient compliance, and in some cases, to lower the cost of medications, a number of combination products for the treatment of HIV are now available. Two-drug combinations include **emtricitabine** with **tenofovir** (Truvada) and **emtricitabine** with **tenofovir** (Descovy). Three-drug combos are available as **emtricitabine** and **tenofovir** with **rilpivirine** (Odefsey), ABC with **dolutegravir** and **lamivudine** (Triumeq), **doravirine** with **lamivudine** and **tenofovir** (Delstrigo), and **bictegravir** with **emtricitabine** and **tenofovir** (Biktarvy).

A new four-drug combination product is available that includes **elvitegravir**, an HIV-1 INSTI, **emtricitabine** and **tenofovir** (NRTIs), and **cobicistat**, a CYP3A inhibitor, is marketed as Genvoya. **Cobicistat** is included in a unique strategy to **increase the plasma levels of elvitegravir** by inhibiting its metabolism at CYP3A. It is also employed in the two-drug combos **darunavir** with **cobicistat** (Prezcobix) and **atazanavir** with **cobicistat** (Evotaz).

DRUGS FOR INFLUENZA

Because **influenza** is one of the most common causes of infectious disease-related deaths, efforts have been made to develop methods to prevent and treat illness caused by this RNA virus. **Vaccines are the primary means of prevention** (see Chapter 46), but neuraminidase inhibitors are useful for prophylaxis during outbreaks and can shorten the duration of illness in infected persons and prevent complications (Box 43.1).

Baloxavir is a very recently approved antiviral for the treatment of the flu virus that works by a new mechanism of action. **Baloxavir** binds to and shuts down the **endonuclease activity** of the polymerase acidic (PA) protein, an enzyme only found in the influenza virus. The inhibition of this enzyme in the **viral RNA polymerase complex** (which is required for viral gene transcription) results in the inhibition of influenza virus replication.

Neuraminidase Inhibitors

Oseltamivir, zanamivir, and **peramivir** inhibit the enzyme **neuraminidase (sialidase)** in **influenza A** and **B** viruses. These drugs were designed to bind to the active site of neuraminidase based on studies of the enzyme's crystalline structure.

Neuraminidase catalyzes reactions that promote viral spreading and infection. First, it enables the **release of virions** from the surface of infected cells after viral replication. Second, it inactivates respiratory tract mucus that would otherwise prevent the **spreading of virions** through the respiratory tract. Neuraminidase accomplishes this by cleaving **sialic acid residues** attached to mucus proteins.

Oseltamivir and zanamivir are active against most current influenza strains, including influenza A 2009 H1N1 and A 2013 H3N2, and the H5N1 avian influenza strain. **Oseltamivir** is given orally and can be used for both **prophylaxis and treatment** of influenza in patients who are at least 1 year of age. For treatment of influenza, oseltamivir

CASE PRESENTATION

A 20-year-old student visits the university health clinic because of chills, fever, sore throat, cough, chest discomfort, severe myalgia, and extreme tiredness that began about 12 h ago. Examination reveals a temperature of 102°F, nonexudative pharyngitis, nasal discharge, and scattered rhonchi on chest auscultation. A nasal aspirate is subjected to a rapid test for influenza nucleoproteins and is found to be positive. The patient is started on oseltamivir and acetaminophen and is sent to the clinic infirmary for bed rest. She is instructed to use an ear-loop face mask in the presence of others. Her symptoms improve over the next 48 h, and she has an uneventful recovery.

CASE DISCUSSION

Influenza is a seasonal respiratory infection caused by influenza type A and type B viruses. Hand washing and influenza vaccines are the primary means of prevention, but the vaccines often fail to include strains that cause influenza outbreaks because vaccine strains must be selected many months before the next flu season begins. The presentation of influenza varies considerably, and it may be difficult to distinguish it from other upper respiratory infections. However, patients with influenza usually have a higher fever and more severe constitutional symptoms, such as myalgia, than patients with other infections. The availability of rapid tests has improved diagnostic accuracy. These tests can be performed in as little as 10 min and usually cost less than $20 (US). The rapid diagnostic tests are highly specific, but their sensitivity, typically 70% to 80%, is less than that of viral culture methods that require more time and expense. Hence, clinical judgment is still important in diagnosing influenza. Treatment of influenza includes antipyretic agents such as acetaminophen, antiviral agents, and bed rest. Oseltamivir and zanamivir are the only drugs that are effective against current strains of influenza, and they are useful for both prophylaxis and treatment.

is administered orally twice a day for 5 days, and it is given once daily for prophylaxis. **Zanamivir** is administered as a nasal spray twice daily for treatment of influenza in persons who are at least 7 years of age and for prophylaxis in persons at least 5 years of age. Because it is administered intranasally, zanamivir should not be used by patients with underlying airway disease, such as asthma or emphysema.

Evidence from previous influenza seasons shows that the neuraminidase inhibitors are most beneficial in reducing **symptom severity and duration** of illness if administered **less than 3 days after the onset** of symptoms, preferably within the first 48 hours. However, the drugs still provide benefit in reducing respiratory failure and death in pregnant women with influenza when started 3 to 4 days after symptom onset. **Neuraminidase inhibitors** also reduce the complications of influenza, such as otitis media and pneumonia. Drug therapy should be started as early as possible for any patient with confirmed or suspected influenza who is hospitalized; has a severe, complicated, or progressive illness; or is at a higher risk of influenza complications.

Neuraminidase inhibitors are 70% to 90% effective in preventing influenza and are useful adjuncts to vaccination. However, the U.S. Centers for Disease Control and Prevention (CDC) does not recommend routine chemoprophylaxis of influenza because of the risk of promoting viral resistance. Instead, the CDC recommends prophylaxis for populations at increased risk of influenza complications and to control outbreaks in institutional settings such as nursing homes. Prophylaxis is appropriate for persons with severe immunodeficiencies who may not respond to vaccination. It is also beneficial to persons at high risk of complications during the first 2 weeks after vaccination who are exposed to an infectious person. To be most effective, prophylaxis must continue throughout the period of potential exposure to influenza and for 7 days afterward.

The **adverse effects** of neuraminidase inhibitors are usually mild and transient, mostly consisting of minor respiratory and gastrointestinal reactions.

Amantadine and Rimantadine

Amantadine and **rimantadine** are synthetic tricyclic amine compounds that block the viral M2 proton channel, and they were formerly used for the prevention and treatment of influenza A. The emergence of **resistant strains** has rendered these agents largely ineffective, and they are **not currently recommended** for prophylaxis or treatment of influenza. Viral resistance to these drugs results from mutations to the M2 proton channel that enables viral acidification required for uncoating viral nucleic acid in host cells. Amantadine is also used occasionally for the **treatment of Parkinson disease** because of its ability to increase neuronal dopamine release (see Chapter 24).

DRUGS FOR HEPATITIS AND OTHER VIRAL INFECTIONS

HBV infection is spread by **contact with body fluids** from an infected person, such as blood and semen, and is most often transmitted by sexual contact in developed countries. The infection may be either acute and self-limiting or chronic. Acute HBV infection does not usually require treatment, and most adults clear the infection spontaneously within weeks to months. Less than 1% of patients require antiviral treatment because they have an aggressive infection or because they are immunocompromised. Patients with chronic HBV infection may need treatment to prevent **cirrhosis and liver cancer**, such as those with persistently elevated serum alanine aminotransferase (AAT) levels that indicate liver damage. Because antiviral **drugs only suppress HBV replication** and do not cure the disease, many patients with a chronic infection will need to continue treatment for life.

The primary drugs for treating HBV infection are **nucleoside and nucleotide RT inhibitors**, including **adefovir, entecavir, lamivudine, telbivudine,** and **tenofovir** (Table 43.5). These drugs inhibit the replication of this **DNA virus**, which depends on the reverse transcription of an RNA intermediate formed during viral replication. RNA transcription produces a negative-sense strand of DNA, which then serves as a template for the synthesis of positive-sense viral DNA. **Tenofovir and entecavir** are recommended as first-line agents for HBV infection by the World Health Organization because they are the most active agents and rarely lead to viral resistance, whereas the use of **lamivudine leads to viral resistance** in about 75% of cases after 5 years. **Tenofovir** and **entecavir provide long-term suppression of HBV** and may reverse hepatic cirrhosis and

TABLE 43.5   Mechanisms of Drugs for Treating Viral Hepatitis and Other Infections

DRUGS	TARGET	MECHANISM OF ACTION	CLINICAL USE
Grazoprevir, paritaprevir, Simeprevir	Nonstructural Protein NS3-4A	Inhibit serine protease and cleavage of HCV polyprotein	Hepatitis C
Daclatasvir, elbasvir, ledipasvir ombitasvir, velpatasvir	Nonstructural Protein NS5A	Inhibit activator of HCV RNA polymerase	Hepatitis C
Dasabuvir, sofosbuvir	Nonstructural Protein NS5B	Inhibits HCV RNA-directed RNA polymerase	Hepatitis C
Entecavir, tenofovir, and others	Reverse transcriptase	Inhibit formation of DNA copy of viral RNA	Hepatitis B
Ribavirin	Inosine monophosphate dehydrogenase	Inhibits guanosine triphosphate and nucleic acid synthesis	Hepatitis C, respiratory syncytial virus
Peginterferon alfa, interferon alfa	Interferon-alpha receptor (IFNAR)	Activate JAK-STAT signaling pathway and T-cells	Hepatitis B and C, condylomata acuminata

achieve viral seroconversion (loss of detectable viral surface antigen). **Peginterferon alfa** has also been used to treat HBV infection but is less used today with the development of better drugs with fewer adverse effects that require careful monitoring.

Hepatitis C virus (HCV) is a virus with an **RNA genome** that is acquired by contact with **contaminated blood** through recreational intravenous drug use or from poorly sterilized medical equipment or needle stick injuries. Most people infected with HCV have mild or no symptoms for many months, but about 75% of those infected eventually develop a **chronic infection** that can lead to cirrhosis, liver failure, or liver cancer. About 130 to 150 million people are infected with HCV worldwide, and an estimated 700,000 people die annually from HCV-related liver disease. Advances in drug treatment for HCV infection are evolving rapidly, and the combined use of so-called **direct-acting antivirals (DAAs)** has reduced, if not eliminated, the need for interferon treatments (see Table 43.5). DAA treatments have the potential to **cure over 90% of patients** with HCV infection in 12 to 24 weeks.

Many of the DAAs used to treat HCV infection block viral proteins responsible for **HCV RNA replication**, and these agents are typically given in combination. The most recent drug combination approved by US and European drug agencies contains sofosbuvir and velpatasvir (EPCLUSA). **Sofosbuvir** inhibits the **HCV RNA polymerase** (nonstructural protein 5B, **NS5B**) that replicates the HCV's genomic RNA, while **velpatasvir** inhibits a key **activator of RNA polymerase** called NS5A. The most important property of velpatasvir is that it is active **against all 6 HCV genotypes**, which may obviate the need for genomic testing before treatment of HCV infections with this agent. In addition, **velpatasvir is active at picomolar concentrations**, making it one of the **most potent antiviral agents ever discovered**. Headache and fatigue are the most common adverse effects reported with sofosbuvir/velpatasvir. The product should not be used concurrently with amiodarone because episodes of bradycardia have been reported with this combination.

VIEKIRA PAK and VIEKIRA XR are different formulations of a recently developed drug combination for treating types 1a and 1b HCV infection. It consists of ombitasvir, paritaprevir, and ritonavir, and tablets containing dasabuvir. **Ombitasvir** inhibits **nonstructural protein 5A** (NS5A), while **dasabuvir** inhibits **nonstructural protein 5B** (NS5B).

Paritaprevir inhibits the **nonstructural protein 3-4A**, a **serine protease enzyme** that catalyzes the cleavage of the HCV polyprotein into mature forms of NS5A, NS5B, and other proteins. **Ritonavir** is not active against HCV and is included in the preparation to inhibit the metabolism of paritaprevir by CYP3A, and thereby increasing its serum levels and prolonging its antiviral activity.

Clinical trials found that the VIEKIRA PAK AND VIEKIRA XR combination can cure over 95% of patients with type 1HCV infection after 12 weeks of therapy. The most **common adverse effects** of this drug preparation are tiredness and weakness, loss of appetite, and nausea and vomiting. The drugs contained in Viekira Pak affect the metabolism and elimination of a large number of other drugs, and **numerous drug interactions** are possible.

In addition to ombitasvir and velpatasvir, several other DAAs inhibit NS5A and viral RNA replication, including **daclatasvir, elbasvir**, and **ledipasvir** (see Table 43.5). The combination of sofosbuvir and ledipasvir (HARVONI) is sometimes used with ribavirin. **Simeprevir** is another agent for HCV infection that inhibits the **NS3-4A protease** that is involved in viral maturation (see earlier). Simeprevir is used in combination with peginterferon alfa and ribavirin, primarily for persons with HCV genotype-1infection who have liver disease such as cirrhosis. Another new drug combination for HCV genotypes 1 and 4 infection consists of **elbasvir and grazoprevir** (ZEPATIER), which is also used alone or in combination with ribavirin. **Elbasvir** joins the growing number of **HCV NS5A inhibitors**, while **grazoprevir** inhibits the NS3-4A viral protease in the same manner as **paritaprevir** and **simeprevir**.

Other new combination drugs for the treatment of hepatitis C infections are **glecaprevir** and **pibrentasvir** (MAVYRET), and **sofosbuvir** with **velpatasvir** and **voxilaprevir** (VOSEVI)

Ribavirin
Mechanism of Action

Ribavirin is a synthetic **guanosine analog** that inhibits viral nucleic acid synthesis. The drug is activated by kinases that phosphorylate the drug. The active metabolites inhibit inosine monophosphate dehydrogenase leading to a deficiency of guanosine triphosphate, a nucleotide precursor to viral nucleic acids (see Table 43.5). Ribavirin can also inhibit the synthesis of host cell nucleic acid, accounting for some of its toxicity.

Pharmacokinetics, Spectrum, and Indications

Table 43.1 outlines the pharmacokinetic properties of ribavirin.

Ribavirin is a **broad-spectrum antiviral** drug and is active in vitro against a wide range of RNA and DNA viruses. These include adenovirus, Colorado tick fever virus, Crimean-Congo hemorrhagic fever virus, Hantaan virus, **hepatitis A and C viruses,** herpesviruses, influenza A and B viruses, Lassa virus, measles virus, Muerto Canyon virus, mumps virus, **respiratory syncytial virus (RSV),** Rift Valley fever virus, and yellow fever virus. Although intravenous ribavirin has been successfully used to treat hemorrhagic fever caused by several of these viruses, the drug is specifically approved for the treatment of **severe RSV infection** and **chronic hepatitis C (HCV).**

For the treatment of hospitalized infants and young children with severe **RSV infection,** ribavirin is administered by aerosol, using a small-particle aerosol generator that serves to localize drug concentrations at the site of the infection. In the treatment of **HCV,** orally administered ribavirin is combined with other agents (see earlier).

Adverse Effects and Interactions

When ribavirin is given by inhalation, it can cause **serious pulmonary and cardiovascular effects,** including apnea, pneumothorax, worsening of respiratory status, and cardiac arrest. When the drug is given orally, it may cause hemolytic anemia, which can worsen cardiac disease and lead to myocardial infarction. Ribavirin is **teratogenic** in animals, and its use is **contraindicated in pregnant or lactating women.** Ribavirin antagonizes the antiviral effect of ZDV, and the two drugs should not be used concurrently.

Palivizumab

Palivizumab is a humanized monoclonal antibody (see Chapter 46) that inactivates the **fusion protein of RSV,** inhibiting viral entry into target cells. The agent is used to **prevent and treat RSV** infection in infants and children under 2 years of age that are at increased risk of severe disease and hospitalization. These include infants with bronchopulmonary dysplasia, congenital heart disease, and neuromuscular, pulmonary, and genetic disorders. Palivizumab reduces the risk of hospitalization due to RSV infection by about 50% and is administered **intramuscularly once a month** until the infection resolves or the agent is no longer needed for prophylaxis.

Interferons
Chemistry and Pharmacokinetics

Interferons are a group of **glycoprotein cytokines** produced by host cell leukocytes in response to viral and bacterial infections. They were named for their ability to *interfere* with viral replication. Interferons are produced by recombinant DNA technology for therapeutic use and designated as **interferons alfa-2a and alfa-2b** (see also Chapter 46). PEGylated derivatives called **peginterferon alfa 2a and alfa 2b** (PEGASYS, PEGINTRON) are available in which polyethylene glycol (PEG) molecules are conjugated with the interferon protein. PEGylation increases the half-life and duration of action of interferons, and these preparations are given **subcutaneously once a week,** whereas non-PEGylated interferons are given 3 times a week. Interferons are not absorbed after oral administration.

Mechanism of Action

Interferons bind to cell surface receptors called interferon-alpha receptors (IFNAR) on leukocytes that are coupled to the **JAK-STAT signaling pathway.** JAK (Janus kinase) phosphorylates IFNAR, leading to activation of STATs (Signal Transducer and Activator of Transcription proteins), and then the activated STATs enter the cell nucleus to activate gene transcription. Gene transcription increase host defenses by activating **cytotoxic T lymphocytes** (CD8+, killer T cells) and by **degrading viral RNA,** and often lead to the destruction of both the virus and infected host cell.

Spectrum and Indications

Interferons are active against **hepatitis viruses** and **papillomaviruses,** and they are used in treating certain **neoplastic diseases** in which they activate tumor cell immunity (see Chapter 46).

Peginterferon alfa is used in combination with ribavirin and DAAs in the treatment of hepatitis B and C (see earlier). In patients with **chronic hepatitis B,** peginterferon treatment results in loss of hepatitis B antigens, normalization of serum aminotransferase activity, sustained hepatic histologic improvement, and a lower risk of liver disease progression.

Interferon alfa is used in the treatment of refractory cases of **condylomata acuminata,** a disorder characterized by papular **anogenital skin eruptions** caused by several types of human epidermotropic **papillomavirus (HPV).** This infection is now the most common **sexually transmitted disease** in western countries. The primary treatments for this condition are cytotoxic agents such as topical podophyllum resin. Refractory cases may respond to interferon alfa injected directly into the lesions three times a week for 3 weeks, then repeated after 12 to 16 weeks.

Adverse Effects

Parenterally administered interferons can cause many serious and unpleasant adverse effects, including hematologic toxicity, cardiac arrhythmias, altered blood pressure, central nervous system dysfunction, gastrointestinal distress, chills, fatigue, headache, and myalgia. Hence, other agents are preferred for treatment whenever available.

DRUGS FOR SMALLPOX INFECTIONS

Due to an unprecedented global immunization campaign, naturally occurring smallpox infection, due to the *variola* virus, was eradicated worldwide by 1980. However, because samples of smallpox virus are kept by the USA and Russia for research purposes, and the smallpox virus or similar virus can be synthesized in the lab, there are concerns that the smallpox virus could be used as a biological warfare agent. A vaccine prevents smallpox, but at present, there is a low risk of exposure to the smallpox virus, so the vaccine is no longer given.

Tecovirimat is the sole FDA-approved drug for the **treatment of smallpox. Tecovirimat** binds to and inhibits the activity of the orthopoxvirus VP37 protein (encoded by and highly conserved in all members of the orthopoxvirus genus) and prevents the formation of egress-competent enveloped virions needed for cell-to-cell and long-range dissemination of the virus.

TREATMENT OF SARS-COV-2 INFECTIONS

The year 2020 opened with a global pandemic produced by the SARS-CoV-2 virus, the causative agent of the disease called COVID-19. SARS-CoV-2 (which stands for Severe Acute Respiratory Syndrome CoronaVirus type 2) is an enveloped, positive-sense, single-stranded RNA *beta*-coronavirus of the family *Coronaviridae*. Previously isolated coronaviruses that infect humans usually produce only mild to moderate upper respiratory tract illness. Unfortunately, in the recent decades, highly pathogenic human coronaviruses arose, including SARS-CoV-1, the Middle East respiratory syndrome coronavirus (MERS-CoV), and the current SARS-CoV-2. At the time of this writing, there are no FDA-approved and highly effective drugs for treating SARS-CoV-2, SARS-CoV-1, or MERS-CoV infections.

One of the first existing drugs tested in COVID-19 patients was **hydroxychloroquine** (Plaquenil). **Hydroxychloroquine** is a drug approved for the treatment of malaria, lupus erythematosus, and rheumatoid arthritis (Chapter 44). Molecular simulation studies suggest that hydroxychloroquine binds to the coronavirus spike protein and prevents virus entry. Although clinical trials are still ongoing, the CDC does not recommend hydroxychloroquine use in COVID-19 patients at this time, and it is not approved for such use by the FDA.

A new drug that was in the clinical development pipeline at Gilead Sciences, **remdesivir** (Veklury), shows some promise in treating COVID-19 patients. Remdesivir is not fully approved by the FDA but is currently available through the Emergency Use Authorization (EUA) mechanism. Remdesivir showed mixed success against the 2014 Ebola virus outbreak in West Africa but is effective *in vitro* tests with SARS-CoV-2 infected cells. Remdesivir works by nucleotide substitution that clogs up the viral RNA polymerase.

Dexamethasone is a **high-potency, long-acting glucocorticoid** (Chapter 33) used in a number of disorders for its **potent immunosuppressive effects** (e.g., allergic states, arthritis, dermatological disorders, and many others). Dexamethasone is thought to combat the ill effects of the "**cytokine storm**" and greater than normal release of immunoreactive substances in response to SAR-CoV-2 virus infection. Dexamethasone is available to treat COVID-19 patients under the EUA mechanism of FDA approval.

In spite of the use of convalescent serum from COVID-19 containing anti-virus antibodies and other monoclonal antibody treatments (see Chapter 46), a successful vaccine against SARS-CoV-2 will be the ultimate answer to the pandemic.

SUMMARY OF IMPORTANT POINTS

- Acyclovir, famciclovir, penciclovir, and valacyclovir are nucleoside analogs used to treat HSV and VZV infections.
- Trifluridine is a nucleoside analog used to treat herpetic keratoconjunctivitis.
- Cidofovir and ganciclovir are nucleoside analogs used for the prevention and treatment of CMV diseases (e.g., retinitis, esophagitis, and colitis).
- Valacyclovir and valganciclovir are prodrugs that are converted to acyclovir or ganciclovir in vivo. The prodrugs have better oral bioavailability and produce higher serum levels of the active metabolites.
- Acyclovir, ganciclovir, and penciclovir are selectively phosphorylated to their monophosphate metabolites by viral kinases, and then host cell kinases convert them to triphosphates. Other nucleoside analogs, including those for treating HIV infection, are phosphorylated only by host cell kinases.
- Acyclovir and most NRTIs cause chain termination when they are incorporated into viral DNA. Ganciclovir and penciclovir inhibit viral DNA polymerase but are not incorporated into viral DNA.
- Foscarnet is a non-nucleoside drug used to treat CMV retinitis and acyclovir-resistant HSV and VZV infections.
- Drugs for HIV infection include agents that inhibit RT, HIV protease, integrase strand transfer (raltegravir and others), and HIV fusion (maraviroc and enfuvirtide).
- Drug combinations act synergistically to reduce viral loads, increase CD4 cells, and ameliorate symptoms. The currently preferred regimens for HIV infection consist of two nucleosides or NRTIs plus an INSTI or a PI.
- Frequently used NRTIs include ABC, tenofovir, emtricitabine, lamivudine, and ZDV. ZDV can cause anemia and neutropenia.
- The currently recommended PIs are darunavir and ritonavir. Ritonavir is also used to increase the serum levels of other drugs by inhibiting their metabolism by CYP450 enzymes.
- NNRTIs include rilpivirine and efavirenz. NNRTIs are used in alternative regimens for patients who do not respond to, or cannot tolerate, a preferred regimen.
- Some PIs and NNRTIs interact with other drugs via inhibition or induction of cytochrome P450 isozymes.
- Oseltamivir and zanamivir are neuraminidase inhibitors that inhibit the release and spreading of influenza A and B virions and are used in prophylaxis and treatment of influenza.
- Entecavir and tenofovir are nucleoside or –tide RT inhibitors and block transcription of viral RNA and are used to treat hepatitis B.
- Grazoprevir, simeprevir, and paritaprevir bind to nonstructural protein NS3-4A, a serine protease that catalyzes the cleavage of hepatitis C polyprotein during viral maturation.
- Dasabuvir and sofosbuvir inhibit the hepatitis C viral RNA polymerase that replicates the viral RNA genome.
- Daclatasvir, elbasvir, ledipasvir, ombitasvir, and velpatasvir bind and inhibit the hepatitis C nonstructural protein NS5A, which is an activator of viral RNA polymerase (NS5B).
- Ribavirin is a broad-spectrum antiviral drug used to treat RSV infection in neonates and hepatitis B and C in combination with other drugs.
- Palivizumab is a monoclonal antibody used to prevent and treat RSV infection in infants who are at increased risk of serious disease and hospitalization. The agent prevents the fusion of the virus and host cell.

- Peginterferon-alfa is used to treat hepatitis B and hepatitis C. Localized interferon alfa injections are used to treat anogenital papular eruptions (condylomata acuminata) due to papillomavirus.

Review Questions

1. A man with HIV infection is taking darunavir, a protease inhibitor. Which adverse effect is associated with this class of drugs?
   (A) anemia
   (B) pancreatitis
   (C) neuropsychiatric reactions
   (D) peripheral neuropathy
   (E) elevated triglyceride and cholesterol levels

2. A patient with shingles receives a drug that is converted to penciclovir in the body. Which antiviral action is exerted by this agent?
   (A) blockade of guanosine triphosphate synthesis
   (B) inhibition of DNA polymerase
   (C) inhibition of viral entry
   (D) DNA chain termination
   (E) prevention of viral maturation

3. A woman with influenza is treated with zanamivir. Which step in viral replication is prevented by this drug?
   (A) entry into host cells
   (B) uncoating of viral nucleic acid
   (C) replication of viral nucleic acid
   (D) maturation of viral proteins
   (E) release of progeny virions

4. Which non-nucleoside drug is used to treat systemic acyclovir and ganciclovir-resistant herpesvirus infections, such as CMV esophagitis?
   (A) foscarnet
   (B) trifluridine
   (C) ribavirin
   (D) rilpivirine
   (E) efavirenz

5. Which drug inhibits nonstructural protein 3-4A and prevents maturation of hepatitis C virus?
   (A) dasabuvir
   (B) ombitasvir
   (C) simeprevir
   (D) ledipasvir
   (E) daclatasvir

CHAPTER 44

Drugs for the Treatment of Parasites

CLASSIFICATION OF ANTIPARASITIC DRUGS

Drugs for Infections Caused by Lumen- and Tissue-Dwelling Protozoa

- Metronidazole (FLAGYL)
- Tinidazole (TINDAMAX)
- Nitazoxanide (ALINIA)
- Paromomycin

Drugs for Infections Caused by Blood- and Tissue-Dwelling Protozoa

Treatment of malaria

- Artesunate
- Primaquine
- Chloroquine (ARALEN)[a]
- Artemether with lumefantrine (COARTEM)[b]

Treatment of toxoplasmosis

- Pyrimethamine (DARAPRIM)

Treatment of other protozoan infections

- Pentamidine (NEBUPENT)
- Nifurtimox (LAMPIT)[c]

Drugs for Helminth Infections

Treatment of nematode infections

- Albendazole (ALBENZA)
- Mebendazole (EMVERM)
- Ivermectin (STROMECTOL)[d]

Treatment of trematode and cestode infections

- Praziquantel (BILTRICIDE)
- Triclabendazole (EGATEN)

Drugs for Ectoparasite Infestations

- Permethrin (NIX)
- Spinosad (NATROBA)
- Abametapir (XEGLYZE)

[a] Also hydroxychloroquine (PLAQUENIL), tafenoquine (ARAKODA, KRINTAFEL), mefloquine, quinine, doxycycline, and clindamycin.
[b] Also atovaquone with proguanil (MALARONE).
[c] Also miltefosine (IMPAVIDO).
[d] Also moxidectin.

OVERVIEW

Parasitism refers to the relationship between two species in which one species, the parasite, benefits from the other species, the host, from which it derives nutrients and other resources. **Endoparasitic infections** are caused by organisms that live within their host—most commonly protozoans and helminths—while **ectoparasitic infections** are due to organisms that live on the skin, primarily **arthropods such as lice and mites**. Parasitic infections affect a large percentage of the population in many parts of the world, particularly in areas where the climate is warm and moist, the sanitation

is poor, and insects and other vectors of disease are prevalent. It is estimated that billions of people in tropical and subtropical regions are infected with **protozoa** (motile, unicellular eukaryotic organisms that dwell in the lumen, tissue, or blood of the host) and **helminths** (worms, including nematodes, trematodes, and cestodes).

Antiparasitic drugs are substances that are **selectively toxic to parasites**, permitting systemic or topical administration to persons with endoparasitic or ectoparasitic infections, respectively. The development of new drugs over the past 50 years has enabled remarkable advances in the treatment of parasitic infections, but more efficacious and less toxic agents are still needed for infections such as trypanosomiasis. **Albendazole** and **mebendazole** have significantly improved the treatment of intestinal nematode infections, whereas **praziquantel** has revolutionized the treatment of trematode and cestode infections. In addition, **metronidazole** and **tinidazole** have provided more effective and less toxic drugs for the treatment of amebiasis, giardiasis, and trichomoniasis. The sites and mechanisms of action of selected antiparasitic drugs are depicted in Fig. 44.1.

Table 44.1 provides information about the causes and treatment of numerous parasitic infections. This chapter focuses on the most commonly used antiparasitic agents and those that represent important advances in the treatment of these infections. Because of increased immigration and international travel, health care providers see **endoparasitic infections** rarely found in their local patient population. A few antibacterial and antifungal agents (e.g., tetracycline or amphotericin B) are listed as a preferred or alternative drug, and these agents are discussed in earlier chapters of this book.

DRUGS FOR INFECTIONS CAUSED BY LUMEN- AND TISSUE-DWELLING PROTOZOA

Amebiasis, balantidiasis, cryptosporidiosis, giardiasis, and **trichomoniasis** are examples of infections caused by protozoan parasites that dwell in the intestines and tissues of their human hosts. Among the agents used to treat these infections are **metronidazole, tinidazole,** and **paromomycin** (see Table 44.1).

Metronidazole and Tinidazole
Chemistry and Pharmacokinetics

Metronidazole and **tinidazole** are synthetic nitroimidazole compounds that are **well absorbed** from the gut and widely distributed to tissues and fluids throughout the body, including the liver and central nervous system (CNS). These compounds are extensively metabolized by CYP3A4 before undergoing renal excretion, and their serum concentrations can be affected by concurrent use of drugs that inhibit or induce this enzyme. **Tinidazole has a considerably longer half-life than metronidazole** (13 hours *versus* 8 hours) and can be given less frequently. Both drugs are usually

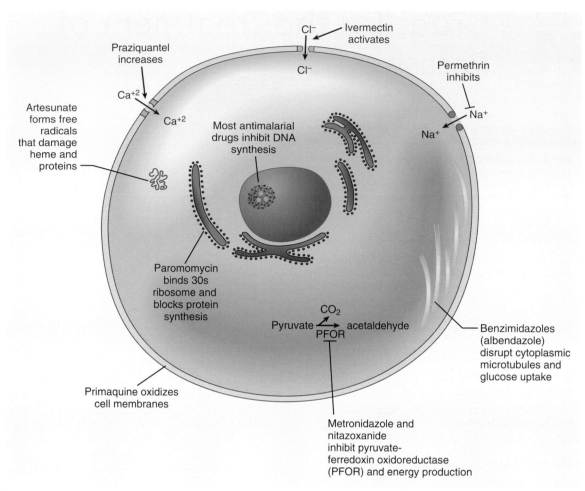

Fig. 44.1 Sites of action and mechanisms of antiparasitic drugs. The sites and mechanisms of antiparasitic agents include cell membranes and ion channels, energy metabolism enzymes, cytoplasmic microtubules, DNA synthesis, ribosomal protein synthesis, and free radical damage.

administered orally, and an intravenous preparation of metronidazole is available for treating severe infections.

Mechanism and Clinical Use

The antiparasitic activity of metronidazole and tinidazole is due to the formation of **nitro free radicals** when the nitro group of these drugs is reduced by **pyruvate-ferredoxin oxidoreductase,** an enzyme found in anaerobic parasites. The free radicals attack DNA and proteins, causing a cytotoxic effect.

Metronidazole and tinidazole are the **preferred agents** for treating infections caused by *Entamoeba histolytica, Giardia intestinalis (Giardia lamblia)*, and *Trichomonas vaginalis.* **Tinidazole** has greater efficacy than metronidazole against most susceptible pathogens, producing a **higher cure rate** in a shorter period of time than metronidazole. Moreover, tinidazole is active against some metronidazole-resistant strains of these parasites. Metronidazole and tinidazole are also used to treat infections due to **anaerobic bacteria,** including *Bacteroides fragilis, Helicobacter pylori,* and *Clostridiodes difficile.*

Amebiasis is transmitted by the fecal-oral route and is usually asymptomatic, though some persons develop mild to severe symptoms. Symptomatic patients typically have an intestinal infection that may be accompanied by dysentery (diarrhea with bloody stools, fever, and abdominal pain).

In some cases, patients develop extraintestinal disease, such as hepatic infection and abscess or peritonitis. The treatment of amebiasis includes **luminal amebicides** that eradicate intestinal organisms and **tissue amebicides** that attack organisms in infected intestinal and body tissues. **Metronidazole and tinidazole** are tissue amebicides that are usually given in combination with a luminal amebicide to treat symptomatic infections. Tinidazole was found to cure about 90% of persons with intestinal or extraintestinal amebiasis with 3 to 5 days of treatment.

Giardiasis is the most common parasitic infection in the United States and is caused by the flagellated protozoan *Giardia intestinalis (lamblia)* found throughout the world. Giardiasis is transmitted by the fecal-oral route and is usually contracted by drinking water from contaminated streams and ponds that contain the cyst form of the parasite. The infection causes abdominal discomfort, bloating, protracted **diarrhea,** and weight loss and is most commonly reported in children. A **single large dose** of tinidazole cures more than 90% of patients with **giardiasis,** whereas metronidazole is given three times daily for 5 days to treat this infection.

Trichomoniasis is a sexually transmitted disease that produces vaginitis in women but is usually asymptomatic in men. To prevent reinfection, it is important to treat both symptomatic patients and their sexual partners with a single

TABLE 44.1 Causes and Treatment of Parasitic Infections and Infestations

CONDITION	COMMON PATHOGENS	PRIMARY DRUGS	ALTERNATIVE DRUGS
Intestinal Protozoan Infections			
Amebiasis, symptomatic with diarrhea, dysentery, or hepatic abscess	*Entamoeba histolytica*	Metronidazole or tinidazole followed by paromomycin	
Amebiasis, asymptomatic cyst passer	*E. histolytica*	Paromomycin	
Balantidiasis	*Balantidium coli*	Tetracycline	Metronidazole
Cryptosporidiosis	*Cryptosporidium parvum*	Nitazoxanide	Fluids and antidiarrheal medication
Dientamoeba infection	*Dientamoeba fragilis*	Metronidazole	Tetracycline, metronidazole, or paromomycin
Giardiasis	*Giardia intestinalis*	Tinidazole or nitazoxanide	Paromomycin or metronidazole
Microsporidiosis	*Encephalitozoon* and *Enterocytozoon* species	Albendazole	Fumagillin
Extraintestinal Protozoan Infections			
Amebic meningoencephalitis	*Naegleria fowleri*	Amphotericin B, azithromycin, or both	
Babesiosis	*Babesia microti*	Atovaquone and/or azithromycin	Clindamycin plus quinine
Leishmaniasis	*Leishmania* species	Visceral: miltefosine or antimony drug (sodium stibogluconate)	Cutaneous: miltefosine, amphotericin B, antimony drug, or fluconazole
Malaria	*Plasmodium vivax* or *Plasmodium ovale*	Primaquine plus chloroquine; primaquine plus artesunate	Primaquine plus quinine and doxycycline
	Chloroquine-sensitive *Plasmodium falciparum*	Chloroquine	Artesunate; quinine plus doxycycline; mefloquine
	Chloroquine-resistant *P. falciparum,* prophylaxis	Atovaquone plus proguanil; also, mosquito nets and repellants	Doxycycline or mefloquine
	Chloroquine-resistant *P. falciparum,* treatment	Artemether plus lumefantrine; artesunate plus mefloquine; atovaquone plus proguanil	Quinine, doxycycline, clindamycin
Toxoplasmosis	*Toxoplasma gondii*	Pyrimethamine plus clindamycin plus folinic acid	Trimethoprim plus sulfamethoxazole; atovaquone
Trichomoniasis	*Trichomonas vaginalis*	Metronidazole or tinidazole	
Trypanosomiasis (African sleeping sickness)	*Trypanosoma brucei*	Pentamidine (early disease); eflornithine (late CNS disease)	
Trypanosomiasis, American (Chagas disease)	*Trypanosoma cruzi*	Nifurtimox	Benznidazole
Intestinal Nematode Infections			
Ascariasis	*Ascaris lumbricoides*	Albendazole or mebendazole	Ivermectin or nitazoxanide
Capillariasis	*Capillaria philippinensis*	Mebendazole	Albendazole
Pinworm infection	*Enterobius vermicularis*	Albendazole or mebendazole	
Hookworm infection	*Ancylostoma duodenale* and *Necator americanus*	Albendazole or mebendazole	
Strongyloidiasis	*Strongyloides stercoralis*	Ivermectin	Albendazole
Whipworm infection	*Trichuris trichiura*	Albendazole	Mebendazole or ivermectin
Extraintestinal Nematode Infections			
Cutaneous or visceral larva migrans	*Ancylostoma braziliense*	Albendazole	Ivermectin
Guinea worm	*Dracunculus medinensis*	Surgical removal	Metronidazole or mebendazole
Filariasis, lymphatic	*Wuchereria bancrofti; Brugia malayi* and *Brugia timori*	Doxycycline 6–8 weeks, then add Ivermectin	Albendazole or ivermectin
Filariasis, cutaneous	*Loa loa*	Ivermectin	Albendazole
River blindness	*Onchocerca volvulus*	Doxycycline followed by ivermectin ± prednisone	
Trichinosis	*Trichinella spiralis*	Albendazole + prednisone	Mebendazole + prednisone

Continued

TABLE 44.1 Causes and Treatment of Parasitic Infections and Infestations—cont'd

CONDITION	COMMON PATHOGENS	PRIMARY DRUGS	ALTERNATIVE DRUGS
Trematode Infections			
Schistosomiasis	*Schistosoma* species	Praziquantel	Oxamniquine for *Schistosoma mansoni*
Chinese liver fluke	*Clonorchis sinensis*	Praziquantel	Albendazole
Sheep liver fluke	*Fasciola hepatica*	Triclabendazole or nitazoxanide	Bithionol
Lung fluke	*Paragonimus westermani*	Praziquantel	Bithionol
Cestode Infections			
Beef tapeworm	*Taenia saginata*	Praziquantel	Niclosamide
Pork tapeworm	*Taenia solium*	Praziquantel	Niclosamide
Dog tapeworm	*Dipylidium caninum*	Praziquantel	Niclosamide
Dwarf tapeworm	*Hymenolepis nana*	Praziquantel	
Fish tapeworm	*Diphyllobothrium latum*	Praziquantel	Niclosamide
Cysticercosis	Larval *T. solium*	Albendazole or praziquantel for CNS disease + dexamethasone	
Echinococcosis (hydatid disease)	*Echinococcus granulosus*	Percutaneous aspiration + albendazole	
Ectoparasite Infestations			
Head lice, crabs	*Pediculus humanus, Phthirus pubis*	Permethrin, spinosad (head lice)	Malathion, ivermectin
Scabies (mites)	*Sarcoptes scabiei*	Permethrin	Ivermectin

CNS, Central nervous system.

large dose of tinidazole or smaller doses of metronidazole for 7 days.

Metronidazole is also used in the management of several disorders that are not caused by protozoa. For example, it is used in the treatment of patients with **dracunculiasis** (guinea worm infection). This infection is caused by *Dracunculus medinensis,* a nematode found in India, Pakistan, and parts of Africa. Although metronidazole is not curative, it reduces inflammation and facilitates manual removal of the worm. Metronidazole is also used for treatment of **enterocolitis** caused by *Clostridioides difficile,* and it is occasionally used to treat infections caused by other anaerobic bacteria. Metronidazole is available in gel or cream form for the topical treatment of **rosacea** (acne rosacea), a skin condition characterized by persistent erythema of the middle third of the face and other areas of the body.

Adverse Effects and Interactions

Metronidazole and tinidazole are usually well tolerated but can cause **gastrointestinal discomfort** as well as nausea, vomiting, a metallic taste, and transient leukopenia or thrombocytopenia. To reduce the gastrointestinal side effects, patients should take these drugs with food. Due to potential adverse effects on the embryo and fetus, these drugs are contraindicated in the first trimester of pregnancy.

Metronidazole and tinidazole can increase the anticoagulant effect of warfarin, and the dosage of warfarin may need to be reduced if therapy is prolonged. Metronidazole also causes a disulfiram-like reaction with ethanol, so patients should avoid drinking alcohol while they are undergoing treatment.

Paromomycin and Nitazoxanide

Paromomycin is a **luminal amebicide** but not a tissue amebicide. A luminal amebicide can be used alone to treat **asymptomatic carriers** of *E. histolytica,* but it must be used in combination **with a tissue amebicide** to treat patients with symptomatic disease, including amebic dysentery and liver abscess. The preferred combination is usually tinidazole or metronidazole followed by paromomycin (see Table 44.1).

Cryptosporidiosis is a diarrheal illness that is usually self-limiting, but it may cause chronic diarrhea in immunocompromised persons, such as those with acquired immunodeficiency syndrome (AIDS). **Nitazoxanide** is a broad-spectrum antiprotozoal agent that is active against several intestinal protozoa, including *Cryptosporidium parvum, Giardia lamblia,* and *Entamoeba histolytica.* The drug is a noncompetitive inhibitor of **pyruvate-ferredoxin oxidoreductase.** Nitazoxanide is indicated for the treatment of **cryptosporidiosis** and **giardiasis** in **immunocompetent persons.** The drug is well tolerated, and a short course of treatment is usually effective. Antidiarrheal medications are also useful in these conditions. Unfortunately, nitazoxanide is **not effective** in treating **cryptosporidiosis in AIDS,** but the use of highly active antiretroviral drugs (see Chapter 43) will improve immune function and usually clear the infection in these patients. Nitazoxanide is also reported to be effective in treating certain helminth infections, including **ascariasis.**

DRUGS FOR INFECTIONS CAUSED BY BLOOD- AND TISSUE-DWELLING PROTOZOA

Babesiosis, leishmaniasis, malaria, toxoplasmosis, and **trypanosomiasis** are examples of infections caused by

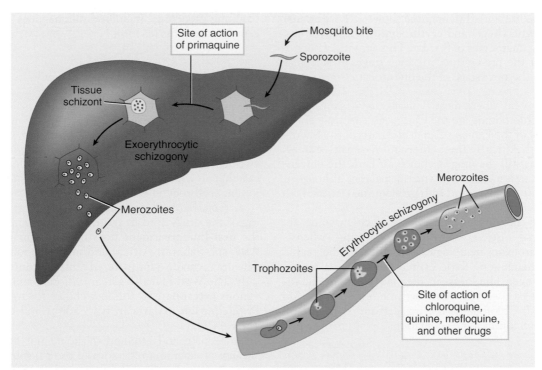

FIG. 44.2 Sites of action of drugs for malaria. When a person is bitten by an infected mosquito, *Plasmodium* sporozoites enter the liver, form tissue schizonts, and undergo exoerythrocytic schizogony to produce merozoites. The merozoites released from the liver invade erythrocytes and form trophozoites that undergo erythrocytic schizogony. Some trophozoites develop into male and female gametocytes, which must subsequently pass back into a mosquito before they can develop into sporozoites and repeat the infection cycle. Primaquine blocks exoerythrocytic schizogony, whereas other antimalarial drugs inhibit erythrocytic schizogony.

protozoan parasites that dwell in the blood and tissues of their human hosts.

Drugs for Malaria

Malaria is one of the **most common infectious diseases** in the world today and is believed to be **responsible for more deaths** than any other infectious disease. Several species of *Plasmodium* cause malaria, including *Plasmodium falciparum*, *Plasmodium malariae*, *Plasmodium ovale*, and *Plasmodium vivax*. Most cases of malaria are caused by *P. falciparum* or *P. vivax*. The disease is spread via the bites of the genus **Anopheles** mosquito and is primarily found in tropical and subtropical areas. Malaria has been largely eliminated from temperate regions, and most infections in North America and Europe are acquired during travel to other countries. Nevertheless, periodic outbreaks of mosquito-borne malaria still occur in the southern United States and Mexico.

Malaria is transmitted when infected mosquitoes inject *Plasmodium* sporozoites into the blood of the host (Fig. 44.2). The sporozoites invade the liver where they undergo **exoerythrocytic schizogony** (asexual multiplication) to form multinucleated tissue **schizonts**. These schizonts then divide their cytoplasm to form thousands of **merozoites** that are released into the blood where they infect erythrocytes and undergo repeated **erythrocytic schizogony** as additional erythrocytes are infected.

The synchronous release of erythrocytic merozoites is responsible for the **episodic fever characteristic of malaria**. During an infection with *P. falciparum* or *P. vivax*, the fever spikes every other day. The disease produced by *P. falciparum* (malignant tertian malaria) is more severe than that produced by *P. vivax* (benign tertian malaria), partly because

P. falciparum causes a **higher level of parasitemia** and produces a persistently higher temperature during the periods between fever spikes.

Whereas both *P. vivax* and *P. ovale* have a **persistent exoerythrocytic stage**, *P. falciparum* and *P. malariae* do not. To eradicate this persistent stage and prevent the relapse of malaria, patients infected with *P. vivax* or *P. ovale* should be treated with the **tissue schizonticide primaquine**.

Sites and Mechanisms of Action

Fig. 44.2 shows the sites of action of drugs for malaria. **Primaquine** inhibits **exoerythrocytic (tissue) schizogony.** All other antimalarial agents **inhibit erythrocytic** schizogony as described in the sections that follow.

Chloroquine and Quinine

Quinine was used for centuries to treat malaria until supplanted by **chloroquine** after World War II. Resistance to chloroquine began to develop in the late 1950s and gradually spread to most areas of the world where malaria was endemic by the 1980s. Newer drugs gradually replaced chloroquine, but malarial resistance to these agents has developed in some areas. Combination drug therapy is often used to treat malaria today.

Chloroquine, hydroxychloroquine, **mefloquine,** tafenoquine, and **quinine** have similar chemical structures. Their mechanisms of action have not been clearly identified. Some evidence indicates that they **prevent the degradation of heme** during the parasite's utilization of hemoglobin in infected erythrocytes. The newest agent, **tafenoquine,** is indicated for prophylaxis and treatment of malaria, with a different brand name and dose for each indivcation

(ARAKODA, KRINTAFEL). **Tafenoquine** shows activity **against pre-erythrocytic** (liver) and **erythrocytic** (asexual) forms, and also the **gametocytes** of *P. vivax*. This activity of tafenoquine against the pre-erythrocytic liver stages of the parasite prevents the next stage of the erythrocytic stage of the parasite.

The only areas where most *P. falciparum* organisms are sensitive to chloroquine are the Caribbean islands, Central America west of the Panama Canal, and parts of the Middle East and North Africa. In these **chloroquine-sensitive areas,** chloroquine is still the drug of choice for both the prevention and the treatment of all types of malaria, although it must be used in combination with **primaquine** (see later) to eradicate *P. vivax* or *P. ovale*.

The most common adverse effects of chloroquine are gastrointestinal distress, nausea, and vomiting, whereas various hematologic, neurologic, and electrocardiographic effects are uncommon. Toxic overdoses can cause **retinal damage** and even **blindness.** In pregnant women, chloroquine should be used cautiously because fetal damage has been reported. Chloroquine may exacerbate psoriasis, and pruritus is common in some populations.

Mefloquine

Mefloquine was a highly effective drug for chloroquine-resistant malaria when it was first introduced in the 1980s, but cure rates have dropped substantially in Southeast Asia. The drug is used for prophylaxis and treatment of **falciparum malaria,** where it is known to be effective, and the combination of **artesunate plus mefloquine** is a first-line therapy in parts of Southeast Asia and South America (see Table 44.1). Mefloquine is given orally, undergoes hepatic metabolism, has a half-life of about 14 days, and is eliminated via the bile and feces.

Mefloquine may cause nausea, vomiting, dizziness, and headache. The higher doses used for treatment of malaria may occasionally cause a **neuropsychiatric syndrome** characterized by hallucinations, anxiety, confusion, seizures, and coma. It can also cause leukopenia and thrombocytopenia as well as bradycardia and arrhythmias.

Primaquine

Primaquine is an aminoquinoline derivative that is active against the **exoerythrocytic tissue stage** of *P. vivax* and *P. ovale*. The mode of action of primaquine is unclear, but it appears to form quinones that oxidize and destroy schizont membranes. By eradicating tissue plasmodia, primaquine prevents the reemergence of organisms from the liver and relapse of the infection. Primaquine is not active against the erythrocytic stage of these organisms and must be used in combination with chloroquine or other drugs to treat *P. vivax* or *P. ovale* infections.

Primaquine may cause **hemolytic anemia** in individuals who have hereditary **glucose-6-phosphate dehydrogenase (G6PD) deficiency,** resulting from the drug's ability to oxidize and destroy erythrocyte membranes. Hemolysis occurs because there is insufficient G6PD to generate enough reduced nicotinamide adenine dinucleotide phosphate (NADPH) to maintain glutathione in its reduced form and prevent oxidation of erythrocyte membranes. Individuals who experience this type of hemolytic anemia are said to have **primaquine sensitivity.** A number of other drugs with oxidizing properties, including sulfonamides and sulfones, can also cause this reaction.

Artesunate and Artemether

The search for new agents to treat multidrug-resistant *P. falciparum* malaria led to the identification of **artemisinin** (*qinghaosu*) as the active ingredient of *Artemisia annua*, a plant used in Chinese medicine for over two millennia. Two derivatives of artemisinin called *artemether* and *artesunate* were subsequently found to have potent activity against the erythrocytic stages of malaria. These drugs form **free radicals** that attack heme and proteins in malarial parasites and inhibit **erythrocytic schizogony.**

Artemether and artesunate are the most **rapidly acting** of the drugs used to treat falciparum malaria and are the **first-line treatment** for this infection in Southeast Asia, sub-Saharan Africa, and much of South America. The drugs can be administered orally, parenterally, or rectally. The World Health Organization recommends **intravenous artesunate** as the first choice for treating **severe *P. falciparum* malaria** in both adults and children (see Table 44.1).

Artesunate and artemether should not be used alone because of emerging resistance of the parasite these drugs. Artesunate-mefloquine is often used in Southeast Asia, whereas artesunate-amodiaquine or artemether plus lumefantrine (COARTEM) are used in many parts of Africa. These drugs are also being used to treat *P. vivax* malaria. For current recommendations, see http://www.cdc.gov/malaria and http://who.int/malaria/en/.

Atovaquone and Proguanil

Atovaquone selectively **inhibits mitochondria electron transport** in plasmodia whereas **proguanil** is converted to an active metabolite that inhibits plasmodial **dihydrofolate reductase** and the formation of tetrahydrofolate required for synthesis of DNA. The combination of atovaquone and proguanil (MALARONE) is considered an alternative drug for prophylaxis and treatment of **chloroquine-resistant falciparum malaria.** Atovaquone is also used in the treatment of *Pneumocystis jiroveci* (*carinii*) infections.

Drugs for Toxoplasmosis

In immunocompromised individuals and congenitally infected neonates, *Toxoplasma gondii* can cause **severe damage** to many organs. For example, *T. gondii* may cause ocular infections and encephalitis in patients with AIDS. *T. gondii* can also cause encephalomyelitis, hydrocephaly, microcephaly, or chorioretinitis in the offspring of women who were infected during pregnancy. Women who were infected with *T. gondii* before pregnancy are not at risk of transmitting the infection to their offspring. In immunocompetent individuals, *T. gondii* infection is common but rarely symptomatic. Even in cases in which it is symptomatic, treatment is not normally required.

Although toxoplasmosis is usually treated with **pyrimethamine** plus **clindamycin** or **dapsone.** Higher doses are required to treat toxoplasmosis in AIDS and lifelong maintenance therapy may be needed to prevent reactivation of the disease. **Leucovorin** (folinic acid) can be added to the treatment regimen to reduce the hematologic effects of these drugs.

Drugs for *Pneumocystis jiroveci* (carinii) Infections

Because *P. jiroveci*, formerly *P. carinii*, was formerly classified as a protozoan parasite, it is discussed in this chapter. However, several studies have shown that it is actually a **yeast-like fungus.** In addition to causing **pneumonia** in premature and malnourished infants, the organism causes pneumonia and other diseases in immunocompromised persons, including those with AIDS.

The treatment of choice for *P. jiroveci* infections is **trimethoprim-sulfamethoxazole**, a drug combination discussed in Chapter 40. Atovaquone and pentamidine are alternatives. **Prednisone**, a corticosteroid drug, is also administered to acutely ill patients to reduce pulmonary inflammation.

The agents used to treat *Pneumocystis* infections are also used for prophylaxis and for posttreatment suppression of this infection. **Pentamidine** is given intravenously for the treatment of *P. jiroveci* infections, but it is administered by inhalation for prevention. The **many adverse effects** of pentamidine include hematologic toxicity, ventricular tachycardia, edema, pancreatitis, bronchospasm, and Stevens-Johnson syndrome (toxic epidermal necrolysis), which is a life-threatening hypersensitivity reaction.

Drugs for Other Protozoan Infections

Pentamidine, given either alone or in combination with **melarsoprol**, is used to treat **African trypanosomiasis** (sleeping sickness), a disease caused by *Trypanosoma brucei* and transmitted by the tsetse fly in sub-Saharan Africa. **Pentamidine** is used for the early stages of the infection (fever, joint pains, swollen lymph nodes in the back of the neck), whereas **eflornithine** is indicated to treat the late CNS manifestations of the disease (confusion, disruption of the sleep cycle). These drugs must be administered intravenously and can cause serious toxicity.

Nifurtimox is the drug of choice for the treatment of **American trypanosomiasis** (Chagas disease), a disease caused by *Trypanosoma cruzi* and transmitted by a group of so-called "assassin" (reduviid) bugs in Central and South America. However, the effectiveness of nifurtimox is limited.

The causes and treatment of babesiosis and leishmaniasis are outlined in Table 44.1. **Miltefosine** is used to treat **cutaneous and visceral leishmaniasis,** which is also known as *kala-azar* (black fever). Miltefosine is a membrane-active phospholipid that inhibits enzymes involved in the metabolism of glycolipids found on the surface of *Leishmania* species. It is well absorbed after oral administration and has a half-life of about 8 days. In the past, antimonial drug treatments for leishmaniasis had to be given parenterally for prolonged periods and caused considerable toxicity. In contrast, miltefosine given orally for 28 days produced a 94% to 97% cure rate of visceral leishmaniasis in children at the end of treatment and at 6-month follow-up. The most common adverse effects have been vomiting and diarrhea, but they usually have been of brief duration and only mild to moderate in severity. A few patients have experienced reversible hepatic and renal toxicity. Because of the high efficacy and relatively low toxicity of miltefosine, it appears to represent a breakthrough in the treatment of visceral and other forms of leishmaniasis (Box 44.1).

DRUGS FOR INFECTIONS CAUSED BY HELMINTHS

Helminths can be classified as **nematodes** (roundworms), **trematodes** (flukes), and **cestodes** (tapeworms). The most

---

BOX 44.1 A CASE OF CUTANEOUS SORES

CASE PRESENTATION

A 42-year-old embassy official in Afghanistan comes to a medical clinic with spreading sores on his left cheek and both arms. The lesions, which developed at the site of insect bites he received several weeks earlier, now measure 2–2.5 cm in diameter. The sores are blistery in appearance with an indurated edge and a central ulceration. A biopsy of the lesions shows *Leishmania* amastigotes (the form of the parasite found in infected tissue), and an indirect immunofluorescence test is positive for *Leishmania*. After a discussion of treatment options, the patient is given oral miltefosine for 4 weeks. The treatment is well tolerated. However, there is a mild increase in serum aspartate aminotransferase and alanine aminotransferase levels during the first week of therapy, which resolves spontaneously. The lesions gradually improve during the course of therapy, and the skin is completely healed 4 months later.

CASE DISCUSSION

Leishmaniasis is a protozoan infection caused by a number of *Leishmania* species and is usually transmitted by the bite of tiny female phlebotomine sandflies. The disease is found in many tropical and subtropical countries, ranging from the rainforests of Central and South America to the deserts of North Africa. It is found in India, Iraq, and Afghanistan, as well as in Mexico and southern Texas, and a few cases have been reported recently in northern Texas. Cutaneous leishmaniasis is the most common form of the disease and often heals spontaneously after several months. Visceral leishmaniasis, which may develop from cutaneous lesions, can cause life-threatening spleen and liver damage if not treated. Cutaneous leishmaniasis often begins with small erythematous lesions that develop weeks to months after a sandfly bite and gradually increase in size to several centimeters in diameter. Frequent use of an insect repellant and sleeping under a bed net are the best methods of preventing sandfly bites and leishmaniasis. Relatively toxic antimony compounds requiring parenteral administration have been the main treatment for leishmaniasis until recently. Miltefosine is a new orally effective drug that appears to be well tolerated, though gastrointestinal disturbances are common, and serum liver enzymes may be elevated by the drug.

---

common parasites are listed in Table 44.1 and infect billions of people throughout the world. Effective drugs are available to treat most helminth infections, but the cost of drug treatment can be high, and many infections go untreated. The World Health Organization and government agencies have sponsored mass treatment programs for some infections, including **onchocerciasis** (river blindness) and **schistosomiasis**.

Drugs used to treat helminth infections are called anthelmintic drugs. Most of these drugs act by **inhibiting metabolism** in the parasite (e.g., albendazole) or by causing **muscle paralysis** (ivermectin, praziquantel, or pyrantel). In many cases, a single dose or a few doses of the drug are curative.

Drugs for Nematode Infections

Albendazole and Mebendazole

Chemistry and Pharmacokinetics. Albendazole and related drugs are benzimidazole compounds that have low water solubility and oral bioavailability. Only about 5% of albendazole and 10% of mebendazole is absorbed from an empty stomach, but absorption is markedly improved if the drug is taken with a high-fat meal. Albendazole is converted to albendazole sulfoxide in the intestinal epithelium and by first-pass hepatic metabolism, and this metabolite accounts for the systemic activity of the drug. The level of albendazole in cerebrospinal fluid is about 40% of the level in plasma. The drugs are eliminated by metabolism and renal excretion.

Mechanisms. The benzimidazoles bind to β-**tubulin** and **inhibit the polymerization of tubulin dimers** and the **formation of cytoplasmic microtubules** in parasites. This action **impairs glucose uptake** and leads to glycogen depletion and decreased energy production, causing immobilization and death.

Spectrum and Indications. Albendazole and mebendazole are primarily used to treat **intestinal nematode infections,** including **ascariasis**, capillariasis, hookworm infection, pinworm infection, and **whipworm infection**. For **trichinosis**, the anthelmintic drug is usually given in combination with a corticosteroid (e.g., prednisone) to relieve the inflammation.

As shown in Table 44.1, albendazole is also used to treat two cestode infections: **cysticercosis** and **echinococcosis**. For echinococcosis, surgical aspiration usually is used in conjunction with albendazole therapy. Treatment is not recommended for cysticercosis outside the CNS, which is benign. For cysticercosis in the CNS, albendazole or praziquantel can be effective along with a corticosteroid (e.g., dexamethasone) to control inflammation caused by cyst death.

Albendazole is also used to treat **microsporidiosis**, an infection caused by several species of intestinal protozoans.

Parasitic Resistance. Resistance to the benzimidazoles is now a worldwide problem in veterinary medicine, but it is not yet a significant problem in human medicine.

Adverse Effects and Contraindications. Albendazole and mebendazole are well tolerated and produce few adverse effects. The most common side effects of albendazole and mebendazole are mild gastrointestinal discomfort and constipation or diarrhea. The high doses of albendazole used to treat echinococcosis can cause hepatitis or hematologic toxicity. All of the benzimidazole drugs are contraindicated during pregnancy because of their potential to inhibit mitosis and impair fetal development.

Ivermectin

Chemistry and Pharmacokinetics. Ivermectin is a semisynthetic derivative of avermectin, an antibiotic containing a macrocytic lactone obtained from *Streptomyces avermitilis*. The drug is well absorbed from the gut, undergoes hepatic biotransformation, and is excreted in the feces with an elimination half-life of about 25 hours.

Mechanisms. Ivermectin increases the **chloride permeability** of invertebrate muscle cells. This hyperpolarizes the cell membrane and causes **paralysis of the pharyngeal muscles** in helminths. Ivermectin is believed to activate the glutamate-gated chloride channel in invertebrate tissue, but it has no effect on chloride ion permeability in mammalian tissue.

Spectrum and Indications. Ivermectin is a **broad-spectrum anthelmintic** drug that is active against a wide range of **nematodes**. It has been used to treat a number of intestinal helminthic infections in domestic and companion animals. In humans, it is used to treat **strongyloidiasis, onchocerciasis,** and **cutaneous larva migrans**. Ivermectin has revolutionized the management of onchocerciasis. It is active against the microfilariae (skin-dwelling, first-stage larvae) of *Onchocerca volvulus*, even at a very low dosage. When a single dose is administered once a year, it can prevent the ocular form of onchocerciasis, which is called **river blindness**. Repeated treatment is necessary because the drug is not active against the adult parasites and only prevents the maturation of filarial offspring.

Ivermectin is active against all stages of the *Loa loa* parasite and is currently used to treat loiasis, a **filarial disease** that can cause both ocular and skin manifestations. Ivermectin is also active against the microfilariae of *Brugia malayi* and *Wuchereria bancrofti*, parasites that cause lymphatic filariasis, though DEC is usually the drug of choice. Studies show that low doses of the drug kill *W. bancrofti*, whereas higher doses are effective against *B. malayi*. Recently, ivermectin has also been used to treat scabies.

Adverse Effects. Ivermectin is usually well tolerated and produces few adverse effects. Uncommonly, it causes constipation, diarrhea, dizziness, vertigo, or sedation.

Moxidectin

Moxidectin is an anthelmintic indicated for the treatment of **onchocerciasis** (river blindness) due to the **nematode** *Onchocerca volvulus*. **Moxidectin** binds to **chloride ion channels** and *gamma*-aminobutyric acid **(GABA) receptors** causing increased membrane permeability, neuronal inhibition by hyperpolarization, and muscle paralysis. Moxidectin also decreases motor movement of all stages of the parasite, and the fertility of both male and female adult worms.

Drugs for Trematode and Cestode Infections
Praziquantel

When praziquantel was introduced in the early 1970s, it revolutionized the treatment of **schistosomiasis**, a disease that can affect a wide range of organs, including the skin, liver, spleen, intestinal and urinary tracts, lungs, brain, and spinal cord. As shown in Table 44.1, it is now the drug of choice for infections caused by several other **tissue flukes** (trematodes) and **tapeworms** (cestodes).

Chemistry and Pharmacokinetics. Praziquantel is an orally effective isoquinoline derivative that is not related to any other antiparasitic drug. In patients taking praziquantel, the drug is widely distributed and enters the brain. It undergoes some first-pass and systemic metabolism, and the parent drug and metabolites are excreted in the urine.

Mechanism of Action. Each schistosome is surrounded by a tegument (outer covering). Praziquantel acts to **increase the calcium permeability** of the tegument and, thereby, cause its depolarization. When the outer bilayer of the tegument is damaged, *Schistosoma* antigens that were previously hidden from host defenses are exposed. This **enables host immune cells to move in and attack the schistosomes**. Thus, praziquantel acts to facilitate host immunity to these flukes. The drug's mechanism of action in other flukes and in tapeworms is unknown but is thought to be similar to that in schistosomes.

Spectrum and Indications. Praziquantel is active against most tissue flukes, including the **Chinese liver fluke**

(*Clonorchis sinensis*), the **lung fluke** (*Paragonimus westermani*), and the various ***Schistosoma*** species that cause human infections. It is also active against the larval form of the **pork tapeworm** (the cause of cysticercosis) and against the adult forms of the **pork, beef, fish, dog,** and **dwarf tapeworms**.

For patients with schistosomiasis or other fluke infections, three doses of praziquantel are administered in a single day. For patients with cysticercosis, three doses of praziquantel are given each day for a period of 2 weeks. If manifestations of neurocysticercosis are present, corticosteroids are given before praziquantel treatment. For patients with adult tapeworm infections, a single dose of praziquantel is usually effective.

Parasitic Resistance. Despite intensive use of praziquantel for more than 40 years, few cases of parasitic resistance to the drug have been documented.

Adverse Effects. Adverse effects are uncommon but include abdominal discomfort, dizziness, drowsiness, and headache.

Other Drugs

Triclabendazole is the drug of choice for the treatment of sheep liver fluke infection (*Fasciola hepatica* infection). Triclabendazole and its active metabolites (sulfoxide and sulfone) are absorbed by the tegument of the immature and mature worms, leading to a **decrease of the resting membrane potential**, inhibition of tubulin function, and protein and enzyme synthesis.

Treatment Considerations

In Africa, Central and South America, and Asia, the use of anthelmintic drugs has evolved from the treatment of individuals to the **treatment of populations.** This has been possible because of the development of broad-spectrum agents that are effective in a single dose. **Albendazole, mebendazole, ivermectin,** and **praziquantel** are examples of drugs that have been successfully used as single-dose therapy to eradicate parasites in a large population.

In most parts of the United States, **pinworm infection** (enterobiasis) is the most common helminthic infection. It is acquired by ingesting eggs deposited by the female parasite on the perianal skin and are then transmitted to the mouth via unwashed fingers or fingernails. Contaminated clothing or bedding can also serve as a source of infection. Pinworm infection is often spread to family members, and outbreaks among children in daycare settings are common.

For this reason, family members and other close contacts of the patient should be treated at the same time. In cases of pinworm infection, a dose of albendazole or mebendazole should be followed 2 weeks later by a second dose of the same drug. In cases of whipworm, hookworm, or *Ascaris* infection, a single dose of an appropriate anthelmintic drug (see Table 44.1) is usually effective.

Drugs for Infestations Caused by Ectoparasites

The most common **ectoparasites** that cause illness in humans are **lice** (wingless insects of the order Phthiraptera) and **mites** (arthropods related to ticks in the class Arachnida). These parasites cause **pediculosis** and **scabies**, respectively.

Permethrin has been the treatment of choice for both types of infestation. The drug is a synthetic pyrethrin-like compound that **blocks sodium currents** in the neurons of parasites and thereby causes paralysis of the organisms. For pediculosis, a liquid preparation is applied to saturate the hair and scalp, and then it is rinsed off after 10 minutes. For scabies, a cream is applied to the skin from head to toe, and it is left on the skin for at least 8 hours before it is washed off. For both types of infestation, a single permethrin treatment may be effective, but it should be repeated in 1 week if parasites are still present. Parasite resistance to permethrin has been increasing.

Spinosad (NATROBA) is a newer drug approved for treating **head lice** in patients ages 4 and older; it is available for topical application to the hair and scalp. Spinosad consists of two compounds (spinosyn A and D) obtained from a soil bacterium (actinomycete). Before being developed for clinical use, the compound was used as an insecticide to control a variety of insects. **Spinosad** activates **nicotinic acetylcholine receptors**, causing muscle contractions followed by paralysis, in a manner similar to the mechanism of **succinylcholine** at the mammalian neuromuscular junction.

In two clinical trials, **spinosad was significantly more effective than permethrin**, with 86% of spinosad subjects being lice-free 2 weeks after the final application versus 44% of permethrin subjects. Moreover, a higher percentage of persons treated with spinosad were lice-free after one application. Spinosad also resulted in a lower incidence of application site erythema. One of the **major advantages of spinosad** is that it is not necessary to comb and remove the nits (lice eggs) after drug application, as it is with permethrin. Hence, spinosad appears to be a major advance in the treatment of this common parasitic infestation.

Abametapir is the newest **ectoparasite elimination agent** targeting head lice. **Abametapir inhibits** the lice enzyme called a **metalloproteinase**. Metalloproteinases are involved in critical biochemical processes in egg development and ultimate survival of lice.

SUMMARY OF IMPORTANT POINTS

- Metronidazole and tinidazole are the drugs of choice for treating symptomatic amebiasis, giardiasis, and trichomoniasis. These agents form nitro free radicals in susceptible anaerobic protozoa.
- Primaquine is the only antimalarial drug that blocks exoerythrocytic schizogony. Artesunate, chloroquine, quinine, and other antimalarial drugs inhibit erythrocytic schizogony.
- Artesunate and artemether are the most active drugs against chloroquine-resistant malaria and act by forming free radicals that damage heme and proteins. They are used in combination with other drugs for this infection, such as artesunate plus mefloquine and artemether plus lumefantrine.
- Chloroquine is used to prevent malaria in geographic regions without chloroquine-resistant plasmodia. Atovaquone plus proguanil, mefloquine, or doxycycline is used to prevent malaria in regions with chloroquine-resistant plasmodia.
- Chloroquine is used to treat all types of malaria caused by chloroquine-sensitive plasmodia. In cases of *P. vivax* or *P. ovale* malaria, chloroquine is given in combination with primaquine.

- Primaquine is active against the persistent tissue phase of *P. vivax* and *P. ovale* and prevents relapses of malaria caused by these organisms.
- Toxoplasmosis can be treated with pyrimethamine and clindamycin.
- Pentamidine (early disease) and eflornithine (late disease) are used to treat African trypanosomiasis. Nifurtimox is used to treat American trypanosomiasis (Chagas disease).
- Miltefosine is used for treating cutaneous and visceral leishmaniasis (kala-azar).
- Most anthelmintic drugs act either by inhibiting microtubule formation (albendazole and mebendazole) or by causing muscle paralysis of the parasite (ivermectin, praziquantel, or pyrantel). Praziquantel exposes parasite antigens to host cell immune mechanisms.
- Albendazole and mebendazole are used to treat intestinal nematode infections.
- Ivermectin are used to treat filarial nematode infections, including river blindness (onchocerciasis). Ivermectin is also used to treat strongyloidiasis and cutaneous larva migrans.
- Praziquantel is the drug of choice for all forms of schistosomiasis and for most tissue fluke and tapeworm infections. It acts to increase the calcium permeability of the tegument of *Schistosoma* species. Triclabendazole is used to treat sheep liver fluke infections.
- Permethrin has been widely used for the treatment of lice and scabies. Spinosad is a new drug for treating head lice that appears to be more effective than permethrin and does not require combing of nits.

Review Questions

1. What is the mechanism of the anthelmintic effect of pyrantel?
   (A) impaired microtubule function
   (B) decreased glucose uptake
   (C) free-radical production
   (D) inhibition of electron transport
   (E) neuromuscular blockade

2. A Peace Corps volunteer experiences severe anxiety and hallucinations while receiving malaria treatment. Which drug is most likely causing this adverse effect?
   (A) primaquine
   (B) artesunate
   (C) mefloquine
   (D) atovaquone
   (E) proguanil

3. A susceptible population is treated with ivermectin to prevent onchocerciasis (river blindness). The permeability of which ion is increased in the parasite by this treatment?
   (A) calcium
   (B) magnesium
   (C) potassium
   (D) sodium
   (E) chloride

4. Nitazoxanide is used to treat which infection in immunocompetent persons?
   (A) leishmaniasis
   (B) malaria
   (C) cryptosporidiosis
   (D) trypanosomiasis
   (E) toxoplasmosis

5. Which drug inhibits erythrocytic schizogony in malarial species by forming free radicals that damage heme and proteins?
   (A) pyrimethamine
   (B) artemether
   (C) atovaquone
   (D) proguanil
   (E) lumefantrine

Antineoplastic Agents

CLASSIFICATION OF ANTINEOPLASTIC AGENTS

Chemotherapeutic Agents

DNA synthesis inhibitors
- Methotrexate (TREXALL)[a]
- Mercaptopurine (6-MP, PURINETHOL)[b]
- Fluorouracil (5-FU, ADRUCIL)[c]

DNA cross-linking and related drugs
- Cyclophosphamide (CYTOXAN)[d]
- Carmustine (BiCNU)[e]
- Cisplatin (PLATINOL)[f]
- Busulfan (MYLERAN)[g]

DNA intercalating drugs
- Doxorubicin (ADRIAMYCIN)
- Bleomycin (BLENOXANE)[h]

DNA topoisomerase inhibitors
- Etoposide (ETOPOPHOS)
- Irinotecan (CAMPTOSAR)[i]

Mitotic inhibitors
- Vincristine (ONCOVIN)
- Paclitaxel (TAXOL)[j]

Other chemotherapeutic agents
- Temsirolimus (TORISEL)
- Thalidomide (THALOMID)[k]

Small Molecule Inhibitors

***EGFR* kinase inhibitors**
- Imatinib (GLEEVEC)
- Erlotinib (TARCEVA)[l]

***HER2* kinase inhibitors**
- Tapatinib (TYKERB)
- Tucatinib (TUKYSA)[m]

***VEGFR/PDGFR* kinase inhibitors**
- Lenvatinib (LENVIMA)
- Pazopanib (VOTRIENT)[n]

Proteasome inhibitors
- Bortezomib (VELCADE)
- Carfilzomib (KYPROLIS)[o]

Other inhibitors
- Palbociclid (IBRANCE)
- Selinexor (XPOVIO)[p]

Hormones and Related Agents

Selective estrogen receptor modulators (SERMs)
- Tamoxifen (SOLTAMOX)
- Toremifene (FARESTON)

Selective estrogen receptor degraders (SERDs)
- Fulvestrant (FASLODEX)

Aromatase inhibitors
- Anastrozole (ARIMIDEX)
- Letrozole (FEMARA)

Antiandrogens
- Finasteride (PROSCAR)[q]
- Flutamide[r]

Gonadotropins and related drugs
- Leuprolide (LUPRON)[s]
- Ganirelix (ANTAGON)[t]

---

[a] Also pemetrexed (ALIMTA).

[b] Also thioguanine (TABLOID), cladribine (LEUSTATIN), clofarabine (CLOLAR), fludarabine (FLUDARA), and nelarabine (ARRANON); also the combination of trifluridine and tipiracil (LONSURF).

[c] Also cytarabine, floxuridine, capecitabine (XELODA), gemcitabine (GEMZAR), azacitidine (VIDAZA), and hydroxyurea (HYDREA); also daunorubicin and cytarabine as a combination liposome injection (VYXEOS), and uridine triacetate (VISTOGARD) as an antidote for fluorouracil or capecitabine toxicity.

[d] Also ifosfamide (IFEX), chlorambucil (LEUKERAN), mechlorethamine (VALCHLOR), and melphalan (ALKERAN); also ifosfamide toxicity preventing drug mesna (MESNEX).

[e] Also lomustine (GLEOSTINE), and streptozocin (ZANOSAR); also carmustine intracranial implant (GLIADEL WAFER).

[f] Also carboplatin (PARAPLATIN), and oxaliplatin (ELOXATIN); mannitol and sodium thiosulfate are used to prevent cisplatin-induced nephrotoxicity.

[g] Also dacarbazine, and temozolomide (TEMODAR).

[h] Also dactinomycin (COSMEGEN), daunorubicin (CERUBIDINE), mitomycin (JELMYTO), idarubicin (IDAMYCIN), and mitoxantrone; also toxicity preventing drug dexrazoxane (ZINECARD).

[i] Also teniposide (VUMON), and topotecan (HYCAMTIN).

[j] Also vinblastine, vinorelbine, and ixabepilone (IXEMPRA), docetaxel (TAXOTERE), and cabazitaxel (JEVTANA).

[k] Also lenalidomide (REVLIMID), and pomalidomide (POMALYST).

[l] Also gefitinib (IRESSA), dacomitinib (VIZIMPRO), ibrutinib (IMBRUVICA), and others (see Table 45.2).

[m] Also neratinib (NERLYNX).

[n] Also sorafenib (NEXAVAR), sunitinib (SUTENT), ripretinib (QINLOCK), selpercatinib (RETEVMO), and avapritinib (AYVAKIT).

[o] Also ixazomib (NINLARO).

[p] Also panobinostat (FARYDAK), abemaciclid (VERZENIO), and others (see Table 45.2)

[q] Also dutasteride (AVODART).

[r] Also bicalutamide (CASODEX), enzalutamide (XTANDI), apalutamide (ERLEADA), darolutamide (NUBEQA), and nilutamide (NILANDRON).

[s] Also goserelin (ZOLADEX), nafarelin (SYNAREL), triptorelin (TRELSTAR), and histrelin (SUPPRELIN LA).

[t] Also cetrorelix (CETROTIDE) and degarelix (FIRMAGON).

OVERVIEW

Cancer is the uninhibited new growth (**neoplasm**) of a cell or tissue. Cancer is the second most common cause of death in the United States and other developed countries. Currently, approximately 2 million new cancer cases and 600,000 cancer deaths occur each year in the United States. About 40% of men and women will be diagnosed with cancer at some point during their lifetime. Listed in descending order according to the number of diagnoses per year, the most **common cancers are breast cancer, lung cancer, prostate cancer, colon cancer, melanoma,** bladder cancer, non-Hodgkin lymphoma, kidney cancer, endometrial cancer, leukemia, pancreatic cancer, thyroid cancer, and liver cancer.

There are two main types of cancer: (1) **solid tumors** that begin as abnormal tissue growths and often spread to other tissues and (2) **hematologic malignancies** that arise in the **bone marrow or lymph nodes** and produce large quantities of **abnormal blood cells.** The most common solid tumor malignancies are those of the **lungs, colon, breast, and prostate.** The hematologic malignancies include **leukemias** consisting of malignant white blood cells (leukocytes), **lymphomas** comprised of malignant lymphocytes, and **multiple myeloma.**

Cancer results from the **transformation** of normal cells into **malignant neoplastic cells** that exhibit **loss of normal function** (de-differentiation), **uncontrolled cell division, invasiveness,** and **metastasis.** The invasiveness of cancer cells enables them to spread into surrounding tissues, while metastasis enables them to spread to other sites in the body through blood vessels and the lymphatic system (lymph nodes). The invasiveness and metastasis of cancer cells depends on the expression of growth factors that promote the formation of new blood vessels to supply the growing tumor. This process is called **angiogenesis** and is a target of several newer anticancer drugs.

Malignant transformation is caused by **genetic mutations** that convert **proto-oncogenes to oncogenes** (cancer forming genes). These genes express proteins that **promote uncontrolled cell proliferation** or that **inactivate tumor suppressor genes.** Some oncogenes encode **growth factors and their receptors,** such as the **receptor tyrosine kinases** coupled with signaling pathways leading to continuous activation of **cyclins** and **cell replication** (Fig. 45.1). These receptor kinases include the **epidermal growth factor receptors** (EGFR) that are over-expressed in lung and breast cancer tumors.

Inactivation of tumor suppressor genes is another important mechanism of cancer development. For example, about half of human solid tumors have a **mutated *p53* gene** that normally suppresses the malignant transformation of cells. In addition, many tumors express one of the *Bcl-2* **genes** that **promote cancer cell survival** by **inhibiting apoptosis** (programmed cell death) that serves to destroy nascent cancer cells.

PRINCIPLES OF CANCER THERAPY

The primary methods of cancer treatment are surgery, radiation, and drug therapy. Surgery and radiation are the preferred treatments for localized solid tumors, and about one-third of cancers are cured with these methods alone. Drug therapy is sometimes used in conjunction with surgery and radiation to eradicate **micrometastases** and locally advanced cancer; about one-half of diagnosed cancers can be cured by the combined use of these modalities. Antineoplastic drugs are also used to treat **hematologic cancers** that cannot be surgically excised, such as leukemia and lymphoma, and to treat **inoperable and advanced metastatic tumors.** However, therapy for metastatic disease is often palliative rather than curative. **Palliative therapy** can prolong life and reduce incapacitating symptoms but does not eradicate the malignancy.

Treatment Regimens and Schedules

Drug regimens for cancer chemotherapy are designed to optimize the **synergistic effects of drug combinations** while minimizing toxicity. The regimens often use drugs that have different toxicities and different mechanisms of action to maximize cytotoxic effects on tumor cells while sparing host tissue.

In the treatment of some types of cancer, specific drug regimens are used for **induction, consolidation,** and **maintenance.** Induction therapy, such as that used in acute lymphocytic leukemia, produces a rapid reduction in the tumor cell burden and symptomatic improvement. Consolidation therapy completes and extends the remission, while maintenance therapy sustains the remission for as long as possible. Chemotherapy regimens often employ multiple drugs administered as intermittent **courses of therapy** rather than as continuous therapy. **Intermittent therapy** allows the bone marrow and other normal host cells to recover between treatment courses and reduces the level of toxicity. According to the **log-kill concept,** each course of therapy eliminates a constant fraction of the remaining tumor cells (e.g., 99.9%), and repeated courses of treatment would ideally reduce the number of tumor cells to the level that the immune system can eradicate. In practice, this seldom occurs because of such factors as **tumor resistance.**

Drug selection has traditionally been based on **clinical trials** comparing the effectiveness of drug combinations in particular stages of a cancer. First-line drugs are employed for the initial treatment of tumors, whereas second-line drugs are indicated for patients who have relapsed after first-line therapy. **Genomic testing** of a patient's tumor cells is now offering a better approach to drug selection by identifying specific oncogenes and genetic mutations susceptible to particular immunotherapy agents and targeted enzyme inhibitors.

Cell Cycle Specificity

The **cytotoxic drugs** can be classified as **cell cycle–specific** and **cell cycle–nonspecific agents.** As shown in Fig. 45.1, the cycle of cell replication includes the G_1, S, G_2, and M phases. DNA is replicated during the S phase, and mitosis occurs during the M phase. Because early cytologists observed no activity between the S and M phases, they referred to the period before S as G_1 (gap 1) and to the period before M as G_2 (gap 2). It is now known that cells are actively preparing for DNA synthesis and mitosis during the G_1 and G_2 phases, respectively. **Cyclins** are growth factors that regulate the progression of cells through the cell cycle and are targets of new drug development. Tumor growth factors often stimulate cyclins and cyclin-dependent kinases. Examples of cyclins are shown in Fig. 45.1.

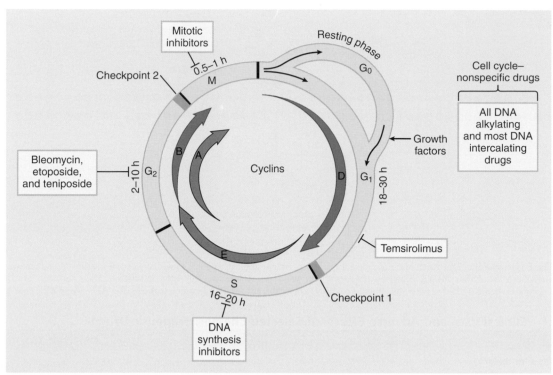

Fig. 45.1 Cell cycle activity of antineoplastic drugs. The cycle of cell replication includes the sequential phases of G_1 (gap 1), S (DNA synthesis), G_2 (gap 2), and M (mitosis). Differentiated cells can enter a resting state called G_0. Growth factors may stimulate resting cells to reenter the cell cycle. Progress through the cycle is promoted by proteins called cyclins (A, B, D, E), which activate cyclin-dependent kinases. Two checkpoints, which often malfunction in cancer cells, control entry into the critical phases of DNA synthesis and mitosis. Cell cycle-specific drugs primarily act during the designated phase of the cycle. Cell cycle-nonspecific drugs act throughout the cell cycle.

Drugs that act during a specific phase of the cell cycle are called **cell cycle–specific drugs,** whereas drugs that are active throughout the cell cycle are called **cell cycle–nonspecific drugs.** Cell cycle–specific drugs include all DNA synthesis inhibitors and mitotic inhibitors. Cell cycle–nonspecific drugs include all DNA alkylating agents and most DNA intercalating agents.

Limitations of Cancer Chemotherapy
Most antineoplastic drugs have three major limitations: susceptibility to **tumor cell resistance,** production of **host toxicity,** and an **inability to suppress metastasis.**

Drug Resistance
Drug resistance is a major cause of **cancer treatment failure.** As with microbial drug resistance, tumor cell resistance can be innate or acquired. **Innate drug resistance** may result from oncogenes that **inactivate tumor suppressor genes,** such as *p53* in cancer cells. These mutations are linked to initial treatment failure with both radiation therapy and a number of anticancer agents. Expression of **anti-apoptotic proteins,** such as *Bcl-2* can produce resistance to drugs by interfering with the cell death signal (apoptosis) normally induced by an antineoplastic agent.

Acquired drug resistance can result from ongoing **genomic mutations** and **abnormal gene expression** as cancer cells evolve. The mechanisms of tumor cell resistance include induction of **drug efflux pumps, decreased affinity** or **overexpression of target enzymes,** and **decreased drug activation** or **increased drug inactivation. Increased tumor cell repair** also lead to drug resistance.

Drug resistance can occur through failure of the drug to reach its target because of **drug efflux from tumor cells.** For example, the **P-glycoprotein** (Pgp) efflux pump expressed by the *MDR1* gene acts to transport many naturally occurring drugs out of tumor cells, including anthracyclines, taxanes, and vinca alkaloids. Induction of Pgp by antineoplastic drugs can lead to multidrug resistance (Fig. 45.2).

Other examples of acquired drug resistance include **topoisomerase mutations** that convey resistance to topoisomerase inhibitors (e.g., **etoposide**). Resistance to methotrexate (MTX) can occur through mutations in its target enzyme, dihydrofolate reductase, or through overexpression of the enzyme so as to overwhelm drug inhibition. Mutations in genes for tubulin or microtubule-associated proteins can cause resistance to the **vinca alkaloids** and **taxane** drugs.

Drug Toxicity
The most common toxicities of antineoplastic drugs (Table 45.1) result from nonspecific inhibition of cell division in normal tissues that undergo continuous rapid cell replication, particularly the bone marrow, gastrointestinal epithelium, and hair follicles. In addition, many antineoplastic drugs stimulate the chemoreceptor trigger zone in the medulla and elicit nausea and vomiting. Some drugs cause toxic effects on the heart, kidneys, nervous system, and other tissues.

The **myelosuppression** (bone marrow suppression) produced by many antineoplastic drugs often results in leukopenia and thrombocytopenia, although anemia can also occur. **Leukopenia** (leukocyte deficiency) predisposes patients to serious infections, whereas **thrombocytopenia** (platelet deficiency) can lead to bleeding. The onset of leukopenia is

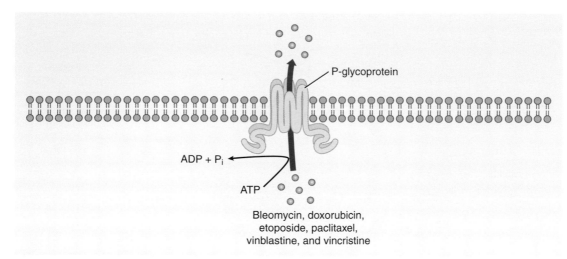

FIG. 45.2 The P-glycoprotein (Pgp) mechanism of drug efflux. Pgp uses adenosine triphosphate to actively export bleomycin and many other naturally occurring antineoplastic drugs from the cell. Because some agents (e.g., verapamil) inhibit the Pgp pump and thereby allow antineoplastic drugs to stay in the cell, these agents are being studied as potential adjuncts to cancer chemotherapy. *ADP,* Adenosine diphosphate; *ATP,* adenosine triphosphate.

TABLE 45.1 Clinical Uses and Adverse Effects of Selected Chemotherapeutic Drugs

DRUG	CLINICAL USE	ACUTE TOXICITY	DELAYED TOXICITY
DNA Synthesis Inhibitors			
Mercaptopurine	AML, ALL, CML	Usually well tolerated	Hepatotoxicity, myelosuppression
Fluorouracil	Breast, colorectal, gastric, and skin cancer	Diarrhea, mild nausea, and vomiting	Alopecia, gastrointestinal and oral ulcers, myelosuppression
Methotrexate	ALL, breast cancer, osteosarcoma, lymphoma, choriocarcinoma, bladder cancer	Diarrhea, nausea	Gastrointestinal and oral ulcers, hepatotoxicity, myelosuppression
Gemcitabine	Pancreatic carcinoma, non-small cell lung cancer, ovarian cancer	Nausea and vomiting, anemia, elevated liver enzymes, proteinuria, edema	Hepatotoxicity, pulmonary toxicity, myelosuppression
DNA Cross-linking and Related Drugs			
Cyclophosphamide	Breast and lung cancer; CLL, ALL, myeloma, neuroblastoma, non-Hodgkin lymphoma	Nausea and vomiting	Alopecia, hemorrhagic cystitis, myelosuppression
Carmustine	Brain cancer, Hodgkin and non-Hodgkin lymphoma	Nausea and vomiting	Myelosuppression, pulmonary fibrosis
Cisplatin	Bladder, breast, lung, ovarian, testicular, non-Hodgkin lymphoma	Renal failure, nausea, and vomiting	Neuropathy, ototoxicity, nephrotoxicity
Busulfan	CML	Diarrhea, nausea and vomiting	Myelosuppression, pulmonary fibrosis
DNA Intercalating Drugs			
Doxorubicin	Breast, lung, ovarian, thyroid, neuroblastoma, sarcoma	Nausea and vomiting	Alopecia, cardiotoxicity, myelosuppression
Bleomycin	Cervical, head, neck, and testicular cancer; Hodgkin and non-Hodgkin lymphoma	Fever, allergic reactions	Alopecia, myelosuppression, mucositis, pulmonary fibrosis
Idarubicin	AML, ALL, CML	Nausea and vomiting	Alopecia, cardiotoxicity, mucositis, myelosuppression
Topoisomerase Inhibitors			
Etoposide	Non-Hodgkin lymphoma, lung, gastric, testicular	Mild nausea and vomiting	Alopecia, myelosuppression
Irinotecan	Colorectal, gastroesophageal, lung	Diarrhea, nausea, and vomiting	Myelosuppression
Mitotic Inhibitors			
Vincristine	ALL; Hodgkin and non-Hodgkin lymphoma, neuroblastoma	Usually well tolerated	Alopecia, mild myelosuppression, neurotoxicity
Paclitaxel	Breast and ovarian cancer, non–small cell lung cancer	Usually well tolerated	Alopecia, myelosuppression, neurotoxicity

ALL, Acute lymphocytic leukemia; *AML,* acute myeloid leukemia; *CLL,* chronic lymphocytic leukemia; *CML,* chronic myeloid leukemia.

delayed because of the time required to clear circulating cells before the effect that drugs have on precursor cell maturation in the bone marrow becomes evident. With many drugs, including MTX, fluorouracil, and cyclophosphamide, the leukocyte count reaches its nadir in about 7 days, and recovery occurs in 2 to 4 weeks. Nitrosourea drugs (e.g., **carmustine**) produce a more delayed and long-lasting suppression of leukocyte production. Bleomycin, cisplatin, and vincristine produce less myelosuppression than other antineoplastic drugs and are sometimes used in combination with myelosuppressive drugs.

The **nausea** and **vomiting** caused by antineoplastic drugs range from mild to severe. Among the antineoplastic drugs, the most emetic are cisplatin and carmustine. Nausea and vomiting can be substantially reduced by pretreatment with a combination of antiemetic drugs, including serotonin antagonists (e.g., ondansetron) and corticosteroids (e.g., dexamethasone). The antiemetics are discussed in greater detail in Chapter 28.

Alopecia is a cosmetically distressing but less-serious adverse effect of chemotherapy. It is generally reversible after treatment ends, although the hair might differ in texture and appearance from its previous condition.

Several antineoplastic drugs have characteristic **organ system toxicities** that appear unrelated to inhibition of cell division. For example, use of doxorubicin and other anthracyclines can cause cardiotoxicity; use of cyclophosphamide and ifosfamide can cause hemorrhagic cystitis; use of cisplatin can cause renal toxicity; use of bleomycin or busulfan can cause pulmonary toxicity; and use of vincristine, paclitaxel, and other vinca alkaloids and taxanes can cause neurotoxicity.

Agents have been developed to prevent some of these organ system toxicities. **Dexrazoxane** was developed to prevent anthracycline-induced cardiotoxicity. Another cytoprotective drug, **mesna,** was developed to prevent **ifosfamide-induced hemorrhagic cystitis. Cisplatin-induced renal toxicity** can be partly prevented by **hydration therapy** (IV fluids), along with **mannitol** and **sodium thiosulfate**. The fluids help dilute the cisplatin concentrations in the kidneys. Mannitol maintains renal blood flow and tubular function, whereas sodium thiosulfate inactivates the drug in the kidneys. Sodium thiosulfate is also part of the antidote treatment for acute cyanide poisoning (see Chapter 11).

No specific agents currently exist to prevent **cisplatin pulmonary toxicity and neurotoxicity**; therefore, patients at risk should be closely monitored so that treatment can be discontinued if these toxicities develop.

ANTINEOPLASTIC DRUGS

Antineoplastic (anticancer) drugs can be divided into two broad categories: (1) **cytotoxic agents** that nonspecifically inhibit cell replication and (2) **targeted and immunotherapy agents** that inhibit specific proteins involved in tumor cell growth. The term *chemotherapy* is often used to designate treatment with traditional **cytotoxic drugs,** whereas targeted agents are called small molecule inhibitors (SMIs). *Immunotherapy* is used to denote treatment with monoclonal antibodies and other biologic agents that enhance tumor immunity.

The introduction of new antineoplastic agents has rapidly accelerated with the development of **small molecular inhibitors** and **monoclonal antibody drugs**. New agents are introduced almost monthly, contributing to an overwhelming abundance of anticancer drugs. These new agents

are having a significant effect on cancer treatment, while increasing the challenge of drug selection. The SMIs are presented later in this chapter while the **monoclonal antibody drugs** are discussed as part of the larger chapter on immunopharmacology (see Chapter 46). Because of the growing number of antineoplastic agents, this chapter focuses on the most important examples in each drug class.

Cytotoxic Agents

DNA Synthesis Inhibitors

The DNA synthesis inhibitors are analogs of folic acid or of the purine or pyrimidine bases found in DNA. They act as **antimetabolites** that inhibit enzymes catalyzing various steps in DNA synthesis. The uses and adverse effects of selected inhibitors are listed in Table 45.1.

Folate Antagonists

MTX was one of the first drugs to be used in cancer treatment after it was found to induce remission in children with childhood leukemia almost 70 years ago. It is still the most widely used antimetabolite in cancer treatment, and it is also used as an **immunosuppressive drug** in the treatment of autoimmune diseases, like rheumatoid arthritis (see Chapter 30).

Chemistry and Mechanisms. **MTX** and **pemetrexed** are structural **analogs of folic acid**. MTX is actively transported into mammalian cells and inhibits **dihydrofolate reductase**, the enzyme that converts dietary folate to the active tetrahydrofolate form required for thymidine and purine synthesis (Fig. 45.3). Pemetrexed is converted to active forms that inhibit several enzymes involved in DNA synthesis, including dihydrofolate reductase and thymidylate synthase.

Pharmacokinetics. MTX can be administered orally or parenterally. The oral bioavailability of MTX is dose dependent, with lower doses absorbed more completely than higher doses. MTX is widely distributed but does not penetrate the central nervous system (CNS). It is partly metabolized and eliminated as the parent compound and metabolites in the urine. In contrast, **pemetrexed** is only given intravenously and is mostly excreted unchanged in the urine.

Indications. The use of MTX in the treatment of **choriocarcinoma**, a trophoblastic tumor, was the first demonstration of curative chemotherapy. Today, MTX has a variety of uses, including the treatment of **trophoblastic tumors**, **breast cancer**, and **osteosarcoma**. It is routinely given by intrathecal administration to prevent **meningeal metastases** during chemotherapy of **acute lymphocytic leukemia**, and it is used similarly with a wide range of other tumors. Pemetrexed is indicated for the treatment of **nonsquamous non-small cell lung cancer** and the treatment of mesothelioma, both in combination with cisplatin.

Adverse Effects. **Myelosuppression** is the primary dose-limiting toxicity MTX and pemetrexed. Administration of activated folic acid (folinic acid, leucovorin) can be used to prevent these effects without impairing drug efficacy. These drugs can also cause **oral ulceration** (stomatitis), and MTX can cause **hepatotoxicity** during long-term therapy for psoriasis and rheumatoid conditions.

Purine Analogs

Mercaptopurine and **thioguanine** are the thio analogs of the purine bases hypoxanthine and guanine, respectively.

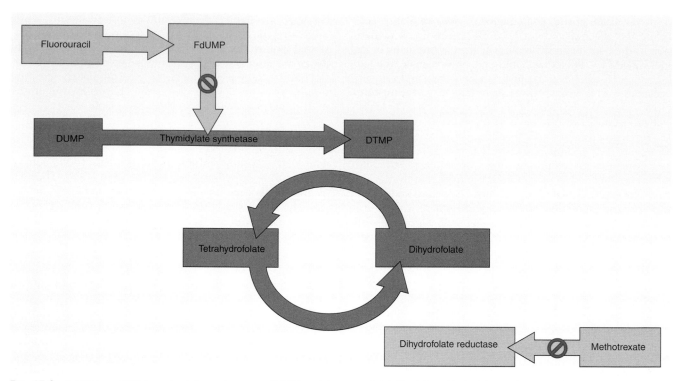

FIG. 45.3 Inhibition of DNA synthesis by methotrexate (MTX) and fluorouracil. MTX inhibits dihydrofolate reductase and the conversion of dihydrofolate to tetrahydrofolate. This reduces the supply of 5,10-methylenetetrahydrofolate, a substance required for the synthesis of deoxythymidine monophosphate (*DTMP*). The conversion of deoxyuridine monophosphate (*DUMP*) to DTMP, a critical step in DNA synthesis, is catalyzed by thymidylate synthetase. This enzyme is inhibited by 5-fluorodeoxyuridine monophosphate (*5-FdUMP*), which is the active form of fluorouracil. Pemetrexed inhibits both dihydrofolate reductase and thymidylate synthetase.

Mercaptopurine was introduced over 60 years ago for the treatment of acute lymphocytic leukemia. Both drugs are converted to nucleotides by the addition of ribose phosphate, a reaction catalyzed by **hypoxanthine guanine phosphoribosyltransferase**. Tumor cells may acquire resistance to these drugs by deleting this enzyme, and cross-resistance is observed between the two drugs. The active metabolites of mercaptopurine and thioguanine inhibit several steps in the biosynthesis of purine bases (adenine and guanine) and in purine recycling pathways that supply purine precursors, thereby impairing DNA synthesis.

Mercaptopurine and thioguanine are given orally, and their bioavailability is variable, incomplete, and reduced by food. Mercaptopurine is given with MTX to maintain remission in patients with **acute lymphocytic leukemia.** Thioguanine is used to maintain remission in patients with acute lymphocytic and **acute myeloid leukemia (AML).** Mercaptopurine is metabolized by xanthine oxidase, whereas thioguanine is degraded by other enzymes.

Mercaptopurine and **thioguanine** are usually **well tolerated**. Myelosuppression is generally mild with mercaptopurine but can be dose-limiting with thioguanine. Long-term mercaptopurine use can cause hepatotoxicity, and both drugs contribute to the development of other cancers (therapy-related cancer). Doses of mercaptopurine must be reduced by at least 50% in patients taking **allopurinol**, which inhibits xanthine oxidase and thereby elevates plasma levels of mercaptopurine. Allopurinol is often given to patients undergoing cancer chemotherapy because it inhibits the synthesis of uric acid and thereby prevents hyperuricemia and gout. Cancer chemotherapy places patients at risk for these problems because the destruction of cancer cells increases purine catabolism and uric acid formation, called **tumor lysis syndrome.** As an alternative to allopurinol, there is a new recombinant formulation of the enzyme **uricase**, which converts uric acid to allantoin (see Chapter 30).

Fludarabine and **cladribine** are halogenated purine nucleoside analogs whose triphosphate metabolites are incorporated into nascent DNA, causing DNA chain termination. Fludarabine is a highly active agent in the treatment of **chronic lymphocytic leukemia (CLL)** and low-grade non-Hodgkin lymphoma. **Cladribine** is primarily used for hairy cell leukemia. **Clofarabine** and **nelarabine** are new purine nucleoside analogs for treating refractory or relapsed acute lymphocytic leukemia.

Pyrimidine Analogs

Fluorouracil (5-FU) and **cytarabine** and are commonly used pyrimidine antimetabolites. Fluorouracil is an analog of thymine in which the methyl group is replaced by a fluorine atom. **Floxuridine** is the deoxyribonucleoside derivative of fluorouracil, whereas **capecitabine** is converted in the body to fluorouracil and its active metabolites.

Fluorouracil has two active metabolites: 5-fluorodeoxyuridine monophosphate (5-FdUMP) and 5-fluorodeoxyuridine triphosphate (5-FdUTP). 5-FdUMP inhibits **thymidylate synthetase** and prevents the synthesis of thymidine, a major building block of DNA (see Fig. 45.3). 5-FdUTP is also incorporated into RNA by RNA polymerase and interferes with RNA function. Fluorouracil and related drugs are extensively metabolized before undergoing renal excretion. **Fluorouracil** is administered intravenously to treat solid tumors, especially **breast, colorectal**, and **gastric carcinoma** and squamous cell tumors of the head and neck. Regional delivery of the drug via the hepatic artery can produce a sustained response in patients whose colorectal cancer has metastasized to the liver. **Topical** application of **fluorouracil** is used to treat **actinic keratoses** and **noninvasive skin cancers**.

Cytarabine is composed of **cytosine** and the sugar arabinose. The active triphosphate metabolite of **cytarabine** blocks DNA synthesis by inhibiting **DNA polymerase** and incorporation into nascent DNA, causing DNA chain termination. **Cytarabine** is administered intravenously or subcutaneously in combination with daunorubicin to treat AML. **Capecitabine** is indicated for colorectal and breast cancer, whereas **floxuridine** is used in the treatment of colorectal cancer.

Gemcitabine, an **S-phase specific inhibitor** of DNA synthesis, is a fluorinated cytidine analog. After conversion to gemcitabine diphosphate and triphosphate, these metabolites inhibit the synthesis of deoxynucleoside triphosphates and their incorporation into DNA. The drug is used as a first-line treatment for **pancreatic carcinoma** and **non–small cell lung cancer** in combination with cisplatin, and for breast and ovarian cancer.

The pyrimidine antimetabolites can cause **myelosuppression** and **oral and gastrointestinal ulceration.** Nausea and vomiting are usually mild. Higher doses of these drugs can damage the liver, heart, and other organs. If toxicity becomes too great, **uridine triacetate (VISTOGARD)** is marketed as an antidote for **fluorouracil or capecitabine overdose** and/or toxicity.

DNA Cross-linking and Related Drugs

The DNA cross-linking drugs form permanent covalent bonds between the drug and DNA bases, primarily guanine (Fig. 45.4). This group of drugs includes the nitrogen mustards, nitrosourea drugs, and platinum compounds, as well as several unique agents that don't fit into one of these categories.

Nitrogen Mustards

The cytotoxic effects of nitrogen mustards were discovered in the early 1940s, leading to their introduction as the first effective anticancer drugs. The nitrogen mustards undergo spontaneous or enzymatic conversion to active metabolites that from covalent bonds with the N7 nitrogen of guanine. The sequential attachment of the drug to two guanine residues results in **cross-linking of DNA strands**, which prevents DNA replication and transcription (see Fig. 45.4A). The alkylating drugs act throughout the cell replication cycle.

Cyclophosphamide and **ifosfamide** are converted to active metabolites that alkylate DNA by hepatic cytochrome P450 enzymes. Both drugs can be administered intravenously, although cyclophosphamide can also be given orally and is completely absorbed after oral administration. **Cyclophosphamide** is the most widely used nitrogen mustard because of its broad spectrum of activity. It is used in the treatment of CLL, non-Hodgkin lymphoma, and for breast, lung, and ovarian cancers (see Table 45.1). Because cyclophosphamide is a potent immunosuppressant, it is used in the management of **rheumatoid disorders** and

autoimmune nephritis, and it is used in preoperative regimens for bone marrow transplantation. **Ifosfamide** is primarily used to treat patients with sarcoma and patients with testicular cancer that is refractory to first-line treatments.

The adverse effects of cyclophosphamide and ifosfamide include alopecia, nausea, vomiting, myelosuppression, and **hemorrhagic cystitis.** Nausea and vomiting are usually mild when cyclophosphamide is given orally but can be severe when given intravenously. The dose-limiting toxicity of cyclophosphamide is myelosuppression, whereas that of ifosfamide is hemorrhagic cystitis. This type of cystitis (bladder inflammation) is characterized by urinary frequency, irritation, and blood loss. Ingestion of large amounts of fluid and administration of **mesna**, a sulfhydryl reagent, can significantly reduce the incidence of cystitis. **Mesna** binds to acrolein, the drug metabolite that causes cystitis, and converts it to an inactive substance.

Chlorambucil, mechlorethamine, and **melphalan** are nitrogen mustards that cross-link DNA strands. Chlorambucil is given orally and is primarily used to treat **CLL** and non-Hodgkin lymphoma. It is well tolerated but can cause dose-limiting leukopenia and thrombocytopenia. Long-term therapy is associated with a high incidence of secondary acute leukemia.

Mechlorethamine is a highly reactive and vesicant drug that is rapidly and spontaneously converted to its alkylating intermediate after intravenous administration. Mechlorethamine is used for treating **Hodgkin and non-Hodgkin lymphoma. Melphalan** is primarily used to treat **multiple myeloma** (plasma cell myeloma) and breast and ovarian cancer.

Nitrosourea Drugs

The nitrosourea drugs include **carmustine, lomustine,** and **streptozocin.** The nitrosoureas are bifunctional alkylating drugs with structures similar to those of the nitrogen mustards. They spontaneously form active intermediates that cross-link DNA.

Nitrosoureas can be given orally or intravenously. They are highly lipophilic and reach **cerebrospinal fluid concentrations** that are about 30% of plasma concentrations. The drugs are extensively metabolized before renal excretion. Because of their excellent **CNS penetration, carmustine** and **lomustine** have been used to treat **brain tumors**, such as astrocytomas. **Carmustine** is also available for **cranial implantation in a wafer** form. **Streptozocin** is used to treat pancreatic islet cell tumor (insulinoma).

The **nitrosoureas** produce delayed and prolonged **myelosuppression** causing leukopenia and thrombocytopenia, with complete recovery taking 6 to 8 weeks. **Pulmonary damage** (interstitial lung disease) and **interstitial nephritis** may also occur.

Platinum Compounds

Cisplatin, carboplatin, and **oxaliplatin** are inorganic platinum derivatives. These drugs react with water to form positively charged metabolites that form **intrastrand cross-links** between neighboring guanine residues. The intrastrand links bend and distort DNA and prevent replication and transcription.

Cisplatin is given intravenously as a first-line drug for treating **testicular, ovarian, cervical, bladder, and lung**

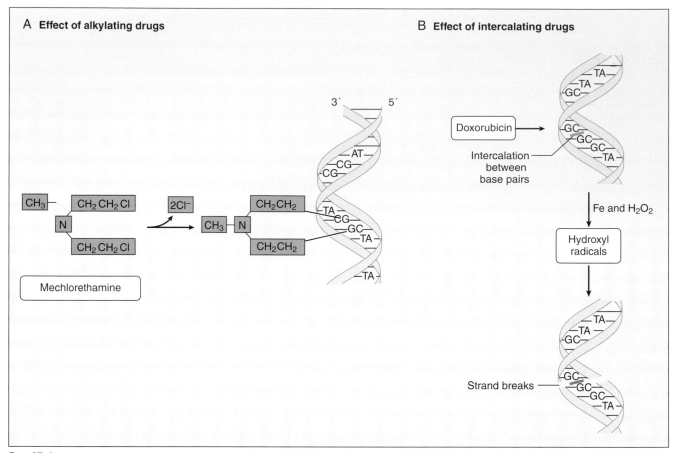

A Effect of alkylating drugs

Mechlorethamine

B Effect of intercalating drugs

Doxorubicin

Intercalation
between
base pairs

Fe and H$_2$O$_2$

Hydroxyl
radicals

Strand breaks

Fig. 45.4   Mechanisms of action of DNA alkylating drugs and DNA intercalating drugs. (A) Mechlorethamine and other bifunctional alkylating drugs form electrophilic intermediates that attack the N7 nitrogen of guanine residues in DNA, thereby cross-linking DNA strands and preventing replication and transcription. (B) Doxorubicin and other anthracycline drugs intercalate between DNA base pairs. Anthracyclines are reduced to intermediates that donate electrons to oxygen to form superoxide. Superoxide then reacts with itself to make hydrogen peroxide, which is cleaved in the presence of iron to form the destructive hydroxyl radical that cleaves DNA.

cancers, and it is useful in the treatment of a number of other solid tumors. **Carboplatin** and **oxaliplatin** are also used to treat several solid tumors.

Cisplatin produces **mild myelosuppression** but can cause severe **nausea, vomiting,** and **nephrotoxicity.** Pretreatment with an antiemetic (e.g., ondansetron) will prevent or significantly reduce the severity of nausea and vomiting. The use of mannitol and sodium thiosulfate will decrease the severity of nephrotoxicity, an adverse effect associated with loss of potassium and magnesium, reduced glomerular filtration, and renal failure. **Mannitol** increases urine flow and can reduce binding of cisplatin to renal tubule proteins. **Sodium thiosulfate** accumulates in renal tubules and neutralizes the cytotoxicity of cisplatin. Renal damage caused by cisplatin is often slowly reversible.

Other DNA Alkylating Drugs

Busulfan is an alkyl sulfonate drug that acts like the nitrogen mustards to cross-link DNA. Busulfan is administered orally and extensively metabolized, and its metabolites are excreted in the urine. Unlike many alkylating drugs, busulfan has greater activity against myeloid cells than lymphoid cells and has been used in the management of **chronic myeloid leukemia** (CML). **Busulfan** causes mild nausea and vomiting and produces dose-limiting myelosuppression. It can also cause fatal **pulmonary fibrosis** ("busulfan lung"),

which is characterized by a nonproductive cough and difficult breathing that occurs in about 4% of patients treated on a long-term basis.

Dacarbazine is converted to active intermediates that can alkylate DNA, although the exact mechanisms are uncertain. Ultimately, the drug inhibits DNA, RNA, and protein synthesis. Dacarbazine is primarily used to treat **Hodgkin lymphoma.**

Temozolomide is an alkylating agent that adds a methyl group to guanine residues of DNA, causing DNA damage and tumor cell death. It is a first-line drug for several **brain tumors,** including **astrocytoma** and **gliomas.**

DNA Intercalating Drugs
Anthracycline Drugs

Doxorubicin, daunorubicin, and **mitomycin** are antibiotics obtained from a *Streptomyces* species, whereas **idarubicin** and **mitoxantrone** are semisynthetic anthracycline compounds. These drugs have a four-member anthracene ring with attached sugars. Two of the four rings are quinone and hydroquinone moieties that enable the compounds to accept and donate electrons and thereby promote the formation of free radicals. The anthracene ring accounts for the intense red color of the drug compounds.

Several mechanisms are responsible for the cytotoxicity of the anthracycline drugs, including **intercalation of DNA,**

inhibition of topoisomerase, and formation of **free radicals**. The drugs bind strongly to DNA by inserting (intercalating) between paired DNA bases, causing deformation and uncoiling of the DNA (see Fig. 45.4B). The anthracyclines cause **DNA strands to break** by blocking topoisomerase II (see later) and by forming destructive hydroxyl free radicals. Free radical formation involves an iron-anthracycline complex that is strongly bound to DNA.

After **intravenous administration**, the anthracyclines are rapidly distributed to all tissues except the CNS and have large volumes of distribution and long half-lives. The drugs are extensively metabolized in the liver, and some metabolites are as pharmacologically active as the parent compounds.

Doxorubicin is one of the most active agents against **breast cancer** and is also used to treat bladder and ovarian cancer, Hodgkin disease, and other hematologic cancers and solid tumors (see Table 45.1). **Daunorubicin and idarubicin** are used in induction and consolidation therapy for AML. **Mitoxantrone** is primarily used in combination with cytarabine for induction of remission in patients with AML.

The primary dose-limiting adverse effects of anthracyclines are **myelosuppression, cardiac damage**, and **nausea and vomiting**. Alopecia and mucosal ulcerations may also occur. **Extravasation** of the drugs during intravenous infusion can lead to localized tissue ulceration and necrosis. These localized reactions can progress over many weeks, and no effective treatment for them currently exists. Hence, exceptional care and specialized training are required for proper administration of anthracycline drugs. It is worth noting that mitoxantrone causes less tissue damage after extravasation, as well as less nausea, vomiting, mucosal ulceration, and alopecia than do other anthracycline drugs.

The anthracyclines cause both **acute and chronic cardiotoxicity**. Acute toxicity presents as sinus tachycardia and ventricular premature beats, which are usually of short duration. Chronic toxicity leads to **congestive cardiomyopathy** and **limits the cumulative dose** of anthracycline that can be given to any patient. The cardiomyopathy appears to result from iron-catalyzed formation of **free radicals** in cardiac tissue. **Mitoxantrone** causes less free radical formation and **cardiac toxicity** than other anthracyclines. **Dexrazoxane** is a chelator of ferric iron that disrupts the iron-anthracycline complex and prevents free radical formation. It is given to women with breast cancer who might benefit from continued doxorubicin therapy. Cardiotoxicity is also reduced by administering **doxorubicin encapsulated in liposomes** (Doxil), which reduces the amount of drug taken up by cardiac tissue.

Several drugs increase doxorubicin toxicity including cyclophosphamide and mercaptopurine. Verapamil, a calcium channel block (see Chapter 11) enhances the cytotoxic effect of anthracycline drugs on cancer cells by inhibiting Pgp efflux.

Bleomycin

Bleomycin is a mixture of two peptides obtained from *Streptomyces verticillus*. The drug has its greatest effect on neoplastic cells in the G_2 **phase** of the cell replication cycle. Although bleomycin intercalates DNA, the major cytotoxicity is believed to result from **iron-catalyzed free radical formation** and DNA strand breakage. The iron-bleomycin complex binds to DNA and reduces molecular oxygen-to-oxygen free radicals that cause DNA strands to break.

Bleomycin is administered intravenously, is widely distributed, and is primarily eliminated by renal excretion. The drug is inactivated in cells by aminohydrolase, whose low levels in skin and lung may partly account for the toxicity of bleomycin in these tissues.

Bleomycin is one of the most widely used antitumor antibiotics. It is useful in Hodgkin and non-Hodgkin **lymphomas**, testicular cancer, and several other **solid tumors**. It is included in the **ABVD** regimen (**Adriamycin, Bleomycin, Vincristine, and Dacarbazine**) for Hodgkin disease.

Bleomycin produces very little myelosuppression and can be combined with myelosuppressive drugs in treatment regimens. The most serious toxicities of bleomycin are **pulmonary and mucocutaneous reactions**. Patients taking the drug can develop pneumonitis that progresses to interstitial fibrosis, hypoxia, and death. Patients should be monitored for manifestations of **pulmonary toxicity**, which include cough, dyspnea, rales, and pulmonary infiltrates on chest x-ray film. Mucocutaneous toxicity manifests as mild stomatitis (inflammation of the oral mucosa), skin hyperpigmentation, erythema, and edema.

Dactinomycin

Dactinomycin (actinomycin D) intercalates DNA and prevents DNA transcription. The drug is given intravenously, and its clinical use is limited to the treatment of **trophoblastic tumors**, such as choriocarcinoma, and treatment of **pediatric tumors**, such as Wilms tumor and Ewing sarcoma.

DNA Topoisomerase Inhibitors

The DNA topoisomerases are enzymes that maintain the normal **structural topology** (spatial characteristics) of DNA. These enzymes relieve the torsional strain that occurs as the two DNA strands unwind during DNA replication or transcription. This is accomplished by producing strand breaks that permit the strands to pass through the gap before the breaks are resealed. Topoisomerase I breaks and reseals single-stranded DNA, whereas topoisomerase II breaks and reseals double-stranded DNA.

Drugs that inhibit topoisomerases cause **permanent strand breaks** by preventing the resealing of the nicked strands of DNA. The two groups of topoisomerase inhibitors are (1) the **podophyllotoxins**, which inhibit topoisomerase II, and (2) the **camptothecin** analogs, which inhibit topoisomerase I.

Podophyllotoxins. **Etoposide** and **teniposide** are analogs of podophyllin, a natural substance obtained from the mandrake or mayapple plant. **Etoposide** has broad activity against hematologic cancers and solid tumors and is especially valuable in the treatment of **testicular carcinoma, lung cancer**, and **non-Hodgkin lymphoma**. The drug is often administered with cisplatin because of its **synergy with platinum compounds**. Etoposide is also used as a preoperative treatment for bone marrow transplantation. **Teniposide** has a more limited anticancer activity and is used to treat **acute leukemias**. Both drugs are given intravenously. Etoposide is primarily eliminated unchanged in the urine, whereas teniposide is extensively metabolized in the liver before excretion.

Etoposide and **teniposide** are fairly well tolerated, though they can produce alopecia, **mild nausea and vomiting, and dose-limiting myelosuppression**. They have also been associated with a low incidence of secondary non-lymphocytic leukemias.

Camptothecin Analogs. **Camptothecin** is an alkaloid obtained from the plant *Camptotheca acuminata.* **Irinotecan** and **topotecan** are semi-synthetic camptothecin analogs that have greater clinical activity and less toxicity than the natural alkaloid. Both drugs are given intravenously for the treatment of cancer. Irinotecan is rapidly metabolized to an active metabolite that has much greater antitumor activity than the parent compound, and which is eliminated in the bile. Topotecan undergoes renal excretion.

Irinotecan is used for the treatment of **colorectal cancer** that has recurred or progressed after fluorouracil therapy. It is also active against lymphomas and breast, cervical, gastric, lung, and other tumors. **Topotecan** is active against glioma, sarcoma, and lung and ovarian tumors.

The dose-limiting toxicity of both camptothecin analogs is **myelosuppression.** Irinotecan produces diarrhea in a significant percentage of patients, and both drugs can cause **alopecia** and **mild nausea** and **vomiting.**

Mitotic Inhibitors

The mitotic spindle that separates the chromosomes during mitosis is made up of hollow tubules called **microtubules.** The microtubules are formed by the polymerization of the structural protein called *tubulin.* During mitosis, microtubules are continuously assembled and disassembled by means of **tubulin polymerization and depolymerization.** As shown in Fig. 45.5, several anticancer drugs inhibit mitosis and cause metaphase arrest by interfering with microtubule function. The **vinca alkaloids** bind to tubulin and block **tubulin polymerization,** whereas the **taxanes** bind to tubulin and prevent **depolymerization.** Microtubules also have important roles in nerve conduction and neurotransmission, which probably explains why mitotic inhibitors cause **neurotoxicity.**

Vinca Alkaloids. **Vincristine** and **vinblastine** are alkaloids obtained from the periwinkle plant, formerly designated *Vinca rosea.* Despite their structural similarity and similar mechanisms of action, the two drugs have different antitumor activities and toxicities. Both drugs are administered intravenously and are extensively metabolized before undergoing biliary excretion. Vinca alkaloids do not enter the CNS in significant amounts.

Vincristine is often used to treat **hematologic cancers,** including acute lymphocytic leukemia and Hodgkin and non-Hodgkin lymphomas, and to treat **solid tumors,** such as rhabdosarcoma, neuroblastoma, and Wilms tumor. Vinblastine is a component of the ABVD regimen described earlier for **Hodgkin disease** and is also used for treating breast cancer (Table 45.2). **Vinorelbine** is a semisynthetic derivative of vinblastine that is used to treat **non-small cell lung cancer,** breast cancer, and ovarian cancer.

Vincristine produces dose-limiting **neurotoxicity** in the form of a **peripheral neuropathy** that affects both sensory and motor function. Suppression of deep tendon reflexes is usually the earliest sign of neuropathy, and paresthesias of the hands and toes are common. Cranial nerve damage can cause hoarseness, facial palsies, or jaw pain, whereas autonomic neuropathies can cause orthostatic hypotension, abdominal pain, and constipation. These effects are usually reversible and do not require discontinuation of vincristine therapy unless they are disabling. **Vincristine** causes **little myelosuppression,** whereas **vinblastine** produces **myelosuppression** but **little neurotoxicity.**

Taxanes. The taxanes are alkaloids obtained from the bark (**paclitaxel**) or needles (**docetaxel** and **cabazitaxel**) of yew trees. The taxanes are given intravenously and are eliminated via metabolism and biliary excretion.

The taxanes have good activity against several types of cancer (see Table 45.1). **Paclitaxel** is indicated as first-line therapy for metastatic **ovarian cancer,** in combination with cisplatin; treatment of **non–small cell lung cancer;**

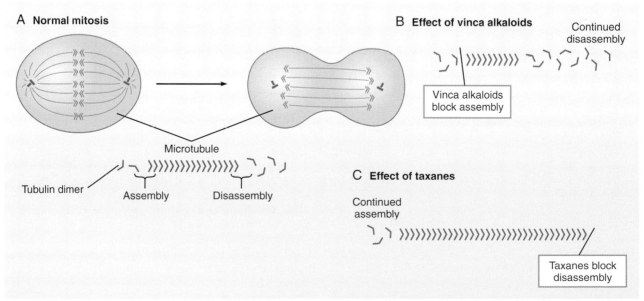

Fig. 45.5 Mechanisms of action of mitotic inhibitors. (A) In normal mitosis, the mitotic spindle is formed by microtubules that continuously undergo assembly and disassembly as a result of tubulin polymerization and depolymerization, respectively. (B) Vincristine and other vinca alkaloids bind to tubulin and prevent the polymerization of tubulin dimers. (C) Paclitaxel and other taxanes bind to tubulin, stabilize the tubulin polymer, and thereby prevent depolymerization. As with vinca alkaloids, taxanes cause metaphase arrest.

TABLE 45.2   Small Molecule Inhibitors Used in Cancer Treatment

CLASS/GENERIC NAME	BRAND NAME	ENZYME(S) INHIBITED	APPROVED INDICATIONS
EGFR Kinase Inhibitors			
Erlotinib	Tarceva	EGFR	Non–small cell lung cancer, pancreatic cancer
Osimertinib	Tagrisso	EGFR (exon 19 deletions/exon 21 mutations)	Non–small cell lung cancer
Gefitinib	Iressa	EGFR (exon 19 deletions/exon 21 mutations)	Non–small cell lung cancer
Dacomitinib	Vizimpro	EGFR (exon 19 deletions/exon 21 mutations)	Non–small cell lung cancer
Ibrutinib	Imbruvica	BTK	Chronic lymphocytic leukemia, small lymphocytic lymphoma
Acalabrutinib	Calquence	BTK	Mantle cell lymphoma, chronic lymphocytic leukemia, small lymphocytic lymphoma
Imatinib	Gleevec	BCR-ABL	Ph+ CML, Ph+ ALL
Nilotinib	Tasigna	BCR-ABL	Ph+ CML, Ph+ ALL
Dasatinib	Sprycel	BCR-ABL	Ph+ CML, Ph+ ALL
Cobimetinib	Cotellic	MAPK/MEK1	Melanoma with a BRAF mutation
Trametinib	Mekinist	MEK1	Melanoma, with BRAF mutation
Binimetinib	Mektovi	MEK1	Melanoma, with BRAF mutation
Selumetinib	Koselugo	MEK1	Inoperable plexiform neurofibromas
Dabrafenib	Taflina	BRAF mutation	Melanoma with BRAF mutation
Vemurafenib	Zelboraf	BRAF mutation	Melanoma with BRAF mutation
Encorafenib	Braftovi	BRAF mutation	Melanoma, colorectal cancer, with BRAF mutation
Midostaurin	Rydapt	multiple receptor tyrosine kinases	Acute myeloid leukemia with FLT3 mutation
Brigatinib	Alunbrig	multiple receptor tyrosine kinases/ALK	Non-small cell lung cancer, ALK-positive
HER2 Kinase Inhibitors			
Lapatinib	Tykerb	EGFR/HER2	Breast cancer, HER2 overexpressing
Tucatinib	Tukysa	HER2/HER3	Breast cancer, HER2 overexpressing
Neratinib	Nerlynx	EGFR/HER2/HER4	Breast cancer, HER2 overexpressing
VEGFR/PDGFR Kinase Inhibitors			
Lenvatinib	Lenvima	VEGFR	Thyroid cancer, renal carcinoma, hepatocellular, endometrial carcinoma
Pazopanib	Votrient	VEGFR/PDGFR	Renal cell carcinoma, soft tissue sarcoma
Sunitinib	Sutent	VEGFR/PDGFR	Renal cell carcinoma, GI stromal tumor
Sorafenib	Nexavar	VEGFR/PDGFR	Thyroid cancer, renal carcinoma, hepatocellular carcinoma
Ripretinib	Qinlock	VEGFR/PDGFR	GI stromal tumors.
Avapritinib	Ayvakit	PDGFR/PDGFR mutant	GI stromal tumors.
Selpercatinib	Retevmo	RET/RET-mutant/ VEGFR	Medullary thyroid cancer, non–small cell lung cancer, with RET-mutant
Proteasome Inhibitors			
Bortezomib	Velcade	26S proteasome	Multiple myeloma, mantle cell lymphoma
Carfilzomib	Kyprolis	26S proteasome	Multiple myeloma
Ixazomib	Ninlaro	26S proteasome	Multiple myeloma

Continued

TABLE 45.2   Small Molecule Inhibitors Used in Cancer Treatment—cont'd

CLASS/GENERIC NAME	BRAND NAME	ENZYME(S) INHIBITED	APPROVED INDICATIONS
Other inhibitors			
Palbociclid	IBRANCE	cyclin-dependent kinase	Breast cancer, ER-positive, HER2-negative
Abemaciclid	VERZENIO	cyclin-dependent kinase	Breast cancer, ER-positive, HER2-negative
Ribociclib	KISQALI	cyclin-dependent kinase	Breast cancer, ER-positive, HER2-negative
Rucaparib	RUBRACA	PARP	Ovarian cancer, primary peritoneal cancer
Niraparib	ZEJULA	PARP	Ovarian cancer, primary peritoneal cancer
Alpelisib	PIQRAY	PI3K	Breast cancer, ER-positive, HER2-negative, PI3K mutation
Copanlisib	ALIQOPA	PI3K	Follicular lymphoma
Venetoclax	VENCLEXTA	BCL2	Chronic lymphocytic leukemia, small lymphocytic lymphoma, acute myeloid leukemia
Enasidenib	IDHIFA	IDH2	Acute myeloid leukemia, with IDH2 mutation
Panobinostat	FARYDAK	Histone deacetylase	Multiple myeloma
Selinexor	XPOVIO	Exportin 1	Multiple myeloma, diffuse large B cell lymphoma
Sonidegib	ODOMZO	Smoothened/HH	Basal cell carcinoma

ALK, Anaplastic lymphoma kinase; *BCL2,* B-cell lymphoma 2; *BCR-ABL, bcr-abl* oncogene; *BRAF, b-Raf* proto-oncogene; *BTK,* Bruton tyrosine kinase; *EGFR,* epidermal growth factor receptor; *ER,* estrogen receptor; *FLT3,* fms like tyrosine kinase 3; *HER2,* human epidermal receptor-2; *HH,* hedgehog protein; *IDH2,* isocitrate dehydrogenase 2; *MAPK,* mitogen-activated protein kinase; *MEK1,* mitogen-activated extracellular signal regulated kinase 1; *PARP,* poly (ADP-ribose) polymerase; *PDGFR,* platelet-derived growth factor receptor; *Ph+ ALL,* Philadelphia chromosome positive acute lymphoblastic leukemia; *Ph+ CML,* Philadelphia chromosome positive chronic myeloid leukemia; *PI3K,* phosphatidylinositol-3-kinase; *RET,* rearrangement during transfection; *VEGFR,* vascular endothelial growth factor receptor.

and treatment of **metastatic breast cancer** unresponsive to first-line therapy. **Docetaxel** is approved for locally advanced or metastatic breast cancer and for metastatic non–small cell lung cancer after failure of cisplatin-based chemotherapy. **Cabazitaxel** is indicated as second-line treatment of metastatic **hormone-refractory prostate cancer**.

The major dose-limiting toxicity of taxanes is **myelosuppression**, particularly neutropenia. Taxanes can also cause alopecia and neurotoxicity.

Ixabepilone is a microtubule inhibitor for the treatment of metastatic or locally **advanced breast cancer** resistant to treatment with other drugs. Ixabepilone has low susceptibility to efflux transporters such as Pgp and multi-drug resistance pump (MRP) and is active against tumors resistant to taxanes, vinca alkaloids, and anthracyclines. The drug is given intravenously and is extensively metabolized before fecal and renal excretion.

Other Chemotherapeutic Agents
Temsirolimus

Temsirolimus is a cell-cycle specific agent that arrests tumor growth in the G_1 phase (see Fig. 45.1). **Temsirolimus inhibits the mTOR** (mammalian target of rapamycin) protein that controls and advances cell division. Inhibition of mTOR activity by temsirolimus results in G_1 growth arrest in tumor cells. **Temsirolimus** is approved for the treatment of **renal cell carcinoma**. Other drugs of this type are used for treatment of organ rejection and include **tacrolimus, sirolimus,** and **everolimus** (see Chapter 46).

Thalidomide

Thalidomide was withdrawn from the market in the 1960s because of its **teratogenic effects**. It was subsequently discovered to have anticancer and immunomodulating effects. It is now used under a strict Risk Evaluation and Mitigation Strategy (REMS) program regulated by the Food and Drug Administration (FDA). Thalidomide is indicated for the treatment of newly diagnosed **multiple myeloma** in **combination with dexamethasone**. Thalidomide exerts a number of immunomodulating actions, including **inhibition of tumor necrosis factor** and an **increase in interleukin-2** (IL-2) production, as well as affecting other cytokines. The drug is also used in the **treatment of leprosy** (see Chapter 41).

Lenalidomide and **pomalidomide** are two new thalidomide-like drugs. **Lenalidomide** is indicated for treatment of **multiple myeloma**, in combination with dexamethasone; mantle cell lymphoma; **follicular lymphoma**, in combination with rituximab product; and **marginal zone lymphoma**. **Pomalidomide** is used for the treatment of **multiple myeloma**, in combination with dexamethasone, and for the treatment of **AIDS-related Kaposi sarcoma**.

SMALL MOLECULE INHIBITORS

SMI block targets such as receptor tyrosine kinase, intracellular kinases, and other proteins. Receptor tyrosine kinase is the key functional component of activated EGRF and human epidermal receptor (HER). Neoplastic cells depend on activation of tyrosine kinase pathways to phosphorylate key proteins to unleash unbridled growth of the cancer. Many cancers are caused by oncogenic mutation in EGRF or HER that allow for ligand-independent (constitutively active) signaling by these receptors. Angiogenesis supports the growth of cancer cells and inhibition of tyrosine kinase activity in vascular endothelial growth factor (VEGF) receptors and platelet-derived growth factor receptors (PDGFR) are also a target for SMI. Other SMI block proteasome enzymes which then causes buildup of undegraded proteins which leads to apoptosis and inhibition of cancer growth.

SMI are suffixed according to the receptor, enzyme, or protein that they inhibit. Drug names that end in -*tinib* means tyrosine kinase inhibitors (e.g., **imatinib**), -*zomib* drugs are proteasome inhibitors (**bortezomib**), -*ciclib* drugs inhibit cyclin-dependent kinase (**palbociclid**), -*rafenib* drugs are b-Raf proto-oncogene (BRAF) kinase inhibitors (**sorafenib**), and generic drug names ending in -*parib* are inhibitors of poly (ADP-ribose) polymerase (PARP) enzymes (**rucaparib**).

SMI act on a number of molecular targets involved in cancer cell transformation and proliferation as shown in Table 45.2. Many of these drugs inhibit tyrosine kinase enzymes that phosphorylate and thereby activate pathways leading to continuous cell proliferation. Other SMI **inhibit proteasomes** that serve to degrade and recycle proteins. The newest SMI inhibit enzymes that have **specific mutations** in cancer cells.

Tyrosine Kinase Inhibitors

Imatinib, **dasatinib**, and **nilotinib** inhibit the **BCR-ABL** (breakpoint cluster region-Abelson) type of **tyrosine kinase** expressed by the Philadelphia chromosome in CML cells (Fig. 45.6). **BCR-ABL tyrosine kinase** is an **oncoprotein** resulting from a reciprocal chromosomal translocation (swap) between chromosomes 9 and 22. This swap inserts ABL from chromosome 9 adjacent to BCR on chromosome 22, forming the **BCR-ABL fusion gene** and leading to expression of an **abnormal tyrosine kinase** and the malignant transformation of hematopoietic stem cells. **Inhibition of the BCR-ABL kinase reduces cell proliferation and induces apoptosis**.

Imatinib has produced remarkable rates of hematologic and cytogenetic remission in CML and is a first-line treatment for this disease. **Imatinib** also **inhibits c-kit**, a tyrosine kinase stem cell receptor, and has been used to treat gastrointestinal stromal tumors (GISTs) associated with c-kit mutations. Both **dasatinib** and **nilotinib** are effective in patients with **imatinib-resistant tumors**, and they appear to and achieve greater cytogenetic responses with less cancer progression in newly diagnosed patients than did imatinib.

Erlotinib and **gefitinib** are specific inhibitors of the **EGFR tyrosine kinase**. They are used as second-line therapies for non-small cell lung cancer and achieve modest increases in survival. Erlotinib is metabolized by CYP3A, and other drugs that inhibit or induce this enzyme can alter its plasma levels.

Sunitinib and **sorafenib** inhibit **several receptor tyrosine kinases**, including VEGF receptors and PDGFR that promote angiogenesis. Both drugs are indicated for advanced renal cell carcinoma. **Sunitinib** is also used for GIST, while **sorafenib** is used to treat hepatocellular carcinoma. **Lapatinib** inhibits the **human epidermal growth factor-2 (HER2)** receptor kinase in breast cancer cells and is used to treat **HER2 receptor-positive breast cancer**.

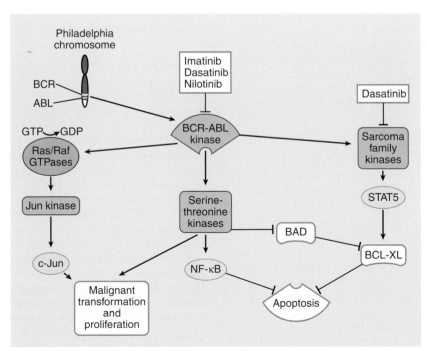

FIG. 45.6 BCR-ABL signal transduction. A simplified illustration of pathways by which the BCR-ABL tyrosine kinase invokes malignant transformation and proliferation by activating small cytoplasmic GTPases (*Ras* and *Raf*) and various serine/threonine kinases, including the Jun kinase and sarcoma family kinases. The activated kinases stimulate transcription factors, including c-Jun, NF-κB (nuclear factor-kappa B), and STAT5 (signal transducer and activator of transcription 5). Some of these factors increase expression of cyclins and other positive regulators of the cell cycle (see Fig. 45.1). The activated kinases and transcription factors also modulate mitochondrial apoptotic regulators, including a proapoptotic caspase (*BAD*) and the antiapoptotic BCL-XL. Together, these effects lead to inhibition of apoptosis (programmed cell death) and promotion of cell replication. BCR-ABL also activates cytoskeletal regulators, leading to altered cell adhesion and motility (not shown). Imatinib and similar drugs inhibit BCR-ABL kinase and induce hematologic and cytogenetic remissions in patients with chronic myeloid leukemia. Dasatinib also inhibits sarcoma family kinases.

The combination of **dabrafenib** and **trametinib** is now available to treat inoperable **metastatic melanoma**. Dabrafenib inhibits the B-raf kinase expressed by the BRAF gene having the V600E mutation. This mutation occurs in about 60% of melanomas and results in continuous B-raf kinase activity, leading to continuous cell proliferation. **Trametinib** is a **MEK** (mitogen-activated protein kinase) **inhibitor** that acts synergistically with dabrafenib to block melanoma cell proliferation. Another B-raf kinase/MEK inhibitor combination for treating metastatic melanoma consists of **vemurafenib** and **cobimetinib**. The most common side effects of this treatment are fever, nausea, vomiting, and diarrhea, though severe adverse effects have also occurred. See Box 45.1 for case example.

The treatment of relapsed CLL has advanced with the introduction of **ibrutinib**, the first **inhibitor of Bruton's kinase** to be developed for cancer treatment. This kinase plays a crucial role in B-lymphocyte maturation. An early study found that the drug reduced disease progression by 80% compared with the standard treatment for relapsed CLL of bendamustine plus rituximab.

Proteasome Inhibitors

Bortezomib was the first small molecule **proteasome inhibitor** to be developed for cancer treatment. The drug prevents the degradation and recycling of proteins by the proteasome of cancer cells, leading to protein accumulation and cell death. Bortezomib is used to treat **multiple myeloma** and **mantle cell lymphoma**. Other small molecule proteasome inhibitors include **carfilzomib** and **ixazomib**. They are both approved for the treatment of multiple myeloma.

Other Inhibitors

Ribociclib is a small molecule inhibitor of cyclin-dependent kinases (CDK 4 and 6). These CDK enzymes are activated upon D-cyclin binding and are crucial kinases that initiate signaling pathways, leading to cell cycle progression and cellular proliferation. **Ribociclib** produces a G_1 growth arrest in breast cancer cells. **Robiciclid** is approved for use in **combination with aromatase inhibitors or fulvestrant** (see below) to treat women with estrogen receptor (ER)-positive, HER2-negative breast cancer. **Abemaciclid** and **palbociclid** are other CDK inhibitors used to treat women with **ER-positive, HER2-negative breast cancer**.

Rucaparib is an **inhibitor** of **PARP** enzymes, namely PARP-1, PARP-2, and PARP-3. The **PARP enzymes are crucial** for **DNA repair** and rucaparib-induced cytotoxicity via inhibition of PARP activity leads to increased formation of PARP-DNA complexes. The increase in PARP-DNA complexes **leads to DNA damage, apoptosis, and cancer cell death**. An increase in rucaparib-induced cytotoxicity and anti-tumor activity was observed in tumor cell lines with mutations in *BRCA* and other DNA repair genes. Rucaparib is approved for use in the treatment of **ovarian, fallopian tube, or primary peritoneal cancer,** and for those women who harbor deleterious *BRCA* mutation-associated epithelial ovarian, fallopian tube, or primary peritoneal cancer. **Niraparib** is a second PARP inhibitor available for the same indications.

Venetoclax is a selective small molecule **inhibitor of BCL-2**, an anti-apoptotic protein. BCL-2 overexpression is observed in cancer cells obtained from patients. Overexpression of BCL-2 is associated with **resistance to chemotherapeutics** and increased tumor cell survival.

Venetoclax reinstates apoptosis by binding directly to the BCL-2 protein, displacing other pro-apoptotic proteins, increasing mitochondrial outer membrane permeability and activating caspases which mediate apoptosis (cell death). **Venetoclax** is approved for the treatment of **CLL, AML,** or small lymphocytic lymphoma (**SLL**).

Selinexor reversibly **inhibits nuclear export** of tumor suppressor proteins (TSPs), growth regulators, and mRNAs of oncogenic proteins by blocking the exportin 1 (XPO1) channel protein, commonly called nuclear pores. **Selinexor inhibition** of XPO1 produces accumulation of TSPs stuck in the nucleus, decreases in several oncoproteins (e.g., *c-myc* and cyclin D1), cell cycle arrest, and apoptosis of cancer cells. **Selinexor demonstrated pro-apoptotic activity** in multiple myeloma cells and showed anti-tumor activity in murine xenograft models of multiple myeloma and diffuse large B cell lymphoma. Accordingly, **selinexor is approved** for use in patients with **multiple myeloma** and diffuse **large B cell lymphoma**.

HORMONAL AGENTS

Several types of hormone-dependent cancer (especially breast, prostate, and endometrial cancers) respond to treatment with their corresponding hormone antagonists. **Estrogen antagonists** are primarily used to treat breast cancer, whereas **androgen antagonists** are used to treat prostate cancer. **Corticosteroids** are particularly useful in treating **lymphocytic leukemias** and **lymphomas**.

The pharmacologic properties of estrogens, androgens, and their antagonists are described in Chapter 34, and those of corticosteroids are described in Chapter 33.

Drugs for Breast Cancer

Breast cancer is usually estrogen-dependent and can be suppressed by the administration of **estrogen antagonists.** **Tamoxifen** is the antagonist of the **SERM** class (see Chapter 34) used most widely. This drug can be given alone to prevent breast cancer in women who have a strong family history of the disease or are otherwise highly predisposed to developing it. Tamoxifen is often used in combination with surgery and other chemotherapeutic drugs for the treatment of breast cancer. In women over 50 years of age, adjuvant use of tamoxifen was found to reduce the annual odds of recurrence by 30%. Long-term survival appears to be greater in women receiving both cytotoxic chemotherapy and tamoxifen.

Tamoxifen

Pharmacokinetics. Tamoxifen is an orally administered **prodrug** that is well absorbed from the gut and then converted to active metabolites in the liver, such as 4-hydroxytamoxifen, that have 30 to 100 times greater affinity for the ER than does tamoxifen. The terminal elimination half-life of tamoxifen is about 7 days. Tamoxifen undergoes enterohepatic cycling and biliary excretion in the same manner as clomiphene.

Mechanisms and Indications. Like other SERMs, the active metabolites of tamoxifen have both estrogenic and antiestrogenic properties. In breast tissue, **4-hydroxytamoxifen** acts as an ER antagonist. After competitively binding to ERs in breast tumor cells, 4-hydroxytamoxifen forms an ER complex that **recruits corepressors** of DNA transcription so as to inhibit expression of **human EGFR 2 (HER2)** and other breast cancer growth factors. Tamoxifen **inhibits breast cancer cell proliferation** and may contribute to the eradication of micrometastases. Tamoxifen is primarily used to prevent or treat **breast cancer** in patients with **tumor cells that are ER positive,** and it is typically used in combination with surgery or other chemotherapy. In cases of advanced or metastatic breast cancer, tamoxifen can be used alone for palliative treatment.

Adverse Effects. Tamoxifen can cause nausea, vomiting, hot flashes, vaginal bleeding, and menstrual irregularities. It can **stimulate proliferation of endometrial cells,** and it increases the risk of **endometrial cancer.**

Toremifene

Toremifene is another ER agonist/antagonist (SERM) that acts as an antagonist in breast tissue and is indicated for the treatment of **metastatic breast cancer** in postmenopausal women. It is administered orally once a day and is converted to less-active metabolites. **Toremifene undergoes enterohepatic cycling** and has an elimination half-life of 5 days. As with tamoxifen, hot flashes, sweating, and nausea are the most common adverse effects.

Selective Estrogen Receptor Degrader

Fulvestrant is a first-in-class ER **antagonist** that acts as a selective ER degrader (SERD). Unlike SERMs which may have agonist or antagonist effects at ERs depending on the tissue, **fulvestrant is a pure ER antagonist** in all tissues tested. It binds to the ER monomer preventing dimerization of the receptor and causes internalization and degradation of the ER

by proteasomes within the tumor cell. **Fulvestrant is indicated for ER+ metastatic breast cancer** and is given by intramuscular injection every 2 weeks for three times then monthly thereafter. Given the success of **fulvestrant** in treating women with **tamoxifen-resistant breast cancer,** there is vigorous development of additional SERDs that will be orally available.

Aromatase Inhibitors

Aromatase inhibitors that prevent estrogen synthesis, including **anastrozole** and **letrozole,** are a first-line therapy for certain forms of breast cancer in postmenopausal women (see Chapter 34). Breast cancer is often hormonally responsive—including breast cancer classified as estrogen and/or progesterone receptor positive. This type of breast cancer has responded to a variety of efforts to decrease estrogen levels (e.g., removal of the ovaries, an oophorectomy) or to inhibit estrogen effects, such as with SERMs. These interventions lead to decreased tumor mass, delayed progression, and improved survival in many patients.

In postmenopausal women, estrogens are derived from adrenal androgens, primarily testosterone and androstenedione, which are **converted to estrogens in peripheral tissues and in cancer tissue** by the **enzyme aromatase** (see Fig. 34.1). **Anastrozole** and **letrozole** are nonsteroidal **aromatase inhibitors** that **reduce circulating levels of estrogen** and are indicated as first-line treatments for locally advanced or **metastatic breast cancer** in postmenopausal women (see Chapter 45). By lowering estrogen levels, these drugs may halt progression of estrogen-sensitive breast cancer. Anastrozole and letrozole are well absorbed after oral administration and have long half-lives of about 2 days. The aromatase inhibitors are well tolerated but can cause hot flashes, nausea, headache, vaginal bleeding, and back pain.

Drugs for Prostate Cancer
Gonadotropin-Releasing Hormone Analogs

When a gonadotropin-releasing hormone (GnRH) analog is administered in a continuous rather than a pulsatile fashion, it reduces LH secretion by the pituitary and thereby reduces testosterone production by the testes.

The GnRH analogs include **leuprolide,** an agent discussed in Chapter 31. Leuprolide has been successfully used in the treatment of inoperable **prostate cancer.** Because leuprolide increases the production of LH and testosterone when it is first administered, the drug is sometimes given in combination with an androgen receptor antagonist (e.g., **flutamide**). Combined androgen blockade with a GnRH analog and an androgen receptor antagonist (see later) prolongs the progression-free period and the length of survival in men with advanced prostate cancer.

Androgen Receptor Antagonists

Flutamide, bicalutamide, enzalutamide, and **nilutamide** are nonsteroidal agents that compete with testosterone for the androgen receptor. These drugs are used in combination with a synthetic GnRH analog to treat inoperable **prostate** cancer. For example, bicalutamide is used with a GnRH analog for treatment of stage D2 metastatic carcinoma of the prostate. In one study, enzalutamide produced a 12-month progression-free survival of 65% versus 14% in those receiving a placebo. After 22 months of treatment, 28% of men receiving enzalutamide had died versus 35% of the placebo group. The adverse effects of these drugs include nausea, gynecomastia, impotence, hot flashes, and hepatitis.

5α-Reductase Inhibitors

Finasteride and **dutasteride** are synthetic testosterone derivatives that block 5α-reductase and decrease the synthesis of DHT in the prostate gland, skin, and other target tissues (see Chapter 34). Finasteride and dutasteride are indicated for the treatment of **benign prostatic hyperplasia (BPH)**. **Finasteride** and **dutasteride** were used off-label to **prevent prostate cancer**. However, studies show that the drugs lower the risk of less aggressive cancers but appear to increase the risk of more aggressive and life-threatening cancers. This effect resulted in one additional case of high-grade prostate cancer for every three to four lower-grade cancers that were prevented. Early detection of prostate cancer using the prostate-specific antigen (PSA) blood test and digital rectal examination, followed by appropriate therapy, may be the best approach to prostate cancer. A limitation of use was specifically added the FDA label in 2011 noting that these agents are **not approved for the prevention of prostate cancer**.

Gonadotropin-Releasing Hormone Agonists

Prostate cancer cell proliferation is stimulated by androgens and suppressed by estrogens. Continuous administration of a **GnRH agonist**, such as **leuprolide**, can be used to inhibit luteinizing hormone secretion and, secondarily, testosterone production in men with advanced prostate cancer, and thereby suppress cancer growth. The GnRH agonists have become the standard of care for **metastatic prostate cancer**. Complete androgen deprivation using a GnRH agonist plus an androgen antagonist (e.g., **flutamide**) can be used to further reduce testosterone stimulation of prostate carcinoma cells and has shown a small survival advantage for these patients in some studies.

Corticosteroids

Corticosteroids (e.g., **prednisone, dexamethasone**) are primarily used because of their lymphocytotoxic effects in the treatment of **lymphocytic leukemias, lymphomas**, and **multiple myeloma**. Corticosteroids are relatively well tolerated and do not produce myelosuppression or other serious organ damage in most patients. They are often combined with cytotoxic and targeted anticancer agents in these treatments.

SUMMARY OF IMPORTANT POINTS

- Most antineoplastic drugs inhibit DNA synthesis or disrupt DNA structure and function.
- DNA synthesis inhibitors include folate antagonists (methotrexate [MTX] and trimetrexate), purine analogs (mercaptopurine, thioguanine, and others), pyrimidine analogs (cytarabine, floxuridine, and fluorouracil), and a ribonucleotide reductase inhibitor (hydroxyurea).
- DNA alkylating drugs that cross-link DNA include nitrogen mustards (cyclophosphamide and others), nitrosoureas (carmustine and others), and miscellaneous drugs (busulfan, dacarbazine). Platinum compounds (cisplatin and others) also cross-link DNA strands.
- DNA intercalating drugs include the anthracycline drugs (doxorubicin and others), bleomycin, and dactinomycin. These agents cause DNA strand breaks and inhibit topoisomerase.

- Inhibitors of mitosis include vinca alkaloids (vincristine and others) and taxane drugs (docetaxel and paclitaxel).
- Topoisomerase inhibitors include podophyllotoxin drugs (etoposide and teniposide) and camptothecin analogs (irinotecan and topotecan).
- Doxorubicin and other anthracycline drugs produce cardiotoxicity; cyclophosphamide and ifosfamide cause hemorrhagic cystitis; bleomycin and busulfan produce pulmonary fibrosis; vincristine, docetaxel, and related drugs cause neurotoxicity; and cisplatin produces renal toxicity.
- Myelosuppression is the dose-limiting toxicity of most chemotherapeutic drugs.
- SMI include imatinib, dasatinib, and nilotinib (BCR-ABL kinases); erlotinib (EGFR); sunitinib and sorafenib (vascular endothelial and PDGFR) and target specific pathways in cancer cells.
- Hormonal agents are used to treat some cancers, especially estrogen antagonists to treat breast cancer, androgen antagonists to treat prostate cancer, and corticosteroids (prednisone) to treat lymphocytic leukemias and lymphomas.

Review Questions

1. A woman being treated for breast cancer develops numbness and tingling in her hands and feet. Which drug most likely caused this adverse effect?
   (A). cyclophosphamide
   (B). docetaxel
   (C). doxorubicin
   (D). tamoxifen
   (E). temsirolimus
2. Which adverse effect may result from cisplatin therapy?
   (A). cardiac toxicity
   (B). liver failure
   (C). muscle toxicity
   (D). nephrotoxicity
   (E). hemolytic anemia
3. A woman with chronic myeloid leukemia responds to imatinib therapy as indicated by a cytologic remission. Which enzyme is inhibited by this drug?
   (A). DNA polymerase
   (B). dihydrofolate reductase
   (C). BCR-ABL tyrosine kinase
   (D). thymidylate synthetase
   (E). hypoxanthine guanine phosphoribosyltransferase
4. Uridine triacetate is given as an antidote to counteract the toxic effects of which one of the following chemotherapeutic agents?
   (A). cyclophosphamide
   (B). doxorubicin
   (C). fluorouracil
   (D). tamoxifen
   (E). doxorubicin
5. Doxorubicin is used to treat breast cancer and other neoplasms. It works by:
   (A). DNA intercalation
   (B). inhibition of ribosomes
   (C). immune checkpoint inhibitor
   (D). DNA alkylation
   (E). targeted antibodies

Immunopharmacology, Biologicals, and Gene Therapy

CLASSIFICATION OF IMMUNOPHARMACOLGICAL, BIOLOGICAL, AND GENETIC THERAPY AGENTS

MONOCLONAL ANTIBODY DRUGS

Antineoplastic Agents

EGFR kinase inhibitors
- Cetuximab (ERBITUX)
- Panitumumab (VECTIBIX)[a]

EGFR kinase inhibitors
- Trastuzumab (HERCEPTIN)
- Pertuzumab (PERJETA)

VEGFR/PDGFR kinase inhibitors
- Bevacizumab (AVASTIN)
- Ramucirumab (CYRAMZA)
- Olaratumab (LARTRUVO)

Immune checkpoint inhibitors
- Ipilimumab (YERVOY)
- Nivolumab (OPDIVO)[b]

Other protein targets
- Rituximab (RITUXAN)
- Obinutuzumab (GAZYVA)[c]

Antibody drug conjugates
- Trastuzumab emtansine (KADCYLA)
- Inotuzumab ozogamacin (BESPONSA)[d]

Antilipidemic Agents

- Evolocumab (REPATHA)
- Alirocumab (PRALUENT)

Antithrombotic and Thrombolytic Reversal Agents

- Abciximab (REOPRO)
- Idarucizumab (PRAXBIND)[e]

Antiasthma Agents

- Omalizumab (XOLAIR)
- Reslizumab (CINQAIR)[f]

Antimigraine Agents

- Galcanezumab (EMGALITY)
- Erenumab (AIMOVIG)[g]

Agents for Inflammatory Bowel Disease/RA

- Adalimumab (HUMIRA)
- Infliximab (REMICADE)[h]

Antipsoriatic Agents

- Ustekinumab (STELARA)

- Secukinumab (COSENTYX)[i]

Antiviral Agents

- Palivizumab (SYNAGIS)
- Ibalizumab (TROGARZO)

Antitoxin Agents

- Bezlotoxumab (ZINPLAVA)
- Obiltoxaximab (ANTHIM)

Other Monoclonal Antibody Drugs

- Alemtuzumab (LEMTRADA)
- Natalizumab (TYSABRI)[j]

BIOLOGICALS

Vaccines for Infants and Children
- Hepatitis B vaccine (RECOMBIVAX HB)
- Diphtheria, tetanus, and acellular pertussis vaccine (DAPTACEL)[k]

Vaccines for Adults and the Elderly

- Pneumococcal 23-valent polysaccharide vaccine (PNEUOMOVAX 23)
- Zoster vaccine recombinant (SHINGRIX)[l]

Passive Immunoglobulins

- Rho(D) Immunoglobulin (RHOPHYLAC)
- Crotalidae Immune Fab (ANAVIP)[m]

Treatment of Organ Rejection

- Cyclosporine (SANDIMMUNE)
- Mycophenolate (CELLCEPT)[n]

Interferon and Related Biologicals

- Peginterferon alfa-2a (PEGASYS)
- Interferon alfa-2b (INTRON A)[o]

GENE THERAPY AGENTS

mRNA Targeting Agents
- Mipomersen (KYNAMRO)
- Eteplirsen (EXONDYS 51)[p]

Gene Modification Agents

- Tisagenlecleucel (KYMRIAH)
- Axicabtagene ciloleucel (YESCARTA)[q]

---

[a] Also necitumumab (PORTRAZZA).
[b] Also pembrolizumab (KEYTRUDA), and others (see Table 46.1).
[c] Also daratumumab (DARZALEX), elotuzumab (EMPLICITI), dinutuximab (UNITUXIN).
[d] Also trastuzumab deruxtecan (ENHERTU), and others (see Table 46.1).

Continued

CLASSIFICATION OF IMMUNOPHARMACOLGICAL, BIOLOGICAL, AND GENETIC THERAPY AGENTS—CONT'D

[e] Also crizanlizumab (ADAKVEO).
[f] Also mepolizumab (NUCALA), and benralizumab (FASENRA).
[g] Also eptinezumab (VYEPTI), and fremanezumab (AJOVY).
[h] Also golimumab (SIMPONI), sarilumab (KEVZARA), and vedolizumab (ENTYVIO).
[i] Also dupilumab (DUPIXENT), tildrakizumab (ILUMYA), and others (see Table 46.2).
[j] Also basiliximab (SIMULECT), Also others (see Table 46.2).
[k] Also many others (see Table 46.3).
[l] Also many others (see Table 46.4).
[m] Also rabies immunoglobulin (BAYRAB), and botulism antitoxin immunoglobulin.
[n] Also azathioprine (IMURAN), belatacept (NULOJIX), tacrolimus (PROGRAF), sirolimus (RAPAMUNE), everolimus (AFINITOR), and basiliximab (SIMULECT).
[o] Also peginterferon alfa-2b (PEGINTRON), interferon beta-1a (AVONEX), interferon beta-1a (REBIF), interferon beta-1b (EXTAVIA), interferon beta-1b (BETASERON), peginterferon beta-1a (PLEGRIDY), interferon gamma-1b (ACTIMMUNE), anakinra (KINERET), and lifitegrast (XIIDRA).
[p] Also nusinersen (SPINRAZA), inotersen (TEGSEDI), golodirsen (VYONDYS 53), and patisiran (ONPATTRO).
[q] Also sipuleucel-T (PROVENGE), brexucabtagene autoleucel (TECARTUS), talimogene laherparepvec (IMLYGIC), voretigene neparvovec (Luxturna), and onasemnogene abeparvovec (Zolgensma).

OVERVIEW

Monoclonal antibody drugs exploded upon the market in the last few years with the discovery of detailed interactions between the immune system and cancer, asthma, rheumatoid arthritis (RA), and other disorders. Monoclonal antibodies (mAb) are limited to targeting cell surface antigens, receptors, and free-floating cytokines and block key protein-protein interactions. While **most immunopharmacology therapeutics are designed to target cancer growth**, a number of new monoclonal antibody drugs also target disorders such as migraine, asthma, hyperlipidemia, and others.

Vaccines are a method to safely present a pathological bacteria or viral antigen to the body so that antibodies (Ab) can be made to counteract the targeted virus or bacteria. Recommended infant, childhood, adult, and elderly vaccines are listed and briefly discussed. Other biologicals discussed include interferons, immunomodulators, and agents used to prevent organ transplant rejection. The chapter closes with an introduction to **messenger RNA (mRNA)-targeting agents** and approved **medications that use genetic modification techniques**.

MONOCLONAL ANTIBODY DRUGS

Monoclonal Ab are a fast-growing class of antineoplastic (anticancer) and other immunotherapy agents. The fragment antigen binding (Fab) portion of monoclonal Ab bind to a specific antigen on a particular type of cancer cell, leading to **blockade or inhibition of an oncogenic pathway**. Some Ab target growth factors or their receptors, whereas others are conjugated with a cytotoxic agent or enhance host immunity (Tables 46.1 and 46.2). Because of their protein structure, these agents must be given **intravenously or intradermally**. As these preparations are protein-based, monoclonal antibody drugs can cause hypersensitivity reactions upon injection.

The names of monoclonal Ab end in *mab* or *monab*. The letters before *mab* indicate the source of the antibody: *o* for mouse, *u* for human, and *xi* for chimeric (two species, usually human–mouse). An internal letter or syllable identifies the therapeutic use of the antibody, for example, *tu* for tumor, *vi* for virus, and *c* or *ci* for circulation. For example, **rituximab** is a chimeric (*xi*) human-mouse *mAb* used to treat tumors (*tu*). **Rituximab was the first monoclonal** antibody drug approved for targeted cancer treatment.

Manufacture of Monoclonal Antibodies

When humans encounter a foreign antigen, such as a bacteria or virus, the foreign antigen binds to a **specific antibody** receptor on a **B lymphocyte** (B cell), which is then stimulated to divide and undergo clonal expansion of identical cells. The B cells mature and become **plasma cells, which secrete millions of the antigen-specific Ab** in the bloodstream and lymph system. These naturally produced Ab (also called immunoglobulins) are a mixture of **polyclonal** Ab because different Ab are produced that **each recognize a specific epitope** or region on the foreign antigen.

mAb are specific for a single epitope on the antigen. They are produced in the laboratory from the injection of a mouse with the targeted antigen, and the B cells from the spleen of the immunized mouse are collected (Fig. 46.1). Because normal B cells are unable to continuous replicate, they are fused with **immortalized myeloma cells** to create hybridoma cells. After placing the cell mixture in **selective medium that only allows hybridoma survival**, the remaining hybridoma cells are screened for the **targeted mAb**. Cells producing the desired mAb are continuously grown in tissue culture, and the culture medium is periodically harvested. The mAbs are purified from the culture medium and prepared as drug formulations.

Monoclonal Antibodies Targeted for Cancer Treatment
Epidermal Growth Factor Receptor Kinase Inhibitors

Cetuximab, panitumumab, and **necitumumab** bind selectively to EGFR on both normal and tumor cells and competitively **inhibit epidermal growth factor (EGF)** and other growth factor ligands. The **EGF receptor** (EGRF) is expressed in many normal tissues and overexpressed in certain human cancers, particularly colon cancer. Overexpression of EGRF is associated with unrestricted cell growth and a poor prognosis. *In vitro* assays and *in vivo* animal studies have shown that **cetuximab binding to EGFR blocks phosphorylation** and activation of receptor associated kinases, which results in **inhibition of cell growth and induction of apoptosis**. Signal transduction through the EGFR results in activation of wild-type Ras proteins, but in cells with **activating Ras mutations**, the resulting **mutant Ras proteins are continuously active** regardless of EGFR activity. The mechanism of these antineoplastic monoclonal antibody agents and others is shown in Fig. 46.2.

Cetuximab is used to treat **colon cancer** in **combination with irinotecan**. Patients receiving this drug combination had better response rates and increased time to tumor progression than patients not receiving cetuximab. The most common adverse effect of cetuximab is an acne-like skin rash, whereas about 3% of patients experience hypersensitivity reactions during drug infusion. It is also approved for **head and neck cancer** in combination with radiation therapy.

TABLE 46.1 Monoclonal Antibody Drugs Used in Cancer Treatment

CLASS/GENERIC NAME	BRAND NAME	ANTIBODY EFFECT	APPROVED INDICATIONS
EGFR Kinase Inhibitors			
Cetuximab	ERBITUX	EGFR antagonist	Colorectal cancer, head and neck cancer
Panitumumab	VECTIBIX	EGFR antagonist	Colorectal cancer
Necitumumab	PORTRAZZA	EGFR antagonist	Non-small cell lung cancer
HER2 Kinase Inhibitors			
Trastuzumab	HERCEPTIN	HER2 antagonist	HER2-overexpressing breast cancer
Pertuzumab	PERJETA	HER2 antagonist	HER2-overexpressing breast cancer
VEGFR Kinase Inhibitors			
Bevacizumab	AVASTIN	VEGF antagonist	Colorectal cancer
Ramucirumab	CYRAMZA	VEGF antagonist	Colorectal cancer, gastric adenocarcinoma, non-small cell lung cancer, hepatocellular carcinoma
PDGFR Kinase Inhibitors			
Olaratumab	LARTRUVO	PDGFR antagonist	Soft tissue sarcoma
Immune Checkpoint Inhibitors			
Ipilimumab	YERVOY	CTLA4 antagonist	Melanoma, renal cell carcinoma, colorectal cancer, hepatocellular carcinoma, non–small cell lung cancer, mesothelioma
Nivolumab	OPDIVO	PD1 antagonist	Non-small cell lung cancer, small cell lung cancer, renal cell carcinoma, Hodgkin Lymphoma, squamous cell carcinoma, urothelial carcinoma, colorectal cancer, and liver cancer
Pembrolizumab	KEYTRUDA	PD1 antagonist	Non–small cell lung cancer, small cell lung cancer, renal cell carcinoma, Hodgkin Lymphoma, squamous cell carcinoma, urothelial carcinoma, colorectal cancer, and liver cancer, and others
Atezolizumab	TECENTRIQ	PD1 antagonist	Urothelial carcinoma, non–small cell lung cancer, small cell lung cancer, triple-negative breast cancer, and others
Durvalumab	IMFINZI	PD1 antagonist	Urothelial carcinoma
Avelumab	BAVENCIO	PD1 antagonist	Merkel cell carcinoma, urothelial carcinoma, renal cell carcinoma
Other Protein Targets			
Rituximab	RITUXAN	CD20 inhibitor	Chronic lymphocytic leukemia, non-Hodgkin lymphoma, leukemia, RA, Wegener'granulomatosis, and pemphigus vulgaris
Obinutuzumab	GAZYVA	CD20 inhibitor	Chronic lymphocytic leukemia
Daratumumab	DARZALEX	CD38 inhibitor	Multiple myeloma
Elotuzumab	EMPLICITI	SLAMF7 activator	Multiple myeloma
Dinutuximab	UNITUXIN	GD2 inhibitor-	High-risk neuroblastoma
Antibody Drug Conjugates			
Trastuzumab emtansine	KADCYLA	HER2 antagonist/ microtubule inhibitor	HER2-positive breast cancer
Trastuzumab deruxtecan	ENHERTU	HER2 antagonist/ topoisomerase inhibitor	HER2-positive breast cancer
Brentuximab vedotin	ADCETRIS	CD30 inhibitor/ microtubule inhibitor	Hodgkin lymphoma
Gemtuzumab ozogamacin	MYLOTARG	CD33 inhibitor/cytotoxic agent	Acute myeloid leukemia
Denileukin diftitox	ONTAK	CD25 inhibitor/cytotoxic agent	T-cell lymphoma
Ibritumomab tiuxetan	ZEVALIN	CD20 inhibitor/ yttrium-90	Non-Hodgkin lymphoma
Inotuzumab ozogamacin	BESPONSA	CD22 inhibitor/ cytotoxic agent	Acute lymphoblastic leukemia

CD, Cluster of differentiation proteins; *CTLA-4,* cytotoxic T-lymphocyte-associated protein-4; *EGFR,* epidermal growth factor receptor; *GD2,* ganglioside type GD2; *HER2,* human epidermal growth factor receptor 2; PD-1, programmed cell death protein 1; *PDGFR,* platelet-derived growth factor receptor; *RA,* rheumatoid arthritis; *SLAMF7,* signaling lymphocytic activation molecule family member 7; *VEGFR,* vascular epidermal growth factor receptor.

TABLE 46.2 Monoclonal Antibody Drugs Used in Non-Cancer Treatment

CLASS/GENERIC NAME	BRAND NAME	ANTIBODY EFFECT	APPROVED INDICATIONS
Antilipidemic Agents			
Evolocumab	Repatha	PCSK9 inhibitor	Primary hyperlipidemia
Alirocumab	Praluent	PCSK9 inhibitor	Primary hyperlipidemia
Antithrombotic and Thrombolytic Reversal			
Abciximab	ReoPro	GP IIb/IIIa receptor antagonist	Patients undergoing percutaneous coronary intervention, unstable angina
Idarucizumab	Praxbind	Dabigatran inhibitor	Uncontrolled bleeding due to dabigatran
Crizanlizumab	Adakveo	P-selectin inhibitor	Vaso-occlusive crises in sickle cell disease
Antiasthma Agents			
Omalizumab	Xolair	IgE inhibitor	Persistent asthma, chronic idiopathic urticaria
Reslizumab	Cinqair	IL5 receptor antagonist	Severe asthma, and with eosinophilic phenotype
Benralizumab	Fasenra	IL5 receptor antagonist	Severe asthma, and with eosinophilic phenotype
Mepolizumab	Nucala	IL5 receptor antagonist	Severe asthma, and with eosinophilic phenotype, hypereosinophilic syndrome
Antimigraine Agents			
Galcanezumab	Emgality	CGRP antagonist	Migraine prevention, cluster headaches
Eptinezumab	Vyepti	CGRP antagonist	Migraine prevention
Erenumab	Aimovig	CGRP antagonist	Migraine prevention
Fremanezumab	Ajovy	CGRP antagonist	Migraine prevention
Drugs for Inflammatory Bowel Diseases/RA			
Adalimumab	Humira	TNFα blocker	Crohn disease, ulcerative colitis, rheumatoid arthritis, psoriatic arthritis, ankylosing spondylitis, plaque psoriasis
Golimumab	Simponi	TNFα blocker	Ulcerative colitis, rheumatoid arthritis, psoriatic arthritis, ankylosing spondylitis
Infliximab	Remicade	TNFα blocker	Crohn disease, ulcerative colitis, rheumatoid arthritis, psoriatic arthritis, ankylosing spondylitis, plaque psoriasis
Certolizumab	Cimzia	TNFα blocker	Crohn disease, rheumatoid arthritis, psoriatic arthritis, ankylosing spondylitis
Vedolizumab	Entyvio	TNFα blocker	Crohn disease, ulcerative colitis
Tocilizumab	Actemra	IL6 receptor antagonist	Rheumatoid arthritis
Sarilumab	Kevzara	IL6 receptor antagonist	Rheumatoid arthritis
Antipsoriatic Agents			
Ustekinumab	Stelara	IL12/IL23 inhibitor	Plaque psoriasis, psoriatic arthritis, Crohn disease, ulcerative colitis
Secukinumab	Cosentyx	IL17A inhibitor	Plaque psoriasis, psoriatic arthritis, ankylosing spondylitis
Ixekizumab	Taltz	IL17A inhibitor	Plaque psoriasis, psoriatic arthritis, ankylosing spondylitis
Brodalumab	Siliq	IL17RA inhibitor	Plaque psoriasis
Guselkumab	Tremfya	IL23 inhibitor	Plaque psoriasis, psoriatic arthritis
Tildrakizumab	Ilumya	IL23 inhibitor	Plaque psoriasis
Risankizumab	Skyrizi	IL23 inhibitor	Plaque psoriasis
Dupilumab	Dupixent	IL4/IL13 inhibitor	Atopic dermatitis (eczema)
Antiviral Agents			
Palivizumab	Synagis	RSV F protein inhibitor	RSV-associated respiratory distress in pediatric patients
Ibalizumab	Trogarzo	CD4 post-attachment HIV inhibitor	HIV infection in heavily treatment-experienced adults, multidrug resistant HIV-1 infection
Other Agents			
Basiliximab	Simulect	CD25/IL2 receptor inhibitor	Organ rejection
Daclizumab	Zinbyta	CD25/IL2 receptor inhibitor	MS
Alemtuzumab	Lemtrada	CD52 inhibitor	MS
Ocrelizumab	Ocrevus	CD20 inhibitor	MS

TABLE 46.2 Monoclonal Antibody Drugs Used in Non-Cancer Treatment—cont'd

CLASS/GENERIC NAME	BRAND NAME	ANTIBODY EFFECT	APPROVED INDICATIONS
Ofatumumab	Kesimpta	CD20 inhibitor	MS
Natalizumab	Tysabri	Integrin inhibitor	MS, Crohn disease
Denosumab	Prolia	RANKL	Osteoporosis
Romosozumab	Evenity	Sclerostin inhibitor	Osteoporosis
Teprotumumab	Tepezza	IGF1R antagonist	Thyroid eye disease
Antitoxin Agents			
Bezlotoxumab	ZINPLAVA	*C. difficile* toxin B inhibitor	*Clostridium difficile* infection
Obiltoxaximab	ANTHIM	anthrax toxin inhibitor	Anthrax infection

CD, Cluster of differentiation; *CGRP,* calcitonin gene-related protein; *GP,* glycoprotein; *HIV,* human immunodeficiency virus; *IgE,* immunoglobulin E; *IGF1R,* insulin growth factor-1 receptor; *IL,* interleukin; *MS,* multiple sclerosis; *PCSK9,* proprotein convertase subtilisin kexin 9; *RA,* rheumatoid arthritis; *RANKL,* receptor activator of nuclear factor *kappa*-B ligand; *RSV,* respiratory syncytial virus; *TNFα,* tumor necrosis factor *alpha.*

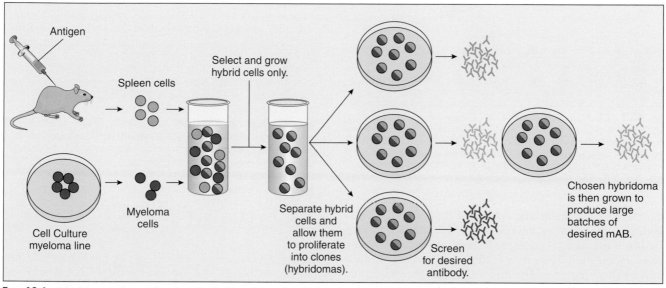

FIG. **46.1** Manufacture of monoclonal antibody drugs. The antigen of interest is injected into mice for development of targeted antibodies. After an immune response occurs, mice are sacrificed, and antibody-producing B cells are removed from the spleen. Immortalized myeloma cells are mixed with the mouse B cells and fused to create hybridoma cells. The hybridoma cells are selected for in the cell culture and unfused cells die off. The remaining cells are screened for those emitting the specific antibody to the antigen of interest. The selected antibody-producing hybridoma cells are grown in vast quantities and the culture media periodically drained off and the monoclonal antibodies purified and packaged for administration.

Panitumumab, and **necitumumab** also inhibit cancer growth by **antagonist action at the EGFR. Panitumumab** is approved for use in treating metastatic **colorectal cancer. Necitumumab** is indicated for the first-line treatment of **non-small cell lung cancer** when used with gemcitabine and cisplatin (Chapter 45).

Human Epidermal Receptor-2 Kinase Inhibitors

Trastuzumab (HERCEPTIN) is a recombinant human monoclonal antibody that binds to the extracellular domain of the human epidermal receptor-2 (HER2) receptor. The HER2 receptor is a tyrosine kinase and a member of the EGRF family involved in stimulating cell proliferation. Trastuzumab is used to treat metastatic **breast cancer** (BC) in the 25% of women whose cancer cells overexpress HER2 (Box 46.1). Trastuzumab is administered once a week, usually in combination with doxorubicin and paclitaxel. Its adverse effects include chills, fever,

nausea, vomiting, chest pain, and dyspnea, and the drug has potential cardiotoxic effects whose long-term consequences are uncertain.

Pertuzumab targets the extracellular dimerization domain of HER2 and blocks ligand-dependent heterodimerization of HER2 with other HER family members. Blocking growth factor binding results in **pertuzumab inhibiting** two major signal pathways; **mitogen-activated protein (MAP) kinase** and **phosphoinositide 3-kinase (PI3K). Pertuzumab** inhibition of MAP kinase pathway results in the arrest of cell growth and inhibition of the PI3K produces apoptosis.

VEGFR/PDGFR Kinase Inhibitors

Bevacizumab is a recombinant humanized antibody to **VEGF.** The drug prevents binding of VEGF to receptors on endothelial cells and thereby inhibits the formation of new blood vessels. It is the first VEGF angiogenesis inhibitor to be approved for cancer chemotherapy and is indicated for

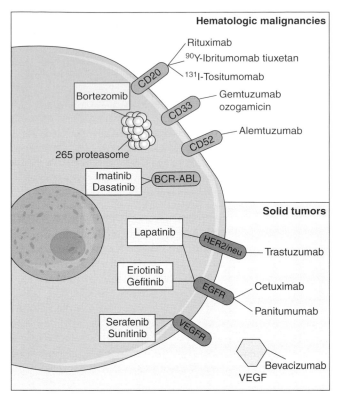

FIG. 46.2 Mechanisms of action of antineoplastic monoclonal antibodies and small molecule inhibitors. Diagram shows targets for select monoclonal antibody drugs and small molecule inhibitors that are used to treat hematologic cancers (top half) or solid tumors (bottom half). Cluster of differentiation (CD) proteins, CD20, CD33, and CD52, the 26S proteasome, the BCR-ABL fusion gene product and receptor kinases are shown.

---

the treatment of **metastatic colorectal cancer, in combination with intravenous fluorouracil**. When bevacizumab is used in a fluorouracil regimen, it increases tumor response rates, progression-free survival time, and overall survival time in these patients. The drug can cause gastrointestinal bleeding and perforation, pulmonary hemorrhage, and other thromboembolic events.

Ramucirumab is a VEGFR antagonist that **specifically binds to the receptor (VEGFR)** and blocks binding of VEGF ligands. As a result, ramucirumab inhibits ligand-stimulated activation of VEGFR, thereby inhibiting proliferation and migration of cancerous endothelial cells. **Ramucirumab** is used for the treatment of **colorectal cancer, gastric adenocarcinoma, non-small cell lung cancer, and hepatocellular carcinoma**.

Olaratumab is a platelet-derived growth factor receptor (PDGFR) kinase inhibitor, which binds to PDGFR *alpha* (PDGFR-α). Olaratumab is used in combination with doxorubicin for the treatment of soft tissue sarcoma.

Immune Checkpoint Inhibitors

In the last decade, there has been a quiet revolution in the cancer treatment arena that has led to real progress in the fight against malignancy. The discovery of **immune checkpoints (i.e., inhibitory signals that decrease T-cell activation)** led to the development of new targets for monoclonal antibody therapy.

Ipilimumab is an anti-CTLA-4 monoclonal antibody drug. Cytotoxic T-lymphocyte-associated protein 4 (CTLA-4) is a negative regulator of T-cell activity. By binding to CTLA-4 ipilimumab blocks the interaction of CTLA-4 with its ligands—CD80 and CD86. Ipilimumab blockade of CTLA-4 augments T-cell activation and proliferation, including the tumor infiltrating T-effector cells. Ipilimumab inhibition of CTLA-4 also reduces T-regulatory cell function, which contributes to an increase in T cell responsiveness and anti-tumor immune responses. Ipilimumab was the first drug to show a survival benefit to patients with metastatic melanoma.

Nivolumab is a monoclonal antibody to the programmed death (PD-1) protein indicated for the treatment of renal cell carcinoma, non-small cell lung cancer, small cell lung cancer, Hodgkin Lymphoma, squamous cell carcinoma, urothelial carcinoma, colorectal cancer, and liver cancer. PD-1 is an immune checkpoint that guards against autoimmunity by increasing apoptosis (programmed cell death) of antigen-specific T-cells and decreasing apoptosis in regulatory (anti-inflammatory, suppressive) T cells. Inhibitors of PD-1 turn up the immune detection of cancer cells and immune mechanisms of their destruction. Nivolumab was recently shown to extend survival in patients with advanced renal cell carcinoma, the most common kidney cancer in adults. Other monoclonal antibody preparations similar to nivolumab are pembrolizumab, atezolizumab, among others listed below in Table 46.1.

BOX 46.1 A CASE OF HER2-POSITIVE BREAST CANCER

CASE PRESENTATION

A 47-year-old woman was seen by her physician after she noted a palpable left breast mass. Diagnostic mammography revealed a 1.9 cm breast mass that was found to be a poorly differentiated invasive ductal adenocarcinoma. Further testing found that 95% of the breast cancer (BC) cells were strongly positive for human EGRF 2 (HER2) but were negative for estrogen receptor and progesterone receptor. Following resection of the breast mass and axillary lymph nodes, a liver metastasis of 2.8 cm was detected radiologically. She then underwent four cycles of paclitaxel and trastuzumab treatments followed by continuous weekly trastuzumab maintenance therapy. The liver metastasis was radiologically negative at 18 months, and she remains in complete remission 5 years later. The patient has not experienced cardiovascular or other adverse effects from the continuing trastuzumab treatments.

CASE DISCUSSION

Approximately 15% to 30% of BCs overexpress HER2, contributing to excessive proliferation and metastasis. Before the development of drugs that target HER2, patients with HER2-positive BC had a poor prognosis. Trastuzumab has improved the clinical outcome of these patients, and survival of women with HER2-positive BC is now greater than with certain types HER2-negative BC. The first-line therapy for metastatic HER2-amplified BC consists of a taxane, such as paclitaxel, and trastuzumab. Recently, it was found dual blockade of HER2 with trastuzumab plus pertuzumab or lapatinib appears to be superior to monotherapy. The optimal duration of trastuzumab maintenance therapy for patients in BC remission is uncertain. Despite some concern about potential adverse effects, women who continue to receive trastuzumab treatments appear to have better survival than those who discontinue therapy after achieving a remission.

Other Protein Targets

Rituximab is an anti-CD-20 cytolytic agent indicated for the treatment of non-Hodgkin lymphoma (NHL), chronic lymphocytic leukemia, RA, Wegener granulomatosis, and pemphigus vulgaris. Rituximab is a monoclonal antibody that targets the CD20 antigen expressed on the surface of pre-B and mature B-lymphocytes. Upon binding to CD20, rituximab mediates B-cell lysis by complement dependent cytotoxicity (CDC) and antibody dependent cell mediated cytotoxicity (ADCC). Other anti-CD20 mAbs include obinutuzumab used in combination with chlorambucil, for the treatment of patients with previously untreated chronic lymphocytic leukemia (CLL), and ofatumumab and ocrelizumab, indicated for the treatment of multiple sclerosis (MS, see Table 46.2).

New immunotherapy agents also provide better options for the treatment of **multiple myeloma,** the third most common hematologic cancer. **Daratumumab** and **elotuzumab** were found to increase progression-free survival significantly compared with standard therapy alone.

Daratumumab is an **antibody directed against CD38,** a transmembrane glycoprotein expressed on the surface of hematopoietic cells, as well as **multiple myeloma cancer cells.** CD38 has multiple functions, such as receptor mediated adhesion, signaling, and modulation of cyclase and hydrolase activity. **Daratumumab** inhibits the growth of CD38 expressing tumor cells by inducing apoptosis directly through Fc mediated cross linking as well as by **immune-mediated tumor cell lysis** through CDC, ADCC and antibody dependent cellular phagocytosis (ADCP).

Elotuzumab is an anti-signaling lymphocytic activation molecule family member 7 (SLAMF7) immunostimulatory antibody used in combination with **lenalidomide** and **dexamethasone** for the treatment of adult patients with multiple myeloma. SLAMF7 is expressed on myeloma cells independent of cytogenetic abnormalities. SLAMF7 is also expressed on natural killer cells, plasma cells, and—at lower levels—on specific immune cell subsets of differentiated cells within the hematopoietic lineage. **Elotuzumab directly activates natural killer cells** through both the SLAMF7 pathway and Fc receptors. Elotuzumab also targets SLAMF7 on myeloma cells and facilitates the interaction with natural killer cells to mediate the killing of myeloma cells through ADCC. In preclinical models, the combination of elotuzumab and lenalidomide resulted in enhanced activation of natural killer cells that was greater than the effects of either agent alone.

Dinutuximab is an anti-GD2 (ganglioside type GD2) monoclonal antibody used in combination with granulocyte-macrophage colony-stimulating factor (GM-CSF), interleukin-2 (IL-2), and 13-cis-retinoic acid (RA) for the treatment of pediatric patients with **high-risk neuroblastoma**

Antibody Drug Conjugates

Antibody drug conjugates combine the **targeting capability** of a monoclonal antibody with the **cytotoxic capability** of a chemotherapeutic agent. The attached chemotherapeutic drugs are either microtubule inhibitors, topoisomerase inhibitors, protein synthesis inhibitors, DNA strand disrupters, or radioactive isotopes.

Trastuzumab emtansine is a **HER2**-targeted antibody and **microtubule inhibitor** (emtansine) used for the treatment of patients with **HER2-positive, metastatic** BC previously treated with trastuzumab and a taxane. **Emtansine binds to tubulin** and disrupts microtubule networks to cause cell cycle arrest and apoptotic cell death. This conjugated antibody-chemotherapeutic drug was the **first targeted chemotherapy agent.** **Trastuzumab deruxtecan** has similar specificity and indications as the previous conjugate, but the deruxtecan is a **topoisomerase inhibitor**.

Brentuximab vedotin is a CD30-directed antibody-drug conjugate for treatment of patients with **Hodgkin lymphoma** after failure of autologous stem cell transplant (ASCT) or two prior multi-agent chemotherapy regimens. The **vedotin is a microtubule disrupting** agent.

Gemtuzumab ozogamicin is a CD33-directed antibody and cytotoxic drug conjugate for the treatment of CD33-positive **acute myeloid leukemia (AML).** The ozogamicin acts as a cytotoxic protein synthesis inhibitor. **Inotuzumab ozogamicin** has an identical cytotoxic conjugate, but it is coupled with a CD22-directed antibody. It is indicated for the treatment in patients with relapsed or refractory B-cell precursor **acute lymphoblastic leukemia (ALL).**

Ibritumomab tiuxetan is a CD20-targeted radiotherapeutic antibody for treatment of relapsed or refractory B-cell NHL. The tiuxetan binds the **radioactive isotope** yttrium-90 and the β-radiation induces cellular damage** by the formation of free radicals in the target cells. Other antibody-drug conjugates are listed in Table 46.1.

Monoclonal Antibodies Targeted for Non-Cancer Treatment

The exquisite targeting ability of monoclonal antibody drugs provides for breakthrough therapy not only for cancer patients but also for those suffering from numerous other maladies. Many of the following agents were introduced in previous chapters, which are referenced herein.

Antilipidemic Agents

Evolocumab is a human monoclonal antibody directed against human **proprotein convertase subtilisin kexin 9 (PCSK9).** Evolocumab locks up PCSK9 and inhibits circulating PCSK9 from binding to the **low-density lipoprotein receptor (LDLR),** preventing PCSK9-mediated LDLR degradation and permitting LDLR to recycle back to the liver cell surface. By inhibiting the binding of PCSK9 to LDLR, **evolocumab increases the number of LDLRs** available to clear LDL from the blood, thereby lowering low-density lipoprotein-cholesterol (LDL-C) levels. **Alirocumab** is a second monoclonal antibody drug that works like evolocumab (see also Chapter 15).

Antithrombotic and Thrombolytic Reversal agents

Abciximab binds to the **platelet GPIIb/IIIa receptor,** which is a member of the integrin family of adhesion receptors and the major platelet surface receptor **involved in platelet aggregation. Abciximab inhibits platelet aggregation** by preventing the binding of fibrinogen, von Willebrand factor, and other adhesive molecules to GPIIb/IIIa receptor sites on activated platelets. **Idarucizumab** (PRAXBIND) is a humanized monoclonal antibody fragment (Fab) indicated in patients treated with dabigatran when **reversal of the anticoagulant effects of dabigatran** is needed for emergency surgery and other urgent procedures and in life-threatening or uncontrolled bleeding (see also Chapter 16).

Crizanlizumab is a humanized monoclonal antibody that binds to P-selectin and blocks interactions with its ligands including P-selectin glycoprotein ligand 1. Binding P-selectin on the surface of the activated endothelium and platelets **blocks interactions between endothelial cells, platelets, red blood cells, and leukocytes**. It is indicated for the treatment of painful **vaso-occlusive episodes in sickle cell disease patients** (see Chapter 17).

Antiasthma Agents

Omalizumab is used for the treatment of acute asthma attacks as it inhibits the binding of IgE to the high-affinity IgE receptor (FcεRI) on the surface of mast cells and basophils. Reduction in surface-bound IgE on FcεRI-bearing cells limits the degree of release of mediators of the allergic response. Treatment also reduces the number of FcεRI receptors on basophils in atopic patients. Reslizumab, mepolizumab, and benralizumab block IL-5 receptor interactions and are approved for the treatment of asthma (see Chapter 27).

Antimigraine Agents

Galcanezumab is a monoclonal antibody targeting **calcitonin-gene related peptide (CGRP)** and indicated in adults for the **preventative treatment of migraine and cluster headaches**. After the initial success of galcanezumab in treating migraine, three other monoclonal antibody drugs were developed: eptinezumab, **fremanezumab**, and **erenumab**. The latest one, **erenumab**, is an antibody **against the CGRP receptor** itself and not the CGRP peptide (see Chapter 29).

Drugs for Inflammatory Bowel Diseases

Immunosuppressive agents may be useful in maintaining remission in patients with **Crohn disease and severe ulcerative colitis**. Adalimumab, golimumab, and **infliximab** are monoclonal Ab to **tumor necrosis factor alpha (TNFα)**, a substance believed to play a role in the pathogenesis of these GI conditions (Chapter 28) as well as in RA (see Chapter 30). Adalimumab and these drugs do not bind or inactivate lymphotoxin (TNFβ). **Vedolizumab** is an **integrin receptor antagonist** indicated for treatment of ulcerative colitis and Crohn disease. It is a monoclonal antibody to the type of integrin expressed on T-lymphocytes and inhibits their migration across the endothelium and into the inflamed GI parenchymal tissue. By blocking integrin on lymphocytes, **vedolizumab reduces the inflammation of the GI tract**. Other monoclonal antibody drugs for Crohn disease and inflammatory bowel disorders are given in Table 46.2.

Antirheumatic Agents

Besides adalimumab, golimumab and infliximab used for both inflammatory bowel disease (above) and for RA, there are two monoclonal antibody drugs specifically indicated for RA. Tocilizumab binds to both soluble and membrane-bound IL-6 receptors (sIL-6R and mIL-6R) and inhibits IL-6-mediated signaling through these receptors. IL-6 is a pleiotropic pro-inflammatory cytokine produced by a variety of cell types including T- and B-cells, lymphocytes, monocytes, and fibroblasts. IL-6 has been shown to be involved

in diverse physiological processes, such as T-cell activation, induction of immunoglobulin secretion, initiation of hepatic acute phase protein synthesis, and stimulation of hematopoietic precursor cell proliferation and differentiation. IL-6 is also produced by synovial and endothelial cells leading to local production of IL-6 in joints affected by inflammatory processes, such as RA. **Sarilumab** is another IL-6 receptor blocker indicated for treatment of adult patients with **moderately to severely active** RA (Chapter 30).

Antipsoriatic Agents

Psoriasis is a chronic autoimmune disease noted by the appearance of red blotches or plaques of abnormal skin. There is a large class of monoclonal antibody drugs developed for the **treatment of psoriasis and atopic dermatitis (eczema)**. Ustekinumab human monoclonal antibody that binds with specificity to the p40 protein subunit of IL-12 and IL-23 cytokines. IL-12 and IL-23 are cytokines that mediate inflammatory and immune responses, such as natural killer cell activation and CD4+ T-cell differentiation and activation. **Ustekinumab blocks IL-12 and IL-23** activation of these pathways. It is indicated for **plaque psoriasis, psoriatic arthritis, Crohn disease, and ulcerative colitis**.

Secukinumab selectively binds to IL-17A cytokine and inhibits its interaction with the IL-17 receptor, which also inhibits IL-stimulated immune and inflammatory responses. **Tildrakizumab** selectively binds to the p19 subunit of IL-23 and inhibits its interaction with the IL-23 receptor. Tildrakizumab inhibits the release of proinflammatory cytokines and chemokines. **Dupilumab**, heavily advertised as DUPIXENT, is a human monoclonal antibody that inhibits IL-4 and IL-13 signaling. Unlike the other agents above, **Dupilumab is used only for the treatment of atopic dermatitis (eczema)**. Other antipsoriatic mAbs for skin autoimmune diseases are given in Table 46.2.

Antiviral Agents

Palivizumab is a monoclonal antibody against the F protein of **respiratory syncytial virus (RSV)**. It is used for the prevention of serious lower respiratory tract disease caused by RSV in pediatric patients. For the treatment of human immunodeficiency virus type 1 (HIV-1) infection in heavily treatment-experienced adults with multidrug resistant HIV-1 infection, **ibalizumab**—a CD4-directed post-attachment HIV-1 inhibitor—is used in combination with other HIV antiretrovirals (see Chapter 43).

Other Monoclonal Antibody Drugs

Basiliximab is an anti-CD25 (IL2 receptor) monoclonal antibody used for the treatment of transplant organ rejection (see below). **Alemtuzumab** binds to **CD52**, a cell surface glycoprotein found on all B and T lymphocytes, natural killer cells, monocytes, and macrophages. Following cell surface binding to T and B lymphocytes, alemtuzumab results in **antibody-dependent cellular cytolysis** and **complement-mediated lysis**. It is indicated for the **treatment of MS**. Alemtuzumab may cause bleeding, hypertension, and kidney failure.

Natalizumab is used for both for MS and Crohn disease. It is an antibody targeting integrin proteins that are expressed on the surface of all leukocytes except neutrophils. **Natalizumab inhibits the integrin-mediated adhesion of**

TABLE 46.3   Child and Adolescent Vaccines, Abbreviations, and Trade Names

VACCINES	ABBREVIATIONS	TRADE NAMES
Diphtheria, tetanus, and acellular pertussis vaccine	DTaP	DAPTACEL, INFANRIX
Haemophilus influenzae type B vaccine	Hib (PRP-T), Hib (PRP-OMP)	ACTHIB, HIBERIX, PEDVAXHIB
Hepatitis A vaccine	HepA	HAVRIX, VAQTA
Hepatitis B vaccine	HepB	ENGERIX-B, RECOMBIVAX HB
Human papillomavirus vaccine	HPV	GARDASIL 9
Influenza vaccine (inactivated)	IIV	*Multiple*
Influenza vaccine (live, attenuated)	LAIV	FLUMIST QUADRIVALENT
Measles, mumps, and rubella vaccine	MMR	M-M-R II
Meningococcal serogroups A, C, W, Y vaccine	MenACWY-D, MenACWY-CRM	MENACTRA, MENVEO
Meningococcal serogroup B vaccine	MenB-4C, MenB-FHbp	BEXSERO, TRUMENBA
Pneumococcal 13-valent conjugate vaccine	PCV13	PREVNAR 13
Poliovirus vaccine (inactivated)	IPV	IPOL
Rotavirus vaccine	RV1, RV5	ROTARIX, ROTATEQ
Tetanus, diphtheria, and acellular pertussis vaccine	Tdap	ADACEL, BOOSTRIX
Tetanus and diphtheria vaccine	Td	TENIVAC, TDVAX
Varicella vaccine	VAR	VARIVAX
Combination Vaccines		
DTaP, hepatitis B, and inactivated poliovirus vaccine	DTaP-HepB-IPV	PEDIARIX
DTaP, inactivated poliovirus, and *Haemophilus influenzae* type B vaccine	DTaP-IPV/Hib	PENTACEL
DTaP and inactivated poliovirus vaccine	DTaP-IPV	KINRIX, QUADRACEL
Measles, mumps, rubella, and varicella vaccines	MMRV	PROQ

leukocytes to vascular cell adhesion molecule-1 (VCAM-1), expressed on activated vascular endothelium, and mucosal addressin cell adhesion molecule-1 (MAdCAM-1), found on vascular endothelial cells of the GI. Disruption of integrin-mediated adhesion **prevents the movement of leukocytes across the endothelium into inflamed parenchymal tissue.**

Ocrelizumab and **ofatumumab** are **anti-CD20** Ab for the treatment of MS. After cell surface binding to the CD-20 on B lymphocytes, both agents cause antibody-dependent cellular cytolysis and complement-mediated lysis.

Denosumab and **romosozumab** are both indicated for the treatment of **osteoporosis** but do so by different mechanisms. **Denosumab** binds and inactivates a **transmembrane protein called RANK Ligand** (RANKL). RANKL augments the formation, function, and survival of osteoclasts and their participation in bone resorption and inactivation of RANKL prevents activation of RANK, the receptor activator of nuclear factor *kappa*-B (NF-κB). **Romosozumab inhibits the action of sclerostin,** a regulatory factor in bone metabolism, increasing bone formation (see Chapter 36).

Teprotumumab binds to insulin growth factor-1 receptor (IGF-1R) and blocks IGFR-1 activation and signaling. It is used for the treatment of patients with **thyroid eye disease,** but teprotumumab's mechanism of action is not fully understood.

Antitoxin Agents

Bezlotoxumab is a human monoclonal antibody that **binds toxin B** produced by *Clostridium difficile*. It is used to reduce recurrence of *Clostridium difficile* infection (CDI) in adult patients. **Obiltoxaximab** is a monoclonal antibody directed against the **protective antigen of *Bacillus anthracis*** (anthrax toxin).

BIOLOGICALS

Biologicals as a drug class refers to many diverse substances that are found in nature; from virus particles, to bacterial toxins, to cytokines that our own cells produce. **Biologicals includes vaccines, blood components, somatic cells, agents for gene therapy, tissues, and recombinant therapeutic proteins.** Development of biologicals is currently undergoing a rapid period of drug discovery and represent the cutting-edge of biomedical research. They are often the **most effective drug** for many medical illnesses and pathological conditions that have **no other treatment available.** This section introduces the reader to vaccines, passive immunoglobulins, agents to treat organ rejection, interferons, and other immunomodulators.

Vaccines

The word "vaccine" is derived from the Greek word for cow (*vacca*) and was coined in 1796 by Edward Jenner, considered the founder of vaccinology, after he inoculated a 13-year-old boy with the cowpox virus and demonstrated that the boy was immune to smallpox infection. **Numerous vaccines now exist for infections** that previously killed much of the population (see Tables 46.3 and 46.4). Although parental acceptance of childhood vaccines has decreased due to unwarranted fears of adverse effects such as autism, vaccine acceptance to acquire immunity to the pandemic **SARS-CoV-2 virus** will likely be greater.

TABLE 46.4   Adult Vaccines, Abbreviations, and Trade Names

VACCINES	ABBREVIATIONS	TRADE NAMES
Haemophilus influenzae type b	Hib	ActHIB, Hiberix
Hepatitis A vaccine	HepA	Havrix, Vaqta
Hepatitis A and hepatitis B vaccine	HepA-HepB	Twinrix
Hepatitis B vaccine	HepB	Engerix-B, Recombivax HB, Heplisav-B
Influenza vaccine, inactivated	IIV	Multiple
Influenza vaccine, live, attenuated	LAIV	FluMist Quadrivalent
Influenza vaccine, recombinant	RIV	Flublok Quadrivalent
Meningococcal serogroups A, C, W, Y vaccine	MenACWY	Menactra, Menveo
Meningococcal serogroup B vaccine	MenB-4C, MenB-FHbp	Bexsero, Trumenba
Pneumococcal 23-valent polysaccharide vaccine	PPSV23	Pneumovax 23
Tetanus and diphtheria toxoids	Td	Tenivac, Tdvax
Zoster vaccine, recombinant	RZV	Shingrix
Zoster vaccine live	ZVL	Zostavax

Vaccines rely on the presentation of foreign antigens to cells of the **adaptive immune system** (e.g., B-cells) so that Ab can be produced. Vaccinations may last for a lifetime (e.g., **measles vaccine**) or may need to be renewed on an annual basis (e.g., **influenza vaccine**). There are four main types of vaccines, which differ on the method of introducing the foreign antigen; (1) **live-attenuated vaccines**, (2) **inactivated vaccines**, (3) **subunit and recombinant vaccines**, and (4) **toxoid vaccines**. Live-attenuated vaccines use a **weakened strain of the virus** and can sometimes cause symptoms of the infection. **Inactivated vaccines use a killed virus** or germ and usually provide a weaker immune response compared to live-attenuated vaccines. **Subunit and recombinant vaccines** use **only a part of the viral protein** to produce an immune response. The subunit may be part of the vaccination like pneumococcal vaccine or may be produced within the body by using an mRNA vaccine, like the SARS-CoV-2 vaccine currently in clinical trials (see below). Finally, **toxoid vaccines** are composed of only the toxin produced by the bacteria or germ, like the **diphtheria and tetanus vaccines**.

Vaccines for Infants and Children

In the USA, numerous vaccines are recommended at regular intervals from birth to adolescence. For example, the **hepatitis B vaccine** is given at birth or as soon as possible afterwards to protect them from exposure to the hepatitis B virus. Infants and young children cannot mount a strong immune reaction to hepatitis B and infection during the first 5 years of life greatly increases the risk of early death from liver disease, failure, or liver cancer. The first dose of the combination vaccine of diphtheria, tetanus, and acellular pertussis vaccine (Daptacel) is also given soon after birth (2 months) to protect against diphtheria, tetanus (lockjaw), and pertussis (whooping cough). Many other vaccines are recommended to be administered throughout infancy until adolescence (see Table 46.3).

Vaccines for Adults and the Elderly

Once the childhood series of vaccines is completed, recommendations for continued vaccinations include the occasional **tetanus booster shots and annual flu vaccines**. In the elderly, additional recommendations for vaccinations include the **pneumococcal vaccine to prevent pneumonia** and the **zoster vaccine to prevent shingles**.

Pneumococcal 23-valent polysaccharide vaccine (Pneumovax 23) is a vaccine indicated for active immunization for the **prevention of pneumococcal disease caused by *Streptococcus pneumoniae*** in patients 65 or older. Pneumovax 23 is an inactivated pneumococcal polysaccharide vaccine, with varied polysaccharide antigens representing 23 of the more than 80 serotypes of pneumococcal bacteria. The vaccination produces **serotype-specific Ab that bind to pneumococci and induce immune cells to kill pneumococci by macrophages** and other leukocytes. However, there is not yet evidence that the levels of Ab correlate with any resistance to pneumococcal disease. Vaccine efficacy rates for up to 1 year after administration range from 77% to 92% in various clinical trials. Adverse effects observed after vaccination in clinical trials included injection-site pain and soreness, headache, and fatigue.

Shingles, known as **herpes zoster**, is the reappearance of the **chicken pox virus** (varicella-zoster) after a lifetime of lying dormant in the dorsal root ganglia along the spinal cord. Shingles is characterized by red, itchy, and painful skin lesions in a dermatomal pattern usually on the trunk of the body. There are two shingles vaccines currently available. The first vaccine, **Zoster vaccine live (Zostavax)** was approved in 2006 for prevention of shingles and complications like postherpetic neuralgia. The second shingles vaccine is **Zoster vaccine recombinant (Shingrix)** is given in two doses, separated by 2 to 6 months, and was 89% to 97% effective against shingles and postherpetic neuralgia. The vaccine still showed 85% effectiveness after 4 years in adults 70 years and older. Many other vaccines are recommended for adults and the elderly (see Table 46.4).

Vaccines for SARS-CoV-2 Infections

Although **no FDA-approved vaccine for SARS-CoV-2** exist at the time of this writing, there are presently numerous vaccines in clinical trials against COVID-19 in the USA and around the world. Two of the most successful

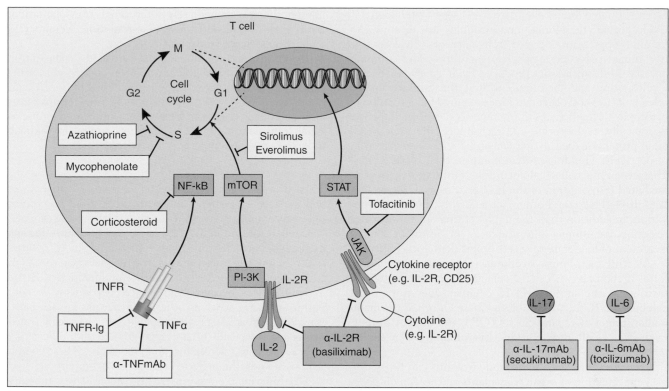

FIG. 46.3 Mechanism of action of drugs used to treat organ rejection. Sites of action for various drugs used for the treatment of organ rejection are shown. See text for further details.

vaccine preparations to date are an **mRNA vaccine** and an **adenovirus-vector vaccine**. The mRNA vaccine encodes an optimized SARS-CoV-2 full-length spike protein, the structure that allows the coronavirus to attack to host cells. The mRNA enters host cells and manufactures the spike protein from the mRNA in the host ribosomes. The host cells **secrete the spike protein, which allows an antibody response and active immunization**. The adenovirus-vector COVID vaccine employs a **replication-incompetent recombinant serotype 5 adenovirus** carrying a **gene encoding the coronavirus spike protein**. The adenoviral DNA does not integrate into the genome and is not replicated during cell division. The host machinery transcribes the viral gene to mRNA and essentially follows the same pathway of viral-directed antibody generation as the mRNA vaccine.

Passive Immunoglobulins

There are a number of polyclonal antibody preparations in common use. Pregnant women are familiar with the Rhesus (Rh) factor. Rh factor is a protein found on the surface of red blood cells. RBCs that express the Rh factor create an Rh-positive (Rh⁺) blood type, otherwise the blood type is Rh-negative (Rh⁻). Rh status is not correlated with health status but becomes a problem if a pregnant patient is Rh⁻ and is delivering an Rh⁺ baby. In that case, the mother could produce Ab to the Rh factor and a second pregnancy could be in peril without the treatment with *Rho(D)* immunoglobulin injections (RHOPHYLAC). **Rhophylac is used to prevent an immune response to Rh⁺ blood** in people with an Rh-negative blood type. Other passive immunoglobulin

treatments include *Crotalidae* Immune Fab (ANAVIP), which is antibody fragments against rattlesnake toxin, rabies immunoglobulin (BAYRAB), and botulism antitoxin immunoglobulin.

Treatment of Organ Rejection

The immune system reacts to foreign proteins (antigens) by inducing immune responses through lymphocyte activation and proliferation, followed by an effector phase in which immune cells and Ab are mobilized to destroy the antigen. Most immunosuppressant drugs act on the induction phase, either by inhibiting IL-2 production (cyclosporine, tacrolimus), by inhibiting DNA synthesis required for lymphocyte proliferation (azathioprine, mycophenolate), or by inhibiting cytokine gene expression (corticosteroids). The mechanism of action of select anti-rejection drugs is shown in Fig. 46.3.

Immunosuppressants are primarily used to **prevent rejection of transplanted organs** and to treat RA and other **autoimmune disorders** (see Chapter 30). This section focuses on agents to **prevent allograft rejection** after organ or bone marrow transplantation. These drugs inhibit the immune response to foreign antigens (alloantigens) contained in an **allograft**, which is a graft (transplant) of tissue between individuals of the same species but of different genotypes. Although donors and transplant recipients are tissue matched with regards to certain markers and blood type, matches are not perfect, and organ rejection can result in **graft versus host disease (GvHD). Cyclosporine and other immunosuppressant** drugs are given to inhibit the immune reactions due to organ rejection.

Calcineurin and Mammalian Target of Rapamycin Inhibitors
Cyclosporine, tacrolimus, and sirolimus are examples of immunosuppressants derived from microbes. Cyclosporine is a fungal polypeptide whereas tacrolimus and sirolimus are macrolide antibiotics produced by *Streptomyces* species. Cyclosporine and tacrolimus inhibit the production and release of IL-2 and other cytokines required for activation of cytotoxic T lymphocytes in response to allogenic challenge. Specifically, cyclosporine and tacrolimus bind to intracellular proteins called *cyclophilin* and *FK12-binding protein*, respectively. The drug-protein complex then binds a phosphatase enzyme called calcineurin and inhibits calcineurin-mediated transcription of the IL-2 gene as well as genes for IL-3, IL-4, TNFα, and other factors involved in T-cell activation. In addition to its use in preventing organ transplant rejection, tacrolimus is available as an ointment for the treatment of moderate to severe atopic dermatitis (eczema).

As with tacrolimus, **sirolimus** (also called rapamycin) forms a complex with *FK12-binding protein*. In contrast to tacrolimus, the sirolimus-FK12 complex **does not inhibit calcineurin**. Rather, it inhibits a kinase known as the **mammalian target of rapamycin** (mTOR), and thereby disrupts IL-driven T-cell proliferation. **Everolimus** has a similar mechanism of action.

Cyclosporine, **tacrolimus**, and **sirolimus** can be used to **prevent rejection of organ transplants** and are usually given in combination with corticosteroids or other drugs. For example, sirolimus is given in combination with mycophenolate and a corticosteroid (e.g., prednisone). Cyclosporine can also be used to treat **psoriasis** and severe autoimmune diseases that are resistant to other therapeutic agents, such as RA that does not respond to MTX. In addition to these indications, everolimus, sirolimus, and tacrolimus have been incorporated into **vascular stents** that slowly release the drugs **(drug-eluting stents)** to inhibit the proliferation of vascular cells that would otherwise cause **restenosis of coronary arteries** after stent placement. The use of drug-eluting stents has reduced the incidence of vascular restenosis after stent placement.

Cyclosporine frequently causes **nephrotoxicity, hypertension, hirsutism, gingival hyperplasia**, and **muscle tremor**. Cyclosporine is metabolized by CYP3A4, a cytochrome P450 enzyme, and interacts with other drugs that inhibit or induce this enzyme. CYP3A4 inhibitors can increase the plasma levels and toxicity of cyclosporine, and these include erythromycin and other macrolide antibiotics, azole antifungal drugs, calcium channel blockers, and grapefruit juice. Drugs that induce CYP3A4, including carbamazepine, phenytoin, and rifampin, can decrease the plasma levels of cyclosporine.

Monoclonal Antibodies Used to Prevent Organ Rejection
Basiliximab is a chimeric (murine/human) monoclonal antibody that functions as an immunosuppressive agent. **Basiliximab** is a monoclonal antibody to the high-affinity **IL-2 receptor** expressed on activated T cells. **Basiliximab** binds to the α-subunit of the receptor and **prevents IL-2 binding**. By this action, IL-2–mediated activation of lymphocytes is prevented, and the response of the immune system to alloantigens (e.g., those present in transplanted allografts) is impaired. A short course of basiliximab is used in combination with other agents as induction immunotherapy immediately after **renal transplantation**. Basiliximab significantly **lowers circulating lymphocytes** and **prevents acute transplant rejection**.

Belatacept is a monoclonal antibody preparation directed against **CD80 glycoprotein** on antigen-presenting cells (APCs) and blocks the costimulation of T cell lymphocytes. The activated T cells are the primary mediators of immunologic rejection. **Belatacept** is indicated for use in **renal transplant** patients in combination with **basiliximab** induction, **mycophenolate**, and **corticosteroids**.

Antiproliferative Agents

These drugs prevent the replication of B and T lymphocytes and are used in combination with other drugs to prevent rejection of organ transplants or treat autoimmune diseases. **Mycophenolate mofetil** inhibits a key enzyme—inosine monophosphate dehydrogenase—in the *de novo* synthesis of **guanosine nucleotide**, a purine precursor to DNA. Mycophenolate selectively blocks the proliferation of **B and T lymphocytes** because lymphocytes depend on *de novo* purine synthesis, whereas other cells can use salvage pathways. Mycophenolate prevents acute rejection of **renal transplants** and is typically used in combination with other drugs such as sirolimus, tacrolimus, and prednisone. These combinations are now the preferred regimens for this purpose.

Azathioprine is a prodrug that is converted to **6-mercaptopurine** and produces immunosuppression by inhibiting purine and DNA synthesis required for **B and T lymphocyte proliferation**. It is given in combination with corticosteroids and cyclosporine or tacrolimus to prevent **rejection of kidney and other organ allografts**.

Corticosteroids

The corticosteroid hormones are discussed in Chapter 33. **Prednisone** and other corticosteroids inhibit the expression of genes encoding various cytokines that stimulate T-cell proliferation. They are used with other immunosuppressive drugs to prevent **organ transplant rejection** and to prevent **graft-versus-host** disease in patients who have undergone bone marrow transplantation. Corticosteroids are also used to treat various **autoimmune disorders** (Chapter 30).

Interferon and Related Biologicals

Interferons are endogenous cytokine proteins that increase the activity of cytotoxic cells in the immune system. Interferon drugs are mainly used in the treatment of cancer, as antiviral agents, and to reduce the frequency of relapses of MS.

Interferon alfa 2b is a recombinant interferon that **suppresses cancer cell proliferation** and has been used to treat hairy cell leukemia, bladder and renal carcinoma, malignant melanoma, and other cancers. It is administered intramuscularly and tends to cause a number of adverse effects, including leukopenia, thrombocytopenia, a flulike syndrome, nausea or vomiting, tiredness, altered taste, and diarrhea. The use of interferons is declining as better agents are developed for treating cancer (see Chapter 45). **Interferon alfa-2b is also used as an antiviral agent** for treatment of genital warts (HPV virus), AIDS-related Kaposi sarcoma, and chronic hepatitis B and C (see Chapter 43).

Peginterferon alfa-2a for injection is an inducer of the innate immune response indicated for the treatment of

chronic hepatitis C in combination therapy with other hepatitis C virus drugs for adults with compensated liver disease. Monotherapy is indicated only if patient has contraindication or significant intolerance to other HCV drugs. It is also used for chronic Hepatitis B infection in adults who have compensated hepatic disease and evidence of viral replication and hepatic inflammation. **Peginterferon alfa-2b** is another **interferon antiviral** approved for the treatment of chronic hepatitis C in patients with compensated liver disease.

Interferon beta-1a, peginterferon beta-1a, and **interferon beta-1b** are all interferon drugs available for subcutaneous injection and indicated for the treatment of **relapsing forms of MS**, including clinically isolated syndromes, relapsing-remitting disease, and active secondary progressive disease (see also Chapter 24).

Interferon gamma-1b is marketed as a subcutaneous injection and used for reducing the frequency and severity of serious infections associated with **chronic granulomatous disease** and for reducing the time to disease progression in patients with severe, **malignant osteopetrosis**.

Two additional drugs are closely related to the above interferon agents. **Anakinra** is a recombinant form of the human **IL-1 receptor antagonist (IL-1Ra)** and blocks the biologic activity of IL-1 by competitively inhibiting IL-1 binding to the IL-1 type I receptor (IL-1RI). It is used for the treatment of RA (see Chapter 30). **Lifitegrast** is a **lymphocyte function-associated antigen-1 (LFA-1) antagonist** formulated in an ophthalmic solution and used to treat **dry eye disease**. The mechanism of action of lifitegrast is thought to be inhibition of inflammatory cytokines.

GENE THERAPY AGENTS
mRNA Targeting agents

There are a number of ways to inhibit production of a specific protein once the mRNA sequence for that protein is known. Synthetic antisense oligonucleotide strands use complementary base-pairing with mRNA to block protein translation of the target protein in the ribosome. **Mipomersen** is an oligonucleotide inhibitor of apolipoprotein B-100 synthesis used along with lipid-lowering medications (e.g., statins) and diet to reduce LDL-C, apolipoprotein B (apo B), total cholesterol (TC), and non-high density lipoprotein-cholesterol (non HDL-C) in patients with homozygous familial hypercholesterolemia. **Mipomersen** binds to the **mRNA for apo B**, preventing synthesis of apo B required for VLDL production in the liver; it is given by weekly injections. The drug may elevate serum hepatic transaminase levels, which must be monitored, and many patients experience injection site reactions, flu-like symptoms, nausea, and headache.

Eteplirsen and golodirsen are both antisense oligonucleotides indicated for the treatment of Duchenne muscular dystrophy (DMD) in patients with confirmed mutations of the DMD gene. Eteplirsen targets the nRNA made from a DMD gene with an exon 51 deletion mutation, whereas golodirsen is selective for the message produced by a DMD mutation with an exon 53 deletion.

Nusinersen is a survival motor neuron-2 (SMN2)-directed antisense oligonucleotide indicated for the treatment of **spinal muscular atrophy (SMA)** in pediatric and adult patients. It is given by the intrathecal route into the spinal cord cavity. **Inotersen** is a transthyretin-directed antisense oligonucleotide indicated for **treatment of the polyneuropathy of hereditary transthyretin-mediated amyloidosis** in adults. **Patisiran** is a transthyretin-directed small interfering RNA and is indicated for the **treatment of the polyneuropathy of hereditary transthyretin-mediated amyloidosis** in adults.

Gene Modification Agents

Direct and selective gene modification in somatic cells can be accomplished using the **CRISPR** technique, a method currently being tested in clinical trials. At present, gene modification agents are approved for *ex vivo* manipulation of leukocytes taken from the patient that are then altered and infused back into the patient.

Tisagenlecleucel is a CD19-directed genetically modified autologous T-cell immunotherapy indicated for the treatment of B-cell precursor **ALL** that is refractory to treatment after two or more lines of systemic therapy. **Axicabtagene ciloleucel** is a second CD19-directed genetically modified autologous T-cell immunotherapy indicated for the treatment of refractory B-cell precursor ALL.

Sipuleucel-T is an autologous cellular immunotherapy procedure indicated for the treatment of **metastatic castrate resistant (hormone refractory) prostate cancer** classified as an autologous cellular immunotherapy. Antigen-presenting cells (APCs, dendritic cells) are harvested from the patient at their first visit, then cells are shipped to the manufacturer's factory for further processing. **Sipuleucel-T** induces an immune response targeted against **prostatic acid phosphatase (PAP)**, an antigen that is highly expressed in most prostate cancer cells. During *ex vivo* culture with PAP-GM-CSF, antigen-presenting cells (APCs, dendritic cells) take up and process the recombinant target antigen into small antigenic peptides that are then displayed on the APC cell membrane. **Cytotoxic T-cells are then activated against the prostate cancer cells.** However, in clinical trials, median survival after 5 years differed only by about 4 to 5 months in the treatment group compared to the controls.

Talimogene laherparepvec is a gene modification oncolytic viral therapy approved for the local treatment of unresectable cutaneous, subcutaneous, and nodal lesions in patients with **melanoma**. It is composed by genetically engineering a strain of herpes simplex virus 1 modified to replicate within tumors and to produce the immune stimulatory protein GM-CSF. **Talimogene laherparepvec** causes lysis of tumors, followed by release of tumor-derived antigens, which together with virally derived GM-CSF, causes an antitumor immune response. The drug is injected directly into the melanoma tumors.

Voretigene neparvovec (LUXTURNA) fixes mutant genes by delivering a new gene by an adenovirus vector. This adeno-associated virus vector-based gene therapy is indicated for the treatment of patients with confirmed **biallelic RPE65 mutation-associated retinal dystrophy**. In order to be effective, patients must have viable retinal cells as determined by the treating physician. **Onasemnogene abeparvovec** is another adeno-associated virus vector-based gene therapy. It is used for the treatment of pediatric patients less than 2 years of age with **SMA** that have bi-allelic mutations in the **survival motor neuron 1 (SMN1) gene.**

SUMMARY OF IMPORTANT POINTS

- Monoclonal antibody drugs are the latest effective treatment for targeted antineoplastic pharmacotherapy. Most monoclonal antibody drugs target receptor kinases in cancer cells and inhibit cell proliferation.
- Immune checkpoint inhibitors unleash the immune system to effectively battle malignant neoplasms.
- Antibody drug conjugates combine the targeted pharmacotherapy of monoclonal antibody drugs with the cytotoxic capability of chemotherapeutic agents.
- Other monoclonal antibody drugs are used in the treatment of hyperlipidemia, asthma, migraine, inflammatory bowel diseases, RA, and other disorders.
- Vaccines are given for a number of childhood diseases and for adult-onset disease like pneumonia and shingles.
- Cyclosporine and other agents are used in the treatment of organ rejection.
- Genetic agents are used to repair and replace defective protein encoded by genetic mutations and target mRNA.

Review Questions

1. Which type of cancer is treated with trastuzumab if the cells overexpress human epidermal growth factor receptors?
   (A). breast cancer
   (B). ovarian cancer
   (C). non-Hodgkin lymphoma
   (D). multiple myeloma
   (E). melanoma

2. Which immunosuppressant drug forms a complex with the FK-binding protein, resulting in inhibition of calcineurin and T lymphocyte activation?
   (A). cyclosporine
   (B). prednisone
   (C). cyclophosphamide
   (D). tacrolimus
   (E). azathioprine

3. The monoclonal antibody, ipilimumab, is an example of which type of immunotherapeutic agent?
   (A). protein inhibitor
   (B). TNFα blocker
   (C). kinase inhibitor
   (D). nuclear pore blocker
   (E). immune checkpoint inhibitor

4. Nivolumab is a monoclonal antibody indicated for the treatment of renal cell carcinoma, non-small cell lung cancer, and small cell lung cancer. Which protein does nivolumab target?
   (A). programmed death (PD-1) protein
   (B). cytotoxic T-lymphocyte-associated protein 4 (CTLA-4)
   (C). signaling lymphocytic activation molecule family member 7 (SLAMF7)
   (D). ganglioside type GD2 (GD2) protein
   (E). epidermal growth factor (EGF) receptor

5. What two types of drugs form the antibody-drug conjugate class of antineoplastic agents?
   (A). mRNA strand and monoclonal antibody
   (B). Cytotoxic antibody and immunosuppressant
   (C). Targeted antibody and cytotoxic agent
   (D). Two cytotoxic agents joined by an antibody linker
   (E). Targeted antibody and IL antagonist

Answers and Explanations

CHAPTER 1

1. **The answer is E:** transdermal. The topical, sublingual, rectal (suppositories), and transdermal routes of administration all avoid first-pass hepatic drug metabolism; however, only the transdermal formulation uses a patch with potent and lipophilic drugs. Orally administered drugs have the highest exposure to first-pass metabolism.

2. **The answer is C:** intravenous. *Drug absorption* refers to the process by which drugs get into the bloodstream. With subcutaneous, intramuscular, sublingual, and inhalation routes of administration, drug molecules have to cross membranes to get into the blood. Direct delivery of drug into the blood by intravenous administration, therefore, has no absorption phase.

3. **The answer is B:** used to administer drug suspensions that are slowly absorbed. After intramuscular injection of a suspension of drug particles, the particles slowly dissolve in interstitial fluid to provide sustained drug absorption over many hours or days. When a drug solution is injected intramuscularly, the drug is usually absorbed rapidly and completely.

4. **The answer is A:** extended release. Using an extended-release tablet or capsule, the patient could most likely reduce the schedule of medication from three times a day to once a day. A suspension for oral administration would not likely reduce the schedule; a suppository would be difficult and reduce patient compliance; and a skin patch for transdermal administration would work only in a few cases with potent and highly lipophilic drugs. Enteric-coated preparations may help absorption or drug stability but would not reduce the schedule of medication.

5. **The answer is E:** trade name. The proprietary name, also known as the *trade name* or the *brand name,* is the name trademarked by the manufacturer and promoted on television, radio, and print ads. The chemical name is rarely seen, being tedious and descriptive only to medicinal chemists, whereas the generic name may be seen in the fine print of the ad but is not usually promoted as extensively as the proprietary name. The nonproprietary name is the same thing as the generic name, and the British Approved Name is an official name that is usually the same as the generic name.

CHAPTER 2

1. **The answer is B:** maximal plasma drug concentration. If the rate of drug absorption is reduced, then the maximal plasma drug concentration will be less because more time will be available for drug distribution and elimination while the drug is being absorbed. Moreover, the time at which the maximal plasma drug concentration occurs will increase. If the extent of drug absorption (fraction absorbed) does not change, then the area under the curve and fractional bioavailability will not change.

2. **The answer is E:** the rate of drug elimination (mg/min) is proportional to the plasma drug concentration. In first-order elimination, drug half-life and clearance do not vary with the plasma drug concentration, but the rate of drug elimination (quantity per time) is proportional to plasma drug concentration at any time.

3. **The answer is B:** 24 hours. The half-life is the time required to reduce the plasma drug concentration by 50%. In this case, it will take four drug half-lives, or 24 hours, to reduce the plasma level from 32 to 2 mg/L.

4. **The answer is D:** 320 mg. The dose required to establish a target plasma drug concentration is calculated by multiplying the clearance by the target concentration and dosage interval. In this case, it is 5 mg/L × 8 L/h × 8 h = 320 mg.

5. **The answer is A:** is more ionized inside cells than in plasma. When a drug is more ionized inside cells, the drug becomes sequestered in the cells, and the volume of distribution can become quite large. This is called *ion trapping*.

CHAPTER 3

1. **The answer is B:** signal transduction pathway. Pharmacodynamics is the study of the detailed molecular pathway starting from the drug (ligand) binding to its receptor, the activation of effector molecules (e.g., G proteins), and the generation of second messengers, which ultimately produce an effect that can be measured at the cell, tissue, or whole animal level. This process is called the *signal transduction pathway.*

2. **The answer is E:** decrease the production of cAMP. Adenylyl cyclase is an enzyme that converts ATP to cyclic AMP (cAMP). GPCRs that activate inhibitory (Gα) subunits are known to inhibit adenylyl cyclase and therefore reduce the generation of cAMP. cAMP is the second messenger in this system even though, in this case, its levels are decreased. Activated Gα subunits also have direct effects on ion channels.

3. **The answer is B:** the concentration of drug and the association or dissociation of drug-receptor complex. The law of mass action is used to derive the affinity of a drug for its receptor and is noted as the K_D. The K_D, which is the equilibrium dissociation constant, comes from the kinetic rate (k_2) of drug-receptor dissociation divided by the rate (k_1) of drug-receptor association.

4. **The answer is D:** position of the curve along the log-dose axis. Potency and efficacy can be determined from a graph of the log dose-response curve by visual inspection. The height of the curve along the effect or y-axis is a measure of efficacy. The placement of the curve along the log-dose axis or x-axis determines potency such that curves to the left represent more potent drugs than curves to the right. This is because curves to the left give rise to smaller doses of a drug needed to reach 50% effect, or ED_{50}. The ED_{50} is a measure of the drug's potency but says nothing of efficacy. Whereas some agents are potent and efficacious, these two characteristics of drug action are not necessarily correlated. It is possible to have an agent that is highly potent but does not have great efficacy.

5. **The answer is D:** cannot produce the full effect, even at high doses. An agonist acts at its receptor to activate the signal transduction pathway and produce an effect. An antagonist binds to its receptor, producing no effect at the receptor but rather blocks the receptor so that agonists cannot bind and produce an effect. A partial agonist binds to the receptor and activates the signal transduction pathway, but not to the maximal degree. Because the degree to which a ligand activates its receptor is called *efficacy*, partial agonists do not have full efficacy.

CHAPTER 4

1. **The answer is B:** Phase II clinical study. Phase II studies are done in a small group of test subjects who have the disease state targeted by the new drug. Phase I studies are done to establish safety and pharmacokinetics in healthy subjects, often students in the health professions. Phase III studies are large, multicenter studies in patients with the disease state. Phase IV studies are postmarketing surveillance, in which physicians report adverse effects to the FDA. There is no Phase V in the drug development process.

2. **The answer is B:** Schedule II. Schedule II controlled drugs have a high degree of abuse potential but are still used by the medical profession. These drugs may still be abused by diversion, the act of illegally obtaining prescription drugs by sale or theft. Schedule I lists the most abused and illegal drugs, including marijuana, mescaline, LSD, and 3,4-methylenedioxymethamphetamine (MDMA, or "ecstasy"). Note that cocaine, although much abused in the form of powder ("coke") and free base ("crack"), is listed as Schedule II, as it does have limited medical use as a local anesthetic and vasoconstricting agent in ear, nose, and throat procedures. Schedules III to V controlled drugs have some degree of abuse potential but less than those of Schedule II.

3. **The answer is C:** fetal malformations. The 4th to 10th week of gestation is the period when fetal organs are developed. Teratogenic drugs may cause fetal malformations if taken by a pregnant woman during this interval. These malformations include cleft palate, malformation of fingers and toes, heart defects, facial abnormalities, and skeletal deformities. Drug-induced labor or jaundice is primarily of concern during the last trimester of pregnancy. Drug-induced cardiac arrest and hemorrhage are not specifically associated with the 4th to 10th week of gestation.

4. **The answer is B:** inhibition of CYP3A4. Inhibition of drug-metabolizing enzymes will increase the half-life and plasma concentrations of affected drugs, thereby posing a risk of toxicity. Induction of these enzymes will reduce half-life and plasma levels. Displacement of a drug from plasma proteins or inhibition of P-glycoprotein might increase plasma levels temporarily until the rate of elimination increases. Acceleration of gastric emptying might increase the rate of drug absorption but would not permanently increase plasma drug levels.

5. **The answer is E:** reduced capacity to oxidize drugs. Conjugative metabolism is relatively unchanged in the elderly, but oxidative drug metabolism is usually reduced. The elderly tend to have a higher percentage of body fat than younger adults and therefore have increased volumes of distribution of fat-soluble drugs. Drug absorption is not typically altered in the elderly, and their blood-brain barrier is not noticeably impaired in most cases.

CHAPTER 5

1. **The answer is A:** lead. Edetate calcium disodium is employed only in the chelation of lead, whereas dimercaprol, unithiol, or succimer are employed in the treatment of mercury (C) and arsenic (D) poisoning. Chelation is not typically used in the treatment of cadmium (B) or beryllium (E) intoxication.

2. **The answer is B:** glyphosate. Glyphosate poisoning can cause skin and ocular irritation, mouth, throat, and esophageal damage, aspiration pneumonia, and renal failure. (A) 2,4-D toxicity is characterized by gastrointestinal distress, hypotension, and neurotoxicity. (C) Paraquat poisoning is manifest as bloody vomiting and stools followed later by respiratory distress and failure due to pulmonary edema. (D) Diquat toxicity is similar to paraquat, although diquat is not as toxic. (E) Diazinon is not an herbicide but rather an organophosphate insecticide.

3. **The answer is D:** anger, depression, and irrational behavior. Neuropsychiatric changes are the hallmark of chronic mercury poisoning, as exemplified by the "mad hatter" in Alice's Adventures in Wonderland because hat makers historically used mercury in felting work. Chronic mercury poisoning does not typically cause hypothermia (A), heart failure (B), biliary obstruction and jaundice (C), or rhabdomyolysis (E).

4. **The answer is B:** activated charcoal. Activated charcoal and Fuller's earth are substances that adsorb various poisons such as paraquat and reduce their gastrointestinal absorption if administered soon after ingestion of the toxic agent. The adsorbent and poison are then eliminated in the feces. Succimer (A), dimercaprol (D), and unithiol (E) are chelating agents used to increase the excretion of absorbed heavy metal poisons. Pralidoxime (C) is used to reactivate acetylcholinesterase after poisoning by an organophosphate insecticide or chemical warfare agent.

5. **The answer is E:** non-Hodgkin lymphoma. Exposure to 2,4-D has been linked in epidemiologic studies with an increased risk of non-Hodgkin lymphoma, a hematologic malignancy. 2,4-D is not typically associated with hypertension (A), hyponatremia (B), pulmonary fibrosis (C), or dementia (D).

CHAPTER 6

1. **The answer is C:** dry mouth. Botulinum toxin inhibits the release of acetylcholine from cholinergic neurons, and it is used to inhibit neuromuscular transmission in persons with dystonia. The drug may also inhibit acetylcholine release from parasympathetic nerves and cause dry mouth and dysphagia, particularly when it is administered to the head and neck. Bradycardia (answer A), urinary incontinence (answer B), diarrhea (answer D), and miosis (constriction of the pupils, answer E) are effects that would be caused by increased release of acetylcholine from parasympathetic nerves.

2. **The answer is B:** increased formation of IP₃. Cevimeline is a muscarinic receptor agonist. In salivary glands, muscarinic M₃ receptor activation leads to stimulation of phospholipase C and the formation of IP₃ and diacylglycerol. IP₃ releases intracellular calcium, which increases secretion of saliva. Activation of M₂ receptors (A) would cause heart rate and conduction to decrease. Increased cyclic AMP levels (C) is not an effect of muscarinic receptor activation. Increased cyclic GMP (D) occurs in vascular smooth muscle after M₃ receptor activation. Increased potassium efflux (E) may follow M₂ receptor activation in cardiac tissue.

3. **The answer is A:** sodium influx. The patient most likely received varenicline, a partial agonist at nicotinic receptors in the brain. Nicotinic receptors are ligand-gated sodium channels, and their activation leads to sodium influx. None of the other options is an effect of nicotinic receptor activation.

4. **The answer is E:** headache. Erectile dysfunction and pulmonary arterial hypertension are treated with sildenafil and other drugs that inhibit breakdown of cGMP by 5-PDE. These drugs cause vasodilation, which may lead to headache. Answers A, B, C, and D (constipation, cough, dry mouth, and sedation) are unlikely to be caused by a phosphodiesterase inhibitor.

5. **The answer is C:** increased neurotransmitter degradation. The patient is experiencing organophosphate toxicity caused by inhibition of cholinesterase and excessive stimulation of muscarinic and nicotinic receptors by acetylcholine. The patient's muscle weakness is caused by prolonged depolarization of skeletal muscle due to high levels of acetylcholine at the neuromuscular junction. Pralidoxime reactivates cholinesterase and leads to increased acetylcholine degradation. Atropine blocks muscarinic receptors (Answer A) and would relieve symptoms of excessive muscarinic receptor stimulation but would not relieve muscle weakness. Activation of nicotinic receptors (B) would increase depolarization and muscle weakness. Induction of drug-metabolizing enzymes (D) and increased excretion of weak acids (E) would have no benefit in this setting.

CHAPTER 7

1. **The answer is D:** succinylcholine. Succinylcholine is the only depolarizing neuromuscular blocking agent in current use. It produces prolonged depolarization of skeletal muscle, thereby causing transient muscle fasciculations followed by paralysis. Cholinesterase inhibitors, acting to increase acetylcholine levels, do not counteract the muscle paralysis produced by succinylcholine and can actually increase the degree of paralysis by augmenting persistent muscle depolarization. Rocuronium (A), cisatracurium (C), and pancuronium (E) are non-depolarizing neuromuscular blocking agents that cause muscle paralysis by competing with acetylcholine and do not produce transient fasciculations. Hyoscyamine (B) is a muscarinic acetylcholine receptor antagonist that has no effect on skeletal muscle.

2. **The answer is B:** bronchospasm. Muscarinic blockers such as atropine and scopolamine cause relaxation of bronchial smooth muscle and bronchodilation and were formerly used to treat asthma. These drugs may also cause hyperthermia (C) by inhibiting sweating, thereby leading to vasodilation and flushing. Scopolamine causes blurred vision (E) by relaxing the ciliary muscle, thereby producing cycloplegia (paralysis of accommodation). Urinary retention (D) occurs when muscarinic blockers relax bladder smooth muscle. Toxic doses of muscarinic blockers may cause central nervous system toxicity, including hallucinations (A), delirium, and seizures.

3. **The answer is D:** relaxation of the iris sphincter muscle. Tropicamide binds to muscarinic receptors and competitively blocks acetylcholine released by the parasympathetic oculomotor nerve. This action leads to relaxation of the iris sphincter muscle and dilation of the pupil (mydriasis), thereby facilitating ophthalmoscopic examination of the peripheral retina. Topical ocular administration of muscarinic receptor blockers does not cause vasoconstriction (D), miosis (constriction of the pupil, answer C), or lacrimation (E). Lacrimation would be inhibited by tropicamide, causing dry eyes.

4. **The answer is B:** relax urinary bladder smooth muscle. Darifenacin is a muscarinic receptor antagonist with some selectivity for bladder smooth muscle. It is used to treat hyperactive bladder and relieve urgency, frequency, and incontinence. It is not used clinically to relax uterine (C), gastrointestinal (E), or bronchial smooth muscle (A), though it would be expected to have these effects to a limited degree. It does inhibit salivary secretions and may cause dry mouth.

5. **The answer is D:** forms an inactive drug complex. Sugammadex is indicated for the rapid reversal of the effects of steroidal neuromuscular blocking agents, like rocuronium and vecuronium. It is a modified γ-cyclodextrin compound that binds with rocuronium or vecuronium to form an inactive drug complex that is rapidly excreted in the urine. Answers (A), agonist at cholinergic acetylcholine receptors, (B) antagonist at cholinergic acetylcholine receptors, (C) antagonist at muscarinic acetylcholine receptors, or (E) inhibits acetylcholinesterase are incorrect.

CHAPTER 8

1. **The answer is D:** inhibits the enteric nervous system. The sympathetic nervous system inhibits the enteric nervous system, whereas the parasympathetic system activates it. Answers A, B, C, and E (discrete activation of specific organs, long preganglionic neurons, action terminated by cholinesterase, activated by increased arterial blood pressure) are attributes of the parasympathetic nervous system.

2. **The answer is D:** decreased heart rate. Metyrosine inhibits tyrosine hydroxylase and norepinephrine synthesis, thereby decreasing sympathetic tone and reducing activation of β₁-adrenoceptors in cardiac tissue. Bronchodilation (answer B) and renin secretion (answer C) result from increased activation of β₂- and β₁-adrenoceptors, respectively. Diarrhea (answer A) and salivation (answer E) primarily result from muscarinic acetylcholine receptor activation.

3. **The answer is C:** midodrine. Midodrine is an alpha-receptor agonist that is used to treat postural (orthostatic) hypotension. Dobutamine (A) is a β₁-adrenoceptor agonist used to treat acute heart failure, while albuterol (B) is a β₂-adrenoceptor agonist employed as a bronchodilator. Clonidine is an α₂-adrenoceptor agonist used to treat hypertension, and isoproterenol (E) is a non-selective beta-adrenoceptor agonist.

4. **The answer is A**: inhibition of adenylyl cyclase. α_2-Adrenoceptor agonists such as apraclonidine are used for short-term control of intraocular pressure before and after ocular surgery and for treatment of glaucoma and ocular hypertension. Activation of α_2-adrenoceptors leads to inhibition of adenylyl cyclase and decreased cAMP levels. Activation of adenylyl cyclase (choice B) is produced by β-adrenoceptor agonists, whereas activation of phospholipase C (choice C) and release of calcium from the sarcoplasmic reticulum (E) are caused by α_1-adrenoceptor activation. None of the adrenoceptor agonists cause inhibition of phospholipase C (choice D).

5. **The answer is B**: rapid heart rate. β_2-Adrenoceptor agonists such as albuterol are used to relax bronchial smooth muscle and prevent bronchospasm in persons with asthma. These drugs also activate β-adrenoceptors in the heart and increase heart rate but do not typically cause sedation (A), muscle weakness (C), low blood pressure (D), or blurred vision (E).

6. **The answer is A**: increased cAMP levels. The preferred treatment for severe hypersensitivity reactions (anaphylaxis) is epinephrine. The drug causes bronchodilation by activation of β_2-adrenoceptors in bronchial smooth muscle, leading to increased cAMP levels and smooth muscle relaxation. cGMP (B) also mediates smooth muscle relaxation, but its levels are not increased by β_2-adrenoceptor activation. Increased IP_3 levels (C) and calcium influx d (D) cause smooth muscle contraction. Sequestration of calcium (E) might cause muscle relaxation but is not an effect of adrenoceptor activation.

CHAPTER 9

1. **The answer is E**: phentolamine. Epinephrine and other adrenoceptor agonists can cause excessive vasoconstriction and ischemia when injected into fingers, toes, or other tissues as a result of activating α_1-adrenoceptors in vascular smooth muscle. Phentolamine is a nonselective α-adrenoceptor antagonist that can be injected directly into affected tissues to counteract the vasoconstrictive effects of adrenoceptor agonists. Phenoxybenzamine (D) is given orally and has a long duration of action. It is not suitable for treatment of acute vasoconstriction. Alfuzosin (A) is a uroselective alpha-blocker with little effect on vascular smooth muscle. Carvedilol (B) and betaxolol (C) are orally administered beta blockers that would not reverse acute vasoconstriction.

2. **The answer is A**: alfuzosin. Alfuzosin is a selective α_1-adrenoceptor blocker that relaxes smooth muscle in the bladder outflow tract and relieves urinary obstruction caused by prostatic hyperplasia. Phentolamine (E) and phenoxybenzamine (D) might relax the urinary bladder but would cause excessive hypotension as well. Carvedilol (B) and betaxolol (C) are beta blockers, which do not relax smooth muscle.

3. **The answer is B**: carvedilol. Carvedilol is a nonselective β-receptor antagonist and a selective α_1-receptor antagonist. It reduces cardiac output by blocking cardiac β_1-receptors and it decreases peripheral vascular resistance by blocking α_1-receptors in vascular smooth muscle. Betaxolol (C) would reduce cardiac output but not peripheral resistance. Phenoxybenzamine (D) and phentolamine (E) would reduce peripheral resistance but

not cardiac output. Alfuzosin (A) would have little effect on either cardiac output or peripheral resistance.

4. **The answer is D**: phenoxybenzamine. The patient most likely has a tumor of the adrenal medulla called *pheochromocytoma*, which secretes large quantities of epinephrine and norepinephrine, thereby causing severe hypertension. Phenoxybenzamine is a long-acting α-receptor antagonist that is used to reduce vascular resistance and blood pressure in patients with this condition. Phentolamine (E) is a short-acting injectable alpha-blocker that is not suitable for treating pheochromocytoma. Carvedilol (B) and betaxolol (C) might reduce cardiac output in this patient but would not reduce peripheral resistance. Hence, blood flow to vital organs might be severely decreased. Alfuzosin (A) would have little effect on blood pressure.

5. **The answer is C**: propranolol. Nonselective β-blockers such as propranolol are most likely to inhibit β_2-receptor–mediated glycogenolysis and slow recovery from hypoglycemia. Selective β_1-blockers such as atenolol (E) and metoprolol (A) are less likely to inhibit glycogenolysis than nonselective blockers, and α-adrenoceptor blockers such as doxazosin and phentolamine are least likely to impair glycogenolysis.

CHAPTER 10

1. **The answer is D**: lisinopril. ACE inhibitors such as lisinopril and angiotensin receptor blockers (ARBs) such as telmisartan have been shown to slow the progression of renal disease in diabetic patients beyond their ability to lower blood pressure. Beta blockers such as metoprolol (A), calcium channel blockers such as nifedipine (C) and diltiazem (E), and thiazide diuretics such as indapamide (D) may slow the progression of renal disease by lowering blood pressure but do not exert the additional renoprotective effects of ACE inhibitors and ARBs.

2. **The answer is C**: nifedipine. CCBs, particularly nifedipine, have been associated with gingival overgrowth or hyperplasia, which occurs in about 10% to 20% of persons taking these drugs. Poor dental hygiene is a strong risk factor for this condition in persons taking CCBs, and good hygiene can often relieve the condition in these patients. Other drugs associated with this condition include cyclosporine and phenytoin. None of the other options are typically associated with gingival overgrowth.

3. **The answer is A**: aliskiren. Aliskiren inhibits renin and the formation of angiotensin I and II. Atenolol (B) acts in part by inhibiting the release of renin from juxtaglomerular cells, while enalapril (C) inhibits the formation of angiotensin II, and valsartan (E) blocks receptors for Angiotensin II. Hydrochlorothiazide (D) has no direct effect on the renin-angiotensin-aldosterone axis.

4. **The answer is B**: blocking angiotensin AT1 receptors. Several drugs inhibit the renin-angiotensin-aldosterone system. Irbesartan blocks angiotensin receptors, while enalapril and similar drugs inhibit angiotensin II formation (D). Aliskiren inhibits renin (A), while spironolactone and eplerenone antagonize aldosterone (E). Amlodipine and nicardipine block the entry of calcium into vascular smooth muscle and thereby produce vasodilation (C).

5. **The answer is A:** carvedilol. Carvedilol is a third-generation β-blocker that blocks alpha-1 and beta adrenoceptors while exerting antioxidant effects that protect the vascular endothelium from damage. Propranolol (C) blocks beta-1 and beta-2 adrenoceptors but does not block alpha receptors or exert antioxidative effects. Doxazosin (E) is an alpha-1 receptor antagonist that has no beta blocking activity, while amlodipine (B) is a calcium channel blocker and hydrochlorothiazide (D) is a diuretic.

CHAPTER 11

1. **The answer is B:** decreased binding of calcium to calmodulin. CCBs reduce calcium influx, decrease formation of the calcium-calmodulin complex, and thereby reduce (rather than increase; answer D) myosin light-chain kinase activity. Organic nitrates release nitric oxide and increase cyclic GMP levels (A), whereas trimetazidine increases metabolic efficiency (E). Alpha-1 adrenoceptor antagonists such as terazosin reduce IP_3 formation (C), though they have no use in the treatment of angina.

2. **The answer is C:** decreased heart rate. Both atenolol, a β_1-adrenoceptor blocker, and diltiazem, a non-dihydropyridine CCB, decrease heart rate and contractility. Option A (decreased cAMP levels) is only caused by atenolol. Option B (increased cGMP levels) is caused by neither atenolol nor diltiazem. Option D (relaxation of arterial smooth muscle) is caused only by diltiazem, whereas neither drug inhibits sodium influx (Option E).

3. **The answer is D:** release of nitric oxide. Organic nitrates release nitric oxide, which activates guanylyl cyclase and increases cGMP levels. Option A (inhibition of phosphodiesterase) is the mechanism by which sildenafil relaxes vascular smooth muscle. Option B (inactivation of aldehyde dehydrogenase) may lead to decreased release of nitric oxide and nitrate tolerance. Options C (blockade of β-adrenoceptors) and E (blockade of calcium channels) are not associated with increased cGMP levels.

4. **The answer is E:** propranolol. Nonselective β-blockers such as propranolol may cause bronchoconstriction by blocking β_2-adrenoceptors. Calcium channel blockers (Options A, B, and D) appear to relax bronchial smooth muscle and are preferred for treating angina in persons with obstructive lung disease. Organic nitrates (Option C) do not significantly affect bronchial smooth muscle and can also be used in patients with obstructive lung disease.

5. **The answer is A:** ranolazine. Ranolazine reduces the late (prolonged) inward sodium current associated with calcium overload and increased ventricular wall tension. Ivabradine (D) blocks the so-called funny current that is responsible for diastolic depolarization in cardiac pacemaker cells in the sino-atrial node. Amlodipine (C) blocks calcium channels in vascular smooth muscle but not significantly in heart tissue. Trimetazidine (E) inhibits fatty oxidation in heart cells, forcing the heart to utilize glucose and thereby reduce oxygen consumption.

CHAPTER 12

1. **The correct answer is C:** both angiotensin II and natriuretic peptide. Neprilysin is an endogenous endopeptidase enzyme that degrades various vasoactive peptides, including angiotensin II, natriuretic peptide, and bradykinin. Increased levels of natriuretic peptide lead to vasodilation and decreased ventricular wall tension in patients with systolic heart failure, whereas increased levels of angiotensin II have undesirable effects on the heart and circulation. Sacubitril inhibits neprilysin and is available in combination with valsartan, an angiotensin receptor blocker. Sacubitril augments natriuretic peptide levels while valsartan blocks elevated levels of angiotensin II. Neprilysin has no direct effect on nitric oxide levels (E).

2. **The correct answer is C:** digoxin. Excessive doses of digoxin may cause nausea and vomiting, visual disturbances, and cardiac arrhythmias. Dobutamine and milrinone (A and D) may also cause cardiac arrhythmias but do not typically cause blurred vision, nausea, and vomiting. Lisinopril and furosemide (B and E) do not usually cause any of these adverse effects. Treatment with the digoxin antidote, Digibind, may be warranted in cases of severe digoxin toxicity.

3. **The correct answer is B:** carvedilol. Carvedilol, a third-generation β-blocker, has been shown to improve cardiac performance, reduce symptoms, slow disease progression, and increase survival in heart failure. Angiotensin inhibitors also increase cardiac output and reduce mortality. Inotropic agents (C and D), diuretics (A), and hydralazine-isosorbide dinitrate (E) improve symptoms but have not been shown to increase survival.

4. **The correct answer is D:** stimulation of guanylyl cyclase. Nesiritide is a recombinant form of type B human natriuretic peptide. This drug activates guanylyl cyclase in vascular smooth muscle and endothelial cells, leading to increased cGMP and vasodilation. Nesiritide is used to treat acutely decompensated heart failure (heart failure in which the stroke volume is no longer proportional to the diastolic fiber length). Vasodilation reduces congestion and dyspnea in these patients. Stimulation of adenylyl cyclase (B) is the mechanism by which dobutamine produces its inotropic effect. None of the drugs used in heart failure inhibit adenylyl cyclase (A) or guanylyl cyclase (C). Inhibition of phosphodiesterase (type 5) leading to increased cyclic GMP levels is the mechanism of sildenafil and related drugs used in treating erectile dysfunction and pulmonary artery hypertension.

5. **The answer is A:** carvedilol. Carvedilol is a non-selective beta-adrenoceptor antagonist and a selective alpha-1 adrenoceptor antagonist. Metoprolol (B) is a selective beta-1 receptor antagonist with little affinity for alpha receptors, while propranolol (C) is a non-selective beta-receptor antagonist. Dobutamine is a selective beta-1 receptor agonist, while phentolamine is a non-selective alpha-1 and alpha-2 adrenoceptor antagonist.

CHAPTER 13

1. **The answer is B:** furosemide. Loop-acting diuretics such as furosemide can cause ototoxicity more frequently than other diuretics. Of the loop-acting diuretics, ethacrynic acid is particularly prone to cause adverse effects such as tinnitus (ringing in the ears), vertigo, hearing impairment, and ear pain. Spironolactone, hydrochlorothiazide, acetazolamide, and mannitol (answers A, C, D, E) are unlikely to cause these adverse effects.

2. **The answer is A:** spironolactone. Potassium-sparing diuretics such as spironolactone can cause hyperkalemia, especially in persons with renal insufficiency. Thiazide diuretics such as hydrochlorothiazide (C) and loop-acting diuretics such as furosemide (B) are more likely to cause hypokalemia. Mannitol (E) and acetazolamide (D) have less effect on potassium excretion and serum potassium levels.

3. **The answer is D:** acetazolamide. Carbonic anhydrase inhibitors such as acetazolamide increase renal sodium bicarbonate excretion and alkalinize the urine. Urine alkalinization increases the ionization of weakly acidic drugs such as amphetamine and thereby increases their renal excretion. Other diuretics do not significantly affect the renal excretion of weakly acidic drugs.

4. **The answer is B:** furosemide. Loop-acting diuretics such as furosemide reduce the paracellular reabsorption of calcium in the loop of Henle and thereby increase renal calcium excretion. Hence, these drugs are used in the treatment of hypercalcemia. Thiazide diuretics such as hydrochlorothiazide (C) decrease calcium excretion and would worsen hypercalcemia. Other diuretics (spironolactone, acetazolamide, and mannitol) have little effect on calcium excretion.

5. **The answer is C:** acetazolamide. Carbonic anhydrase inhibitors such as acetazolamide have been used for the prevention and treatment of high-altitude sickness. Their beneficial effects partly result from inhibition of carbonic anhydrase in the brain and cerebrospinal fluid (CSF) that leads to decreased CSF pressure and altered pH and may partly result from a mild metabolic acidosis produced by the drugs that counteract respiratory alkalosis resulting from hyperventilation during high altitude exposure. None of the other diuretics have been useful in treating this condition.

CHAPTER 14

1. **The answer is E:** amiodarone. Amiodarone is a thyroxine analog that can cause hypothyroidism and, less commonly, hyperthyroidism. Dronedarone (B) is a non-iodinated analog of amiodarone that does not affect thyroid function. None of the other options is associated with thyroid dysfunction. Procainamide (A) may cause a lupus-like syndrome. Dofetilide (C) prolongs the QT interval and may cause torsades de pointes. Verapamil (D) may cause hypotension and aggravate heart failure.

2. **The answer is C:** prolonged QRS duration. The woman was most likely taking a Class IC antiarrhythmic agent such as flecainide. These drugs dissociate very slowly from sodium channels and, therefore, slow ventricular depolarization and increase QRS duration. A prolonged or shortened PR interval (A or B) result from slower or faster impulse conduction, respectively, in the AV node. A prolonged QT interval (D) results from delayed ventricular repolarization. Sinus bradycardia (E) results from decreased a decreased rate of depolarization of the SA node pacemaker.

3. **The answer is A:** QT prolongation. The man is most likely receiving dofetilide, ibutilide, or sotalol, which block potassium channels that repolarize ventricular tissue. Because of this drug's tendency to prolong the QT interval, the ECG must be monitored during dosage titration. Potassium channel blockade is not associated with changes in the PR interval (C), QRS duration (B), T-wave inversion (D), or the heart rate (E).

4. **The answer is D:** increased potassium efflux. Adenosine activates G protein–coupled adenosine receptors that mediate potassium efflux and hyperpolarization of supraventricular tissue, thereby preventing rapid atrial depolarization. Adenosine does not increase chloride influx (A), cyclic guanosine monophosphate levels (B), or calcium influx (C), and it does not decrease sodium influx (E).

5. **The answer is A:** sotalol. In addition to having Class III antiarrhythmic activity, sotalol is a non-selective β-adrenoceptor antagonist. It may cause bronchospasm and precipitate asthma in susceptible persons by blocking $β_2$-adrenoceptors in bronchial smooth muscle. Hence, the drug should be avoided in persons with asthma and chronic obstructive lung disease. Diltiazem (B), flecainide (C), quinidine (D), and lidocaine (E) do not typically cause bronchospasm.

CHAPTER 15

1. **The answer is C:** ezetimibe. Ezetimibe is the only drug choice that inhibits the intestinal absorption of cholesterol. Colesevelam (A) and colestipol (D) inhibit the intestinal reabsorption of bile acids, but they do not significantly affect cholesterol absorption. Fenofibrate (B) and niacin (E) have no direct effect on cholesterol absorption and act in part by reducing VLDL secretion or increasing VLDL clearance.

2. **The answer is D:** colestipol. Drugs that are associated with skeletal muscle pain, inflammation, and destruction (myopathy) include statins (A and E), fibrates (C), and niacin (B). Bile acid-binding resins such as colestipol do not typically cause myopathy.

3. **The answer is D:** inhibits apolipoprotein B synthesis. Mipomersen is an antisense oligonucleotide to the messenger RNA for apolipoprotein B (apo B). Antisense oligonucleotides are complementary single-stranded RNA molecules that bind to the target RNA to form a double-stranded molecule that is unable to serve as template for protein synthesis. Inhibition of microsomal triglyceride transport (A) is the mechanism by which lomitapide inhibits VLDL production. Ezetimibe inhibits cholesterol absorption (B), and statins inhibit cholesterol synthesis (C). None of the available drugs directly increases cholesterol excretion (E), though bile-acid binding resins indirectly increase cholesterol excretion in the form of bile acids.

4. **The answer is A:** triglycerides. Fibrate drugs such as fenofibrate increase the expression of lipoprotein lipase via activation of PPAR-α. Lipoprotein lipase catalyzes the release of triglycerides from VLDL for uptake by adipose tissue and thereby lowers serum triglyceride levels. Lipoprotein lipase has no direct effect on serum levels of HDL or LDL-cholesterol (B, C), apolipoprotein B (D), or phospholipids (E).

5. **The answer is E:** colesevelam. Bile acid-binding resins such as colesevelam and colestipol increase the intestinal excretion of bile acids and necessitate increased utilization of cholesterol to replace those excreted. Niacin (A), rosuvastatin (B), gemfibrozil (C), and ezetimibe (D) do

not affect bile acid excretion significantly or increase utilization of cholesterol to synthesize bile acids.

CHAPTER 16

1. **The answer is C**: dabigatran. Dabigatran is an orally effective direct thrombin inhibitor. Eptifibatide (A) and prasugrel (B) are antiplatelet drugs that have no direct effect on thrombin activity. Enoxaparin (E) is a low-molecular-weight heparin that primarily inhibits active factor X (Stuart factor) by potentiating antithrombin III and must be given parenterally. Rivaroxaban (D) is an orally administered active factor X inhibitor.

2. **The answer is B**: prasugrel. Prasugrel and clopidogrel are irreversible antagonists of adenosine diphosphate P2Y receptors in blood platelets and thereby reduce activation of GP IIb/IIIa receptors required for platelet aggregation, whereas ticagrelor is a reversible antagonist. Eptifibatide (A) blocks GP IIb/IIIa receptors, whereas dabigatran (C), rivaroxaban (D), and enoxaparin (E) are inhibitors of thrombin or active factor X.

3. **The answer is D**: rivaroxaban. Rivaroxaban is an orally administered active factor X inhibitor. Enoxaparin (E) inhibits active factor X by potentiating antithrombin III, and it must be given parenterally. Prasugrel (B) is an antiplatelet drug, whereas dabigatran (C) is an orally administered direct thrombin inhibitor.

4. **The answer is A**: eptifibatide. Eptifibatide and tirofiban are reversible GP IIb/IIIa receptor antagonists that prevent fibrinogen cross-linking of these receptors and platelet aggregation. Prasugrel (B) is an ADP P2Y receptor antagonist that prevents activation of GP IIb/IIIa receptors. Dabigatran (C), rivaroxaban (D), and enoxaparin (E) are anticoagulants that inhibit thrombin or active factor X.

5. **The answer is B**: heparin. Heparin can induce thrombocytopenia in up to 5% of treated patients. Argotroban (A) is a direct-acting thrombin inhibitor that can be used in treating thrombosis in patients with heparin-induced thrombocytopenia. Tirofiban (C) has a low risk of causing thrombocytopenia, while bivalirudin (D) and rivaroxaban (E) are not usually associated with thrombocytopenia.

6. **The answer is D**: dabigatran. Idarucizumab (Praxbind) is a monoclonal antibody that inactivates dabigatran and can be used to treat bleeding caused by this anticoagulant. The treatment of bleeding caused by alteplase (A) is aminocaproic acid. Warfarin-induced bleeding (B) can be treated with vitamin K_1 (phytonadione). Bleeding caused by dalteparin (C) can be inhibited with protamine sulfate, but there is no specific antidote for bleeding caused by apixaban and other active factor X inhibitors.

CHAPTER 17

1. **The answer is C**: ferrous fumarate. Iron deficiency anemia is a hypochromic (low erythrocyte hemoglobin concentration) and microcytic (low erythrocyte corpuscular volume) anemia. Several months of treatment with oral ferrous sulfate or another ferrous salt is usually required to correct the iron deficiency and restore hemoglobin concentrations to normal. Patients should also consume a diet containing adequate amounts of folic acid (E) and vitamin B_{12} (A) to ensure adequate erythropoiesis, but the primary treatment is iron replacement. Epoetin (B) and filgrastim (D) are not indicated or effective for treating iron deficiency anemia.

2. **The answer is D**: filgrastim. Filgrastim is a recombinant G-CSF that is used to treat cancer chemotherapy–induced neutropenia in patients with neoplasms, such as breast cancer. Sargramostim has similar indications. Folic acid (E) and vitamin B_{12} (A) are required for normal leukopoiesis but will not by themselves accelerate leucopoiesis caused by drug-induced myelosuppression. Epoetin (B) and ferrous fumarate (C) are not used to treat neutropenia.

3. **The answer is A**: cyanocobalamin. Pernicious anemia usually results from inadequate vitamin B_{12} absorption because of decreased production of intrinsic factors by gastric parietal cells. Vitamin B_{12} deficiency causes a megaloblastic anemia characterized by an abnormally high mean corpuscular volume. Persons with pernicious anemia will also have a low serum level of vitamin B_{12} and a high serum concentration of methylmalonic acid because B_{12} is required to convert methylmalonyl CoA to succinyl CoA. Folic acid (E) may partially correct the anemia caused by B_{12} deficiency but should not be used alone. Epoetin (B) and filgrastim (D) have no specific role in treating pernicious anemia. Ferrous fumarate (C) would be useful if dietary iron intake is inadequate.

4. **The answer is B**: epoetin. Epoetin is a recombinant form of erythropoietin. Patients with end-stage renal disease often require epoetin treatment to prevent anemia because their kidneys are unable to produce sufficient erythropoietin to maintain erythropoiesis. Ferrous fumarate (C) is given to support erythropoiesis stimulated by epoetin but will not correct the anemia by itself. Cyanocobalamin (A) and folic acid (E) are not required to treat anemia due to chronic renal disease, and filgrastim (D) has no role in this condition.

5. **The answer is C**: increasing duration of action. The addition of polyethylene glycol moieties to recombinant colony-stimulating factors (pegylation) serves to reduce their metabolism or excretion and thereby increase their duration of action so that they can be given less frequently. Pegylation does not increase oral bioavailability (A), decrease excretion rate (B), increase binding to receptors (D), or decrease adverse effects (E).

CHAPTER 18

1. **The answer is B**: heteroreceptor. A heteroreceptor is a type of presynaptic receptor that is also located on the neuronal terminal but binds a different neurotransmitter than the one being released from the terminal. The signaling through this type of receptor usually causes decreased release of the neurotransmitter. Answer A, presynaptic receptor, is a general term for any type of receptor located on the neuronal terminal. Answer C, postsynaptic receptor, is incorrect because this receptor is located on the postsynaptic membrane. Answer D, autoreceptor, is a type of presynaptic receptor in which the binding of the same neurotransmitter released from the neuronal terminal decreases further release of that neurotransmitter. Answer E, ionotropic receptor, is the term for a receptor associated with an ion channel and could be located on either the presynaptic or postsynaptic membrane.

2. **The answer is E:** exocytosis. Fusion of the neurotransmitter vesicle is triggered with an influx of Ca^{2+} into the presynaptic terminal. This process is called exocytosis. Answer A, apoptosis, is incorrect as this means programmed cell death. Answer B, phagocytosis, means the engulfing of cellular debris or bacteria by another cell, usually a macrophage. Answer C, endocytosis, is the process whereby receptors and other membrane proteins are recycled back into the neuron. Answer D, pinocytosis, refers to is a form of endocytosis in which small particles of liquids are brought into the cell within small vesicles formed from the membrane.

3. **The answer is A:** neuropeptides are synthesized in the cell body. Unlike classical neurotransmitters that are synthesized in vesicles en route or at the neuronal terminal from precursor substances, neuropeptides arise from the transcription of a neuropeptide gene, processing of the neuropeptide messenger RNA (mRNA), and translation of the mRNA into a neuropeptide product in the endoplasmic reticulum in the cell body of a neuron. Answer B, classical neurotransmitters have a longer duration of action, is not true in general, and many studies show that neuropeptides act more as neuromodulators with longer duration of action than classical neurotransmitters. Answer C, neuropeptides undergo rapid reuptake into the presynaptic terminal, is incorrect as there are no known transport proteins in presynaptic membranes to facilitate the reuptake of neuropeptides back into the terminal. Answer D, classical neurotransmitters are packaged into vesicles, is true but does not differentiate between the two types of substances because neuropeptides are also packaged into vesicles for release, albeit into different types called *dense-core vesicles*. Answer E, neuropeptides are degraded by acetylcholinesterase in the synapse, is incorrect because other enzymes called peptidases are responsible for the degradation of neuropeptides after release into the synapse.

4. **The answer is D:** opioid receptors are downregulated. Chronic administration of an agonist, such as the opioid agonists morphine and oxycodone, will cause a decrease in the number of receptor proteins expressed by the neuron in an attempt to decrease the signaling through that pathway and establish homeostasis. Answer A, the metabolism of morphine is upregulated, could be true because the metabolism of some CNS agents, most notably the barbiturates, self-induce metabolic enzymes, but this mechanism is not known to occur with opioid analgesics. Answer B, pain intensity has greatly increased, could also be true, but there is no information given in the question to assume that this might be the case. Answer C, the efficiency of G protein coupling is decreased, is a mechanism more noted for acute changes after agonist administration, whereas down-regulation is more likely with long-term or chronic administration of an agonist. Answer E, the patient is a "drug seeker" and addicted to opioid medications, is very unlikely because metastatic lung cancer can be a very painful condition and less than 4% of patients treated with opioid analgesics develop substance abuse disorders.

5. **The answer is C:** fluoxetine. Fluoxetine, with the trade name of Prozac, is one of the classes of antidepressants called *selective serotonin reuptake inhibitors*, or SSRIs.

Answer A, lithium, is incorrect as this agent to treat bipolar disorder acts at the level of signal transduction. Answer B, morphine, is incorrect as this opioid agonist acts by receptor activation. Answer D, levodopa, is an antiparkinsonian agent that acts by a strategy known as *precursor loading*, which feeds the biosynthetic pathway for the synthesis of dopamine. Answer E, donepezil, is incorrect as this drug to treat Alzheimer disease acts by inhibiting the breakdown of acetylcholine, the neurotransmitter that is reduced in Alzheimer disease.

CHAPTER 19

1. **The answer is A:** potentiating the effect of GABA at chloride ion channels. Benzodiazepines bind to an allosteric site on the $GABA_A$ receptor–ion channel complex to increase the affinity of GABA. GABA action increases the conductance of chloride ion into the neuron, thereby hyperpolarizing the membrane and making it harder to reach depolarization threshold and fire action potentials. Answer B, blocking glutamate excitation, is the mechanism of action of N-methyl-d-aspartate receptor antagonists. Answer C, blocking the inactivation of sodium ion channels, is the mechanism of action of certain antiepileptic agents. Answer D, binding to opioid receptors to produce sedation, refers to the site of opioid analgesic action. Answer E, potentiating the action of the inhibitory amino acid, glycine, is incorrect because benzodiazepines do not have significant binding affinity for the glycine receptor.

2. **The answer is D:** decreasing the REM stage of sleep. Benzodiazepines are noted for decreasing the time spent in REM sleep, an effect that is unmasked by REM rebound after the administration of the benzodiazepine is stopped. Answer A, increasing the time to sleep onset, is the opposite effect of sedative-hypnotics, which decrease the latency to sleep. Answer B, decreasing stage 2 NREM sleep, is not correct because studies do not show a consistent effect of benzodiazepines on stage 2 NREM sleep. Answer C, increasing slow-wave sleep, may be beneficial to a restful sleep, but no evidence suggests that benzodiazepines produce this effect. Choice E, increasing sleep awakenings, occurs in patients with insomnia, a symptom that benzodiazepines and other sedative-hypnotic agents aim to treat.

3. **The answer is E:** is a selective benzodiazepine antagonist. Flumazenil is a competitive antagonist of the benzodiazepine receptor. The availability of flumazenil to reverse benzodiazepine action is useful in cases of drug overdose or in outpatient procedures to bring patients back to normal wakefulness. Answer A, does not produce withdrawal seizures, is certainly true; however, it is not the best statement describing flumazenil. Answer B, has the longest elimination half-life, is not true because often flumazenil must be given in repeated administrations to reverse the effects of a longer-lasting benzodiazepine such as diazepam. Answer C, is not metabolized into an active agent, is also true but is not the best choice. Answer D, is also used for the treatment of epilepsy, is incorrect regarding the indicated uses of flumazenil.

4. **The answer is B:** has a shorter elimination half-life. Zaleplon, like zolpidem, has a more selective action than

benzodiazepines. It has the advantage of a shorter half-life and therefore is approved for patients who awaken in the middle of the night and cannot return to sleep. Answer A, produces withdrawal seizures, does not appear to be true for both agents but is noted on cessation of chronic doses of alprazolam. Answer C, has a different chemical structure than benzodiazepines, and answer D, shows less tolerance to sedative effects, is also true for both agents. Answer E, produces greater morning sedation, is not true, and neither agent produces much sedation after its initial hypnotic effect.

5. **The answer is E:** buspirone. Buspirone is a unique, nonsedating anxiolytic agent mediating its effects by way of the 5-HT receptor. No sedative effects are associated with its action, although it differs in that it may take 2 to 4 weeks of daily administration for clinical effectiveness. Answers A through D are all sedating drugs, including the antihistamine hydroxyzine and the benzodiazepines diazepam, oxazepam, and alprazolam.

CHAPTER 20

1. **The answer is B:** prolonging the inactivation of the Na^+ ion channel. Both these agents bind to the Na^+ channel protein and prolong the state of inactivation. This leads to a decrease in repetitively firing neurons. Answer A, inhibiting low-threshold Ca^{2+} ion channels, is the mechanism of action of ethosuximide and valproic acid, particularly useful in controlling absence seizures. Answer C, potentiating the release of GABA by inhibiting GABA reuptake, is the mechanism of action of tiagabine. Answer D, increasing the release of GABA by vesicular fusion, is the action of gabapentin, although the precise mechanisms are unknown. Answer E, blocking glutamate receptor excitation, is part of the mechanism of action of topiramate.

2. **The answer is D:** carbamazepine. This agent has also gained approval for the use as an antimanic agent or mood stabilizer for treatment of bipolar disorder and for trigeminal neuralgia. Answer A, ethosuximide, is the drug of choice for treating absence seizures in children. Answers B, zonisamide, and C, levetiracetam, are approved only for adjunct treatment of partial seizures. Answer E, phenytoin, has gained some acclaim as a mood stabilizer but has not been mentioned for use in trigeminal neuralgia.

3. **The answer is A:** ethosuximide. Ethosuximide acts by inhibiting the low-threshold Ca^{2+} channels thought to be active during absence seizures. Answers B, zonisamide, and C, levetiracetam, are newer agents for the treatment of partial seizures. Answers D, carbamazepine, and E, phenytoin, are classic drugs used to treat partial seizures and generalized tonic-clonic seizures.

4. **The answer is A:** increases Na^+ channel inactivation, increases GABA, blocks glutamate. Topiramate is a newer agent with three known mechanisms of action. The other answers, B through E, contain at least one mechanism of action that would produce greater excitation of neurons or is not a mechanism of topiramate.

5. **The answer is E:** increases release of neurotransmitters. Gabapentin is an analog of GABA and is known to cause greater release of GABA from neurons, but the precise mechanism is unknown. Answer A, inhibits monoamine oxidase, is an action of certain types of antidepressant drugs. Answer B, agonist effect at dopamine receptors, is an action of some antiparkinsonism agents. Answer C, increases Na^+ channel inactivation, and answer D, blocks reuptake of neurotransmitters, describe the action of the newer antiepileptic agent tiagabine.

CHAPTER 21

1. **The answer is B:** blocking the Na^+ channels in nerves. Local anesthetics produce a block of voltage-gated sodium channels needed to conduct action potentials along nerve fibers. The unprotonated form of the local anesthetic molecule passes through the neuronal membrane and is changed to the protonated form in the cytoplasm. This form then binds to the inside of the sodium channel protein. Answer A, increasing K^+ conductance and hyperpolarizing nerves would cause inhibition of firing but not total blockade of action potentials because they are not dependent on potassium channels for nerve fiber conduction. Answer C, inactivating the Na^+,K^+-adenosine triphosphatase (ATPase) pump, is the action of some cardiovascular agents used for congestive heart failure. Answer D, blocking excitation at postsynaptic receptors, is the action of a receptor antagonist. Answer E, blocking by a direct action only at the synapse, again, is not the action of a local anesthetic, which can block all along the nerve fiber.

2. **The answer is A:** to decrease the rate of absorption of the local anesthetic. Epinephrine causes vasoconstriction acting at α_1 receptors and thus decreases the amount of systemic absorption of the local anesthetic. Answer B, to decrease the duration of action of the local anesthetic, is wrong because epinephrine actually prolongs the duration of action by reducing absorption away from the nerve fiber. Answer C, to block the metabolism of ester-type local anesthetics, and E, to act synergistically with local anesthetic at the nerve ion channel, are wrong because no evidence exists for epinephrine having this effect. Answer D, to enhance the distribution of local anesthetic, is incorrect because epinephrine affects the pharmacokinetic property of absorption directly.

3. **The answer is B:** minimal alveolar concentration. The minimal alveolar concentration value, which is used for inhalational agents to determine potency, is defined as the percent concentration in the administered air that produces no response to surgical incision in 50% of the subjects. Answers A, C, and D are measures of the characteristics of anesthetics but do not give the potency. Answer E, relative analgesic potency, is a term used when comparing analgesic agents.

4. **The answer is B:** nitrous oxide. Although nitrous oxide has the fastest rate of induction and is safe to use, the potency is such that one would have to administer the gas under hyperbaric conditions for it to be the sole inhalational agent. It is often used in dental procedures for its analgesic effects and as an adjunct in other procedures.

5. **The answer is A:** fentanyl. Fentanyl is a potent opioid agonist given as part of balanced anesthesia. It can cause chest wall (truncal) rigidity because of interactions in the striatum. This effect has not been noted for B, midazolam, C, ketamine, D, propofol, or E, thiopental.

CHAPTER 22

1. **The answer is A:** dopamine D_2 receptors. Antipsychotic agents are classified as typical, generally the older agents with actions at dopamine receptors, and the atypical antipsychotics, which can have multiple receptor action but primarily interact at 5-HT receptors. Answers B, α_2-adrenergic receptors (α_2-adrenoceptors), and C, muscarinic receptors, mediate some of the adverse effects of typical antipsychotic agents. There is no evidence for answer D, histamine receptors, in the clinical effects of typical antipsychotics, but they can be involved in sedative effects of the older, less-selective agents. Answer E, serotonin receptors, is correlated to the efficacy of the atypical agents and not the typical ones.

2. **The answer is D:** risperidone. Risperidone is a unique dual-acting antipsychotic agent that is an antagonist at both D_2 receptors and 5-HT_2 receptors and is effective in treating both positive and negative symptoms of schizophrenia. Answers A, chlorpromazine, B, haloperidol, C, thiothixene, and E, thioridazine, are all older, typical antipsychotics that block dopamine receptors (among other receptors) but with no appreciable affinity for 5-HT receptors.

3. **The answer is D:** acetylcholinesterase inhibitors. Acetylcholinesterase inhibitors, also known as *indirect-acting cholinergic agonists*, increase the synaptic concentration of acetylcholine. This has utility in the treatment of the dementia of Alzheimer disease but does not have antidepressant activity. The other answers are types of antidepressants.

4. **The answer is E:** sexual dysfunction. Whereas the older TCAs can cause all of the adverse effects listed from A through D, it is the newer SSRIs, such as fluoxetine, that are noted for sometimes causing sexual dysfunction, including priapism and impotency.

5. **The answer is B:** MAOIs. The MAOIs irreversibly inhibit monoamine oxidase, the enzyme that degrades biogenic amine neurotransmitters. This elevates the levels of the amine neurotransmitter available for synaptic release. Tyramine in food is not degraded because the MAO enzyme is blocked, and a hypertensive crisis might ensue. Answers A and C through E are agents that do not interfere with the catabolism of dietary amines.

CHAPTER 23

1. **The answer is D:** μ (mu) receptors. Although there are three homologous opioid receptor proteins, most clinical opioid analgesics are agonists at the μ receptors. Answer A, κ (kappa), is also a type of opioid receptor that can mediate analgesia but plays only a minor role in the action of some mixed agonist-antagonist opioids. Answer B, α (alpha), is part of the adrenoceptor family. Answer C, β (beta), is a type of adrenoceptor. Answer E, δ (delta), is also a type of opioid receptor and does mediate analgesia in preclinical models, but δ-selective agents have not surfaced in the clinic.

2. **The answer is A:** codeine undergoes less first-pass metabolism. Codeine is methylmorphine with the methyl group at the 3 position. As this is the principal site of glucuronide metabolism of morphine, the codeine molecule is somewhat protected from the first-pass effect of hepatic metabolism. Answer B, morphine is conjugated more quickly, is true but is not the best answer because codeine is not conjugated initially but first metabolized to morphine. Answers C, morphine directly passes into systemic circulation, D, codeine is available only in liquid formulation, and E, codeine is metabolized more by hepatic enzymes, are not accurate statements.

3. **The answer is E:** opioids increase vestibular sensitivity. Ambulatory patients report more instances of nausea and vomiting than recumbent patients administered morphine. In vitro studies show that opioids modulate the inner ear vestibular complex to increase its sensitivity. Answers A, morphine inhibits chemoreceptor trigger zone neurons, and B, morphine sensitizes medulla cough center neurons, are both wrong because morphine has the opposite effects and stimulates the chemoreceptor trigger zone neurons in the medulla and inhibits cough center neurons. Answer C, opioids cause sedation, which makes walking more difficult, may be true but does not affect the onset of nausea and vomiting. Answer D, patients on opioids eat more, has no support from the literature, although fasting does appear to increase endogenous opioid peptides in the CNS and has been implicated in the pathology of the eating disorder anorexia nervosa.

4. **The answer is E:** fentanyl. This potent opioid is available as a transdermal patch for the treatment of chronic pain. Answer A, morphine, is not so lipophilic to allow transdermal administration. Answer B, naltrexone, is an opioid antagonist that does come in a patch formulation but would not help with chronic pain. It is used to treat opioid and alcohol dependence. Answer C, scopolamine, does also come in a patch but is used for motion sickness. Answer D, methadone, is a long-acting opioid agonist but is not available in a patch.

5. **The answer is A:** may have a shorter half-life than the opioid agonist. Treatment of opioid overdose often requires repeated doses of naloxone or continuous infusion to compete with the agonist at the receptor. Answer B, is effective only at high cumulative doses, is not true, and even the first dose of naloxone may provide miraculous reversal of opioid overdose. Answers C through E are not true.

CHAPTER 24

1. **The answer is E:** selective dopamine reuptake inhibition. Although this mechanism of action would be beneficial in the treatment of parkinsonism because it would lead to an increase in synaptic levels of dopamine, no such agents are currently available. Answer A, direct dopamine agonist, is a mechanism used by dopamine agonists such as bromocriptine. Answer B, precursor loading, is the mechanism of L-dopa. Answer C, dopamine metabolism inhibition, is used by selegiline. Answer D, cholinergic receptor blocking, is a mechanism also used for the treatment of parkinsonism by such agents as benztropine.

2. **The answer is C:** direct β-adrenoceptor stimulation. Metabolism of L-dopa in the periphery to dopamine can lead to cardiac arrhythmias by direct action of dopamine on cardiac β-adrenoceptors. Administration of L-dopa with carbidopa will decrease the formation of dopamine in the periphery and decrease the likelihood of cardiac abnormalities. Answer A, direct action on cardiac dopamine receptors, may be a possible mechanism

if there were significant dopamine receptors in the heart modulating cardiac rhythm, but there are not. Answer B, decreased release of catecholamines, would decrease cardiac stimulation. Answer D, increased release of dopamine, is not the best answer because increased peripheral formation is not the same as increased neuronal release. Answer E, interaction with vagal cholinergic receptors, might affect cardiac function, but dopamine or L-dopa has no interaction with cholinergic receptors.

3. **The answer is C:** neurotransmitter imbalance in the basal ganglia. The decrease of dopamine projections to the striatum results in a relative abundance of acetylcholine activity in the striatum. Acetylcholine (muscarinic) antagonists rebalance this abnormality. Answer A, decreased levels of acetylcholine from loss of neurons, would not be a reason to give an antagonist to correct this condition. Answer B, the continuing degeneration of dopamine neurons, is a fact of the progression of the disease state, but antimuscarinic agents do not retard the progression of parkinsonism. Answer D, increased activity of acetylcholinesterase, is not correct because no evidence of enzyme up-regulation in parkinsonism exists. Answer E, increased release of dopamine in basal ganglia, is clearly wrong because the disease is caused by the degeneration of dopamine neurons.

4. **The answer is A:** it is a selective MAO-B inhibitor. Selegiline retards the progress of parkinsonism by inhibiting the formation of free radicals from the action of MAO-B on dopamine. Answer B, it blocks the reuptake of dopamine, would be a possible treatment, but no drug like this has been tried in the treatment of parkinsonism. Answer C, it irreversibly binds to COMT, may cause increased dopamine, but this is not the mechanism of selegiline. Answer D, it increases release of dopamine vesicles, is the mechanism of amantadine. Answer E, it blocks muscarinic cholinergic receptors, is the mechanism of anticholinergic agents used for the treatment of parkinsonism.

5. **The answer is A:** is a receptor agonist at $GABA_B$ receptors. Baclofen is presently the only $GABA_B$-receptor agonist approved for the treatment of spasticity. Answers B through E are incorrect because they are the mechanisms of anticholinergics, amantadine, memantine, and sedative-hypnotic agents, respectively.

CHAPTER 25

1. **The answer is C:** increasing circulating acetaldehyde concentrations. Disulfiram inhibits the acetaldehyde dehydrogenase, a step in the metabolism of alcohol. Concurrent administration of disulfiram and ethanol causes increased acetaldehyde blood levels, which is associated with flushing, nausea and vomiting, and other ill effects. Answer A, increasing plasma ethanol concentration, would not be a good ethanol treatment plan because disulfiram is approved for the treatment of alcohol dependence. Answer B, preventing the conversion of ethanol to methanol in the liver, is simply not true, and answer D, blocking the action of ethanol at its cell membrane receptor, is also incorrect. Answer E, stabilizing the cell membrane to prevent ethanol disruption, refers to an older hypothesis of ethanol action in which it was thought that ethanol fluidizes neuronal membranes and thereby disrupts ion channels and neurotransmission. This is clearly not an action of disulfiram.

2. **The answer is E:** heroin is distributed more rapidly to the brain. Heroin is an illicit opioid made by the addition of two acetyl groups at the 3 and 6 positions of the morphine molecule. Because of this, diacetylmorphine (heroin) is more lipophilic and crosses the blood-brain barrier quite rapidly to exert its reinforcing effects. Although answer A, morphine is a partial agonist, and answer B, heroin binds more tightly to opioid receptors, are wrong, answer C, morphine is metabolized faster than heroin, may be generally true because heroin has extra groups to demethylate, but the degree of reinforcement is greater with more rapidly acting agents. Answer D, morphine is first metabolized to heroin, is simply wrong.

3. **The answer is B:** LSD. This potent ergot derivative is noted for synesthesia, the phenomenon whereby the perception of sensory modalities crosses over; for example, sounds can be seen, and sights can be heard. The drugs of abuse listed as answers A and C through E are not known to have this CNS effect.

4. **The answer is E:** increased intraocular pressure. This is not an effect of marijuana use, and indeed, THC, the active ingredient in marijuana, shows promise as a treatment for glaucoma, which is increased intraocular pressure. The other adverse effects listed as answers A through D are true concerning the chronic use of marijuana.

5. **The answer is C:** reinforcement is greater with inhalation versus insufflation. The crack epidemic was caused by the switch from insufflation (snorting) to inhalation (smoking) because of the change in cocaine formulation from powder to the free base forms (crack). Answer A, cocaine in crack is more potent than cocaine in powder form, is not true; the cocaine molecule itself has the same potency regardless of form. Answers B, crack cocaine is not metabolized in humans, and D, powder cocaine reaches the brain more rapidly than crack cocaine, are simply not true. Answer E, coca plants in the 1990s were bred for greater cocaine content, may be true, but the cocaine molecule itself would not have been altered.

CHAPTER 26

1. **The answer is E:** meclizine. Meclizine is a first-generation antihistamine with higher antiemetic activity than other agents and is also less sedating. Answers A through C are second-generation antihistamines and gain little access to the CNS and thus are nonsedating and ideal for treating allergies but would be little help for motion sickness. Answer D, diphenhydramine, has antiemetic effects but is more sedating than meclizine and thus is not the ideal treatment agent. Dimenhydrinate, which is a mixture of diphenhydramine and 8-chlorotheophylline, is used for motion sickness, however.

2. **The answer is B:** ability to cross the blood-brain barrier. The major problem with treatment of allergies with the first-generation antihistamines is the adverse effects of sedation. Answer A, selectivity at H_1 receptors, may be the case for select first-generation versus second-generation agents but is not the major difference between the classes. Answer C, effectiveness in treating allergies, is not correct because both can effectively treat the symptoms of allergies, but second-generation agents can do so without significant sedation. Answer D, potency at blocking H_1 receptors, is another measure of antagonist

affinity and is not correct for the same reasons that A is not correct. Answer E, indications for use, is not correct because both types of agents are used for allergies.

3. **The answer is D:** 5-HT$_3$. This type of receptor for serotonin is famous as the only biogenic amine receptor that is ionotropic. The other answers, A through C and E, are all types of metabotropic receptors, also known as G protein-coupled receptors.

4. **The answer is C:** epoprostenol. Epoprostenol is the same substance as PGI$_2$ (prostacyclin) and is used for the treatment of pulmonary hypertension. Answer A, misoprostol, is a synthetic PGE$_1$ analog that is available in an orally administered formulation for the prevention of NSAID-induced gastric ulcers and duodenal ulcers. Answer B, alprostadil, is a naturally occurring prostaglandin but is known as PGE$_1$. Answer D, treprostinil, is also used for pulmonary hypertension but is a stable analog of prostacyclin, not the same as prostacyclin itself. Answer E, travoprost, is a PGF$_{2\alpha}$ analog and an agonist at FP receptors. It is used for the treatment of open-angle glaucoma.

5. **The answer is B:** ocular hypertension and open-angle glaucoma. Latanoprost, like bimatoprost and travoprost, is an agonist at the PGF$_{2\alpha}$ receptors and is among the most prescribed classes of antiglaucoma agents. Answer A, cornea abrasions, might call for the use of an ocular antihistamine. Answer C, ocular albinism, might make sense considering the bizarre adverse effect of latanoprost in darkening the color of the iris but is not approved by the U.S. Food and Drug Administration as an indication for latanoprost. Answer D, closed-angle glaucoma, is usually treated by carbonic anhydrase inhibitors (e.g., acetazolamide) because the pressure rises very high inside the eye and needs to be dropped rapidly. Answer E, allergic conjunctivitis, is best treated by one of the ocular antihistamines.

CHAPTER 27

1. **The answer is A:** Montelukast blocks receptors for leukotrienes C$_4$, D$_4$, and E$_4$. It does not inhibit cytochrome P450 enzymes (B) or leukotriene synthesis (D). Monteleukast is taken as a single daily dose in the evening and not twice daily (C). It is not excreted unchanged (E) but is extensively metabolized before excretion.

2. **The answer is B:** zileuton. Zileuton inhibits 5-lipoxygenase and decreases formation of all leukotrienes, including leukotrienes LTB$_4$, LTC$_4$, LTD$_4$, and LTE$_4$. Theophylline (A) is a nonspecific phosphodiesterase inhibitor, whereas roflumilast (E) is a specific type IV phosphodiesterase inhibitor. Zafirlukast (C) blocks receptors for cysteinyl leukotrienes, and fluticasone (D) is a corticosteroid.

3. **The answer is E:** blockade of calcium influx. The patient is most likely using an ophthalmic solution of lodoxamide or nedocromil, which are drugs related to cromolyn. These drugs block calcium influx into mast cells and thereby prevent degranulation and release of histamine and other allergy mediators. Lodoxamide does not activate β$_2$-adrenoceptors (A), decrease cytokine production (B), block muscarinic receptors (C), or inhibit 5-lipoxygenase (D).

4. **The answer is A:** immunoglobulin E. The patient is most likely taking omalizumab, a monoclonal antibody that inactivates immunoglobulin E and thereby prevents

asthma attacks induced by allergies. Antibodies to leukotriene C$_4$ (B), major basic protein (C), histamine (D), or interleukin-2 (E) are not used in treating asthma.

5. **The answer is C:** formoterol. Formoterol is a long-acting β$_2$-agonist that may cause tachycardia and death in asthmatic patients. Although ipratropium (B) may occasionally cause tachycardia, the drug is poorly absorbed after inhalation and is less likely to cause severe tachycardia than are the β$_2$-agonists. Budesonide, cromolyn, and montelukast (A, D, and E) are even less likely to cause tachycardia.

CHAPTER 28

1. **The answer is E:** dry mouth. The woman is most likely taking scopolamine, a muscarinic receptor antagonist that may cause dry mouth. Scopolamine is more likely to cause constipation than diarrhea (D), and it is unlikely to cause flatulence, heartburn, or headache (A, B, and C).

2. **The answer is B:** ischemic colitis. Alosetron is used to treat diarrhea-predominant IBS, but it may rarely cause ischemic colitis. It is not associated with pulmonary fibrosis, ischemic heart disease, gastric ulcer, or muscle rigidity and tremor (A, C, D, and E). However, tegaserod is a 5HT$_4$ agonist used for treating constipation-predominant IBS that slightly increases the risk of ischemic heart disease (angina and myocardial infarction).

3. **The answer is D:** a proton pump inhibitor (PPI, pantoprazole) plus two or three antimicrobial agents provide the most rapid and effective treatment for *H. pylori* infection. Combinations that include sucralfate or histamine H$_2$ blockers such as famotidine (A and C) require longer durations of treatment than combinations containing a PPI. Likewise, a bismuth compound plus tetracycline (B) is not the best antimicrobial drug combination for this infection, and antimicrobial agents used alone (E) have not been as effective as regimens that include an acid inhibitor.

4. **The answer is C:** dopamine D$_2$ receptor blockade. Metoclopramide increases lower esophageal sphincter tone by blocking dopamine D$_2$ receptors and increasing acetylcholine release, thereby activating muscarinic receptors in esophageal muscle. Metoclopramide does not block muscarinic or histamine receptors (A and B), and it does not activate α-adrenoceptors or chloride channels (D and E).

5. **The answer is A:** palonosetron, dexamethasone, and aprepitant. Current guidelines recommend a three-drug combination to prevent acute emesis with highly emetogenic drugs such as cisplatin. The combination should include a serotonin 5-HT$_3$ antagonist, dexamethasone, and aprepitant (or rolapiptant). Single- and dual-drug therapies are less effective for this purpose (B, C, D, and E).

CHAPTER 29

1. **The answer is A:** zolmitriptan. The triptan agents are effective only in the acute treatment of a migraine headache. They are agonists at 5-HT$_{1B/1D}$ receptors in cerebral blood vessels that produce vasoconstriction on trigeminal nerve endings, inhibiting the release of inflammatory substances and in the brain stem to prevent activation

of trigeminal nerves. Answers B through E have shown various degrees of effectiveness in preventing migraines in controlled studies.

2. **The answer is B:** patients with uncontrolled hypertension. Triptans can increase blood pressure by constriction of peripheral smooth muscle. This is also a contraindication for using ergot agents such as DHE and ergotamine. Answers A, C, D, and E are not conditions warranting contraindications for triptan use.

3. **The answer is B:** stimulation of serotonin 5-HT$_{1D}$ receptors. These agents are agonists at 5-HT$_{1B/1D}$ receptors. Answers A and C through E are mechanisms of other agents unrelated to the clinically used triptan drugs.

4. **The answer is E:** blocks calcium channels. Verapamil is used for the treatment of migraine or, better stated, the prophylactic treatment to prevent migraine attacks because of its ability to block calcium channels and cause vasodilation. Other answer choices are not the primary mechanism of action of verapamil.

5. **The answer is C:** dihydroergotamine. DHE is an ergot alkaloid, and these agents are known to cause vasoconstriction and paresthesia in the extremities, especially at high doses. Answer A, butorphanol, is an opioid analgesic and not associated with the woman's symptoms. Answer B, sumatriptan, is a triptan also used for acute attacks and can cause vasoconstriction, but not as commonly as observed with DHE. Answer D, tramadol, is a dual-action opioid-antidepressant agent, helpful in the acute treatment of migraine but not producing the patient's constellation of adverse effects. Answer E, naproxen, is an NSAID agent that can cause increased release of norepinephrine and possible vasoconstriction, but it does not produce these effects as commonly as DHE.

CHAPTER 30

1. **The answer is C:** thromboxane A$_2$. Aspirin binds irreversibly to COX enzymes in platelets, and because the platelets do not have a nucleus and cannot synthesize new COX protein, the effect of aspirin persists until the platelet is taken out of circulation. Thromboxane A$_2$ produces vasoconstriction and promotes the formation of clots; therefore, aspirin can prevent clot formation and coronary thrombosis. Answer B, prostacyclin (prostaglandin I2 [PGI2]), is also inhibited by aspirin because it is a COX product, but the particular enzyme to synthesize PGI2 is not found in platelets. The other agents are not affected by aspirin administration.

2. **The answer is D:** it is selective for a newly discovered isozyme of COX. This isozyme, called COX-3, appears to be a splice variant of COX-1 (from the same gene, but with different posttranscriptional processing of the RNA). It is also sometimes mentioned that the peroxide formation at sites of inflammation inhibits the activity of acetaminophen, but this may be less of a factor now that COX-3 is recognized. Answers A through C are not correct, and answer E is not true to a greater degree than other NSAIDs that do have antiinflammatory action.

3. **The answer is E:** anakinra. Anakinra, a recombinant form of the human IL-1Ra protein, blocks the biologic activity of IL-1 by competitively inhibiting IL-1 binding to IL-1RI. Answer A, adalimumab, is a human IgG1 monoclonal antibody specific for human TNF. Answer B,

leflunomide, is an immunosuppressive drug that inhibits mononuclear and T-cell proliferation. Answer C, etanercept, is a protein formed by recombining human p75 TNF receptors with Fc fragments of human IgG1. Answer D, infliximab, is a chimeric human-murine (mouse) monoclonal antibody that inactivates TNF and is approved for the treatment of Crohn disease and RA.

4. **The answer is D:** leukocyte migration. The invasion of leukocytes (macrophages and so on) into the joint capsule and subsequent release of inflammatory cytokines are parts of a key process in the progression of gout. The agent that disrupts tubulin formation is colchicine. Other processes given as answers are not important regarding colchicine action.

5. **The answer is B:** allopurinol. The two main strategies for treating gout are to increase the excretion of uric acid with a uricosuric agent (probenecid or lesinurad) or decrease the production of uric acid by inhibiting xanthine oxidase with allopurinol. The 24-hour rate of uric acid excretion provides a guideline for which therapy to use: if less than 800 mg, use a uricosuric because there is too little excretion of uric acid; and if more than 800 mg, use allopurinol because there is too much uric acid being made.

CHAPTER 31

1. **The answer is C:** leuprolide. Leuprolide is an agonist at pituitary receptors for gonadotropin-releasing hormone (GnRH). When administered continuously, rather than in a physiologically pulsatile manner, leuprolide and other GnRH agonists cause down-regulation of GnRH receptors, leading to decreased secretion of gonadotropins (luteinizing hormone [LH] and follicle-stimulating hormone [FSH]). This action reduces secretion of gonadal steroids and thereby slows the onset of puberty in children with precocious puberty.

2. **The answer is A:** pegvisomant. Pegvisomant is used in the treatment of acromegaly and acts by blocking receptors for growth hormone and thereby reduces the formation of insulin-like growth factors (IGFs) that mediate the growth-stimulating and other effects of growth hormone. Other drugs used to treat acromegaly act by reducing growth hormone secretion: octreotide (C) and cabergoline (E). Somatropin (B) is a recombinant form of human growth hormone, while leuprolide (D) is a GnRH agonist.

3. **The answer is D:** activates receptors for prolactin-inhibiting hormone. Prolactin secretion is ordinarily restrained by tonic secretion of prolactin-inhibiting hormone (PIH or dopamine). Cabergoline and bromocriptine are dopamine receptor agonists that act to mimic the effect of endogenous prolactin-inhibiting hormone and thereby reduce excessive prolactin secretion in persons with prolactin-secreting pituitary adenomas. The other choices (A, B, C, and E) are plausible mechanisms for reducing prolactin secretion or activity but are not actions of currently available drugs for this indication.

4. **The answer is D:** It is a more potent inhibitor of growth hormone secretion than is somatostatin. Octreotide contains only eight amino acids and is not identical to somatostatin (A and E). It is not administered orally (C), and it is not used to treat growth hormone

deficiency (B). In fact, octreotide is used to treat acromegaly caused by excessive growth hormone secretion (as is pegvisomant).

5. **The answer is B:** follitropin alfa then lutropin alfa. Follitropin alfa is an FSH preparation used to stimulate maturation of the ovarian follicle. It is given for 9 to 12 days, followed by a dose of the LH preparation, lutropin alfa. Choice A (choriogonadotropin alfa and lutropin alfa) and choice D (hCG and lutropin alfa) both consist of two LH preparations. Choice C (choriogonadotropin alfa and follitropin beta) is incorrect because the FSH and LH preparations are given in the wrong sequence. Choice E (follitropin alfa and follitropin beta) consists of two FSH preparations.

CHAPTER 32

1. **The answer is D:** inhibition of thyroid hormone release. Potassium iodide reduces the release of thyroid hormone and is given before thyroid surgery to reduce the size and vascularity of the gland and facilitate surgical removal. It does not inhibit TSH secretion (C), inhibit the sodium/iodide symporter (A), reduce synthesis of thyroid hormones by thyroperoxidase (B), or cause destruction of thyroid tissue (E).

2. **The answer is C:** pruritic rash. The most common adverse effect of thioamide drugs such as methimazole and propylthiouracil is a maculopapular pruritic (itchy) rash. These drugs cause agranulocytosis (E) and liver failure (D) only rarely. Propranolol and other beta blockers may cause hypotension and bradycardia (A), but thioamide drugs do not. Thromboembolism (B) is also not associated with methimazole and propylthiouracil.

3. **The answer is A:** partly converted to T_3 in the body. About 35% of levothyroxine is converted to triiodothyronine in various tissues. Levothyroxine is administered once a day, rather than several times (B), and it has a half-life of 7 days, rather than 1 day (D). and is not as potent as liothyronine (synthetic T_3). Its oral bioavailability is about 80% rather than 95% (E). Liothyronine (T_3) is the most potent synthetic thyroid hormone preparation (C).

4. **The answer is D:** potassium iodide. After a nuclear reactor accident, uptake of radioactive iodide may destroy thyroid tissue. Potassium iodide competes with radioactive iodide for uptake by the thyroid gland, and sufficient doses can prevent thyroid gland destruction. Liothyronine (A), methimazole (B), propranolol (C), and levothyroxine (E) would have no effect on radioactive iodide uptake by the thyroid gland.

5. **The answer is B:** inhibiting enzymes forming T_3 and T_4. PTU and Methimazole and are thioamide drugs that inhibit peroxidase-catalyzed steps in the synthesis of thyroid hormone. PTU also inhibits the peripheral conversion of T_4 to T_3. The drug effects are not observed until after the depletion of thyroid hormone already in the thyroid. Answer (A) is the mechanism of action of beta-blockers that are used sometimes during a thyroid storm. (C) destroying thyroid tissue is how radioactive iodine (RAI) works. (D) inhibiting release of T_3 and T_4 is one of the actions of potassium iodide, which also reduces the vascularity and size of the thyroid gland before surgery. Answer (E), acting on thyroid hormone receptors,

is the action of the substitution drugs, levothyroxine and liothyronine.

CHAPTER 33

1. **The answer is D:** Cushing syndrome. In healthy persons, a dose of dexamethasone should suppress cortisol secretion the next morning, and cortisol levels should be less than 5 mcg/dL. In this case, the patient's cortisol level was elevated, suggesting the presence of Cushing syndrome. Congenital adrenal hyperplasia, chronic adrenal insufficiency, 11β-hydroxylase deficiency, and pituitary insufficiency are all associated with decreased cortisol secretion.

2. **The answer is D:** gradually decreasing doses over several days. For the treatment of acute allergic reactions, the most effective regimens are those in which glucocorticoids are given in large doses initially and then gradually tapered over 5 to 7 days. This produces the most rapid improvement in symptoms while causing relatively little adrenal suppression.

3. **The answer is B:** fludrocortisone. Fludrocortisone is approximately 100 times more potent as a mineralocorticoid than is cortisol and is the most potent mineralocorticoid available for clinical use. It acts to increase sodium retention and potassium excretion, thereby lowering serum potassium levels. Aldosterone (E), an endogenous mineralocorticoid, is not available as a drug. Dexamethasone (A), triamcinolone (C), and prednisone (D) are potent glucocorticoids that would cause excessive glucocorticoid effects in a person already receiving adequate doses of hydrocortisone.

4. **The answer is D:** aldosterone. Exogenous administration of glucocorticoid drugs causes feedback inhibition of the secretion of corticotropin-releasing hormone, corticotropin, cortisol, and cortisone. Secretion of the mineralocorticoid aldosterone is primarily under the influence of the renin-angiotensin axis and is not suppressed greatly by exogenous glucocorticoid administration.

5. **The answer is A:** desonide. Desonide is a low-potency topical corticosteroid appropriate for treating conditions of the face and eyes. Prednisone (B) is not administered topically. Clobetasol (C) is a very high-potency topical steroid, and fluocinonide (D) and desoximetasone (E) are high-potency topical steroids. Medium- to high-potency steroids are used on areas of the body with thicker skin than on the face and eyes.

CHAPTER 34

1. **The answer is B:** osteoporosis. Raloxifene has antiestrogen effects on breast and uterine tissue but estrogenic effects on bone, and it is used to prevent osteoporosis. It is also used to reduce the risk of breast cancer in postmenopausal women. It is not indicated for the treatment of thromboembolism (A), menopausal symptoms (C) or endometriosis (D), or for contraception (E). In fact, raloxifene increases the risk of thromboembolism.

2. **The answer is B:** endometrial cancer. Postmenopausal women receiving HRT should receive a progestin for 10 to 13 days each month to suppress endometrial hyperplasia that would otherwise be produced by unopposed estrogen therapy. A progestin is not required in women who have had a hysterectomy. Inclusion of a progestin will

not prevent (A) breast cancer, (C) myocardial infarction, (D) stroke, or (E) elevated cholesterol levels.

3. **The answer is E:** hot flashes. Bicalutamide, flutamide, and nilutamide are androgen receptor antagonists that prevent feedback inhibition of hypothalamic GnRH secretion in men, leading to hot flashes. These drugs do not cause (A), breast tenderness, (B) alopecia, (C) glaucoma, or (D) deep vein thrombosis.

4. **The answer is B:** irregular menstrual cycles. Progestin contraceptives act in part by thickening cervical mucus and decreasing sperm penetration. An irregular or unpredictable menstrual cycle is one of the main reasons women discontinue progestin-only contraceptives. Progestins do not typically cause (A) venous thromboembolism, (C) hot flashes, (D) breast enlargement, or (E) hypertension.

5. **The answer is A:** aldosterone. Drospirenone is a synthetic progestin used in an estrogen-progestin oral contraceptive. It blocks both androgen and aldosterone receptors and lowers blood pressure by decreasing salt and water retention due to aldosterone antagonism. Drospirenone does not block estrogen, progestin, gonadotropin, or glucocorticoid receptors (B, C, D, and E).

CHAPTER 35

1. **The answer is A:** closing of potassium channels. The meglitinide drugs such as nateglinide are taken 30 minutes before meals to control postprandial glycemia. These drugs increase insulin secretion in the same manner as sulfonylureas by inhibiting ATP-sensitive potassium channel in pancreatic beta cells. This leads to closing of potassium channels, membrane depolarization, and insulin secretion. Slowed gastric emptying (B), is caused by an amylin analog (pramlintide) and by incretin mimetics such as exenatide. Inhibition of α-glucosidase (C) is the mechanism of acarbose and miglitol. Inhibition of DPP-4 (D) is produced by sitagliptin. Insertion of glucose transporters in cell membranes (E) results from pioglitazone administration.

2. **The answer is B:** nausea and anorexia. Pramlintide is an amylin analog that slows gastric emptying and the delivery of carbohydrates to the intestines, but it can cause nausea, vomiting, and anorexia. Increased appetite (A) and weight gain (D) are adverse effects of sulfonylurea drugs such as glyburide. Flatulence and bloating (C) are side effects of α-glucosidase inhibitors such as acarbose. Increased risk of heart failure (E) is associated with pioglitazone.

3. **The answer is D:** insertion of glucose transporters in cell membranes. Pioglitazone activates peroxisome proliferator-activated receptor-γ (PPAR-γ) and causes insertion of GLUT 4 glucose transporter molecules into cell membranes of muscle and adipose tissue. Pioglitazone tends to raise HDL cholesterol rather than lower it (B), and to lower triglyceride levels rather than increase them (C). It may cause weight gain rather than weight loss (E).

4. **The answer is D:** it is slowly absorbed over 24 hours. Insulin glargine is a type of long-acting insulin injected once a day to meet the basal insulin requirement of diabetics. It is not injected at mealtimes (A), and it does not have proline and lysine transposed in the B chain (B), as does insulin lispro. Insulin glargine does not have aspartate substituted for proline (C), as in insulin aspart. Insulin glargine is not administered by inhalation (E), as

is a preparation of powdered recombinant regular human insulin (Afrezza).

5. **The answer is C:** diarrhea. Diarrhea occurs in about one-third of patients taking metformin, though it usually can be controlled by taking psyllium or polycarbophil. Metformin is not associated with an increased risk of heart failure (A) as is pioglitazone, and it tends to cause weight loss rather than weight gain (B), which is associated with sulfonylurea drugs such as glipizide. Metformin only rarely causes lactic acidosis (D), and it does not typically cause hypoglycemia (E), as do insulin secretagogues such as glipizide and repaglinide.

CHAPTER 36

1. **The answer is D:** raloxifene. Raloxifene activates estrogen receptors in bone and reduces osteoclast activation. It acts as an estrogen antagonist in breast and other tissues and can increase the incidence and severity of estrogen withdrawal symptoms such as hot flashes. Alendronate (A), denosumab (B), and calcitonin (C) reduce osteoclast activation but do not interact with estrogen receptors and cause hot flashes. Teriparatide (E) promotes osteoblast activity rather than inhibiting osteoclast production, and it does not cause hot flashes.

2. **The answer is D:** zoledronic acid. Zoledronic acid is a potent bisphosphonate drug that is given intravenously to prevent bone loss and hypercalcemia in persons with malignancies. It is not indicated for the treatment of osteoporosis. Calcitonin (A) and ibandronate (B) are used to treat osteoporosis but not osteolytic bone lesions. Calcitriol (C) is the active form of vitamin D and is used to prevent hypocalcemia and its various manifestations, but it does not prevent osteolytic bone lesions. Cinacalcet (E) increases the sensitivity of calcium receptors in the parathyroid gland and is used to treat hyperparathyroidism and parathyroid cancer.

3. **The answer is D:** increased activity of osteoblasts. Teriparatide stimulates bone formation by promoting differentiation of preosteoblasts to osteoblasts and is given by daily subcutaneous injection. Teriparatide does not increase absorption of dietary calcium (A), increase serum levels of vitamin D (B), decrease activation of osteoclasts (C), or adsorb to bone (E).

4. **The answer is B.** decreased urine hydroxyproline levels. The man most likely has Paget disease of bone and was treated with calcitonin. Calcitonin decreases bone resorption and markers of abnormal bone turnover, such as elevated urine hydroxyproline levels by stimulating a G-protein coupled receptor leading to increased cyclic AMP levels. Calcitonin decreases, rather than increases, serum alkaline phosphatase activity (A), and it decreases, rather than increases, bone turnover (C). Calcitonin decreases, rather than increases, serum calcium levels (D). Calcitonin does not increase osteoblast activity (E).

5. **The answer is A:** risedronate. Risedronate, as well as alendronate, and ibandronate are approved for treatment of osteoporosis. These drugs adsorb to hydroxyapatite and remain in bone for years. The other choices, teriparatide (B), calcitonin (C), denosumab (D), and vitamin D_3 (E), are employed in the prevention and treatment of osteoporosis, but none of them adsorb to hydroxyapatite and remain in bone for years.

CHAPTER 37

1. **The answer is E:** P-glycoprotein. P-glycoprotein is a cell membrane protein that pumps antibiotics and other drugs out of mammalian and microbial cells. It prevents accumulation of drugs in target cells and is one of the mechanisms that confer resistance to chemotherapeutic agents. Plasmids (A) contain extra-chromosomal DNA that may contain transferable resistance genes. Porins (B) are outer membrane proteins in gram-negative bacteria that permit entry of antibiotics. Resistance factor (C) usually refers to a gene encoding a mechanism of bacterial resistance. β-lactamase (D) is an enzyme that inactivates penicillins and cephalosporin antibiotics.

2. **The answer is B:** postantibiotic effect. The *postantibiotic effect* (PAE) refers to a period of time during which bacterial growth continues to be inhibited after an antibiotic has been removed from a bacterial culture or eliminated from the body. The PAE increases the effective duration of action of antimicrobial agents and enables less-frequent administration of some antibiotics. Bacteriostatic (A) refers to an antibiotic that inhibits but does not kill a bacteria. Time-dependent killing (C) is a property of antibiotics whose bactericidal effect depends on the length of time a microbe is exposed to the drug, whereas concentration-depending killing (D) refers to a killing effect that is proportional to drug concentration. Synergistic effect (E) describes an antimicrobial effect of two drugs that is greater than the sum of their individual effects.

3. **The answer is C:** synergism. A synergistic effect occurs when the combined effect of two drugs is greater than the sum of their individual effects. Several antibiotic combinations show synergism against susceptible organisms, such as gentamicin and ampicillin against enterococci. Mutual antagonism (A) refers to two drugs that both inhibit the effect of the other drug. Indifference (B) refers to a drug combination in which neither drug has an effect on the other drug's antimicrobial activity. Additive (D) describes the effect of two antibiotics whose combined effect is the sum of their individual effects. Competition (E) occurs when a drug inhibits the effect of another drug or an endogenous substance.

4. **The answer is D:** plasmid exchange. *Transferable drug resistance* refers to the transfer of genes conferring resistance to other bacteria. Most commonly, this occurs by bacterial conjugation followed by the exchange of plasmids containing resistance genes. Transduction (transfer of bacterial DNA by a bacteriophage; choice A) and transformation (uptake of naked DNA; choice B) are not common mechanisms of transferable drug resistance. Mutation and selection (E) is not a type of transferable resistance.

5. **The answer is A:** E-test strip method. The E-test strip is a semiquantitative antibiotic diffusion device for determining the MIC of an antibiotic. It is based on visualization of the point of intersection between the zone of bacterial growth inhibition and the concentration scale on the test strip. The E-test method is more convenient and economical than broth dilution methods (B). The disk diffusion method (C) enables the determination of microbial sensitivity but does not determine the MIC. Growth rate method and turbidity method (D and E) are not procedures used to determine a MIC.

CHAPTER 38

1. **The answer is D:** *Pseudomonas aeruginosa*. Aztreonam is a monobactam antibiotic that does not bind to penicillin-binding proteins in gram-positive bacteria, and it is not effective for the treatment of infections due to *Staphylococcus aureus* (A), *Enterococcus faecium* (B), *Streptococcus pneumoniae* (C), or *Bacillus anthracis* (E). Aztreonam is used to treat serious infections due to gram-negative bacteria, including *P. aeruginosa*. Infections due to methicillin-sensitive *S. aureus* can be treated with an anti-staphylococcal penicillin (nafcillin) or a first-generation cephalosporin (cephalexin). Methicillin-resistant S. aureus infections can be treated with vancomycin and agents listed in Table 39.4. Enterococcal infections are treated with ampicillin, vancomycin, linezolid, or quinupristin-dalfopristin (see Chapter 39). Pneumococcal infections can be treated with a penicillin, a cephalosporin, a macrolide antibiotic, tigecycline (see Chapter 39), or a fluoroquinolone (see Chapter 40). Anthrax (*B. anthracis*) can be treated with a fluoroquinolone.

2. **The answer is A:** avibactam. Avibactam is the only currently available β-lactamase inhibitor that is active against some Class C and other extended-spectrum β-lactamases. It is available in combination with ceftazidime for treating complicated infections. Clavulanate (B), sulbactam (C), and tazobactam (D) are only active against Class A beta-lactamases. Monobactam is the name of the class of antibiotics represented by aztreonam, which is not a β-lactamase inhibitor.

3. **The answer is E:** impaired hearing. Higher doses of vancomycin may cause ototoxicity, including both vestibular effects such as vertigo and ataxia and cochlear effects such as impaired hearing. Vancomycin is not typically associated with hepatitis (A), alopecia (B), hallucinations (C), or hypertension (D).

4. **The answer is C:** urinary tract infection. Fosfomycin is a unique bacterial cell wall inhibitor that is given as a single large dose to treat uncomplicated urinary tract infections. It is not used to treat gonorrhea (A), syphilis (B), impetigo (D), or traveler's diarrhea (D). Gonorrhea may be treated with ceftriaxone in combination with azithromycin or doxycycline. Syphilis can be treated with a single dose of long-acting benzathine penicillin. Traveler's diarrhea is treated with a fluoroquinolone or rifaximin (see Chapter 40). Impetigo can be treated with topical mupirocin, amoxicillin-clavulanate, or a first-generation cephalosporin.

5. **The answer is B:** imipenem. Imipenem is degraded by renal dehydropeptidase, and cilastatin is administered in combination with imipenem to inhibit this enzyme. Ceftazidime (A), piperacillin (C), vancomycin (D), and bacitracin (E) are not degraded by dehydropeptidase or given with cilastatin. Ceftazidime is used alone or in combination with the β-lactamase inhibitor avibactam, while piperacillin is often administered in combination with tazobactam. Bacitracin is only active against gram-positive organisms and can be administered with other antibiotics that inhibit gram-negative organisms to treat or prevent skin infections.

CHAPTER 39

1. **The answer is C:** thrombocytopenia. Linezolid binds the 23S RNA component of the 50S ribosomal subunit and prevents formation of the 70S initiation complex

required for bacterial protein synthesis. It may cause bone marrow suppression leading to thrombocytopenia, anemia, or leukopenia. It is not typically associated with myalgia and arthralgia (A), which may be caused by quinupristin-dalfopristin. Nystagmus and vertigo (B) may be caused by aminoglycosides such as gentamicin, whereas discoloration of body fluids (D) is most likely due to rifampin. Flushing and hypotension (E) may result from administration of vancomycin.

2. **The answer is A:** initiation. Gentamicin and other aminoglycosides bind the 30S ribosomal subunit. Aminoglycosides prevent formation of the protein synthesis initiation complex and cause misreading of messenger RNA. Peptide bond formation (B) catalyzed by peptidyl transferase is blocked by macrolides such as erythromycin, chloramphenicol, and dalfopristin. Isoleucine t-RNA synthesis (C) is inhibited by mupirocin. Peptide translocation on the ribosome (D) is prevented by macrolides and clindamycin, while t-RNA binding to the 30S ribosomal subunit (E) is blocked by tetracyclines.

3. **The answer is C:** doxycycline. Doxycycline is used to treat chlamydial urethritis and may cause photodermatitis after sun exposure. Azithromycin (A) and erythromycin (D) are also used to treat chlamydial infections but do not typically cause photodermatitis. Clindamycin (B) and mupirocin (E) are not used to treat chlamydial infections and do not cause photodermatitis.

4. **The answer is D:** tobramycin. Aminoglycoside antibiotics such as tobramycin are ionized in body fluids and must be given parenterally for systemic infections. Doxycycline (A), azithromycin (B), clindamycin (C), and linezolid (E) exhibit good oral bioavailability and can be given orally or parenterally to treat infections.

5. **The answer is E:** quinupristin-dalfopristin. Antibiotics active against vancomycin-resistant strains of *E. faecium* include quinupristin-dalfopristin and linezolid. Azithromycin (A), doxycycline (B), chloramphenicol (C), and clindamycin (D) are not active against *E. faecium*. Gentamicin is sometimes used to treat enterococcal endocarditis in combination with other drugs, though its activity against vancomycin-resistant strains is uncertain.

CHAPTER 40

1. **The answer is D:** ciprofloxacin. Fluoroquinolones such as ciprofloxacin may cause tendonitis and tendon rupture. Trimethoprim (A) may rarely cause megaloblastic anemia in persons with inadequate folate intake, while daptomycin (B) may cause muscle toxicity. Sulfonamides such as sulfacetamide (C) may cause skin rash, gastrointestinal reactions, headache, hepatitis, and hematologic effects. Polymyxin B (E) is primarily used topically because systemic administration can cause nephrotoxicity and neurotoxicity.

2. **The answer is B:** polymyxin B and daptomycin. These two agents disrupt cell membrane function leading to loss of potassium and other effects. Trimethoprim and sulfamethoxazole (A) inhibit bacterial folate synthesis. Rifaximin and fidaxomicin (C) impair RNA synthesis by inhibiting RNA polymerase. Ciprofloxacin and moxifloxacin (D) inhibit DNA topoisomerases. Nitrofurantoin

(E) is believed to form reactive intermediates in bacterial cells that damage various cell constituents, while fosfomycin inhibits bacterial cell wall synthesis.

3. **The answer is C:** glucose-6-phosphate dehydrogenase deficiency. Sulfonamides may cause hemolytic anemia in persons with glucose-6-phosphate dehydrogenase deficiency. Trimethoprim-induced folate deficiency (B) may lead to megaloblastic anemia but not to hemolytic anemia. Immunodeficiency (A) predisposes to *Nocardia* infections but not to hemolytic anemia. Iron and thiamine deficiencies (D and E) are not specifically related to hemolytic anemia.

4. **The answer is B:** rifaximin. Rifaximin is a rifampin derivative that is not absorbed from the gut and is used to treat diarrhea caused by susceptible organisms. Ciprofloxacin (A) and trimethoprim-sulfamethoxazole (TMP-SMX) (B) have also been used to treat traveler's diarrhea, but they are both well absorbed from the gut. Moreover, TMP-SMX is not a reliable therapy for this condition in many countries. Daptomycin and nitrofurantoin (D and E) are not used to treat traveler's diarrhea.

5. **The answer is B:** gatifloxacin. Fluoroquinolones such as gatifloxacin inhibit bacterial DNA topoisomerases, including DNA gyrase. Mutations to DNA gyrase may reduce drug binding and effects. Bacterial resistance to trimethoprim (A) and sulfamethoxazole (C) may result from mutations to the genes for their target enzymes, dihydropteroate synthase and dihydrofolate reductase, respectively. The mechanisms of resistance to daptomycin (D) and nitrofurantoin (E) are uncertain but unlikely to involve DNA gyrase.

CHAPTER 41

1. **The answer is B:** isoniazid. Isoniazid is the preferred drug for treating persons with latent TB. If isoniazid is not tolerated, rifampin (A) can be given in its place. Streptomycin (C), ethambutol (D), and pyrazinamide (E) are not recommended for treatment of latent TB.

2. **The answer is A:** rifampin. Rifampin and related antibiotics inhibit DNA-dependent RNA polymerase in bacteria and thereby reduce the formation of ribonucleic acids. Ethambutol (B) produces a bacteriostatic effect by preventing arabinogalactan synthesis required for cell wall formation. Isoniazid (C) inhibits the formation of mycolic acid. Amikacin (D) is an aminoglycoside antibiotic that interferes with protein synthesis in bacteria. Pyrazinamide (E) is believed to inhibit fatty acid synthesis and translation of messenger RNA in susceptible mycobacteria.

3. **The answer is D:** Ethambutol. Ethambutol produces a dose-dependent optic neuritis leading to impaired red-green discrimination, whereas isoniazid (A) produces peripheral neuritis (paresthesia, numbness) due to drug-induced pyridoxine (vitamin B_6) deficiency. Rifampin (B) may occasionally impair liver function. Amikacin (C) and streptomycin (E) may cause hearing impairment and renal dysfunction, while pyrazinamide (D) can cause hyperuricemia and gout, hepatitis, and hematologic toxicity.

4. **The answer is A:** isoniazid. Isoniazid is activated by the enzyme catalase-peroxidase, which is expressed by the *kat*G gene in M. *tuberculosis*. Mutations to this gene may

confer resistance to isoniazid but not to other antimycobacterial drugs. Resistance to pyrazinamide (B) is usually due to a mutation in the gene for pyrazinamidase, the bacterial enzyme that converts pyrazinamide to pyrazinoic acid, which is the active form of the drug. Resistance to amikacin (C) appears to result from mutations to the ribosomal target site of the antibiotic. Resistance to rifampin (D) is most often due to mutations to the DNA-dependent RNA polymerase, the antimicrobial target of rifampin. Resistance to ethambutol (E) may result from mutations to the gene that encodes the arabinosyl transferase enzyme that is the drug's target in mycobacteria.

5. **The answer is E:** dapsone. Dapsone and isoniazid are both metabolized in humans by conjugation with acetate catalyzed by acetyltransferase. Genetic polymorphism of this enzyme gives rise to slow and fast acetylation phenotypes. Persons with the fast phenotype metabolize these drugs more rapidly and have lower levels of unmetabolized drugs. Acetyltransferase is not involved in the elimination of other antimycobacterial drugs (A, B, C, and D).

CHAPTER 42

1. **The answer is C:** primarily excreted in the urine. Fluconazole is excreted in the urine unchanged and can be used to treat renal candidiasis. It has good oral bioavailability (not choice A), high cerebrospinal fluid concentrations (not choice B), a long elimination half-life (not choice D), and can be given orally or parenterally (not choice E).

2. **The answer is A:** micafungin. Micafungin, caspofungin, and anidulafungin are echinocandin drugs that inhibit the synthesis of β-(1,3)-D-glucan, a component of the fungal cell wall. Posaconazole (B) and other azole drugs inhibit a P450 enzyme that catalyzes the formation of the lanosterol component of the fungal membrane. Flucytosine (C) prevents the formation of fungal RNA, while nystatin (D) and amphotericin B bind to ergosterol and create pores in fungal membranes. Terbinafine (E) inhibits squalene epoxidase and the formation of the precursor to lanosterol, squalene-2, 3-oxide.

3. **The answer is E:** itraconazole. Ketoconazole and itraconazole inhibit human cytochrome P450 enzymes that may lead to a number of drug interactions. Fluconazole (B) has a greater affinity for fungal P450 enzymes than for human P450 enzymes and causes fewer drug interactions than ketoconazole and itraconazole. Likewise, amphotericin B (A), caspofungin (C), and naftifine (D) are unlikely to cause drug interactions due to inhibition of P450 enzymes.

4. **The answer is E:** headache and dizziness. Griseofulvin inhibits microtubule function and mitosis in fungi and has been used to treat tinea capitis. It may occasionally cause dizziness, headache, and insomnia, but it is unlikely to cause sedation (A), constipation (B), nausea and vomiting (C), or blurred vision (D).

5. **The answer is B:** invasive aspergillosis. Caspofungin and other echinocandin drugs are indicated for the treatment of systemic candidiasis and invasive aspergillosis. They are not indicated for treatment of pulmonary blastomycosis (A), systemic histoplasmosis (C), cryptococcal meningitis (D), or mucormycosis (E). Pulmonary blastomycosis is usually treated with itraconazole, systemic histoplasmosis with itraconazole or amphotericin B, cryptococcal meningitis with amphotericin B, and flucytosine followed by fluconazole, and mucormycosis (*Rhizopus* species and others) with amphotericin B or posaconazole.

CHAPTER 43

1. **The answer is E:** elevated triglyceride and cholesterol levels. Protease inhibitors such as darunavir and atazanavir are associated with dyslipidemia, drug-induced hepatitis, and cardiac electrocardiogram abnormalities. Anemia (A) is most often caused by zidovudine. Pancreatitis (B) and peripheral neuropathy (D) are associated with didanosine and stavudine. Neuropsychiatric reactions (C) may be caused by efavirenz.

2. **The answer is B:** inhibition of DNA polymerase. The patient received famciclovir, which is converted to penciclovir in the body. The active triphosphate metabolite of penciclovir inhibits viral DNA polymerase, but it is not incorporated into nascent DNA to cause chain termination (D). Penciclovir does not block guanosine triphosphate synthesis (A), which is inhibited by ribavirin. Viral entry (C) can be blocked by enfuvirtide and maraviroc. Viral maturation (E) is prevented by protease inhibitors such as darunavir, grazoprevir, paritaprevir, and simeprevir.

3. **The answer is E:** release of progeny virions. Zanamivir and oseltamivir inhibit viral neuraminidase and the release and spread of progeny virions. They do not affect entry into host cells (A), uncoating or replication of viral nucleic acid (B and C), or maturation of viral proteins (D). Viral nucleic acid replication can be inhibited by a large number of nucleoside and nucleotide analogs, including ganciclovir, emtricitabine, and tenofovir, as well as by nonnucleoside drugs such as foscarnet and rilpivirine.

4. **The answer is A:** foscarnet. Foscarnet is an alternative drug for treating herpesvirus infections caused by strains that are resistant to nucleoside analogs such as acyclovir and ganciclovir. The drug is reserved for resistant infections because it may cause renal failure, cardiac arrhythmias, hematologic deficiencies, and other adverse effects. Trifluridine (B) is only used for topical ocular administration to treat herpes simplex keratitis. Ribavirin (C) is used to treat severe respiratory syncytial virus infections and hepatitis. Rilpivirine (D) and efavirenz (E) are nonnucleotide reverse transcriptase inhibitors for treating HIV infections.

5. **The answer is C:** semiprevir. Semiprevir inhibits nonstructural protein 3-4A in hepatitis C virus, preventing cleavage of the viral polyprotein and viral maturation. Dasabuvir (A) inhibits nonstructural protein 5B, a viral RNA polymerase that replicates the viral genome. Ombitasvir (B), ledipasvir (D), and daclatasvir (E) inhibit nonstructural protein 5A, which is believed to activate RNA polymerase in hepatitis C virus.

CHAPTER 44

1. **The answer is E:** neuromuscular blockade. Activation of nicotinic acetylcholine receptors by pyrantel causes persistent muscle depolarization and neuromuscular

blockade in nematodes. Albendazole and mebendazole impair microtubule formation (A) and glucose uptake (B) in nematodes. Formation of nitro free radicals (C) results from interaction of metronidazole and tinidazole with an enzyme in anaerobic parasitic amoeba. Atovaquone inhibits electron transport (D) in plasmodial species causing malaria.

2. **The answer is C:** mefloquine. Neuropsychiatric reactions are most likely caused by mefloquine. Primaquine, artesunate, atovaquone, and proguanil (A, B, D, E) are unlikely to cause these reactions.

3. **The answer is E:** chloride. Onchocerciasis is an ocular filarial infection that may be prevented by annual administration of ivermectin, a drug that increases chloride permeability and causes hyperpolarization of nematode tissues. Ivermectin does not have any direct effect on sodium, potassium, calcium, or magnesium permeability (A through D). However, praziquantel increases the calcium permeability of susceptible trematodes, including *Schistosoma* species.

4. **The answer is C:** cryptosporidiosis. Several antiprotozoan agents inhibit pyruvate-ferredoxin oxidoreductase, including metronidazole, tinidazole, and nitazoxanide. Nitazoxanide is used to treat giardiasis and cryptosporidiosis. It is not used to treat leishmaniasis (A), malaria (B), trypanosomiasis (D), or toxoplasmosis (E).

5. **The answer is B:** artemether. Artesunate and artemether are believed to inhibit erythrocytic schizogony of plasmodial species by forming free radicals that damage heme and proteins. Pyrimethamine (A) and proguanil (D) inhibit dihydrofolate reductase and the formation of tetrahydrofolate. Atovaquone (C) inhibits electron transport and energy production, while the mechanism of lumefantrine, which is combined with artemether in COARTEM, is unknown.

CHAPTER 45

1. **The answer is B:** docetaxel. Drugs that inhibit microtubule function, such as docetaxel and vincristine, are associated with peripheral neurotoxicity due to their effects on neuron microtubules. Docetaxel is used to treat breast cancer, whereas vincristine is not. Cyclophosphamide, doxorubicin, tamoxifen, and temsirolimus (A, C, D, and E) do not inhibit microtubule function.

2. **The answer is D:** nephrotoxicity. Cisplatin may cause nephrotoxicity leading to loss of potassium and magnesium, reduced glomerular filtration, and renal failure. Administration of mannitol and sodium thiosulfate may prevent or reduce this adverse effect. Cisplatin is not typically associated with cardiac toxicity (A), liver failure (B), muscle toxicity (C), or hemolytic anemia (E).

3. **The answer is C:** tyrosine kinase. Imatinib inhibits the BCR-ABL tyrosine kinase in cancer cells that is coupled with pathways promoting myeloid cell proliferation. DNA polymerase (A) is inhibited by cytarabine, while dihydrofolate reductase (B) is blocked by methotrexate and pemetrexed. Thymidylate synthetase (D) is inhibited by fluorouracil. Thioguanine and mercaptopurine are activated by hypoxanthine guanine phosphoribosyltransferase (E), which converts the drugs to nucleotides.

4. **The answer is C:** fluorouracil. Fluorouracil (5-FU) is a pyrimidine antimetabolite chemotherapeutic agent. The pyrimidine antimetabolites can cause myelosuppression and oral and gastrointestinal ulceration. Higher doses of these drugs can damage the liver, heart, and other organs. If toxicity becomes too great, uridine triacetate (VISTOGARD) is marketed as an antidote for fluorouracil or capecitabine overdose and/or toxicity.

5. **The answer is A:** doxorubicin. **Doxorubicin** is an antibiotic obtained from a *Streptomyces* bacteria species that is used for treatment of breast cancer. It works by binding strongly to DNA by inserting (intercalating) between paired DNA bases, causing deformation and uncoiling of the DNA, which causes cytotoxicity and cancer cell death.

CHAPTER 46

1. **The answer is A:** breast cancer. Trastuzumab is a monoclonal antibody to the human epidermal growth factor receptor-2 (HER2) receptor and is used to treat metastatic breast cancer if tumor cells overexpress this receptor. Trastuzumab is not used to treat ovarian cancer (B), non-Hodgkin lymphoma (C), multiple myeloma (D), or melanoma (E).

2. **The answer is D:** tacrolimus. Tacrolimus forms a complex with an immunophilin known as FK12-binding protein, resulting in inhibition calcineurin and decreased activation of T lymphocytes. Cyclosporine (A) binds to a different immunophilin called cyclophilin, resulting in inhibition of calcineurin. Prednisone (B) is an adrenal steroid that suppresses T cell proliferation and immunity. Cyclophosphamide (C) is a cytotoxic agent that destroys lymphoid cells, while azathioprine (E) is converted to mercaptopurine and thereby inhibits purine biosynthesis required for the proliferation of lymphoid cells.

3. **The answer is E:** immune checkpoint inhibitor. The discovery of immune checkpoints, i.e., inhibitory signals that decrease T-cell activation, led to the development of new targets for monoclonal antibody therapy to turn on the T-cells by inhibiting these checkpoints. Ipilimumab is an anti-CTLA-4 monoclonal antibody drug which by binding to CTLA-4, blocks the interaction of CTLA-4 with its ligands. Ipilimumab was the first drug to show a survival benefit to patients with metastatic melanoma.

4. **The answer is A:** programmed death (PD-1) protein. PD-1 is an immune checkpoint that guards against autoimmunity by increasing apoptosis (programmed cell death) of antigen-specific T-cells and decreasing apoptosis in regulatory (anti-inflammatory, suppressive) T cells. Inhibitors of PD-1 like nivolumab turn up the immune detection of cancer cells and immune mechanisms of their destruction. Nivolumab was recently shown to extend survival in patients with advanced renal cell carcinoma, the most common kidney cancer in adults.

5. **The answer is C:** targeted antibody and cytotoxic agent. Antibody-drug conjugates (ADCs) combine the targeting capability of monoclonal antibodies with the cancer-killing ability of chemotherapeutic agents (cytotoxic agents) to provide successful treatment of a number of cancers. The attached chemotherapeutic drugs are either microtubule inhibitors, topoisomerase inhibitors, protein synthesis inhibitors, DNA strand disrupters, or radioactive isotopes.

Index

Page numbers followed by "*f*" indicate figures, "*t*" indicate tables, and "*b*" indicate boxes.